Periodontal therapy

Periodontal therapy

HENRY M. GOLDMAN, D.M.D., F.A.C.D., F.I.C.D.

Professor of Oral Pathology and Dean Emeritus,
Henry M. Goldman School of Graduate Dentistry,
Boston University; Professor of Stomatology,
Boston University School of Medicine,
Boston, Massachusetts

D. WALTER COHEN, D.D.S., F.A.C.D., F.I.C.D.

Dean, University of Pennsylvania School of Dental Medicine;
Professor of Periodontics, University of Pennsylvania School
of Dental Medicine; Professor of Dental Medicine, Medical
College of Pennsylvania, Philadelphia, Pennsylvania;
Visiting Professor of Periodontology, Boston University,
Henry M. Goldman School of Graduate Dentistry,
Boston, Massachusetts

SIXTH EDITION

with 3452 illustrations and 2 color plates

The C. V. Mosby Company

ST. LOUIS • TORONTO • LONDON   1980

SIXTH EDITION

Printed in the United States of America

The C. V. Mosby Company
11830 Westline Industrial Drive, St. Louis, Missouri 63141

Library of Congress Cataloging in Publication Data

Goldman, Henry Maurice, 1911-
   Periodontal therapy.

   Includes bibliographies and index.
   1. Periodontics. I. Cohen, David Walter,
1926-   joint author. II. Title.
[DNLM: 1. Periodontal diseases—Therapy.
WU240 G619pe]
RK361.G597 1979   617.6′32   79-13055
ISBN 0-8016-1875-4

GW/CB/B 9 8 7 6 5 4 3 2 1   03/A/303

Contributors

LEONARD ABRAMS, D.D.S., P.C., F.A.C.D.

Associate Professor in Periodontics, University of Pennsylvania School of Dental Medicine, Philadelphia, Pennsylvania

MORTON AMSTERDAM, D.D.S., F.A.C.D.

Professor of Periodontics and Periodontal Prosthesis, University of Pennsylvania School of Dental Medicine, Philadelphia, Pennsylvania

DAVID BEAUDREAU, D.D.S.

Professor of Crown and Bridge and Periodontology; Dean, Georgetown University School of Dentistry, Washington, D.C.

ARTHUR A. BLOOM

Associate Professor, Department of Oral Histology, Boston University, Henry M. Goldman School of Graduate Dentistry, Boston, Massachusetts

NEAL W. CHILTON, D.D.S., M.P.H., F.A.C.D.

Research Professor of Oral Medicine, University of Pennsylvania School of Dental Medicine, Philadelphia, Pennsylvania

HERMAN CORN, D.D.S., F.A.C.D.

Professor, Department of Periodontics, University of Pennsylvania School of Dental Medicine, Philadelphia, Pennsylvania

J. GEORGE COSLET, D.D.S., M.Sc.D.

Associate Professor of Periodontics and Director, Division of Advanced Education, University of Pennsylvania School of Dental Medicine, Philadelphia, Pennsylvania

JOHN C. DERBYSHIRE, D.D.S., M.S.

Clinical Associate, University of Oregon School of Dentistry, Portland, Oregon

SPENCER N. FRANKL, D.D.S., M.S.D.

Dean and Professor of Pedodontics, Boston University, Henry M. Goldman School of Graduate Dentistry, Boston, Massachusetts

ROBERT J. GENCO, D.D.S., Ph.D.

Chairman, Department of Oral Biology, State University of New York at Buffalo, Buffalo, New York

PAUL GOLDHABER, D.D.S., M.A. (Hon.)

Professor of Periodontology and Dean, Harvard School of Dental Medicine, Boston, Massachusetts

JOHN C. GREENE, D.M.D., M.P.H.

Deputy Surgeon General and Chief Dental Officer, Public Health Service, Washington, D.C.

SAMUEL V. HOLROYD, B.S., D.D.S., M.S., F.A.C.D.

Professor and Chairman of Periodontics, Washington University School of Dentistry, St. Louis, Missouri

GERALD A. ISENBERG, D.D.S., M.Sc.D.

Associate Professor of Periodontics, Boston University, Henry M. Goldman School of Graduate Dentistry, Boston, Massachusetts

ANTHONY JONG, D.D.S., M.P.H., D.Sc.D.

Professor and Chairperson, Department of Public Health and Community Dentistry, Boston University, Henry M. Goldman School of Graduate Dentistry, Boston, Massachusetts

SIMAO KON, C.D., M.Sc.D.

Professor of Periodontics, Faculdade de Odontologia, Universidade de Sao Paulo, Sao Paulo, Brazil

GERALD M. KRAMER, D.M.D., F.A.C.D.

Professor and Chairman, Department of Periodontology, Boston University, Henry M. Goldman School of Graduate Dentistry, Boston, Massachusetts

MAX A. LISTGARTEN, D.D.S., M.A. (Hon.)

Professor of Periodontics, University of Pennsylvania, Center for Oral Health Research and School of Dental Medicine, Philadelphia, Pennsylvania

HARALD LÖE, D.D.S., Dr. Odont.

Dean, University of Connecticut School of Dental Medicine, Farmington, Connecticut

JAMES A. McMULLEN, D.D.S., M.Sc.D., F.I.C.D.

Associate Clinical Professor and Director of Postgraduate Clinical Periodontics, State University of New York at Buffalo, School of Dentistry, Buffalo, New York

MANUEL H. MARKS, D.D.S., F.A.C.D.

Associate Professor of Periodontics, University of Pennsylvania School of Dental Medicine, Philadelphia, Pennsylvania

GARRY MERRILL MILLER, D.D.S.

Assistant Professor of Periodontics, University of Pennsylvania School of Dental Medicine, Philadelphia, Pennsylvania

CLAUDE L. NABERS, D.D.S., M.S.D.

Visiting Lecturer, Department of Periodontics, University of Pennsylvania School of Dental Medicine, Philadelphia, Pennsylvania

TIMOTHY J. O'LEARY, D.M.D.

Professor of Periodontology and Chairman, Department of Periodontics, Indiana University School of Dentistry, Indianapolis, Indiana

R. EARL ROBINSON, D.M.D., F.A.C.D., F.I.C.D.

Lecturer, Post-Graduate Division, University of California School of Dentistry, San Francisco, California

LOUIS F. ROSE, D.D.S., M.D.

Associate Professor of Periodontics, University of Pennsylvania School of Dental Medicine; Chief, Division of Dental Medicine and Surgery, Medical College of Pennsylvania, Philadelphia, Pennsylvania

MORRIS P. RUBEN, D.D.S., F.A.C.D., F.I.C.D., F.A.D.S.

Professor and Chairman of Oral Biology and Professor of Periodontology, Boston University, Henry M. Goldman School of Graduate Dentistry, Boston, Massachusetts

SIDNEY M. SCHULMAN, D.D.S.

Associate Professor of Periodontology, Boston University, Henry M. Goldman School of Graduate Dentistry; Attending Dental Surgeon, Beth Israel Hospital; Attending Dental Surgeon, University Hospital, Boston, Massachusetts

JAY S. SEIBERT, D.D.S., M.Sc.D.

Professor of Periodontics and Chairman of Department, University of Pennsylvania School of Dental Medicine, Philadelphia, Pennsylvania

IRWIN I. SHIP, D.M.D., M.Sc.

Professor of Oral Medicine and Director of the Clinical Research Center, University of Pennsylvania School of Dental Medicine, Philadelphia, Pennsylvania

ALAN SHUMAN, D.M.D.

Associate Professor of Periodontology, Boston University, Henry M. Goldman School of Graduate Dentistry, Boston, Massachusetts

HYMAN SMUKLER, B.D.S., D.M.D., H. Dip.

Associate Professor of Periodontology and Chairman, Department of Oral Diagnosis and Radiology, Boston University, Henry M. Goldman School of Graduate Dentistry, Boston, Massachusetts

S. SIGMUND STAHL, D.D.S., M.S.

Professor and Chairman, Department of Periodontics, and Associate Dean for Academic Affairs, New York University College of Dentistry, New York, New York

ROBERT L. VANARSDALL, D.D.S.

Assistant Professor of Periodontics and Orthodontics, University of Pennsylvania School of Dental Medicine, Philadelphia, Pennsylvania

ARNOLD S. WEISGOLD, D.D.S.

Professor and Chairman, Form and Function of the Masticatory System, and Director of Postdoctoral Periodontal Prosthesis, University of Pennsylvania School of Dental Medicine, Philadelphia, Pennsylvania

Preface

Since the last edition of *Periodontal Therapy,* basic and clinical research have demonstrated data concerning not only the etiology of periodontal disease but clinical approaches to it as well. The indications and contraindications for periodontal procedures have been defined. The excisive and reconstructive reparative techniques have become firmly established in periodontal practice. This new material has been included in this edition. Preventive methodologies have also been stressed.

This text is intended for the undergraduate, the graduate student, and the practitioner with the understanding that the basis of a healthy dentition forms the foundation of dental disease prevention and therapy. This philosophy of general practice is aided by the specialist when needed. In this way the general public receives the best of care.

We are extremely grateful to all who have contributed to this and past editions.

Henry M. Goldman
D. Walter Cohen

Contents

COLOR PLATES

1 Anatomy and histology

Part 1
GINGIVA
Anatomy

The gingiva is that part of the oral mucous membrane that covers the alveolar processes and the cervical portions of the teeth. It has been divided traditionally into the *free* and the *attached gingivae*. The line of division between the two is an imaginary line between the bottom of the *gingival sulcus* and the gingival surface opposite to it. The attached gingiva then extends apically from this point to the *mucogingival junction*. Apical to this line the alveolar mucosa is continuous without any demarcation into the mucous membrane of the cheek, lip, and floor of the oral cavity (Figs. 1-1 to 1-3). It should be noted here that the gingival sulcus as observed in histologic sections of well-preserved tissue blocks is not necessarily the same entity as the gingival sulcus determined by sounding with a clinical probe.

In fully erupted teeth the gingival margin is located on the enamel approximately 0.5 to 2 mm coronal to the cervix (Fig. 1-4). In human teeth the gingival margin seldom forms a knife-edge termination against the tooth, but is rounded. A shallow furrow is usually found between the gingival margin and the tooth surface. This is the entrance to or orifice of the *gingival sulcus*. The clinically healthy *gingival sulcus* rarely exceeds 2 to 3 mm. However, the depth of the gingival sulcus, which is obtained by measurement with a periodontal probe, may differ significantly from that of the gingival sulcus as observed in well-preserved histologic specimens. Since the depth of the *histologic* gingival sulcus at strictly normal sites is a negligible fraction of the total width of the attached gingiva, it has been suggested that the use of the qualifying terms ''free'' and ''attached'' in reference to the gingiva be discontinued. Furthermore, since periodontal probing does not accurately reflect the depth of the *histologic sulcus,* the readings provided by the periodontal probe would be more accurately described by a term such as ''probing depth'' or ''probeable depth'' of the gingival sulcus, rather than by the current terminology ''sulcus depth.'' The term ''pocket'' should be reserved for pathologically altered sulci, the probing depth of which exceeds 3 mm. In fully developed and erupted teeth the gingival sulcus is lined coronally with *sulcular epithelium,** the nonkeratinized extension of the *oral epithelium* into the sulcus. The bottom of the sulcus is formed by the coronal surface of the *junctional epithelium.* The junctional epithelium unites the gingival connective tissue to the enamel surface from the cervix or neck of the

---

*This term is used interchangeably with *oral sulcular epithelium,* as defined by H. E. Schroeder and M. A. Listgarten: In Wolsky, A., editor: Monographs in developmental biology, vol. 2, Basel, 1971, S. Karger.

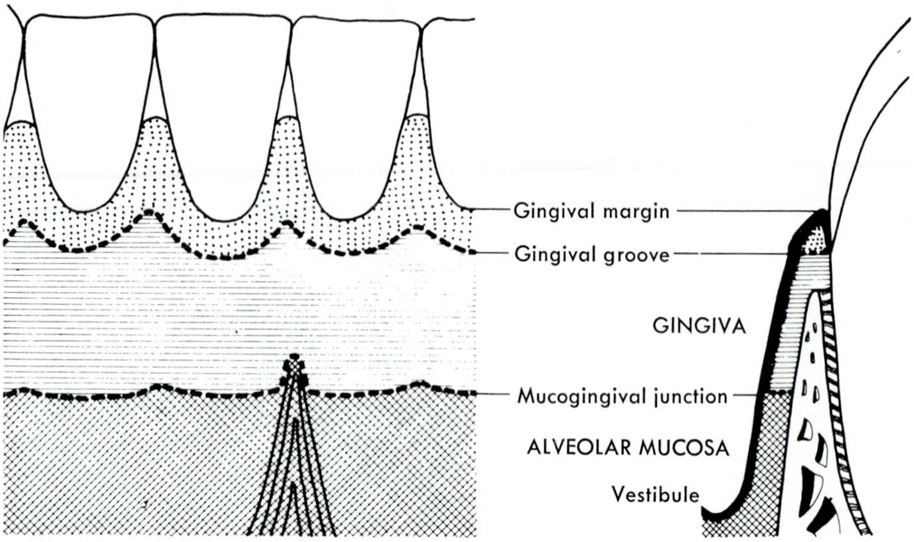

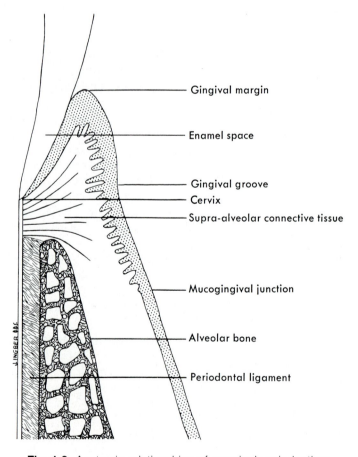

Fig. 1-1. Anatomic relationships of normal gingiva.

Gingival margin
Gingival groove
GINGIVA
Mucogingival junction
ALVEOLAR MUCOSA
Vestibule

Gingival margin

Enamel space

Gingival groove
Cervix
Supra-alveolar connective tissue

Mucogingival junction

Alveolar bone

Periodontal ligament

Fig. 1-2. Anatomic relationships of marginal periodontium.

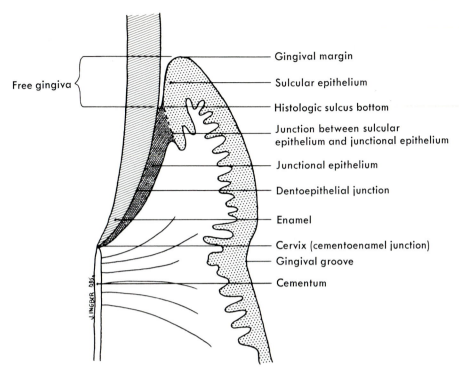

Free gingiva {

— Gingival margin

— Sulcular epithelium

— Histologic sulcus bottom

— Junction between sulcular epithelium and junctional epithelium

— Junctional epithelium

— Dentoepithelial junction

— Enamel

— Cervix (cementoenamel junction)

— Gingival groove

— Cementum

J. INGBER 006

Fig. 1-3. Histologic relationships of marginal gingiva.

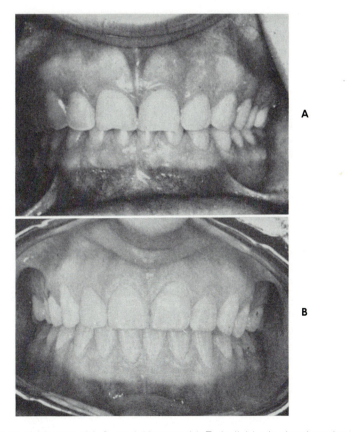

A

B

Fig. 1-4. Dentitions of 38-year-old, **A,** and 40-year-old, **B,** individuals showing physiologic form of gingival tissue.

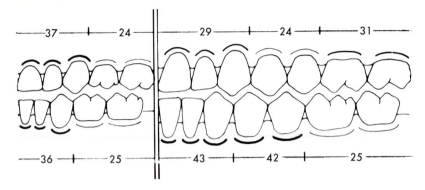

Fig. 1-5. Frequency of occurrence (%) of gingival groove on different teeth in deciduous (left) and permanent (right) dentition. (From Ainamo, J., and Löe, H.: J. Periodontol. **37**:5, 1966.)

tooth to the bottom of the gingival sulcus (Fig. 1-3). The length of the junctional epithelium rarely exceeds 2 to 3 mm.

The margin of the gingiva describes a wavy course around the four surfaces of the tooth, with the gingival margin on the interdental surfaces constituting the most occlusally located part of the gingiva. The steepness of the arcate form varies in accordance with the course of the cementoenamel junction in different teeth. In anterior teeth the gingival papilla is the interdental extension of the gingiva; the form and size are determined by the contact relationships of the adjacent teeth, the course of the cementoenamel junction, and the width of the interdental surfaces. The interdental papillae of anterior teeth have the shape of a pyramid, the base of which is an imaginary horizontal plane through the region of the cementoenamel junction. From this base the facial and oral parts of the marginal gingiva and the mesial and distal surfaces attached to the tooth form the steep sides of the pyramid. The four surfaces join at the tip of the papilla. In the premolar and the molar regions the papilla is more rounded in the facio-oral direction.

In some instances the interdental gingiva may consist of two papillae, one facial to and one oral to the contact point or contact area. This configuration of the interdental gingiva has been described as a saddle, or a *col*, in the facio-oral dimension. Such a smooth saddlelike depression of the interdental gingiva is frequently found in children. In the normal periodontium the tip of the interdental papilla is always that part of the gingiva located nearest the incisal or occlusal surface of the tooth.

The *gingival groove* is a shallow groove that runs parallel to and at a distance of 0.5 to 2 mm from the margin of the gingiva. It may be found both on the facial and on the oral aspects of the gingiva. Less than half of all normal gingivae show a gingival groove (Fig. 1-5). Its presence or absence does not seem to depend on whether the gingival margin is located on the enamel, since the gingival groove frequently occurs in teeth where the gingival margin is confined to various levels below the cementoenamel junction. Measurements indicate that the distance from the gin-

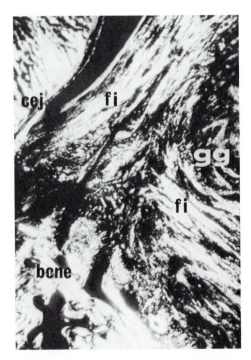

Fig. 1-6. Histologic section of marginal epithelium of a monkey. Well-defined fan-shaped fiber bundles emerge from cementum between cementoenamel junction, *cej,* and alveolar crest, *bone.* Epithelial ridge corresponding to gingival groove, *gg,* is situated in angle produced by fiber arrangements, *fi.* (From Ainamo, J., and Löe, H.: J. Periodontol. **37**:5, 1966.)

gival margin to the gingival groove roughly corresponds to the distance from the gingival margin to the apical extension of the junctional epithelium.

The presence or absence, as well as the location of the groove, is dependent on the distinctness of the fan-shaped arrangement of the supraalveolar collagenous fibers running from the cementum into the gingiva. There seems to be no correlation between the occurrence of a gingival groove and the mechanical effects of mastication. It is believed that the special configuration of the fiber systems arises when a certain number of dimensional relationships exist between the different anatomic features of the marginal periodontium (Fig. 1-6). The facts that the gingival groove persists during mild and moderate inflammation and that less than half of all normal gingivae exhibit a gingival groove indicate that a

groove is not directly related to the health of the marginal gingiva. Consequently, the presence of a gingival groove cannot be used as a criterion for normal gingiva.

The oral and vestibular surfaces of the healthy marginal gingiva, including the tip of the interdental papilla, are covered with keratinized or parakeratinized epithelium. They are firm, frequently stippled, and pink. The gingiva extends from the gingival margin to the level of the mucogingival junction. It comprises an epithelial lining and the supra-alveolar connective tissue. The *gingival epithelium* has three components: the *oral, sulcular,* and *junctional* epithelia. The connective tissue core attaches the gingiva to the cementum and the alveolar bone (Figs. 1-2 and 1-6).

Except for the hard palate, which is entirely covered with masticatory mucosa, the width of the gingiva varies between 1 and 9 mm. The widest

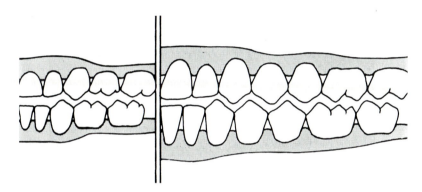

Fig. 1-7. Variation in width of attached gingiva in primary (left) and permanent (right) teeth. (From Ainamo, J., and Löe, H.: J. Periodontol. **37**:5, 1966.)

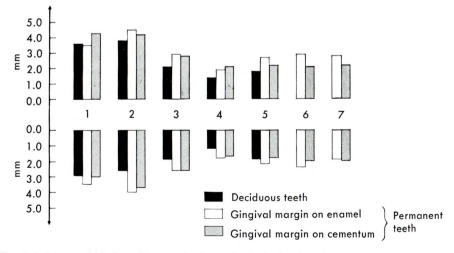

Fig. 1-8. Mean width (in millimeters) of attached gingiva in primary and permanent dentitions. (From Ainamo, J., and Löe, H.: J. Periodontol. **37**:5, 1966.)

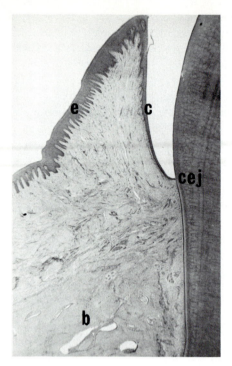

Fig. 1-9. Histologic section of marginal periodontium. *e,* Surface epithelium; *c,* junctional epithelium; *cej,* cementoenamel junction; *b,* alveolar bone.

area found on the maxillary and mandibular incisors decreases toward the canine region and the lateral segments (Fig. 1-7). The narrowest zone of gingiva is found in the region of the maxillary and mandibular first premolars and usually in connection with frenum and muscle attachments. The pattern of variation is approximately the same in deciduous and permanent teeth (Fig. 1-8).

The gingiva is firm and resilient because of the tight attachment of the fibers of the supraalveolar connective tissue and the lamina propria to the cementum and bone (Fig. 1-9). The gingiva is covered by a keratinized or parakeratinized epithelium, the surface of which presents minute depressions and elevations, giving the surface an orange-peel appearance. This stippling of the gingiva may vary considerably within the normal. It varies with age, being less conspicuous in childhood than in adult life. It is more common on the facial than on the lingual surfaces.

The alveolar mucosa is relatively sharply delineated from the attached gingiva at the mucogingival junction. It covers the basal part of the alveolar process and continues without demarcation into the vestibular fornix or the floor of the mouth. In contrast to the attached gingiva, the alveolar mucosa is but loosely attached to the periosteum and is therefore highly movable. The surface of the alveolar mucosa is smooth. It is covered by nonkeratinized epithelium and is markedly redder than the attached gingiva.

Gingival epithelium

The gingival surface is covered with a stratified squamous epithelium. In humans this epithelium (oral epithelium of the gingiva) is normally of the keratinizing type. The epithelium of the dentogingival junction is not keratinized.

The oral epithelium of the gingiva is fairly uniform in thickness and character. The border between the epithelium and the underlying lamina propria of the connective tissue is uneven and characterized by deep epithelial ridges that surround fingerlike connective tissue papillae (Fig. 1-10, *A*). These ridges and papillae, as they appear in histologic preparations, represent interdigitating pegs or folds that tend to run horizontally and parallel to the surface of the gingiva (Fig. 1-10, *B*).

The oral epithelium of the gingiva is, like epidermis, subdivided into several layers of cells (Fig. 1-11). In the *basal layer (stratum basale, stratum germinativum)* all cells are adjacent to the connective tissue, from which they are separated by a *basement lamina (basal lamina).* The cells are relatively small and more or less cuboidal. This is the layer in which mitotic figures are most commonly noted. The next several layers of cells constitute the *prickle cell layer (stratum spinosum),* so named because the relatively large, polyhedral cells in this layer have short cytoplasmic processes resembling spines, which connect with the processes of adjacent cells. These connecting cytoplasmic projections were formerly called intercellular bridges (Fig. 1-18). However, electron microscopy has shown the lack of any cytoplasmic continuity between these cell processes, making this term inappropriate. The cellular processes are merely connected to one another by specialized junctions. Superficial to the stratum spinosum are several layers of flattened cells that form the *granular layer (stratum granulosum).* The cytoplasm of these cells characteristically displays *keratohyaline granules* that have been associated with keratin formation. The most superficial layer is the *cornified layer (stratum corneum),* which consists of closely packed, flattened cells that have lost their nuclei and most other organelles as they became keratinized. These cells contain primarily densely packed tonofilaments enclosed by a thickened plasmalemma.

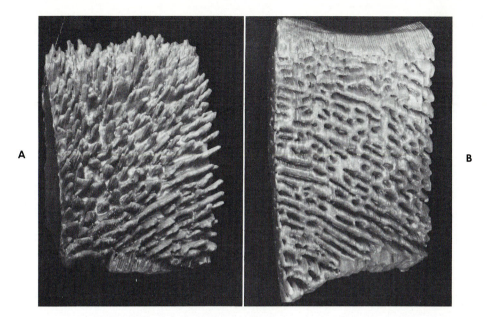

Fig. 1-10. Three-dimensional models of epithelium–connective tissue boundary of gingiva. Connective tissue papillae, **A,** are arranged in rows running predominantly parallel to gingival margin (top). In some areas papillae tend to fuse and form horizontal ridges (lower right corner). Epithelium, **B,** shows a pattern corresponding to that of connective tissue. Smooth parallel ridges running horizontally are connected by vertical cross ridges. Ridges are pitted at intervals corresponding to distribution of connective tissue papillae. (× 200.) (From Löe, H., and Karring, T.: J. Periodontol. **2:**71, 1967.)

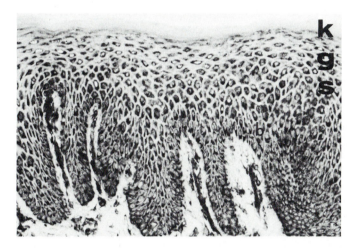

Fig. 1-11. Frozen sections of human attached gingiva (5μm thick) incubated to show glutamic dehydrogenase activity. *b,* Basal layer; *s,* spinous layer; *g,* granular layer; *k,* keratinized surface layer. (From Löe, H., and Nuki, K.: J. Periodont. Res. **1:**43, 1967.)

Electron microscopic studies have shown that the basal cells rest on a basement lamina consisting of an amorphous, moderately dense layer, the *lamina densa,* approximately 40 to 60 nm thick, separated from the epithelial cell membrane by a space 25 to 45 nm wide, the *lamina lucida.* The basement lamina is a structural entity of epithelial origin visible only with the electron microscope; the basement lamina should not be confused with the *basement membrane,* a region identified with the light microscope that in addition to the basement lamina probably also includes connective tissue elements. The cytoplasmic membrane of the basal cells covers the numerous fingerlike extensions of the cell that protrude into the underlying connective tissue (Figs. 1-12 and

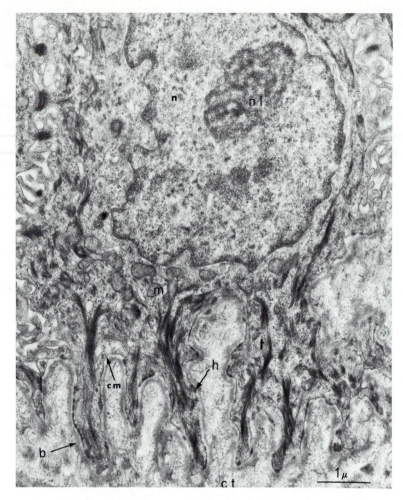

Fig. 1-12. Basal epithelial cell resting on basement lamina. Basement lamina consists of an electron-dense lamina densa, *b,* separated from cytoplasmic membrane, *cm,* of basal cell by an electron-lucent zone, lamina lucida. At intervals cytoplasmic membrane is attached to basement lamina through hemidesmosomes, *h.* Numerous projections of basal cell extend into connective tissue, *ct.* Cytoplasm contains a nucleus, *n,* with nucleolus, *nl,* numerous mitochondria, *m,* and other organelles and inclusions such as tonofilaments, *t.* (From Schroeder, H., and Theilade, J.: J. Periodont. Res. **1:**95, 1966.)

1-13). The cytoplasm of the basal cells generally contains a relatively high concentration of organelles and other cytoplasmic constituents. *Tonofibrils* are regularly seen in the basal cells. They are comprised of finer elements, the *tonofilaments,* which measure approximately 5 nm in diameter.

Specialized connective tissue fibrils have been described in close association with a variety of basement laminae, including those of the gingival epithelium. These so-called *anchoring fibrils* are believed to connect the lamina densa to the underlying connective tissue (Fig. 1-13).

The cells of the spinous layer (stratum spinosum) are generally larger than the basal cells. They contain fewer cytoplasmic organelles and relatively more tonofibrils than the basal cells (Fig. 1-14). In the superficial layers the tonofibrils become concentrated on the periphery of the cell and increase in number. In the stratum corneum the cells are densely packed with tonofilaments. The peripheral cytoplasm tends to become condensed against the inner leaflet of the cell membrane, thereby giving the latter a thickened appearance. Lipid droplets may be present within the cell, but other cytoplasmic organelles are infrequently recognized.

Both basal and spinous cells have an irregular contour. Numerous cytoplasmic processes protrude from the entire cell periphery, giving the cell surface a jagged appearance (Fig. 1-15). The

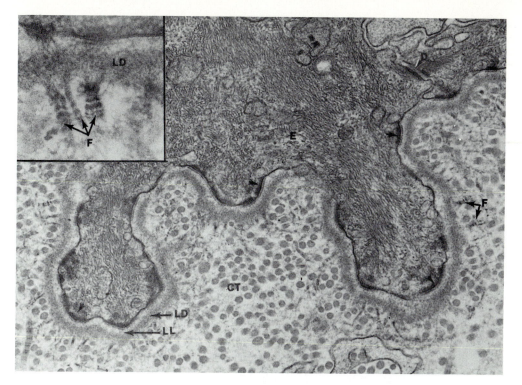

Fig. 1-13. Gingiva. Basement lamina joining epithelial cell, *E,* to underlying connective tissue, *CT,* consists of finely granular lamina densa, *LD,* separated from cell membrane by clear lamina lucida, *LL.* Hemidesmosomes *(arrows)* connect epithelial cell to basement lamina. Anchoring fibrils, *F,* may participate in joining basement lamina to underlying connective tissue. *D,* Desmosome joining adjacent epithelial cells. (× 33,000.) Inset: higher magnification of anchoring fibrils, *F,* and their relationship to lamina densa, *LD.* (× 110,000.) (From Listgarten, M.: Unpublished data, 1967.)

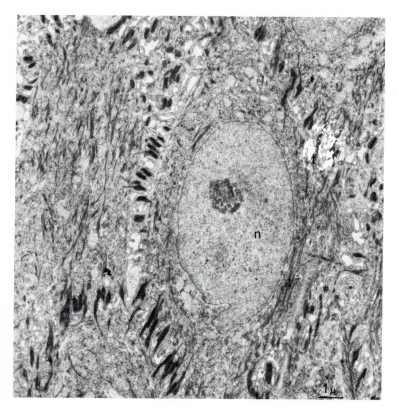

Fig. 1-14. Spinous epithelial cells. Tonofilaments, *t,* are seen in cytoplasm around nucleus, *n,* and extending toward periphery of cytoplasm. (From Schroeder, H., and Theilade, J.: J. Periodont. Res. **1:**95, 1966.)

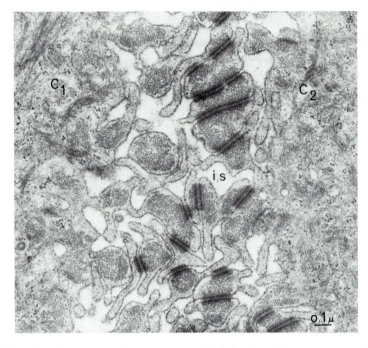

Fig. 1-15. Relationship between two adjacent cells, c_1 and c_2. Numerous cytoplasmic processes protrude from cell periphery into intercellular space, *is,* giving cell surface a jagged appearance. (From Schroeder, H., and Theilade, J.: J. Periodont. Res. **1:**95, 1966.)

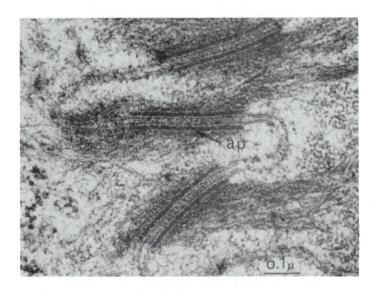

Fig. 1-16. Typical desmosomes consisting of attachment plaque areas of two adjacent cells separated by a 20 nm to 30 nm wide laminated space. Attachment plaques, *ap,* from two adjacent cells and laminated intercellular space constitute desmosome. (From Schroeder, H., and Theilade, J.: J. Periodont. Res. **1:**95, 1966.)

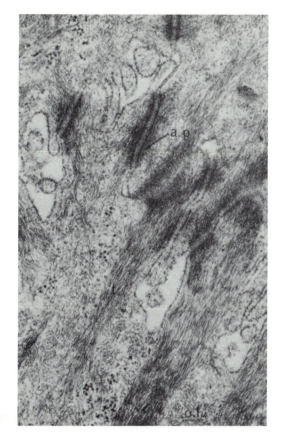

Fig. 1-17. At intervals cell membrane is thickened, and adjacent intracellular cytoplasm is condensed. Such areas are designated attachment plaques, *ap.* Intracellular tonofibrils, *t,* terminate at internal aspect of attachment plaque. (From Schroeder, H., and Theilade, J.: J. Periodont. Res. **1:**95, 1966.)

cell membranes of adjacent cells are generally found in close apposition to each other. This results in narrow and irregular intercellular spaces between the cells.

Adjacent cells are attached to each other by specialized portions of the cell membrane. The most common type of junction is the *desmosome* (Fig. 1-16). It consists of two adjacent attachment plaques, one from each cell, that are separated by an interval approximately 30 nm wide that contains three dense lamellae. Intracellular tonofilaments converge toward the internal surface of the attachment plaques (Fig. 1-17). The desmosome and a portion of the cytoplasm from each of the adjacent cells constitute the "intercellular bridge" of classic histology (Fig. 1-18). *Tight junctions (maculae occludentes)* which are also found in the gingival epithelium, are formed by fusion of the external leaflets of adjacent cell membranes. The area of fusion appears to be of a size and shape similar to that of a desmosome (Fig. 1-19). The connection of one cell to another depends on the chemical and physical forces that determine the properties of various cell junctions. It is possible that the intercellular substance, which contains polysaccharides, proteins, and some lipid, may also play a part in the adhesion of adjacent cells (Fig. 1-20).

In the granular layer (stratum granulosum) the cells become flattened in a plane parallel to the gingival surface. The tonofibrils become more prominent than in the stratum spinosum. Keratohyaline granules, up to 1 μm in diameter, round in shape, and electron dense, appear in the cytoplasm (Fig. 1-21). There is a further decrease in the number of mitochondria. Smaller *membrane-coating granules,* approximately 0.1 μm in diameter, can be observed in close proximity to the

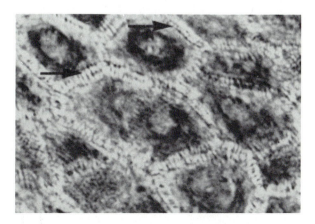

Fig. 1-18. Intercellular bridges *(arrows)* crossing between prickle cells.

most superficial cell membrane. The content of these granules appears to contribute to the material within the narrow intercellular spaces characteristically noted at this level. The desmosomes become oriented more or less parallel to the cell surface.

At the inferior border of the cornified layer (stratum corneum) the cells undergo a sudden transition into keratinized cells. This is characterized by an increased prominence of the tono-

filaments that are closely packed together and form the predominant morphologic constituent of the cell. Clear, rounded bodies probably representing lipid droplets appear within the cytoplasm. The remaining organelles and the nucleus disappear. Concomitant with these alterations, the cell membrane appears to undergo a marked thickening of the inner leaflet of the membrane, which becomes about as thick as the attachment plaque of the desmosomes with which it is continuous (Fig.

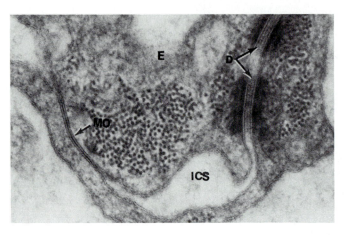

Fig. 1-19. Desmosomes, *D,* and tight junction (macula occludens, *MO*) connecting adjacent portions of gingival epithelial cells, *E.* Note relationship of inner and outer leaflet of cell membranes to each type of junction. *ICS,* Intercellular space. (×67,000.) (From Listgarten, M.: Unpublished data, 1967.)

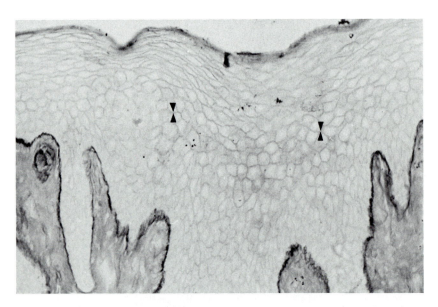

Fig. 1-20. Keratinized epithelium of attached gingiva (5µm thick) stained in periodic acid–Schiff (PAS). Note heavy PAS-positive material of basement membrane and PAS-positive material of intercellular substance of epithelium *(arrows).*

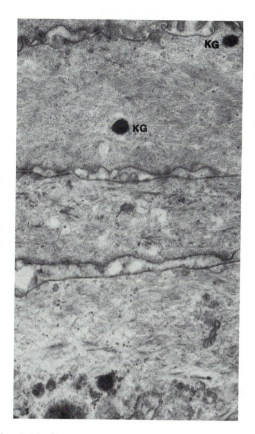

Fig. 1-21. Stratum granulosum. Note diminution of cytoplasmic organelles from bottom of illustration to top and appearance of keratohyaline granules, *KG*. Membrane-coating granules are not apparent in this section. Note thickening of cell membranes. (×10,000.) (From Listgarten, M.: Unpublished data, 1964.)

1-22). The outer leaflet is frequently interrupted and difficult to identify. The superficial cells desquamate as a result of intradesmosomal disruption.

Gingival sulcus and dentogingival junction

The soft tissue wall of the gingival sulcus is lined coronally with *sulcular epithelium*. The apical part of the soft tissue wall and the bottom of the sulcus are formed by the coronal surface of the *junctional epithelium* (Fig. 1-3).

The junctional epithelium consists of a thin layer of epithelium that joins the gingival connective tissue to the tooth surface. In recently erupted teeth, this epithelium extends from the bottom of the gingival sulcus to the apical border of the enamel. It consists of a band varying in thickness from 15 to 30 cells in the vicinity of the gingival sulcus to as few as one cell at its apical extension in the cervical area. The cells immediately adjacent to the gingival connective tissue and the cells located in the most apical portion of the junctional epithelium have characteristics in common with basal epithelial cells, including the ability to divide. The remaining cells that are oriented in a plane parallel to the long axis of the tooth are morphologically similar to cells of the lower stratum spinosum.

The histologic appearance of junctional epithelium is different from that of the keratinized oral epithelium. It is thinner and lacks well-developed epithelial ridges. Consequently, the basement membrane bordering on the subepithelial connective tissue follows a relatively straight course. However, in the normal gingiva of adult individuals, epithelial ridges and connective tissue

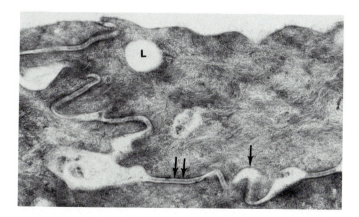

Fig. 1-22. Superficial cell of stratum corneum. Densely packed tonofilaments and lipid droplets, *L,* are prime constituents of cell interior. Thickened inner leaflet of plasmalemma *(single arrow)* is nearly as broad as attachment plaque of desmosomes *(double arrow).* (×30,000.) (From Listgarten, M.: Unpublished data, 1966.)

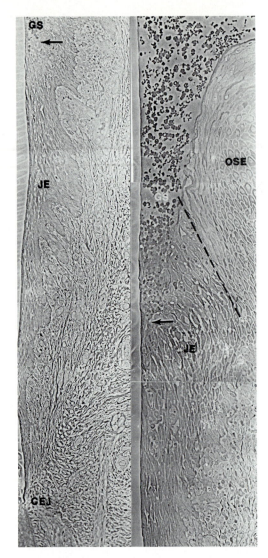

Fig. 1-23. Gingival sulcus, *GS,* and junctional epithelium, *JE.* Epithelial attachment extends from bottom of gingival sulcus *(arrow)* to apical border of enamel, *CEJ.* Dotted line indicates junction of oral sulcular epithelium, *OSE,* and junctional epithelium, *JE.* Phase-contrast micrograph. (From Schroeder, H. E., and Listgarten, M. A.: In Wolsky, A., editor: Monographs in developmental biology, vol. 2, Basel, 1971, S. Karger.)

papillae are frequently encountered beneath the sulcular epithelium lining the coronal portion of the sulcus. Provided that no signs of inflammation or other pathologic conditions are present, this should be regarded as normal. Junctional epithelium does not contain a stratum granulosum or stratum corneum. Histochemical stains also show that cells of the normal junctional epithelium do not show any tendency toward keratinization. The cells of the junctional epithelium are oriented with their long axis parallel to the tooth surface. The coronal surface of the junctional epithelium represents its free surface, since it is the surface from which desquamation takes place. This surface forms the floor and part of the apical portion of the lateral wall of the gingival sulcus (Fig. 1-23).

Whereas the orifice of the gingival sulcus is bound by the tooth surface on one side and sulcular epithelium on the other, the bottom of the sulcus is frequently surrounded by epithelium on all sides. This is due to the persistence of junctional epithelial cells on the tooth surface for a distance of approximately 100 μm coronal to the sulcus bottom (Fig. 1-24).

The epithelium lining the coronal portion of the lateral wall of the gingival sulcus resembles the gingival epithelium covering the external surface of the gingiva in all respects with the exception that it does not become fully keratinized. Unlike junctional epithelium, which is composed almost entirely of stratum spinosum-type cells, this epithelium is stratified in the pattern generally observed in other oral epithelia. The surface cells are flattened and exhibit a tendency toward partial keratinization (Figs. 1-24 and 1-25).

Electron microscopically, the junctional epithelial cells are moderately rich in rough-surfaced endoplasmic reticulum and mitochondria. They have well-developed Golgi regions and relatively few tonofibrils. The intercellular spaces are relatively larger and the number of desmosomes fewer than in the stratum spinosum of the gingival epithelium.

The sulcular epithelium is ultrastructurally similar to the oral epithelium of the gingiva described previously, except that the superficial cells may retain some organelles and exhibit focal accumulations of glycogen in addition to the lipid droplets typically found in the superficial cells of oral epithelium (Fig. 1-25). The compacted tonofilaments characteristically noted in keratinized epithelial cells are also present, but more loosely arranged in the superficial cell layers of the sulcular epithelium.

Supra-alveolar connective tissue

The supra-alveolar connective tissue comprises the mesodermal structures of the gingiva coronal to the crest of the alveolar bone. It consists primarily of cells, fibers, and blood vessels embedded in an amorphous ground substance. The main cell is the fibroblast, which produces the basic elements of the connective tissue. Other cells normally found include undifferentiated mesenchymal cells, mast cells, and macrophages. The predominant

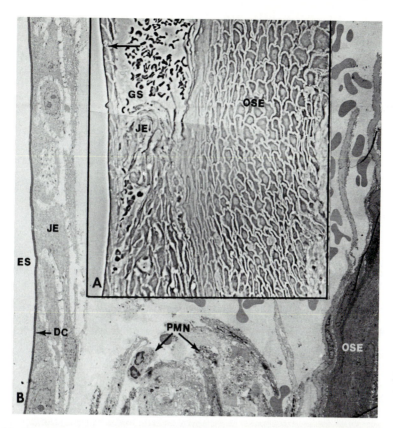

Fig. 1-24. Gingival sulcus. **A,** Phase-contrast micrograph illustrating bottom of gingival sulcus, *GS,* bound by oral sulcular epithelium, *OSE,* laterally; free surface of junctional epithelium, *JE,* beneath; and junctional epithelial cells still clinging to enamel surface *(arrow).* **B,** Electron micrograph of serial section showing tendency of *OSE* to keratinize and presence of a dental cuticle, *DC,* between junctional epithelial cells, *JE,* still clinging to tooth and enamel space, *ES.* Bottom of sulcus consists of desquamating junctional epithelial cells and polymorphonuclear leukocytes, *PMN,* in various stages of disintegration. (**A** ×360; **B** ×2,400.) (From Schroeder, H. E., and Listgarten, M. A.: In Wolsky, A., editor: Monographs in developmental biology, vol. 2, Basel, 1971, S. Karger.)

connective tissue fibers are of two distinct types: *collagen* and *elastic fibers. Reticular fibers,* which are young collagen fibers, are numerous beneath the basement lamina in a narrow area adjacent to the epithelium. Reticular fibers are also found in loose tissue investing blood vessels. They appear to be composed of a special variety of collagen designated as type III collagen, whereas most of the remaining collagen fibers are composed of type I collagen.

Oxytalan fibers, so named because of their resistance to acid digestion, are found throughout the periodontal connective tissue, but do not seem to contribute significantly to the attachment of the teeth. Their origin, chemical composition, and function are as yet not known. They probably represent a form of immature elastic fiber, consisting of the microfibrillar component of the mature elas-

tic fiber without the amorphous elastin. *Anchoring fibrils,* which have been described in close association with the connective tissue side of epithelial basement laminae, constitute an entity, the composition of which still requires clarification (Fig. 1-13).

The most conspicuous parts of the gingival connective tissue are the collagen fibers. Some of these fibers are distributed in a haphazard arrangement throughout the connective tissue ground substance. Others are arranged in coarse bundles that exhibit a distinct orientation (Fig. 1-26). The fiber bundles have been given names according to their general direction and coarseness. Each of the fiber arrangements consists of collagenous fiber bundles built up from numerous fibers. According to current nomenclature these fiber systems should not be termed "fibers." The terms "circular fibers,"

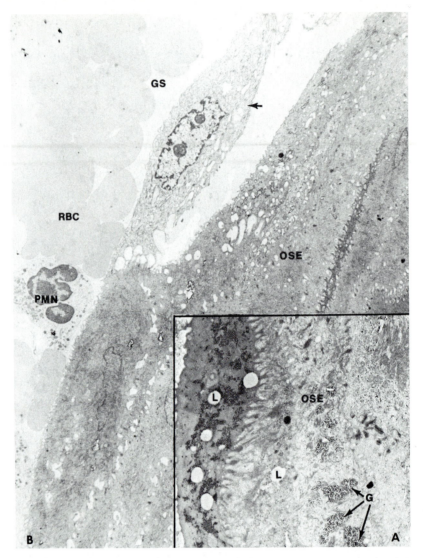

Fig. 1-25. Oral sulcular epithelium, *OSE,* that lines lateral wall of gingival sulcus, *GS,* shows partially keratinized surface cells, one of which *(arrow)* is desquamating into sulcus. Inset: glycogen particles, *G,* are present in surface cells as well as deeper layers. *RBC,* Red blood cells from surgical hemorrhage; *PMN,* polymorphonuclear leukocyte; *L,* lipid droplets. (**A** ×4,300; **B** ×6,000.) (From Schroeder, H. E., and Listgarten, M. A.: In Wolsky, A., editor: Monographs in developmental biology, vol. 2, Basel, 1971, S. Karger.)

"transseptal fibers," and so on, however, have been adapted into the professional language and will also be used in the following description with the understanding that they are systems of collagen fiber bundles.

The *circular fibers* (Fig. 1-26) belong to the free gingiva and encircle the tooth in a ringlike fashion.

The *dentogingival fibers* (Fig. 1-26) are part of a fan-shaped fiber system that emerges from the supra-alveolar part of the cementum of the entire circumference of the tooth. The dentogingival branch of this system sweeps outward and upward and terminates in the marginal gingiva. Another group emerges from the same area, but it passes outward beyond the alveolar crest in an apical direction into the mucoperiosteum of the attached gingiva. These are the *dentoperiosteal fibers.*

An *interpapillary* group of fibers has also been described that runs in an orovestibular direction from the vestibular to the oral interdental papillae of posterior teeth.

The architecture of the gingival and interdental ligaments of clinically healthy young adult marmosets was studied by Page et al. (1974). The gin-

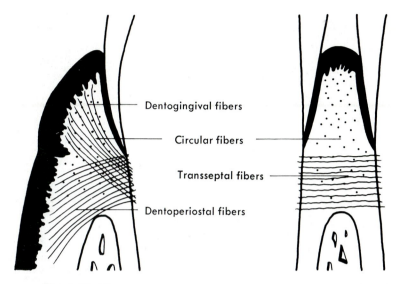

Fig. 1-26. Fiber arrangements of gingival connective tissue.

givae were free of histologic manifestations of inflammatory gingival disease. In addition to the fiber groups previously described, *semicircular fibers* were found to arise from the cementum near the cementoenamel junction, traverse the free marginal, facial, and lingual gingivae, and insert into a comparable position on the opposite side of the tooth at a level just apical to the circular fibers. *Intergingival fibers* course in the free marginal gingiva on both the facial and lingual surfaces of the teeth; also *transgingival fibers* arise from the cementum of one tooth and extend into the marginal gingiva of an adjacent tooth.

The *transseptal fibers* (Fig. 1-26) extend from the supra-alveolar cementum of one tooth mesiodistally through the interdental gingiva above the septum of the alveolar bone to the cementum of the adjacent tooth.

The *lamina propria* of the attached gingiva is a layer of dense connective tissue into which most of the above-mentioned fiber systems enter but which, in addition, contains numerous other bundles of fibers of more or less well-defined orientation. Some of the latter fibers provide for the firm attachment of the lamina propria to the periosteum of the alveolar process.

The gingival fibers as well as the principal fibers of the periodontal ligament consist mainly of bundles of collagen fibrils embedded in a ground substance. The fibrils are composed of aggregated collagen molecules.

The basic structure of the collagen molecule is a rodlike molecule approximately 300 nm long and 1.5 nm in diameter. It is composed of three polypeptide chains, the α-chains, each approximately 100,000 mol w, wrapped together in a right-handed helix.

There are at least four types of collagen, which are differentiated according to their α-chain composition. The α-chains are currently classified as $\alpha 1$ or $\alpha 2$ chains depending on their elution position from chromatography columns. In addition, the $\alpha 1$ chains are subdivided further, according to the sequence of the amino acids along their length, into "types" I to IV.

The most common form of collagen in the body is the collagen of skin, mucous membranes, bone, dentin, and cementum. Under the electron microscope it appears as well-defined fibrils with a characteristic axial periodicity of approximately 70 nm (see Fig. 1-48). This form of collagen is referred to as type I collagen. Type I collagen molecules are composed of two $\alpha 1$ type I and one $\alpha 2$ chains. The structural formula for type I collagen is $[\alpha 1(I)]_2 \alpha 2$.

Other types of collagen that have been recognized include collagen from cartilage, which is designated as type II, with the structural formula $[\alpha 1(II)]_3$; collagen from fetal skin and reticular fibers, which contains type III $[\alpha 1(III)]_3$ collagen; and type IV collagen, which is found in basement membranes, with the structural formula $[\alpha 1(IV)]_3$.

Type I collagen is the only form that has been shown to contain both $\alpha 1$ and $\alpha 2$ chains. It is able to form, by lateral aggregation of the collagen molecules, striated collagen fibrils with a distinct periodicity (see Fig. 1-48, *A*).

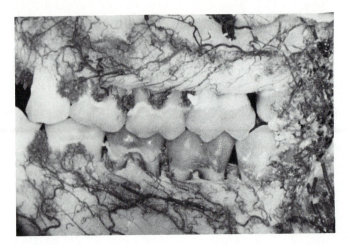

Fig. 1-27. Corrosion preparation of left buccal maxillary and mandibular segments of a monkey injected with cold-setting colored acrylic through carotid artery. Gingival branches of buccal and facial arteries are shown. (From Karring, T., and Löe, H.: J. Periodont. Res. **2**:74, 1967.)

Two unusual amino acids characterize the collagen protein: hydroxyproline and hydroxylysine. The hydroxyproline content of tissues in general is taken as a measure of their collagen content.

Between the collagenous elements is found an interfibrillar, amorphous ground substance. Histochemical and chemical analyses have disclosed that the ground substance is characterized by the presence of certain polysaccharide-protein complexes or proteoglycans. Proteoglycans that contain a relatively high proportion of protein are also called "glycoproteins." When carbohydrates predominate, the proteoglycans are called "mucopolysaccharides" or "glycosaminoglycans," the latter term having largely replaced the former. Glycosaminoglycans consist of linear carbohydrate chains linked by covalent bonds to a protein core. Some of these molecules are sulfated (e.g., chondroitin sulfates); others do not contain sulfate (e.g., hyaluronic acid).

It is difficult to precisely specify the function of the ground substance. But its important role in the maintenance of normal tissue physiology is probably best demonstrated by the fact that the ground substance constitutes the immediate environment of the cells. Any substance vital to cells must pass from the blood vessels through this substance to reach the cells.

Deviations from normal as to chemical composition and physical state of the ground substance will consequently reflect on both the cellular physiology and the rheology.

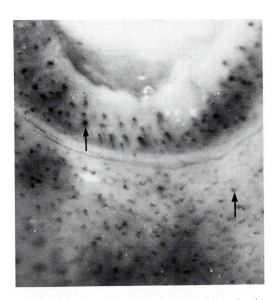

Fig. 1-28. Small blood vessels *(arrows)* terminating in loops at connective tissue–epithelium interface of buccal gingiva. (From Glavind, L., and Löe, H.: J. Periodont. Res. **2**:74, 1967.)

Blood supply of gingiva

The blood supply of the gingival tissues is derived mainly from supraperiosteal vessels originating from the lingual, mental, buccinator, and palatine arteries. These vessels give off branches along the facial and oral surfaces of the alveolar bone (Fig. 1-27). The superficial portions of these vessels are readily seen through the vestibular and oral mucosa (Fig. 1-28). Also branches of

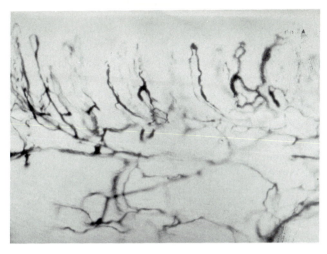

Fig. 1-29. Terminating vessels immediately below basement membrane in attached gingiva. Animal was injected with carbon serum. (From Karring, T., and Löe, H.: J. Periodont. Res. **2:**74, 1967.)

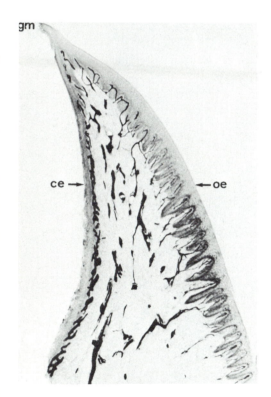

Fig. 1-30. Clinically healthy gingiva of a dog (buccolingual section) showing a layer of blood vessels in close apposition to junctional epithelium, *ce. gm,* Gingival margin; *oe,* oral epithelium. Animal was injected with carbon gelatin. (From Egelberg, J.: J. Periodont. Res. **1:**63, 1966.)

the alveolar arteries penetrating the interdental septa or emerging from the periodontal ligament contribute to the gingival blood supply. These branches anastomose with the periosteal ones and form the vascular bed of the gingiva. Due to the keratinized surface layer of the gingiva, blood vessels are not commonly seen with the naked eye.

The nutritional supply to the gingival epithelium is via capillaries terminating in groups immediately below the basement membrane (Fig. 1-29). Microscopic studies of the gingival surface in vivo have shown that there are approximately 50 capillaries per square millimeter, each of which terminates in a loop in the peripheral part of the connective tissue papillae adjacent to the epithelial border. Wide variations in number exist, however, between teeth as well as between different individuals. However, longitudinal studies show that within a particular gingival region the same vascular pattern persists over a long period of time. This indicates that under normal conditions the blood supply is quite consistent with respect to the number, distribution, and size of the blood vessels.

Next to the sulcular and junctional epithelia, the terminal blood vessels form a plexus that extends under the epithelial surface from the gingival margin to the apical extension of the junctional epithelium (Fig. 1-30).

Most of the vessels in the gingival connective tissue are arterioles, capillaries, and small veins. Occasionally small arteries are seen in the connective tissue of oral mucosa. The overall diameter of an arteriole is of the order of 100 μm. The walls of the arterioles consist of three more or less well-defined layers. The *intima* is a simple layer of endothelial cells. Sometimes a small amount of connective tissue may be interposed between this and the *media,* which is made up of circularly arranged smooth muscle fibers. Occasionally in the larger arterioles the *adventitia* may consist of collagenous and elastic fibers forming an external elastic lamina.

The change from arteriole to capillary is a gradual one, during which both the diameter and the thickness of the wall of the arteriole decrease. The capillary wall is made up of a single layer of endothelial cells arranged end to end and held together by specialized junctions and an intercellular cementing substance. The diameter of the capillary is approximately 10 μm. The endothelial cells as observed in electron micrographs are surrounded by an amorphous basement lamina. The basement lamina is too thin to be observed by the light microscope. However, a layer containing thin connective tissue filaments surrounds the basement lamina and separates the blood vessel from the surrounding collagenous matrix. It is probable that the basement lamina, together with this adjacent region, constitutes what at the level of the light microscope is termed the basement membrane.

Normally the transport of substances between the circulatory system and the tissues takes place across the capillary wall at a rate that meets the requirements of the particular part of the tissue at any given moment. For a long time it was believed (1) that the transfer of fluid as well as particulate matter from the inside of the capillary to the surrounding tissue occurred exclusively at the regions between endothelial cells and (2) that the

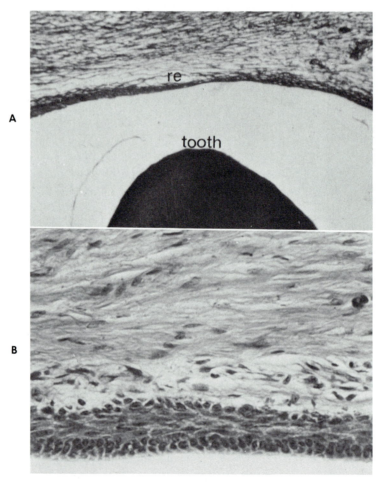

Fig. 1-31. Unerupted tooth during formation. **A,** Note reduced enamel epithelium, *re,* encircling crown. **B,** Reduced enamel epithelium consists of shortened ameloblasts and cellular derivatives from other cell layers of enamel organ.

nature of the intercellular cementing substance would facilitate such a process. Recent research, however, has indicated that the endothelial cells themselves also take part in transport activity through their cytoplasm. Under normal conditions water and electrolytes diffuse through the capillary wall. This diffusion is made possible by the slightly higher hydrostatic pressure within the vessel as compared to that outside. Normally, high-molecular-weight substances from plasma do not leak out into the tissue fluid. Nevertheless, it is evident that plasma proteins under physiologic conditions are found in the extravascular compartment. The necessary adjustment of capillary circulation and the alteration of the capillary wall

to allow for this transfer are controlled by indirect and direct mechanisms. Although the capillaries are indirectly controlled by nervous mechanisms to some degree, the major regulation of permeability is dependent on general and local chemical mechanisms. Accumulation of locally formed metabolites (e.g., histamine), as well as lack of oxygen, increased carbon dioxide tension, and corresponding change in pH, causes dilatation and increased permeability. For shorter periods of oxygen deprivation the rate of filtration through the capillary wall may be increased several times, and the endothelium may be so permeable that protein molecules may also pass through with ease. As the capillaries dilate, fresh blood flows through

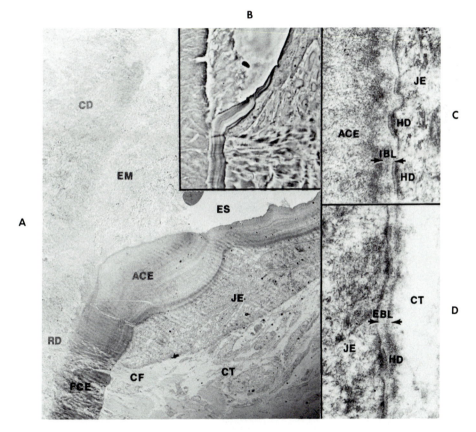

Fig. 1-32. Cervical region of tooth. **A,** Electron micrograph illustrating fibrillar root cementum, *FCE,* covering root dentin, *RD.* Cervical enamel surface is covered by a layer of afibrillar cementum that does not contain collagen fibrils, *ACE.* Junctional epithelium, *JE,* is attached to outer surface of *ACE* "spur" and extends apically up to fibrillar cementum of root. A collagen fiber, *CF,* immediately below it extends from gingival connective tissue, *CT,* into *FCE. CD,* Crown dentin; *EM,* enamel matrix; *ES,* enamel space. **B,** Phase-contrast micrograph of a serial section of **A** for orientation. **C,** Junction of *JE* with *ACE.* Note presence of hemidesmosomes, *HD,* and an internal basement lamina, *IBL.* **D,** Junction of *JE* with *CT.* This region is similar to **C** and contains hemidesmosomes and an external basement lamina, *EBL.* (**A** × 1,800; **B** × 420; **C** × 45,000.) (From Schroeder, H. E., and Listgarten, M. A.: In Wolsky, A., editor: Monographs in developmental biology, vol. 2, Basel, 1971, S. Karger.)

the area removing the waste material and bringing a new supply of oxygen. The attraction of metabolites into the venous blood is made possible through the fact that the osmotic pressure of blood is somewhat greater than the osmotic pressure of tissue fluid.

Histogenesis of dentogingival junction

Recent evidence indicates that after the enamel matrix is deposited the ameloblasts become shortened, but continue to function for a period of time in a resorptive capacity during maturation of the enamel. The epithelial cells derived from the enamel organ, including the reduced ameloblasts and cells adjacent to their proximal (external) surface, form the *reduced enamel epithelium* (Fig. 1-31). In normal human teeth prior to eruption, the reduced enamel epithelium forms an almost complete covering over the external surface of the enamel. In the cervical region of the crown, minor interruptions in the lining may occur that allow the formation of relatively thin, irregularly shaped layers of cementum over the exposed enamel surface. These afibrillar cementum patches are frequently devoid of typical collagen fibrils. In sections they may appear as cementum "spurs" that overlap the apical border of the enamel (Fig. 1-32) or as "islands" of afibrillar cementum on the cervical enamel surface.

The reduced enamel epithelium is normally composed of several layers of cells that are arranged with their long axes parallel to the enamel surface. As the tooth erupts and approaches the oral epithelium covering the alveolar ridge, the outer cell layers of the reduced enamel epithelium covering the tip of the crown begin to divide. The reduced ameloblasts cannot divide, since they have lost the ability to do so shortly after their differentiation from preameloblasts. As the crown is about to break into the oral cavity, the reduced enamel epithelium appears to fuse with the oral epithelium.

At this stage the enamel surface is partly covered with epithelium, the coronal part of which may be morphologically similar to junctional epithelium and the apical portion to reduced enamel epithelium (Fig. 1-33). Shortly after the crown enters the oral cavity, the epithelium over the

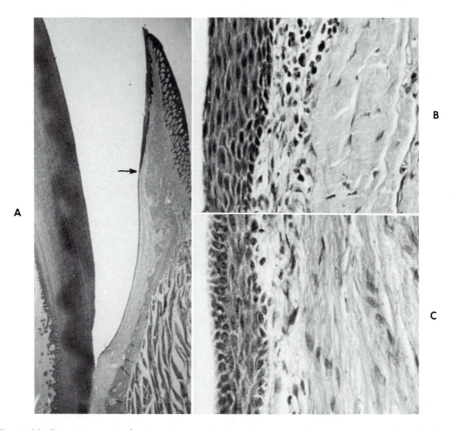

Fig. 1-33. Erupting tooth, **A,** showing gradual replacement of reduced enamel epithelium, **C,** by junctional epithelium, **B.**

enamel becomes entirely composed of junctional epithelium, which may form a band several millimeters wide around the crown. With further eruption the crown is gradually uncovered until the tooth has reached the plane of occlusion.

As the crown surface is uncovered, the width of the junctional epithelial band diminishes, since in the normal state the apical extension remains more or less stabilized at the level of the cervical region.

Some investigators have claimed that the reduced enamel epithelium is displaced by cells derived primarily from oral epithelial cells that proliferate in an apical direction and replace the reduced enamel epithelium. Electron microscopic and autoradiographic data suggest that the junctional epithelium is produced primarily by proliferation of the outer cells of the reduced enamel epithelium. The reduced ameloblasts become flattened and assume the morphologic characteristics of squamous epithelial cells. Because they have lost the ability to divide, they are eventually displaced by the outer cells of the reduced enamel epithelium that give rise to most of the junctional epithelium. This occurs as part of the normal physiologic turnover of the cells in junctional epithelium. Oral epithelium may initially contribute to the formation of only the most coronal portion of the junctional epithelium. In some erupted teeth a *dental cuticle* may be noted between the junctional epithelium and the adjacent tooth surface (Fig. 1-34). The origin and nature of this structure are not clear. As the junctional epithelium assumes a more apical position in relation to the tooth surface during the years that follow tooth emergence into the oral cavity, the dental cuticle

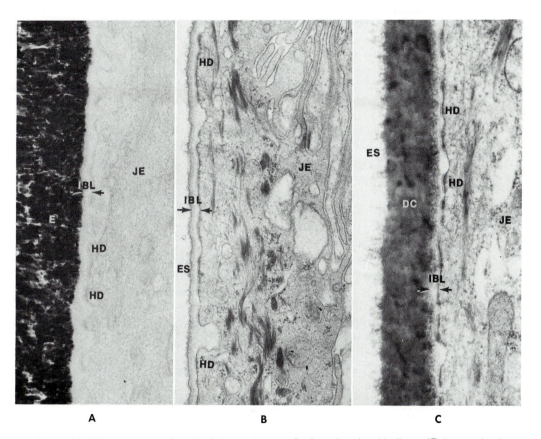

A   B   C

Fig. 1-34. Ultrastructure of epithelial attachment. **A,** Junctional epithelium, *JE,* is attached to undemineralized enamel, *E,* by internal basement lamina, *IBL,* and hemidesmosomes, *HD.* **B,** Similar section to that shown in **A** except that tissue was first demineralized. *ES,* Enamel space; *IBL,* internal basement lamina; *HD,* hemidesmosomes; *JE,* junctional epithelium. **C,** Dental cuticle, *DC,* is interposed between enamel space, *ES,* and internal basement lamina, *IBL,* of junctional epithelium, *JE. HD,* Hemidesmosomes. (×14,000.) (From Schroeder, H. E., and Listgarten, M. A.: In Wolsky, A., editor: Monographs in developmental biology, vol. 2, Basel, 1971, S. Karger.)

may become exposed to the oral environment, while remaining attached to the tooth surface in the vicinity of the gingival sulcus. In this location it may subsequently become colonized by bacteria or worn off.

Although the oral epithelium may play a limited role in the initial formation of the junctional epithelium, it is capable, when called upon, of regenerating a completely new junctional epithelium (e.g., after gingivectomy).

Connection between epithelium and enamel

The nature of the relationship between epithelium and enamel has been the subject of controversy for many years. Until 1921 the epithelium was not believed to be connected to the enamel surface. The gingival sulcus was thought of as a space lined by an extension of the oral epithelium into the sulcus, the epithelium tapering toward the cervix of the tooth where it ended in the form of a linear junction. In 1921 Gottlieb reported that the epithelium was attached to the enamel surface. Gottlieb stated that during completion of enamel formation the ameoloblasts produce a specialized layer of material that he named the "primary enamel cuticle." Subsequently, the ameloblasts were thought to degenerate, followed by the cells of the stratum intermedium and stellate reticulum. The outer enamel epithelium was believed to change from a simple epithelium into a stratified squamous keratinizing epithelial layer; the keratin layer formed an "organic union" between the epithelium and the primary enamel cuticle covering the enamel surface. Gottlieb referred to the keratinized layer as the "secondary enamel cuticle." Subsequently, this name was changed to "dental cuticle." Although Gottlieb originally postulated the presence of a keratinized cuticle between the epithelium and the enamel surface, subsequent histochemical and electron microscopic studies have indicated that this material is not composed of keratin.

Another view, proposed by Weski and by Becks, postulated that the odontogenic epithelium does not persist but degenerates and becomes replaced by epithelial cells proliferating from the oral epithelium. The degenerating odontogenic epithelium was thought to keratinize and form the secondary cuticle, which established a firm union with the primary cuticle. A later theory rejected the concept of a secondary cuticle as a medium of structural continuity between the two tissues and suggested that the new epithelial cells arising from the oral epithelium attach themselves to the enamel by means of tonofibrils inserted into the primary cuticle. This was not corroborated by subsequent electron microscopic data.

Based on the consideration that Gottlieb's histologic concept of the epithelial attachment did not coincide with clinical observations, Waerhaug set out to investigate the discrepancy. Waerhaug noted that thin steel blades could be inserted through the gingival sulcus to the region of the cementoenamel junction with relative ease. On the basis of these and related experiments Waerhaug restated the view held to be valid prior to Gottlieb that no structural continuity exists between gingiva and enamel, and that the bottom of the gingival sulcus is located at the cementoenamel junction. Waerhaug believed that the epithelium was only weakly adherent to the enamel surface and described the epithelium surrounding the neck of the tooth as an "epithelial cuff."

Electron microscopic and autoradiographic studies have provided a clearer understanding of the nature of the dentoepithelial interface. Toward the end of enamel maturation, the plasmalemma of the ameloblasts in contact with the enamel surface develops *hemidesmosomes*. The space between the cell membrane and the enamel surface is occupied by a *basement lamina* joining the cells to the enamel surface. The hemidesmosomes and the basement lamina are believed to form the attachment apparatus joining the epithelium to the tooth. A similar attachment apparatus is also found between the external surface of the reduced enamel epithelium and the surrounding connective tissue. The basement lamina facing the tooth surface is referred to as the *internal basement lamina*, whereas the basement lamina facing the connective tissue is called the *external basement lamina*. The biologic mechanism that unites epithelial cells to the tooth surface may be properly described as the *epithelial attachment*. This term should not be used to describe an epithelium such as the junctional epithelium or reduced enamel epithelium. Its morphologically recognizable components consist of hemidesmosomes and the internal basement lamina.

Electron microscopic studies have revealed the presence of hemidesmosomes and a basement lamina at the interface of a large variety of epithelial membranes and the underlying connective tissue. It has been shown that epithelial cells grown in tissue culture are also capable of synthesizing such an apparatus against the surface on which they are cultured. It has also been demonstrated that junctional epithelial cells are able to attach to artificial endosseous tooth implants by means of hemidesmosomes and a basement lamina. The basement lamina consists of a carbohydrate-protein complex, the exact composition of which may vary in different sites of the body. The main protein component of basement laminae has been identified as a form of collagen peculiar to basement laminae. It is one of at least four different types of collagen, which have been previously defined. It is known as type IV collagen, whereas the collagen fibrils commonly observed in the connective tissue of the periodontium and in the organic matrix of bone, dentin, and cementum are composed of type I collagen. The basement lamina material serves as a glue that attaches the epithelial cell to the underlying surface. The strength of this attachment may be greater in the immediate vicinity of hemidesmosomes. Despite the presence of an epithelial attachment, the cells appear to be capable of moving in relation to the underlying stratum. An analogous situation exists when two glass plates are held together by a film of water. They cannot be readily pulled apart, although they slide easily over each other.

As the tooth erupts into the oral cavity, the enamel surface is covered with a layer of reduced enamel epithelium characterized by the presence of recognizable ameloblasts in contact with the enamel surface. Ultrastructurally, these cells may be identified by the presence of large numbers of mitochondria, invaginated nuclei frequently surrounded by pigmentlike granules in the perinuclear cytoplasm, and their attachment to the enamel surface via hemidesmosomes and the internal basement lamina. After eruption most of the reduced ameloblasts undergo a morphologic change so that they begin to resemble squamous epithelial cells. Most of the mitochondria are lost and the nucleus assumes a more ovoid shape. The cytoplasm with its tonofibrils, Golgi region, and other cytoplasmic components becomes indistinguishable from that of typical squamous epithelial cells. In addition to their cytoplasmic reorganization these cells become flattened and indistinguishable from the epithelial cells found in the mature junctional epithelium. At the same time the cells external to the transformed ameloblasts proliferate, thereby causing an increased thickening of the epithelium. These cells eventually displace the transformed ameloblasts and become in turn attached to the enamel surface through hemidesmosomes and an internal basement lamina.

When reduced ameloblasts can no longer be recognized as such within the epithelium lining the enamel surface, the epithelium becomes known as the *junctional epithelium*. The morphology of the attachment apparatus of the junctional epithelium to the enamel surface is identical to that connecting the reduced enamel epithelium to the enamel. In erupted teeth an electron-dense *dental cuticle* may be found in close association with the junctional epithelium. When present, it is generally found between the enamel surface and the junctional epithelium (Fig. 1-34). It may also appear as an intervening layer between the surface of afibrillar cementum patches and the junctional epithelium. Its origin and nature are not known at the present time. It is clear, however, that this material is not a keratinized layer as originally suggested by Gottlieb.

The nature of the connection between the junctional epithelium and the tooth surface is such that mechanical stresses to this region result in tears within the epithelium, rather than in a clean separation of the epithelium from the tooth surface. Because the cell turnover rate in this region is relatively high (the junctional epithelium replaces itself approximately every 7 days), minor tears can be readily repaired within that period of time. Cells in the junctional epithelium pass from the basal layer through the epithelium lining to become desquamated in the gingival sulcus.

In ideal situations the junctional epithelium may be attached to the tooth all the way from the most apical border of the enamel to a level approaching the gingival margin. In such cases the depth of the histologic sulcus may approach 0 mm. The clinical sulcus depth as determined with periodontal probing may considerably disagree with the histologic sulcus depth. This is apparently due to tearing of the epithelium by the periodontal probe. The depth of such tears may vary with such factors as width of the junctional epithelium, local inflammation, contour of the dentoepithelial junction, size of the probe, and direction and force applied to it. It should be clear at this point that the probeable depth of a sulcus and histologic sulcus depth are two distinct entities that should not be equated with each other, particularly in the presence of an inflammatory infiltrate.

Sulcular fluid

Flow of tissue fluid through the sulcular epithelium and the possible biologic function of this fluid have been the object of considerable research during the last 15 years. After intravenous injection or oral administration of fluorescein, which labels plasma proteins, Brill et al. recovered the dye at the orifice of the gingival sulci. The fluid was col-

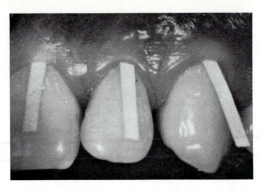 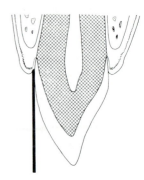

Fig. 1-35. Intrasulcular sampling of exudate. Note that strip is placed at entrance of sulcus. (From Löe, H., and Holm-Pedersen, P.: Periodontics **3:**171, 1965.)

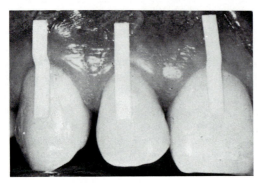 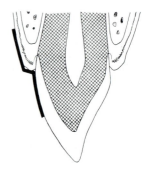

Fig. 1-36. Extrasulcular sampling method. (From Löe, H., and Holm-Pedersen, P.: Periodontics **3:**171, 1965.)

lected on filter paper strips that were either inserted into the sulci or adapted to bridge the orifice of the facial aspect of the gingival sulci (Figs. 1-35 to 1-37). The results indicated that a fluid containing small molecules might pass from the subepithelial tissues into the gingival crevice and out into the oral cavity. Other epithelial surfaces of the mouth did not allow the passage of tissue fluid.

Immunoelectrophoretic analyses have disclosed that at least seven different plasma proteins are present in this fluid. Both α_1- and α_2-globulins as well as beta and gamma globulins were identified.

A series of similar experiments tended to show that flow of fluid has an intimate relationship with capillary permeability and that it passes from the subepithelial connective tissues between or through the cells of the junctional epithelium.

The amount of fluid from normal gingivae is scanty. It increases after mechanical stimulation of the gingivae or after intravenous injection of histamine. If bacteria or other particulate materials are introduced into the sulcus, they are expelled with the fluid within minutes, provided that they are not mechanically retained. Also, in these in-

stances the flow of fluid is increased. The suggestion has been made that the flushing effect that is in this way produced may form an important part of the local defense mechanism, since the outward flow can normally prevent the penetration of foreign particulate matter into the gingival sulcus.

In gingival inflammation the rate of outward flow is markedly increased. Obviously this fluid must be considered not simply as a filtrate from tissues with normal metabolism, but as an inflammatory exudate. Because of the almost invariable presence of an inflammatory reaction at the gingival margin, and the regular finding of neutrophilic leukocytes in the sulcular fluid, it has been difficult to accept the presence of sulcular fluid as part of the normal noninflamed gingiva. In fact, a recent investigation has shown that strictly normal human gingiva does not exhibit a flow of fluid. Nor does mechanical stimulation of the periodontium produce a flow of fluid from normal sulci. Inflamed gingiva, on the other hand, regularly shows the presence of fluid, the amount of which varies with the severity of the inflammation. These results tend to show that the fluid

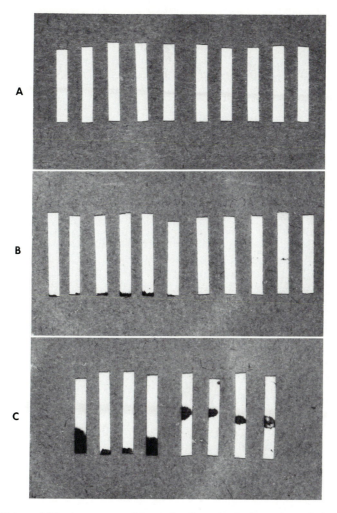

Fig. 1-37. Strips of filter paper used for collecting gingival exudate. Strips on left half of illustrations were used to collect intrasulcular samples. Treating strips with ninhydrine shows absence of fluid in teeth with clinically normal gingiva, **A,** traces or small amounts of exudate in teeth with slightly inflamed gingiva, **B,** and increased amount of exudate in teeth with moderate gingival inflammation, **C.** (From Löe, H., and Holm-Pedersen, P.: Periodontics **3:**171, 1965.)

which oozes out between the gingiva and the tooth is closely related to tissue changes in the area.

This relationship has been confirmed in a longitudinal study of the development of gingivitis (Fig. 1-38). During this experiment, gingivae that at the start did not exhibit any flow of fluid began to do so as soon as increased bacterial activity developed in the region. The amount of fluid increased steadily throughout the experimental period, and maximal flow occurred shortly before clinically observable gingivitis developed. As soon as gingival inflammation lessened as a result of local treatment, a corresponding decrease in flow of fluid occurred. Finally, a few days after gingival

inflammation had resolved, the flow of fluid ceased.

Together with the facts that (1) inflammatory cells are regularly present in sulcular fluid, (2) the chemical composition is different from tissue fluid, and (3) the passage of fluid is closely related to the area of inflammation, the sulcular fluid should be considered as an inflammatory exudate rather than as a physiologic secretion. The relatively narrow intercellular spaces of the sulcular epithelium, which are generally free of leukocytes, and the tendency demonstrated by the surface cells toward keratinization suggest that the coronal portion of the sulcus lined by sulcular epithelium is relatively more impermeable to the passage of sulcular fluid

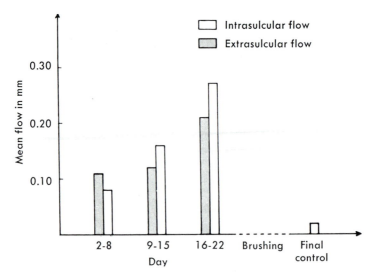

Fig. 1-38. Mean flow of gingival exudate of 15 teeth after withdrawal of all oral hygiene measures in eight individuals. Teeth showed no flow at start of experiment. During period of no cleansing all teeth developed flow of exudate, amount of which increased throughout experimental period. As soon as tooth cleansing was reintroduced, flow of fluid decreased and finally disappeared. (From Löe, H., and Holm-Pedersen, P.: Periodontics **3:**171, 1965.)

or leukocytes than the apical portion lined by junctional epithelium.

The finding that the flow of fluid regularly starts before structural changes can be ascertained at the clinical level and persists some time after clinical inflammation has subsided means that exudation is discernible before gingival inflammation can be clinically assessed. It is possible, therefore, that the absence or presence of fluid may represent the best available clinical means of establishing the distinction between normal and subclinically inflamed gingivae.

Defense mechanism of gingiva

Recent periodontal research has furnished substantial evidence that bacterial irritation is essential for the development and maintenance of marginal periodontal inflammation. As in any other infection, the clinical manifestations of the disease are dependent on the aggressive properties of the microorganisms and the capability of the host to withstand the aggression.

Although particulate material may not find ready ingress into the sulcular and junctional epithelia, it is likely that soluble products originating in the gingival sulcus can diffuse into the connective tissue via the junctional epithelium. The role played by the epithelium in protecting the underlying connective tissue from damaging substances originating in the oral cavity appears to be less dependent on the so-called seal at the dentoepithelial junction (epithelial attachment) than on the permeability of the junctional epithelium (Fig. 1-39). Although bacterial plaque may extend to the very bottom of the gingival sulcus, individual microorganisms may not necessarily be able to penetrate the epithelial barrier. However, their soluble products may enter the connective tissue via the large intercellular spaces of the junctional epithelium and give rise to an inflammatory response in the region immediately subjacent to the permeable portion of the junctional epithelium. This would explain the localization of the earliest inflammatory lesion in close proximity to the junctional epithelium.

Besides structural protection, the local defense against exogenous attack generally rests on mechanical, chemical, and cellular mechanisms. The efficacy of the mechanical factor is probably best illustrated by the lubricating action of saliva and the continuous desquamation of superficial epithelial cells, which prevent bacteria from settling en masse on the oral mucosa. The cleansing effect of the saliva on the gingival area seems rather insignificant. Recent experiments actually indicate that an effective self-cleansing of the marginal parts of human teeth does not occur, not even during prolonged mastication of a diet comprised of hard food. Some cleansing effect has been ascribed to the sulcular fluid inasmuch as it has

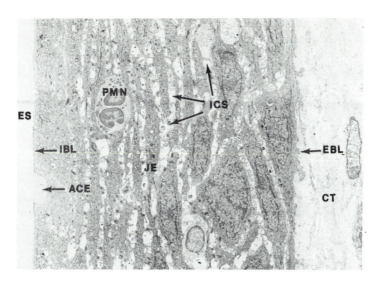

Fig. 1-39. Junctional epithelium, *JE.* Intercellular spaces, *ICS,* are wider than in normal gingival epithelium and may contain polymorphonuclear leukocytes, *PMN,* particularly in close proximity to sulcus. Cells are attached to each other by relatively few desmosomes. Sulcular exudate probably percolates through intercellular spaces rather than internal basement lamina, *IBL,* joining epithelium to tooth surface. *ACE,* Afibrillar cementum island; *ES,* enamel space; *EBL,* external basement lamina; *CT,* gingival connective tissue. (×2,000.) (From Schroeder, H. E., and Listgarten, M. A.: In Wolsky, A., editor: Monographs in developmental biology, vol. 2, Basel, 1971, S. Karger.)

been shown that the fluid is able to expel bacteria and particles that have gained entrance into the sulcus. From this it has been inferred that the fluid to some extent may also resist the introduction of foreign material into the gingival sulcus.

The presence of immunoglobulins in the sulcular fluid may indicate that it possesses antibacterial properties, but the effectiveness of this immunologic factor must be determined through further study. It has also been demonstrated that polymorphonuclear leukocytes are consistently found in this fluid. There can be little doubt about the phagocytic properties of these cells as long as they are lodged in the epithelium or the connective tissue. However, since microorganisms are frequently deposited in comparatively large numbers outside the gingival tissues on the tooth or gingival surface, phagocytosis at this site may not be clinically significant.

It is likely that the most important defense mechanism of the dentoepithelial junction resides in the inflammatory reaction that manifests itself initially as a gingivitis. It remains to be shown whether the resulting sulcular exudate and the leukocytes it contains possess any immunologic or phagocytic properties that may be of significance in this process. Variations in the protective efficacy of the inflammatory process and the composition of the

microbial flora may be the chief causes of differences in susceptibility to periodontal disease.

Apical shift of dentogingival junction

When the tooth has reached the occlusal plane, the gingival sulcus is located approximately over the gingival third of the crown. The junctional epithelium extends from this point apically to the region of the cervix. Apical to this point and along the entire circumference of the root the Sharpey fibers anchored into the cementum attach the tooth to the jaw. This is the ideal arrangement of the periodontium.

Many authorities, starting with Gottlieb, hold that this state of affairs is merely a transitional stage and that the epithelium, as age progresses, is apt to proliferate in an apical direction. In so doing it establishes a new firm union (epithelial attachment) with the cementum surface. This apical shift of the dentogingival junction has been termed *passive eruption*. Passive eruption is thought to continue at a varying rate throughout life.

The apical shift of the bottom of the gingival sulcus may be accompanied by an increase in sulcus depth. In other instances a shallow sulcus may remain, in which case a recession of the marginal gingiva has taken place concomitantly with the downgrowth of the epithelium. Why marginal atrophy occurs in some instances, whereas in others deepening of the sulcus takes place, has not been explained. In any event, downgrowth of the sulcular epithelium below the cementoenamel junction, with or without gingival recession, represents a significant change in the periodontium that, from a functional point of view, results in a loss of fibrous attachment and functional support of the teeth.

Gottlieb and others have considered passive eruption as a physiologic process that is continuous throughout life at a rate corresponding to the occlusal movement of the teeth in compensation for attrition. The latter process is known as *active eruption*. Active and passive eruptions have been thought to occur simultaneously; the purpose of passive eruption is to keep the clinical crown at an adequate length.

Basically, any apical proliferation of cells of the junctional epithelium along the cemental surface presupposes a breakdown of the uppermost Sharpey's fibers. According to Gottlieb, loss of fiber attachment occurs as a result of a devitalization of the cementum. In his opinion, attached fibers were believed to live and function for a certain length of time and then die, leaving behind a devitalized cementum. The vitality of the cementum was con-

sidered to be a matter of age of the tissue. The evidence to support this view has never been substantiated.

As will be shown shortly, the fate of the fiber attachment seems to be entirely dependent on the state of the supra-alveolar connective tissue. A simple degeneration of its fibers as part of a physiologic process has not been demonstrated and seems very unlikely. On the other hand, collagen from any location in the body has a certain turnover; i.e., collagen fibrils and fibers are dissolved and replaced by new ones at corresponding rates. The turnover of periodontal collagen has not been studied sufficiently, but there seems to be no reason to believe that this collagen generally differs in any respect from similar collagen elsewhere in the body. These processes are physiologic processes that aim at the maintenance of tissue, and they cannot be held responsible for the permanent destruction of periodontal fibers.

It has been suggested that a permanent dissolution of the collagen fibers may be brought about by an enzymatic action of the epithelial cells; but so far there is no evidence to substantiate such an activity on the part of the sulcular or junctional epithelium.

It is well known that endocrine function affects

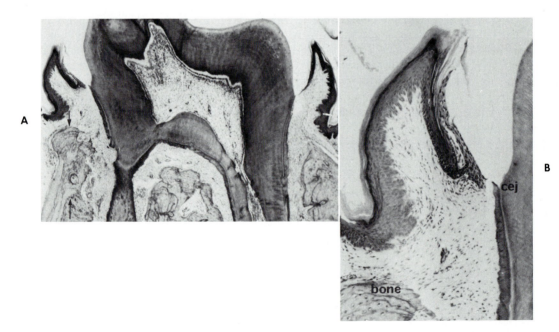

Fig. 1-40. Histologic section of mandibular rat molar after extraction of corresponding maxillary molars, allowing lower molars to move in occlusal direction. **A,** Injections with 1% lead acetate at day 0, 7, 33, and 62 show that new bone (between *arrows*) has been laid down at alveolar crest. **B,** Although tooth has moved occlusally, bottom of sulcus is still located at cementoenamel junction. (From Löe, H.: Unpublished data.)

connective tissue physiology and that sex hormones in particular have specific effects on the synthesis and maintenance of the fibrous collagen of the reproductory organs during pregnancy and after parturition. There is, however, no information to suggest that a clinical or subclinical imbalance of the female or male sex hormones during or outside pregnancy produces appreciable changes of the periodontal collagen fibers.

Variations of specific dietary components do not seem to cause downgrowth of sulcular epithelium. Not even in vitamin C deficiency, where connective tissue metabolism is seriously altered, are these fibers destroyed to the extent that a downgrowth of epithelium can take place.

The concept of passive eruption as a physiologic process seems to derive mainly from microscopic examination of human teeth of different ages, in which it is regularly seen that the bottom of sulci in the teeth of adults are situated at varying levels below the cementoenamel junction. In view of the fact that nearly all civilized adult patients have or have had a history of periodontal tissue inflammation, the use of specimens without a known history may be of doubtful value as a basis for investigating this problem.

The most obvious cause of apical migration of the cells of the sulcular epithelium is that the uppermost fibers have been destroyed as a result of gingival inflammation. Indeed, histologic preparations of teeth may be encountered where the epithelium is found below the cementoenamel junction and where histologic signs of inflammation are absent. However, appearances like these

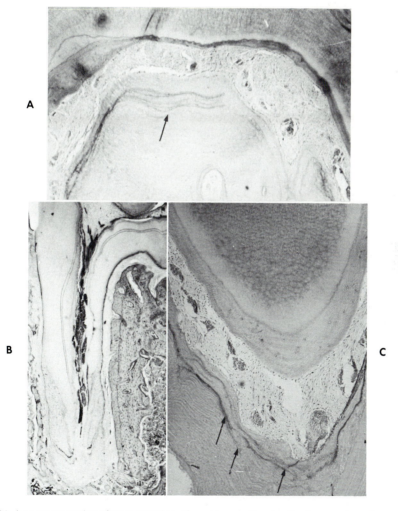

Fig. 1-41. Lower rat molar after extraction of corresponding teeth of upper jaw. Appositional lines in bone *(arrows)* are found at bifurcation area, **A,** at apical area, **C,** and in pulp cavity, **B,** according to labeling with lead acetate during experimental period. (From Löe, H.: Unpublished data.)

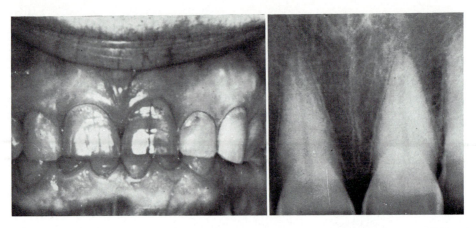

Fig. 1-42. Anterior teeth of a 78-year-old woman without periodontal disease. Although there is a great deal of occlusal wear, there is no recession of gingival margin or reduction in height of alveolar crest; that is, passive eruption has not occurred.

do not exclude the presence of inflammatory reactions at the moment of dissolution of the fibers and apical migration of the eipthelium. Histologic sections represent static pictures of the morphologic relationship at a particular moment in time. Unless the specimens are part of an experimental series, such preparations do not usually demonstrate the events that lead up to the situation that is pictured at the moment of examination.

Experimental results have shown that active eruption may take place without any movement of the junctional epithelium below the neck of the tooth (Figs. 1-40 and 1-41). Several teeth of monkeys were ground out of occlusion so that approximately 2 mm separated the opposing teeth. In the course of 9 months, occlusal movement brought these teeth into occlusion again. New cementum and bone formed to compensate for the eruption. The most apical extension of the junctional epithelium was still located at the cervix, and the relationship between this and the margin of the alveolar bone was normal due to apposition of bone tissue at the alveolar margin.

In other words, occlusal movement of teeth does not necessarily imply an apical shift of the dentogingival junction. The observation that in the dentition of Eskimos the gingival margin usually covers the cervical border of the enamel even in the presence of extreme occlusal wear corroborates these experimental findings. Similar conditions may also be found in civilized individuals who have escaped periodontal disease (Fig. 1-42).

Therefore the apical shift of the dentogingival junction, or passive eruption, does not appear to be a physiologic process. Migration of the junctional epithelium onto root cementum is possible

only after dissolution of the uppermost Sharpey's fibers. This destruction is effected at the stage where the marginal inflammation has reached into the supra-alveolar connective tissue. The clinical picture is characterized by recession of the gingival margin and a shallow gingival sulcus or by retention of the original level of the gingiva and a deepening of the sulcus.

It should be noted, however, that in either case the process can be arrested. If good oral hygiene is established, a normal junctional epithelium can reform at the existing level on the root surface, in the same relationship that existed originally over the enamel.

Clinical criteria of normal gingiva

It is widely held that clinically normal gingiva always exhibits a low degree of chronic inflammation and that the border between a normal and a pathologically changed gingiva is rather vague. Consequently, the term "clinically healthy gingiva" appears to be a highly arbitrary concept, and what appears to be normal gingiva to one examiner may not fulfill the requirements of another.

Recent experimental results indicate, however, that a strictly healthy gingiva at the clinical level may also show absence of inflammation when examined in microscopic preparations. In such specimens the sulcular epithelium is almost entirely free of inflammatory cells, and the underlying connective tissue shows no leukocytes or other blood cells in an extravascular location. To achieve freedom of gingival inflammation such as this, an extremely regimented program of oral hygiene must be instituted. It is of interest to note that germ-free beagles raised in the complete absence of bacteria, but not subject to any regimen of oral hygiene, may demonstrate the presence of polymorphonuclear leukocytes in junctional epithelium and of lymphocytes and plasma cells in the underlying connective tissue.

The clinical counterpart to this state of induced normality is a gingiva that complies with the qualitative criteria of a healthy gingiva as to color, surface, form, consistency, and gingival sulcus.

Color. The color of the healthy gingiva is pale pink. This pale appearance as compared with that of the redder oral mucosa is due to the thickness and keratinized state of the surface epithelium. The overall color may be modified by the presence of pigmentation in persons of dark complexion and the blood flow through the tissues.

Surface. The surface of the dried gingiva should be matt. Ordinarily it presents an uneven, stippled surface that resembles an orange peel. However, the degree of stippling may vary considerably within the normal.

Form. The form of the gingiva is dependent on the shape and size of the interdental areas, which again may depend on the shape and position of the teeth. The tip of the gingival papilla is the most incisally or occlusally located part of the gingiva. The gingival margin should be thin. The gingiva may terminate against the tooth in a knife-edge fashion, although in most human teeth the gingival margin is rounded.

Consistency. On palpation with a blunt instrument the gingiva should be firm. The gingiva is resilient and tightly bound to the underlying hard tissues. The marginal gingiva, although slightly movable, should be closely adapted to the tooth surface.

Gingival sulcus. The probing depth of the gingival sulcus may vary between 1 and 3 mm. Probing with a blunt probe should not cause bleeding. Normal gingiva exhibits no flow of sulcular fluid.

Part 2

ATTACHMENT APPARATUS (DENTOALVEOLAR UNIT)*

The mode of attachment of the tooth to the alveolus consists of numerous bundles of collagenous tissue (principal fibers) arranged in groups, which are separated by loose connective tissue containing blood vessels, lymph vessels, and

*The terms "attachment apparatus" and "dentoalveolar unit" are synonyms. Both are used in this text.

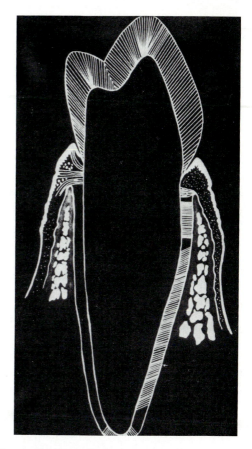

Fig. 1-43. Buccolingual aspect of periodontium: gingiva, alveolar process, dentoalveolar unit (cementum, periodontal ligament, bone). Fibers of periodontal ligament are divided into four groups: alveolar crestal, horizontal, oblique, and apical. Difference in epithelium covering gingiva in attached, keratinized zone to that of alveolar mucosa should be noted. Marginal fiber apparatus is also depicted.

nerves (Fig. 1-41). This ligament functions as the investing and supportive mechanism for the tooth. It is termed the *periodontal ligament* (Fig. 1-43). The dentoalveolar unit comprises the *cementum,* the *periodontal ligament,* and the *alveolar bone.* The periodontal ligament is the tissue that surrounds the roots of the tooth and attaches it to the bony alveolus. Cementum is the hard bonelike tissue covering the anatomic roots of the teeth. The *alveolar bone proper* is a plate of compact bone, the radiographic image of which is termed "*lamina dura.*"

The main function of the dentoalveolar unit is supportive, but it also has formative, nutritive, and sensory roles. The supportive function consists of maintaining and retaining the tooth. The formative function is necessary for the replacement of tis-

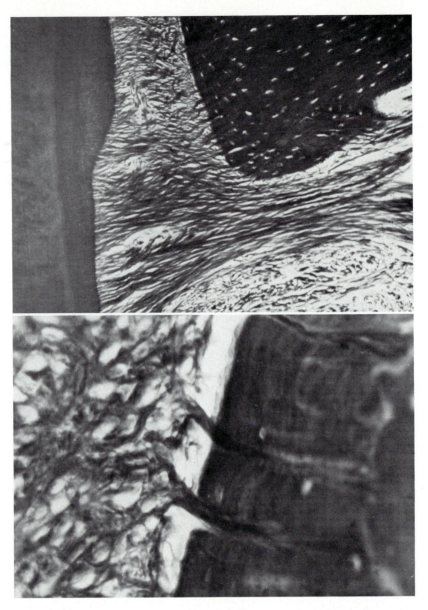

Fig. 1-44. Photomicrograph of a mesiodistal section of alveolar crest, periodontal ligament, and transseptal fibers. High power shows Sharpey's fibers entering alveolar bone.

sue—cementum, periodontal ligament, and alveolar bone. Three specialized cells are associated
with this function: *cementoblasts, fibroblasts,*
and *osteoblasts.* The nutritive and sensory functions are accomplished by the blood vessels and
nerves, respectively. Thus the attachment apparatus serves as a suspensory mechanism for
the tooth, as a pericementum for the maintenance of the root covering, and as periosteum
for the alveolar bone (Figs. 1-44 and 1-45).

Root cementum

Cementum is a hard tissue whose intercellular
substance is calcified. It is arranged in layers
around the tooth root. There are two types of root
cementum: *acellular* and *cellular.* The acellular
type is clear and structureless, being formed by
cementoblasts that deposit the substance but do not
become embedded in it, as is the case when the
cellular type is formed. During tooth formation,
as the cementum is formed, collagen fibers become incorporated in it. These are known as
Sharpey's fibers (Fig. 1-46). Acellular cementum
always covers the cervical portion of the root,
extending at times over almost all of the root except for the apical portion where cellular cementum is seen. Cellular cementum is bonelike in
character. It may later form over the acellular type.

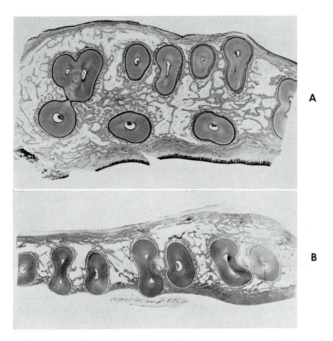

Fig. 1-45. Cross section of molar region of maxilla and mandible. **A,** Roots of molars surrounded by bone. Note contour of roots, formation of alveolar bone, and supporting bone. **B,** Roots of mandibular molars. Alveolar bone surrounding these roots is evident, and character of supporting bone is easily distinguished. These photomicrographs illustrate topography of attachment apparatus around molars.

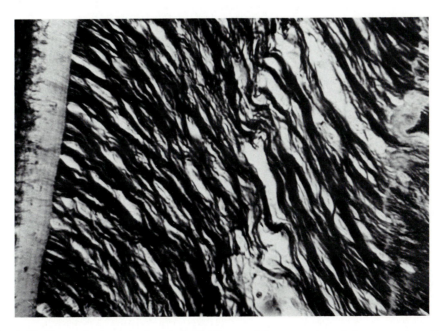

Fig. 1-46. Photomicrograph of periodontal ligament, bone, and acellular cementum. Note homogeneous appearance of acellular cementum; however, careful scrutiny shows a fibrillar appearance.

Cementocytes are found within *lacunae*. Cementum contains fewer embedded cells than bone tissue and fewer anastomosing canaliculi. It is devoid of vascular elements. Cementocyte processes anastomose with one another. Cementocytes have the same relationship to the matrix of the cementum as osteocytes to bone. Unlike bone, cementum does not remodel, although it may continue to grow by apposition of new layers. Evidence of apposition can be determined by darkly staining lines in sections stained with hematoxylin and eosin. These lines represent periods of nonformation. However, cemental apposition is slow, since teeth in later adult life normally show only relatively few appositional layers. Electron microscopic studies of specimens from young and old mice have suggested that adult cementum formation could be described as a slow apposi-

tional mineralization of the periodontal ligament. It must be stressed, however, that changes in function will have a great influence on the activity of cemental growth. Cementoblasts lining the root surface may exhibit the cytology of cells actively synthesizing protein or may take on the appearance of resting cells.

Acellular cementum

Acellular cementum forms a thin layer covering the dentin surface, the thickness of which varies from 20 to 50 μm near the cervix to 150 to 200 μm near the apex. In transmitted light it exhibits numerous appositional lines. In microradiographs the innermost zone nearest to the dentin appears less well mineralized than the remaining cementum. Recent studies by microradiography and electron microscopy have confirmed that acellular ce-

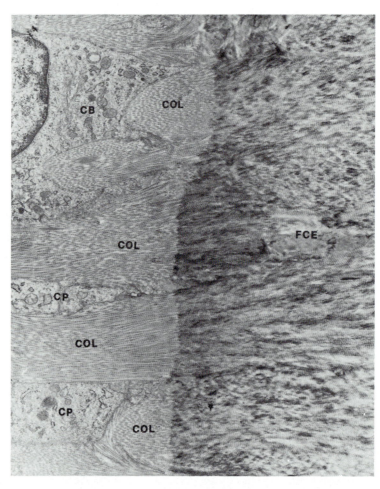

Fig. 1-47. Junction between acellular cementum, *FCE,* and periodontal ligament in which cementoblastic processes, *CP,* and collagen fiber bundles, *COL,* are visible. Collagen fiber bundles lose their identity as individual fibers after incorporation into cementum. *CB,* Cementoblast. (×5,000.) (From Listgarten, M.: Unpublished data, 1968.)

mentum is more highly calcified than cellular cementum. Electron microscopically, the acellular cementum consists of densely packed collagen fibrils with the typical collagen bands in register between adjacent fibrils. The fibrils are continuous with the collagen fibrils of the periodontal ligament (Figs. 1-47 and 1-48). Although the periodontal ligament consists of collagen fibrils running in distinct bundles, the latter frequently lose their identity as individual bundles when they become incorporated into the acellular cementum covering the coronal part of the root. This is particularly evident in the cementum just beneath the cervix (Fig. 1-44).

In mineralized preparations the normal banding of the collagen fibrils is obscured by the densely packed crystals of apatite that form the mineral phase of cementum (Fig. 1-45). The mineral component of cementum is an apatite that is deposited in the form of thin crystals (maximum size is 40 $\times$ 20 $\times$ 2nm); the long axis is generally parallel to the collagen fibrils. The crystals at the cementum surface tend to form small projections along the insertion of individual collagen fibrils from the periodontal ligament. Near the dentinocemental junction, some fibril bundles are incompletely mineralized, thereby making this region more radiolucent.

The dentinocemental junction may be identified by the different orientation and organization of the collagen fibrils. Whereas the collagen fibrils in dentin are arranged haphazardly, each fibril running an independent course, in acellular cementum the fibrils generally run in the same direction and more or less perpendicularly to the cementum surface (Fig. 1-49).

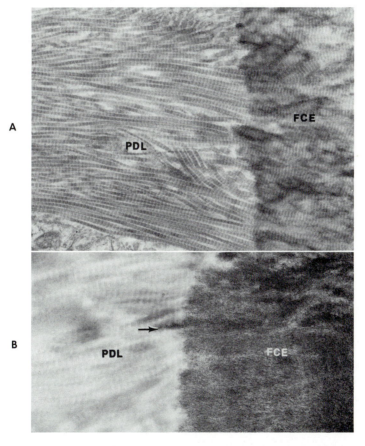

Fig. 1-48. Junction between collagen fibrils of periodontal ligament, *PDL,* and cementum, *FCE.* **A,** Demineralized specimen. Note incorporation of periodontal ligament collagen into cementum without any alteration of natural periodicity of collagen fibrils. **B,** Mineralized specimen. Banding of collagen fibrils in cementum is obliterated by crystals of apatite. Arrow indicates mineralized portion of a single fibril that forms a small spur extending into periodontal ligament. (**A** ×16,500; **B** ×28,000.) (From Listgarten, M.: Unpublished data, 1968.)

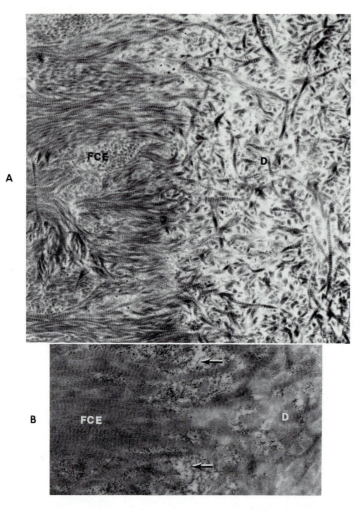

Fig. 1-49. A, Dentinocemental junction can be recognized by haphazard arrangement of collagen fibrils in dentin, *D,* bordering on relatively parallel bundles of collagen fibrils in cementum, *FCE.* **B,** Deposits of granular, interfibrillar matrix *(arrows)* occur at junction of cementum, *FCE,* and dentin, *D.* **(A** ×10,500; **B** ×20,000.) (From Listgarten, M.: Unpublished data, 1968.)

The organic matrix of cementum consists of the collagenous component already described and an interfibrillar component that at the ultrastructural level appears finely granular. This material probably represents the mucoprotein portion of the organic matrix. It is more readily demonstrable near the dentinocemental junction.

Cellular cementum

Cellular cementum appears less regularly organized than its acellular counterpart. It may reach a thickness of 1 to several millimeters, the thickness increasing with age. The more rapid rate of formation of cellular cementum probably explains the incorporation of cementum-forming cells into typical lacunae from which canaliculi containing cellular processes radiate through the adjacent calcified matrix. Cementocytes are usually absent from the deeper portions of the cellular cementum. With transmitted light appositional lines can also be noted in cellular cementum.

Electron microscopically the organic and inorganic components appear similar to those observed in acellular cementum. Some differences exist, however, in their organization.

Usually the periodontal fiber bundles continue within the cementum as well-defined Sharpey's fibers (Figs. 1-50 and 1-51). Although their orientation is generally perpendicular to the cementum surface, some bundles of fibers run in different directions as well. The central core of Sharpey's fibers may be incompletely mineralized. However,

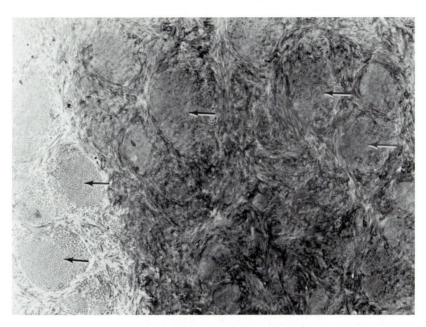

Fig. 1-50. Apical root cementum. Note that in this tangential section collagen fiber bundles *(arrows)* retain their individual organization in periodontal ligament as well as in cementum. (×5,700.) (From Listgarten, M.: Unpublished data, 1970.)

the relationship of the apatite crystals to individual collagen fibrils remains the same.

Alveolar process

The tissue elements of the alveolar process are no different from those of bone elsewhere. The alveolar bone portion of the alveolar process lines the sockets into which the roots of the teeth fit. It is thin, compact bone that is pierced by many small openings through which blood vessels, lymphatics, and nerve fibers pass. The alveolar bone fuses with the cortical plates of the labial and lingual sides at the crest of the alveolar process. The alveolar bone contains the embedded ends of the connective tissue fibers of the periodontal membrane (Sharpey's fibers, Figs. 1-52 and 1-53). The cancellous portion of the process occupies the area between the cortical plates and the alveolar bone. It is continuous with the spongiosa of the body of the jaws. The spongiosa occupies most of the interdental septum, but a relatively small portion of the labial or lingual plate. In these areas the incisal region has less spongiosa than it has in the molar areas. The architectural arrangement of the trabeculae and their characteristics are related to the demands of function.

Bone tissue is continually undergoing change. Characteristically, bone apposition and resorption may occur simultaneously on neighboring bone surfaces. In the alveolar bone, adjacent lamellae

can be identified by the presence of so-called *cementing lines.* When a bony surface is inactive for a period of time, a basophilic line forms. These lines are seen over sections where apposition or resorptive phases have occurred previously. If resorption was followed by apposition, the line is known as a *reversal line,* and thus reveal the changes that have previously taken place.

Thus bone is a relatively active tissue, whereas cementum is relatively inactive. This difference can easily be seen microscopically in tissue of adult individuals. Very little apposition of cementum is seen, whereas a definite remodeling of the alveolar bone is apparent. This observation is of great significance, since the periodontal ligament unites these tissues. It can be reasoned, therefore, that there is a need for some mechanism to allow for the independent behavior of these two hard tissues. This will be discussed later.

Bone is a highly specialized mesodermal tissue, consisting of organic matrix and inorganic matter. The matrix is composed of a network of osteocytes and intercellular substance. The inorganic portion consists chiefly of calcium, phosphate, and carbonate in the form of apatite crystals. Bone is first laid down as an open framework of spongy bone, some of which becomes compact later on. The spaces in the spongiosa are termed marrow spaces. Under normal conditions bone is constantly subject to simultaneous tissue growth and re-

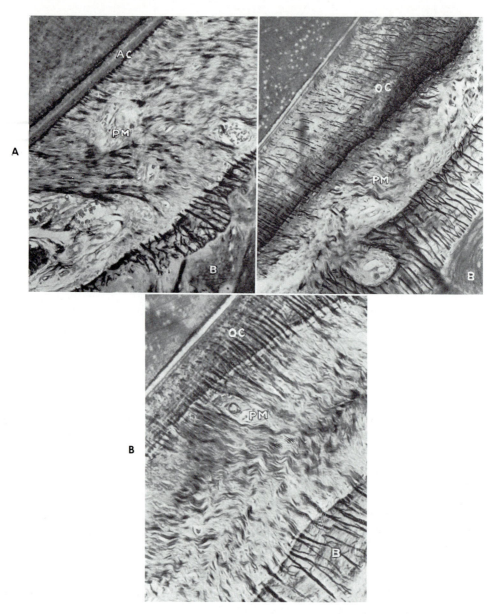

Fig. 1-51. A, Periodontal ligament fibers connected to acellular cementum, *AC* (upper left photomicrograph). Sharpey's fibers are seen in osteocementum, *OC*, and bone, *B* (upper right photomicrograph). **B,** Sharpey's fibers in osteocementum and bone with wavy fibers of periodontal ligament (dog material). *PM*, periodontal ligament.

sorption, which are finely coordinated. Microscopically, bone surfaces may exhibit areas of bone apposition, areas where bone is undergoing resorption, and other areas where the status quo is being maintained. Under normal conditions, as in the other portions of the skeleton, the physiologic status of the bone is dependent on age and function.

Ritchey and Orban have pointed out that in the absence of periodontal disease the configuration of the crest of the interdental alveolar septum is deter-mined by the relative position of the adjacent cementoenamel junctions and also that the width of the interdental alveolar bone is determined by the tooth form present. Relatively flat approximal tooth surfaces call for narrow septa, whereas in the presence of extremely convex tooth surfaces wide interdental septa with flat crests are found.

Alveolar bone is deposited next to the periodontal ligament and is itself supported by supporting bone. One or more large arteries, veins, and nerve bundles run through in the interradicular bony

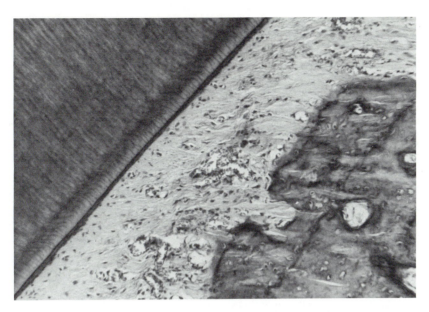

Fig. 1-52. Photomicrograph of periodontal ligament. Root is covered with a thin layer of cementum; a cementoblastic layer is evident. Note also that an osteoblastic layer is present, denoting bone formation. These findings are consistent with formative aspects of dentoalveolar unit and result from slight tension on tooth.

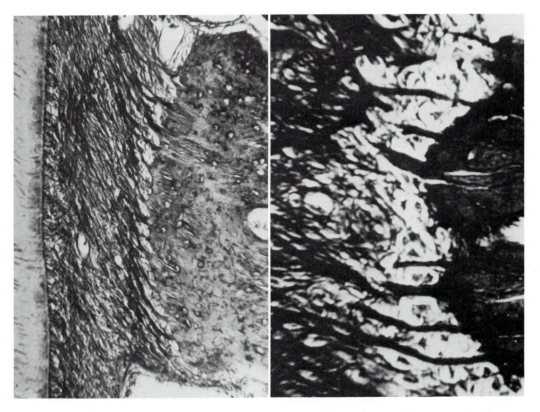

Fig. 1-53. Photomicrographs of low- and high-power of a periodontal ligament, showing an active osteoblastic layer adjacent to bone. High power is a silver staining. Note Sharpey's fibers. There is active bone formation; yet cementum is thin and no cementoid can be observed.

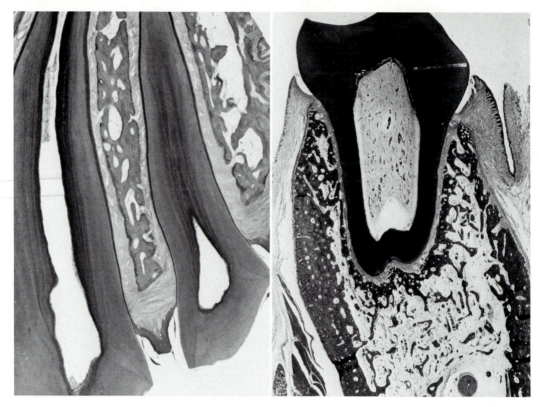

Fig. 1-54. Photomicrographs of a low-power mesiodistal section of maxillary anterior teeth and buccolingual section of a mandibular molar (dog). Pictured are gingiva, alveolus, and periodontal ligament.

process, and branches from them enter the periodontal ligament through the many openings in the cribriform plates (Fig. 1-54).

Functional relationship of alveolar and supporting bone. The bone housing the tooth is dependent on the function exerted on the tooth to maintain its structure. The changes in the supporting bone and in the periodontal ligament when stress to the teeth is withdrawn, as in the case where antagonists are lost, attest to the dependence of these tissues on functional stimulation. In fact, after long-standing loss of function, changes in the alveolar bone may be noted. In jaws in which the teeth are subjected to intense stress it is usual to find the spongy or supporting bone composed of thicker and more numerous trabeculae. Although bone tissue is dependent on function for the maintenance and arrangement of the trabeculae, other factors may be involved, for example, disturbances in bone metabolism. Such an experiment has been described by Anderson et al. They have shown that the bony changes around the mandibular molars in rats after the extraction of the maxillary molars are more pronounced in rats on a low inorganic salt diet.

Metabolism of alveolar bone. Of interest is the rate of metabolism of the alveolar bone in contrast to other bone tissue elsewhere. Rogers and Weidman have conducted a metabolic study involving the use of tracer elements with respect to the isotopes of calcium, iodine, nitrogen, and phosphorus. They have shown that not only do individual animals appear to exhibit variations in rate of skeletal metabolism, but also that different species have different rates. It was found that the rate of metabolism of mandibular alveolar bone is slower than that of metaphyseal bone but more rapid than that of diaphyseal bone. This seems to be true for all the animals examined. Studies that have been made of dogs with renal osteodystrophy show marked changes in the alveolar and supporting bone in contrast to changes elsewhere in the skeleton. The more rapid rate of metabolism of bone tissue in the jaws than that in other skeletal areas may be a factor in those cases of periodontal disease in which local etiologic factors are at a minimum but where the alveolar bone exhibits marked destructive changes.

Microscopic appearance. Bone is composed of organic and inorganic components. The organic portion is composed of cells, fibers, and amorphous cementing substance. The fibers and the cementing substance form the bone matrix. Between adjacent structural units of bone, narrow bands of fiber-free matrix are found, and these are referred to as cement lines. The inorganic component is composed of mineral salts.

Microscopically, bone is composed of osteocytes embedded in a calcified intercellular matrix, each cell within a lacuna. Extending from a lacuna are minute canals called canaliculi. These communicate with canaliculi of adjacent lacunae. Through this system of canals, nutrient material reaches the osteocyte, and the canals are also avenues for removal of waste products of metabolism.

Bone tissue of the jaws undergoes a constant exchange (as does the tissue of the entire skeleton). Bone formation and resorption are going on continually, but a physiologic equilibrium exists between the two. Bone formation is seen as a marginal layer of osteoid in relation to a layer of polyhedral osteoblasts, whereas resorptive phases are generally characterized by the presence of multinucleated osteoclasts or connective tissue cells in irregular concavities in the bone margin. This process, termed "osteoclastic resorption," involves the participation of lysosomal enzymes.

The method by which resorption of bone occurs has been a controversial subject for many years. Essentially there are two mechanisms. The first, called osteoclastic resorption, was just described. The second involves osteocytes, which are claimed to have the capacity to resorb the bone surrounding the lacunae and canaliculi. The process is known as *osteolysis*. Recently, polymorphonuclear leukocytes have been reported to be present near osteoclasts in areas of bone resorption at the alveolar crest in periodontal disease in monkeys. It has been suggested that they may contribute to rapid bone destruction through release of prostaglandins or other factors that might stimulate osteoclastic activity.

Bone may be classified according to the character and pattern of the incorporated fibers and cells. Three types of bone can be distinguished on this structural basis: *woven bone, lamellar bone,* and *bundle bone.*

When numerous bundles of collagen fibers become incorporated in the bone, the term "bundle bone" is applied. The alveolar bone adjacent to the periodontal ligament contains numerous fibers, the mineralized portion of the collagen fibers of the periodontal ligament. These are referred to as *Sharpey's fibers.* Bundle bone, because it forms

the immediate bone attachment of the periodontal ligament, is of intense interest to the periodontist.

The changes in alveolar bone associated with age are essentially a more osteoporotic structure and a reduction of periosteal cells on the bone surface. Aging osteoblasts become smaller and fusiform. Matrix production ceases.

Two types of cells that can differentiate into osteoblasts have been described: *osteogenic precursor cells* and *inductible osteogenic precursor cells.* The inductible cells normally do not differentiate, but can do so by appropriate stimuli. Of clinical importance is the discovery by Melcher and Accursi that periosteum elevated from the bone of adult animals is not osteogenic, whereas periosteum adjacent to a wound and periosteum from an osteoperiosteal flap is. Goldman has found that injury to the periosteum results in proliferation of osteoblasts.

The bones of the cranial vault and facial skeleton and the shafts of the clavicles begin to ossify directly in mesenchyma without any preceding cartilaginous stage. Clusters of osteoblasts differentiate from mesenchymal precursor cells. The osteoblasts begin the formation of bone matrix, which soon calcifies. Some of the mesenchymal cells remain undifferentiated to form a reservoir of cells from which osteoblasts can later arise. In the jaws there is a covering periosteum.

Oxytalan fibers

The oxytalan fiber, a distinct type of connective tissue fiber, was initially described by Fullmer; this fiber has been demonstrated to be a normal constituent of the periodontal ligament. Oxytalan fibers generally follow the course of the collagen fibers and seemingly are related to the amount of stress placed on the ligament. They are found in increased numbers in the ligament of teeth used for bridge abutments and less frequently around nonfunctioning teeth. Interestingly they are found in the ligament adjacent to the cementum in greater numbers than on the bone side.

Neural supply

The neural control of the muscles of mastication is derived primarily from the motor centers within the brain. However, this activity is modified by proprioceptive impulses originating within the muscles themselves, within the temporomandibular joints, and within the gingiva and periodontal ligament. The proprioceptive nerves within the periodontal ligament have been shown to be directional. It is in this way that under normal circumstances the dentoalveolar unit is protected from damage from excessive forces being brought to play by the muscles of mastication. The neural density in the human is said to be much higher in the intermediate region than in the apical region of the root; however, there is great dispute about this, with some investigators reporting the apical portion to contain more nerve endings. Also the morphology of the neural endings varies from animal to animal according to different investigators.

Gingival innervation. The innervation of the gingiva is derived from fibers of the labial or lingual branches of the second and third divisions of the trigeminal nerve and to a much lesser extent from anastomosing fibers from the periodontal ligament. The major nerves, coursing with the blood vessels in the supraperiosteal area of the alveolar plate, form a rete, which has been termed the "deep plexus." As these fibers pass through the connective tissue of the gingiva, branches are given off to terminate as a "superficial plexus" in the lamina propria of the dermal papillae and on occasion continue into the epithelium as fine ultraterminal fibers. The interproximal gingiva is innervated by coronal extensions of the nerve plexii of the periodontal ligament as well as from supracrestal ramifications of the interdental nerves terminating in the transseptal fiber systems of adjacent teeth. Bernick has reported that he did not observe specialized endings such as Krause's or Meissner's corpuscles in his 1% pepsin preparations of the gingiva. Simpson has also noted this negative observation. Other writers, however, have reported observing these corpuscles and other complex end organs in the gingival tissues. Such absence or sparsity of organized and specialized nerve endings is not unusual as it has also been observed in areas of skin and mucous membrane that exhibit varying degrees of sensibility.

Innervation of periodontal ligament. The function of the periodontal ligament nerves is to transmit impulses of resultant forces of occlusion and mastication (touch, pressure, and pain) to higher neurologic centers where appropriate responses can be transmitted to the effector muscle groupings to elicit protective reactions. The prime sources of this afferent innervation are periodontal branches of the dental nerve after it perforates the alveolar plate before entering the tooth and from the intra-alveolar nerve as it courses crestally and its lateral branches perforate the cribriform plate. In the alveolar phase of the periodontal ligament the two groups anastomose and send branches both apically and occlusally to form a complex rete

parallel to the long axis of the tooth. From this network branches are given off to terminate in the connective tissue. Rapp and co-workers have felt that the larger neural branches run in association with the blood vessels while the smaller nerve fibers may not. The intraseptal nerves provide the major portion of the ligament innervation, and as a consequence, surgery at the apical area of the tooth or inflammatory destruction of the tissues of this region does not greatly compromise the nerve supply of the rest of the periodontal ligament. The nerves may pass close to the cementum and alveolar bone, and their peripheral endings may form fine arborizations. Sicher has described three types of observed endings: knoblike structures, rings or loops around principal fiber bundles, and free nerve endings. Simpson has commented that definite end organs are seldom seen in the periodontal ligament and that fine endings are the predominating terminal feature. Studies by Bernick (1959) also have reported the finding that Meissner's, Ruffini's, or Pacini corpuscles are not observed. In the apical third of the periodontium of a human tooth, myelinated nerves have been seen to lose their sheath and terminate as spindlelike structures. Brashear felt that as the coarse nerve fibers travel occlusally in the alveolar phase, sensations are mediated by the varying caliber of myelinated and nonmyelinated fibers present: pain conducted by small diameter nerves of both types; temperature by intermediate medullated fibers; and touch by the large myelinated nerves. Nerves may form rings or loops around principal fiber bundles or may terminate between them so as to function in proprioception and localization. In the cemental phase, Rapp, Avery, and Rector (1959) have observed that most neurofibrils approach the cementum to form loops and then turn back toward the midportion of the ligament. Berkelbach van der Sprenkle has described a rete of nonmedullated fibers coursing radially from the central area of the periodontal ligament to penetrate the cementum.

The coronal termination of the nerve fibers of the periodontal ligament has been reported in the circular fiber group of the gingiva where they anastomose with nerve fibers of adjacent teeth to contribute to the total innervation of the area.

Periodontal ligament

The fibers of the periodontal ligament proper, attaching the tooth to the alveolar housing, are arranged in the following groups: (1) the *alveolar crestal group,* extending from the cervical area of the root to the alveolar crest; (2) the *horizontal*

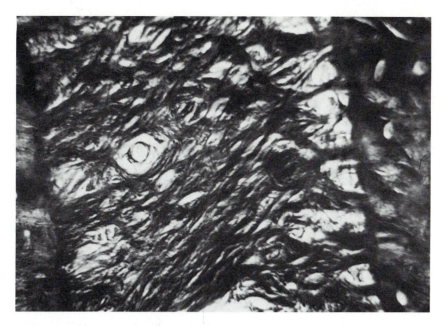

Fig. 1-55. High-power photomicrograph of the periodontal ligament. Course and arrangement of principal fibers and their insertion into cementum and bone as well as small blood vessels should be noted. Fibers on cementum side are relatively more numerous and thin, whereas on bone side they are fewer in number and of greater diameter.

group, running perpendicularly from the tooth to the alveolar bone; (3) the *oblique group,* oriented obliquely with insertions in the cementum, and extending more occlusally in the alveolus (approximately two thirds of the fibers fall into this group); and (4) the *apical group,* radiating apically from tooth to bone. The arrangement of the groups of fiber bundles is designed to sustain the tooth against forces to which it is subjected. The structure of the periodontal ligament, however, continuously changes as a result of functional requirements. Crumley has reported that the periodontal ligament of rat molars normally demonstrates a remarkably high rate of collagen production.

The periodontal ligament is composed primarily of collagen fibrils generally arranged in bundles (Fig. 1-55). The fibrillar bundles unite the cementum to the alveolar bone surface. Collagen accounts for approximately 50% of the dry weight of the whole periodontal ligament; approximately 90% of the collagen of the ligament in fully erupted teeth is insoluble. The finding of collagenase and the fact that there are marked changes in the fibers of the periodontal ligament in animals maintained on diets deficient in protein suggest that there is a rapid turnover of collagen.

The course and arrangement of the principal fibers of the periodontal ligament show insertion of these fibers in the cementum and bone. It has

been demonstrated that in the mouse, hamster, and marmoset the cementoalveolar fibers pass through the interdental septum and are continuous with similar fibers of adjacent teeth. The perforating fibers show frequent branching anastomoses. In man, however, the interdental septa contain marrow spaces, and this arrangement of fibers has not been demonstrated. Selvig has demonstrated that Sharpey's fibers in both alveolar bone and cellular cementum are composed of an uncalcified core surrounded by a calcified sheath.

Bernick, Levy, Dreizen, and Grant reported findings of the course of the fibers of the periodontal ligament of one tooth to its adjacent neighbor. Sections of the jaws from marmosets were stained with silver nitrate to demonstrate the intrabony course of the alveolar fibers of the periodontal ligament. They found that as the interseptal bone underwent a period of resorption and apposition, the intrabony alveolar fibers were also lost, and re-formed. A continuum of fibers traversing the alveolar septum could not be determined. In one illustration showing the crest area of the interdental bone the mesial and distal alveolar fibers terminated in the midregion of the bone where the ends formed an intermeshing network. In another illustration the interdental region between a first premolar and a canine from a mature marmoset was shown. The distal periodontal ligament was wider than that of the mesial surface. A serpentine resting line was seen traversing the length of the bone. The mesial and distal alveolar fibers within the bone terminated at the resting line. With advancing age there was a marked change in the depth of bony penetration of the alveolar fibers of the periodontal ligament. In these old animals the alveolar bone proper in both maxilla and mandible was reduced to a thin layer of darkly stained acellular calcification directly adjacent to the osteons filling the spongiosa. Insertion of the alveolar fibers within the alveolar bone proper was limited to this narrow area and did not extend into the haversian systems. The periodontal fibers originate on the cementum side as numerous relatively thin bundles separated by the cellular elements of the cementoblastic layer. These bundles spread out and the individual fibers of adjacent bundles become interwoven into a network that occupies the greatest width of the ligament. On the bone side, the origin of the fibrils from bone is similar to that noted on the cementum side, except that individual fiber bundles are fewer in number and of greater diameter than on the cementum side. These fiber bundles spread out, and their fibrillar elements become part of the network of fibers that course through the ligament.

The ligament is traversed by channels of loose connective tissue that contain blood and lymph vessels as well as nerve bundles (Fig. 1-56). These channels are located approximately in the midportion of the ligament.

The blood vessels found in the periodontal ligament arise mainly from the bone marrow of the supporting bone through lateral perforations of the alveolar bone and to some extent from the periapical vessels. They form an elaborate anastomosing network (Figs. 1-57 and 1-58). These vessels are supplied with their own sympathetic nervous system. The lymphatics form a complicated pattern. The nerves are both myelinated and naked. Their endings have been described as knoblike swellings, rings or loops around fiber bundles, and as free endings between fibers. Free endings are sensitive to pain. Some endings are proprioceptive in nature. They permit localization of masticatory stimuli and control masticatory muscle function.

In addition to the fibrous portion of the ligament and the neurovascular channels, certain cellular elements are regularly found in the ligament structure. These include cementoblasts, fibroblasts, osteoblasts, osteoclasts, and epithelial cell rests. Ultrastructurally, epithelial rests are readily identified by the presence of prominent tonofibrils

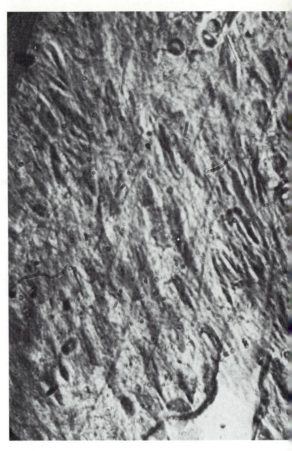

Fig. 1-56. Neural elements in periodontal ligament.

in their cytoplasm, desmosomes connecting adjacent cells, and hemidesmosomes and a basal lamina surrounding the entire cell rest. These characteristics help to distinguish epithelial cells from vascular elements, the cells of which do not contain such well-defined tonofibrils, and the intercellular junction of which consist primarily of close or tight junctions. Furthermore, the pinocytotic vesicles characteristically observed in endothelial cells are not nearly as prominent in epithelial cell rests.

The osteoblasts frequently demonstrate well-developed Golgi regions and a densely arranged rough-surfaced endoplasmic reticulum, characteristic of cells actively engaged in protein synthesis for extracellular use. The cementoblasts, on the other hand, seldom contain these organelles in such a well-developed manner (Fig. 1-59). These observations fit the autoradiographic data that indicate a greater degree of protein synthesizing activity on the bone side of the periodontal ligament, with little activity on the cementum side. When these cells become enclosed in the lacunae characteristically noted in bone or cellu-

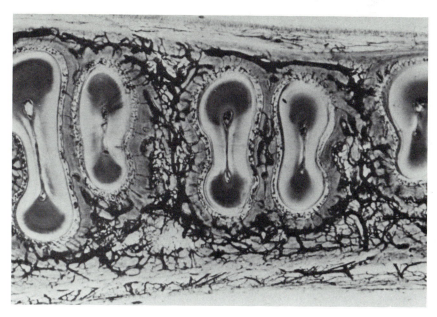

Fig. 1-57. Lower power photomicrograph of a mandibular occlusal section of a dog, showing vascularity of alveolus. Note large blood vessels feeding into periodontal ligament through nutrient canals.

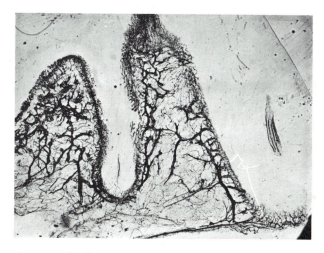

Fig. 1-58. Vascular network of periodontal ligament in a perfused dog. Note large vessel running parallel to periodontal ligament, from which are leadoffs to smaller vessels of periodontal ligament.

lar cementum, the cytoplasmic volume and the number of organelles markedly. Osteoclasts, when noted, are characterized by one or more nuclei, a cytoplasm containing numerous vesicles and mitochondria, with interspersed strands of rough-surfaced endoplasmic reticulum, and a markedly convoluted cell surface on the side of the cell facing the bone surface.

Fibroblasts morphologically resemble osteoblasts and cementoblasts. These cells can only be distinguished from one another with any degree of certainty because of their location in relation to the mineralized tissue surfaces. Fibroblasts usually possess thin cytoplasmic extensions that course between fiber bundles. The long axis of the cell usually extends in a plane parallel to the general direction of the fiber bundles.

The fibroblasts of the periodontal ligament frequently contain intracytoplasmic vacuoles that enclose one or more collagen fibrils. The vacuoles may demonstrate lysosomal enzyme activity, which suggests that fibroblasts contribute to col-

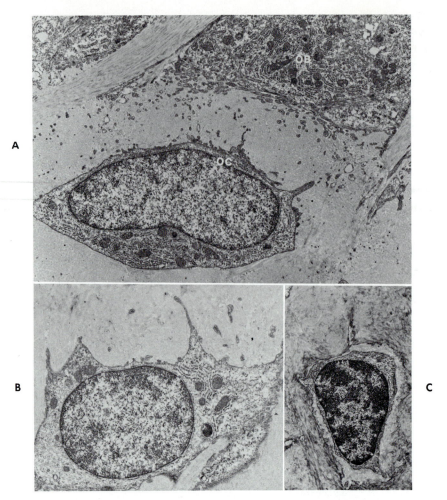

Fig. 1-59. A, Osteoblast, *OB,* and cell about to become an osteocyte, *OC,* with relatively high concentrations of mitochondria and rough-surfaced endoplasmic reticulum in cytoplasm. **B,** Cementoblast with relatively few cytoplasmic organelles. **C,** Cementocyte within a lacuna demonstrating cytoplasmic shrinkage and loss of most cytoplasmic organelles. (**A** ×6,400; **B** ×8,000; **C** ×4,600.) (From Listgarten, M.: Unpublished data, 1969.)

lagen removal by endocytosis of fibrils. Thus fibroblasts may serve not only as a source of new collagen, but also in the destruction of already formed collagenous fibrils.

To explain relative movements of the tooth in relation to the alveolar bone, e.g., during rapid eruption, the concept of an "intermediate plexus" was introduced by Sicher. This concept provided for a zone in the periodontal ligament where fibers originating from bone could mesh with fibers originating from cementum. This was in contrast with the concept existing previously, according to which fibers were believed to run from one side of the ligament to the other, each fiber end being anchored in bone as well as cementum. The essentially mechanical nature of the concept underlying the function of the "intermediate plexus"

should be integrated with the results of autoradiographic studies, which have demonstrated regions of high collagen turnover in association with the bone side of the ligament. A number of investigators, utilizing H^3-proline as a label, have offered evidence to support the concept of differential rates of fiber formation. The fibers in the middle of the ligament and those on the alveolar side appeared to be labeled more heavily than those on the cemental side. Carneiro showed that the periodontal ligament is the site of a high rate of synthesis and rapid turnover of collagen, particularly in the crestal and apical fibers. It is likely that turnover and remodeling occurs at a molecular level. Such a state of events would not necessarily be reflected in a morphologically distinct zone, that is, the "intermediate plexus."

Deporter and Ten Cate reported that examination at the hard surfaces adjacent to the periodontal ligament revealed fibroblast-like cells engaged in phagocytosis of anchored ligament fibrils. It is suggested that in this way there can be organization of the ligament.

PHYSIOLOGY
Relationship of dental anatomy to physiology of supporting structures

The anatomic form of the occlusal surfaces of the teeth is designed in such a manner that the force required for masticatory function is minimal and yet effective. In this way the mandibular teeth move against the maxillary teeth without excessive vertical or lateral stresses to the supporting structures during normal masticatory function. Cuspal anatomy changes with age in that the degree of cusp height decreases; however, this altered form still functions physiologically.

Mesial movement of teeth

Because of slight buccolingual movement of the teeth normally possible in the masticatory process, the contact areas between the teeth show progressive abrasion with age. As a result of this wear the mesiodistal width of the teeth becomes narrower. It has been estimated that this interproximal abrasion causes the loss of 1 cm in the antero-posterior length of the total arch by the age of 40 years. Thus, to maintain a protective contact relation for the gingival tissue and also to preserve proximal contact for support against external forces, the teeth move mesially. With the wearing of the cusps of the teeth this compensatory mesial migration of the teeth can go on uninhibited. With the physiologic attrition of the occlusal surface the resultant direction of tooth movement is in a mesio-occlusal path.

Physiologic forces influencing dentition

Various forces of physiologic phenomena influence the fully developed dentition. Some forces are developed by the muscles of mastication, other forces originate from facial muscles, and others originate from the tongue. Thus there is a functional equilibrium, with all of the forces counteracting one another. Breitner has described some of the antagonistic forces acting upon the masticatory apparatus, e.g., the force of the lips counteracting that of the tongue and the force of the cheeks also equalizing that of the tongue. Fig. 1-60 illustrates these counterbalancing influences.

Tooth suspension. The transmission of masticatory forces to the supporting structures of the tooth is the function of the attachment apparatus. Three factors operate: (1) the principal fiber apparatus of the periodontal ligament, (2) the shape and size of the root of the tooth, and (3) the fluid content of the periodontal ligament.

Gottlieb believed that the number of fiber bundles of the periodontal ligament per unit area and the square area of the root surface are most important, since the fiber apparatus sustains the masticatory force. On the other hand, Boyle has described the mechanism of tooth suspension as hydraulic pressure on the walls of the alveolus. Escape of fluid by means of vascular channels communicating with the bone marrow spaces allows for a gradual extension of the periodontal fibers by which the full force of occlusion is ultimately transmitted as tension to the alveolar bone. He has also stated that further efficiency in the absorption of occlusal forces is secured by the special form of the teeth themselves and the resiliency of the dentin of which they are composed, showing the cross sectional form of the tooth root to be efficiently designed to resist forces tending to flatten the arc of longitudinal curvature of the tooth. He explains that this form also offers efficiently shaped surfaces for the transmission of pressures on the labial and mesial sides, which furnish maximum surface for attachment of the periodontal fibers on the lingual and distal sides.

Churchill also has indicated that a hydraulic mechanism operating via the fluid content of the blood of the periodontal ligament acts as a means for absorbing force on the tooth.

It is most likely that the connective tissue fiber apparatus of the periodontal ligament, arranged with a predominance of oblique fibers and a fluid displacement mechanism, is the method of suspension of the tooth.

Physiologic occlusion

Normal occlusion, according to Strang, may be defined as ''the normal relationship of the occlusal inclined planes of the teeth when the jaws are closed, accompanied by the correct proximal contacts and axial positioning of all teeth, and the normal growth, development, location and correlation of the various associated tissues and parts'' (Strang, 1933) (Fig. 1-61). According to this definition the teeth have a relationship to each other in the same jaw and to those in the opposing jaw. The first molars are designated as the keys to occlusion, and their relationship denotes whether

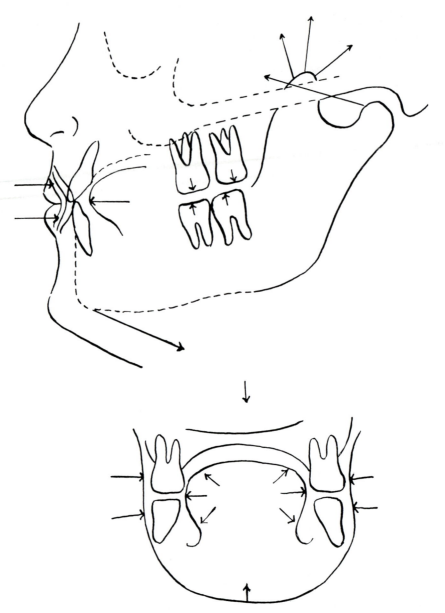

Fig. 1-60. Some antagonistic forces acting on masticatory apparatus. Lips ↔ tongue; cheeks ↔ tongue; eruption (growth of teeth) ↔ masticatory muscles (masseter, temporalis, internal pterygoid); air pressure on skin and nasal cavity ↔ tongue in closed mouth, air pressure in open mouth; masseter ↔ elasticity of periodontal ligament, particularly of molars and suprahyoid muscles; internal pterygoid in vertical movement ↔ same as masseter; in lateral movement ↔ internal pterygoid of other side; external pterygoid in anterior movement ↔ posterior third of temporalis, suprahyoid group, digastricus, muscles of neck; in lateral movement ↔ external pterygoid of other side. (Modified from Breitner, C.: J. Periodontol. **13:**72, 1942.)

that of the mandible to the maxilla is correct. It should be as follows: the mesial inclined plane of the mesiobuccal cusp of the upper first molar occludes with the distal inclined plane of the mesiobuccal cusp of the lower first molar, whereas the distal inclined plane of the distobuccal cusp of the upper first molar occludes with the mesial inclined

plane of the distal cusp of the lower first molar.

Next in importance to the molar relationship as a key to contact by a normal inclined plane is the occlusion of the upper canine. This tooth should lie between and labial to the lower canine and the first premolar. Then the mesial incline of the cusp of the upper canine will harmonize in position with

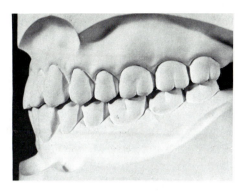

Fig. 1-61. Models showing relationships of posterior teeth. Cuspid and first molar landmarks are evident.

the distal incline of the cusp of the lower canine. The ideal relationship of incline planes of the mandibular to the maxillary teeth, however, is but seldom encountered. We interpret occlusion as a broad concept that embraces maxillomandibular jaw relationship and the positions, forms, and dentofacial contact relationships of teeth as they are related to function, integrity of the supporting tissues of the teeth, the temporomandibular articulation, and aesthetics.

The term "occlusion" is usually thought of as a static position — the arrangement of the teeth to one another and of one jaw to the other. However, since the function placed on the jaws is a dynamic one, it is not the occlusion in its static position that is important but the relationship that the teeth assume during function. A seemingly normal occlusion in its static position may, during function, be capable of producing an irritation on a single tooth or on a group of teeth. Thus in lateral excursions of the mandible a premolar or a premolar and a molar may be traumatized by being exposed to the total force exerted. This is dependent, however, on the function of the masticatory muscles and on the length of time during which the force is brought to play.

A physiologic occlusion therefore is one that operates in harmony and presents no pathologic manifestation in the supporting structures of the teeth. The stresses placed on the teeth are dissipated normally, and there is a balance between the stresses and the adaptive capacity of the supporting tissues. Thus the occlusion must be examined as it functions as an integral part of a dynamic masticatory apparatus. This apparatus includes not only the teeth but also their supporting tissues, the mandible and maxilla proper, the musculature, the temporomandibular joints, the tongue,

and the nerve and vascular supply to the parts, in accord with the basic principles of neuromuscular physiology and the physiology of the temporomandibular joints.

Thus, during physiologic function there should be no deflecting interference of one tooth against another; the teeth should make contact in a stable relationship, the stress on the tooth being directed axially in the posterior teeth.

There is marked disagreement over how the teeth of the dentition should function in relation to one another and how the mandible should function against the maxilla. A wide range of functional and static relationships are seen functioning in health with neither subjective or objective symptoms. For these individuals the dentition is physiologically acceptable. Thus the mandibular position of centric relation occlusion can coincide with centric relation or these mandibular positions need not coincide, and yet the teeth can be seen functioning without damage being produced.

During normal function the mandible is moved by the muscles with the condyles of the mandible moving in the glenoid fossae in a rotation and translation pattern. The pathways of the mandible against the maxilla are determined by the limits set by the ligaments and structures of the temporomandibular joints. A characteristic pattern outlining the border positions has been described by Posselt; he demonstrated that these positions were constant and reproducible for the particular individual and that these positions could be traced in both sagittal and horizontal planes. These movements are called the envelope of motion when the mandible opens; the first range is a pure rotation like a hinge; soon after the lateral pterygoid muscles react and cause a forward translation.

Theoretically, maximum intercuspation of the teeth should occur when the mandible is in the centric relation position. However, most people exhibit an anterior shift from centric relation (jaw-to-jaw position) to maximum contact of the teeth. As stated before, this factor does not always indicate dysfunction. It is said that if the shift is over a millimeter or so and if a lateral component is present, then the cuspal relationships will result in damage to the attachment apparatus, especially under parafunctional circumstances.

Temporomandibular joints. The temporomandibular joint consists of four parts: the glenoid fossa of the temporal bone, the interarticular disc, the condyle of the mandible, and the articular tubercle of the zygomatic process of the temporal bone. The joint is enclosed in an articular capsule.

The temporomandibular articulation allows for a wide range of jaw movement and different degrees of mouth opening. Some investigators believe the joint to work on a hingelike movement, whereas others claim that there is only a translatory motion involved. During mastication of small bits of food or during speech there is a slight opening of the jaws. This action is said to take place in the lower half of the joint, with the head of the condyle rotating on the undersurface of the interarticular disc. When further opening takes place, the upper half of the joint is employed. Then a gliding movement or translation occurs. In this action the head of the condyle, the interarticular disc, and the lower half of the joint move forward and downward over the articular tubercle.

There is a general agreement on the importance of the relationship existing between the occlusion of the teeth and the relation of the mandible to the temporomandibular joint. Some authorities believe this latter position to be unalterable, whereas others claim that it is changeable. Review of the literature indicates wide divergence of opinion with regard to temporomandibular joint physiology. There is still need for further and more extensive study.

Rest position of mandible. In the absence of mastication, deglutition, or speech, the mandible occupies a resting position unrelated to the presence or absence of teeth. In this resting position the teeth are not normally in occlusion but rather are separated by what has been called the freeway space. The resting position is maintained reflexly by a balance in which there is a resting point on the mild contractions of the muscles that tend to elevate or depress the mandible. These mild muscular contractions are expressions of activity based on muscle tonus. It should be kept in mind that this rest position of the mandible is a postural one and is subject to slight variations depending on the position and inclination of the head.

Centric relation (retruded occlusal position, posterior border movement) and centric occlusion (intercuspal position). The following represents a point of view agreed upon by some investigators. In a consideration of jaw relationship it must be recognized that the fundamental anatomic positon for physiologic movement of the mandible is established by the musculature and not the teeth. Centric relation is best understood when it is interpreted as a physiologic concept and as a jaw-to-jaw relationship that is inherent in each individual. It has been defined as the most posterior relation of the mandible to the maxilla at the established vertical dimension; the condyles are in the most posterior position in the glenoid fossa, and unstrained lateral movements can be made.

Centric relation in the natural dentition is not to be confused with position of the teeth, relationship of tooth to tooth, or as a precise relationship of condyles to fossae. Rather it should be thought of as a practiced, learned, neuromuscular pattern, as a position of mandible to maxilla based on a pathway to terminal tooth contact when the most posterior, unstrained, hingelike movement of the mandible is effected.

Physiologically functioning occlusions are characterized by a harmonious interaction of the periodontium, the temporomandibular joint, and their associated musculature. Preferably, centric relation and the maximum intercuspation and contact of the teeth should coincide; however, in most individuals an anterior position of the mandible is seen where maximum cuspal contact is present. Many investigators question whether it is necessary for centric relation and habitual relationship to coincide.

The current accepted beliefs concerning ''occlusion'' are that there should be a free-way space at the postural resting position of the mandible. Preferably, centric relation—the jaw-to-jaw position—should coincide with maximum cuspal contact. During function there should be no deflecting interference upon closure; the teeth should make contact in a stable fashion. A canine contact should result in a noncontact of all teeth, both working and balancing sides, during lateral excursion of the mandible. In protrusive position of the mandible, when the anterior teeth occlude, the posterior teeth from the mandibular first premolar back should not come into contact.

Physiology of mastication

The physiology of mastication has been a subject of much dispute. The movements of the mandible in the chewing cycle have been relegated to a neuromusculr phenomenon by one group and to the dictates of the temporomandibular joint by another. Evidence by new methods of research such as electromyography points to the fact that the chewing act is controlled by a neuromuscular action. The physiology of mastication may be divided into three steps: incision of food, mastication of the bolus, and swallowing.

Manly, investigating the physiology of the natural dentition, has shown that very slight differences in thickness and hardness of plastic discs can be detected by individuals with a natural dentition. The teeth can detect very small changes in texture of foods. He has shown that foods consumed on the average diet may vary widely in their resistance to pulverization from a study of 35 foods. The toughest foods, raw vegetables and meats, require as much as ten times the number of chewing strokes to produce the same degree of pulverization as do the softer foods such as nuts, cooked vegetables, and fish.

From these studies Manly has concluded that the maximum forces that can be exerted by natural teeth are ten times as great as those normally used during mastication (5 to 10 pounds). A decrease in the maximum force available is still more than adequate. Persons lacking only third molars are considered to have an efficiency of 100%. In comparison to this, the average 6-year-old child with a complete dentition has 30% efficiency. His efficiency doubles by the age of 10 years, falls during the transitional years of 11 and 12, and rises again to a 60% efficiency at the age of 14 years.

From his experiments Manly has shown that the rate of pulverization decreases rapidly from the first few chewing strokes to the act of swallowing. Right and left sides of the mouth are separate masticating organs, with preference given to the side free of pain, the one most efficient, or the one corresponding to the side of the preferred hand. Children generally prefer the right side of the mouth and adults the more efficient side. An important finding was that the chewing ability for the whole mouth is equivalent to that of the preferred side. The size of the mouthful of food does not affect the chewing ability if the test is based on a certain number of strokes per gram of food.

In the incisive phase the mandible is depressed and projected forward so that the protrusive motion is produced. The amount of opening of the mouth depends on the amount and type of food to be incised. As the food is placed by the hand between the lips to a position between the anterior teeth, the lower jaw is elevated and retracted, separating the bolus of food. Whether the anterior teeth occlude during this act is dependent on the character of the food and the tearing mechanism by the hand. In the incision of tough foods there may be sufficient retraction and elevation of the mandible to bring the edges of the lower teeth toward slight contact with the incisal edge or the lingual surfaces of the maxillary teeth, depending on the consistency of the food and the positional relationship of the teeth.

In these tougher foods there may be some rotation of the mandible during the act, especially if the food is placed in the cuspid region, the action being a lateral protrusive motion. The softer the food, the more this action is mitigated, the bolus being separated not only by the teeth but also by a tongue-and-groove action.

When a mass of food of satisfactory size has been incised or has been placed in the mouth after having been previously cut, it is picked up by the tongue and deposited on the occlusal surfaces of the posterior teeth, with the help of the cheek muscles. The chewing act at this time is dependent on the size and character of the bolus of food. Hard, dry foods are easily crushed, quickly absorb saliva, and are softened rapidly. Thus little chewing is required for these foods. For tougher foods sufficient chewing is necessary to prepare the bolus for swallowing. Small portions of the total mass may be separated, individually mixed with saliva, and crushed and swallowed while the remainder of the bolus is being held or chewed intermittently.

Kurth studied the physiology of mandibular movement by recording stroboscopic photographs of gliding and masticatory movements. The light source was a stroboscopic lamp that flashed intermittent rays of light with no afterglow. A pin with a head capable of reflecting this light was cemented between the lower central incisors. The patient was instructed to glide and chew, and the movement of the pin, which duplicated the mandibular movements, was photographed by a clinical camera. The picture of three-dimensional movements of the mandible was obtained and referred to any one plane as horizontal, frontal, or sagittal. This study revealed no indication of spherical movement of the mandible during mastication.

According to the studies of Jankelson et al. with the oscillograph, chewing is not rhythmic, and tooth contact during mastication is absent or negligible during the chewing act up to the swallowing stage. Contact often does not occur, even during the first swallow, since there is sometimes residual bolus between the teeth that prevents contact. Chewing is continued, followed by swallowing, after which tooth contacts may occur. The teeth do not slide up the buccal cusps of the maxillary teeth, into the sulcus, and down the lingual cusps. They vary their movements in accordance with the job they have to do. In other words, their action is governed by the condition of the food at a particular instant of time, and, since the character of the food is constantly changing in consistency, position, size, shape, and infiltration with saliva during each stroke, the action also changes. The movement of the teeth therefore is determined by the location, size, and resistance of the bolus.

Jankelson et al. have shown that the masticatory cycle depends almost entirely on the character of the food being chewed, modified to some extent by the patient's pain threshold. It does not necessarily start from or return to any particular place. It starts from a wider open position for a larger morsel of food and ends whenever the pressure on the teeth builds up so that tactile sense warns the individual to let up on the pressure. When food has no resistance, it is either mushed or chewed slightly in preparation for swallowing. The terminal stroke of chewing here may approach tooth contact, and even slight tooth contacts may be made.

Graf and Zander's work has seemingly reconciled these findings in that they have shown that contact occurs during masticatory cycles in the intercuspal or habitual closure but not in the retruded position of the mandible (centric relation). Thus the difference could depend on the jaw relation in which the records were made.

On the other hand, Anderson and Picton have stated that the teeth come into contact for more than half the chewing strokes and that in some individuals every thrust makes contact.

The response of the dentoalveolar unit to masticatory forces has been studied. Castelli and Dempster computed a force of 3 g/cm as sufficient to occlude the blood supply. Goldman showed, however, that occlusion of the periodontal ligament did not alter the vascularity of the gingiva. Brewer measured actual contact of the teeth by the use of miniaturized radio transmitters in full dentures and found that mastication accounted for 5 minutes of contact. Sheppard and Markus, using cinefluorographic techniques, reported a total time of 8 minutes. Graf, employing telemetry and electromyographic recordings, reported a total time of 17½ minutes over a 24-hour span with an average contact of 0.3 second. In contrast to the time contact recorded above it has been estimated that in bruxators, the contact of teeth is much longer; the intensity of the contact is also much greater.

Although the function of the teeth is thought to be the most important part of mastication, there are many interrelated processes that are equally significant. The masticatory process not only includes the preparation and segmentation of food for swallowing but also allows for the mixing of the foodstuff with saliva to facilitate the passage of the food to the stomach. It is well known that without adequate salivary flow swallowing cannot take place, and thus it is perhaps this function of mixing saliva and food that is the most important process of mastication. Another consideration is the comminution of food for the purpose of increasing the exposed surface area of the foodstuff to the digestive fluids. This comminution also allows for enhancement of the mechanical functions of the stomach. The palatability of food is determined by taste and smell. The mixing of food with saliva allows for the dissolving of the taste stimulants contained in the food and facilitates the spread of these stimulants to the taste buds. The segmentation of food into small bits also releases volatile components that are picked up by the olfactory area, and thus the sense of smell is enhanced by the process of mastication.

Tongue function. The tongue plays an important role in the masticatory process. For some foods the tongue has a direct crushing effect, pressing them against the hard palate. This function is assisted by the surface texture of the tongue and the rugae of the palate. Many foods need no additional mastication and are ready for deglutition. Others are formed into a compact bolus by this action and are then placed on the occlusal platform for tooth action.

Saliva. The functions of saliva are (1) digestive, (2) to aid in swallowing, (3) cleansing, (4) lubricative, (5) bactericidal, and (6) excretory. The quantity of saliva secreted is variable but on the average is between 1,000 and 1,500 ml per 24-hour period. Of this, over 99% is water, with solids comprising the rest. Human saliva normally has a slightly acid reaction, and the pH is usually between 6.3 and 6.9. The saliva is probably buffered principally by the carbonic acid and sodium bicarbonate systems, but it is thought that the proteins and phosphates present in saliva also play a role.

That increased salivation takes place during mastication is a well-established fact. This is necessary since food cannot be swallowed when dry. Thus a most important physiologic function of mastication is to mix saliva with food for deglutition. The food is separated, which allows it to become lubricated. Salivary flow also has some ability to cleanse the teeth and the oral cavity. In the absence of saliva, food and debris collect around the necks of the teeth. Experiments in laboratory animals in which the salivary glands have been removed show a marked increase in the incidence of caries. Saliva lubricates the oral mucosa, a property necessary to maintain the health of the tissue. In cases of xerostomia, changes in the oral mucosa, as well as in the composition of the oral microbial flora, are evident. For example, the proportions of *Streptococcus mutans* tend to rise. The bactericidal effect of saliva has been demonstrated by Bibby et al., who have shown that saliva destroys or inhibits the growth of a wide variety of microorganisms.

Deglutition

Food is transferred from the mouth to the stomach by the act of deglutition or swallowing. In this process the bolus of food is projected past the pharynx into the esophagus. The jaws are closed and the tongue is raised so as to press against the palate, the raising of the tongue being caused by a contraction of the mylohyoid muscle aided by the intrinsic muscles of the tongue itself (Fig. 1-62). At the same time the base of the tongue is drawn slightly backward by the contraction of the styloglossus and palatoglossus muscles. While the bolus is in the pharynx, the soft palate is raised so as to prevent the passage of food into the nares. The saliva, by its mixture with the food, assists not only in mastication but also in deglutition.

The currently accepted theory of deglutition may be divided into four phases. These phases actually merge into one another since the swallowing reflex is a continuous process. The first phase is a preparatory phase, which starts after preparation of the bolus. The liquid or bolus is positioned on the dorsum of the tongue with the oral cavity sealed by the lips and by the tongue. As far as is presently known, the size of the bolus seemingly is constant for each subject. The second phase is the oral phase. This phase is started by the withdrawal of the soft palate from its rest position against the base of the tongue. The soft palate moves upward, and the tongue drops downward and back. The bolus is pushed from the oral cavity by the tongue while fluids flow ahead of the lingual contractions. During the third phase the oral cavity maintains an anterior seal. The cheeks form a lateral border seal. The fourth phase be-

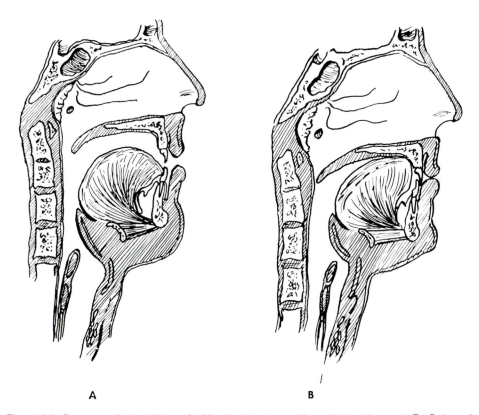

A **B**

Fig. 1-62. Process of deglutition. **A,** Mouth at rest position with teeth apart. **B,** Bolus of food has been projected past pharynx and into esophagus, jaws are closed, and mandibular teeth are pressed against maxillary teeth.

gins as the bolus passes through the fauces and then by the cricopharyngeal sphincter. While peristaltic movement carries the food through the esophagus, the soft palate and tongue return to their original positions.

When a large section of food has been taken into the mouth, it is chewed, but prior to swallowing it is sectioned by the tongue into smaller parts and is swallowed consecutively until the oral cavity is empty.

In one study an average individual swallows once per minute between meals, but nine times per minute while eating. Swallowing also occurs at infrequent intervals during sleep. During a 24-hour period, approximately 2,400 somatic and visceral swallows occur. In another study an overall mean of 7½ swallows per hour have been computed, whereas a mean of 296 swallows per hour has been recorded during eating.

REFERENCES

Ainamo, J., and Löe, H.: Anatomical characteristics of gingiva. I. A clinical and microscopic study of the free and attached gingiva, J. Periodontol. **37:**5, 1966.

Aisenberg, M. S.: Histology and physiology of the supporting structures, J. Am. Dent. Assoc. **44:**628, 1952.

Allstrom, R., Graf de Beer, M., and Schroeder, H.: Clinical and histological characteristics of normal gingiva in dogs, J. Periodont. Res. **10:**115, 1975.

Anderson, B. J., Smith, A. H., Arnim, S. S., and Orten, A. V.: Changes in molar teeth and their supporting structures in rats following extraction of the upper right first and second molars, Yale J. Biol. Med. **49:**145, 1929.

Anderson, D. J.: Measurement of stress in mastication, J. Dent. Res. **35:**664, 1956.

Anderson, D. J., and Picton, D. C. A.: Tooth contact during chewing, J. Dent. Res. **36:**21, 1957.

Arnim, S. S., and Hagerman, D. A.: The connective tissue fibers of the marginal gingiva, J. Am. Dent. Assoc. **47:**271, 1953.

Attström, R.: Presence of leukocytes in crevices of healthy and chronically inflamed gingivae, J. Periodont. Res. **5:**42, 1970.

Attström, R., and Egelberg, J.: Emigration of blood neutrophils and monocytes into the gingival crevices, J. Periodont. Res. **5:**48, 1970.

Baer, P. M., and Bernick, S.: Age changes in the periodontium of the mouse, Oral Surg. **10:**430, 1957.

Barker, B. C. W.: Relation of the alveolus to the cemento-enamel junction following attritional wear in aboriginal skulls. An enquiry into the normality of cementum exposure with aging, J. Periodontol. **46:**357, 1975.

Barnett, M. L.: Mast cells in the epithelial layers of human gingiva, J. Ultrastruct. Res. **43:**247, 1973.

Barnett, M. L., and Szabo, G.: Gap junctions in human gingival keratinized epithelium, J. Periodont. Res. **8:**117, 1973.

Bass, C. C.: A demonstrable line in extracted teeth indicating location of the outer border of the epithelial attachment, J. Dent. Res. **25:**401, 1947.

Bass, C. C., and Fullmer, H. M.: The location of the zone of disintegrating epithelial attachment cuticle; relation to the cemento-enamel junction and to the outer border of the periodontal fibers on some tooth specimens, J. Dent. Res. **27:**623, 1948.

Beagrie, G. S.: An autoradiographic study of the gingival epithelium of mice and monkeys with thymidine-H³, Dent. Pract. Dent. Rec. **14:**18, 1963.

Beagrie, G. S., and Skougaard, M. R.: Observations on the life cycle of the gingival epithelial cells of mice as revealed by autoradiography, Acta Odontol. Scand. **20:**15, 1962.

Becks, H. V.: Normal and pathologic pocket formation, J. Am. Dent. Assoc. **16:**2167, 1929.

Beertsen, W.: Migration of fibroblasts in the periodontal ligament of the mouse incisor as revealed by autoradiography, Arch. Oral Biol. **20:**659, 1975.

Beertsen, W., and Snijder, J.: Histologic difference between the periodontal membranes of teeth with a continuous and a limited eruption, Ned. Tandheilk. **76:**542, 1969.

Belanger, L. F.: Resorption of cementum by cementocyte activity ("cementolysis"), Calcif. Tissue Res. **2:**229, 1968.

Belting, C. M., Schour, I., Weinman, J. P., and Shepro, M. J.: Age changes in the periodontal tissues of the rat molar, J. Dent. Res. **32:**332, 1953.

Berkelbach van der Sprenkel, H.: Microscopical investigations of the innervation of the tooth and its surroundings, J. Anat. **70:**233, 1936.

Bernick, S., Levy, B. M., Dreizen, S., and Grant, D.: Course of alveolar fibers on periodontal ligament, J. Dent. Res. **56:**1409, 1977.

Bernick, S.: Innervation of the primary tooth and supporting tissues of monkeys, Anat. Rec. **113:**215, 1952.

Bernick, S.: Silver impregnation of nerves after enzymatic removal of collagenous elements, Stain Tech. **30:**253, 1955.

Bernick, S.: The innervation of the teeth and periodontium of the rat, Anat. Rec. **125:**185, 1956.

Bernick, S.: Innervation of teeth and periodontium after enzymatic removal of collagenous elements, Oral Surg. **10:**323, 1957.

Bernick, S.: Innervation of the teeth and periodontium, Dent. Clin. North Am., pp. 503-514, July 1959.

Berwick, L., and Coman, D. R.: Some chemical factors in cellular adhesion and stickiness, Cancer Res. **22:**982, 1962.

Bevelander, G., and Nikahara, H.: The fine structure of the periodontal ligament, Anat. Rec. **162:**313, 1968.

Bien, S. M.: Hydrodynamic damping of tooth movement, J. Dent. Res. **45:**907, 1966.

Bjorn, H.: The vascular supply of the periodontal membrane, J. Periodontol. **1:**51, 1966.

Bloom, W., and Fawcett, D. W.: A textbook of histology, ed. 9, Philadelphia, 1970, W. B. Saunders Co.

Bodecker, C. F.: A consideration of some of the changes in the teeth from youth to old age, Dent. Cosmos **67:**543, 1925.

Box, H. K.: Evidence of lymphatics in the periodontium, J. Can. Dent. Assoc. **15:**8, 1949.

Boyle, P. E.: The structure and function of the tooth supporting tissues. In Boyle, P. E., editor: Kronfeld's histopathology of the teeth and their surrounding structures, ed. 4, London, 1955, Henry Kimpton.

Boyle, P. E.: Tooth suspension; a comparative study of the paradental tissues of man and the guinea pig, J. Dent. Res. **17:**37, 1938.

Bradlaw, R.: The innervation of teeth, Proc. R. Soc. Med. **29:**507, 1936.

Bradlaw, R.: The histology and histopathology of dental innervation, Proc. R. Soc. Med. **32:**1040, 1939.

Brashear, A. D.: The innervation of the teeth, J. Comp. Neurol. **64:**169, 1936.

Breitner, S. C.: Tooth supporting apparatus under occlusal changes, J. Periodontol. **13:**72, 1942.

Brill, N.: Effect of chewing on rate of flow of tissue fluid into human gingival pockets, Acta Odontol. Scand. **17:**277, 1959.

Brill, N.: Gingival pocket fluid, Acta Odontol. Scand. **20:** Supp., 1962.

Brill, N.: Influence of capillary permeability on flow of tissue fluid into gingival pocket, Acta Odontol. Scand. **17:**23, 1959.

Brill, N.: Removal of particles and bacteria from gingival pockets by tissue fluid, Acta Odontol. Scand. **17:**432, 1959.

Brill, N., and Bjorn, H.: Passage of tissue fluid into human gingival pockets, Acta Odontol. Scand. **17:**11, 1959.

Brill, N., and Brönnestam, R.: Immuno-electrophoretic study of tissue fluid from gingival pockets, Acta Odontol. Scand. **18:**95, 1960.

Brill, N., and Krasse, B.: The passage of tissue fluid into the clinically healthy gingival pocket, Acta Odontol. Scand. **16:**233, 1958.

Browne, R. M.: Some observations on the fluid flow from the gingival crevice, Dent. Pract. Dent. Rec. **14:**470, 1964.

Browne, R. M.: A preliminary study of the fluid flow from the gingival sulcus, Proc. R. Soc. Med. **55:**486, 1962.

Brudevold, F., Steadman, L. T., and Smith, F. A.: Inorganic and organic components of tooth structure, Ann. N.Y. Acad. Sci. **85:**110, 1960.

Carmichael, G. C., and Fullmer, H. M.: The fine structure of the oxytalan fiber, J. Cell Biol. **28:**33, 1966.

Carneiro, J.: Synthesis and turnover of collagen in periodontal tissues; use of radioautography investigation of protein synthesis, New York, 1965, Academic Press, Inc.

Carranza, F. A., Jr., and Cabrini, R. L.: Histochemical reactions of periodontal tissues; a review of the literature, J. Am. Dent. Assoc. **60:**464, 1960.

Castelli, W. A., and Dempster, W. T.: The periodontal vasculature and its responses to experimental pressures, J. Am. Dent. Assoc. **70:**890, 1965.

Churchill, H. R.: Meyer's normal histology and histogenesis of the human teeth and associated parts, Philadelphia, 1935, J. B. Lippincott Co., pp. 104-157.

Cimasoni, G.: The crevicular fluid. In Myers, H. M., editor: Monographs in oral science, vol. 3, Basel, 1974, S. Karger.

Cimasoni, G., Fiore-Donno, G., and Held, A. J.: Mucopolysaccharides in human epithelial reattachment, Helv. Odontol. Acta **7:**60, 1963.

Cohen, L.: The intercellular cement substance of oral epithelium in man and Macacus irus, Arch. Oral Biol. **13:**163, 1968.

Cohn, S. A.: A new look at the orientation of cementoalveolar fibers of the mouse periodontal ligament, Anat. Rec. **166:**292, 1970.

Collins, A. A., and Gavin, J. B.: An evaluation of the antimicrobial effect of the fluid exudate from the clinically healthy gingival crevice, J. Periodontol. **32:**99, 1961.

Coolidge, E. D.: The thickness of the human periodontal membrane, J. Am. Dent. Assoc. **24:**1260, 1937.

Cowley, G. C.: Application of fluorescent protein tracing to the study of gingival inflammation, J. Dent. Res. **43:**947, 1964.

Crumley, P. J.: Collagen formation in the normal and stressed periodontium, Periodontics **2:**53, 1964.

Deporter, D. A., and Ten Cate, A. R.: Collagen resorption by periodontal ligament fibroblasts at the hard tissue–ligament interfaces of the mouse periodontium, J. Periodontol. In press.

Diab, M. A., Stallard, R. E., and Zander, H. A.: The life cycle of the epithelia elements of the developing molar, Oral Surg. **22:**241, 1966.

Dixon, A. D.: Nerve plexuses in the oral mucosa, Arch. Oral Biol. **8:**435, 1963.

Dodson, J. W., and Hay, E. D.: Secretion of collagenous stroma by isolated epithelium grown *in vitro,* Exp. Cell Res. **65:**215, 1971.

Dummett, C. O.: Physiologic pigmentation of the oral and cutaneous tissue in the Negro, J. Dent. Res. **25:**422, 1946.

Dummett, C. O.: Clinical observations on pigment variations in healthy oral tissues of the Negro, J. Dent. Res. **24:**7, 1945.

Egelberg, J.: Blood vessels of the dento-gingival junction, J. Periodontol. **1:**163, 1966.

Egelberg, J.: Cellular elements in gingival pocket fluid, Acta Odontol. Scand. **21:**283, 1963.

Egelberg, J.: Diffusion of histamine into the gingival crevice and through the crevicular epithelium, Acta Odontol. Scand. **21:**271, 1963.

Egelberg, J., and Cowley, G. C.: The bacterial state of different regions within the clinically healthy gingival crevice, Acta Odontol. Scand. **21:**289, 1963.

Eley, B. M., and Harrison, J. D.: Intracellular collagen fibrils in the periodontal ligament of man, J. Periodont. Res. **10:**168, 1975.

Engler, W. D., Ramfjord, S. P., and Hiniker, J. J.: Development of epithelial attachment and gingival sulcus in rhesus monkeys, J. Periodontol. **36:**44, 1965.

Farquhar, M. G., and Palade, G. E.: Junctional complexes in various epithelia, J. Cell Biol. **17:**375, 1963.

Fawcett, D. W.: An atlas of fine structure; the cell, its organelles, and inclusions, Philadelphia, 1966, W. B. Saunders Co.

Fearnhead, R. W.: Histological evidence for the innervation of human dentine, J. Anat. **91:**267, 1957.

Flaxman, B. A., Lutzner, M. A., and van Scott, E. J.: Ultrastructure of cell attachment to substratum in vitro, J. Cell Biol. **36:**406, 1968.

Forssland, G.: The structure and function of the capillary system in the gingiva in man, Acta Odontol. Scand. 17 (suppl. 26):1959.

Frank, R., and Cimasoni, G.: Electron microscopic study of the human epithelial attachment, J. Dent. Res. **49:**691, 1970.

Frank, R., and Cimasoni, G.: Ultrastructure de l'epithélium cliniquement normal du sillon et de la jonction gingivo-dentaires, Z. Zellforsch. **109:**356, 1970.

Freeman, E., and Ten Cate, A. R.: Development of the periodontium: an electron microscopic study, J. Periodontol. **42:**387, 1971.

Fullmer, H. M.: A critique of normal connective tissues of the periodontium and some alterations with periodontal disease, J. Dent. Res. **41:**223, 1962.

Fullmer, H. M.: Observations on the development of oxytalan fibers in the periodontium of man, J. Dent. Res. **38:**510, 1959.

Fullmer, H. M., and Lillie, R. D.: The oxytalan fiber; a previously undescribed connective tissue fiber, J. Histochem. Cytochem. **6:**425, 1958.

Furseth, R.: The fine structure of the cellular cementum of young human teeth, Arch. Oral Biol. **14:**1147, 1969.

Gairns, F. W.: The sensory nerve endings of the human gingiva, palate and tongue, J. Dent. Res. **35:**958, 1956.

Gavin, J. B.: A study of the permeability of gingiva using intravenous colloidal thorium dioxide, N.Z. Dent. J. **68:** 201, 1972.

Gavin, J. B., and Collins, A. A.: Occurrence of bacteria within the clinically healthy gingival crevice, J. Periodontol. **32:**198, 1961.

Gibson, W. A., and Fullmer, H. M.: Histochemistry of the periodontal ligament. II. The phosphatases, Periodontics **5:**226, 1967.

Gibson, W. A., and Fullmer, H. M.: Histochemistry of the periodontal ligament. I. The dehydrogenases, Periodontics **4:**63, 1966.

Glavind, L., and Löe, H.: Capillary microscopy of the gingiva in pregnant and nonpregnant individuals, J. Periodont. Res. **2:**74, 1967.

Glavind, L., and Zander, H. A.: Dynamics of dental epithelium during tooth eruption, J. Dent. Res. **49:**549, 1970.

Glickman, I.: Clinical periodontology, ed. 3, Philadelphia, 1964, W. B. Saunders Co., p. 15.

Goldhaber, P.: Collagen and bone, J. Am. Dent. Assoc. **68:** 825, 1964.

Goldman, H. M.: Discussion of connective tissues, J. Dent. Res. **41:**230, 1962.

Goldman, H. M.: The effects of dietary protein deprivation and of age on the periodontal tissue of the rat and spider monkey, J. Periodontol. **25:**87, 1954.

Goldman, H. M.: The topography and role of the gingival fibers, J. Periodontol Res. **30:**331, 1951.

Goldman, H. M., Millsap, J. S., and Brenman, H.: Origin of registration of the architectural pattern, the lamina dura, and the alveolar crest in the dental radiograph, Oral Surg. **10:**749, 1957.

Gottlieb, B.: Histologic consideration of the supporting tissues of the teeth, J. Am. Dent. Assoc. **30:**1872, 1943.

Gottlieb, B.: Zur Biologie der Epithelansatzes und des Alveolarrandes, Dtsch. Zahnaerztl. Wochenschr. **25:**434, 1922.

Gottlieb, B.: Aetiologie und Prophylaxe der Zahnkaries, Z. Stomat. **19:**129, 1921.

Gottlieb, B.: Der Epithelansatz am Zahne, Dtsch. Mschr. Zahnheilk. **39:**142, 1921.

Gottlieb, B.: Zur aetiologie und Therapie der Alveolar-pyorrhoe, Z. Stomat. **18:**59, 1920.

Graf, H.: Occlusal tooth contact patterns in mastication, Thesis, University of Rochester, Rochester, N.Y., 1968.

Graf, H., and Zander, H. A.: Tooth contact patterns in mastication, J. Prosthet. Dent. **13:**1055, 1963.

Grant, D., and Bernick, S.: The formation of the periodontal ligament, J. Periodontol. **43:**17, 1972.

Grant, D., and Bernick, S.: The periodontium of ageing humans, J. Periodont. Res. **43:**660, 1972.

Grant, D., Bernick, S., Levy, B. M., and Dreizen, S.: A comparative study of the periodontal ligament development in teeth with and without predecessors in marmosets, J. Periodontol. **43:**162, 1972.

Greene, A. H.: A study of the characteristics of stippling and its relation to gingival health, J. Periodontol. **33:**176, 1962.

Greulich, R. C.: Cell proliferation and migration in the epi-

thelial attachment collar of the mouse molar, Int. Assoc. Res. (abstract), **40:**80, 1962.

Griffin, C. J., and Harris, R.: Innervation of the human periodontium. I. Classification of periodontal receptors, Aust. Dent. J. **19:**51, 1974.

Gross, J.: Collagen, Sci. Am. **204:**121, 1961.

Hanson, M. L., Logan, W. B., and Case, J. L.: Tongue thrust in pre-school children, Am. J. Orthod. **57:**15, 1970.

Heijl, L., Rifkin, B. R., and Zander, H. A.: Conversion of chronic gingivitis to periodontitis in squirrel makeup, J. Periodont. **47:**710, 1976.

Hillman, D. G.: Stresses in the periodontal ligament, J. Periodont. Res. **8:**51, 1973.

Hodson, J. J.: A critical review of the dental cuticle with special reference to recent investigations, Int. Dent. J. **16:**350, 1966.

Howell, A. H., and Manly, R. S.: An electronic strain gauge for measuring oral forces, J. Dent. Res. **27**(6):705, 1948.

Hunt, A. M., and Paynter, K. J.: The role of cells of the stratum intermedium in the development of the guinea pig molar. A study of cell differentiation and migration using tritiated thymidine, Arch. Oral Biol. **8:**65, 1963.

Ito, H., Enomoto, S., and Kobayashi, K.: Electron microscopic study of the human epithelial attachment, Bull. Tokyo Med. Dent. Univ. **14:**267, 1967.

Jande, S. S., and Belanger, L. F.: Electronmicroscopy of osteocytes and the pericellular matrix in rat trabecular bone, Calcif. Tissue Res. **6:**280, 1971.

Jankelson, B., Hoffman, G. M., and Hendron, J. A.: The physiology of the stomatognathic system, J. Am. Dent. Assoc. **46:**375, 1953.

Jerge, C. R.: Comments on the innervation of the teeth, Dent. Clin. North Am., pp. 117-127, March 1965.

Johnson, P. L., and Bevelander, G.: The role of the stratum intermedium in tooth development, Oral Surg. **10:**437, 1957.

Kameyama, Y.: Autoradiographic study of ^{3}H-proline incorporation by rat periodontal ligament, gingival connective tissue, and dental pulp, J. Periodont. Res. **10:**98, 1975.

Karring, T., Lang, N. P., and Löe, H.: The role of gingival connective tissue in determining epithelial diferentiation, J. Periodont. Res. **10:**1, 1975.

Karring, T., and Löe, H.: The three-dimensional concept of the epithelium-connective tissue boundary of gingiva, Acta Odontol. Scand. **28:**917, 1970.

Karring, T., and Löe, H.: Blood supply to the periodontium, J. Periodont. Res. **2:**74, 1967.

Keller, G. J., and Cohen, D. W.: India ink perfusion of the vascular plexus of oral tissues, Oral Surg. **8:**539, 1955.

Kenney, E. B., and Ramfjord, S. P.: Cellular dynamics in root formation of teeth in rhesus monkeys, J. Dent. Res. **48:**114, 1969.

Kohl, J. T., and Zander, H. A.: Morphology of the interdental gingival tissues, Oral Surg. **14:**287, 1961.

Kramer, I. R. H.: Alveolar bone in health and disease, Dent. Pract. Dent. Rec. **12:**327, 1962.

Krasse, B., and Egelberg, J.: The relative proportions of sodium, potassium and calcium in gingival pocket fluid, Acta Odontol. Scand. **20:**143, 1962.

Kronfeld, R.: Biology of cementum, J. Am. Dent. Assoc. **25:**1451, 1938.

Kronfeld, R.: Increase in size of the clinical crown in human teeth with advancing age, J. Am. Dent. Assoc. **23:**382, 1936.

Kronfeld, R.: Structure, function and pathology of the human periodontal membrane, N.J.J. Dent. **6:**112, 1936.

Kronfeld, R., and Ulik, R.: Brechen auch bei wilden Tieren die Zahne Kontinuierlich durch? Z. Stomat. **26:**84, 1928.

Kurth, L. E.: Physiology of mandibular movement related to prosthodontia, N.Y. Dent. J. **12:**323, 1949.

Kurth, L. E.: Mandibular movements in mastication, J. Am. Dent. Assoc. **29:**1729, 1942.

Lamberg, S. I., and Stoolmiller, A. C.: Glycosaminoglycans. A biochemical and clinical review, J. Invest. Dermatol. **63:**433, 1974.

Lear, C. S. C., Flanagan, J. B., and Moorres, C. F. A.: The frequency of delutition in man, Arch. Oral Biol. **10:**83, 1965.

Lefkowitz, W.: The formation of cementum, Am. J. Orthod. **30:**224, 1944.

Lewinsky, W., and Stewart, D.: The innervation of the periodontal membrane of the cat, with some observations on the function of the end organs found in that structure, J. Anat. **71:**232, 1937.

Lewinsky, W., and Stewart, D.: An account of our present knowledge of the innervation of the teeth and their related tissues, Br. Dent. J. **65:**687, 1938.

Listgarten, M. A.: Structure of surface coatings on teeth. A review, J. Periodontol. **47:**139, 1976.

Listgarten, M. A.: Afibrillar dental cementum in the rat and hamster, J. Periodont. Res. **10:**158, 1975.

Listgarten, M. A.: Similarity of epithelial relationships in the gingiva of rat and man, J. Periodontol. **46:**677, 1975.

Listgarten, M. A.: Normal development, structure, physiology and repair of gingival epithelium, Oral Sci. Rev. **1:**3, 1972.

Listgarten, M. A.: Changing concepts about the dento-epithelial junction, J. Can. Dent. Assoc. **36:**70, 1970.

Listgarten, M. A.: A light and electron microscopic study of coronal cementogenesis, Arch. Oral Biol. **13:**93, 1968.

Listgarten, M. A.: A mineralized cuticular structure with connective tissue characteristics on the crown of unerupted teeth in amelogenesis imperfecta. A light and electron microscopic study, Arch. Oral Biol. **12:**877, 1967.

Listgarten, M. A.: Electron microscopic features of the newly formed epithelial attachment after gingival surgery, J. Periodont. Res. **2:**46, 1967.

Listgarten, M. A.: Phase-contrast and electron microscopic study of the junction between reduced enamel epithelium and enamel in unerupted human teeth, Arch. Oral Biol. **11:**999, 1966.

Listgarten, M. A.: Electron microscopic study of the gingivodental junction of man, Am. J. Anat. **119:**147, 1966.

Listgarten, M. A.: The ultrastructure of human gingival epithelium, Am. J. Anat. **114:**49, 1964.

Listgarten, M. A., and Kamin, A.: The development of a cementum layer over the enamel surface of rabbit molars — a light and electron microscopic study, Arch. Oral Biol. **14:**961, 1969.

Löe, H.: Bone tissue formation; a morphological and histochemical study, Acta Odontol. Scand. **17:**311, 1959.

Löe, H.: Periodontal changes in pregnancy, J. Periodontol. **36:**209, 1965.

Löe, H.: Epidemiology of periodontal disease; and evaluation of the relative significance of the aetiological factors in the light of recent epidemiological research. Odont. Tskr. **71:**479, 1963.

Löe, H.: Nyere undersokelser over emaljens organiske komponent (Recent investigations on the organic component of dental enamel), Odont. Tskr. **70:**483, 1962.

Löe, H.: Physiological aspects of the gingival pocket — an experimental study, Acta Odontol. Scand. **19:**387, 1961.

Löe, H.: and Holm-Pedersen, P.: Absence and presence of fluid from normal and inflamed gingiva, Periodontics **3:**171, 1965.

Löe, H.: and Nuki, K.: Observations on the peracetic acid-aldehyde fuchsin (oxytalan) positive tissue elements in the periodontium, Acta Odontol. Scand. **22:**579, 1964.

Löe, H.: and Nuki, K.: Oxidative enzyme activity in keratinizing and non-keratinizing epithelium of normal and inflamed gingiva, J. Periodont. Res. **1:**43, 1966.

Löe, H.: and Silness, J.: Tissue reactions to a new gingivectomy pack, Oral Surg. **14:**1305, 1961.

Löe, H.: and Silness, J.: Tissue reactions to string packs used in fixed restorations, J. Prosthet. Dent. **13:**318, 1963.

Löe, H.: Theilade, E., and Jensen, S. B.: Experimental gingivitis in man, J. Periodontol. **36:**177, 1965.

Mandel, I. D.: Dental plaque: nature, formation and effects, J. Periodontal. **37:**357, 1966.

Manly, R. S., and Braley, L. C.: Masticatory performance and masticatory efficiency, J. Dent. Res. **29:**448, 1950.

Manly, R. S., and Vinton, P.: A survey of the chewing ability of denture wearers, J. Dent. Res. **30:**314, 1951.

Mann, W. V., Jr.: The correlation of gingivitis, pocket depth and exudate from the gingival crevice, J. Periodontol. **34:**379, 1963.

Manson, J. D.: The lamina dura, Oral Surg. **16:**432, 1963.

Marsland, E. A., and Fox, E. C.: Some abnormalities in the nerve supply of the oral mucosa, Proc. R. Soc. Med. **51:**951, 1958.

Maxwell, G. H.: Biologic-mathematical formula for ideal occlusion, J. Am. Dent. Assoc. **24:**238, 1937.

Maxwell, G. H.: Structural functional elements of normal occlusion, Int. J. Orthod. **23:**1182, 1937.

McDougall, W. A.: The effect of topical antigen on the gingiva of sensitized rabbits, J. Periodont. Res. **9:**153, 1974.

McDougall, W. A.: Penetration pathways of a topically applied foreign protein into rat gingiva, J. Periodont. Res. **6:**89, 1971.

McHugh, W. D.: The keratinization of gingival epithelium, J. Periodontol. **35:**338, 1964.

McHugh, W. D.: Some aspects of the development of gingival epithelium, Periodontics **1:**239, 1963.

McHugh, W. D.: The development of the gingival epithelium in the monkey, Dent. Pract. Dent. Rec. **11:**314, 1961.

McHugh, W. D., and Zander, H. A.: Cell division in the periodontium of developing and erupted teeth, Dent. Pract. Dent. Rec. **15:**451, 1965.

MacKenzie, I. C.: Does toothbrushing affect gingival keratinization? Proc. R. Soc. Med. **65:**1127, 1972.

McLean, D. W.: Physiology of mastication, J. Am. Dent. Assoc. **27:**226, 1940.

McLean, F. C., and Urist, M. R.: Bone, Chicago, 1955, University of Chicago Press.

Melcher, A. H.: Gingival reticulin: identification and role in histogenesis of collagen fibers, J. Dent. Res. **45:**426, 1966.

Melcher, A. H.: The architecture of human gingival reticulum, Arch. Oral Biol. **9:**125, 1964.

Melcher, A. H.: The interpapillary ligament, Dent. Pract. **12:**461, 1962.

Melcher, A. H.: The interpapillary ligament, Dent. Pract. Dent. Rec. **12:**461, 1962.

Melcher, A. H., and Accursi, G. E.: Osteogenic capacity of periosteal and osteoperiosteal flaps elevated from the parietal bone of the rat, Arch. Oral Biol. **16:**573, 1971.

Melcher, A. H., and Bowen, W. H.: Biology of the periodontium, London, 1969, Academic Press, Inc.

Meyling, H. A.: Structure and significance of the peripheral extension of the autonomic nervous system, J. Comp. Neurol. **99:**495, 1953.

Miles, A. E. W.: Aging in the teeth and oral tissues. In Bourne, G. H., and Wilson, E. M. H., editors: Structural aspects of aging, London, 1961, Sir Isaac Pitman & Sons, Ltd.

Mongkollugsana, D., and Edwards, L. F.: The extra-osseous innervation of the gingivae, J. Dent. Res. **36:**516, 1957.

Morris, M. L.: The position of the margin of the gingiva, Oral Surg. **11:**969, 1958.

Moyers, R. E.: An electromyographic analysis of certain muscles involved in temporomandibular movement, Am. J. Orthod. **36:**48, 1950.

Nakata, T. M., Stepnick, R. J., and Zipkin, I.: Chemistry of human dental cementum: the effect of age and fluoride exposure on the concentration of ash, fluoride, calcium, phosphorus and magnesium, J. Periodontol. **43:**115, 1972.

Newman, H. N.: Ultrastructure of the apical border of dental plaque. In Lehner, T., editor: The borderland between caries and periodontal disease, New York, 1977, Grune & Stratton, Inc., pp. 79-103.

Nigra, T. P., Friedland, M., and Martin, G. R.: Controls of connective tissue synthesis: collagen metabolism, J. Invest. Dermatol. **59:**44, 1972.

Nimni, M. E.: Metabolic pathways and control mechanisms involved in the biosynthesis and turnover of collagen in normal and pathological connective tissues, J. Oral Pathol. **2:**175, 1973.

Niswonger, M. E.: Rest position of the mandible and centric relation, J. Am. Dent. Assoc. **21:**1572, 1934.

Noyes, F. B., Schour, I., and Noyes, H. J.: Dental histology and embryology, Philadelphia, 1938, Lea & Febiger.

Nuki, K., and Hock, J.: The organization of the gingival vasculature, J. Periodont. Res. **9:**305, 1974.

O'Leary, J. L., Petty, J., Harris, A. B., and Inukai, J.: Supravital staining of mammalian brain with intraarterial methylene blue followed by pressurized oxygen, Stain Tech. **43:**197, 1968.

O'Leary, T. J., and Rudd, D. K.: An instrument for measuring horizontal tooth mobility, Periodontics **1:**249, 1963.

Orban, B.: Oral histology and embryology, ed. 4, St. Louis, 1957, The C. V. Mosby Co., p. 231.

Orban, B.: Current concepts concerning gingival anatomy, Dent. Clin. North Am., p. 705, November, 1960.

Orban, B.: Clinical histologic study of the surface characteristics of the gingiva, Oral Surg. **1:**827, 1948.

Orban, B.: Study of surface characteristics of gingiva, Oral Surg. **1:**827, 1948.

Orban, B.: Contribution to the knowledge of physiological processes in the periodontium, J. Am. Dent. Assoc. **16:**405, 1929.

Orban, B., Bhatia, H., Kollar, J. A., Jr., and Wentz, F. M.: Epithelial attachment (the attached epithelial cuff), J. Periodontol. **27:**167, 1956.

Orlowski, W. A.: The incorporation of H³-proline into the collagen of the periodontium of a rat, J. Periodont. Res. **11:**96, 1976.

Page, R., Ammons, W., Schechtman, L., and Billingham, L.: Collagen fiber bundles of the normal marginal gingiva, Arch. Oral Biol. **19:**1039, 1974.

Palade, G. E., and Farquhar, M. G.: A special fibril of the dermis, J. Cell Biol. **27:**215, 1965.

Picton, D. C. A.: On the part played by the socket in tooth support, Arch. Oral Biol. **10:**945, 1965.

Pierce, G. B., Jr.: Basement membranes. VI. Synthesis by epithelial tumors of the mouse, Cancer Res. **25:**656, 1965.

Pierce, G. B., Jr., and Nakane, P. K.: Antigens of epithelial basement membranes of mouse, rat and man, Lab. Invest. **17:**499, 1967.

Pierce, G. B., Jr., Beals, T. F., Sri Ram, J., and Midgley, A. R.: Basement membranes. IV. Epithelial origin and immunologic cross reactions, Am. J. Pathol. **45:**929, 1964.

Pierce, G. B., Jr., Midgley, A. R., and Sri Ram, J.: The histogenesis of basement membranes, J. Exp. Med. **117:**339, 1963.

Quigley, M. B.: Perforating Sharpey's fibers of the periodontal ligament and bone, Ala. J. Med. Sci. **7:**336, 1970.

Rapp, R., Avery, J. K., and Rector, R. A.: A study of the distribution of nerves in human teeth, J. Can. Dent. Assoc. **23:**447, 1957.

Rapp, R., Kirstine, W. D., and Avery, J. K.: A study of neural endings in the human gingiva and periodontal membrane, J. Can. Dent. Assoc. **23:**637, 1957.

Rebstein, F.: La jonction entre l'épithélium et l'émail chez l'homme. Étude histologique et histochimique, Parodont. Acad. Rev. **1:**207, 1967.

Reith, E. J.: The stages of amelogenesis as observed in molar teeth of young rats, J. Ultrastruct. Res. **30:**11, 1970.

Reith, E. J.: The ultrastructure of ameloblasts during early stages of maturation of enamel, J. Cell Biol. **18:**691, 1963.

Reith, E. J.: The ultrastructure of ameloblasts during matrix formation and the maturation of enamel, J. Biophys. Biochem. Cytol. **9:**825, 1961.

Reith, E. J., and Cotty, V. F.: The absorptive activity of ameloblasts during the maturation of enamel, Anat. Rec. **157:**577, 1967.

Retief, D. H.: Adhesion in biological systems, J. Dent. Assoc. S. Afri. **30:**101, 1975.

Rippin, J. W.: Collagen turnover on the periodontal ligament under normal and altered functional forces. 1. Young rat molars, J. Periodont. Res. **11:**101, 1976.

Ritchey, B. and Orban, B.: The crests of the interdental alveolar septa, J. Periodontol. **24:**75, 1953.

Rogers, H. J., and Weidman, S. M.: Metabolism of alveolar bone, Br. Dent. J. **90:**7, 1951.

Rose, S. T., and App, G. R.: A clinical study of the development of the attached gingiva along the facial aspect of the maxillary and mandibular anterior teeth in the deciduous, transitional and permanent dentitions, J. Periodontol. **44:**131, 1973.

Ross, R.: The ultrastructure of fibrinogenesis, J. Dent. Res. **45:**449, 1966.

Ross, R., and Bornstein, P.: Elastic fibers in the body, Sci. Am. **224:**44, 1971.

Saglie, R., Johansen, J. R., and Fløtra, L.: The zone of completely and partially destructed periodontal fibres in pathological pockets, J. Clin. Periodontol. **2:**198, 1975.

Saglie, R., Johansen, J. R., and Tollefsen, T.: Plaque-free zones on human teeth in periodontitis, J. Clin. Periodontol. **2:**190, 1975.

Sakada, S., and Maeda, K.: Characteristics of innervation and nerve endings in cat's mandibular periosteum, Bull. Tokyo Dent. Coll. **8:**77, 1967.

Salkind, A., Oshrain, H. I., and Mandel, I. D.: Observations on gingival pocket fluid, Periodontics **1:**196, 1963.

Schroeder, H. E.: Histopathology of the gingival sulcus. In Lehner, T., editor: The borderland between caries and periodontal disease, New York, 1977, Grune & Stratton, Inc., pp. 43-78.

Schroeder, H. E.: Transmigration and infiltration of leukocytes in human junctional epithelium, Helv. Odontol. Acta **17:**16, 1973.

Schroeder, H. E.: Melanin containing organelles in cells of the human gingiva. I. Epithelial melanocytes, J. Periodont. Res. **4:**1, 1969.

Schroeder, H. E.: Ultrastructure of the junctional epithelium of the human gingiva, Helv. Odontol. Acta **13:**65, 1969.

Schroeder, H. E.: Melanin containing organelles in cells of the human gingiva. II. Keratinocytes, J. Periodont. Res. **4:**235, 1969.

Schroeder, H. E., and Listgarten, M. A.: Fine structure of the developing epithelial attachment of human teeth. In Wolsky, A., editor: Monographs in developmental biology, vol. 2, Basel, 1971, S. Karger.

Schroeder, H. E., and Munzel-Pedrazzoli, S.: Morphometric analysis comparing junctional and oral epithelium of normal human gingiva, Helv. Odontol. Acta **14:**53, 1970.

Schroeder, H. E., and Theilade, J.: Electron microscopy of normal human gingival epithelium, J. Periodont. Res. **1:**95, 1966.

Schultz-Haudt, S. D., and Aas, E.: Dynamics of periodontal tissues. II. The connective tissues, Odontol. Tskr. **70:**397, 1962.

Schultz-Haudt, S. D., and From, S.: Dynamics of periodontal tissues. I. The epithelium, Odontol. Tidskr. **69:**431, 1961.

Schultz-Haudt, S. D., Waerhaug, J., From, S. H., and Attramadal, A.: On the nature of contact between the gingival epithelium and the tooth enamel surface, Periodontics **1:**103, 1963.

Seipel, C. M.: Trajectories of jaws, Acta Odontol. Scand. **8:**81, 191, 1948.

Selvig, K. A.: Non-banded fibrils of collagenous nature in human periodontal connective tissue, J. Periodont. Res. **3:**169, 1968.

Selvig, K. A.: Ultrastructural changes in cementum and adjacent connective tissue in periodontal disease, Acta Odontol. Scand. **23:**459, 1966.

Selvig, K. A.: The fine structure of human cementum, Acta Odontol. Scand. **23:**423, 1965.

Selvig, K. A.: An ultrastructural study of cementum formation, Acta Odontol. Scand. **22:**105, 1964.

Selvig, K. A.: Electron microscopy of Hertwig's epithelial sheath and of early dentin and cementum formation in the mouse incisor, Acta Odontol. Scand. **21:**175, 1963.

Shackleford, J. M.: Scanning electron microscopy of the dog periodontium, J. Periodont. Res. **6:**45, 1971.

Shackleford, J. M.: The indifferent fiber plexus and its relationship to principal fibres of the periodontium, Am. J. Anat. **121:**427, 1971.

Sheetz, J. H., Fullmer, H. M., and Narkates, A. J.: Oxytalan fibers: identification of the same fiber by light and electron microscopy, J. Oral Pathol. **2:**254, 1973.

Sheppard, I. M., and Markus, N.: Total time of tooth contacts during mastication, J. Prosthet. Dent. **9:**220, 1959.

Sicher, H.: Orban's oral histology and embryology, ed. 6, St. Louis, 1966, The C. V. Mosby Co., pp. 184-203.

Simpson, H. E.: The innervation of the periodontal membrane as observed by the apoxestic technique, J. Periodontol. **37:**374, 1966.

Skougaard, M.: Turnover of the gingival epithelium in marmosets, Acta Odontol. Scand. **23:**623, 1965.

Skougaard, M., and Beagrie, G. S.: The renewal of gingival epithelium in marmosets (Callithrix jacchus) as determined through autoradiography with thymidine-H³, Acta Odontol. Scand. **20:**467, 1962.

Skougaard, M., Levy, R., and Simpson, J.: Collagen metabolism in skin and periodontal membrane of the marmoset, Scand. J. Dent. Res. **78:**256, 1970.

Skougaard, M. R., Levy, B. M., and Simpson, J.: Collagen metabolism in skin and periodontal membrane of the marmoset, J. Periodont. Res. **4:**28, 1969.

Soni, N. N., Silberkweit, M., and Hayes, R. L.: Histologic characteristics of stippling in children, J. Periodontol. **34:**427, 1963.

Squier, C. A.: The permeability of keratinized and nonkeratinized oral epithelium to horseradish paroxidase, J. Ultrastruct. Res. **43:**160, 1973.

Stahl, S. S., and Person, P.: Reattachment of epithelium and connective tissue following gingival injury in rats, J. Periodontol. **33:**51, 1962.

Stallard, R. E.: The utilization of H³-proline by the connective tissue elements of the periodontium, Periodontics **1:**185, 1963.

Stallard, R. E., Diab, M. A., and Zander, H. A.: The attaching substance between enamel and epithelium—a product of the epithelial cells, J. Periodontol. **36:**130, 1965.

Stern, I. B.: Electron microscopic observations of oral epithelium. I. Basal cells and the basement membrane, Periodontics **3:**224, 1965.

Stern, I. B.: An electron microscopic study of the cementum, Sharpey's fibers and periodontal ligament in the rat incisor, Am. J. Anat. **115:**377, 1964.

Stewart, D., and Lewinsky, W.: A comparative study of the innervation of the gum, Proc. R. Soc. Med. **32:**1054, 1939.

Strahan, J. D.: The relation of the mucogingival junction to the alveolar bone margin, Dent. Pract. Dent. Rec. **14:**72, 1963.

Strang, R. H. W.: Textbook of orthodontia, Philadelphia, 1933, Lea & Febiger.

Sueda, T., Cimasoni, G., and Held, A. J.: High levels of acid phosphatase in human gingival fluid, Arch. Oral Biol. **12:**1205, 1967.

Susi, F. R.: Anchoring fibrils in the attachment of epithelium to connective tissue in oral mucous membranes, J. Dent. Res. **48:**144, 1969.

Susi, F. R., Belt, W. D., and Kelly, J. W.: Fine structure of fibrillar complexes associated with the basement membrane in human oral mucosa, J. Cell Biol. **34:**686, 1967.

Synge, J. L.: The theory of an incompressible periodontal membrane, Int. J. Orthod. **19:**567, 1933.

Ten Cate, A. R., and Syrbu, S.: A relationship between alkaline phosphatase activity and the phagocytosis and degradation of collagen by the fibroblast, J. Anat. **117:**351, 1974.

Theilade, J.: The ultrastructure of the gingival crevicular epithelium, J. Ultrastruct. Res. **14:**420, 1966.

Thoma, K., and Goldman, H. M.: The pathology of dental cementum, J. Am. Dent. Assoc. **26:**1943, 1939.

Thonard, J. C., and Scherp, H. W.: Histochemical demonstration of acid mucopolysaccharides in human gingival epithelial intercellular spaces, Arch. Oral Biol. **7:**125, 1962.

Tolman, D. E., Winkelmann, R. K., and Gibilisco, J. A.:

Nerve endings in gingival tissue, J. Dent. Res. **44:**657, 1965.

Tonna, E. A.: Factors (aging) affecting bone and cementum, J. Periodontol. **47:**267, 1976.

Toto, P. D., and Sicher, H.: The epithelial attachment, Periodontics **2:**154, 1964.

Trelstad, R. L.: The developmental biology of vertebrate collagens, J. Histochem. Cytochem. **21:**521, 1973.

Trott, J. R., and Gorenstein, S. L.: Mitotic rates in the oral and gingival epithelium of the rat, Arch. Oral Biol. **8:**425, 1963.

Waerhaug, J.: Current concepts concerning gingival anatomy; the dynamic epithelial cuff, Dent. Clin. North Am., p. 715, November, 1960.

Waerhaug, J.: Tissue reaction around acrylic root tips, J. Dent. Res. **36:**27, 1957.

Waerhaug, J.: Gingival pocket; anatomy, pathology, deepening and elimination, Odontol. Tskr. **60:**Supp. 1952.

Weinreb, M. M.: Epithelial attachment, J. Periodontol. **31:**186, 1960.

Weinstein, E., and Mandel, I. D.: The fluid of the gingival sulcus, Periodontics **2:**147, 1964.

Weinstein, E., Mandel, I. D., Salkind, A., Oshrain, H. I., and Pappas, G. D.: Studies of gingival fluid, Periodontics **5:**161, 1967.

Weiss, L.: The adhesion of cells, Int. Rev. Cytol. **9:**187, 1960.

Weiss, L., and Neiders, M. E.: A biophysical approach to epithelial cell interactions with teeth, Adv. Oral Biol. **4:**179, 1970.

Weiss, M. D., Weinmann, J. P., and Meyer, J.: Degree of keratinization and glykogen content in the uninflamed and inflamed gingiva and alveolar mucosa, J. Periodontol. **30:**208, 1959.

Weiss, P.: Cell contact, Int. Rev. Cytol. **7:**391, 1958.

Wentz, F. M., Maier, A. W., and Orban, B.: Age changes and sex differences in clinically normal gingiva, J. Periodontol. **23:**13, 1952.

Wertheimer, F. W., and Fullmer, H. M.: Morphologic and histochemical observations on the human dental cuticle, J. Periodontol. **33:**29, 1962.

Williams, C. H. M.: Investigation concerning the dentition of Canada's Eastern Arctic, J. Periodontol. **14:**34, 1943.

Wright, D. E.: The source and rate of entry of leucocytes in the human mouth, Arch. Oral Biol. **9:**321, 1964.

Yurkstas, A.: Compensation for inadequate mastication, Br. Dent. J. **91:**261, 1951.

Yurkstas, A., and Manly, R. S.: Value of different test foods in estimating masticatory ability, J. Appl. Physiol. **3:**45, 1950.

Yurkstas, A., and Manly, R. S.: Measurement of occlusal contact area effective in mastication, Am. J. Orthod. **35:**185, 1949.

Zajicek, G.: Fibroblast cell kinetics in the periodontal ligament of the mouse, Cell Tissue Kinet. **7:**479, 1974.

Zwarych, P. D., and Quigley, M. G.: The intermediate plexus of the periodontal ligament; histology and further observations, J. Dent. Res. **44:**383, 1965.

2 Epidemiology of periodontal disease

SCOPE AND DEFINITIONS

The science of epidemiology originally referred to the study of epidemics. An epidemic is a frequency of case occurrence beyond that which is usual for the particular season, place, and population group (Santwell, 1973). Today this concept has been broadened, so that contemporary epidemiology describes the distribution of human health problems and seeks to establish the causes of these problems in order to discover and formulate effective preventive measures (Goerke and Stebbins, 1968). Various definitions in current use differ largely in their degree of inclusiveness: it is ''the study of the distribution and determinants of disease prevalence in man'' (MacMahon et al., 1960); it is ''concerned with measurements of the circumstances under which diseases occur, where diseases tend to flourish, and where they do not'' (Paul, 1966). More broadly, epidemiology includes ''the various factors and conditions that determine the occurrence and distribution of health, disease, defect, disability, and death among groups of individuals'' (Clark, 1965) or is ''concerned with the study of the processes which determine or influence the physical, mental, and social health of people'' (Cassel, 1965). In general, these definitions of epidemiology—whether the focus is on disease or on the total health-disease spectrum—share an emphasis on process and a recognition of the involvement of

a multiplicity of influencing factors (Goerke and Stebbins, 1968). As H. Trendly Dean stated:

> The term *epidemiological method* refers to the procedure employed in the study of a disease or a condition as a mass phenomenon. It is distinctly opposed to the clinical method in which the individual, rather than a population of individuals, is the unit of investigation. In an epidemiological inquiry all observations are related to the group; in a clinical study the observations are related to the group; in a clinical study the observations remain related to the specific individuals under study. The epidemiological method requires a population of individuals for study, and any disease, communicable or non-communicable, or condition may be the subject of investigation. The method is essentially quantitative and the disease or condition being investigated may be actual, suspected, or assumed. (Dean, 1942)

In the past, *descriptive* epidemiologic methods provided data from surveys, giving characteristics of various diseases based on various population surveys. Thus levels of disease states were obtained that sometimes gave insight into the etiology, severity, and distribution of the disease entity in various population groups. Such information will be presented in the discussion on Prevalence of Periodontal Disease.

At the same time that attempts were being made to evaluate the relative efficacy of various treatment methods (''treatment'' refers to various therapeutic regimens, including drugs), which became known as ''clinical trials,'' *experimental* epidemiology came into being. In recent year: the importance of the carefully conducted clinical trial has received greater recognition in dental research. This was first acknowledged in the area of dental caries (ADA, 1955, 1972) and now has received attention in periodontal disease research. In fact, two conferences (Cohen and Ship, 1967; Chilton, 1974) have been held on this subject, and the Federation Dentaire Internationale has published guidelines for the conduct of both caries

63

Table 1. Comparison of the clinical trial and the epidemiologic survey in periodontal diseases*

Clinical trial	Epidemiologic survey
Experimental and control group(s) are usually specially constituted as representative samples from appropriate populations	Naturally occurring samples of target populations are usually studied
Sample sizes are usually small, particularly when the "treatments" are more complicated	Fairly large sample sizes are employed
Trials are conducted over a period of time usually varying from 1 week to 6 months, depending on treatment involved, to compare treatment effects	Surveys are usually cross sectional in design, utilizing only one time period, although longitudinal designs are occasionally used
While assessment methods may be indices, the methodologies used should have greater acuity and clinical significance	Indices used for assessment serve to establish disease levels in selected populations. These indices should be in general use to enable comparison of data for different populations
Data generated from clinical trials should be applicable for specific hypothesis testing	Data generated from surveys are used to establish underlying etiologic factors and derive possible preventive methods, leading to development of hypotheses to be tested by controlled clinical trials
Informed human consent forms are required	Informed human consent forms are usually not required

*From Chilton, N. W., and Miller, M. F.: Paper presented at International conference on research in the biology of periodontal disease, Chicago, 1977.

and periodontal disease clinical trials (FDI, 1974, in preparation).

While descriptive epidemiologic studies of periodontal disease predate controlled clinical trials, there is still a great deal of confusion in the minds of many between these two research activities. The principles of experimental designs of clinical trials in periodontal diseases have recently been described by Chilton (1977). These two research methodologies do overlap, but they are, in reality, two different approaches. Table 1 attempts to compare them.

INDICES

In order to describe gingival and periodontal disease in large populations, it is necessary to use descriptive methods that lend themselves to quantitative evaluation and electronic data processing. These are known as indices. While there are indices dealing with assessment of soft and hard tissue deposits, these do not deal primarily with periodontal disease and will not be discussed here. For excellent reviews and assessments, the reader is referred to the papers by Mandel and Volpe in the Proceedings of the International Conference on Agents used in the Prevention/Treatment of Periodontal Diseases (Chilton, 1974). An outstanding review and assessment of the various

indices used in the assessment of periodontal diseases was prepared by Mumma (1975) for the World Health Organization, on which we have extensively relied.

Gingivitis indices

In the hierarchy of periodontal diseases it is assumed that almost all cases of periodontitis are preceded by gingivitis, although the converse that all cases of gingivitis do not necessarily go on to periodontitis does not always hold true. There are basically two methods, with some overlap, that have been developed for assessing the presence and extent of gingivitis. They are (1) grading the inflammation according to how many gingival units are judged to be inflamed (grading by extension) and (2) grading the inflammation according to qualitative changes that are observed in the gingival tissues (qualitative grading).

The rationale behind grading the severity of gingivitis by extension of the lesion relies on the belief that as the severity of the condition increases, a greater number of gingival units will be affected. This approach was adopted by Massler and Schour (PMA index) (1967) and Russell (PI—gingivitis portion) (1967) in the development of their indices. The PMA index, as originally conceived, requires only the summing of inflamed papillary,

marginal, and attached gingival units, while the PI requires judgment with regard to whether none, part, or all the gingiva encircling the tooth is inflamed.

The second category, that of qualitative grading of gingivitis, is best exemplified by Löe and Silness's Gingival Index (1963) and by Mühlemann and Mazor's Sulcus Bleeding Index (PM index) (1958). The gingival index of Löe and Silness scores gingivitis according to normal gingiva and mild, moderate, and severe inflammation, with the three grades of inflammation being characterized by —

1. Slight change in color and slight edema, without bleeding on probing
2. Redness, edema, and glazing, with bleeding on probing
3. Marked redness and edema, with ulceration and a tendency to spontaneous bleeding

The PM index of Mühlemann and Mazor assesses gingivitis at four levels:

1. No inflammation
2. Bleeding from the gingival sulcus on gentle probing, with the tissue otherwise appearing normal
3. Bleeding on probing plus a change in color due to inflammation, without swelling or edema
4. Ulceration or additional symptoms

Both these indices, unlike the PMA and PI, do not use extension of the disease to assess severity, but rather depend upon the tendency of the gingiva to bleed as the decisive criterion.

A third group of indices combine the features of grading gingivitis by extension of the lesion and by qualitative changes: Parfitt's modification of the PMA (1957), Ramfjord's PDI (gingival portion) (1967), and O'Leary's GPI (gingivitis portion) (1967).

Parfitt's modified PMA index severity rating is as follows:

1. A detectable hyperemia in the papilla, marginal, or attached mucosa
2. A loss of stippling, redness, swelling, or bleeding on pressure
3. The presence of symptoms such as bleeding, sensitivity, itching sensation, or tenderness, of which the patient is usually aware
4. The presence of severe hyperemia or hemorrhage occurring spontaneously at the slightest touch of food or toothbrush

Four grades of gingivitis are recorded in the gingivitis portion of Ramfjord's PDI:

1. Absence of inflammation

2. Mild to moderate inflammatory gingival changes not extending all around the tooth
3. Mild to moderately severe gingivitis extending all around the tooth
4. Severe gingivitis characterized by marked redness, tendency to bleed, and ulceration

The following criteria are employed in the gingivitis portion of O'Leary's GPI:

1. No gingivitis, characterized by tight adaptation of the gingival tissue to the teeth, showing firm consistency and physiologic architecture
2. Slight to moderate gingivitis, characterized by less than complete encirclement of one or more teeth in the segment by color changes from pink to various shades of red, retraction of the gingival margin by more than 1 mm when the tissue is dried with a firm blast of compressed air, or blunting and slight enlargement of the marginal or papillary tissue when associated with color change or loss of consistency
3. One or more of the same changes, but completely encircling one or more teeth in the segment
4. Marked inflammatory or gingival contour changes characterized by acute gingival inflammation, ulceration, hemorrhage on light probing or thorough compressed air drying, and marked deviation from normal gingival contour

The reader must always bear in mind that the scores used in these indices are not based on a ratio scale; that is, a score of 2 does not necessarily denote twice as much inflammation as a score of 1, nor does the difference between 0 and 1 have the same clinical significance as the difference between 2 and 3. This has led Ainamo and Bay (1975) to advocate site prevalence (the number of teeth or tooth surfaces affected in one individual) over mean severity scores (a return to the "all or nothing" approach), and Jackson (1965) to use only mouth prevalence because he found that measures of extent and degree were shown to vary only slightly with age. In epidemiologic surveys and indeed in many clinical trials the use of scores of selected tooth areas rather than total mouth scores will yield representative data and allow for larger samples to be employed. The anterior teeth or the teeth selected by Ramfjord are usually employed: (1) maxillary right first molar, (2) maxillary left central incisor, (3) maxillary left first premolar, (4) mandibular left first molar, (5) mandibular right central incisor, and (6) mandibular right first molar. It should always be kept in mind that data derived from surveys involving selected tooth areas cannot be compared with data derived from other tooth areas, even though data from these areas correlate highly with total mouth scores (Chilton et al., in press).

Periodontal indices

Most indices of periodontitis combine elements of both site prevalence and mouth prevalence. Ramfjord's PDI and O'Leary's GPI rely on periodontal pocket depth, while Russell's PI, Sandler and Stahl's PDR (Periodontal Disease Rate) (Sandler and Stahl, 1959), Stahl and Morris's Gingival Recession (Stahl and Morris, 1955), and Dunning and Leach's Gingival-Bone Count index (Leach, 1960) employ other criteria. A brief description of several of these indices follows.

The PI developed by Russell requires that for moderate periodontitis the examiner must discover a break in the epithelial attachment and the presence of a periodontal pocket and that for advanced destruction the examiner must determine that the tooth may—

1. Be loose
2. Have drifted
3. Sound dull on percussion with a metallic instrument
4. Be depressed in its socket

Sandler and Stahl's PDR employs what its authors describe as minimal but unmistakable signs of periodontal disease. According to this index, periodontal disease is indicated if one or more of the following criteria are met:

1. Gingival necrosis, hypertrophy, or inflammation encircling the tooth or a purulent exudate from the gingival crevice
2. A gingival crevice depth of 3 mm or more
3. Tooth mobility greater than 1 mm in any direction
4. Roentgenographic evidence of resorption of alveolar bone extending more than 3 mm apically from the cementoenamel junction

The Gingival-Bone Count index of Dunning and Leach weights gingivitis and bone loss on a three-to-five basis; thus the periodontitis portion of this index is determined primarily by a bone loss determination, modified somewhat by its authors' definition for moderate and severe gingivitis as being characterized by involvement of attached gingiva, hypertrophy, and easy hemorrhage. The bone loss is identified through the use of radiographs, revealing the loss in quarters of

root length, with the assignment of appropriate scores.

Waerhaug (1977) has recently described an index for evaluating subgingival plaque and loss of attachment in extracted teeth. The purposes of this index are (1) to estimate the speed of the apical growth of subgingival plaque, (2) to establish the correlation between subgingival plaque and loss of attachment, and (3) to evaluate the result of various treatment procedures. Using this index, Waerhaug has concluded "that what has been diagnosed as periodontosis is in fact a highly destructive juvenile periodontitis. The high destructiveness depends on a host parasite imbalance rather than on a degenerative basis" (Waerhaug, in press). This is a good example of the use of an epidemiologic tool to establish the etiology of a disease.

PREVALENCE OF PERIODONTAL DISEASE

Periodontal disease accounts for the greatest loss of teeth in humans. Because it is a chronic, painless condition, it develops so gradually that the afflicted person lives unaware of the pathologic changes. Moreover, lack of public concern and general unawareness of the consequences of periodontal disease have contributed to its broad prevalence. Since only in its later stages, with deep pocket formation and mobility, does the disease become bothersome, treatment is often sought too late to be able to save sufficient teeth. The public health significance of such neglect, both in terms of the health of the population as well as the economic burden, is staggering. Since early forms of periodontal disease are seen in young children, particularly with the eruption of the permanent dentition, efforts at eradicating or controlling the continued incidence of periodontal disease should be directed at this age group, where extensive therapeutic measures are not required to prevent the disease.

Geographic considerations

Results from the last United States National Health Survey (1969) indicate that almost four of every ten children 6 to 11 years old have periodontal disease in some form. This percentage increases with age, so that in the adult age group (18 to 79 years) almost 74% of the population has periodontal disease in one stage of progression or another (DHEW, 1972) (Table 2).

Even higher ratios have been documented in various African (Sheiham, 1968; Poulsen, 1972;

Table 2. Periodontal status of adults by sex and age, United States, 1960 to 1962*

Sex and age (years)	Average PI	Average OHI-S†	Without disease	Percent distribution	
				With disease	
				Without pockets	With pockets
Both sexes					
18-79	1.13	1.5	26.1	48.5	25.4
Men					
18-24	0.62	1.5	29.0	60.6	10.3
25-34	0.92	1.6	26.3	51.7	22.0
35-44	1.27	1.7	22.1	48.1	29.7
45-54	1.62	1.9	15.0	48.1	36.9
55-64	2.15	2.1	15.3	39.1	45.6
65-74	2.50	2.5	5.6	36.0	58.4
75-79	2.91	2.2	6.2	33.7	60.0
TOTAL, 18-79	1.34	1.8	20.9	49.0	30.1
Women					
18-24	0.48	1.2	36.8	53.6	9.6
25-34	0.60	1.2	37.6	50.2	12.3
35-44	0.82	1.2	33.3	46.2	20.5
45-54	1.23	1.5	26.6	43.7	29.6
55-64	1.56	1.6	20.8	43.6	35.5
65-74	1.62	1.6	15.2	52.0	32.8
75-79	2.94	1.9	11.0	35.3	53.8
TOTAL, 18-79	0.93	1.3	31.0	47.9	21.0

*From National Center for Health Statistics Series 11, no. 7.
†Simplified Oral Hygiene Index.

Table 3. Mean PI scores returned in series of studies sponsored by the World Health Organization

Age (years)	Ceylon			Sudan	Iran	Rural India
	Anuradhapura villages	Jaffna villages	Colombo Secretariat			
5-9				0.99		
10-14	0.97	0.65		1.40	1.49	
15-19	0.89	0.84		1.23	1.30	
20-29	2.06	1.64	1.38	1.76	1.94	1.53*
30-39	3.86	3.06	2.34	2.42	3.00	
40-49	5.06	4.36	3.49		3.37	
50-59	5.99	5.23	4.07			
60 and over	5.36	5.97				

*Ages 19 to 30 years.

Enwonwu, 1970) and Asian nations (Day and Shourie, 1949; Chirangeevi and Wade, 1972). In India periodontal disease caused the loss of 11,960 teeth (6.3% of the total) for all patients of all ages and was responsible for the loss of 79.2% of all teeth in all patients over 30 years of age (Mehta et al., 1958). Data from South America indicates that ulcerated gingiva were present in 36% of male and 28% of female school children averaging about 15 years of age, while 20% to 32% of the adult population was afflicted (Vivone, 1956). Levels of periodontal disease such as those found in the United States have also been recorded in the Scandinavian countries (Shei et al., 1959).

Because many studies have not been performed

Table 4. Percentages of children with severe gingivitis (Great Britain) or with one or more obvious periodontal pockets (United States)

Age (years)	Great Britain		United States	
	Number examined	**Percent with "severe" gingivitis**	**Number examined**	**Percent with obvious pockets**
4	85	0	18	0
5	378	0	668	0
6	408	0.3	1439	0.07
7	439	0.2	1567	0.13
8	413	0	1714	0
9	460	0.3	1907	0.16
10	409	0.7	2525	0.12
11	440	0.9	2978	0.42
12	424	1.2	6391	0.66
13	445	2.7	7110	1.05
14	109	4.6	5856	1.76
15			2892	2.59
16			1838	2.99
17			1042	3.17

Table 5. Mean PI scores in civilian groups aged 40 to 49 years, surveyed by examiners of Epidemiology and Biometry Branch, National Institute of Dental Research

Place	Mean score
Baltimore (Caucasians)	1.03
Colorado Springs	1.04*
Alaska (primitive Eskimos)	1.17†
Ecuador	1.85
Ethiopia	1.86
Baltimore (Negroes)	1.99
Vietnam (Vietnamese)	2.18
Colombia	2.21
Alaska (urban Eskimos)	2.31†
Chile	2.74
Lebanon (Lebanese)	2.98
Thailand	3.30
Lebanon (Palestinian refugees)	3.52
Burma	3.58
Jordan	3.96
Vietnam (hill tribesmen)	3.97
Trinidad	4.21
Jordan (Palestinian refugees)	4.41
Nigeria	5.14

*Ages 40 to 44 only.
†Males only.

Table 6. Average PI findings for Caucasian and Negro persons by educational attainment, Birmingham, Ala., 1957*

Age in years	Numbers of years of school completed			
	8 or less	**9-11**	**12**	**13 or more**
Caucasian				
All ages	1.42	0.93	0.52	0.29
15-29	1.23	0.59	0.48	0.26
30-49	1.31	1.13	0.53	0.29
50 and over	2.06	1.42	0.82	0.39
Negro				
All ages	2.18	1.09	0.80	0.41
15-29	1.16	0.67	0.55	0.32
30-49	2.15	1.26	1.09	0.62
50 and over	2.72	3.41	2.97	1.23

*From Russell, A. L., and Ayers, P.: Am. J. Public Health **50:**206, 1960.

on randomly selected populations representative of the population as a whole (Kristofferson and Bang, 1973; Nash and Fishman, 1971; Smith and Buchner, 1973; Suomi and Doyle, 1972; Fishman, 1974; Camrass, 1974; Ainamo and Holmberg, 1974), care should be given when abstracting or generalizing the data for an entire country or when comparing one country or population with another. In spite of this fact, however, the data do support the hypothesis that periodontal disease is geographically widespread and that in most populations over 50% of adults have some form of the disease. Tables 3, 4, 5, and 6 present data for different population groups.

Socioeconomic status

Data both from the United States National Health Survey and other sources continue to support the findings that periodontal disease is negatively correlated with increasing education and increasing family income (DHEW, 1972; Enwonwu and Edozien, 1970; Lordal et al., 1963; Mobley and Smith, 1963; Moore and Muhler, 1964; Russell, 1957; Russell and Ayers, 1970).

In the United States periodontal disease decreases by over 50% with increasing family income in both white and black youths 12 to 17 years of age. Similarly, if the educational level of the head of the family is correlated with periodontal disease levels in this same age group of children, periodontal disease decreases from a high of 0.61 PI units (head of household having only a grade school education) to a low of 0.16 PI units (head of household with 17 or more years of education), a decrease of approximately 75% (DHEW, 1972).

Race

In Waerhaug's (1966) review of periodontal disease he noted that no racial differences in levels of periodontal disease can be detected if the groups are balanced for age, sex, or socioeconomic status. Moreover, any differences observed are largely attributable to oral hygiene status rather than to actual racial differences (Hansen, 1973). In the United States, blacks have been observed to have more periodontal disease than whites, including 50% more serious periodontal pockets (DHEW, 1960). This must be balanced, however, by the fact that blacks have fewer than half as many visits to the dentist and a much lower rate of extraction than whites (DHEW, 1969). Because of these data, it would be wrong to assume that the prevalence of periodontal disease in blacks

is higher than in whites from a purely racial standpoint; obviously other factors must be taken into account.

Other factors

Findings similar to those reported by Waerhaug (1966) have been demonstrated in the direct correlation of periodontal disease to age (Roper et al., 1972; Hansen, 1973), sex (DHEW, 1972), oral hygiene (Suomi and Doyle, 1972; Fishman, 1974), tobacco (Lee and van der Werf, 1974; Chawla et al., 1971; Hazen, 1968), systemic disease (e.g., diabetes [Rose, 1973; Cohen et al., 1970; Campbell, 1972; Tuckman, 1970]), nutritional factors (Lee and van der Werf, 1974; Hazen, 1968; Chawla et al., 1971), fluoride (Birkeland et al., 1973; Murray, 1972; Murray, 1973), malocclusion (Lewin and Lemmer, 1974; Karlsen, 1972; Paunio, 1973; Geiger et al., 1974; Buckley, 1972; Geiger et al., 1973), and mental retardation (Rosenstein et al., 1971; Cutress, 1971; Kroll, 1970; Miller, 1977).

CONCLUSION

The prevalence of periodontal disease is worldwide. It is present from the first decade of life to old age. It accounts for over 50% of missing teeth in adults and results in tremendous economic and social burdens both to the individual and society. The effect of missing teeth or a totally edentulous mouth upon the nutritional status of an individual can only be estimated, but surely its effects go well beyond the slight inconvenience of not being able to eat corn on the cob or apples. Prevention is the only answer, since numerous studies support the fact that the world's population of dentists is inadequate to meet even a fraction of the need, much less the demand. National preventive programs are long overdue, and even wealthier nations such as the United States have failed to place periodontal disease at the head of the list of chronic diseases to be eradicated. And it is not even present on some lists.

REFERENCES

ADA: Principles for the clinical testing of cariostatic agents: adapted from a conference held at the American Dental Association, Chicago, 1972.

ADA: Clinical testing of dental caries preventives: report of a conference to develop uniform standards and procedures in clinical studies of dental caries, Chicago, 1955, American Dental Association.

Ainamo, J., and Bay, I.: Problems and proposals for recording gingivitis and plaque, Int. Dent. J. **25:**229, 1975.

Ainamo, J., and Holmberg, S.: The oral health of children of dentists, Scand. J. Dent. Res. **82:**574, 1974.

Birkeland, J. M., Jorkjend, L., and von der Fehr, F. R.: The influence of fluoride mouth rinsing on the incidence of gingivitis in Norwegian children, Community Dent. Oral Epidemiol. **1:**17, 1973.

Buckley, L. A.: The relationship between malocclusion and periodontal disease, J. Periodontol. **43:**415, 1972.

Campbell, M. J.: Epidemiology of periodontal disease in the diabetic and the non-diabetic, Aust. Dent. J. **17:**274, 1972.

Camrass, R.: An oral health survey of western Samoans, Community Dent. Oral Epidemiol. **2:**12, 1974.

Cassel, J. M.: Potentialities and limitations of epidemiology. In Katz, A. H., and Felton, J. S., editors: Health and community, New York, 1965, The Free Press.

Chawla, T. N., Kapoor, K. K., Teotia, S. P., et al.: Anemia and periodontal disease—a correlative study, J. Indian Dent. Assoc. **43:**67, 1971.

Chilton, N. W.: Experimental design of clinical trials in periodontics. In Rowe, N. H., editor: The scientific basis for evaluation of periodontal therapy, Ann Arbor, 1977, University of Michigan Press, pp. 3-25.

Chilton, N. W., editor: International conference on clinical trials of agents used in the prevention/treatment of periodontal disease, J. Periodont. Res. **9**(suppl. 14) 1974.

Chilton, N. W., Fertig, J. W., and Talbott, K.: Correlation between partial and full mouth gingivitis scores, Pharmacol. Therap. Dent. **3:**39, 1978.

Chirangeevi, K., and Wade, A. B.: Periodontal effects of a national health service on an immigrant population, J. Periodontol. **43:**718, 1972.

Clark, E. G.: The epidemiologic approach and contributions to preventive medicine. In Leavell, H. R., and Clark, E. G., editors: Preventive medicine for the doctor in his community, ed. 3, New York, 1965, McGraw-Hill Book Company.

Cohen, D. W.: Conference on clinical methods in periodontal diseases. Introduction and purpose of conference, J. Periodontol. **38**(suppl.):582, 1967.

Cohen, D. W., Friedman, L. A., Shapiro, J., Kyle, G. C., and Franklin, S.: Diabetes mellitus and periodontal disease. I. Two year longitudinal observations, J. Periodontol. **41:**709, 1970.

Cutress, T. W.: Periodontal disease and oral hygiene in trisomy 21, Arch. Oral Biol. **16:**1345, 1971.

Dean, H. T.: The investigation of physiological effects by the epidemiological method in fluorine and dental health. In F. R. Moulton, editor: pub. no. 19, Washington, D.C., 1942, American Association for the Advancement of Science.

DHEW: Periodontal disease and oral hygiene among children, DHEW pub. no. (HSM) 72-1060, Washington, D.C., 1972, U.S. Government Printing Office.

DHEW: Dental visits: volume and interval since the last visit, DHEW pub. no. (HSM) 72-1066, Washington, D.C., 1969, U.S. Government Printing Office.

DHEW: Selected dental findings in adults by age, race, and sex: United States, 1960-1962, DHEW pub. no. (HRA) 74-1274, Washington, D.C., 1962, U.S. Government Printing Office.

Dunning, J. M., and Leach, L. B.: Gingival-bone count: a method for epidemiological study of periodontal disease, J. Dent. Res. **39:**506, 1960.

Enwonwu, C. O., and Edozien, J. C.: Epidemiology of periodontal disease in western Nigeria in relation to socio-economic status, Arch. Oral Biol. **15:**1231, 1970.

FDI Technical Report no. 1: Principal requirements for controlled clinical trials of caries preventive agents and procedures. London, 1974, Federation Dentaire Internationale.

FDI Technical Report: Principal requirements for controlled clinical trials in periodontal diseases, London, Federation Dentaire Internationale. In preparation.

Fishman, S. L.: Oral health in the Republic of Paraguay, Community Dent. Oral Epidemiol. **2:**12, 1974.

Geiger, A., Wasserman, B. H., and Turgeon, L. R.: Relationship of occlusion and periodontal disease. VIII. Relationship of crowding and spacing to periodontal destruction and gingival inflammation, J. Periodontol. **45:**43, 1974.

Geiger, A. M., Wasserman, B. H., and Turgeon, L. R.: Relationship of occlusion and periodontal disease. VI. Relation of anterior overjet and overbite to periodontal destruction and gingival inflammation, J. Periodontol. **44:**150, 1973.

Goerke, L. S., and Stebbins, E. L.: Mustard's introduction to public health, ed. 5, New York, 1968, MacMillan, Inc.

Hansen, G. C.: An epidemiologic investigation of the effect of biologic aging on the breakdown of periodontal tissue, J. Periodontol. **44:**369, 1973.

Hazen, S. P.: The role of nutrition in periodontal disease, Ala. J. Med. Sci. **5:**328, 1968.

Jackson, D.: The measurement of gingivitis, Br. Dent. J. **118:**521, 1965.

Karlsen, K.: Traumatic occlusion as a factor in the propagation of periodontal disease, Int. Dent. J. **22:**387, 1972.

Kristofferson, T., and Bang, G.: Periodontal disease and oral hygiene in an Alaskan Eskimo population, J. Dent. Res. **52:**791, 1973.

Kroll, R. G., Budnick, J., and Kobren, A.: Incidence of dental caries and periodontal disease in Down's syndrome, N.Y. State Dent. J. **36:**151, 1970.

Lee, L. B., and van der Werf, K.: Nutrition in periodontal disease, N.M. Dent. J. **24:**14, 1974.

Lewin, A., and Lemmer, J.: Occlusion and periodontal disease: new light on an old problem, J. Prosthet. Dent. **31:**403, 1974.

Löe, H., and Silness, J.: Periodontal disease in pregnancy, Acta Odontol. Scand. **21:**533, 1963.

Lordal, A., Arno, A., and Waerhaug, J.: Incidence of clinical manifestations of periodontal disease in light of oral hygiene and calculus formations, J. Am. Dent. Assoc. **66:**486, 1963.

MacMahon, B., Pugh, T. F., and Ipsen, J.: Epidemiologic methods, Boston, 1960, Little, Brown and Company.

Marshall-Day, C. D., and Shourie, K. L.: Roentgenographic survey of periodontal disease in India, J. Am. Dent. Assoc. **39:**572, 1949.

Massler, M.: The P-M-A index for the assessment of gingivitis, J. Periodontol. **38:**592, 1967.

Mehta, F. S., Sanjana, M. K., Shroff, B. C., and Doctor, R. H.: Relative importance of the various causes of tooth loss, J. All-India Dent. Assoc. **30:**211, 1958.

Miller, M. F., and Ship, I. I.: Periodontal disease in the institutionalized mongoloid, J. Oral Med. **32:**9, 1977.

Mobley, E., and Smith, S. H.: Some social and economic factors relating to periodontal disease among young negroes, J. Am. Dent. Assoc. **66:**486, 1963.

Moore, R. M., Muhler, J. C., and McDonald, R. E.: Study on the effect of water fluoride content and socio-economic status on the occurrence of gingivitis in school children, J. Dent. Res. (Suppl.) **43:**782-783, 1964.

Mühlemann, H. R., and Mazor, A. S.: Gingivitis in Zürich school children, Helv. Odontol. Acta **2:**3, 1958.

Mumma, R. D., Jr.: Criteria employed for the assessment of periodontal diseases: a literature review. Report to World Health Organization, 1975.

Murray, J. J.: Gingival recession in tooth types in high fluoride and low fluoride areas, J. Periodont. Res. **8:**243, 1973.

Murray, J. J.: Gingivitis and gingival recession in adults from high fluoride and low fluoride areas, Arch. Oral Biol. **17:** 1269, 1972.

Nash, D., and Fishman, S. R.: Selected dental findings of a rural county in Appalachia, J. Public Health Dent. **31:**243, 1971.

O'Leary, T.: The periodontal screening examination, J. Periodontol. **38:**617, 1967.

Parfitt, G. J.: Five year longitudinal study of the gingival condition of a group of children in England, J. Periodontol. **28:** 26, 1957.

Paul, J. R.: Clinical epidemiology, rev. ed., Chicago, 1966, The University of Chicago Press.

Paunio, K.: The role of malocclusion and crowding in the development of periodontal disease, Int. Dent. J. **23:**470, 1973.

Poulsen, S., Møller, I. J., Naerum, J., and Pedersen, P. O.: Periodontal disease and oral hygiene in 2383 Moroccan school children aged eight to twelve years, Arch. Oral Biol. **17:**1513, 1972.

Ramfjord, S. P.: The periodontal disease index, J. Periodontol. **38:**602, 1967.

Roper, R., Knerr, G. W., Gocka, E. F., et al.: Periodontal disease in aged individuals, J. Periodontol. **43:**304, 1972.

Rose, H.: The relationship of hyperglycemia to periodontal disease, J. Periodontol. **44:**303, 1973.

Rosenstein, S. N., Bush, C. R., Jr., and Gorlick, J.: Dental and oral conditions in a group of mental retardates attending occupation day centers, N.Y. State Dent. J. **37:**416, 1971.

Russell, A. L.: The periodontal index, J. Periodontol. **38:** 585, 1967.

Russell, A. L.: A social factor associated with the severity of periodontal disease, J. Dent. Res. **36:**922, 1957.

Russell, A. L., and Ayers, P.: Periodontal disease and socioeconomic status in Birmingham, Ala., Am. J. Public Health **50:**206, 1970.

Samson, E.: Editorial: nicotine-agers beware, Br. Dent. J. **136:**249, 1974.

Sandler, H. C., and Stahl, S. S.: The measurement of periodontal disease prevalence, J. Am. Dent. Assoc. **58:**93, 1959.

Santwell, P. E., editor: Maxcy-Rosenau's Preventive medicine and public health, ed. 10, New York, 1973, Appleton-Century-Crofts, Inc.

Schei, O., Waerhaug, J., Loudal, A., and Arno, A.: Alveolar bone loss as related to oral hygiene and age, J. Periodontol. **30:**7-16, 1959.

Schwartz, D. M., and Baumhammers, A.: Smoking and periodontal disease, Periodont. Abstr. **20:**103, 1972.

Sheiham, A.: The epidemiology of chronic periodontal disease in western Nigerian school children, J. Periodont. Res. **3:**257, 1968.

Sheiham, A.: Periodontal disease and oral cleanliness in tobacco smokers, J. Periodontol. **42:**259, 1971.

Smith, P., and Buchner, A.: Periodontal disease prevalence in young adult Israelis, Isr. J. Dent. Med. **22:**94, 1973.

Stahl, S. S., and Morris, A. L.: Oral health conditions among army personnel at the Army Engineer Center, J. Periodontol. **20:**180, 1955.

Suomi, J., and Doyle, J.: Oral hygiene and periodontal disease in an adult population in the U.S., J. Periodontol. **43:** 677, 1972.

Tuckman, M. A., Kaslick, R. S., Shapiro, W. B., et al.: The relationship of glucose tolerance to periodontal status, J. Periodontol. **41:**513, 1970.

Vivone, R. A.: Prevalence of periodontal (parodontal) disease, S. Am. Int. Dent. **6:**26-30, March 1956.

Waerhaug, J.: Epidemiology of periodontal disease—review of literature. In Ramfjord, S. P., Kerr, D. A., and Ash, M. M., editors: Proceedings of the World Workshop in Periodontics, Ann Arbor, 1966, University of Michigan Press.

Waerhaug, J.: Subgingival plaque and loss of attachment in periodontosis as evaluated on extracted teeth, J. Periodontol. **43:**125, 1977.

Waerhaug, J.: An index for the evaluation of subgingival plaque and loss of attachment, Community Dent. Oral Epidemiol. In press.

3 Microbiologic and host response factors in periodontal disease

ORAL FLORA

Many areas of the body support a microbial flora in a state ordinarily called health. This indigenous microflora of man and other macroorganisms are in many respects useful to the host. For example, microbes of the intestinal flora produce nutrients that the host absorbs and utilizes. Some animal species have come to depend on the intestinal flora for certain essential vitamins, an observation supported by the failure of these animals to survive in the gnotobiotic state unless vitamins are provided in the diet.

The oral cavity supports one of the most dense and varied of the indigenous flora. The emphasis in discussion of the oral flora has been on the potential of this flora to overgrow and cause dental diseases. Krasse has pointed out that the oral flora does not represent a homogeneous collection of organisms throughout the oral cavity, but rather is localized in three main foci: on the dorsum of the tongue, in the gingival crevice, and on those areas of the teeth not cleaned by mastication.

An early experiment by Krasse (Fig. 3-1) shows that *Streptococcus salivarius* represents a mean of about 1% of the total streptococci in plaque, whereas on the dorsum of the tongue this organism represents a mean of 70% of the total streptococci. The frequency of *S. salivarius* in paraffin-stimulated saliva was nearly as high as that on the tongue and much higher than that in plaque, suggesting that many of the bacteria found in saliva are probably derived from the tongue. Krasse has also shown that 1 mg of plaque contains twice as many lactobacilli and 300 times as many streptococci as 1 mg of saliva. These experiments and other recent studies provide strong evidence for the existence of several foci of heavy aggregations of various combinations of microbes in the oral cavity, each representing a separate "ecologic niche," or microbial community. The source of bacteria for each of these colonies is unknown. Dental scientists are now asking important questions as to the interdependence of these foci. Van Houte et al. (1970) have described selective bacterial adherence as one of the factors that may be operative in determining the microbial composition of the various foci of oral flora. In a series of experiments these researchers showed that *S. salivarius,* a predominant tongue organism, adheres to a much greater extent to the tongue than it does to enamel. On the other hand, *S. sanguis,* which is a major organism on the tooth surface in young plaque, adheres to a much greater extent to the tooth surface than it does to the tongue. Selective bacterial adherence may explain the difference in bacterial composition of early dental plaque as compared to the tongue flora. Other factors such as oxygen tension, pH, availability of nutrients, and host antibacterial factors as well as adherence may deter-

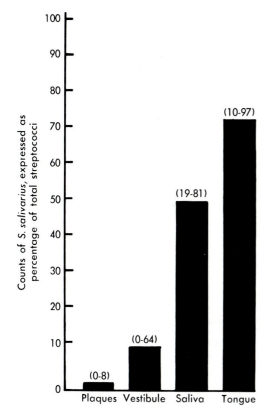

Fig. 3-1. Distribution of *Streptococcus salivarius* in oral cavity. (Adapted from Krasse, B.: Odontol. Rev. **5**:203, 1954.)

mine the microbial composition of the later developing mature plaque.

The origin of the normal flora of the body is not completely known, but it appears that most organisms in the oral cavity come from the immediate environment of the infant. During the process of delivery the mouth, as well as the skin, the nose, and the conjunctiva, become colonized with organisms from the genital passage of the mother, and within a few hours after birth these microorganisms proliferate within the oral cavity and the alimentary canal. Once the normal oral flora is established, organisms become adapted to specific sites in the mouth, and it is difficult to displace them. In healthy persons, potentially pathogenic organisms are prevented from free multiplication by the normal flora as well as by defense mechanisms of the host. For further information on the oral flora, see Rosebury (1962), Burnett et al. (1976), and Skinner and Carr (1974).

ROLE OF BACTERIA

The periodontal tissues are subject to a variety of pathoses that can be classified in several ways. Clinical entities such as gingivitis, periodontitis, gingivosis (chronic desquamative gingivitis), juvenile periodontitis (periodontosis), acute necrotizing ulcerative gingivitis (ANUG), and occlusal traumatism are operationally convenient. Epidemiologically, the predominant pathoses of the periodontal tissues are seen as a gradual series of inflammatory involvements, and generally further differentiations are not made. Etiologic classification of periodontal diseases can be based only on general factors at the present, since distinctive etiologic agents have not been related to particular periodontal syndromes. The most common forms of periodontal disease, gingivitis and periodontitis, and the less frequently occurring ANUG and juvenile periodontitis can be classified as infectious processes, requiring the presence of microbial cells.

It is quite clear that trauma from occlusion per se can aggravate destruction of periodontal tissues, yet this process is not often seen in its pure form. The course of periodontal destruction occurring as a result of occlusal traumatism is thought to be markedly accelerated by concurrent infectious gingivitis and periodontitis.

The influence of trauma from occlusion on the progression of periodontitis in the beagle dog has been studied by Lindhe and Svanberg (1974). In these experiments it was shown that experimental periodontal infection alone induced significant horizontal bone loss. When infectious periodontitis was combined with a cap splint and bar device that caused repetitive occlusal trauma, both horizontal as well as vertical bone loss resulted. These results suggest that repetitive occlusal trauma combined with infectious periodontitis results in more bone loss than comparable infectious periodontitis alone. Alternatively, one may conclude that repetitive occlusal trauma induces an adaptive response, which appears as a vertical bony defect. The role of occlusal trauma in alveolar bone loss is thus not resolved, but trauma from occlusion can lead to greater bone loss and more rapid apical migration of the epithelial attachment when there are coexisting plaque-induced inflammatory changes. In the absence of a plaque-induced infectious process it appears that there is little or no significant bone loss from occlusal trauma alone.

It appears then that in most forms of periodontal disease, bacteria play an important role, either as primary or secondary etiologic agents. Evidence that bacteria do play a role in periodontal disease can be discussed under two headings: studies of periodontal syndromes in animals and studies of human periodontal disease.

Studies of periodontal syndromes in animals

Periodontal disease does not occur spontaneously in many species of experimental animals. Keyes and Likins in 1946 made the important observation that a type of periodontal pathosis does occur spontaneously in Syrian hamsters. This observation led to a series of experiments using the Syrian hamster as an experimental model for periodontal disease. From these experiments the following important information has been obtained:

1. There was an infectious and transmissible component of the hamster periodontal disease syndrome. The disease could be transmitted from "infected" golden hamsters to the "noninfected" albino hamsters (in which the disease did not occur spontaneously) by inoculation with plaque or fecal paste from the infected hamsters (Keyes and Jordan, 1964).

2. The microbial agent responsible for this transmissibility was an aerobic, gram-positive filamentous bacterium, originally named *Odontomyces viscosus* and now called *Actinomyces viscosus* T 6 (serotype 1, rodent) (Jordan and Keyes, 1964; Howell et al., 1965). Other strains of hamster plaque organisms, including *Streptococcus, Sarcina,* gram-negative rods, and various gram-negative oval or spindle-shaped cells were isolated from the infected hamsters and failed to produce significant pathology when inoculated into the uninfected albino hamsters (Table 7).

3. Filament-forming bacteria, including *Rothia dentocariosa,* and strains of *Actinomyces* resembling *A. naeslundii, A. viscosus* (serotype 2, human), *A. viscosus* (serotype 1, rodent), and *A. odontolyticus* have been isolated from the carious dentin of human teeth with root surface caries. These organisms were found by Jordan and Hammond (1971) to induce the periodontal syndrome as well as cervical caries in the hamster model system.

The findings listed above lend considerable support to the concept that filamentous microorganisms resembling *Actinomyces* and *Rothia* species play a role in the pathology of human periodontal disease and in the root surface caries that frequently accompany this condition.

Studies of periodontal disease in *mice* have led to the conclusion that this species loses alveolar bone slowly in the absence of microorganisms. The presence of large numbers of microorganisms in the gingival crevice region markedly accelerates this alveolar bone loss. It has been suggested that a similar situation exists in humans.

Table 7. Induction of periodontal syndrome in albino hamsters with pure cultures of bacteria isolated from golden hamsters suffering from the periodontal syndrome*

Bacterial type	Strains	Gingival plaque	Alveolar bone resorption
Controls	—	—	—
Streptococ-cus	10 strains	—	—
Filaments	T 6	+	+
	BA 8	+	+
	BA 3	+	+
	T 9	+	+
	BA 5	—	—
Gram-nega-tive rods	T 10	+	—
	T 2	+	—
	BA 11	+	—
	4 other strains	—	—
Sarcina	2 strains	—	—

*Adapted from Jordan, H. V., and Keyes, P. H.: Arch. Oral Biol. **9:**401, 1964.

The *rice rat* is another experimental animal in which a periodontal syndrome consisting of gingival distortion, periodontal pockets, alveolar resorption, and tooth mobility occurs spontaneously. This syndrome can be dramatically reduced by administration of antibiotics. Dick and Shaw (1966) demonstrated the essential role of bacteria in the rice rat periodontal syndrome by transmitting the disease with plaque bacteria taken from "susceptible" individuals to those who were bred for their "resistance."

Gnotobiotic *rats* of the Sprague-Dawley strain are valuable in demonstrating the essential role of bacteria in periodontal disease. Socransky (1970) lists several bacterial species isolated from the human oral cavity that, when used as monocontaminants in the rat, lead to severe alveolar bone loss. These microorganisms include certain strains of "cariogenic" streptococci, gram-positive rods resembling *Actinomyces naeslundii,* and a strain of *Bacillus.* Irving and co-workers (1975) described bone loss occurring in Sprague-Dawley rats monoinfected with a gram-negative surface-translocating organism isolated from subjects with juvenile periodontitis (periodontosis). Listgarten and co-workers (1977) have described bone loss occurring in rats monoinfected with *Eikenella corrodens.* Socransky (1977) has tested a number of organisms in the rat model and found that several representatives of the gram-negative anaerobic surface-translocating rod group of organisms isolated from pockets of juvenile periodontitis patients cause bone resorption when used as contaminants in gnotobiotic Sprague-Dawley rats. On the other hand, a series of organisms including strains of *Veillonella, Fusobacterium, Campylobacter, Escherichia coli, Selenomonas, Bacteroides* and *Treponema* showed no potential to cause bone resorption when tested as monocontaminants in the rat model. The failure of an organism to cause a periodontal syndrome in rats is not readily interpreted, however, since simple failure to colonize the teeth as monocontaminants could account for failure to cause disease. The pathogenic potential of many organisms hence cannot be tested in this model because they cannot colonize the gnotobiotic rats. Some of these organisms that failed to cause bone resorption when used singly may well colonize the tooth and cause periodontal destruction as combined infections with other organisms. Experiments with gnotobiotic rats provide direct proof that bacteria can cause periodontal destruction. In the rat experiments many different species of bacteria, including streptococci, filaments, and bacilli, led to periodontal destruction, whereas in the hamster model only the filaments caused periodontal destruction (Table 7). This difference may simple represent a species difference. However, it may also mean that an organism can implant, form dental plaque, and cause periodontal destruction with relative ease in a gnotobiotic animal as compared to a conventional animal (e.g., the hamster used for study of periodontal disease), in which microbial antagonism is possible and in which host defense mechanisms may be more vigorous.

Beagle *dogs* have been shown to develop spontaneous periodontal disease by Saxe and co-workers (1967). In a well-controlled study they showed that periodontal disease in the beagles could be prevented by control of plaque accumulation and regular removal of mineralized deposits. Lindhe and co-workers (1975) showed that beagle dogs placed on a soft diet and allowed to freely accumulate plaque rapidly developed signs of gingivitis. Over a period of 4 years they developed clinical, radiographic, and histologic signs of periodontitis including alveolar bone loss. These studies provide evidence that plaque can lead to periodontitis. They were also able to prevent the progression of gingivitis to periodontitis by subjecting control dogs to twice-daily toothbrushing, which prevented calculus and plaque accumulation.

A model of acute necrotizing ulcerative gingivitis has been described in beagle dogs by Van Campen and co-workers (1977). These investigators found a condition resembling ANUG occurring spontaneously in a beagle dog colony. They also reported that by transferring the flora (from a dog with ANUG) to a group of dogs treated with corticosteriods, they were able to induce ANUG in the treated dogs in 2 weeks. This may provide a much needed model for ANUG; however, further experiments will be needed to determine its fidelity to human acute necrotizing ulcerative gingivitis.

Taken as a whole the animal experiments lend strong support to the concept that periodontal diseases, characterized by gingival inflammation and alveolar bone loss, are caused by certain strains of bacteria associated with the periodontal tissues.

Studies of human periodontal disease

A review of the epidemiologic studies of human periodontal disease by Russell (1967) led to the conclusion that there is a direct relationship between the amount of plaque, oral debris, and calculus and the severity of periodontal disease. He further adds that the linear correlation between mouth cleanliness (plus age) and the periodontal disease index values is so strong as to leave little variation in disease scores to be accounted for by any factors other than age or hygiene. This strong, positive correlation between oral debris and periodontal disease does not establish a cause-and-effect relationship between these factors.

A direct cause-and-effect relationship between dental plaque and gingivitis has been demonstrated, however, by the very interesting experiments of Löe et al. (1965) and Theilade et al. (1966). In these longitudinal experiments a group of dental students were given dental prophylaxis and practiced plaque removal procedures until they exhibited little or no measurable dental plaque or gingivitis. All oral hygiene procedures were then withdrawn, and in a few days the subjects developed accumulations of dental plaque. Clinically measurable gingivitis was observed in most subjects after 2 to 3 weeks of no oral hygiene, at which time a dense and complex plaque flora had developed. When oral hygiene procedures were reinstituted, the dental plaque material was removed and gingivitis subsided.

Similar longitudinal experiments in human beings demonstrating a cause-and-effect relationship between bacterial plaque and alveolar bone loss have not as yet been reported and may not be feasible. However, cross-sectional studies of over

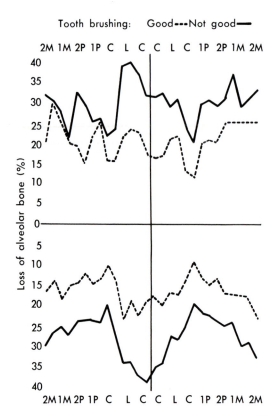

Tooth brushing: Good---Not good—

Fig. 3-2. Alveolar bone loss in man as related to oral hygiene. (Adapted from Schei, O., Waerhaug, J., Lovdal, A., and Arno, A.: J. Periodontol. **30:**7, 1959.)

700 adults reported in 1959 by Schei et al. show that loss of alveolar bone increases with poor oral hygiene (Fig. 3-2). These authors measured bone loss radiographically and classified toothbrushing efficiency by visual estimation of bacterial deposits on the teeth. It is clear from these studies that alveolar bone loss is most severe in individuals judged to have poor oral hygiene, that is, in those having the largest accumulation of bacterial plaque at the gingival margin.

Human epidemiologic studies, the experimental gingivitis studies, and cross-sectional studies cited clearly implicated *dental plaque* as the *major causative* agent in *periodontal diseases* that are characterized by gingival inflammation and alveolar bone loss.

A considerable body of clinical information suggests modern periodontal therapy is effective in markedly reducing the destruction of periodontal tissues in man. Over the years clinical observations strongly suggest that successful periodontal therapy hinges on regular removal of the bacterial masses that grow at or near the gingival margin. Lindhe and co-workers (1975), for example, show

in well-controlled human clinical experiments that it is possible to treat periodontal disease successfully, even in advanced stages, by traditional therapy plus postsurgical professional tooth cleaning every 2 weeks. Over a 2-year period they were able to keep plaque levels very low and obtained remarkable healing of periodontal defects. Many therapeutic procedures used in periodontics are directed to removing sites in which bacteria may multiply, since they are inaccessible to present-day oral hygiene devices. These clinical observations and experiments are consistent with the primary role of dental plaque in periodontal disease that has been demonstrated in animal and human experiments.

Although the evidence is strong concerning the primary etiologic role of dental microbial accumulation in periodontal disease, there is less information regarding the role of systemic factors in periodontal disease. This information will be discussed in detail in another chapter; however, some effects of hormonal and neutrophil disorders will be discussed here. It is well known that there are hormonal influences on periodontal disease manifested in pregnancy (Cohen et al., 1970; Löe and Silness, 1963). These studies show that the effect of local irritants on gingival inflammation is accentuated during pregnancy. There is also evidence that hormonal oral contraceptives lead to an exaggerated gingival response to dental plaque (Pearlman et al., 1974).

Hormonal alterations also occur in individuals with hyperparathyroidism. In this condition, decalcification of the skeleton may occur, and it was thought that periodontal disease should be more severe. However, based upon the contrary findings of Svanberg and Lindhe (1973), caution has to be exerted in this seemingly logical explanation of the potential effects of altered calcium metabolism on periodontal disease. These authors question the importance that the degree of mineralization of the alveolar process has for resistance against progression of periodontitis, since they found that plaque control in dogs in which nutritional hyperparathyroidism was induced prevents progression of periodontitis.

In addition to hormonal influences it is well established that diseases such as diabetes and Down's syndrome are associated with a greater severity of periodontal disease. Also, in neutrophil disorders such as agranulocytosis, neutropenia, the Chediak-Higashi syndrome, and chronic granulomatous disease, periodontal disease is more severe.

The role of neutrophil function in periodontal

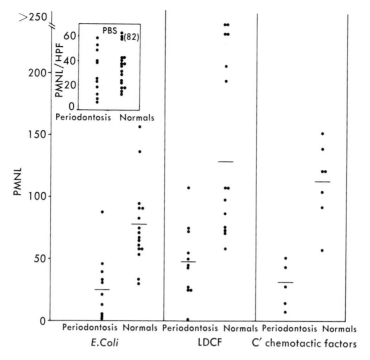

Fig. 3-3. Chemotactic response of polymorphonuclear leukocytes from individuals with juvenile periodontitis (periodontosis) compared to normal individuals. Purified neutrophils from peripheral blood of subjects were compared in chemotactic assay using three standard chemotactic agents: culture filtrate from *Escherichia coli,* leukocyte-derived chemotactic factor, *LDCF,* and chemotactic components of complement system. Random migration is shown in insert. Nonchemotactic phosphate-buffered saline, *PBS,* was used in place of standard chemotactants *HPF,* high-powered fields. (From Cianciola, L. J., Genco, R. J., Patters, M. R., McKenna, J., and van Oss, C. J.: Nature **265:**445, 1977b.)

disease, suggested by the experiments of nature mentioned above, has been brought into perspective by Cianciola and co-workers (1977). These workers found that patients with idiopathic juvenile periodontitis localized to molars and incisors (periodontosis) have depressed neutrophil chemotaxis and phagocytosis (Fig. 3-3). The monocytes responded normally in these patients. Depressed neutrophil function appears to be common in subjects with diabetes and Down's syndrome as well as in subjects with idiopathic juvenile periodontitis. Neurtophil alterations are severe in patients with neutropenia and agranulocytosis, the Chediak-Higashi syndrome, and chronic granulomatous disease. In all these conditions periodontal disease is much more severe than can be accounted for by bacterial factors alone, suggesting an important *protective role* for the *neutrophil.* According to this concept, diseases or conditions that depress neutrophil protective functions would likely result in more severe periodontal disease. Conversely, enhancing depressed neutrophil function may help in the control of periodontal disease in these patients.

Clearly, then, systemic factors such as hormones and neutrophils do play a role in periodontal diseases, but it is unlikely that they alone can cause the common forms of periodontal disease. Systemic factors may influence the course of periodontal disease, but without dental plaque there would likely be little or no periodontal disease for these factors to affect.

MICROBIAL DENTAL PLAQUES

With the importance of plaques in mind we will discuss their structure, development, and mechanisms of formation and their inhibition and dispersion.

Dental plaque, bacterial plaque, or perhaps most accurately microbial dental plaques vary microbiologically from surface to surface and are defined as a product of microbial growth, tenaciously attached to the surfaces of the teeth and adjacent gingiva, which exhibit a definite microscopic architecture. Kleinberg (1970) views plaques as aggregates of bacterial cells (although a few inflammatory and epithelial cells are also found) that are bridged by intercellular substances. Fluids such as saliva, gingival fluid, and liquids from the diet can percolate through this structure to a greater or lesser extent, depending on the porosity. The porosity in turn depends on the specific arrangement of cells and intercellular material and the extent to which the intercellular spaces are filled with salivary or serum components, polysaccharides, and other matrix substances synthesized by plaque bacteria.

Microbial dental plaques are conveniently classified according to location into coronal, gingival, and subgingival. *Coronal plaques* refer to those microbial aggregations found on the tooth surfaces but not in contact with the gingiva; *gingival*

plaques refer to those aggregates in contact with the marginal gingiva; and *subgingival plaques* refer to those aggregations found within the gingival crevice or periodontal pockets. Periodontal pockets contain a thin layer of attached plaque on the tooth surface and a layer of loosely arranged bacterial cells at the tissue interface. There are also aggregations of bacteria that represent a form of dental plaque in the fissures of the tooth crown. Many bacteria in *fissure plaque* are nonviable, and it may be that this plaque is associated with fissure caries.

Dental plaque should be distinguished from other accumulations or accretions on the tooth surface such as (1) *materia alba,* an amorphous bacterial accumulation, which, unlike dental plaque, is easily removed with a dental water spray, (2) *pellicle,* which is an organic film deposited on the tooth surface and which contains no bacteria, and (3) *calculus,* which represents calcified dental plaque. Plaque, pellicle, and calculus can stain various colors depending upon the diet or habits of the subject.

Structure. Dental plaque consists mainly of microbial masses and a cuticle or pellicle interposed between these masses and the tooth surface. Total microscopic counts indicate the presence of about 250 million organisms per milligram of wet weight of plaque. Since a centrifuged pellet of a pure culture of streptococcus has about the same number of cells per milligram wet weight, it is reasonable

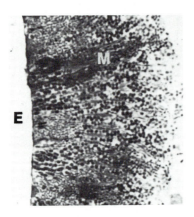

Fig. 3-4. Normal. Note coccoid flora on enamel surface. *E,* enamel space; *M,* columnar microcolony. (× 1325.) (Adapted from Listgarten, M.: J. Periodontol. **47:**1, 1976.)

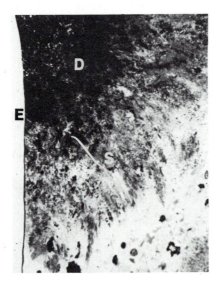

Fig. 3-5. Gingivitis. Note apical extension of microbial layer. (× 400.) (Adapted from Listgarten, M.: J. Periodontol. **47:**1, 1976.)

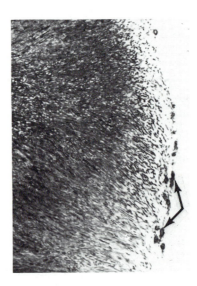

Fig. 3-6. Gingivitis. Note dense filamentous bacteria with corncob formations at surface. (× 550.) (Adapted from Listgarten, M.: J. Periodontol. **47:** 1, 1976.)

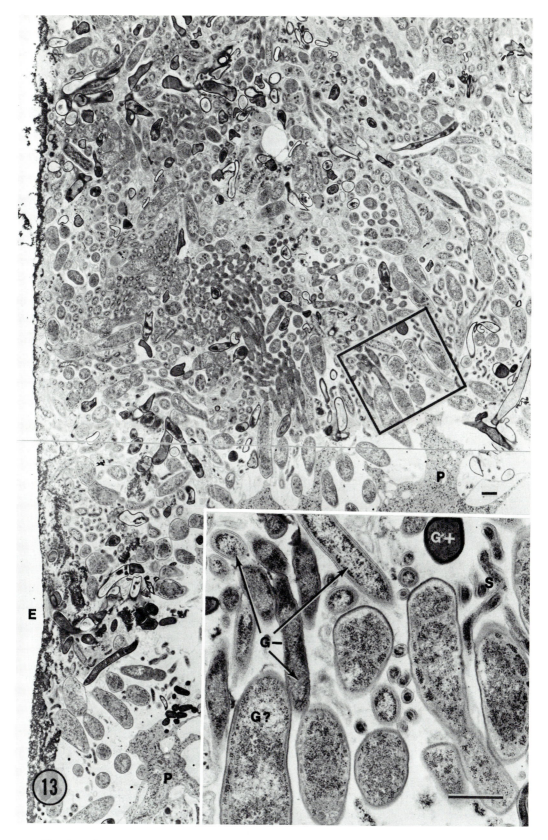

Fig. 3-7. Gingivitis sample; higher powered view of apically located microbial mass with details in insert. *E,* enamel space; *P,* projections from adjacent polymorphonuclear leukocytes. (×4500.) In insert note presence of small spirochetes, *S,* and gram-positive, *G+,* gram-negative, *G−,* and atypical cells, *G?.* (Adapted from Listgarten, M.: J. Periodontol. **47:**1, 1976.)

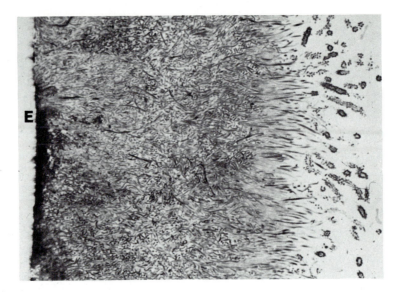

Fig. 3-8. Periodontitis. Dense, predominantly filamentous bacterial mass adherent to enamel surface. Corncob formations extend from surface. *E,* enamel space. (× 850.) (Adapted from Listgarten, M.: J. Periodontol. **47**:1, 1976.)

to assume that most of the weight of plaque is due to bacteria.

McDougall (1963) has published an interesting histologic study of dental plaque and pellicle formed on teeth. He found that fully formed plaque is seen under the light microscope as a mass of filamentous bacteria at right angles to the pellicle near the tooth surface. Closer to the periphery the filaments curve and are irregular. In the outer, younger portion of plaque many cocci and other small bacterial forms are found. Roughly two thirds of the plaque is gram positive.

The ultrastructure of the microbial flora associated with the tooth and periodontal tissues in various states of health and disease have been reported by Listgarten (1976). These studies will be discussed under four categories: *normal, gingivitis, periodontitis,* and *juvenile periodontitis* (periodontosis).

In the *normal* state of periodontal health the microbial flora is mostly supragingival and mostly confined to the enamel surface. The microbial flora consists of a relatively thin layer of adherent bacterial cells. The arrangement varies from isolated single cells to cells that are densely packed or arranged in columnar microcolonies (Fig. 3-4). At the interface between the enamel surface and the plaque bacteria is an electron-dense cuticle called the "dental pellicle." Cells of this plaque are predominantly cocoid in shape with a majority exhibiting cell-wall features of gram-positive microorganisms. Filamentous forms and gram-nega-

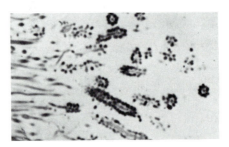

Fig. 3-9. Magnified view of corncob formations in Fig. 3-8. Corncobs consist of a central filamentous microorganism surrounded by adherent coccoid cells. (× 1500.) (Adapted from Listgarten, M.: J. Periodontol. **47**:1, 1976.)

tive organisms are present in small numbers, frequently on the outer surface of the microbial layer rather than in contact with the teeth. No flagellated cells or spirochetes are observed in the microbial flora associated with the normal state.

The microbial flora found in the *gingivitis samples* is associated with the enamel and sometimes the cemental surface of the tooth since the epithelial attachment frequently extends apically to the cementum. A variety of microorganisms including coccoid as well as filamentous forms and cells with gram-positive and a variety of gram-negative cell-wall patterns are noted (Fig. 3-5). Bacterial deposits may reach a thickness of 0.4 mm or more, considerably thicker than those found in the normal. The deeper layers of the adherent bacterial mass have undergone lysis, and mineralization of

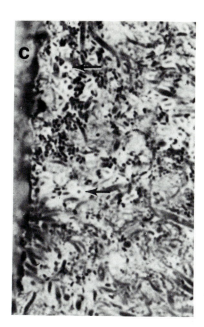

Fig. 3-10. Periodontitis. Microbial layer adherent to cementum, *C*, in transitional zone between supragingival and subgingival microbial flora. *Arrows* point to cross sections of large filaments surrounded by a clear zone. (×3100.) (Adapted from Listgarten, M.: J. Periodontol. **47**:1, 1976.)

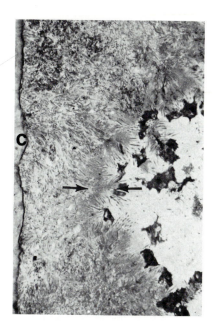

Fig. 3-11. Periodontitis. Subgingival flora. Surface of adherent flora is covered by a palisading layer of test-tube brush formations and spirochetes (between *arrows*). Adherent flora is less filamentous than supragingival flora and shows no particular orientation with respect to cementum surface, *C*. (×600.) (Adapted from Listgarten, M.: J. Periodontol. **47**:1, 1976.)

cells is common. Filamentous bacteria are relatively more numerous than in the normal samples, and there are dense masses of filaments occasionally covered with "corncob" formations (Fig. 3-6). In the gingivitis samples, flagellated bacteria and spirochetes are observed in the apical portion of the plaque distributed among the other bacteria (Fig. 3-7). Epithelial cells and polymorphonuclear leukocytes are also found adherent to the most apical portion of the microbial mass (Figs. 3-5 and 3-7).

In *periodontitis* the epithelial attachment is located on the root surface, and the surface area occupied by the microbial deposits is greater than in teeth from normal or gingivitis subjects. Filamentous forms are prominent; however, all the cell types encountered in the gingivitis sample are observed in the periodontitis sample (Fig. 3-8). *Leptotrichia buccalis* can be identified because of the characteristic appearance of its cell wall. Corncob formations are common at the surface of the supragingival deposits (Figs. 3-8 and 3-9). There is a transition zone noted between the predominant filamentous supragingival plaque and the largely motile-appearing subgingival plaque (Fig. 3-10). In the transition zone there is a substantial increase in the number of flagellated bacteria and

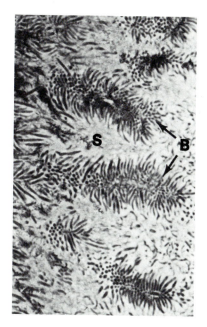

Fig. 3-12. Longitudinal section through test-tube brush formations, *B*, the base of which is surrounded by a spirochete-rich flora, *S*. (×1500.) (Adapted from Listgarten, M.: J. Periodontol. **47**:1, 1976.)

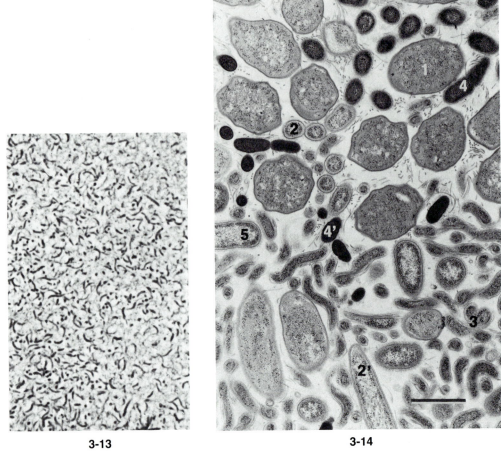

3-13

3-14

Fig. 3-13. Predominantly gram-negative flora with curved microorganisms resembling *Selenomonas sputigena.* (× 1500.) (Adapted from Listgarten, M.: J. Periodontol. **47:**1, 1976.)

Fig. 3-14. Periodontitis. Representative subgingival flora. *1,* large, irregularly contoured filament (shown in cross section) with peritrichous flagellation; *2,* and *2',* thin, gram-negative filaments resembling fusiforms; *3,* spirochetes; *4,* and *4',* small, electron-dense coccoid bacteria; *5,* gram-negative rod. (× 15,000.) (Adapted from Listgarten, M.: J. Periodontol. **47:**1, 1976.)

a few large filaments. The most distinct features of the periodontitis plaque samples are noted in the portion of the deposits that occupy the periodontal pocket (Fig. 3-11). A thin layer of varied thickness adherent to the root surface is seen in this subgingival area. On the surface of this adherent layer, at the bacterial-tissue interface, there is a layer of distinctive microorganisms, many of which are flagellated. In this superficial layer of bacteria there are many "bristle-brush" or "test tube–brush" formations surrounded by a spirochete-rich flora (Fig. 3-12). Also on the tissue side of the subgingival flora are other cell types including gram-negative bacteria with concave bodies and multiple flagella resembling the species *Sele-*

nomonas sputigena (Fig. 3-13). There are also very narrow coccoid organisms and a variety of rods with gram-negative cell walls in this superficial layer (Fig. 3-14). The surface of the subgingival microbial mass facing the pocket epithelium is generally covered with polymorphonuclear leukocytes and a few macrophages, and these phagocytes occasionally contain phagocytosed bacteria.

The surfaces of the teeth extracted from *juvenile periodontitis (periodontosis)* patients are remarkable for their lack of grossly detectable surface deposits. The surfaces of these teeth are frequently covered with cuticle that exhibits an irregular contour (Fig. 3-15). Small clumps of gram-

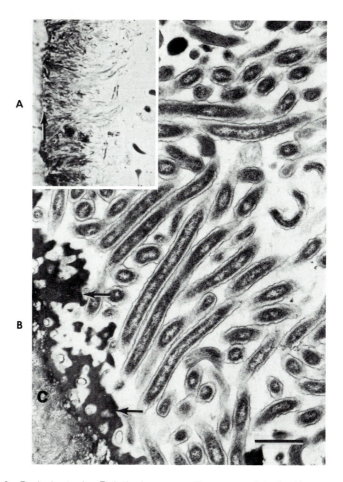

Fig. 3-15. A, Periodontosis. Relatively sparse flora associated with cementum surface *(arrow).* (×1100.) **B,** Electron micrograph of **A.** Thin filaments with loosely adapted gram-negative cell walls are oriented more or less perpendicularly to dense cuticle *(arrows)* covering cementum surface, C. (×13,000.) (Adapted from Listgarten, M.: J. Periodontol. **47:**1, 1976.)

negative coccoid bacteria and polymorphonuclear leukocytes in varying stages of disintegration are frequently associated with this lobulated cuticle material. Thin filaments with loosely adapted gram-negative cell walls form deposits covering the cementum surface (Fig. 3-15). The bacterial population associated with these teeth is a sparse gram-negative flora and relatively simple when compared to the populations seen in periodontitis and gingivitis. The predominant bacteria observed in situ in juvenile periodontitis are comparable to the predominant cultivable flora of these lesions as reported by Newman et al. (1976).

It is quite clear from these studies that there are many types of microbial flora associated with periodontal tissues in health and disease. There are certainly tenaciously attached dental plaques both supragingivally and subgingivally; however, subgingivally in periodontitis and periodontosis there is a loosely attached flora found at the advancing

front of the lesion. The microbes in the area of the advancing front are likely to be of major importance in the destructive events occurring in periodontal disease. It is also clear that there is a flora, predominantly coccoid, compatible with periodontal health.

The flora changes occurring over 2 months in humans with artificial crowns are documented by Listgarten et al. (1975). Deposits of less than 1 week are predominantly a coccoid flora very similar to the normal flora described on natural teeth. In 1 to 3 weeks, during which time gingivitis develops, a flora is found resembling that seen in gingivitis described above on natural teeth. After 2 months the flora is similar to that seen in periodontitis, with a spirochete-rich subgingival layer at the tissue interface. These studies show that changes in the microbial flora from normal to periodontitis occurs in a fairly characteristic manner. The flora in juvenile periodontitis appears to be unique. It is relatively simple and composed mainly of gram-negative coccoid and thin filamentous cells.

Several authors have described what appears grossly to be a *plaque-free zone* on extracted teeth and at the gingival margins in vivo.

Chemical composition. The chemical composition of dental plaque is difficult to determine because it varies with age and diet. In general, however, plaque is about 80% water and 20% solids. The solids include the cells that make up about 35% of the dry weight and the extracellular portion that comprises the remaining 65% of the dry weight. Polysaccharides in plaque have been extensively studied, and dextran appears to be the major (95%) hexose-containing polysaccharide. Most of the remaining 5% of plaque hexose-containing polysaccharide is levan. Both dextran and levan are formed by bacterial enzymes from sucrose. Dextran has been implicated in plaque formation, and levan may function as a storage polysaccharide. There are very low levels of sialic acid and fucose in plaque, which may be of some significance in understanding plaque formation.

Development. Dental plaque development on exposed tooth surfaces is generally thought to begin with the laying down of an acquired pellicle on the tooth surface. Chemical studies of human pellicle provide strong evidence that it mainly consists of glycoproteins derived from the submandibular gland. The acquired pellicle appears to form on artificial tooth surfaces and dentures as well as on natural teeth and is clearly distinct from the primary cuticle (Nasmyth's membrane).

Bacterial colonization of the surface of the acquired pellicle appears to be the next step in plaque formation. Microbiologic studies of developing plaque formation have shown that bacterial attachment takes place very rapidly. Manganiello et al. (1977) found that within 5 minutes after carefully pumicing the surface of a molar, approximately 1 million organisms were deposited per square millimeter of enamel surface. The two major groups of organisms represented in the first few hours were gram-positive facultative pleomorphic rods and strains of *S. sanguis.* Few or no gram-negative organisms were detected in very early plaque.

Studies of plaque formation over a period of 2 to 3 weeks have led Löe et al. (1966) to describe three phases of microbial maturation of plaques associated with experimental gingivitis, starting with a cleaned tooth surface.

The *first phase* occurs within 2 days without oral hygiene. During this phase there is a proliferation of gram-positive cocci and rods. The *second phase* (1 to 4 days) is characterized by the appearance and increase in numbers of fusobacteria and filaments. The *third phase* (4 to 9 days) is characterized by the appearance of spirilla and spirochetes.

Ritz (1967) cultured bacteria from plaque allowed to develop over a similar time period. He found that during early stages of plaque formation, *Streptococcus, Neisseria,* and *Nocardia* were predominant, whereas after 9 days, *Streptococcus, Actinomyces, Veillonella,* and *Corynebacterium* predominate. Fusobacteria were present in greater portions in 9-day plaque than in earlier plaque. Ritz (1967) suggests "growth of anaerobic organisms such as veillonella and fusobacteria are dependent upon prior growth of aerobic and facultative organisms with a resultant increase in plaque thickness yielding conditions suitable for anaerobic growth."

Mechanisms of formation. The term "colonization" is used to describe dental plaque formation. There are at least two sets of processes involved in colonization of a surface by a microbial flora. Considerable attention has been given to these processes, with the hope that in better understanding the mechanisms of dental plaque formation we may be better equipped to disperse or inhibit the formation of these deposits.

One set of processes results in the attachment, adhesion, or implantation of free-living microorganisms on the surface to be colonized. The other set of processes affects the multiplication and growth of these organisms once they have become attached to the surface. The possible mechanisms involved in dental plaque formation are listed in Table 8.

Inhibition and dispersal. Our understanding of the essential role of dental plaque in smooth surface caries and periodontal disease, the "odontopathic" infections, has led to the widespread realization that regular plaque dispersal or inhibition of plaque formation will lead to the eradication of these infections. Clearly, one of the most important methods of presently available plaque control involves mechanical self-removal at regular intervals, with toothbrushes, dental floss, and other aids described in Chapter 5. Unfortunately, for many individuals the mechanical removal of dental plaque may be difficult to accomplish, and for many others individual motivation to carry out mechanical plaque control is lacking. With these problems in mind, attempts are being made to inhibit or disperse dental plaque by means that are

Table 8. Possible factors in formation of microbial dental plaque

Attachment or adhesion	Multiplication and growth
Adhesion to pellicle or tooth surface mediated by extracellular polysaccharide (i.e., dextran or levan) or by "receptors" on cell surface	Availability of nutrients
	Secretion of metabolites
	Physical crowding limiting growth
Cell-to-cell adhesion, either dextran induced or salivary induced	Change in oxidation-reduction potential
	Host factors (i.e., antibodies) and phagocytotic cells may inhibit plaque formation
Interbacterial agglutination	

simpler to carry out and that may be usable as public health measures for large population groups. The following approaches have been studied for widespread microbial dental plaque control: enzyme mouth rinses and antimicrobial agents.

Enzyme mouth rinses. One of the mechanisms of bacterial cell adhesion to the tooth and to other cells involves the adhesive bacterial polysaccharide dextran (Table 8). Initial experiments in animals using dextranase, an enzyme capable of hydrolyzing the glycoside linkages of the large dextran molecule, showed considerable plaque reduction. Subsequent human experiments (Keyes et al., 1971) have shown only partial success with dextranase used in mouthwashes to disperse dental plaque. This limited success is explained by the fact that there are other mechanisms for adhesion of plaque bacterial cells to the tooth surface and to themselves. Dextranase only interferes with those mechanisms that depend on dextran as the adherent polymer. Since dextranase mouthwashes do not appear to be very successful in plaque dispersal in humans, it is reasonable to assume that these alternate adhesive mechanisms are clinically important in plaque formation.

Many other enzymes or combinations of enzymes have been administered topically or incorporated into dentifrices or chewing gums in an attempt to control plaque. These preparations include various proteolytic and carbohydrate-hydrolyzing enzymes, and they have been largely ineffective.

Antimicrobial agents. Since plaque is composed mainly of living bacteria, antimicrobial agents have been tested for their plaque-inhibiting capacity. Several antibiotics, including penicillin, tetracycline, vancomycin, and spiramycin, when added to the diet, drinking water, or applied topically to experimental animals, inhibit dentogingival plaque. Among the antibiotics tested on human beings, an adhesive paste containing 1% vancomycin was found to reduce plaque in mentally retarded children (Mitchell and Holmes,

1965). Löe et al. reported in 1967 that three daily rinses with 0.25% tetracycline prevented plaque from forming. Stallard et al. in 1969 found that a macrolide antibiotic (CC 10232), obtained from a strain of *Streptomyces*, reduced the formation of plaque and calculus in humans. Several antibiotics can inhibit plaque formation, but there is no doubt of the potential danger in the use of such drugs. The production of resistant strains, sensitization, and other undesirable side effects of long-term antibiotic administration limit the use of these antiplaque agents to special circumstances. Present-day antibiotics do not appear to offer a practical solution to lifelong plaque control. Perhaps lifelong disease control can be achieved with judicious use of antibiotics at intervals when pathogenic organisms begin to accumulate.

Numerous antimicrobial agents other than true antibiotics have been used for many years in mouthwashes. The emphasis in many studies of these agents (see comprehensive review by Schroeder, 1969) has been the prevention or dissolution of calculus. Some of these chemical disinfectants have recently been reinvestigated for their effects on plaque formation. One of the agents, chlorhexidine gluconate (Hibetane), has been shown by Löe and Schiott (1970) to be very effective in preventing the formation of dental plaque. These authors had subjects use a 0.2% solution of chlorhexidine twice a day as a mouthwash. Undesirable side effects included disturbance of taste sensation and brown staining of the teeth.

To what extent this and similar antimicrobial agents can be used in long-term control of plaque will depend on studies of possible toxicity and effects on the gastrointestinal flora. This appears to be a promising approach.

ORGANISMS OF GINGIVAL CREVICE REGION AND THEIR PATHOGENIC POTENTIAL

Very large amounts of plaque accumulate in patients with periodontitis; for example, Shawary et al. (1966) have found that from 100 to 200 mg of plaque can be recovered from the dentition of subjects with periodontitis. This consists mainly of bacteria. It has been estimated that a 10 to 15 cm^2 area of gingival pocket epithelial is exposed to the plaque and pocket flora, and much of this gingival pocket epithelium may be ulcerated. It is clear that the accumulation of plaque can expose the gingiva to large numbers of bacteria; however, in spite of this exposure bacteria are rarely found within viable gingival tissues. The only periodontal disease (aside from periodontal abscesses) in which bacteria have been found regularly in the periodontal tissues is ANUG (Listgarten et al. 1964). In ANUG there are intermediate and large spirochetes and other bacteria within viable gingival tissues at the base of the ulcers. In most other forms of periodontal disease the subgingival flora is walled off by a layer of neutrophils and some macrophages that are interposed between the flora and the sulcular or pocket epithelium.

Enumeration of various microorganisms that inhibit the gingival crevice area of humans and are cultivable was carried out in 1963 by Socransky et al. and by Gibbons and co-workers. Approximately 10% to 20% of the microorganisms counted microscopically in these early studies were cultivated from gingival debris and dental plaque. Recent studies employing better media and continuous anaerobic techniques have markedly improved the recoveries of plaque microorganisms to levels approximating 60% to 85% of the microscopic count (Loesche et al., 1972; Poole and Gilmour, 1971; Manganiello et al., 1977). The techniques used are adaptations of those described for cultivation of anaerobic microflora from other parts of the body by Moore (1966) and from rumen by Hungate (1969). In these techniques organisms are samples from the tooth in prereduced media flushed with oxygen-free gases. The suspension is anaerobically dispersed and diluted prior to plating onto prereduced media and then incubated under strict anaerobic conditions. Anaerobic maintenance of the specimen from the time of sampling throughout culture has increased the yield of cultivable organisms, and many previously unrecognized species have been recovered. This should be kept in mind in evaluating future clinical studies where cultivation of the oral flora is attempted.

In early studies of the oral microflora, plaque on the various teeth was thought to be reasonably constant in its microbial content, and most studies were performed on pooled plaque samples. The results indicated that the bacterial profile from diseased and normal teeth was similar, and the conclusion was drawn that little or no microbial specificity was involved in periodontal disease. It later became clear that the microbial flora taken from different teeth and from different areas on the teeth (e.g., supragingival vs. subgingival) differed in content of various organisms. This led to the development of techniques that could sample discrete sites. From these studies a remarkable specificity of flora was revealed. This specificity is best exemplified in the studies of Newman and Socransky (1977, 1976) and Slots (1976), who showed that the organisms cultivated from the advancing front of lesions in patients with juvenile periodontitis consist of relatively few types of bacteria, which include several groups of gram-negative surface-translocating anaerobic rods, some of which had not previously been described. Irving and co-workers (1975) found that a representative of these gram-negative surface-translocating anaerobic rods was able to cause a periodontal syndrome in monoinfected rats, suggesting that they play an etiologic role in the lesions of juvenile periodontitis. Darwish and co-workers (1975), sampling from disease-associated sites, found that the predominant cultivable organisms in lesions of patients with early periodontitis were distinct from those found in juvenile periodontitis (periodontosis). They report that asaccharolytic species of *Bacteroides melaninogenicus* are predominant organisms in periodontitis.

A detailed listing of microorganisms found in gingival areas of normal as well as diseased individuals is presented in Table 9. Comments regarding pathogenicity and occurrence of the organism are given when known. No attempt is made to give the percent occurrence of various groups since this varies markedly with state of disease, location, and age of microbial flora.

Many of the organisms listed in Table 9 are organisms that can be cultivated with present techniques with the notable exception of the spirochetes. Only the smaller spirochetes are able to be cultivated, and unfortunately the hard-to-cultivate intermediate and larger spirochetes are prominent in electron microphotographs of subgingival plaque as well as in viable gingival tissues in ANUG. Other organisms of the periodontal flora are also not able to be cultivated; hence our knowledge of this flora is incomplete.

Detailed studies of the flora by Darwish and co-workers (1973), Crawford and co-workers (1975), Newman and Socransky (1977, 1976), Slots (1977a and b, 1976), Loesche et al. (1973), Williams et al. (1974), and Mouton et al. (1977) as well as ultrastructural studies by Schroeder and DeBoever (1970) and Listgarten (1976) have led to the concept that there are different constellations of organisms associated with health and various forms of periodontal disease. The predominant flora in these conditions can be summarized as follows:

1. *The normal:* mainly thin supragingival plaque; the major organisms are *S. sanguis, A. viscosus* and *A. naeslundii; S. mitis, R. dentocariosa,* and *A. israelii.*

2. *Gingivitis:* plaque is thickened and there is an increase in absolute numbers as well as percentage of members of the genus *Actinomyces.* Members of the genera *Fusobacterium, Haemophilus, Campylobacter,* and *Veillonella* are observed. A complex flora is observed at the tissue-plaque interface and is rich in filaments, flagellated bacteria, and spirochetes. At the external surface of supragingival plaques are seen corncob configurations, the central core of which is *Bacteroides matruchotti.*

3. *Periodontitis:* the flora found in the depths of deep periodontal pockets in periodontitis in adults is mainly gram negative. The types of organisms seen vary from individual to individual; however, the prominent organisms seen include intermediate-sized spirochetes, *Bacteroides melaninogenicus,* ss. *asaccharolyticus, Fusobacterium nucleatum,* anaerobic vibrios, ''corroding'' *Bacteroides* species, *Eikenella corrodens,* and gram-negative capnophilic surface-translocating organisms.

4. *Juvenile periodontitis:* the flora of the thin adherent and nonadherent bacterial masses in the depths of pockets from subjects with juvenile periodontitis is mainly gram negative. Many of the isolates do not fit into recognizable species; however, gram-negative rods capable of surface translocation whose growth is stimulated by carbon dioxide are prominent. These organisms have been tentatively called members of the genus *Capnocytophaga* by Socransky and co-workers. Other isolates from juvenile periodontitis lesions are members of the genus *Bacteroides,* but of no known species. Spirochetes are also seen in these pockets.

5. *Acute necrotizing ulcerative gingivitis:* this appears to be the only form of periodontal disease in which organisms are seen to invade the periodontal tissues. Spirochetes of the intermediate type are observed in the tissues while other organisms, especially fusiform-shaped bacteria, are seen in necrotic zones superficial to the zone infiltrated with spirochetes.

It should be added that although the above-listed organisms are numerous at the advancing front of the respective lesions and likely important in these lesions, it is also possible that some of them are prominent *because* of the disease. That is, the growth conditions found in the pockets are conducive to their proliferation. Also numerically minor organisms may be important in periodontal disease if they have potent virulence.

Criteria for determining that a microorganism bears a causative relationship to a disease were set forth over a century ago. These criteria are known as Koch's postulates and can be paraphrased as follows:

1. The organism must be found in the disease. The location of the organism must correlate with the lesions observed.

2. The organism introduced into a suitable host must reproduce the disease.

3. The organism must be recovered from the experimental infection.

Koch's postulates have been fulfilled for periodontal disease by several strains of *Actinomyces* in the Syrian hamster model. With use of the gnotobiotic rat model and a number of organisms, including cariogenic streptococci, *Actinomyces,* and gram-negative rods, have been shown to cause alveolar bone destruction. The relevance of this model and in the Syrian hamster model to human periodontal disease is still to be resolved.

Having several organisms satisfy Koch's criteria does not provide full evidence that one or another of these endogenous organisms is actually involved in a particular individual with periodontal disease. Socransky (1970) has suggested another criterion that should be fulfilled before we can say definitely that a microbial agent or process is significant in the etiology of human periodontal disease; that is, ''it must be shown to actually have an effect on the periodontal tissues in the course of human periodontal disease.'' This criterion has not yet been satisfied; hence it is not clear *which* group or species of plaque microorganism causes periodontal disease. However, it should be remembered that there is substantial evidence that *some* microorganisms in microbial dental plaque are responsible for most forms of human periodontal disease.

Table 9. Organisms found in gingival sulcus or periodontal pocket region of man*

Group	Genera or Species	Comment
Gram-positive cocci	Staphylococcus epidermidis	Facultative; catalase positive
	Streptococci	Facultative; catalase negative
	Enterococci	Grow in unfavorable environments
	S. mutans	Forms dextran and acid from sucrose; ferments mannitol and sorbitol; cariogenic; several serotypes
	S. sanguis	Forms dextran; early colonizer of teeth
	S. mitis	Poorly defined species
	S. salivarius	Forms levan; numerous on tongue and in saliva; few in plaque
	Peptostreptococcus	Anaerobic; some are proteolytic
Gram-negative cocci	Neisseria	Facultative; diplococcus; N. sicca forms plaque; may be cariogenic
	Veillonella	Possess endotoxins; several serotypes; found in lesions of advanced periodontitis
	V. alcalescens	
	V. parvula	
	Simonsiella	
Gram-positive rods	Corynebacterium	
Facultative	Lactobacillus	Acidogenic; may be important in fissure and recurrent caries
	Nocardia	
	Rothia	Catalase positive; may be involved in cervical caries
	Arachnia	
	Actinomyces (Odontomyces) viscosus	Filament-forming diphtheroid; serotype 1 (e.g., strain T 6) associated with rodent periodontal syndrome; serotype 2 (human strains) may be associated with periodontitis and cervical caries; virulent and avirulent strains of A. viscosus with plasmid-determined virulence factors have been described
	Bacterionema matruchotii	May be important in calculus formation; central filament in many corncob configurations
Anaerobic	Actinomyces	
	A. naeslundii	Strain from humans forms plaque and causes periodontal syndrome in rodents
	A. israelii, A. bovis, A. odontolyticus, A. propionicus, A. eriksonii, and others	Role in periodontal disease suspected for some species
	Propionibacterium intermedius	Prominent member of flora in early periodontitis
	Eubacterium saburreum	Strict anaerobe; commensal relationship demonstrated with Veillonella
	Corynebacterium acnes	
Gram-negative rods		
Facultative	Eikenella corrodens	"Pitting" organism; found in advanced periodontitis; shown to cause periodontal disease in rats

*Data from Crawford et al., 1975; Darwish et al., 1973; Darwish et al., 1977; Gibbons et al., 1963; Hammond et al., 1976; Irving et al., 1975; Jordon and Keyes, 1964; Lambe and Jerris, 1976; Listgarten et al., 1977; Loesche et al., 1973; Manganiello et al., 1977; Newman and Socransky, 1977; Slack and Gerenger, 1970; Slots, 1976, 1977; Socransky et al., 1963; Socransky, 1970; Socransky et al., 1971; Williams, Pantalone, and Sherris, 1976; Murayama and Mashimo, 1977; Mouton et al., 1977.

Table 9. Organisms found in gingival sulcus or periodontal pocket region of man—cont'd

Group	Genera or species	Comment
Anaerobic	*Leptotrichia buccalis*	Obligate anaerobe; prominent spindle-shaped cells seen in old plaque
	Bacteroides	
	B. melaninogenicus	Marked pathogenic potential; requires hemin and some require menadione; essential component of mixed infection; isolated from abscesses, peritonitis, appendicitis; produce array of potentially tissue-destroying substances
	ss. melaninogenicus	Serotype A
	ss. intermedius	Serotype C (saccharolytic), prominent in early periodontitis lesions
	ss. asaccharolyticus (or *B. asaccharolyticus*)	Serotype B (assacharolytic), prominent in advanced periodontitis lesions, notably lacking in gingivitis and juvenile periodontitis
	B. oralis	Biochemically similar to *B. melaninogenicus,* ss. *melaninogenicus* but *not* pigmented; numerous in oral flora
	B. corrodens	Forms colonies that "pit" agar surface
	B. fragilis	Prominent member of intestinal flora, may be found in pocket
	Campylobacter sputorum	Motile, curved, formerly called "vibrio"
	Selenomonas sputigena	Motile spirillum, also called *Spirillum sputigenum,* found in lesions of advanced periodontitis
	Fusobacterium	Can cause skin abscesses after intracutaneous injection and show anachoresis and synergistic enhancement of spirochetal abscesses; *F. nucleatum* prominent in advanced periodontitis lesions
	F. polymorphum	
	F. nucleatum	
	Others exhibiting surface translocation—"Capnocytophaga" or *Bacteroides ochraceus*	Thin (0.2-0.4 μm diameter) rods prominent in juvenile periodontitis; cause periodontal disease syndromes in germ-free rats
Spirochetes	*Treponema*	
	T. denticola	
	T. macrodentium	
	T. oralis	
	Borrelia vincentii	
	Larger spirochetes	Observed in ANUG

Another approach to the study of the pathogenicity of oral organisms utilizes the *experimental mixed infection.* For these studies various combinations of pure cultures of oral microorganisms are introduced into or under the skin of experimental animals such as the guinea pig or rabbit. These experiments have led to the following information (some of which is summarized in Table 9) regarding the pathogenic potential of oral microorganisms.

Bacteroides

Bacteroides melaninogenicus is commonly found in large numbers in the gingival crevice region and produces a large array of potentially damaging substances such as collagenase, fibrinolysin, endotoxin, hydrogen sulfide, ammonia, and a variety of organic acids. This organism has been repeatedly isolated from lesions such as appendicitis, peritonitis, brain and lung abscesses, cellulitis, and gangrene. Some strains of *B. melaninogenicus* grow well both in vitro and in vivo in the presence of microorganisms that can provide a vitamin K growth factor. *B. melaninogenicus* may not initiate periodontal disease; yet once the disease is begun it is likely that the toxic products of this organism play a role in the progression of the disease.

Recently, Holdeman and Moore (1975) have proposed separation of *Bacteroides melanino-*

genicus into three subspecies based upon biochemical differences. Serologic grouping reported by Lambe and Jerris (1976) follows this biochemical grouping. These three subspecies (ss) are:

    B. melaninogenicus, ss. melaninogenicus, serotype A
    B. melaninogenicus, ss. asaccharolyticus, serotype B
    B. melaninogenicus, ss. intermedius, serotype C

In the subgingival flora in early periodontitis *B. melaninogenicus, ss. intermedius* is prominent, whereas in advanced periodontitis *B. melaninogenicus, ss. asaccharolytic* is prominent (Slots, 1977a). The significance of the difference in flora from the saccharolytic to the *asaccharolytic* subspecies of *B. melaninogenicus* in development of periodontitis is not clear. It is not known whether the *asaccharolytic* subspecies is more virulent or simply grows better in periodontal pockets found in advanced periodontitis.

Fusospirochetal infections

Investigations begun 30 to 40 years ago showed that mixtures of oral organisms, usually containing fusobacteria and spirochetes as well as various other organisms, produced a transmissible mixed infection in animals. A wide variety of human diseases, such as acute necrotizing ulcerative gingivitis, Vincent's angina (essentially an extension of ANUG to the fauces and tonsils), cancrum oris, tropical ulcer, and some pulmonary abscesses, are called fusospirochetal diseases. They are characterized as necrotizing ulcerative processes, in which fusobacteria are abundant on the surface. Spirochetes are found deeper in the lesion, and they characteristically invade normal tissue at the base of the lesions. All these diseases can be abated with penicillin and leave varying amounts of tissue destruction depending on the severity of the disease. These clinical infections, along with the experimentally induced fusospirochetal infections, lend support to the pathogenicity of oral fusobacteria and spirochetes. However, little is understood about the transmissibility, mechanism of pathogenesis, role of the host, or particular species or strains of microorganisms involved in the fusospirochetal infections.

Virulence factors associated with periodontopathic organisms

Recently Hammond and co-workers (1976) have described several molecular aspects related to the virulence of *Actinomyces viscosus* in rodent periodontal disease syndromes. They found a virulent strain and an avirulent strain of *A. viscosus* to differ in several properties. The virulent strain has a supercoiled circular species of extrachromosomal DNA, resembling a plasmid of about 4.5×10^6 daltons. The virulent strain also has proteinaceous surface appendages with the ultrastructural characteristics of pili, as well as a virulence-related cell-wall antigen containing the sugar 6-deoxy-L-talose (6-DOT). The nonvirulent strain on the other hand, lacks the pili and 6-DOT antigen, but it produces copious amounts of an extracellular heteropolysaccharide slime consisting of n-acetyl-glucosamine, glucose, and galactose (Hammond, 1977). The precise role of these strain differences in determining virulence is not clear at present; however, the virulent strain changes to the avirulent strain with reversion of the above properties and loss of pathogenicity.

Pathogenic potential of oral organisms in systemic diseases

Many strains of oral streptococci (e.g., "viridans" streptococci) have been implicated as colonizing organisms on damaged heart tissues in subacute bacterial endocarditis (SBE). There are also many anaerobic infections of oral and dental structures that may extend locally to the jaws, face, neck, and sinuses, or disseminate widely to the meninges or the bloodstream to produce serious infections or septicemias. A large number of oral organisms have been isolated from infections of the head and face, and these include many Bacteroides species such as *B. melaninogenicus, B. oralis, B. fragilis,* and *B. corrodens* and others such as *Actinomyces, Fusobacterium nucleatum, Spirillum sputigenum, Leptotrichia, Veillonella, Corynebacterium,* peptostreptococci, and anaerobic oral streptococci (Finegold, 1977). It is clear from the cultural data demonstrating oral organisms in many dental (facial as well as systemic) infections that they possess considerable pathogenic potential. Many oral organisms are potentially serious pathogens that in the state of health are kept in check by the flora and host defense mechanisms operative in the oral cavity. In the event of trauma or if a dental infection is untreated these organisms may enter the circulation or travel through tissues where they can and often do cause serious infections.

PATHOGENESIS OF PERIODONTAL DISEASE

The pathologic aspects of inflammatory gingival and periodontal disease have been studied in detail, and the overall features of the pathogenesis have been conveniently subdivided into four stages by Page and Schroeder (1976). These are the *initial* lesion, the *early* lesion, the *established* lesion, and the *advanced* lesion. The *initial* lesion exhibits features resembling an acute vasculitis in which the vessels subjacent to the junctional epithelium show evidence of increased permeability and a large number of polymorphonuclear leukocytes are found migrating through the vessels and junctional epithelium into the gingival crevice. These manifestations may be associated with the generation of vasoactive and chemotactic substances in the region of the gingival sulcus either through the complement system or mast cells or derived from bacteria directly. The next stage is termed the *early* lesion and is characterized by the presence of a dense infiltrate of small- and medium-sized lymphocytes immediately subjacent to the gingival sulcus. Also found are pathologic alterations in fibroblasts and loss of connective tissue substance beginning subjacent to the gingival epithelium. Subsequently the disease progresses to the third stage defined as the *established* lesion. In this stage plasma cells predominate but extensive bone destruction has *not* yet occurred. Some features of acute inflammation continue to persist. The nature of the cellular infiltrate and the presence of extravascular immunoglobulins and complement (Genco et al., 1974) at this stage have led to the concept that humoral immune mechanisms may play an important role in the observed tissue alterations. The *advanced* lesions are exceedingly complex and resemble in some respects those in other longterm chronic inflammatory diseases in which immune mechanisms are considered to play a major role. In the advanced lesion there are many of the features of the established lesions with plasma cells predominating and some acute inflammatory cells present. In addition there is marked alveolar bone resorption and continuing collagen destruction.

The common forms of periodontal disease, plaque-associated gingivitis and marginal periodontitis, can thus be considered to be both acute and chronic inflammatory processes.

It is clear from the evidence discussed previously in this chapter that microbial dental plaque that accumulates at the gingival margin serves as the source of inciting agents for periodontal tissue destruction. We will now discuss the possible mechanisms by which these microbial inciting agents bring about destruction of the periodontal tissues. Before discussing the mechanisms of tissue destruction several points should be kept in mind.

Role of dental calculus

There are most likely some factors involved in the *initiation* of periodontal disease and other factors involved in the *progression* of periodontal disease. For example, it is frequently suggested that the occurrence of subgingival calculus in periodontal pockets is a result and not a cause of periodontal disease. Certainly mineralization of dental plaque is not necessary for the induction of gingivitis. However, there is considerable clinical evidence that complete removal of subgingival calculus is necessary for resolution of periodontal pockets. It may well be that subgingival calculus is involved in the progression of a periodontal pocket providing a persistent nidus for the accumulation of more microbial plaque from which agents are released that cause tissue damage. Calculus is almost always covered with a noncalcified layer of microbial plaque.

Role of inflammatory processes

Gingivitis and marginal periodontitis are classified as inflammatory processes. Inflammation is a complex set of local changes that occur in living tissue after injury. The features of the inflammatory response depend on many factors, including the nature and intensity of the inciting agent, the anatomic location, and the condition of the host. There are, however, a limited number of ways in which the host can react to injury, and many events that occur in periodontal inflammation are similar to those that occur in inflammation in other parts of the body. Inflammation is generally regarded as a protective mechanism involving the events of vascular reaction, exudation, resolution, and repair. However, it is becoming apparent that many of the events occurring in inflammation are capable of causing considerable damage to the host tissues. For example, a microbial antigen that may not cause much tissue damage per se may gain access to the periodontal tissues and provoke an allergic inflammatory response that is markedly exaggerated in comparison to the inflammatory response that the antigen itself is capable of eliciting. This exaggerated inflammatory response may lead to considerable tissue breakdown and, if of a chronic nature, would *preclude* resolution and repair.

Studies of human gingiva in what is generally agreed to be a state of health, that is, freedom from grossly visible signs of disease such as erythema, edema, and tendency to hemorrhage, show evidence of certain inflammatory processes. It has been recognized for many years that the so-called clinically normal gingiva is infiltrated with varying numbers of inflammatory cells, with the mononuclear cells predominant in the gingival connective tissue and neutrophils predominant in the epithelial tissue. Rigorous plaque removal will result in the disappearance of most of these inflammatory cells, but this ''supernormal'' condition probably rarely exists except under experimental conditions where plaque removal is zealously performed.

Protective factors. There is evidence that the inflammatory elements present in the crevicular epithelium of normal gingiva can exert protective functions. Schroeder (1970) has shown that the epithelium of normal human gingiva contains large numbers of neutrophils that appear to be migrating between the epithelial cells of the junctional epithelium (but not the oral epithelial portion of the crevicular lining) into the gingival crevice, possibly in response to bacterial and complement-derived chemotactic factors. He presents morphologic evidence of neutrophils engaging in phagocytosis of crevicular bacteria. Using immunofluorescence, Genco and Krygier (1974) demonstrated immunoglobulin of the IgG class localized in the connective tissue and between the cells of the junctional epithelium of clinically normal gingiva (Fig. 3-16). There are few neutrophils and little or no immunoglobulin detectable in the oral epithelium that borders pars of the gingival crevice. It appears that both serum antibodies and neutrophils are passing between the cells of the junctional epithelium to come in contact with the crevicular bacteria.

Often sections of diseased gingival units with their content of subgingival bacteria and adjacent tooth surface intact show a layer of neutrophils interposed between the pocket or crevicular epithelium and the subgingival microbial flora. Bacteria and bacterial products from this subgingival flora must travel through this layer of neutrophils to gain access to the periodontal connective tis-

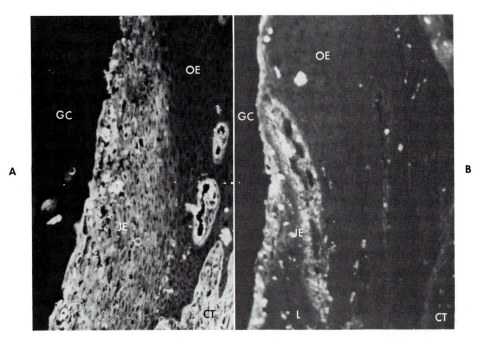

Fig. 3-16. Localization of immunoglobulin G in epithelium lining crevice of normal human gingiva. **A,** Area of junctional epithelium, *JE,* and oral epithelium, *OE,* treated with fluorescein-labeled antibodies to human IgG. Immunoglobulin is localized mainly in junctional epithelium and connective tissue, *CT,* no immunoglobulin is detectable in oral epithelium that lines part of gingival crevice, *GC,* in health. **B,** Another section of same gingiva as in **A.** Tissue was stained with same fluorescein-conjugated antibodies to IgG, except that reaction with tissue IgG is blocked by adding excess soluble IgG to reactions. Staining in junctional epithelium and connective tissue is specifically blocked, demonstrating specificity of staining in **A.** It should be noted that some bright spots in junctional epithelium represent nonspecific fluorescence of leukocytes, *L,* that are abundant in junctional epithelium. (**A** × 100; **B** × 100.)

sues and alveolar process. For example, bone-resorbing factors derived from bacteria such as endotoxin or lipoteichoic acid must travel through the neutrophil layer and the epithelium into the connective tissue before they get to the area of the alveolar process to exert their bone-resorbing effects. This is a long and involved pathway, and the neutrophils can be thought to act as the *first line of defense,* preventing not only whole bacteria but their products from entering the periodontal tissues. It is reasonable to expect that the crevicular or pocket neutrophils perform a neutralizing or barrier function; that is, they intercept or inactivate bacteria or bacterial products, preventing their entrance in toxic form into the periodontal tissues. This may explain why patients who do not have adequate numbers of or adequate functioning neutrophils have much more severe periodontal disease.

A protective role of the neutrophil is suggested by description of defective polymorphonuclear leukocyte functions in subjects with idiopathic localized juvenile periodontitis (periodontosis) by Cianciola and co-workers (1977) described above. These findings are of special importance since it appears that they are consistent with the experiments of nature in which neutrophil numbers or function are reduced and the periodontal disease is more severe. Cianciola, Genco, Patters, and McKenna (1977) have described a family with juvenile periodontitis in which both diseased (three sisters) and nondiseased (a younger brother and sister) siblings have similar neutrophil dysfunctions. This family study suggests that the neutrophil defects in juvenile periodontitis are inherited and predispose individuals in these families to early rapid alveolar bone loss. It is likely then that the polymorphonuclear leukocytes, especially the neutrophil, play a major role in protecting the host against severe periodontal insult by subgingival bacteria. The role of accessory factors such as antibody and complement, which enhance neutrophil protective functions, are also important but as yet largely undefined in periodontal disease. By better understanding the role of the neutrophil and its accessory factors in periodontal disease and the nature of defects in neutrophil function which occur in juvenile periodontitis, we may be able to intervene to restore neutrophil function with immunopotentiating substances and thereby increase host resistance to periodontal disease.

The state of ''health'' in the periodontal tissues can be represented, then, as a constant struggle between the host and the microbial flora that is attempting to accumulate in the gingival crevice. The host, by exerting local defense reactions, is able to cope with a low level of potentially damaging crevicular bacteria. If the crevicular bacteria increase in number or shift to a more virulent population of bacteria, then the host may not be able to cope with the inciting agents, and periodontal tissue destruction will occur. On the other hand, if the host's defenses are compromised as seen in individuals with depressed neutrophil function, periodontal infections may be more severe.

Oral hygiene

There appears to be a *threshold level* of microbial dental plaque that most individuals can tolerate without suffering destructive periodontal diseases. There is recent evidence to support the concept of a threshold from epidemiologic studies of Sheiham (1977). When relating oral hygiene scores to increments in periodontal disease there appears to be a low level of oral hygiene tolerated, which leads to little or no periodontal disease. However, once this level of oral hygiene is exceeded, there is a definite increment in periodontal disease. One might predict that if one or more of the important elements of the local defense mechanism were defective or absent in an individual, then this individual might have a *low* threshold level of plaque tolerance that would be clinically manifested as an exaggerated form of periodontal disease. Indeed, the severe periodontal disease seen in individuals with cyclic neutropenia and agranulocytosis may well result in part from their inability to cope with even small accumulations of subgingival plaque resulting from a lack of neutrophils.

Mechanisms of tissue destruction

The possible mechanisms that have been put forth over the years to explain periodontal tissue destruction can be divided into two categories: (1) factors elaborated by organisms that damage tissues directly and (2) factors that damage tissues indirectly by inciting host-mediated tissue destruction (Table 10).

The factors elaborated by microorganisms of dental plaque that can damage tissues directly are histolytic enzymes and cytotoxic agents. Collagenase, which is produced by *Bacteroides melaninogenicus,* is capable of hydrolyzing native collagen and may well lead to destruction of collagen in periodontal disease. Other enzymes such as hyaluronidase (which can hydrolyze hyaluronic acid and is produced by strains of diphtheroids,

Table 10. Possible mechanisms of tissue destruction in periodontal disease

Microbial dental plaque accumulation	
Direct effects	**Indirect effects**
Bacterial enzymes	Host enzymes
Collagenase	Collagenase
Hyaluronidase	Hyaluronidase
Chondroitin sulfatase	Antibody-mediated pathogenic effects
Proteases	Anaphylactic
Deoxyribonuclease	Cytotoxic
Ribonuclease	Arthus-type
Neuraminidase	Delayed hypersensitivity
Others	(lymphokines)
"Cytotoxic" agents	Activation of complement (chemo-
Endotoxin (gram negative)	tactants, vasoactive peptides, bone
Mucopeptides (gram positive)	resorption)
Ammonia	Kinin system
Hydrogen sulfide	Clotting system
Toxic amines	
Organic acids	
Bone resorption	
Stimulatory products	
Endotoxin	
Lipoteichoic acid	
Actinomyces factor(s)	

*Host mediated.

enterococci, *S. mitis,* and *S. salivarius*) and chondroitin sulfatase (which is produced by diphtheroids) may lead to destruction of the amorphous ground substance in periodontal disease. Several workers have shown that introduction of hyaluronidase into the gingival crevice will increase the permeability of the crevicular epithelium, presumably by hydrolyzing the ground substance between the epithelial cells, and thus facilitate passage of materials through this barrier. Other bacterial lytic enzymes such as neuraminidase, proteases, deoxyribonuclease, and ribonuclease have been shown to be present in dental plaque, and some have been shown to be produced by certain strains of plaque bacteria. The precise role of these bacterial histolytic enzymes in the pathogenesis of periodontal disease has not been established. They may cause considerable tissue alteration leading to increased epithelial and connective tissue permeability, which in turn allows other potent inciting agents access to the periodontal tissues.

Another group of bacterial substances have a direct cytotoxic effect on tissue cells. Cobb and Brown showed in 1967 that debris, or bacteria-free filtrates of debris from normal sulci or periodontal pockets, can induce degenerative changes in mammalian cells grown in culture. Among the plaque substances that exhibit cytotoxicity are endotoxins, mucopeptides derived from the cell walls of gram-positive organisms, ammonia, hydrogen sulfide, indole, toxic amines, and organic acids such as formic, acetic, and butyric acids. (For references to these substances, consult Socransky, 1970.) The potential for damage to periodontal tissues resulting from prolonged exposure to these cytotoxic factors is apparent. As yet, however, their exact role in human periodontal disease has not been established.

Another group of mechanisms that lead to tissue destruction are termed "indirect," since the bacterial component, which acts as the inciting agent, activates host effector systems, which in turn lead to the destruction of periodontal tissues. The inciting agent may lead to the production or activation of *endogenous histolytic enzymes*. It has been well established, for example, that the gingival tissue itself can produce collagenase and hyaluronidase, which may act to alter the integrity of the periodontal tissues.

INFLAMMATION

Inflammation has long been postulated as the mechanism for a considerable portion of periodontal tissue destruction. Certain microbial metabolites are capable of initiating inflammatory processes in the gingiva. For example, Temple et al. have described a potent chemotactic factor produced by many plaque bacteria, including *Actinomyces viscosus*. This factor is chemotactic for neutrophils and is relatively small, with a molecular weight of about 2,000. Its small size likely facilitates entry into the gingival crevice through enzyme altered crevicular epithelium. This factor and others, such as the chemotactic factors released upon activation of the complement system by endotoxin or by antigen-antibody reactions, probably account for the neutrophils seen in the gingiva (Schenkein and Genco, 1977a and b). As discussed earlier many of these neutrophils may be involved in protective functions; however, there is evidence that neutrophils can also lead to tissue destruction. They contain lysosomal enzymes that will digest phagocytosed microorganisms. If these lysosomal enzymes are released into the tissues they can cause considerable tissue destruction. Studies from the laboratories of Taichman and colleagues (1976) have shown that bacteria or clumps of dental plaque can cause release of polymorphonuclear leukocyte–lysosomal enzymes, and that this enzyme release can be enhanced if complement and antibody directed to the bacteria are present. They have shown that lysosomal release can occur in the absence of phagocytosis. This is of special interest in the gingival crevice region where only occasional neutrophils are observed to have phagocytosed bacteria. Phagocytosis of clumped bacteria such as found in plaque is a relatively rare event whereas bacteria free in suspension are more readily phagocytosed.

Endotoxin. Endotoxin, a lipopolysaccharide obtained from gram-negative organisms, including *Veillonella, Bacteroides, Fusobacterium, Leptotrichia, Selenomonas,* and spirochetes, is a potent inducer of inflammation. It appears that many of its toxic effects result from its ability to activate a number of host effector systems such as complement, the clotting system, and the kinin system. Rizzo and Mergenhagen (for review see Mergenhagen et al., 1969) have shown that submicrogram amounts of endotoxin injected into the skin or mucosa of an animal leads to a prompt increase in vascular permeability, vascular dilation, and accumulation of polymorphonuclear leukocytes followed by accumulation of small lymphocytes and mononuclear leukocytes. Their careful experiments give substantial support to the concept that many of these effects result from activation of the complement system by endotoxin. When endotoxin reacts with complement, activated components are released that lead to enhanced vascular permeability, chemotaxis, and smooth muscle contraction. The end result of activation of the complement system on the surface of a cell is cell lysis and death (see Simon et al., 1971).

Endotoxin purified from *Bacteroides melaninogenicus,* as well as from *Salmonella* and *Escherichia coli,* was found by Hausmann et al. to stimulate bone resorption in tissue cultures. The mechanism by which endotoxin stimulates bone resorption is not yet known; however, it appears from their experiments that complement and known inflammatory processes are not involved.

Other bacterial substances also have been shown by Hausmann and co-workers (1977, 1974) to stimulate bone resorption. These include lipoteichoic acid from gram-positive organisms and soluble substances from *Actinomyces viscosus* and *Actinomyces naeslundii*.

IMMUNOPATHOLOGIC MECHANISMS

Immunopathologic mechanisms have been put forth as contributing to tissue destruction in some forms of periodontal disease. A number of bacterial antigens when applied to the periodontium will induce so-called allergic inflammation in animals. Human studies have shown that periodontal patients have circulating antibodies and immediate hypersensitivity to a number of oral organisms, and the studies of Ivanyi and Lehner (1970) have shown evidence of delayed hypersensitivity to antigens of several oral organisms in patients with gingivitis and moderate periodontitis. The potential for immunopathologic mechanisms to play a role in periodontal pathology is clear. Antigens are abundant in dental plaque; periodontal tissues can exhibit immunologic reactivity; and experimental periodontal disease has been induced in animal models by immunologic means.

ALLERGIC REACTIONS

Allergic (hypersensitivity) reactions capable of inducing tissue damage have been classified by Gell and Coombs into four categories. The first three, *anaphylactic, cytotoxic,* and *Arthus-type* (or antigen-antibody complex) reactions, require some form of detectable serum antibody, whereas the fourth type, *delayed* (or *cell-mediated*) *hypersensitivity,* occurs in the absence of circulating antibody. This classification was proposed several years ago but it still represents a useful, if simplified, accounting of events in immunopathologic

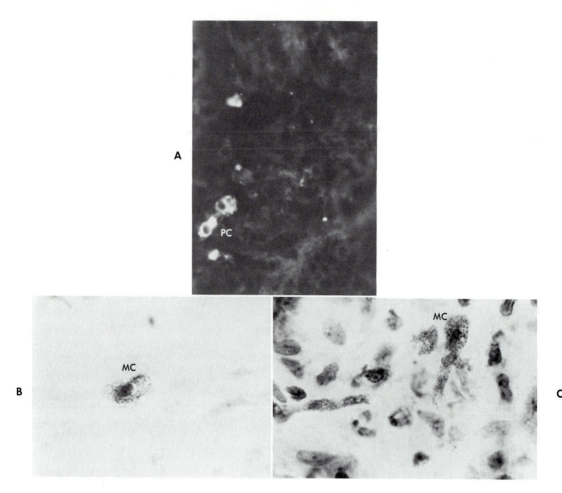

Fig. 3-17. Connective tissue of inflamed human gingiva. **A,** Plasma cells, *PC,* containing immunoglobulin E or reagin as detected by immunofluorescent technique. **B** and **C,** Mast cells, *MC,* of different shapes whose granules are stained with methyl green–thionin stain. (**A** × 500; **B** × 1000.)

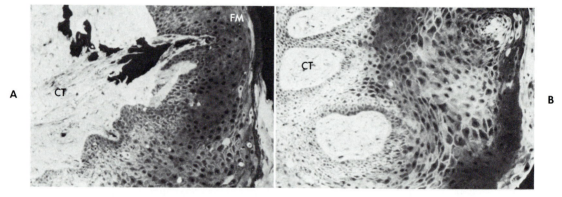

Fig. 3-18. Localization of immunoglobulin G in epithelium and connective tissue of inflamed human gingiva. **A,** Keratinized free marginal gingiva, *FM,* blending into crevicular epithelium. **B,** Inflamed crevicular epithelium lining periodontal pocket. **A** and **B,** Localization of immunoglobulin G between cells of inflamed crevicular epithelium and in connective tissue. Little or no immunoglobulin G is detectable in keratinized epithelium at margin of gingiva. (× 100.)

reactions. It should be kept in mind, however, that there are many interactions among the various immunopathologic reactions, and that it is rare for any one of these reactions to occur alone.

Anaphylactic or reagin-dependent reactions. In the anaphylactic type of reaction, reaginic antibodies, mainly of the IgE class of immunoglobulins, fix strongly to cells. Upon subsequent challenge with antigen, pharmacologically active substances such as histamine, slow-reacting substance of anaphylaxis (SRS-A), bradykinin, and eosinophil chemotactic factor of anaphylaxis are released from these cells. The substances released induce vascular and smooth muscle changes, some of which are inhibited by antihistamines. It appears that basophil leukocytes and tissue mast cells are the main cell types that are capable of binding the IgE reaginic antibodies. The presence of IgE-containing cells in human gingiva and the evidence of a decrease in numbers of gingival mast cells with inflammation (Fig. 3-17) suggest that anaphylactic reactions may occur in human periodontal tissues.

It should be noted that there are other ways by which mast cells can be made to degranulate. For example, C5a, an activation product of the fifth component of complement, will cause mast cells to degranulate and release their contents. Also factors released from neutrophils upon ingestion of immune complexes or phagocytosis of bacteria will also cause mast cells to release their contents.

Cytotoxic reactions. Antibodies react directly in cytotoxic reactions with antigens that are bound to tissue cells. These antigens may be natural components of the cell, or they may be foreign antigens bound to tissue cells. These foreign antigens may be derived from bacteria, drugs, or altered tissue components. So-called cytotoxic antibodies react with the cell-associated antigens and lead to tissue damage by cell lysis or release of lysosomal antigens from cells coated with antigens. Tissue damage in the area would then result. Cytotoxic antibodies may be of the IgG or IgM class, and complement is usually activated when these antibodies bind to the cell-associated antigens. There is little direct evidence for the occurrence of cytotoxic reactions in the gingival tissues. Antigen and extravascular IgG (Fig. 3-18) have been found in the connective tissue and epithelium of inflamed gingival tissues. Complement, IgG, and IgM have been demonstrated in gingival crevicular fluid by Brandtzaeg (1965). Schenkein and Genco (1977) have measured the levels of immunoglobulins, complement components, and other proteins im-

portant in inflammatory reactions such as α-2-HS-glycoprotein, α-1 antitrypsin, transferrin, and α-2 macroglobulin in the gingival fluid and serum of patients with advanced periodontal disease (Table 11). They found that the gingival fluid concentrations of these macromolecules ranges from 65% to 85% of the serum concentration. However, the one substance that is markedly different from all of the others is C3, the third component of complement. Native C3 is present in gingival fluid at only 25% of its serum concentration, suggesting that C3 and likely the terminal components of the complement system (C5 to C9) are activated. In addition, they found that C3d, an activation product of C3, is present in gingival fluid in substantial amounts. They also showed that C3 proactivator, a component of the alternate complement pathway, was activated in gingival fluids. An interesting difference in complement activation between periodontitis and periodontosis was also found. They found that the fourth component of complement C4 is activated *only* in gingival fluid of juvenile periodontitis patients but *not* in gingival fluid from those with periodontitis.

These studies imply that the alternate as well as classic pathways of the complement system may be activated in gingival fluid. Alternatively, the fragments detected may have resulted from proteolytic degradation. It is likely that the components of the complement system found in gingival fluid come mainly from the blood vessels of the

Table 11. Gingival fluid inflammatory macromolecules*

Component	Gingival fluid concentration as a percent of serum concentration ($\overline{X} \pm 1$ SEM)†
IgG	85.4 ± 6.6
IgA	71.8 ± 4.5
IgM	75.3 ± 9.0
Transferrin	70.0 ± 7.6
α-1 antitrypsin	71.4 ± 5.19
α-2 macroglobulin	65.7 ± 3.5
α-2-HS-glycoprotein	79.0 ± 5.3
C3 proactivator	85.2 ± 1.0
C4	62.4 ± 4.3
C3	23.0 ± 1.8

*Adapted from Schenkein, H. A., and Genco, R. J.: J. Periodontol. In press.
†Measurements made by radial immunodiffusion. Gingival fluid taken from deep infrabony pockets from subjects with advanced periodontitis; note marked reduction in native C3 levels.

gingiva. They travel through the connective tissue and crevicular or pocket epithelium into the gingival crevice or pocket and somewhere along this pathway are activated. Complement activation may occur in cytotoxic reactions, with the antigen-antibody complexes on cells such as fibroblasts. or epithelial cells activating complement. There are many other possibilities for complement activation, including activation of the alternate pathway by endotoxin and carbohydrates of bacteria, immune complexes, or proteolytic enzymes.

Arthus or antigen-antibody complex reactions. The Arthus-type of immunopathologic reaction is dependent on the formation of complexes of antigen and antibody usually in slight antigen excess. These complexes form microprecipitates in and around small blood vessels that lead to activation of complement and subsequent tissue damage. The Arthus reaction, unlike anaphylaxis, is not inhibited by antihistamines, and it appears that the release of pharmacologically active mediators is not important for tissue destruction. Inflammation, hemorrhage, and later necrosis characterize the experimentally induced Arthus reaction in skin. Tissue damage appears to be a consequence of the liberation of histolytic enzymes from the large number of neutrophils that migrate to the area. Immune complement activation with release of leukocyte chemotactic factors may account for the neutrophil infiltration.

Freedman et al. (1968) demonstrated extracellular lysosomal bodies in connective tissue and in the dilated intercellular spaces of inflamed human gingiva. Although many mechanisms lead to lysosomal release, it is not unreasonable that neutrophil lysosomes are released into human gingival tissues as a result of an Arthus-type reaction.

Delayed or cell-mediated hypersensitivity. In delayed hypersensitivity, classic serum antibody has not been shown to participate; instead, the sensitized lymphocyte appears to be essential for the pathologic effects seen. When lymphocytes taken from an individual who manifests delayed hypersensitivity are challenged with antigen, they undergo blast transformation and produce several soluble factors with marked biologic activity. One of these factors, called macrophage-inhibiting factor (MIF), prevents the migration of macrophages in vitro and when injected in vivo intradermally produces a mononuclear reaction typical of delayed hypersensitivity. Another factor that is chemotactic for monocytes has been found to be produced by lymphocytes. This factor, along with MIF, may play a role in the accumulation and persistence of mononuclear cells at a site of delayed hypersensitivity. Lymphotoxin is elaborated by lymphocytes after stimulation by antigen, and this protein may be responsible for much of the tissue damage at sites of delayed hypersensitivity. There are other lymphokines produced by lymphocytes that may result in capillary vasodilation, edema, and neutrophilic infiltration. Ivanyi and Lehner (1970) and Horton et al. (1974) present evidence for the presence of circulating lymphocytes sensitive to oral microbial antigens in humans with periodontal disease. Patters and co-workers (1976) have shown that cell-mediated immunity as measured by lymphocyte stimulation induced by substances in dental plaque, as well as various organisms isolated from plaque including *Actinomyces naeslundii, Bacteroides melaninogenicus,* and *Leptotrichia buccalis,* appears to follow the pattern expected for infecting antigens. For example, normal lymphocytes from individuals who have little or no periodontal disease react weakly to the above antigens in the lymphocyte blastogenesis assay (Table 12). Patients with gingivitis react to *Actinomyces* and *Leptotrichia* but seldom react to *Bacteroides,* whereas those with periodontitis react to all three organisms. Edentulous sub-

Table 12. Cell-mediated immunity as measured by the lymphocyte blastogenic response to oral bacterial antigens*†

	Percent with positive lymphocyte blastogenic response			
Stimulating antigen	Normal	Gingivitis	Periodontitis	Edentulous
Actinomyces viscosus	20	92	77	67
Bacteroides melaninogenicus	0	14	62	0
Leptotrichia buccalis	29	43	75	0

*Adapted from Patters, M. R., Genco, R. J., Reed, M. J., and Mashimo, P. A.: Infect. Immun. **14:**1213, 1976.
†Subjects' lymphocytes were cultured with the appropriate antigenic mixture. The incorporation of tritiated thymidine was measured as an indication of blastogenesis induced by the antigen.

jects (who have no periodontal disease) only react to *Actinomyces*. This is consistent with the bacteriologic picture where *B. melaninogenicus* is found in the subgingival flora in periodontitis but in small numbers in the flora of gingivitis patients. *Actinomyces* is found in both conditions as well as in the edentulous mouth. It appears that the lymphocyte blastogenic assay, as a measure of cellular immunity, parallels the microbial findings in various states of periodontal disease and health and may be a reflection of antigenic stimulation through the gingival epithelium by prominent gingival organisms. Sensitized lymphocytes observed in the peripheral blood likely migrate to the gingival region. Here they may come into subsequent contact with antigens diffusing from the plaque. The antigens then stimulate the local sensitized lymphocytes to differentiate into plasma cells or produce lymphokines or do both. Some of these lymphokines such as lymphotoxin or osteoclast-activating factor can cause local periodontal tissue destruction.

Ivanyi and co-workers (1973) have reported specific serum factors that enhance lymphocyte blastogenesis in patients with gingivitis and serum factors that suppress blastogenesis in patients with severe periodontitis. These observations raise the possibility of humoral control of cellular immunity in periodontal disease.

The extent to which cell-mediated immunity plays a role in periodontal disease is suggested by several studies of periodontal disease in immunologically deficient or immunologically suppressed individuals. Individuals who have lymphocyte function suppressed such as those who have T- or B-lymphocyte deficiencies are found to have less periodontal disease than immunologically competent controls matched for age and oral hygiene (Robertson et al., 1977). These results suggest that lymphocyte-mediated immunity contributes to the pathogenesis and the chronicity of periodontal lesions. This is in marked contrast to the more severe periodontal syndromes observed in individuals with neutrophil deficiencies. It appears then that lymphocyte-mediated responses may contribute to the *pathogenesis* of periodontal disease, whereas the net effect of neutrophils is *protective*.

It should be noted that although anaphylactic, cytotoxic, Arthus-type, and delayed hypersensitivity reactions can be demonstrated as discrete processes in certain diseases and in experimental models, it is possible that various combinations of these reactions account for some of the pathology seen in periodontal disease. One of the striking features of the chronic inflammatory infiltrate in periodontal disease is the numerous lymphocytes and plasma cells that accumulate in the gingival connective tissue (Fig. 3-19). Exogenous microbial antigens, although reportedly present in inflamed gingival tissues, are not prominent. It is possible that the immunocompetent gingival inflammatory cells are responding to autologous material usually inaccessible or that has been altered by the inflammatory response and is functioning as antigen.

Comment regarding role of bacteria in alveolar bone loss

Two lines of evidence suggest that the bacteria of dental plaque are necessary for periodontal bone loss. One is the demonstration of alveolar bone re-

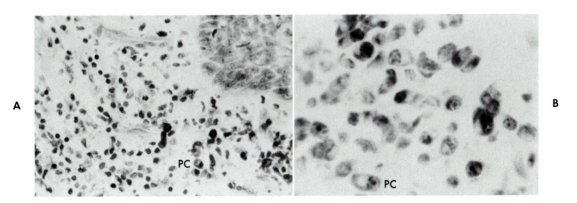

Fig. 3-19. Inflammatory cells in chronically inflamed human gingiva. **A,** Accumulation of lymphocytes and plasma cells, *PC,* beneath crevicular epithelium. **B,** Area of plasma cells found in gingival connective tissue. Note typical cartwheel eccentric nucleus, prominent Golgi area, and abundant cytoplasm. (Methyl green–thionin stain; **A** × 100; **B** × 1000.)

sorption in the hamster and gnotobiotic rat models of periodontal disease, and the other consists of the cross-sectional studies of human periodontal disease that show a direct correlation between the amount of dental debris and alveolar bone loss. Neither of these approaches gives a very good indication of the mechanism of microbially induced bone resorption. Rizzo and Mergenhagen (1964) demonstrated the attraction of osteoclasts to bone in response to injections of endotoxin. As mentioned, Hausmann et al. (1970) demonstrated that endotoxin is a potent stimulus to bone resorption even in the absence of inflammation. Another mechanism of bone resorption that may be operative in alveolar bone resorption has recently been described. Complement-sufficient serum but not complement-deficient serum has the capacity to induce bone resorption (Hausmann et al., 1973). Complement activation leads to increased prostaglandin levels in bone culture, and this parallels increased bone resorption (Raisz et al., 1974). Both prostaglandin production and bone resorption

in organ culture can be prevented by the addition of indomethacin, an inhibitor of prostaglandin synthetase. Immune complexes and endotoxin and other bacterial components through the alternate pathway may activate complement, stimulating bone resorption by this mechanism.

Another immune mechanism that can stimulate bone resorption is production of the lymphokine osteoclast–activating factor by lymphocytes upon stimulation of either mitogens or antigens as described by Horton et al. (1972). These findings lead to the concept that bacterial endotoxin or bacterial antigens could, either alone (as in the case of endotoxin) or in the presence of specific antibody and complement, stimulate alveolar bone resorption.

SUMMARY

Most forms of gingivitis and periodontitis are of bacterial etiology. Some species of bacteria cause a periodontal syndrome in gnotobiotic animals.

It is clear that a prerequisite for most forms of

Table 13. Immunologic profile of subjects with periodontal diseases

Test	Subject group		
	Gingivitis	Periodontitis	Juvenile periodontitis (periodontosis)
Antibodies	Present to most oral organisms; may enhance lymphocyte blastogenic response (Ivanyi et al., 1973; Mashimo et al., 1976)	Present to most oral organisms; may be elevated to certain organisms e.g., *A. viscosus* (Nisengard, 1974) May suppress lymphocyte blastogenic response in severe cases (Ivanyi et al., 1973; Mashimo et al., 1976)	IgG and IgM levels may be elevated in some (Lehner et al., 1974)
Gingival fluid complement		C3 and C3pa are activated; C4 is *not* activated (Schenkein and Genco, 1977a and b)	C3, C3pa and C4 are activated (Schenkein and Genco, 1977a and b)
Cellular immunity	Strong blastogenic response to *Actinomyces;* weak to *Bacteroides melaninogenicus* (Patters et al., 1976)	Strong blastogenic response to *Actinomyces* and to *Bacteroides melaninogenicus* (Patters et al., 1976)	Strong blastogenic response to *Actinomyces*
Polymorphonuclear leukocytes Chemotaxis and phagocytosis	Normal	Normal	Reduced (Cianciola et al., 1977)

periodontal disease is the accumulation of microbial dental plaque in the area of the gingival crevice, and hence procedures directed to preventing periodontal disease must result in regular removal of plaque.

The mechanisms by which microbial dental plaque leads to destruction of the gingiva, cementum, periodontal ligament, and alveolar bone and changes in the cementum are not completely elucidated. It appears that bacteria can exert direct effects on the periodontal tissues by production of histolytic enzymes and cytotoxic agents. Agents from microbial dental plaque are also capable of stimulating host-mediated responses that can lead to destruction of the periodontal tissues. Some host-mediated effects include the release of endogenous histolytic enzymes, activation of the complement, clotting, and kinin systems, and induction of immunopathologic process.

Table 13 presents a summary of immunologic tests that differentiate various forms of periodontal disease. Based upon these differences we have developed an immunologic profile of subjects with periodontal disease that aids in diagnosis and understanding of host responses. In the future these profiles may also have prognostic significance. For example, the role of the neutrophil is emerging from the understanding of experiments of nature in which neutrophil numbers or defects are noted and also from studies of neutrophil function in juvenile periodontitis. It is clear from these studies that alterations in neutrophil protective function or reduction in neutrophil numbers, either grossly as occurs in agranulocytosis or intermittently as occurs in cyclic neutropenia, leads to increased susceptibility to periodontal infections.

From our present understanding of the role of the neutrophil and the lymphocyte and of the mechanisms of bone resorption it is clear that there are several avenues of intervention possible that might be pursued in restoring or enhancing host responses or intercepting pathogenic mechanisms. For example, if neutrophil defects can be corrected, then one might increase resistance to periodontal disease. If, as it appears, lymphocyte hypersensitivity (cellular immunity) contributes to the destructive aspects of periodontal disease, then suppressing this response may decrease the pathology seen in periodontal disease. Present methods to suppress lymphocyte-mediated immunity have multiple and serious side effects that may preclude their use in managing periodontal disease. Interfering with the mechanism of release of mediators from cells, particularly those that cause bone resorption, appears to be another valid approach. One such mediator is prostaglandin. The synthesis of this mediator by prostaglandin synthetase can be interfered with by the use of indomethacin and related salicylates such as aspirin. These approaches in the future may prove beneficial in moderating inflammatory pathologic changes seen in periodontal disease.

At the present time regular removal of microbial dental plaque is the most practical method of preventing both the initial occurrence and progression of periodontal disease. Careful analysis of the mechanisms by which microbial dental plaque leads to tissue destruction may lead to the future development of specific agents capable of blocking these mechanisms; alternatively, a better understanding of host defense mechanisms may allow us to restore these when defective or augment them when normal to prevent periodontal diseases.

REFERENCES

Araujo, W. C., de, Varah, E., and Mergenhagen, S. E.: Immunochemical analysis of human oral strains of Fusobacterium and Leptotrichia, J. Bacteriol. **86**:837, 1963.

Brandtzaeg, P.: Local factors of resistance in the gingival area, J. Periodont. Res. **1**:19, 1966.

Brandtzaeg, P.: Immunochemical comparison of proteins in human gingival pocket fluid, serum, and saliva, Arch. Oral Biol. **10**:796, 1965.

Brandtzaeg, P., and Kraus, F.: Autoimmunity and periodontal disease, Odontol. Tskr. **73**:285, 1965.

Brill, N.: The gingival pocket fluid, Acta Odontol. Scand. **20**(suppl. 32):1, 1962.

Burnett, G. W., Scherp, H. W., and Schuster, G.: Oral microbiology of infectious diseases, ed. 4, Baltimore, 1976, The Williams & Wilkins Company.

Cianciola, L. J., Genco, R. J., Patters, M. R., and McKenna, J.: A family study of neutrophil chemotaxis in idiopathic juvenile periodontitis (periodontosis), A.A.D.R. Program and Abstract of papers, J. Dent. Res. **56B**(abstr. 155):90, 1977.

Cianciola, L. J., Genco, R. J., Patters, M. R., McKenna, J., and van Oss, C. J.: Defective polymorphonuclear leukocyte function in a human periodontal disease, Nature **265**:445, 1977.

Cobb, C. M., and Brown, L. R.: The effects of exudate from the periodontal pocket on cell culture, Periodontics **5**:5, 1967.

Cohen, D. W., Friedman, L. A., Shapiro, J., Kyle, G. C., and Franklin, S.: Diabetes mellitus and periodontal disease. I. Two-year longitudinal observations, J. Periodontol. **41**:709, 1970.

Crawford, A., Socransky, S., and Bratthall, G.: Predominant cultivable microbiota of advanced periodontitis, Abstract no. 209, A.A.D.R. Program and Abstract of papers, 1975.

Darwish, S., Hyppa, T., Manganiello, A. D., and Socransky, S.: Predominant cultivable microorganisms in periodontitis and periodontosis, Abstract no. 289, I.A.D.R. Program and Abstract of papers, 1973.

Darwish, S., Hyppa, T., and Socransky, S.: Predominant cultivable organisms in early periodontitis, J. Periodont. Res. In press.

Dick, D. S., and Shaw, J. R.: The infectious and transmissible nature of the periodontal syndrome of the rice rat, Arch. Oral Biol. **11:**1095, 1966.

Finegold, S. M.: Anaerobic bacteria in human disease, New York, 1977, Academic Press, Inc.

Freedman, H. L., Listgarten, M. A., and Taichman, N. S.: Electron microscope features of chronically inflamed human gingiva, J. Periodont. Res. **3:**313, 1968.

Gell, P. G. H., and Coombs, R. R. A., editors: Clinical aspects of immunology, ed. 2, Philadelphia, 1968, F. A. Davis Co.

Genco, R. J.: Immunoglobulins and periodontal disease, J. Periodontol. **41:**6, 1970.

Genco, R. J., Evans, R. T., and Ellison, S. A.: Dental research in microbiology with emphasis on periodontal disease, J. Am. Dent. Assoc. **78:**1016, 1969.

Genco, R. J., and Krygier, G.: Localization of immune cells, immunoglobulins and complement in human gingiva, J. Periodont. Res. (suppl. 10):30, 1972.

Genco, R. J., Mashimo, P. A., Krygier, G., and Ellison, S. A.: Antibody-mediated effects on the periodontium, J. Periodontol. **45:**330, 1974.

Gibbons, R. J., Socransky, S. S., Sawyer, S., Kapsimalis, B., and Macdonald, J. B.: The microbiota of the gingival crevice area of man. II. The predominant cultivatable organisms, Arch. Oral Biol. **8:**281, 1963.

Hammond, B. F.: Personal communication, 1977.

Hammond, B. F., Steel, C. F., and Peindl, K. S.: Antigens and surface components associated with virulence of *Actinomyces viscosus,* J. Dent. Res. **55:**A19, 1976.

Hausmann, E.: Potential pathways for bone resorption in human periodontal disease, J. Periodontol. **45:**338, 1974.

Hausmann, E., Genco, R. J., Weinfeld, N., and Sacco, R.: Effects of serum on bone resorption in tissue culture, Calcif. Tissue Res. **13:**311, 1973.

Hausmann, E., Levine, M. J., and Chen, P.: Factor(s) from *Actinomyces viscosus* and *naeslundii* which stimulate bone resorption in organ culture, Abstract no. 106, I.A.D.R. Program and Abstract of papers, 1977.

Hausmann, E., Raisz, L. B., and Miller, W. A.: Endotoxin: stimulation of bone resorption in tissue culture, Science **168:**862, 1970.

Hausmann, E., Weinfeld, N., and Miller, W. A.: Effects of lipopolysaccharides on bone resorption in tissue culture, Calcif. Tissue Res. **9:**272, 1972.

Holdeman, L. V., and Moore, W. L. C.: Anaerobe Laboratory Manual, ed. 3, Anaerobe Laboratory, Virginia Polytechnical Institute and State University, Blacksburg, Virginia, 1975.

Horton, J. E., Oppenheim, J. J., and Mergenhagen, S. E.: A role for cell-mediated immunity in the pathogenesis of periodontal disease, J. Periodontol. **45:**351, 1974.

Horton, J. E., Raisz, L. G., Simmons, H. A., Oppenheim, J. J., and Mergenhagen, S. E.: Bone resorbing activity in supernate fluid from cultured human peripheral blood leukocytes, Science **177:**793, 1972.

Howell, A. J., Jordan, H. V., Georg, L. K., and Pine, L.: Odontomyces viscosus, Gen Nov, Spec Nov: a filamentous microorganism isolated from periodontal plaque in hamsters, Sabouraudia **4:**65, 1965.

Hungate, R. E.: A roll tube method for cultivation of strict anaerobes. In Norris, J. R., and Ribbons, D. W., editors: Methods in Microbiology, 3B, New York, 1969, Academic Press, Inc., p. 117.

Irving, J. T., Newman, M. G., Socransky, S. S., and Heeley, J. D.: Histologic changes in experimental periodontal disease in rats monoinfected with a gram-negative organism, Arch. Oral Biol. **20:**219, 1975.

Irving, J. G., Socransky, S. S., Newman, M., and Savit, T. E.: Periodontal destruction induced by capnocytophagia in gnotobiotic rats, J. Dent. Res. **55:**abstract no. 783, 1976.

Ivanyi, L., Challacombe, S. J., and Lehner, T.: The specificity of serum factors in lymphocyte transformation in periodontal disease, Clin. Exp. Immunol. **14:**491, 1973.

Ivanyi, L., and Lehner, T.: Stimulation of lymphocyte transformation by bacterial antigens in patients with periodontal disease, Arch. Oral Biol. **15:**1089, 1970.

Ivanyi, L., Wilton, J. M. A., and Lehner, T.: Cell-mediated immunity in periodontal disease: cytotoxicity, migration inhibition in lymphocyte transformation studies, Immunology **22:**141, 1972.

Jordan, H. V., and Keyes, P. H.: Aerobic, gram-positive, filamentous bacteria as etiologic agents of experimental periodontal disease in hamsters, Arch. Oral. Biol. **9:**401, 1964.

Jordan, H. V., and Hammond, B. F.: Filament-forming bacteria in human cervical caries, Abstract no. 193, I.A.D.R. Program and Abstract of papers, 1971.

Keyes, P. H., Hicks, M. A., Goldman, B. M., McCabe, R. M., and Fitzgerald, R. J.: Dispersion of dextranous bacterial plaques on human teeth with dextranase, J. Am. Dent. Assoc. **82:**136, 1971.

Keyes, P. H., and Jordan, H. V.: Periodontal lesions in the Syrian hamster. III. Findings related to an infectious and transmissible component, Arch. Oral Biol. **9:**377, 1964.

Keyes, P. H., and Likins, R. C.: Plaque formation, periodontal disease and dental caries in Syrian hamsters, J. Dent. Res. **25:**166, 1946.

Kleinberg, I.: Biochemistry of the dental plaque, Adv. Oral Biol. **4:**43, 1970.

Klinkhamer, J. M.: Human oral leukocytes, Periodontics **1:**109, 1963.

Krasse, B.: Oral aggregations of microbes, J. Dent. Res. **42:**521, 1963.

Lambe, D. W., Jr., and Jerris, R. C.: Description of a polyvalent conjugate and new serogroup of *Bacteroides melaninogenicus* by fluorescent antibody staining, J. Clin. Microbiol. **3:**506, 1976.

Lehner, T., Wilton, J. M. A., Ivanyi, L., and Manson, J. D.: Immunological aspects of juvenile periodontitis (periodontosis), J. Periodont. Res. **9:**261, 1974.

Lindhe, J., Hamp, S. E., and Löe, H.: Plaque-induced periodontal disease in beagle dogs: a four-year roentenographical and histometrical study, J. Periodont. Res. **10:**243, 1975.

Lindhe, J., and Nyman, S.: The effect of plaque control and surgical pocket elimination on the establishment of maintenance of periodontal health: a longitudinal study of periodontal therapy in cases of advanced disease, J. Clin. Periodontol. **2:**67, 1975.

Lindhe, J., and Svanberg, G.: Influence of trauma from occlusion on progression of experimental periodontics in the beagle dog, J. Clin. Periodontol. **1:**3, 1974.

Listgarten, M. A.: Structure of the microbial flora associated with periodontal health and disease in man, J. Periodontol. **47:**1, 1976.

Listgarten, M. A.: Electron microscopic observations on the bacterial flora of acute necrotizing ulcerative gingivitis, J. Periodontol. **36:**328, 1965.

Listgarten, M. A., Johnson, D., Nowotny, A., Crawford, A., and Socransky, S.: Pathogenesis of periodontal disease in rats monoinfected with *E. corrodens,* Abstract no. 120, I.A.D.R. Program and Abstract of papers, 1977.

Löe, H.: A review of the prevention and control of plaque. In McHugh, W. D., editor: Dental plaque, Edinburgh, 1970, E. & S. Livingstone.

Löe, H., and Silness, J.: Periodontal disease in pregnancy. I. Prevalence and severity, Acta Odontol. Scand. **21:**533, 1963.

Löe, H., and Schiott, C. R.: The effect of suppression of the oral microflora upon the development of dental plaque and gingivitis. In McHugh, W. D., editor: Dental plaque, Edinburgh, 1970, E. & S. Livingstone.

Löe, H., Theilade, E., Jensen, S. B., and Schiott, C. R.: Experimental gingivitis in man. III. The influence of antibiotics on gingival plaque development, J. Periodont. Res. **2:**282, 1967.

Löe, H., Theilade, E., and Jensen, S. B.: Experimental gingivitis in man, J. Periodontol. **36:**177, 1965.

Loesche, W. J., Hockett, R. N., and Syed, S. A.: The predominant cultivable flora of tooth surface plaque removed from institutionalized subjects, Arch. Oral Biol. **17:**1311, 1973.

Mandel, I. D.: Dental plaque: nature, formation and effects, J. Periodontol. **37:**357, 1966.

Manganiello, A. D., Socransky, S., Smith, C., Propas, D., Oram, V., and Dogon, I. L.: Attempts to increase viable count recovery of human supergingival dental plaque, J. Periodont. Res. **12:**107, 1977.

Mashimo, P., Genco, R. J. and Ellison, S. A.: Antibodies reactive with *Leptotrichia buccalis* in human serum from infancy to adulthood, Arch. Oral Biol. **21:**277, 1976.

McDougall, W. A.: Studies on the dental plaque. I. The histology of the dental plaque and its attachment, Aust. Dent. J. **8:**261, 1963.

Mergenhagen, S. E., Snyderman, R., Gewarz, H., and Shin, H. S.: Significance of complement to the mechanism of action of endotoxin, Curr. Top. Microbiol. Immunol. **50:**37, 1969.

Mitchell, D. F., and Holmes, L. A.: Topical antibiotic control of dentogingival plaque, J. Periodontol. **36:**202, 1965.

Moore, W. E. C.: Techniques for routine culture for fastidious anaerobes, Int. J. Syst. Bact. **16:**173, 1966.

Mouton, C., Nisengard, R. J., Mashimo, P. A., Evans, R. T., and Genco, R. J.: Immunofluorescent identification of the filamentous component of the "corn-cob" configuration in supragingival human plaque, A.A.D.R. Program and Abstract of papers, J. Dent. Res. **56B**(abstr. 286):123, 1977.

Murayama, Y., and Mashimo, P. A.: Commensal relationship between oral strains of Eubacterium and Veillonella, A.A.D.R. Program and Abstract of papers, J. Dent. Res. **56B**(abstr. 285):123, 1977.

Newman, M., and Socransky, S. S.: Predominant cultivable microbiota in periodontosis, J. Periodont. Res. **12:**120, 1977.

Nisengard, R. J.: Immediate hypersensitivity and periodontal disease, J. Periodontol. **45:**344, 1974.

Nisengard, R. J., Beutner, E. H., and Gauto, M.: Immunofluorescence studies of IgE in periodontal disease, Ann. N.Y. Acad. Sci. **177:**39, 1971.

Page, R. C., and Schroeder, A. G.: The pathogenesis of chronic inflammatory periodontal disease, Lab. Invest. **34:**235, 1976.

Patters, M. R., Genco, R. J., Reed, M. J., and Mashimo, P. A.: Blastogenic response of human lymphocytes to oral bacterial antigens: comparison of individuals with periodontal disease to normal and edentulous subjects, Infect. Immun. **14:**1213, 1976.

Pearlman, B. A.: An oral contraceptive drug in gingival enlargement: the interrelationship between local and systemic factors, J. Clin. Periodontol. **1:**1, 1974.

Poole, A. E., and Gilmour, M. N.: The variability of unstandardized plaques obtained from single or multiple subjects, Arch. Oral Biol. **16:**681, 1971.

Raisz, L. G., Sandberg, A. L., Goodson, J. M., Simmons, H. A., and Mergenhagen, S. E.: Complement dependent stimulation of prostaglandin synthesis and bone resorption, Science **185:**789, 1974.

Ritz, H. L.: Microbial population shifts in developing human dental plaque, Arch. Oral Biol. **12:**1561, 1967.

Rizzo, A. A.: Absorption of bacterial endotoxin into rabbit gingival pocket tissue, Periodontics **6:**65, 1968.

Rizzo, A. A., and Mergenhagen, S. E.: Histopathologic effects of endotoxin injected into rabbit oral mucosa, Arch. Oral Biol. **9:**659, 1964.

Robertson, P. B., Wright, T. L., Mackler, B. F., Lenertz, D. M. and Levy, B. M. Oral status of patients with abnormality of the immune system, J. Dent. Res. **56B**(abstr. 160): 93, 1977.

Rosebury, T.: Microorganisms indigenous to man, New York, 1962, McGraw-Hill Book Company.

Russell, A. L.: Epidemiology of periodontal disease, Int. Dent. J. **17:**282, 1967.

Sacco, R., Hausmann, E., and Genco, R. J.: Immunologically activated factors: stimulation of bone resorption in tissue culture, J. Dent. Res., Int. Assoc. Dent. Res., Abst., 370, 140, 1972.

Saxe, S. R., Greene, J. C., Bohannan, H. M., and Vermillion, J. R.: Oral debris, calculus and periodontal disease in the beagle dog, Periodontics **5:**217, 1967.

Schei, O., Waerhaug, J., Lovdal, A., and Arno, A.: Alveolar bone loss as related to oral hygiene and age, J. Periodontol. **30:**7, 1959.

Schenkein, H. A., and Genco, R. J.: Gingival fluid and serum in periodontal disease. I. Quantitative study of immunoglobulins, complement components and other plasma proteins, J. Periodontol. **48:**772, 1977.

Schenkein, H. A., and Genco, R. J.: Gingival fluid and serum in periodontal disease. II. Evidence for activation of complement components C3, C3 proactivator and C4 in gingival fluid, J. Periodontol. **48:**778, 1977.

Schroeder, H. E.: The structure and relationship of plaque to the hard and soft tissues: electron microscopic interpretation, Int. Dent. J. **20:**353, 1970.

Schroeder, H. E.: Formation and inhibition of dental calculus, Berne, 1969, Hans Huber Medical Publisher.

Schroeder, H. E., and DeBoever, J.: The structure of microbial dental plaque. In McHugh, W. D., editor: Dental plaque, Edinburgh, 1970, E. & S. Livingstone.

Schuldtz-Haudt, S., Bruce, M. A., and Bibby, B. G.: Bacterial factors in non-specific gingivitis, J. Dent. Res. **33:**454, 1954.

Sharawy, A. M., Sabharwal, K., Socransky, S. S., and Lobene, R. R.: A quantitative study of plaque and calculus formation in normal and periodontally involved mouths, J. Periodontol. **37:**495, 1966.

Sheiham, A.: Personal communication, 1977.

Simon, B. I., Goldman, H. M., Ruben, M. P., and Baker, E.: The role of endotoxin in periodontal disease. III. Correlation of the amount of endotoxin in human gingival exudate with the histologic degree of inflammation, J. Periodontol. **42:**210, 1971.

Skinner, F. A., and Carr, J. G.: The normal microbial flora of man, London and New York, 1974, Academic Press, Inc.

Slack, J. M., and Gerenger, M. A.: Two new serological groups of Actinomyces, J. Bacteriol. **103:**265, 1970.

Slots, J.: The predominant cultivable microflora of advanced periodontitis, Scand. J. Dent. Res. **85:**114, 1977a.

Slots, J.: Microflora in the healthy sulcus of man. Scand. J. Dent. Res. **85:**247, 1977b.

Slots, J.: The predominant cultivable organisms in juvenile periodontitis, Scand. J. Dent. Res. **84:**1, 1976.

Socransky, S. S.: Personal communication, 1977.

Socransky, S. S.: Relationship of bacteria to the etiology of periodontal disease, J. Dent. Res. **49**(suppl. 2):203, 1970.

Socransky, S. S., Gibbons, R. J., Dale, A. C., Bortnick, L., Rosenthal, E., and Macdonald, J. B.: The microbiota of the gingival crevice area of man. I. Total microscopic and viable counts of specific organisms, Arch. Oral Biol. **8:** 275, 1963.

Socransky, S. S., Manganiello, A. D., Oram, J. V., Propas, D., Dogan, I. L., and Van Houte, J.: Development of early dental plaque, J. Dent. Res., Int. Assoc. Res. Abst., 502, 178, 1971.

Stallard, R. E., Volpe, A. R., Orban, J. E., and King, W. J.: The effect of an antimicrobial mouthrinse on dental plaque, calculus, and gingivitis, J. Periodont. Res. suppl. 4, abst. no. 32, 1969.

Svanberg, G., Lindhe, J., Hugoson, A., and Grondahl, H. G.: The effect of nutritional hyperparathyroidism on experimental periodontitis in the dog, Scand. J. Dent. Res. **81:**155, 1973.

Taichman, N. S.: Inflammation and tissue injury. I. The response to intradermal injections of human dentogingival plaque in normal and leukopenic rabbits, Arch. Oral Biol. **11:**1385, 1966.

Taichman, N. S., and McArthur, W. P.: Interaction of inflammatory cells on oral bacteria: release of lysosomal hydrolases from rabbit polymorphonuclear leukocytes exposed to gram-positive plaque bacteria, Arch. Oral Biol. **21:**257, 1976.

Temple, T. R., Snyderman, R., Jordan, H. V., and Mergenhagen, S. E.: Factors from saliva and oral bacteria, chemotactic for polymorphonuclear leukocytes: their possible role in gingival inflammation, J. Periodontol. **41:**3, 1970.

Theilade, E., Wright, W. H., Jensen, S. B., and Löe, H.: Experimental gingivitis in man. II. A longitudinal clinical and bacteriological investigation, J. Periodont. Res. **1:**1, 1966.

Van Campen, G. J., Wouters, S. L. J., Mikx, F. H. M., and Van der Hoeven, J. S.: The occurrence of ANUG in a beagle dog colony, J. Dent. Res., Int. Assoc. Dent. Res. Abst. no. 12, 56, A45, 1977.

Van Houte, J., Gibbons, R. J., and Banghart, S. B.: Adherence as a determinant of the presence of *Streptococcus salivarius* and *Streptococcus sanguis* on the human tooth surface, Arch. Oral Biol. **15:**1025, 1970.

Williams, B. C., Pantalone, R. M., and Sherris, J.: Subgingival microflora and periodontitis, J. Periodont. Res. **11:**1, 1976.

Zachrisson, B. V.: Mast cells of the human gingiva. IV. Experimental gingivitis, J. Periodont. Res. **4:**55, 1968.

4 Inflammatory periodontal disease: etiology and additional local influences

Unlike many chronic diseases with acute variances, periodontal disease is not a single entity nor is there a single causative factor that elicits a consistent periodontal response. The term encompasses a host of periodontopathies, each presenting definite clinical and histologic profiles and each resulting from a melange of etiologic factors. To evaluate the various inflammatory and degenerative periodontal lesions one must first have a thorough understanding of the embryology, anatomy, histology, and biology of the periodontal tissues in health. The practitioner is charged with assisting in maintaining that degree of normality. In order to accomplish this goal it is essential to have an awareness of the potential factors that contribute to periodontal disease and to prevent, arrest, control, or eliminate such factors before they are able to provoke irreversible disease changes.

We are faced with a multitude of primary and secondary local contributory factors, each having the capability to act as a coantagonist to periodontal health. Furthermore, the general systemic state of the host will influence the periodontal response and repair potential.

CLASSIFICATION

Historically, etiologic factors affecting periodontal health have been classified as local, occlusal, and systemic. The *local factors* present an environmental alteration that predisposes to inflammatory periodontal disease. *Occlusal factors* also present an environmental alteration but they predispose to degenerative periodontal disease. *Systemic factors* occur as (1) oral manifestations such as dermatologic diseases, (2) altered host response as seen in some endocrinopathies, or (3) an extension of a systemic dysfunction as seen in blood dyscrasias. Rarely will one find a clinical periodontopathy where there is only a single etiologic factor operating. Local factors are responsible for the majority of periodontal diseases affecting both the gingival unit and the attachment apparatus. Occlusal factors have the attachment apparatus alone as their primary target. There are a host of local, occlusal, and systemic factors working in consort to produce the clinical entity. Although this chapter is divided into specific discussions for a systematic presentation, the reader must constantly be aware of the interdependence of local, occlusal, and systemic etiology.

PREVENTION

Many of the coantagonists to be reviewed have iatrogenic overtones. Therefore the therapist has a degree of control over many factors contributing to inflammatory periodontal disease, while having less influence over factors contributing to degenerative lesions. With this understanding in mind the dentist's role in preventive periodontics becomes obvious.

Prevention is the ultimate goal in health sciences, and it has come of age in dentistry with the disclosure of etiology. Yet our dependence upon patients as cotherapists in maintaining health still exists, and their vulnerability is ever present. To achieve success in preventive periodontics as it is practiced today we require a behavioral change in our patients. If this change could be made so that optimum plaque control could be achieved, then we could direct our attention toward establishing an environment suitable for health maintenance: one that would prevent the initiation of periodontal disease and promote the maintenance of oral health.

PRIMARY FACTOR IN INFLAMMATORY PERIODONTAL DISEASE: PLAQUE

The classic work of Löe et al. (1965) showed that the sine qua non of inflammatory periodontal disease is dentobacterial plaque. The causal relationship of plaque as the covert antagonist to periodontal health has been thoroughly demonstrated in Chapter 3. Host reaction to this etiologic factor presents a wide range of response. In the adaptation syndrome proposed by Selye (1951) the constant or repeated exertion of a series of etiologic factors on the host eventually exceeds the tolerance. The coup de grace (i.e., irreversible damage) follows in inflammatory periodontal disease when etiologic factors remain undetected or ignored. Their effect over a period of time passes beyond the capacity of the host to resist. It is of paramount importance to disclose and reverse the factors producing the histopathologic changes early in the genesis of the disease process.

Additional local factors contributing to inflammatory and degenerative results include (1) factors propagating plaque retention and accumulation, (2) anatomic aberrancies (3) habits, and (4) mechanical, thermal, and biochemical factors.

Factors propagating plaque retention and accumulation

For their role in enhancing plaque retention and accumulation the following factors are the most frequently found contributors to inflammatory periodontal disease. Our understanding of these factors has improved so that the age-old beliefs that overhangs and calculus cause gingivitis by mechanical injury have given way to the knowledge that they enhance plaque accumulation and retention, which in turn initiate inflammation.

Root surfaces. The topography of the root is important in maintaining plaque control. On gross evaluation, coronal or radicular niches and concavities become harbors for plaque accumulation and cannot be reached with present-day therapeutic aids.

The relative smoothness of the root surface has been demonstrated utilizing the profilometer and scanning electron microscope (Kerry, 1967; van Valkenburg, 1976). Yet there is conflict in the literature concerning the effect of root roughness on the accumulation of accretions. Several authors (Taylor and Campbell, 1972; Turesky and Glickmen, 1961; Waerhaug, 1956) suggest that root roughness contributes to increased deposition while another team (Rosenburg and Ash, 1974) found that root roughness could not be related to plaque or inflammatory indices.

The modes of attachment of deposit proposed by Zander (1954) and by Moskow (1969) and presented later in this discussion deal with rough or broken surfaces. Therefore it appears probable that a smoother surface is easier to maintain.

Inadequate restorations. Restorative procedures can affect the periodontal tissues in several ways: (1) destruction can occur during tooth preparation, (2) restorations can initiate periodontal response from inadequacies in contours, contacts, and marginal adaptation, (3) materials can elicit allergic tissue response, and (4) faulty restorations can cause plaque accumulation and induce degenerative periodontal disease from poor occlusal relationships. Probably the greatest single cause of a restorative procedure evoking an adverse periodontal response is the failure to obtain periodontal health prior to restorative involvement. Restorative procedures in the presence of periodontal disease preclude proper marginal finish and contours. Tissue preparation and management are essential prior to definitive restorative dentistry.

The selection of restorative material is often considered essential when the preparation approaches the gingival tissues. Larato (1971) found that silicate restorations approximating the gingival margin caused an increase in plaque accumulation and a concomitant increase in periodontal inflammation. Sotres et al. (1969) in a histologic and clinical study comparing amalgam, silicate, and resin restorations found an elevated inflammatory response related to unfinished margins. There was an increase in dentobacterial plaque associated with rough margins regardless of the restorative material. Myers (1975), evaluating stainless steel crowns, and Frank et al. (1975), in an ultrastructural study of gold foils, report that the inflammatory responses increased with an increase in plaque indices coincident with rough margins. The evidence suggests that the manner in which a restoration is finished is more important than the choice of material.

The position of a restorative margin as it relates to preventive dentistry has been the subject of controversy. Richter and Ueno (1973) evaluated the gingival response of gold crowns when one half the margin was placed subgingivally and the other half placed supragingivally. After a 2-year period no difference was found in the periodontal response, and they concluded that the fit and finish of the margin were more important than its location. Noble et al. (1973) report that subgingival margins are more difficult to finish and thus lead to plaque retention. Mörmann et al. (1974) supported this finding in comparing rough subgingival inlays to those that had been polished. In a series of papers Silness (1970, 1974) and Silness and Ohm (1974) report a consistent increase in the plaque index, gingival index, and pocket depth when margins were placed subgingivally. Supragingival margins had a peri-odontal response that equaled controls. Newcomb (1974) found that inflammatory responses increase the closer a margin is to the base of the gingival crevice. He suggests that margins should terminate at the gingival crest or just into the sulcus.

When caries or aesthetics are not factors that demand additional extention, restorative margins should be kept at the coronal portion of the sulcus. At this location they can be adequately finished and maintained in daily hygiene.

Overhangs. One of the most frequently found factors enhancing plaque accumulation is overhanging restorations. Regardless of the type or choice of material used, overhangs become reservoirs for the accumulation and retention of dento-

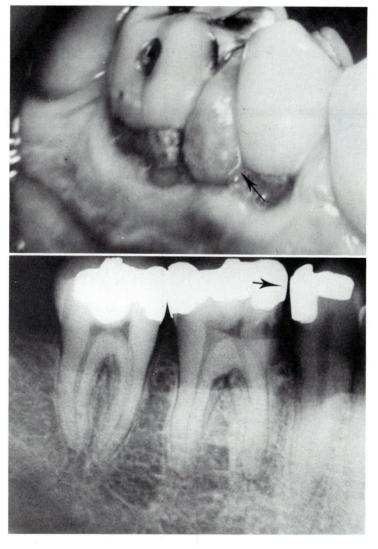

Fig. 4-1. Clinical and radiographic evidence of an inadequate contact with impaction and retention of debris with resultant gingival response.

bacterial plaque. They create a defective surface, difficult if not impossible to maintain. Björn et al., evaluating metal restorations (1969) and gold restorations (1970) statistically showed an increase in alveolar bone loss in areas directly associated with overhanging margins. Gilmore and Sheilam (1971) report finding a greater severity of periodontal destruction in subjects with overhanging restorations. Plaque, gingival, and periodontal indices including bone loss increase proportionately with an increase in defective or overhanging margins (Fig. 4-1).

The restored *contours, contacts,* and *marginal ridge levels* also play a role in the accumulation and retention of dentobacterial plaque. The ultimate goal in an isolated restorative procedure is

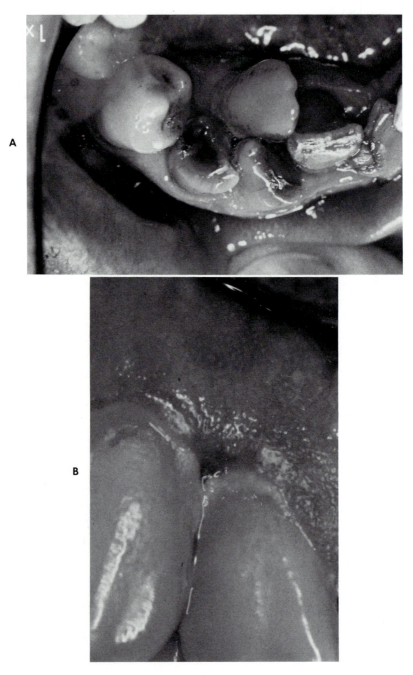

Fig. 4-2. A, Overcrowding, facilitating plaque accumulation and retention. **B,** Long, crowded contact requiring special attention in plaque control.

an attempt to replace that which has been lost so that this area can continue to contribute to the total unit. Many authors have presented papers on the so-called ideal anatomic considerations in restorative dentistry (Burch, 1971; Hazen and Osborne, 1967).

Interdental contours should be designed to join their proximal counterparts in a circumscribed area at the midcoronal third of the tooth. This position allows interdental cleansing, and the firm contact area will prevent food impaction and retention.

The buccal, lingual, mesial, and distal contours should follow the principles of pro re nata (i.e., that which is needed to maintain health). There is an overwhelming tendency to overcontour coronal architecture in restorative dentistry regardless of the reduction used in the preparation. Such overcontouring leads to plaque accumulation and potential periodontial breakdown. Recent studies by Townsend (1976), Sackett and Gildenhuys (1976), and Parkinson (1976) show that the cause of inflammatory disease associated with overcontours is not from gingival stagnation as often reported, but from increased accumulations of dental plaque in such areas.

A fact that becomes sadly evident in reviewing the aforementioned literature on the relationship of restorations to inflammatory periodontal disease is the percentage of inadequate restorations: 31% to 83%. The reasons for such inadequacies are varied, but the figures do emphasize the degree of control that the dentist has and must maintain in preventive periodontics.

Tooth position. Overcrowding of teeth often contributes to the accumulation of plaque and hampers its removal (Fig. 4-2). Gould and Picton (1966) reported that spacing rather than over-crowding caused more severe periodontal breakdown. However, Buckley (1972) and Paunio (1975) studied the periodontal response to overcrowding and found an increase in deposit and inflammation when compared with controls.

Tooth position relative to the dental arch, that is, buccal or lingual version, or mesial or distal tipping, create plaque traps. Osseous ledges, present in osteophytic protrusions, exostoses, odontomas, or oblique ridges also form regions where accretions tend to remain (Fig. 4-3). It is important that areas of compromised topography be disclosed; oral hygiene can then be altered to accommodate plaque control.

Removable partial dentures can affect periodontal health adversely in three ways (Bissada et al., 1974; Christidou et al., 1973; Nordquist and McNeill, 1975; Rudd, 1972; Weintraub and Goual, 1976):

1. Mechanical irritation (pressurized impingement) from dentures can cause gingival sloughing and even osseous destruction (Figs. 4-4 and 4-5). Irritation can occur on a lingual surface associated with base material, a facial surface where a retainer is present, or on the edentulous ridge associated with an abutment tooth.

2. Dentures can cause plaque niches where denture materials approximate gingival tissues.

3. Occlusal and retentive denture designs can become traumatogenic to the attachment apparatus.

Bissada et al. (1974) have shown that the degree of relief and the choice of metal base material evoke a reduced gingival response when compared with partial dentures having no relief or those made with acrylic base materials.

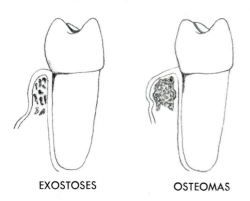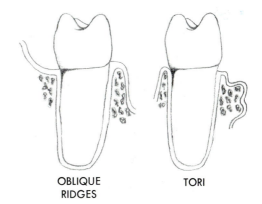

EXOSTOSES   OSTEOMAS   OBLIQUE RIDGES   TORI

Fig. 4-3. Underlying topography creating dentogingival junctions with distorted architecture.

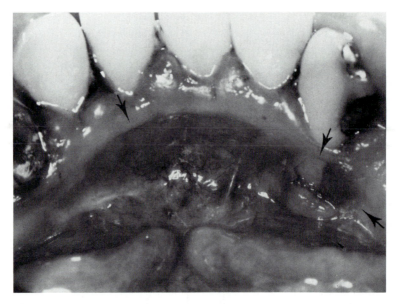

Fig. 4-4. Partial denture trauma with pressure necrosis from lingual bar.

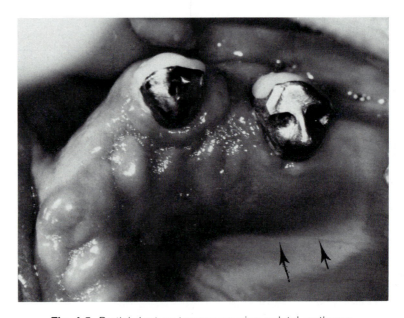

Fig. 4-5. Partial denture trauma causing palatal erythema.

Of specific consideration is the use of the Dolber or Baker's bar under partial dentures. It is essential that this be placed out of contact with marginal gingiva and designed to allow complete cleansing of the area (Fig. 4-6).

The amount of adherence of plaque to partial dentures and removable orthodontic appliances makes it essential for the dentist to instruct patients with appliances about plaque control.

Food impaction. Contours and contacts lacking minimal required anatomic topography predispose to food impaction and retention. Hirschfeld (1930) defined food impaction as the ''forceful wedging of food against the gum tissue through occlusal

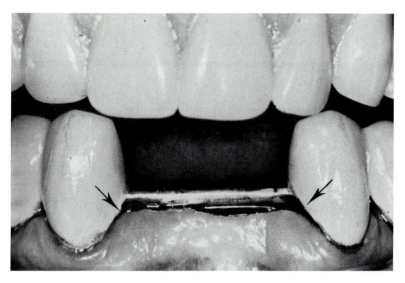

Fig. 4-6. Dolber or Baker's bar used in a combination fixed-removable prosthesis must be designed to allow cleansing at dentogingival junctions *(arrows)*.

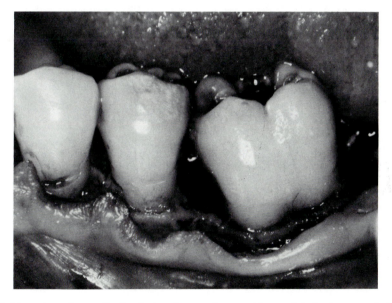

Fig. 4-7. Unreplaced mandibular first molar predisposed to mesial displacement of second molar and creating (1) an inadequate interdental contact, (2) a poor marginal ridge relationship (both enhancing food impaction), (3) an occlusal abnormality, and (4) a pseudo-vertical osseous defect that parallels cementoenamel junctions of approximating teeth.

pressure.'' He furthermore classified vertical food impaction relative to etiologic factors:

Class I   Occlusal wear
Class II   Loss of proximal support
Class III Extrusion of a tooth beyond the occlusal plane
Class IV   Congenital morphologic abnormalities
Class V   Improperly constructed restorations

Areas of interproximal contact and marginal ridge relationships can be altered by occlusal wear and supraeruption (Barker, 1975; Williams, 1949). Open proximal surfaces result from caries, inadequate restorations, and drifting of periodontally involved teeth. Unreplaced teeth create both inter-arch and intra-arch alteration. The resultant supra-

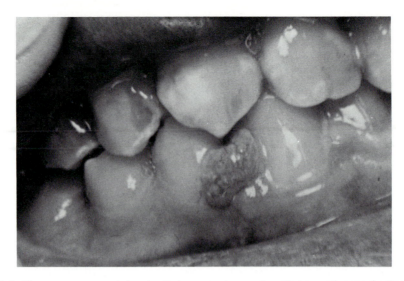

Fig. 4-8. Plunger cusp wedging teeth in opposing arch with impaction and retention of debris. Note tissue response.

eruption alters both the interproximal contact and marginal ridge relationship in the involved arch; it predisposes to occlusal factors in its relationship to the opposing arch. Furthermore, mesial or distal drifting of teeth into an edentulous site alters the contact area and marginal ridge relationships. It also establishes a crestal bone pattern parallel to the cementoenamel junctions of the approximating teeth (Ritchey and Orban, 1953). This pseudovertical defect can become an etiologic factor in the propagation of periodontal disease (Fig. 4-7).

Plunger cusps. A pronounced cusp with steep, inclined planes can initiate a wedging effect on the interproximal area in the opposing arch. Receptive axial forces become pathogenic torquing forces, and the etiologic factor has been called a "plunger cusp" (Fig. 4-8). A similar situation occurs when a Class II division II occlusal exists and there are minimum maxillary incisal cingula. Here a wedging effect is established on the palatal aspect of maxillary anteriors and on the labial aspect of mandibular anterior teeth.

There is horizontal or lateral component to food impaction. This can occur when there are large interdental areas existing naturally or resulting from periodontal disease, dental caries, abrasion, erosion, or surgical pocket elimination. In addition there is a narrow band of attached gingiva with its adjacent shallow vestibule. Food is directed into the fornix where muscular activity from the tongue, lips, and cheeks can force sections of the bolus into the interproximal areas, where they are retained.

The modus operandi of periodontal disease re-sulting from food impaction was usually attributed to mechanical trauma. Although this explanation should not be completely discounted (Larato, 1975), more recent findings suggest that the retention of impacted food acts as a medium for bacterial metabolism. It therefore becomes a nutritional cofactor in the etiology of inflammatory periodontal disease. Resultant symptoms of food impaction such as pressure, vague pain, and occlusal complaints suggest a functioning mechanical component. Chronic inflammation, abscess formation, foul taste and odor, bone destruction, and caries support the position that food retention enhances bacterial colonization.

Orthodontic appliances. Fixed appliances alter the coronal anatomy of a tooth in such a way that most of the functional attributes of the dentition are impaired. Mechanical plaque control is grossly changed, and tissue reaction is universal. In a series of papers Kloehm and Pfeifer (1974) and Zachrisson and Zachrisson (1972a and b) demonstrated that fixed appliances increased gingival and plaque indices and produced marked tissue hyperplasia especially in the interproximal areas. However, these changes were reversible, and tissue returned to normal 4 months after removing the bands. Zachrisson (1972) extended this same study to a histologic evaluation and reported a reversal of inflammatory cell infiltrate and proliferative epithelial changes after termination of orthodontic treatment. The articles support the fact that plaque and not mechanical irritation is the provocateur of gingival health although mechanical irritation should not be entirely discounted.

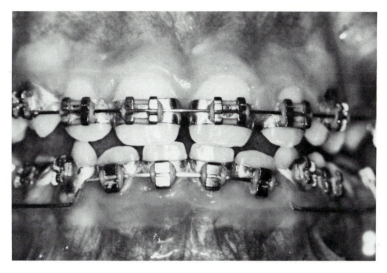

Fig. 4-9. Orthodontic appliances act as debris traps and require alterations in oral hygiene for effective plaque control.

Oral hygiene. The prevalence of inflammatory dental disease would change drastically with the use of a suitable antiplaque agent. Until that time we are charged with motivating our patients to adopt and practice mechanical plaque removal. This would include the thorough disengagement of accumulation on five surfaces of every tooth. It must be impressed upon dentulous individuals that it is their obligation to remove deposits consistently to prevent adverse tissue response. The primary cause of plaque accumulation is the lack of knowledge, skill, and desire on the part of the patient to remove such deposits (Fig. 4-9). It is our duty to alter those three variables. The techniques and the effect of oral hygiene in controlling gingival and periodontal indices are covered in Chapter 18.

Nutrition. Food acts as a local contributory factor in three ways: (1) it acts regionally as a medium for bacterial growth of supragingival microorganisms, (2) it contributes systemically as a medium for subgingival bacteria via the serum, and (3) it has recently been shown that some food extracts are capable of causing a cellular immune response and thus initiating periodontal disease.

Physical consistency. There is no foundation for the statement that fibrous foods either remove plaque or prevent its formation. Screebny (1975) showed that physical consistency of food does not alter oral cleanliness nor degree of keratinization. Studies by Lindhe and Wicen (1969) and by Longhurst and Berman (1973) using carrots or apples as the source of fibrous food failed to show any significant plaque reduction. Arnim (1963) reported a 3% to 19% plaque reduction when subjects chewed fibrous foods. However, the gingival margins and interdental areas showed no reduction in accumulation.

Self-cleansing. The previously mentioned studies would suggest a reevaluation of the highly accepted term "self-cleansing area." An examination of a subject undergoing an experimental gingivitis study (Arnim, 1963; Hazen and Osborne, 1967; Löe et al., 1965) shows that there is little or no natural cleansing activity below the coronal third of the tooth. The apical two thirds and pits and fissures are areas of plaque accumulation and retention when avoided in daily hygiene. *Self-cleansing* should be used to denote the methods used by an individual in contrast with *professional cleansing,* or the methods employed by the dentist (Fig. 4-10).

Substrate. Ingested foods act as a medium for the generation of bacteria and the development of plaque. Egelberg (1965) and Loesche (1968) in tube-feeding studies demonstrated that when food bypassed the oral cavity the metabolism of supragingival plaque was altered. Some bacterial types increased, some decreased, but no specific pattern was presented. In Loesche's study as well as in a report by Geddes and Jenkins (1974) carbohydrates, proteins, fats, and the frequency of eating influenced the constituency of the flora. Caldwell (1962) suggested that food has to be reduced in solution before it can be metabolized by resident organisms and form toxic products of etiologic significance.

Several papers have demonstrated the role of specific foodstuffs on the oral flora. Sugars appear to be of utmost importance for normal plaque

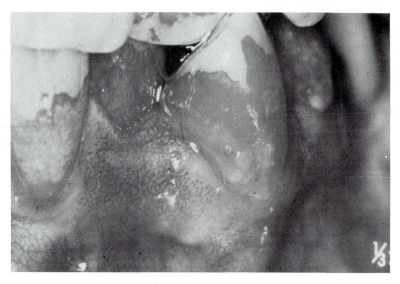

Fig. 4-10. Experimental gingivitis studies show that there is no self-cleansing mechanism in interdental or apical third of dentition.

metabolism. Glucose increases the rate of plaque formation (Critchley and Bowen, 1970) and the number of cariogenic bacteria (Drucker, 1970). Sucrose causes a drastic reduction in the pH of plaque (Mühlemann and DeBoever, 1970). Both sugars increase the formation of extracellular polysaccharides. The medium for plaque is complex. Eliminating one amino acid at a time does not affect bacterial composition (Inward et al., 1970).

The second method, when food acts as a local contributory cofactor, utilizes a systemic pathway (Alfano, 1976). The components of the diet can affect the subgingival microflora by its systemic assimilation and distribution in the bloodstream. It contributes to the local media via the gingival fluids that bathe the sulcular environment.

• • •

Once plaque begins to form, all factors leading to its development contribute to continued deposition. In addition to the above-mentioned factors calculus, caries, and the periodontal pocket support additional plaque accumulation.

Calculus. With an increase in the specificity of experimental parameters in recent years dentobacterial plaque and host response have replaced calculus as the primary etiologic factor in inflammatory periodontal disease. The role of calculus deposits in initiating periodontal disease by means of mechanical trauma is not valid. However, the ability of calculus to propagate plaque accumulation and the toxicity of these accretions cannot be overemphasized. It is for these reasons and the fact that calcification occurs where plaque already exists that the lithogenic processes should be studied (Löe et al., 1965; Schroeder and Bambauer, 1966). Mineralization of dental plaque begins 4 to 8 hours after deposition of the bacterial deposit (Tibbetts and Kashiwa, 1970). All dental plaque, however, does not undergo calcification, and gnotobiotic studies have shown that a calculus deposit can be found in the absence of plaque (Heneghan and Listgarten, 1973; Theilade et al., 1964). However, this germ-free calculus results when calcium salts are deposited in an organic salivary precipitate. This chalky, scalelike substance forms rapidly and crumbles quite easily.

Classification. Clinically, calculus has been classified as to its position relative to the gingival margin. *Supragingival calculus* relies on salivary minerals for its calcification. Although stains from tobacco, food, and bacterial metabolism can cause alterations, supragingival calculus is usually grey-white to grey-yellow. It can be found in any plaque-forming area on the tooth or appliance although it is most common in areas of salivary pooling. These would include the lingual aspect of lower anterior teeth, the labial and interproximal surfaces of the lower anterior teeth in tongue thrusters, and the baccal and interproximal surfaces of maxillary molars proximal to the orifice of Stensen's duct (Fig. 4-11).

Subgingival calculus varies in color and texture. It is harder, tenacious, and darker. It varies from green-brown to grey-black and is not affected by ingested food or tobacco at the local level. Differences between the two types of calculus

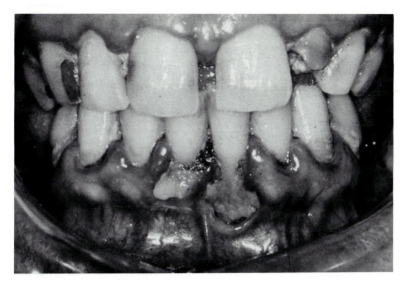

Fig. 4-11. Supragingival calculus acting as nidus for continued accumulation of materia alba and plaque.

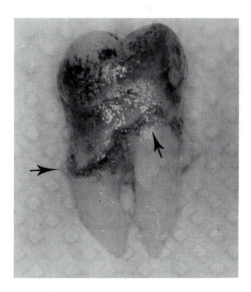

Fig. 4-12. Centric layer of subgingival deposit that lined periodontal pocket coronal to epithelial attachment (junctional epithelium).

suggest separate origins. It is the current consensus that subgingival calculus derives its components from gingival fluid and not from saliva (Stewart and Radcliff, 1966). It is therefore termed "serumnal calculus" in distinction from supragingival or salivary calculus. Differences in the supragingival and subgingival floras may also explain the differences in color and texture of the two deposits. Although their sources of inorganic salts are different they share a common mechanism of formation. Since subgingival deposit is found as a by-product of gingival fluid,

this accretion is probably a resultant and a propagator rather than an initiating factor in inflammatory periodontal disease (Fig. 4-12).

Composition. Calculus is composed of varying amounts of inorganic salts deposited in an organic matrix. The organic components of mature calculus consist essentially of carbohydrates and proteins in complexes of glycoproteins, mucoproteins, and acid mucopolysaccharides. Desquamated epithelial cells, bacteria, and leukocytes complete the organic content. Proteins from saliva contain most if not all amino acids. Lipids are present as cholesterol ester, phospholipids, free fatty acids, and neutral fats. Percentage composition of each food group varies as to location and chronicity of the deposit. Carbohydrates account for 1% to 9%, protein occupies 30% to 40%, and lipids account for 0.2% to 0.5% of the major organic matter (Little et al., 1966, 1964).

The inorganic segment of calculus contains calcium phosphate, calcium carbonate, magnesium phosphate, and many trace elements. Calcium accounts for 40% phosphorous and 20% magnesium for 0.8% of the major inorganic complex.

Leung and Jensen (1958) have demonstrated that approximately 70% of the inorganic structure is crystalline. Electron microscopy and x-ray diffraction studies demonstrate a combination of four distinct phosphate crystals. In descending order of percentage composition they are—

Hydroxyapatite
Brushite
Whitlockite
Octocalcium phosphate

The proportion of crystal present in a deposit is influenced by the age of the calculus, the location in the oral cavity, the location relative to the gingival margin, and the mineral component in the subject's oral cavity and systemic circulation (Schroeder, 1969; Schroeder and Bambauer, 1966; Schwartz and Masler, 1971). Early calculus and supragingival deposits consist primarily of brushite and octocalcium phosphate. Whitlockite is more common in posterior and subgingival deposits. These differences have been attributed to protein and mineral differences when comparing gingival fluid with saliva.

Development. The process of calculus formation has been described by a host of authors (Listgarten, 1975; Mandel, 1974a and b; Mislowsky and Mazella, 1974; Schroeder and Bambauer, 1966; Tibbetts and Kashiwa, 1970). Plaque acts as a scaffold for calcification when calcium ions bind to the organic matrix and precipitate calcium phosphate salts. Intercellular zones and bacterial surfaces are the first sites of crystallization. Later, crystals form within bacteria. Formation studies using mylar strips (Mandel et al., 1957; Zander et al., 1960) show that calcification is initiated at the internal or dental interface of plaque. Mineral layers are formed and interspaced by a thin cuticular substrate that becomes part of the deposit during calcification.

Theories of calculus formation. Over the past 50 years a series of proposals have been suggested in attempting to explain calculus precipitation.

1. The *bacteriologic theory* suggests that the metabolic activity of microorganisms initiate the deposition of calcium salts when introduced to a calcium phosphate–rich substrate such as saliva or gingival fluid (Naeslund, 1926).

2. The *physicochemical theory* advances the proposal that salivary colloids maintain the normal supersaturated state of saliva relative to calcium and phosphorus. When saliva pools or stagnates surface tension and colloidal properties are altered, the colloidal protective action is thus reduced, and calcium and phosphate salts are precipitated (Prinz, 1928).

3. In the *salivary pH theory* an elevation in salivary pH causes a precipitation of calcium phosphate salts. This rise is brought about by the formation of ammonia by dental plaque or by the loss of carbon dioxide (Bibby, 1935; Leung and Jensen, 1958). There is a volatilization of carbon dioxide from fresh saliva. The loss of carbon dioxide results in a decreased hydrogen ion concentra-

tion and an increase in pH. This alteration favors precipitation of calcium salts.

4. The *enzymatic theory* suggests that the inorganic phosphate radical is liberated when phosphatases hydrolyze organic phosphate compounds in saliva. Such an increase in phosphate would favor precipitation of inorganic phosphate salts. The enzymes could originate from saliva, serum, or microorganisms.

5. The *epitactic theory* establishes that the concentration of calcium and phosphate ions is not high enough in serum and saliva to precipitate spontaneously. However, it is high enough to support crystal growth once an initial crystal (seed) is formed. It postulates that the initial crystal involves the intercellular matrix of plaque (Mandel et al., 1957; Neuman and Neuman, 1958; Wasserman et al., 1958) but the mechanism is as yet unknown. Perhaps in this seeding mechanism, portions of mucopolysaccharide molecules may selectively remove calcium and phosphate ions from a supersaturated solution (chelation). The calcium ions then bind with glycoprotein chains to form nuclei for further deposition of minerals.

The epitactic theory is an active concept of calculus formation. The physicochemical, salivary pH, and enzymatic theories are passive: a local elevation in the degree of calcium on phosphate ions predisposes to mineral precipitation.

The bacterial theory of Naeslund and the physicochemical theory proposed by Prinz both require salivary stagnation as a prerequisite to precipitation of calcium salts. In the salivary pH theory salivary flow is essential. These theories as well as the enzymatic theory require an overt environmental alteration prior to the formation of crystalline structures.

Today the epitactic theory is best supported as the method of initiating deposition of calcium salts. However, the earlier contributions by Naeslund, Prinz, and Bibby should not be dismissed, for the possibility of salt precipitation with multifactoral control still exists.

Modes of attachment. Zander (1954) described four methods in which calculus attaches to root surfaces. Moskow (1969) suggested a fifth method.

1. Attachment of the organic matrix of calculus into minute irregularities that were previously insertion locations of Sharpey's fibers

2. Attachment into cemental defects where resorptive and appositional changes occurred during function

3. Penetration of microorganisms into the ce-

mental surface with resultant formation of a calculus matrix within the root

4. Attachment mediated by a secondary cuticle

5. Attachment to cemental tears and separations

Since plaque in the absence of mineralized deposit can initiate the marginal lesion the role of calculus in the etiology of inflammatory disease becomes secondary. Its presence induces additional plaque accumulation, and it harbors toxic products that contribute adversely to host response.

Caries. Epidemiologists have presented statistics on the location and prevalence of caries relative to the periodontal lesion, but their interrelationship is speculative. They should be considered as two separate and distinct processes. Caries do, however, act to further inflammatory periodontal disease in two ways: (1) carious interdental areas predispose to food impaction and retention and (2) cervical caries create harbors for continued accumulation of dentobacterial plaque. The sequelae of both entities in contributing to inflammation have been discussed earlier (Fig. 4-13).

The periodontal pocket. Recent studies have been presented that begin to question the need for pocket reduction in maintaining periodontal health (Lindhe and Nyman, 1975; Ramfjord et al., 1973; Rosling et al., 1976). The obvious fact is that these longitudinal studies require frequent and repeated maintenance treatment by the dentist and place the responsibility of the health-disease equation on him alone. Although the study is informative and workable in a controlled and limited number of subjects it would be harmful to generalize and assign the same results to groups. We are still acting in consort with our patients in controlling periodontal disease. Our treatment plan must include securing a dentogingival relationship that a patient can maintain on a daily basis. Orban and Mueller (1929) and Toller (1948) have demonstrated that a shallow sulcus has less chance of becoming pathologic.

When a pocket is present the result of pathogenicity becomes a cause. The pocket becomes a reservoir for the retention of subgingival plaque and continued periodontal destruction.

Anatomic aberrancies enhancing the pathogenesis of plaque

The anatomy of the periodontal tissues exerts a guiding influence on the pathogenesis of inflammation. Keller and Cohen (1955) diagramed vascular patterns supplying the various parts of the periodontium. Their work clearly demonstrated separate sources of blood supply between the gingival unit and the attachment apparatus. Goldman (1957) showed that lesions arising in the gingival unit do not extend into the periodontal ligament but follow vascular channels into the interseptal and periosteal areas of supporting bone.

These earlier works describing anatomic pathways of gingival inflammation are further supported in several additional papers (Kennedy, 1974; Nuki and Hock, 1974; Polson et al., 1974a and b; Safavi et al., 1974). The anatomic makeup of the periodontium dictates that degenerative periodontal disease (occlusal traumatism) does not exert a discernible influence on either the severity of gingival inflammation or the transfer of ex-

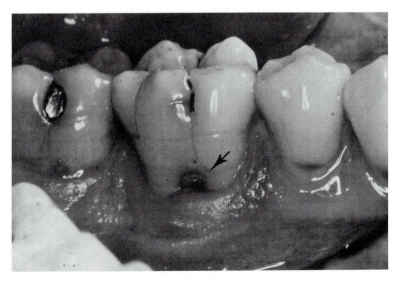

Fig. 4-13. Suprafurcation caries acting as reservoir for dentobacterial plaque.

udates to the attachment apparatus. Several anatomic variances do, however, enhance inflammatory disease to the degree that there is loss of attachment and irreversible damage.

Enamel projections and other anomalies. There exists a unique attachment of soft tissue to cementum, described in Chapter 1. That same histologic relationship does not exist when the epithelial attachment is in contact with enamel. If enamel were to transcend cementum there would be an extremely poor adaptation of gingival tissues to the tooth surface. Such is the case when enamel projections, gingivopalatal grooves, enamel pearls, and enamelomas are located in an area of inflammatory periodontal disease.

In 1964 Masters and Hoskins renewed interest in

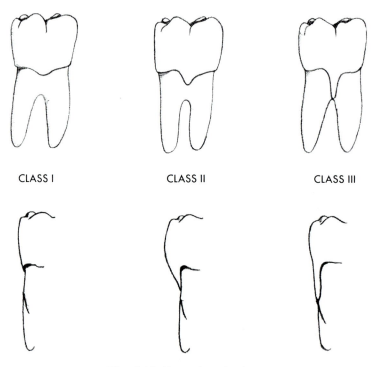

CLASS I   CLASS II   CLASS III

Fig. 4-14. Enamel projections.

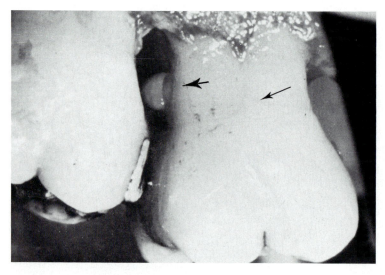

Fig. 4-15. Enamel pearl 1.5 mm below cementoenamel junction. Also note enamel projection. (Courtesy Dr. A. Goldstein, SUNY at Buffalo.)

the *enamel projection* as an anomaly that may affect periodontal stability. They classified projections (Fig. 4-14) and found the highest incidence of occurrence on the buccal aspect of lower second molars. This was supported by Andrews (1975) and Tsatsas et al. (1973) and related to localized extension of periodontal destruction by Bissada et al. (1973) and Simon et al. (1971). The enamel projection cannot be visualized on a radiograph.

Enamel pearls can be found on any lateral surface of the root. They differ from enamel projections in that they are isolated islands of ectopic enamel rather than extensions of coronal enamel. Furthermore, they differ from *enamelomas* in that enamelomas are not bonded to the root but are found in the periodontal ligament. Moskow (1971) described the histology of these formations and found that radicular pearls have a cementumlike coating. Cavanha (1965, 1967) described the pearl in two papers, and one would conclude that the only situation when they become contributors to periodontal breakdown occurs when the inflammatory process contacts their coronal aspect. Therefore the closer the enamel pearl is to the cementoenamel junction, the greater is its chance of becoming a contributory factor (Fig. 4-15).

Palatogingival grooves. The palatogingival groove is also described as a distal lingual groove. It has as its origin the cingulum and can extend the entire length of the root surface. Although most commonly described as a localized invagination affecting maxillary lateral incisors it can be found on any maxillary anterior tooth (Everett and Kramer, 1972; Lee et al., 1966). It begins as an enamel structure but can be seen displaying radicu-

lar histology at its more apical portion. It contributes to localized periodontal destruction in that it offers a weak barrier to extension of inflammation and also acts as a plaque trap (Fig. 4-16). The gross anatomy of the gingival tissues can contribute to the host's response to plaque. The *adequate zone of attached gingiva* has historically been listed among the requisites of healthy periodontal tissues. Lang and Löe (1972) demonstrated that 2 mm of keratinized gingiva, 1 mm being attached, was sufficient to maintain gingival health. However, the demands of adequate attached gingiva have to be evaluated on (1) the adjacent dental anatomy, (2) the presence of restorations, and (3) an individual's plaque index.

The anatomic variance, when we see the least amount of attached gingiva with its concommitant shallow vestibule, is associated with an *aberrant frenum attachment*. Mirko et al. in a two-part article (1974) concluded that the most common finding in periodontal breakdown associated with the high frenum attachment was inflammation related to plaque accumulation. This supports the findings of Lovdal et al. and of Löe in that the anatomic defect supports plaque accumulation that probably results from compromised hygiene in the area. The suggestion that the frenum instigates local recession by marginal pull is difficult to accept unless the stress used to activate a frenum in diagnosis was used habitually. Henry et al. (1976) were unable to demonstrate any muscle fibers in the frenum proper. Localized areas of gingival recession present the clinician with an anatomic aberrancy that requires special attention. Maynard and Ochsenbein (1975) in studying mucogingival problems in children concluded that insufficient keratinized gingiva was developmentally related to either a thin buccolingual alveolar process, eruptive patterns of permanent teeth, or a combination. Parfitt and Mjör (1964) found that gingivitis is more severe in areas of localized recession.

The area of localized recession as well as the area of high attachment present the patient with the challenge of special care in order to prevent plaque accumulation and inflammatory disease (Figs. 4-17 and 4-18).

Protective contours. When the protective contours of the tooth or gingiva are absent or altered the dentogingival junction can be affected by inadequate food deflection. Enamel hypoplasia, amelogenesis imperfecta, and congenital anodontia alter coronal form. The ideal knifelike marginal gingiva is no longer protected by the greater contour of the tooth in altered passive erup-

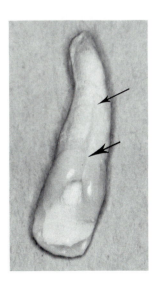

Fig. 4-16. Gingivopalatal groove.

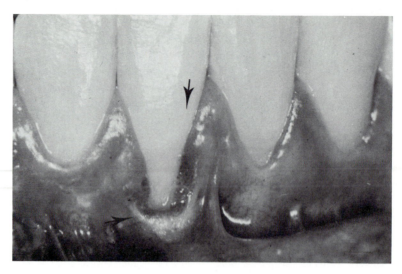

Fig. 4-17. Inadequate keratinized gingiva with recession and creation of a plaque-retention area.

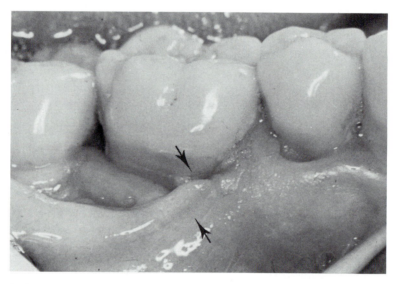

Fig. 4-18. Aberrant frenum on mesiobuccal aspect of mandibular first molar creates an area that challenges adequate sulcular cleansing.

tion, familial hyperplasia, and so-called Dilantin hyperplasia. In each instance the environment becomes receptive to food impaction and retention (Fig. 4-19). In addition to creating plaque traps there can be traumatic irritation to the gingival tissues (see discussion on Mechanical Factors).

Cysts, foreign bodies, and rugae. There are many alterations in gingival architecture that result from traumatic injury or odontogenic maladies. Most of these abnormalities are symptomless, and the individual is unaware of their presence. The most benign and passive lesion is the gingival cyst (Moskow and Weinstein, 1975). It is odontogenic in origin and presents a problem in its disruption of gingival form. The recurrent ossifying fibroma, pyogenic granulomas, and epulides also distort gingival architecture (Eversole and Rovin, 1973, 1972; Hayward, 1973) and allow plaque accumulation when present at the dentogingival junction (Fig. 4-20). Foreign body reaction to impression and filling materials and sutures initiates a more granulomatous or chronic tissue reaction (Cataldo and Santis, 1974; Lilly et al., 1973). Palatal rugae whose pedunculated bases approxi-

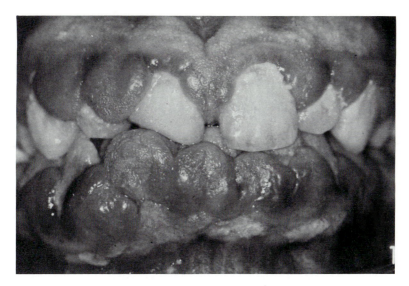

Fig. 4-19. Gingival hyperplasia that interferes with masticatory function. Note impaction and retention of debris as well as mechanical trauma from incisal contact with gingival tissue.

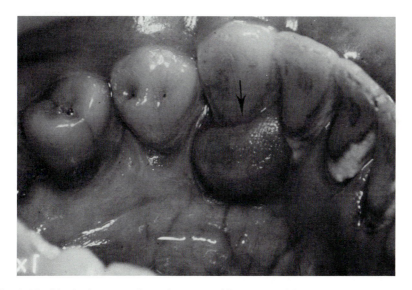

Fig. 4-20. Gingival cyst on lingual aspect of lower cuspid creating a plaque trap.

mate marginal tissue can also act as plaque traps. These situations can occur developmentally but more often result from periodontal flap surgery (Fig. 4-21). A rugoplasty performed prior to the flap incision can prevent this unacceptable tissue architecture.

Mouth breathing and the lip line. Anatomic variances in the lip line can predispose to erythematous gingival tissues. When a lip rests at a position that allows gingival exposure the normally moist mucous membrane becomes superficially dehydrated. The gingival response mimics the clin-

ical entity of habitual mouth breathing. Mouth breathing is usually found in recurrent osteitis associated with nasopharyngeal tonsils and adenoids. It also is a frequent finding in epilepsy, but it has not been determined whether epileptics are mouth breathers because of the entity or as a result of antiepileptic medications. Individuals with recurrent sinusitis or those on decongestants should be suspected of being transient mouth breathers. When gingival tissues dehydrate because of a high lip line or mouth breathing they appear swollen and edematous and are in sharp contrast to the

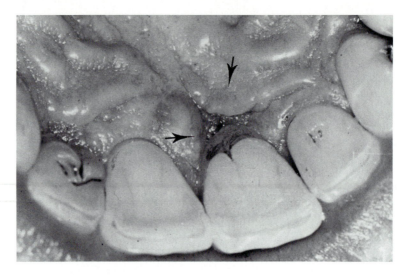

Fig. 4-21. Rugae forming a plaque-retentive area at dentogingival margin. Rugoplasty is indicated to create physiologic form.

neighboring areas covered by the lips and cheeks. Jacobson (1973) found an increase in the gingival index in mouth breathers, but the plaque index was not significantly higher. He suggests that dehydrated plaque may be more pathogenic.

The root canal. The anatomy of the root canal is such that there is direct communication with the periodontal tissues. Although the apex is the most consistent site of this union the demonstration of lateral or auxiliary canals stimulated investigations into a combined origin of a pathogenic processes. Burch (1974) and Lowman et al. (1973) studied extracted teeth for the incidence of accessory canals and found a high percentage of these canals in the furcation and the coronal third of the root. However, the greatest incidence was found in the apical third. Simon et al. (1972) and Chacker (1974) described periodontal inflammation arising from inflammatory pulpal lesions via lateral canals and dentinal tubules. In a series of papers Seltzer and Bender (1965), Seltzer et al. (1963), and Bhaskar (1976) demonstrated the interaction of pulpal and periodontal inflammation across lateral canals. They found that the passage of toxin from pulpal degeneration through the canal system can initiate periodontal lesions and bone loss. This finding was further supported in several investigations (Blair, 1972; Ruback and Mitchell 1965; Sinai and Soltanoff, 1973), as was the reverse, that is, pulpal lesions arising from inflammatory periodontal lesions (Ruback and Mitchell, 1965; Seltzer et al., 1963). Kirkham (1975) found a low incidence of actual periodontal lesions associated with lateral canals. The anatomic presence of the canal suggests, however, the potential of transference of disease from the periodontium to the endodontium (Fig. 4-22).

Root topography. The concavities and convexities of the tooth present a challenge in hygiene to the most dexterous individual. Once periodontal disease begins and there is apical migration to the epithelial attachment this challenge is even greater. The cervical lip where enamel and cementum join, buccolingual concavities, and cul-de-sacs created by open furcations are potential areas of plaque accumulation and retention (Fig. 4-23). When destruction proceeds even further and reverse architecture results or when a concave intermediate bifurcation ridge (Fig. 4-24) is present it is highly unlikely that plaque can be controlled. Here the practitioner must make the necessary anatomic changes to create an environment that is in harmony with cleaning procedures.

The *position of the furcation* relative to the cementoenamel junction is also a factor to be considered. The closer the furcation is to the crown, the greater the chance of furcation involvement in the periodontally involved mouth (Larato, 1975). The presence of a high or low furcation is important from a prognostic point of view (Fig. 4-25). The anatomic relationship of roots is also important in the pathogenesis of periodontal disease. The closer the proximity roots, the more likely one finds labile, corticallike bone similar to that on the labial aspect of anterior teeth. The greater the interroot spacing, the greater the chance of having stable cancellous bone with its multifaceted repair potential.

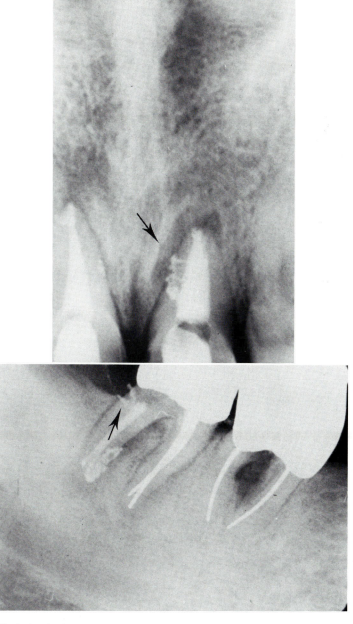

Fig. 4-22. Endodontic lesions displaying accessory canals, which exit into periodontal ligament.

Split or fractured teeth. A completely or incompletely fractured tooth presents a challenge to the diagnostician. In its incipient stages the symptoms include an intermittent, sharp, shooting pain resulting from specific stimuli (Cameron, 1974, 1966; Hiatt, 1973). In the more chronic forms one can see all the clinical and radiographic signs of periodontal disease (Polson, 1977). The fracture line acts as a funnel of communication between the oral ecology and the attachment apparatus (Fig. 4-26).

Diseased cementum. Just as a pocket resulting from disease becomes a contributing factor, cementum, the mineralized wall lining the chronic pocket, becomes a source of pathogenesis in the disease cycle. In periodontitis there are morphologic and biochemical changes that take place within cementum, and they perpetuate tissue destruction (Saglie et al., 1974; Saxton, 1976; Selvig, 1966; Stahl, 1975). Recent studies have explored the nature of diseased roots. Morris (1975) concluded that the organic component of

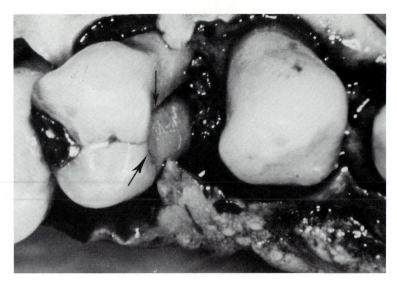

Fig. 4-23. Buccolingual concavity and high furcation present radicular anatomy that is difficult to maintain.

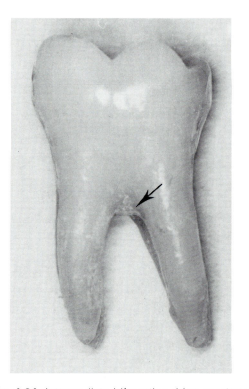

Fig. 4-24. Intermediate bifurcation ridge creates a series of concavities and convexities that harbor plaque when attachment has been lost in area.

cementum has an inhibitory influence on repair. The biochemical change in the collagenous structure of cementum (Selvig, 1966) may initiate an autoimmune response as suggested in biologic models. Further animal studies by Register and Burdick (1976, 1975) demonstrated an anabolic response of diseased cementum (cementogenesis and reattachment) when it was demineralized in situ. Whether the result occurred from the acids' effect on the organic or inorganic component requires further study. Aleo (1975) and co-workers studied teeth extracted because of periodontal disease. In culture, human fibroblasts would not grow over the portion of the root that lined the periodontal pocket. If the diseased cementum is removed or undergoes phenol-water extraction, fibroblasts then attach. They earlier found that a diseased root harbors the lipopolysaccharide endotoxin, which contributes to the propagation of the periodontal wound. Endotoxins are capable of many toxic immune reactions (see Chapter 3).

SECONDARY FACTORS INITIATING PERIODONTAL BREAKDOWN

Many precipitous factors affect their target prior to inflammation or degeneration from plaque and occlusal trauma, respectively. These factors, once regarded as primary etiologic agents, are presently discussed as secondary factors propagating plaque retention and accumulation. However, habits and mechanical, chemical, and thermal factors do operate in initiating periodontal breakdown.

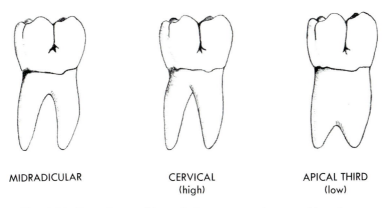

MIDRADICULAR   CERVICAL   APICAL THIRD
                        (high)   (low)

Fig. 4-25. Furcation position relative to cementoenamel junction.

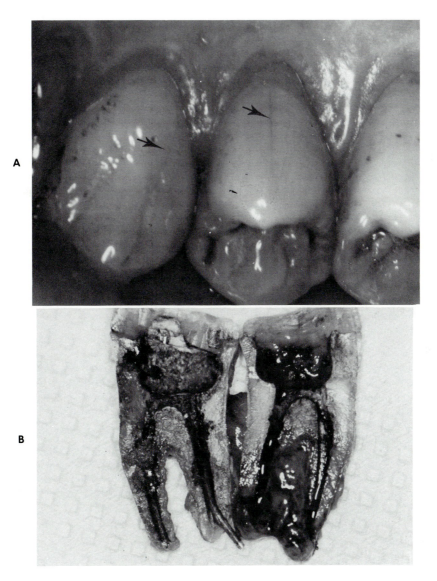

A

B

Fig. 4-26. Root fracture. **A,** Incomplete fractures on maxillary cuspid and first bicuspid. **B,** Complete mesiodistal, vertical fracture of an endodontically treated molar.

Mechanical factors

Mechanical factors can be subdivided into those that initiate inflammation, those that initiate degeneration, or those that provoke a combination of responses. They include (1) orthodontic therapy, (2) restorative techniques, (3) oral hygiene techniques, and (4) habits.

Orthodontic therapy. The contribution of some forms of orthodontic therapy to gingival inflammation was presented in the discussion on Factors Propagating Plaque Retention and Accumulation. Orthodontic therapy can also induce mechanical etiology and damage the attachment apparatus. This is not to be critical of the methods used in orthodontics. Orthodontists are presented with cases when clinical crowns are only partially erupted, bands are difficult to fit and adapt, and often their patients are undergoing pubertal changes with all their ramifications. In more recent years there has been an increase in the acceptance of adult orthodontics as an adjunct to preventive periodontics and restorative dentistry. Although the majority of reports on tooth movement techniques as they apply to the periodontium concern children, data presented on tooth position and the attachment apparatus can be applied to all age groups. Zachrisson and Alnaes (1974, 1973) compared the periodontal condition in orthodontically treated teeth with untreated controls. In their first paper (1973) they reported an increase in loss of attachment in the orthodontic group. In a second article (1974) they reported an increase in bone loss in the test group. The loss was greatest on the pressure side of retracted cuspids in closed extraction cases. O'Leary et al. (1974) and Pritchard (1975) report finding an increase in interdental irregularities and uneven marginal ridge relationships in postorthodontic cases.

Since Reitan's (1947) description of the histology of the periodontium during bodily tooth movement, much has been learned about the orthodontic micropathology. Ten years later this same author (1957) reported that facial tipping could cause horizontal protrusion of the radicular surface outside of the alveolar bone (dehiscence). This was due to a lack of compensatory bone formation on labial surfaces of teeth. Rygh (1973) applied the electron microscope to study changes in the ultrastructure of periodontal tissues undergoing orthodontic tooth movement. He reported that pressure zones exhibited extensive alterations in areas of hyalinization within the periodontal ligament. When forces were maintained at a clinical range, degenerations and necrosis were limited to small, circumscribed areas of the attachment apparatus.

Orthodontic wires, bands, and elastics can contribute to the initiation of periodontal inflammation by first acting as mechanical irritants. Judicious and select use of each appliance can prevent these hazards. Bands should be placed as far from the gingiva as retentive requirements will allow. They should be thoroughly adapted and contoured, and care should be exercised to removal all residual cement from the sulcular area. Wire should be contoured so as not to impinge on the gingival tissues and should allow plaque control although it will be compromised. There have been several reports demonstrating the traumatogenic effects of orthodontic elastics that migrate subgingivally (Hogeboom and Stephens, 1965; Vandersall, 1971; Zager and Barnett, 1974). The elastic initiating mechanical irritation then becomes a plaque-retentive factor and produces a lesion similar to one found in rapid periodontitis (Fig. 4-27).

A loss of attachment from the apex toward the crown can result when forces of movement exceed repair. The root resorption that results leaves the tooth with a reduced surface area of periodontal attachment (Fig. 4-28).

Restorative techniques. Tissue preparation prior to definitive restorative techniques and meticulous operating procedures would eliminate most iatrogenic mechanical damage to the periodontal tissues (Fig. 4-29 to 4-31).

Preventive approaches should be utilized during all dental procedures. Periodontal destruction can result when too much or too rapid adrenalized anesthesia is injected. There is both a mechanical and a chemical response. A localized microcirculatory collapse follows, and the gingival tissues then slough.

The rubber dam and its clamp are excellent safeguards for the periodontal tissues. However, the clamp can injure both the marginal tissue and crestal bone if incorrectly placed on those tissues (Fig. 4-32). If pieces of dam are left in the gingival sulcus they become plaque-retentive factors.

Several authors have reported on damage occurring during restorative impressions. O'Leary et al. (1973), Price and Whitehead (1972), and Glenwright (1975) have reported on cases with severe periodontal response when rubber base material was forced into the subcrevicular tissues. It was suggested that preparatory procedures using epinephrine (Adrenalin)-coated string or electrosurgery may have initiated a pathway for material to ooze into the deeper structures. The clinical reaction to this phenomenon results in a periodontal abscess. The authors show that repair and regeneration follows the removal of the rubber base material.

Coelho and associates (1975) examined teeth receiving full coverage 6 months after insertion of the restorations. Recession was found to be generalized when compared with the heights of the preoperative gingival margins. The authors concluded that the electrosurgery used when taking

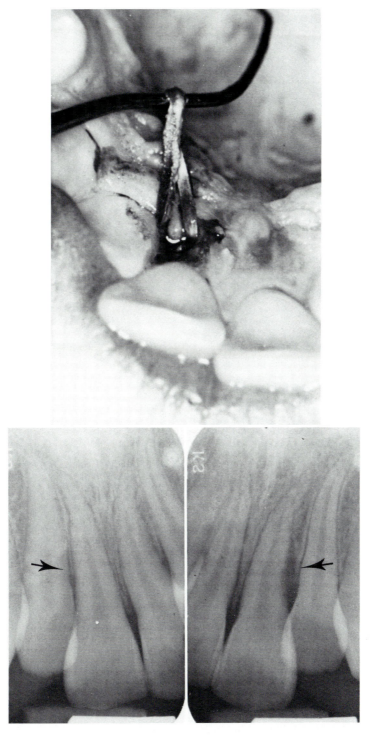

Fig. 4-27. In an attempt to close a central incisor diastema, an orthodontic elastic was retained, migrated apically, and caused a severe periodontal lesion.

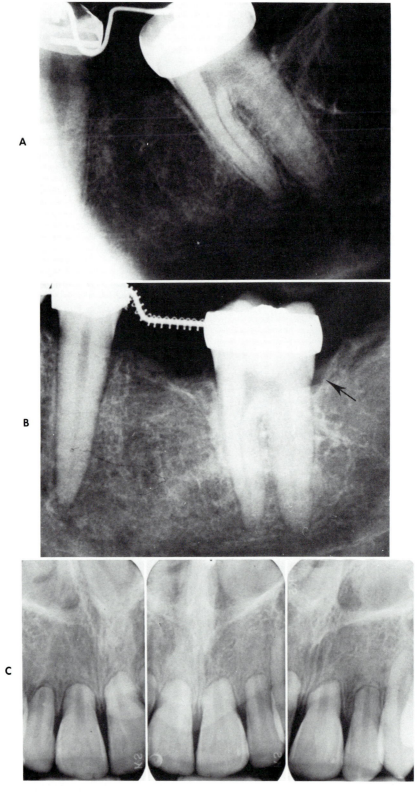

Fig. 4-28. A and **B,** Uprighting of a distal abutment created a supracervical pseudoosseous defect. **C,** Loss of surface area of attachment from apex coronally in postorthodontic case.

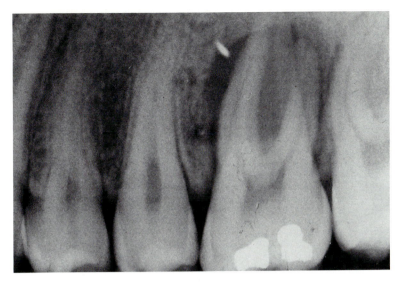

Fig. 4-29. Fractured tip of curet approximating periapex in otherwise healthy young mouth. Tooth is vital, and modus operandi of this result could not be obtained.

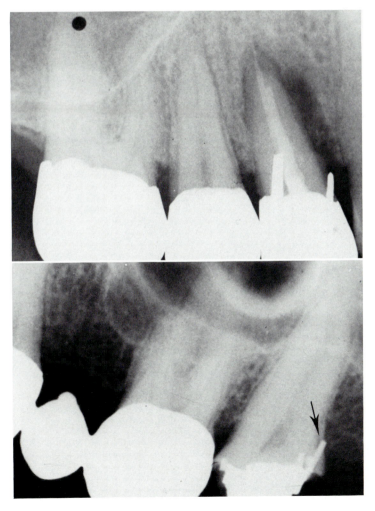

Fig. 4-30. Retentive pins used in restorative dentistry exiting into periodontal ligament space.

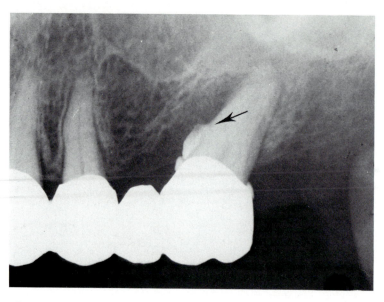

Fig. 4-31. Cement within a periodontal pocket obviously ignored during restorative therapy. In addition to chemical irritation, cement facilitates plaque accumulation.

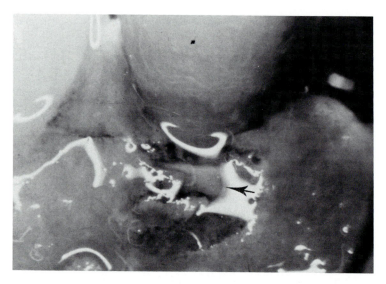

Fig. 4-32. Four days following a restorative procedure this patient complained of pain and roughness where rubber dam clamp rested. Examination disclosed gingival slough and osseous exposure.

impressions was the factor producing the gingival entity. Donaldson (1974) studied areas of recession following restorative procedures and the use of temporary coverage. He reported that the periodontal lesion, that is, the gingival recession, was caused by mechanical pressure and overextension of the temporary restoration. Informative as they may be, neither report includes plaque indices.

In a given array of circumstances any instrument, hand or rotary, and many materials have the potential of initiating a periodontopathy. It is

well to be aware of the indications as well as the limitations of our armamentarium in order to prevent such episodes.

Oral hygiene techniques. Used properly the toothbrush and dental floss are the two most beneficial adjuncts in maintaining periodontal health. Used improperly they can be contributory factors in periodontal disease. Not only will their inadequate use allow for plaque accumulation, but their misuse can contribute to mechanical trauma to the gingival and dental structures (Fig. 4-33).

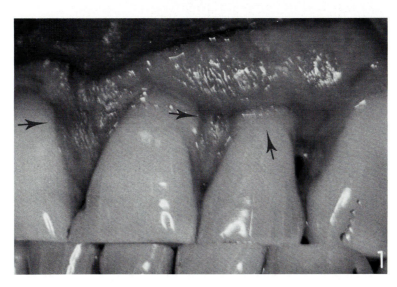

Fig. 4-33. Bonafide toothbrush trauma. Note that papillary gingiva as well as tooth displays traumatogenic effects.

Toothbrushing: trauma, abrasion, gingival recession. It has been shown that the toothbrush can cause traumatic effects on the gingiva. Gingival recession in the absence of clinical inflammation and plaque is frequently referred to as an area resulting from toothbrush trauma. Eroded cementoenamel junctions and root surfaces that have become exposed are often cited as areas of toothbrush abrasion. However, it is difficult to establish a modus operandi for a clinical situation that has developed, matured, and ended before the diagnostician has examined it.

In addition to periodontitis many factors can contribute to the clinical entity of recession other than improper toothbrushing techniques. When the labial or lingual radicular surfaces of teeth are positioned outside facial or lingual osseous tissue either developmentally or from tooth positioning they are likely to display recession. Gingival recession is not uncommon when associated with deeply cuspate teeth. The occlusal traumatic lesion can affect the buccal or lingual attachment apparatus in such a way as to cause loss of osseous support. A gingival inflammatory lesion then encourages loss of integrity of the epithelial attachment and apical migration of the epithelial attachment with resultant clinical recession.

In 1921 Stillmen described areas of localized recession and concluded that they resulted from occlusal trauma. Thirteen years later Hirschfeld (1934) reported on these soft tissue irregularities and concluded that they were caused by

toothbrush trauma. If the vast number of areas of recession with associated destruction of tooth structure were caused by the toothbrush, how could the interdental facial papillae, located coronal to the labial dentogingival entity, escape traumatization (Fig. 4-33)? Gingiva is much less resistant to mechanical trauma, and it too is in the pathway of the toothbrush. Rarely can one elicit a history of sore gingival tissues in the so-called toothbrush trauma case (Fig. 4-34). It is difficult to accept that gingival and tooth destruction can be provoked mechanically without some semblance of discomfort.

Several animal studies were designed to evaluate the causes of localized gingival recession. Bass in 1948 and Anneroth and Poppelman in 1967 showed a positive correlation between toothbrushing and recession in dogs. Baker and Seymour (1976) in rat experimentation and Hopps and Johnson (1974) in studying monkey tissues concluded that areas of recession were accompanied by subclinical inflammation. They report that recession is the result of localized inflammation, which produces a breakdown of connective tissue leading to proliferation of the epithelium into the area of connective tissue destruction. In a discussion on the development of the periodontal cleft, Novaes et al. (1965) support the fact that inflammation is constant.

In addition to inflammation several anatomic factors that influence localized recession are (1) prominent roots with thin vestibular osseous plates or alveolar dehiscence (Fig. 4-35), (2) the

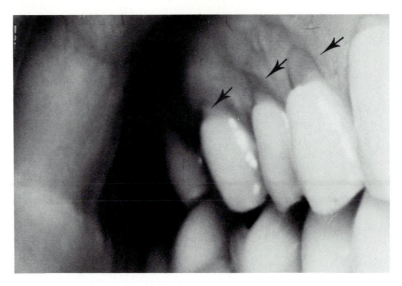

Fig. 4-34. Toothbrush abrasion?

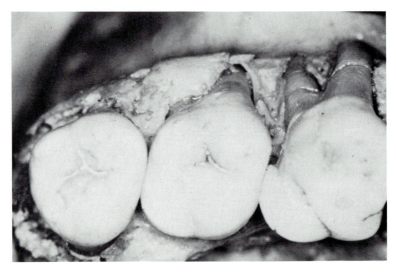

Fig. 4-35. Tooth position relative to alveolus. Third molar, located in midbuccolingual alveolus, as is distal half of second molar, displays adequate levels of buccoradicular support. Mesial aspect of second molar and first molar are positioned outside buccal alveolus with resultant dehiscence. If gingival tissue were to follow osseous form, one would expect to see recession on buccal aspect of first molar and on mesiobuccal root of second molar.

presence of a thin or narrow band of attached gingiva, (3) prominent version of a tooth relative to the dental arch, (4) a traumatic occlusion, and (5) orthodontic forces exceeding the repair potential of radicular facial osseous tissues.

The roles of the inflammatory lesion and plaque as they relate to the clinical entity of recession have been the topic of several reports. Gorman (1967) and O'Leary et al. (1971) reported that in areas of recession gingival and plaque scores were reduced. It was suggested as a result of their observations that faulty toothbrushing and tooth position were responsible for gingival recession. In their investigation in children, however, Parfitt and Mjör (1964) reported that gingivitis is more severe in areas of recession. Wolfram et al. (1974) demonstrated that toothbrushing may even be responsible for pocket formation. When subjects substituted the antiplaque agent chlorhexidine for a toothbrush the gingival sulcus was reduced and in

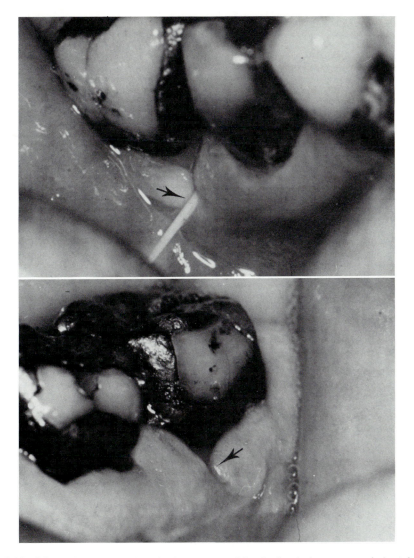

Fig. 4-36. Bilateral mucogingival lesions created by indiscriminate use of dental floss.

some cases disappeared. When toothbrushing was resumed the sulcus increased in depth.

Abrasion, often seen with gingival recession, has drawn the attention of several investigators. Radentz et al. (1975) separate traumatic, noncarious abrasions from erosions. Erosion results when a lowered pH from medicaments or foods causes a chemical demineralization of tooth surfaces. Use of the right or preferred hand is also a factor in that additional force can be applied to the opposite side of the favored hand (Kenney et al., 1976). Padbury and Ash (1974) report that the scrub method of brushing produced a greater localized abrasion.

Dentifrices. In addition to abrasion produced by toothbrushing, two studies (Manly and Foster, 1967; Sangnes, 1976) concerned themselves with the abrasiveness of dentifrices. A third (Saxton,

1976) applied the scanning electron microscope to the subject. They concluded that abrasive dentifrices as well as hard toothbrushes and excessive brushing correlate well with destruction of the root surfaces in the form of abrasion.

Other hygienic modalities. Any hygiene modality used inordinately can contribute to the inflammatory lesion. Taylor and Campbell (1972) have suggested that the epithelial attachment (junctional epithelium) is weak in nature and readily disturbed by careless use of dental floss and toothbrushing. Sconyers et al. (1973) evaluated the incidence of bacteremia resulting from the mechanical action of the toothbrush on bacteria-laden crevicular gingiva. They found a positive correlation in patients with periodontitis. This was also the finding when Lineberger and DeMarco (1973) studied bacteremias resulting from the use of Stim-u-dents in cases of active periodontal disease. The inadvertent trauma of dental floss can sever gingival tissue (Fig. 4-36).

The oral lavage has reappeared in the last decade as a therapeutic adjunct to oral hygiene. Used properly it is reported safe (Hoover and Robinson, 1968; Krajewski et al., 1964; Lainson, 1972; Meklas and Stewart, 1972) in its effectiveness in removing loose accumulations surrounding the dentition. When dealing with inflamed gingiva, pressure above 8 g elicited pain (Lobene, 1971). Furthermore, in patients with gingivitis and periodontitis the irrigating device produced bactermias 60 seconds after use in 50% of the tested subjects (Felix et al., 1971; Romans and App, 1971). O'Leary et al. (1970a) introduced carbon particles, comparable to the size of oral bacteria, to inflamed gingival crevices. As demonstrated histologically the mechanical action of the irrigating devices forced the particles into crevicular tissues. The same result could not be obtained when using a toothbrush on carbon-lined sulci (O'Leary et al., 1970b). Since these reports show that material can be forced into a diseased sulcus with an oral lavage, it is possible that some local damage can result. Arnim (1967) and Sumner (1965) have reported that acute periodontal abscesses can occur with the injudicious use of these devices.

The effectiveness of the oral lavage in the removal of plaque in inflammatory periodontal disease has been questioned. Lobene (1969) reported that they do not reduce plaque and Toto et al. (1969) found the toothbrush to be more effective than the irrigation device. Arnim (1976) concluded that these instruments do not remove all deposit but are capable of altering the environment to make it less desirable for bacterial inhabitation.

Removal of unattached deposit and the dilution of concentrated media appear to be the most favorable indications in using an oral lavage. The dentist is charged with the duty of seeing that patients follow proper instructions in its use to prevent untoward effects. The aforementioned studies should alert the clinician to the possibility of subacute bacterial endocarditis. Bacteremia production during oral hygiene procedures in the periodontally involved mouth is a very real possibility. In the susceptible individual it is paramount to take proper medical precautions and control or eliminate inflammatory disease while being abreast of his response to your detailed oral hygiene instructions.

· · ·

In conclusion, mechanical factors can incite acute trauma, but rarely cause tooth loss from their effect alone. They do, however, contribute to tooth loss by provoking or initiating an entrance for inflammation or degeneration of the periodontal tissues.

Habits. A repeated static or functional exercise or ritual is defined as a habit. Society tends to accept good habits, for example, altruism and good hygiene, at face value and reject bad habits as flaws in character. Bad habits seem to be the easiest to develop and the most difficult to correct. Habits contribute to periodontopathies by contributing to both inflammatory and degenerative lesions.

Bruxism, clenching, doodling. A very common form of oral habit concerns the parafunctional movements of the mandible, that is, movements other than those used in speech, deglutition, and mastication. Bruxism, clenching, and doodling induce parafunctional forces on the periodontal tissues. *Clenching* has been defined as the fluctuating and repetitive force exerted on teeth in opposing arches when the dentition is in a fixed or locked position. It represents isometric contractures in the muscles of mastication. *Bruxism* is the repetitive grinding or gritting of the teeth that can occur both nocturnally and at daytime (Robinson et al., 1969). This represents isotonic contractures. *Doodling* is the repetitive toying, tapping, or clenching on an isolated tooth or group of teeth when the mandible is in an eccentric position. The three parafunctional habits will be discussed as one because of their apparent similarities in origin and their resultant effect on the periodontium.

It is generally reported that two factors operate in the etiology of these habits: premature contacts and neuroses. First, the habit develops as a subconscious attempt to eliminate the occlusal interference. The fact that occlusal disharmony is involved is supported by changes in electromyographic findings. Occlusal habits show increased masticatory muscle activity. Ramfjord's (1961) experiments showing that bruxism and elevated muscular activity disappear by establishing a harmonious occlusion further supports premature contacts as etiologic factors. The second causative factor is more highly disputed but its importance should not be dismissed (Lindquist, 1974, 1972). Stress and emotional tension play a role in the genesis of these three habits (Nadler, 1968; Thaller et al., 1976) It is for this reason that Goldman and Cohen suggest the term ''occlusal neurosis'' in defining bruxism, clenching and doodling. Thaller and associates (1976) define the profile of the bruxistic patient as a person who tends to be anxious, with intrinsic hostility, and unable to vent frustration outwardly. Psychiatrists explain these neuroses as the oral outlet for subconscious aggression. Further support for psychogenic etiology is reported in a recent article by Goodman et al. (1976). The authors found approximately one third of the subjects engaging in bruxism abandoned the habit after a mock occlusal adjustment. The percentage, however, rises abruptly with definitive occlusal adjustment. Recognition of these habits requires the knowledge of a gamut of signs and symptoms. One may expect to see polished tooth facets, flat incline planes, mobility, radiographic evidence of occlusal trauma, muscle fatigue, muscles sensitive to palpation, eccentric occlusion, mandibular deviation, and temporomandibular joint dysfunction. Clenching and doodling, due to their locked position, have their impact on the attachment apparatus. Bruxism, in addition to its effect on the periodontium, also causes tooth wear. Alveolar bone is not always lost from these habits. Frank mobility in the absence of loss of alveolar support should make the diagnostician suspicious of an operating habit.

Occlusal habits can cause cuspal wear, broadening the occlusal table, and supraeruption, altering interdental contacts and marginal ridge relationships. Bruxism and doodling can also cause tooth displacement with all its ramifications. These habits can initiate the occlusal traumatic lesion. Treatment for bruxism, clenching, and doodling include occlusal therapy (bite appliances, selective grinding, orthodontics, restorative therapy, or combinations), use of psychotherapeutic drugs, or psychotherapy. The patient's physician should be consulted on the latter two approaches.

Occupations. The previous discussion centered on habits that deal with tooth-to-tooth relationships. There is magnification of the periodontal response to parafunctional forces when there is a third factor added, that is, a tooth-object-tooth or lip continuum.

A farmer jolted around in his tractor as he cultivates a dry field has abrasive dusts to facilitate occlusal wear when bruxing. Carpenters and cobblers with nails or tailors and seamstresses with pins temporarily stored between their teeth can induce incisal wear or provoke an occlusal traumatalike response in the attachment apparatus (Fig. 4-37).

Smoking stems. The individual who smokes a pipe, cigarette, or cigar with a wooden or plastic filter directs hot smoke to a target area in the oral cavity (see discussion on Tobacco). If he "wears" the pipe or holder he can induce a pathogenic response in the attachment apparatus. The tooth or teeth involved can be intruded, and those that remain, loosing the occlusal support of affected teeth, can show evidence of hyperfunction (Fig. 4-38).

Nail biting. Using incisors to redesign or shorten fingernails or cuticles can lead to displacement in

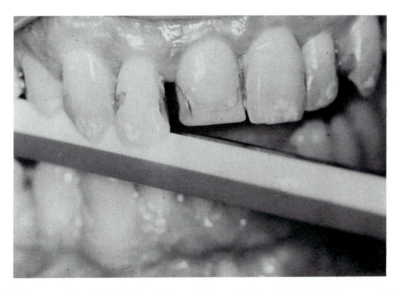

Fig. 4-37. Occupational habit. Dispatcher with pen-biting habit displacing maxillary right lateral incisor.

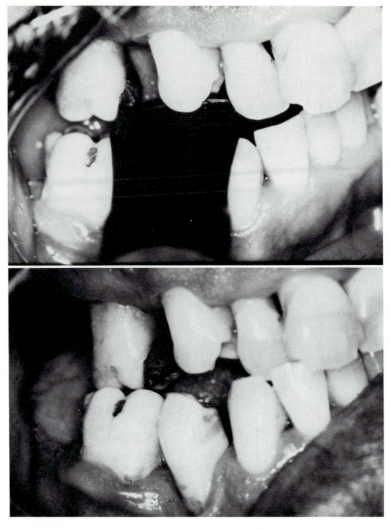

Fig. 4-38. Pipe stem habit. Involved teeth are intruded. Other teeth accept occlusal load when pipe is out of mouth.

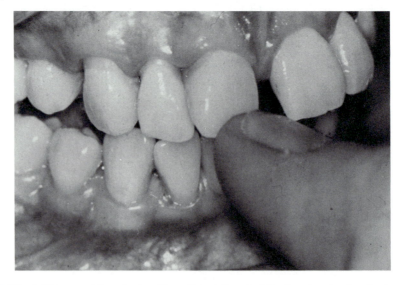

Fig. 4-39. A 27-year-old patient with cuticle-biting habit showing tooth displacement.

the form of rotation and diastema of the involved teeth. The maxillary anteriors are the most common sites of loss of arch integrity from this habit. This voluntary habit is one that must be controlled if one is to expect successful tooth positioning to correct the migrated and unaesthetic result (Fig. 4-39).

Lips, cheeks, tongue. The inadvertent habit of biting or chewing on the lips, cheek, or tongue can affect periodontal health. Chewing the mucosa on the interior lip or cheek usually results in a keratinized bite line in the affected area. Frequency and repetition of this action will determine the effect on the supporting structures. In a Class II Division I occlusion the degree of overjet frequently carries the incisal edges of maxillary incisor past the vermilion border of the lower lip. This establishes a wedging force from the labial and circumoral musculature against the lingual aspects of maxillary anteriors. Migration, mobility, and degeneration of the labial attachment apparatus can occur (Fig. 4-40).

Thumbsucking. Thumb or handsucking (Anderson et al., 1974) can be a problem in periodontics only if it (1) continues into the postchildhood years as seen in some congenital diseases or retardation or (2) had a profound effect in childhood and contributed to arch displacement and malocclusion. The periodontal result would be similar to that discussed directly above.

Reed instruments. There are two popular types of reed instruments: single reed and double reed. The clarinet and the saxophone are examples of the single reed instrument, in which the mouthpiece is placed at an angle behind the maxillary incisors and compression is developed by sealing the lower part of the mouthpiece with the lower lip (Fig. 4-41). The double reed instrument (for example, the oboe) is sealed by both lips. Instead of eliciting an anterior component of force on the maxillary incisors as in the single reed instrument, it places pressure on both lips and can induce anterior crowding. It has been suggested that the proper wind instrument could be used to position

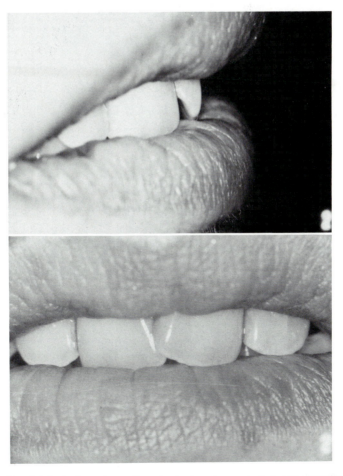

Fig. 4-40. Overjet that placed maxillary incisal surfaces anterior to vermilion border.

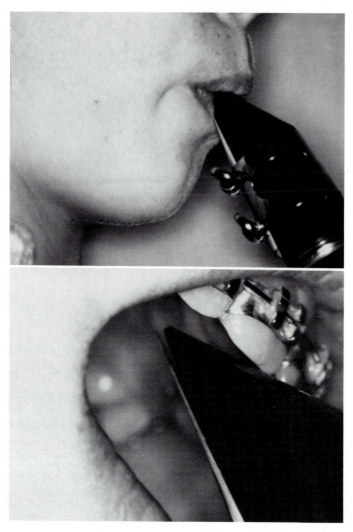

Fig. 4-41. Single-reed instrument exerts a wedging effect on lingual aspect of maxillary incisors. Maxillary circumoral musculature must counteract this force.

anterior malaligned teeth. Yet others oppose the use of these instruments as potentially traumatogenic to anterior teeth. Pang (1976), following a study involving 84 schoolchildren who played reed instruments, concluded that on an individual basis there was no predictable result of the effect the instrument exerted on the anterior teeth.

Tongue thrust (pressure). Tongue habits present themselves in two ways. First, pressurized force against the lingual aspects of the dentition can exert a traumatogenic effect if frequency and pressure are intense (Winders, 1958). Usually, however, the destruction is evident along the lateral borders of the tongue and is seen as crenation markings with or without hyperkeratosis. Second, tongue thrusting or reverse swallowing are commonly present but not usually recognized (Straub, 1961). There is an incipient or transient form of

thrusting whereby an individual glides his tongue over the incisal edges of his anterior teeth and across the vermilion border of the lips. At this stage the tongue habit is passive, and if the periodontal tissues are healthy there will be no adverse reaction. The more advanced stage of tongue thrusting accompanies the deviate swallow. Its etiology is developmental, and its effect on the periodontium can be destructive. There are two philosophies of the cause of tongue thrusting: (1) it results when there is a developmental open bite; the tongue is thrust into this opening to seal the oral cavity and facilitate swallowing and (2) the deviate swallow is a complex mechanism characterized by overdevelopment and exertion of the lingual muscles and passive restraint of the circumoral muscles. It is postulated that during infancy too much milk gets into the child's mouth or the

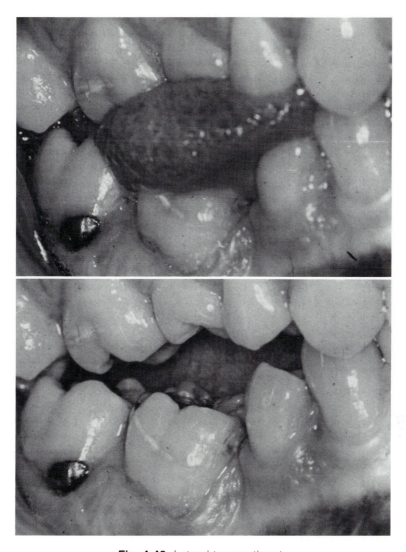

Fig. 4-42. Lateral tongue thrust.

nipple protrudes too far distally. The child, in an attempt to halt this assault, forces the liquid or nipple anteriorly with a thrust of the tongue. The repeated enactment of this phenomenon causes overdevelopment and overactivity of the glossal musculature and a weakening of the circumoral muscles during a period of active development (Picard, 1959). There is a third clinical expression of tongue thrusting that is rarely discussed and whose etiology has not been defined, that is, the lateral tongue thrust (Fig. 4-42).

Anterior tongue thrusting presents several classic signs. The tongue is often enlarged (macroglossia), and the upper lid is flaccid, suggestive of Picard's bottle mouth. An anterior open bite is often found, and the patient may be a mouth breather. There is an atypical grimace when swallowing, and often dental deposit is found on the

anteriointerdental surfaces of lower anterior teeth where saliva forms a pool. Also a high palatal vault is present, and the rugae are pronounced due to their lack of contact with the tongue. There can be fanning of the teeth, and this individual may have a lisp.

The tongue thrust presents a problem to dentistry in many aspects. Left untreated in the adult it can cause relapse of orthodontically treated cases (Garliner, 1971). The force of the tongue can cause flaring and the development of diastema. That same force initiates a torquing vector with a traumatic, occlusionlike result. The most severe periodontopathy is the trauma from occlusion in the teeth that are not involved in the thrust. In advanced cases the thrust can produce an open bite from the molars anteriorly. That would leave isolated molar teeth to carry the entire occlusal load

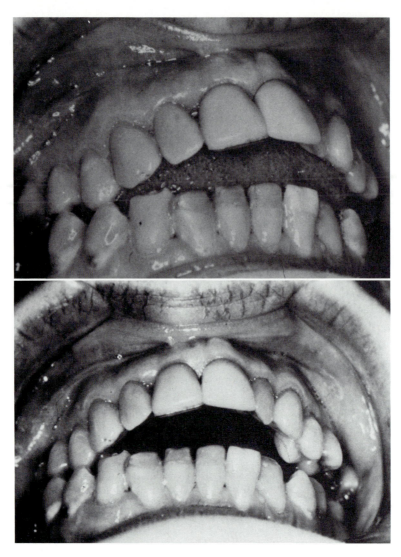

Fig. 4-43. Anterior tongue thrust.

(Fig. 4-43). Mobility and all the clinical and radiographic signs of occlusal trauma result.

Treatment of tongue thrust can be performed with appliances therapy, myofunctional and speech therapy, or a combination (Chaikin, 1972; Garliner, 1971). Restorative therapy alone will not resolve the damage caused by tongue thrusting. An individual can continue to move teeth that have been splinted and repeatedly unseat a denture with a tongue habit. The treatment of the overt anterior thrust must include comprehensive attention to the circumoral as well as the glossal musculature, for both systems are involved in the etiology.

Factitial habits. A self-inflicted injury of the periodontal tissues can occur with repeated voluntary trauma to a localized area. This injury can be caused by pacifiers, fingernails, pens, pen-

cils, eyeglass stems, and many other provocative objects (Baer and Archard, 1974; Blanton et al., 1977; Stewart, 1976; Stewart and Kernohan, 1973, 1972). Factitial habits, as they are called, can cause a local mechanical injury that invites bacterial contamination and results in inflammatory disease (Figs. 4-44 and 4-45). Stewart and Kernoham (1973) showed that these habits can proceed from localized recession to bone loss if left unattended. The psychologic profile of an individual with a factitial habit should be considered in the treatment plan.

Summary. Although many individuals have potentially destructive oral habits, the aforementioned results are not predictable. Often the periodontal tissues do not show any change from a habit until they are first weakened by periodonti-

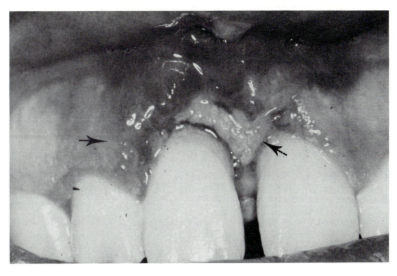

Fig. 4-44. Factitial habit with fingernail showing gingival slough, exposed osseous tissue, and secondary inflammation.

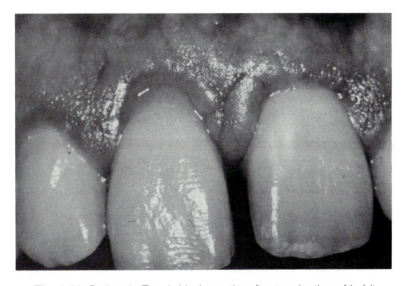

Fig. 4-45. Patient in Fig. 4-44, 4 months after termination of habit.

tis. Habitual etiology, frequency of habit, force exerted, and the degree of periodontal health will dictate response.

Thermal and radiant factors

Like mechanical factors thermal and radiant stimulants can initiate a periodontal response as well as contribute to tissue breakdown in consort with other factors. Although liquids and foods such as soup, coffee, and pizza commonly cause tissue burns (especially on palatal mucosa) the lesions eventually revert to normal. The incidence of thermal and radiant etiology causing irreversible damage is low when compared with the other etiologic factors in periodontal disease.

Several reports deal with the response of the periodontium to electrosurgery (heat) and cryotherapy (freezing). Extreme care must be used and treatment well defined when using *electrosurgery*. Several reports (Glickman and Imber, 1970; Nixon et al., 1975; Schneider and Zaki, 1974; Simon et al., 1976) demonstrate the histologic and ultrastructural changes in the periodontal tissues using this technique. In shallow resections of gingiva one might create a trough acting as a reservoir for bacterial plaque (Hazen and Osborne, 1967). The most common findings in deep electrosurgical resections include slow healing, pain, and loss of alveolar height.

The most frequently reported gingival response

to *cryotherapy* is irreversible injury to epithelial cells (Hurt et al., 1972; Mayers et al., 1971). When considering the use of this instrument in the treatment of tumors, especially vascular tumors, its purpose is catabolic at the cellular level.

Radiation is a popular method for treating oral facial malignancies. Like antimetabolites its purpose is to inhibit or destroy the reproduction of abnormal cellular activity. In so doing it adversely affects normal cellular metabolism and host response to exogenous agressors. Studies of the jaws of rats exposed to therapeutic radiation and cobalt 60 (Meyer et al., 1962) as well as studies on marginal periodontal tissue exposed to radiation in humans (Schüle and Betzhold, 1969) show a gradient of responses. They report that gingival hemorrhage, ulcerations, recession, necrosis of bone, looseness and devitalization of teeth, and loss of teeth can be demonstrated. Brown et al. (1975) reported on changes in the oral flora in individuals with xerostomia after being irradiated. The alteration in flora, the reduced anabolic response of the host, and the increased catabolic response to plaque often present a bizarre clinical entity leading to osteoradionecrosis.

Biochemical factors

The toxicity of plaque and calculus to the periodontium is the most frequently occurring chemical factor in the etiology of inflammatory disease (see Chapter 3). There are several other agents that evoke a pathologic response that is mediated biochemically.

Dental materials. Dental materials used today have in the main passed the rigorous steps for approval by the Council on Therapeutics of The American Dental Association. However, many of these materials are designed to contact mineralized surfaces. Any contact with the gingival tissue can initiate an adverse tissue response. One must be ever mindful that organic solvents, etching suspensions, cavity liners, and some desensitizing agents have the potential of initiating chemical destruction to periodontal tissue. The use of the rubber dam when working with these materials is an excellent preventive technique.

Several reports reveal the effect of specific restorative materials in isolated situations. Acrylic, in the form of a temporary crown (Giunta and Zablotsky, 1976), copper (Trachtenberg, 1972), and amalgam (Feuerman, 1975; Goldschmidt et al., 1976) have been shown to initiate a cytotoxic response with resultant gingival lesions and, in one case, facial edema. Careful history taking can reduce the chance of contributing to this phenomenon in individuals with known allergies to particular materials.

Tobacco. There is a threefold effect of tobacco on the periodontal tissues: (1) chewing tobacco elicits a biochemical effect, (2) smoking initiates a thermal and biochemical effect, and (3) the effect of tobacco on tooth surfaces is accompanied by

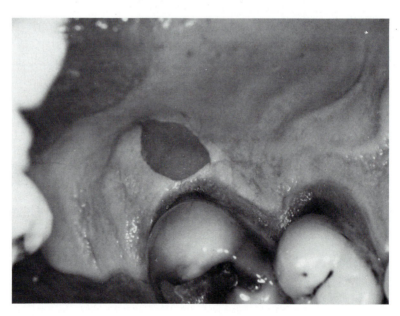

Fig. 4-46. Smoker's palate with ulcerated lesion approximating area where pipe stem terminates.

higher plaque scores. Individuals who chew tobacco develop the habit of retaining the material in a specific area in the facial vestibule of the mandibular arch. Adjacent tissues present a response similar to a hyperkeratotic lesion. Clinically there are white folded lesions in the alveolar mucosa, and the attached gingiva is gnarled in appearance. Frequently both recession and erosion can be seen where the tobacco wad rests. Arno et al. (1959) reported on a higher incidence of alveolar bone loss in individuals who were chronic tobacco consumers.

Smoking causes thermal changes in the tissues it contacts. The chronic irritation from heat causes alterations in vascular flow and salivary secretions. Habitually the pipe or the mouthpiece used with cigars and cigarettes directs a steady stream of heat to an isolated area where an ulcerative or hyperkeratotic lesion may develop (Figs. 4-46 and 4-47).

Understanding host response to the biochemical effect of nicotine, tars, and other factors will shed light on the oncogenic potential of smoking. This is a parameter of current research. The frequency of smoking correlates positively with periodontal disease (Arno et al., 1958; Sumners and Oberman, 1968). Preber and Kant (1973), studying the effect of smoking on 15-year-old school children, reported finding an elevated oral hygiene index in smokers when compared with nonsmoking controls. Bandtzaeg (1964), Solomon et al. (1968), and Sheiham (1971) reported on increased peri-

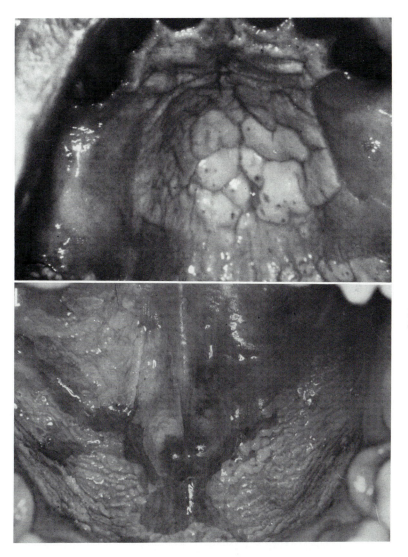

Fig. 4-47. White hyperkeratotic lesions affecting palate, floor of mouth, and attached gingiva in heavy cigarette smoker. Note absence of lesion in areas covered by partial denture.

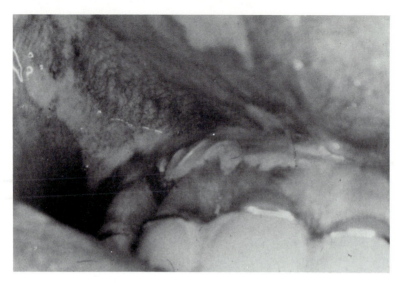

Fig. 4-48. Mucosal burn following repeated application of aspirin.

odontal disease scores in smokers. Plaque scores increased considerably in smokers, and their degree of oral cleanliness was significantly decreased. Frandsen and Pindborg (1949) found that pipe smokers accumulated more deposit than cigarette smokers. Kenney et al. (1975) were unable to demonstrate a statistically significant alteration in the anaerobic flora of individuals who were heavy smokers.

Missing from the aforementioned reports is evidence supporting reasons for increased plaque scores in smokers. Does the thermal or chemical alteration in the environment affect the growth of pathologic microbes or influence their media? Does the smoker have a retarded sense of taste and oral sensitivity resulting in an ignorance of oral cleanliness, or does the psychologic profile of the smoker include a lack of personal regard for oral hygiene? If this latter question is answered affirmatively, then smoking per se would not contribute to increased plaque accumulation.

Chemical desiccants. Much of the folklore that was historically a segment of the basic healing arts is being replaced by more reasonable approaches to treatment. This, however, is not the case when we see the repeated misuse of acetylsalicylic acid. The topical application of aspirin to oral mucosa will produce a circumscribed area of tissue necrosis (Fig. 4-48). Applied frequently for "toothache" and discomfort after therapy the chemical response is great and the therapeutic result is negligible. "Aspirin burn," as it is called, is a self-limiting lesion that heals adequately when the etiologic factor is removed. The effects of chemical

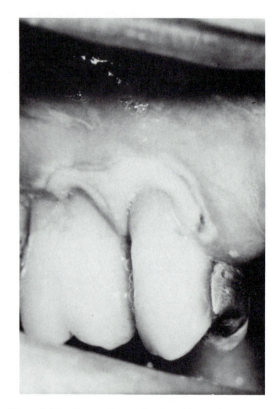

Fig. 4-49. Necrosis and sloughing of marginal gingiva following application of fluoride-desensitizing agent to adjacent root surfaces. (Courtesy Dr. M. Barnett, SUNY at Buffalo.)

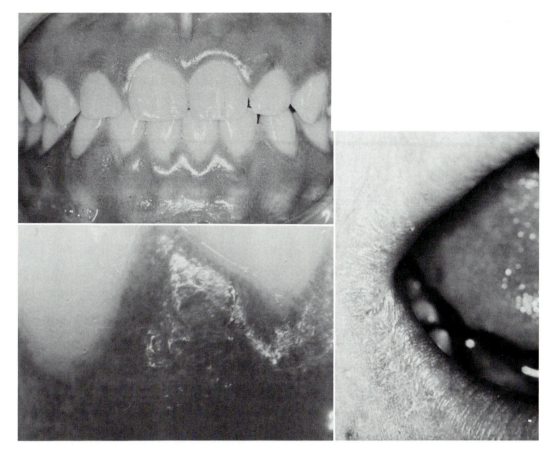

Fig. 4-50. Allergic gingivostomatitis resulting from chewing gum. Attached gingiva is hyperemic, distorted, and sore. Tongue is coated, and there are areas of filiform depapillation. Angular cheilitis is a common finding.

desiccants on gingival tissues was exemplified by Löe (1961) in reporting on chemical gingivectomy. He applied potassium hydroxide to chemically reduce hypertrophic tissues.

Dentrifrices have been presented in their role as abrasives in the discussion on Mechanical Factors. They can also affect periodontal health by initiating an allergiclike response to their ingredients. Allen et al. (1975) and Kowitz et al. (1973) reported on gingival lesions ranging from erythemia to ulceration and peeling of epithelium in susceptible individuals. Allen et al. conclude that the response is not one of individual hypersensitivity. The erythematous lesions are the result of a chemical response to one or more components of the dentrifrice.

Fluorides. The fluoride ion can affect gingival tissues in limited cases (Fig. 4-49). Murray (1972) found that fluoride in drinking water had no effect on the development or progression of gingivitis or recession. Guam et al. (1973) reported on several cases of epithelial sloughing when acidulated fluo-

ride phosphate gel contacted the gingiva. This was most commonly found when the gingival tissues were inflamed prior to application. Bronemark studied the effects of topical sodium fluoride application on gingival tissues in humans (1967) and in dogs (Lindhe et al., 1971). There was no evidence of tissue response in clinically healthy gingiva. When a preexisting ulcerated sulcular epithelium was present the gingival response was accentuated. This was probably due to a dysfunction in the microcirculation caused by the sodium fluoride.

Allergic gingival and oral lesions. There is an atypical form of gingival response to certain base materials found in chewing gum, candies, and dentifrices. It does not have the clinical appearance of inflammatory periodontal disease, and its diagnosis can be challenging. Several authors (Greer and Popper, 1975; Hamner and Croft, 1973; Kerr et al., 1971; Perry et al., 1973) have reported on cases of allergic response to such stimuli. Kerr et al. (1971) first introduced this phenomenon to the periodontal literature in 1971. Later Hamner and Croft (1973) and Perry et al. (1973) supported Kerr's paper in describing a triad of cyclic clinical signs and symptoms that accompany allergic gingival stomatitis; (1) angular cheilitis, (2) burning glossitis with loss of the filiform papillae, and (3) fiery red hyperemia of the attached gingiva (Fig. 4-50). The blood chemistry in these patients is essentially normal with a slight eosinophilia. The histologic picture is dominated by a plasma cell infiltrate, dilated capillaries, and a thin hyperplastic epithelium. Unless superimposed, the histopathology of typical inflammatory periodontal disease is absent. The allergic response is chemically mediated by base materials and essential oils used in the provocative product.

It is important to differentiate allergic gingivostomatitis from bacterial or fungal infections, manifestations of endocrinopathies, oral psoriasis, and desquamative gingival lesions. A positive history of contact is important information in establishing a diagnosis. There is complete remission of the clinical and histologic signs and symptoms 4 months after the etiologic agent is removed.

• • •

Etiologic factors associated with the occlusion, systemic profile, and specific entities, that is, acute necrotizing ulcerating gingivitis and periodontosis, will be discussed in later chapters.

REFERENCES

Aleo, J. J., DeRenzis, F. A., and Farber, P. A.: In vitro attachment of human gingival fibroblasts to root surfaces, J. Periodontol. **46:**639, 1975.

Aleo, J. J., DeRenzis, F. A., Farber, P. A., and Varboncoeur, A. P.: The presence and biologic activity of cementum-bound endotoxin, J. Periodontol. **45:**672, 1974.

Alfano, M.: Controversies, perspectives and clinical implications of nutrition and periodontal disease, Dent. Clin. North Am. **20:**519, 1976.

Allen, A. L., Hawley, C. E., Cutright, D. E., and Herbert, J. S.: An investigation of the clinical and histologic effects of selected dentifrices on human palatal mucosa, J. Periodontol. **46:**102, 1975.

Anderson, D. L., Thompson, G. W., and Popovich, F.: Contributory factors in oral debris removal and thumb sucking, J. Periodontol. **45:**230, 1974.

Andrews, N. H.: Periodontal significance of cervical enamel projections, J. Can. Dent. Assoc. **41:**50, 1975.

Anneroth, G., and Poppelman, A.: Histologic evaluation of gingival damage by toothbrushing. An experimental study in dogs, Acta Odontol. Scand. **33:**119, 1967.

Arnim, S. S.: Dental irrigators, J. Am. Soc. Prev. Dent. **6:**10, 1976.

Arnim, S. S.: Dental irrigators for oral hygiene, periodontal therapy and prevention of dental disease, J. Tenn. Dent. Assoc. **47:**65, 1967.

Arnim, S. S.: The use of disclosing agents for measuring tooth cleanliness, J. Periodontol. **34:**227, 1963.

Arno, A., Schei, O., Lovdal, A., and Waerhaug, J.: Alveolar bone loss as a function of tobacco consumption, Acta Odontol. Scand. **14:**3, 1959.

Arno, A., Waerhaug, J., Lovdal, A., and Schei, O.: Incidence of gingivitis as related to sex, occupation, tobacco consumption, toothbrushing and age, Oral Surg. **11:**587, 1958.

Baer, P. N., and Archard, H. O.: Factitial disease of gingiva and buccal mucosa. Report of a Case, N.Y. State Dent. J. **40:**33, 1974.

Baker, D. L., and Seymour, G. L.: The possible pathogenesis of gingival recession. A histologic study of induced recession in the rat, J. Clin. Periodontol. **3:**208, 1976.

Barker, B. C. W.: Relation of the alveolus to the cemento-enamel junction following attritional wear in aboriginal skulls. An enquiry into the normality of cementum exposure with aging, J. Periodontol. **46:**357, 1975.

Bass, C. C.: The optimum characteristics of toothbrushes for personal oral hygiene, Dent. Items Interest **70:**697, 1948.

Bhaskar, S. N., editor: Orban's oral histology and embryology, ed. 8, St. Louis, 1976, The C. V. Mosby Co.

Bibby, B. G.: The formation of salivary calculus, D. Cosmos **77:**668, 1935.

Björn, A. L., Björn, H., and Grkovic, B.: Marginal fit of restorations and its relation to periodontal bone level. II. Crowns, Odontol. Revy **21:**337, 1970.

Björn, A. L., Björn, H., and Grkovic, B.: Marginal fit of restorations and its relation to periodontal bone level. I. Metal fillings, Odontol. Revy **20:**311, 1969.

Bissada, N. F., and Abdelmalek, R. G.: Incidence of cervical enamel projections and its relationship to furcation involvement in Egyptian skulls, J. Periodontol. **44:**583, 1973.

Bissada, N. F., Ibrahim, S. I., and Barsoum, W. M.: Gingival response to various types of removable partial dentures, J. Periodontol. **45:**651, 1974.

Blair, H. A.: Relationship between endodontics and periodontics, J. Periodontol. **43:**209, 1972.

Blanton, P. L., Hurt, W. C., and Largent, M. D.: Oral factitious injuries, J. Periodontol. **48:**33, 1977.

Brandtzaeg, P.: The significance of oral hygiene in the prevention of dental diseases, Odontol. Tksr. **72:**460, 1964.

Brönemark, P-I.: Local tissue effects of sodium fluoride, Odontol. Revy **18:**273, 1967.

Brown, L. R., Dreizen, S., Handler, S., and Johnston, D. A.: Effect of radiation induced xerostomia on human oral microflora, J. Dent. Res. **54:**740, 1975.

Buckley, L. A.: The relationship between malocclusion and periodontal disease, J. Periodontol. **43:**415, 1972.

Burch, J. G.: Ten rules for developing crown contours in restorations, Dent. Clin. North Am. **15:**611, 1971.

Burch, J. G.: A study of the presence of accessory foramina and the topography of molar furcations, Oral Surg. **38:**451, 1974.

Caldwell, R. C.: Adhesion of foods to teeth, J. Dent. Res. **41:**821, 1962.

Cameron, C.: Cracked tooth syndrome: additional findings, J. Am. Dent. Assoc. **93:**971, 1976.

Cameron, C.: Cracked tooth syndrome, J. Am. Dent. Assoc. **68:**405, 1964.

Cataldo, E., and Santis, H.: Response of oral tissues to exogenous foreign materials, J. Periodontol. **45:**93, 1974.

Cavanha, A. O.: A new rare type of enamel pearl, Oral Surg. **23:**213, 1967.

Cavanha, A. O.: Enamel pearls, Oral Surg. **19:**373, 1965.

Chacker, F. M.: The endodontic-periodontic continuum, Dent. Clin. North Am. **18:**393, 1974.

Chaikin, B. S.: Analysis of the therapy of an open bite due to tongue thrusting, J. Periodontol. **43:**362, 1972.

Christidou, L., Osborne, J., and Chambelain, J. B.: The effects of partial denture design on the mobility of teeth, Br. Dent. J. **135:**9, 1973.

Coelho, D. H., Cavallaro, J., and Rothschild, E. A.: Gingival recession with electrosurgery for impression making, J. Prosthet. Dent. **33:**422, 1975.

Critchley, P., and Bowen, W. H.: Correlation of the biochemical composition of plaque with the diet. In McHugh, W. D., editor: Dental plaque, Dundee, Scotland, 1970, Thomson and Co. Ltd.

Donaldson, D.: The etiology of gingival recession associated with temporary crowns, J. Periodontol. **45:**468, 1974.

Drucker, D. B.: Optimum pH values for growth of various plaque streptococci. In McHugh, W. D., editor: Dental plaque, Dundee, Scotland, 1970, Thomson and Co. Ltd., p. 241.

Egelberg, J.: Local effect of diet on plaque formation and development of gingivitis in dogs. III. Effect of frequency of meals and tube feeding, Odontol. Revy **16:**50, 1965.

Everett, F. G., and Kramer, G. M.: The distro-lingual groove in the maxillary lateral incisor: a periodontal hazard, J. Periodontol. **43:**352, 1972.

Eversole, L. R., and Rovin, S.: Diagnosis of gingival tumefactions, J. Periodontol. **44:**429, 1973.

Eversole, L. R., and Rovin, S.: Reactive lesions of the gingiva, J. Oral Pathol. **1:**30, 1972.

Felix, J. E., Rosen, S., and App, G. R.: Detection of bacteremia after the use of an oral irrigation device in subject with periodontitis, J. Periodontol. **42:**785, 1971.

Feuerman, E. J.: Recurrent contact dermatitis caused by mercury in amalgam dental fillings, Int. J. Dermatol. **14:**657, 1975.

Frandsen, A. M., and Pindborg, J. J.: Tobacco and gingivitis. III. Difference in the action of cigarette and pipe smoking, J. Dent. Res. **46:**464, 1949.

Frank, R. M., Brion, M., and DeRouggignac, M.: Ultrastructural gingival reactions to gold foil, J. Periodontol. **46:**614, 1975.

Garliner, D.: Abnormal swallowing habits, New York, 1971, Bartel Dental Book Co.

Gaum, E., Cataldo, E., and Shiere, F.: The reaction of the gingiva to acidulated fluoride gel, J. Dent. Child. **40:**22, 1973.

Geddes, D., and Jenkins, G. N.: Intrinsic and extrinsic factors influencing the flora of the mouth. In Skinner, F. A., and Carr, J. G., editors: The normal microbial flora, New York, 1974, Academic Press, Inc., p. 85.

Gilmore, N., and Sheiham, A.: Overhanging dental restorations and periodontal disease. J. Periodontol. **42:**8, 1971.

Giunta, J., and Zablotsky, N.: Allergic stomatitis caused by self-polymerizing resin, Oral Surg. **41:**631, 1976.

Glenwright, H. D.: Bone regeneration following damage by polysulphide impression material. A case report, J. Clin. Periodontol. **2:**250, 1975.

Glickman, I., and Imber, L.: Comparison to gingival resection with electrosurgery and periodontal knives—a biometric and histologic study, J. Periodontol. **41:**142, 1970.

Goldman, H. M.: Extension of exudate into the supporting structures, J. Periodontol. **28:**175, 1957.

Goldschmidt, P. R., Cogen, R. B., and Taubman, S. B.: Effects of alloy amalgam corrosion products on human cells, J. Periodont. Res. **11:**108, 1976.

Goodman, P., Greene, C. S., and Laskin, D. M.: Response of patients with myofasical pain-dysfunction syndrome to mock equilibration, J. Am. Dent. Assoc. **92:**755, 1976.

Gorman, W. J.: Prevalence and etiology of gingival recession, J. Periodontol. **38:**316, 1967.

Gould, M. S., and Picton, D. C.: The relationship between irregularities of the teeth and periodontal disease, Br. Dent. J. **121:**20, 1966.

Greer, R. O., and Popper, H.: Gingivostomatitis syndrome; current etiologic considerations and report on two cases, Am. Dent. J. **34:**24, 1975.

Hamner, J. E., and Croft, L. K.: Clinical, endocrinological and histopathological findings in allergic gingivostomatitis, J. Periodont. Res. **8:**192, 1973.

Hayward, J. R.: Multiple recurrent fibro-osseous epulides. Int. J. Oral Surg. **2:**115, 1973.

Hazen, S., and Osborne, J.: Relationship of operative dentistry to periodontal health, Dent. Clin. North Am., p. 245, March, 1967.

Heneghan, J. B., and Listgarten, M. A.: Observations on the periodontium and acquired pellicle of adult germfree dogs, J. Periodontol. **44:**85, 1973.

Henry, S. W., Levine, M. P., and Tsakis, P. J.: Histologic features of the superior labial frenum, J. Periodontol. **47:**25, 1976.

Hiatt, W. H.: Incomplete crown-root fracture in pulpal-periodontal disease, J. Periodontol. **44:**369, 1973.

Hirschfeld, I.: Traumatization of soft tissues by toothbrush, Dent. Items Interest **55:**529; **56:**159, 1934.

Hirschfeld, I.: Food impaction, J. Am. Dent. Assoc. **17:**1504, 1930.

Hogeboom, F. E., and Stephens, K. A.: The dangerous rubber band, J. Dent. Child. **32:**199, 1965.

Hoover, D. R., and Robinson, H. B.: The comparative effectiveness of the Water Pik in a non-instructed population, J. Periodontol. **39:**43, 1968.

Hopps, R. M., and Johnson, N. W.: Relationship between the histological degree of inflammation and epithelial proliferation in macque gingiva, J. Periodont. Res. **9:**273, 1974.

Hurt, W. C., Nabers, C. L., and Rose, G. S.: Some clinical and histologic observations of gingiva treated with cryotherapy, J. Periodontol. **43:**151, 1972.

Inward, P. W., Upstone, D., and Van Houte, J.: Nutritional requirements of oral streptococci. In McHugh, W. D., editor: Dental plaque, Dundee, Scotland, 1970, Thomson and Co. Ltd., p. 217.

Jacobson, T.: Mouthbreathing and gingivitis, J. Periodont. Res. **8:**269, 1973.

Keller, G. J., and Cohen, D. W.: India ink profusions of the vascular plexus of oral tissues. Oral Surg. **8:**539, 1955.

Kennedy, J. E.: Effects of inflammation on collateral circulation of the gingiva, J. Periodont. Res. **9:**147, 1974.

Kenney, E. B., Saxe, S. R., and Bowles, R. D.: The effect of cigarette smoking on anaerobiosis in the oral cavity, J. Periodontol. **46:**82, 1975.

Kenney, E. B., Saxe, S. R., Lenox, J. A., Cooper, T. M., Caudill, J. S., Collins, A. R., and Kaplan, A.: The relationship of manual dexterity and knowledge to performance of oral hygiene, J. Periodont. Res. **11:**67, 1976.

Kerr, D. A., McClatchey, K. D., and Regezi, J. A.: Allergic gingivostomatitis (due to chewing gum), J. Periodontol. **42:**709, 1971.

Kerry, G. J.: Roughness of root surfaces after use of ultrasonic instruments and hand curettes, J. Periodontol. **38:**340, 1967.

Kirkham, D. B.: The location and incidence of accessory pulpal canals in periodontal pockets, J. Am. Dent. Assoc. **91:**353, 1975.

Kloehm, J. S., and Pfeifer, J. S.: The effect of orthodontic treatment on the periodontium, Angle Orthod. **44:**127, 1974.

Kowitz, G.: Effects of dentifrices on soft tissues of the oral cavity, J. Oral Med. **28:**105, 1973.

Krajewski, J., Giblink, J. and Gargiulo, A.: Evaluation of water pressure cleansing device as an adjunct to periodontal treatment, J. Am. Soc. Periodont. **2:**76, 1964.

Lainson, P. A., Bergquist, J. J., and Fraleigh, C. M.: A longitudinal study of pulsating water pressure devices, J. Periodontol. **43:**444, 1972.

Lang, N. P., and Löe, H.: The relationship between the width of keratinized gingiva and gingival health, J. Periodontol. **43:**623, 1972.

Larato, D. C.: Some anatomical factors related to furcation involvements, J. Periodontol. **46:**608, 1975.

Larato, D. C.: Influence of silicate cement restorations on gingiva, J. Prosthet. Dent. **26:**186, 1971a.

Larato, D. C.: Relationship of food impaction to interproximal intrabony lesions, J. Periodontol. **42:**237, 1971b.

Lee, K. W., Lee, E. C., and Poon, K. Y.: Palatogingival grooves in maxillary incisors, Br. Dent. J. **124:**14, 1968.

Leung, S. W., and Jensen, A. T.: Factors controlling the deposition of calculus, Int. Dent. J. **8:**613, 1958.

Lilly, G. E., Osborn, D. B., Hutchinson, R. A., and Henflich, R. H.: Clinical and bacteriological aspects of polyglycolic acid sutures, J. Oral Surg. **31:**103, 1973.

Lindhe, J., Hansson, B. O., and Brönemark, P. I.: The effect of topical application of fluoride on the gingival tissues, J. Periodontol. Res. **6:**211, 1971.

Lindhe, J., and Nyman, S.: The effect of plaque control and surgical pocket elimination on the establishment and maintenance of periodontal health. A longitudinal study of periodontal therapy in cases of advanced disease, J. Clin. Periodontol. **2:**67, 1975.

Lindhe, J., and Wicen, P. O.: The effects on the gingival of chewing fibrous food, J. Periodont. Res. **4:**193, 1969.

Lindquist, B.: Bruxism in twins, Acta Odontol. Scand. **32:**177, 1974.

Lindquist, B.: Bruxism and emotional disturbance, Odontol. Revy **23:**231, 1972.

Lineberger, L. T., and DeMarco, T. J.: Evaluation of transient bacteremia following routine periodontal procedures, J. Periodontol. **44:**757, 1973.

Listgarten, M. A.: Structure of surface coatings on teeth. A review, J. Periodontol. **47:**144, 1975.

Little, M. F., Bowman, L., Casciani, C. A., and Rowley, J.: The composition of dental calculus. III. Amino acid and saccharide component, Arch. Oral Biol. **11:**385, 1966.

Little, M. F., Bowman, L., and Dirkson, T. R.: The lipids of supragingival calculus, J. Dent. Res. **43:**836, 1964.

Lobene, R. R.: The effect of a pulsed water pressure cleansing device on oral health, J. Periodontol. **40:**667, 1969.

Lobene, R. R.: A study of the force of water jets in relation to pain and damage to gingival tissues, J. Periodontol. **42:**166, 1971.

Löe, H.: Chemical gingivectomy — effect of potassium hydroxide on periodontal tissues, Acta Odontol. Scand. **19:**517, 1961.

Löe, H., Theilade, E., and Jensen, I. B.: Experimental gingivitis in man, J. Periodontol. **36:**177, 1965.

Loesche, W. J.: Importance of nutrition in gingival crevice microbial ecology, J. Periodontol. **36:**177, 1968.

Longhurst, P., and Berman, D. S.: Apples and gingival health, Br. Dent. J. **134:**475, 1973.

Lowman, J. V., Burke, R. S., and Pelleu, G. B.: Patent accessory canals: incidence in molar furcation region, Oral Surg. **36:**580, 1973.

Mandel, I. D.: Biochemical aspects of calculus formation. I. Comparative studies of plaque in heavy and light formers, J. Periodont. Res. **9:**10, 1974a.

Mandel, I. D.: Biochemical aspects of calculus formation. II. Comparative studies of saliva in heavy and light calculus formers, J. Periodont. Res. **9:**211, 1974b.

Mandel, I. D., Levy, B. M., and Wasserman, B. H.: Histochemistry of calculus formation, J. Periodontol. **28:**132, 1957.

Manly, R. S., and Foster, D. H.: Importance of factorial designs in testing abrasion by dentifrices, J. Dent. Res. **46:**442, 1967.

Masters, D., and Hoskins, S.: Projection of cervical enamel in molar furcations, J. Periodontol. **35:**49, 1964.

Mayers, P. D., Tussing, G., and Wentz, F. M.: The histologic reaction of clinically normal gingiva to freezing, J. Periodontol. **42:**346, 1971.

Maynard, J. G., Jr., and Ochsenbein, C.: Mucogingival problems, prevalence and therapy in children, J. Periodontol. **46:**543, 1975.

Meklas, J. F., and Stewart, J. L.: Investigation of the safety and effectiveness of an oral irrigating device, J. Periodontol. **43:**441, 1972.

Meyer, I., Shklar, G., and Turner, J.: A comparison of the effects of 200 K V radiation and cobalt 60 radiation on the jaws and dental structures of the white rat. A preliminary report, Oral Surg. **15:**1098, 1962.

Mirko, P., Miroslav, S., and Lubor, M.: Significance of the labial frenum attachment in periodontal disease in man. I. Classification and epidemiology of the labial frenum attachment, J. Periodontol. **45:**891, 1974a.

Mirko, P., Miroslav, S., and Lubor, M.: Significance of the labial frenum attachment in periodontal disease in man. II. An attempt to determine the resistance of periodontium, J. Periodontol. **45:**895, 1974b.

Mislowsky, W. J., and Mazzella, W. J.: Supragingival and subgingival plaque and calculus formation in humans, J. Periodontol. **45:**822, 1974.

Mörmann, W., Regolati, B., and Renggli, H. H.: Gingival reaction to well-fitted subgingival proximal gold inlays, J. Clin. Periodontol. **1:**120, 1974.

Morris, M. L.: An inhibitory principle in the matrix of periodontally diseased roots, J. Periodontol. **46:**33, 1975.

Moskow, B. S.: Some observations on radicular enamel, J. Periodontol. **42:**92, 1971.

Moskow, B. S.: Calculus attachment in cemental separations, J. Periodontol. **40:**125, 1969.

Moskow, B. S., and Weinstein, M. M.: Further observations on the gingival cyst, J. Periodontol. **46:**178, 1975.

Mühlemann, H. R., and DeBoever, J.: Radiotelemetry of the pH of interdental areas exposed to various carbohydrates. In McHugh, W. D., editor: Dental plaque, Dundee, Scotland, 1970, Thomson and Co. Ltd.

Murray, J. J.: Gingivitis and gingival recession in adults from high fluoride and low fluoride areas, Arch. Oral Biol. **17:** 1269, 1972.

Myers, D. R.: A clinical study of the response of the gingival tissue surrounding stainless steel crowns, J. Dent. Child. **42:**281, 1975.

Nadler, S. C.: The importance of bruxism, J. Oral Med. **23:** 142, 1968.

Naeslund, C.: A comparative study of the formation of concentrations in the oral cavity and in the salivary glands and ducts, Dent. Cosmos **68:**1137, 1926.

Neuman, W. F., and Neuman, M. W.: The chemical dynamics of bone mineral, Chicago, 1958, University of Chicago Press, p. 209.

Newcomb, G. M.: The relationship between the location of subgingival crown margins and gingival inflammation, J. Periodontol. **45:**151, 1974.

Nixon, K. C., Adkins, K. F., and Keys, D. W.: Histological evaluation of effects produced in alveolar bone following gingival incision with an electrosurgical scalpel, J. Periodontol. **46:**40, 1975.

Noble, W. H., Tueller, V. M., and Douglass, G. D.: Margin placement in restorative dentistry, J. Am. Soc. Prev. Dent. **3:**49, 1973.

Nordquist, G. G., and McNeill, Wm.: Orthodontic vs. restorative treatment of the congenitally absent lateral incisor—long term periodontal and occlusal evaluation, J. Periodontol. **46:**139, 1975.

Novaes, A. B., Ruben, M. P., Kon, S., Goldman, H. M., and Novaes, A. B., Jr.: The development of the periodontal cleft, J. Periodontol. **46:**701, 1965.

Nuki, K., and Hock, J.: The organization of the gingival vasculature, J. Periodont. Res. **9:**305, 1974.

O'Leary, T. J., Bladell, M. C., and Bloomer, R. S.: Interproximal contact and marginal ridge relationships in periodontally healthy young males classified as to orthodontic status, J. Periodontol. **46:**6, 1974.

O'Leary, T. J., Drake, R. B., Crump, P. P., and Allen, M. F.: The incidence of recession in young males: a further study, J. Periodontol. **42:**264, 1971.

O'Leary, T. J., Shafer, W. G., Swenson, H. M., Nesler, D. C., and Van Dorn, P. R.: Possible penetration of crevicular tissue from oral hygiene procedures. I. Use of oral irrigating devices, J. Periodontol. **41:**158, 1970a.

O'Leary, T. J., Shafer, W. G., Swenson, H. M., Nesler, D. C., and Van Dorn, P. R.: Possible penetration of crevicular tissue from oral hygiene procedures. II. Use of the toothbrush, J. Periodontol. **41:**163, 1970b.

O'Leary, T. J., Standich, S. M., and Bloomer, R. S.: Severe periodontal destruction following impression procedures, J. Periodontol. **44:**25, 1973.

Orban, B., and Mueller, E.: The gingival crevice, J. Am. Dent. Assoc. **16:**1206, 1929.

Padbury, A. D., and Ash, M. M.: Abrasion caused by three methods of toothbrushing, J. Periodontol. **45:**434, 1974.

Pang, A.: Relationship of musical wind instruments to malocclusion, J. Am. Dent. Assoc. **92:**565, 1976.

Parfitt, G. S., and Mjör, I. A.: Clinical evaluation of local gingival recession in children, J. Dent. Child. **31:**257, 1964.

Parkinson, C. F.: Excessive crown contours facilitate endemic plaque niches, J. Prosthet. Dent. **35:**424, 1976.

Paunio, K.: The role of malocclusion and crowning in the development of periodontal disease, Int. Dent. J. **23:**470, 1973.

Perry, H. O., Deffner, N. F., and Sheridan, P. J.: Atypical gingivostomatitis, Arch. Dermatol. **107:**872, 1973.

Picard, P. J.: Bottle feeding as preventive orthodontics, J. Calif. Dent. Assoc. and Nevada Dent. Soc. **35:**90, 1959.

Polson, A. M.: Periodontal destruction associated with vertical root fracture-report of four cases, J. Periodontol. **48:**27, 1977.

Polson, A. M., Kennedy, J. E., and Zander, H. A.: Trauma and progression of marginal periodontitism in squirrel monkeys. I. Co-destructive factors of periodontitis and thermally produced injury, J. Periodont. Res. **9:**100, 1974a.

Polson, A. M., Kennedy, J. E., and Zander, H. A.: Trauma and progression of marginal periodontitism in squirrel monkeys. II. Co-destructive factors of periodontitis and mechanically-produced injury, J. Periodont. Res. **9:**108, 1974b.

Preber, H., and Kant, T.: Effect of tobacco smoking on periodontal tissue of 15-year-old school children, J. Periodont. Res. **8:**278, 1973.

Price, C., and Whitehead, F.: Impression material as foreign bodies, Br. Dent. J. **133:**9, 1972.

Prinz, N.: Diseases of the soft structures of the teeth and their treatment, Philadelphia, 1928, Lea & Febiger, chapter 33.

Pritchard, J. F.: The effect of bicuspid extraction orthodontics on the periodontium, J. Periodontol. **46:**534, 1975.

Radentz, W. H., Barnes, G. P., and Cutright, D. E.: A survey of factors possibly associated with cervical abrasion of tooth surfaces, J. Periodontol. **47:**148, 1975.

Ramfjord, S. P.: Bruxism: a clinical and electromyographic study, J. Am. Dent. Assoc. **62:**21, 1961.

Ramfjord, S. P., Knowles, J. W., Nissle, R., Shick, R. A., and Burgeth, F. G.: Longitudinal study of periodontal therapy, J. Periodontol. **44:**66, 1973.

Register, A. A., and Burdick, F. A.: Accelerated reattachment with cementogenesis to dentin, demineralized in situ. II. Defect repair, J. Periodontol. **47:**497, 1976.

Register, A. A., and Burdick, F. A.: Accelerated reattachment with cementogenesis to dentin, demineralized in situ, J. Periodontol. **46:**646, 1975.

Reitan, K.: Some factors determining the evaluation of forces in orthodontics, Am. J. Orthod. **43:**32, 1957.

Reitan, K.: Continuous bodily movement and its histologic significance, Acta Odontol. Scand. **6:**115, 1947.

Richter, W. A., and Ueno, H.: Relationship of crown margin placement to gingival inflammation, J. Prosthet. Dent. **30:** 157, 1973.

Ritchey, B., and Orban, B.: The crests of interdental alveolar septa, J. Periodontol. **24:**75, 1953.

Robinson, J., Reding, G., Zepelin, H., Smith, V., and Zimmerman, S.: Nocturnal teeth grinding, J. Am. Dent. Assoc. **78:**1308, 1969.

Romans, A. R., and App, G. R.: Bacteremia, a result from oral irrigation in subjects with gingivitis, J. Periodontol. **42:**757, 1971.

Rosenberg, R. M., and Ash, M. M., Jr.: The effect of root roughness on plaque accumulation, J. Periodontol. **45:**146, 1974.

Rosling, B., Nyman, S., and Lindhe, J.: The effect of systemic plaque control on bone regeneration in infrabony pockets, J. Clin. Periodontol. **3**:38, 1976.

Ruback, W. C., and Mitchell, D. F.: Periodontal disease, accessory canals and pulp pathosis, J. Periodontol. **36**:34, 1965.

Rudd, K. D.: Tissue injury from removable partial dentures, Dent. Clin. North Am. **16**:805, 1972.

Rygh, P.: Ultrastructural changes in pressure zones of human periodontium incident to orthodontic tooth movement, Acta Odontol. Scand. **31**:109, 1973.

Sackett, B. P., and Gildenhuys, R. R.: The effect of axial crown overcontour on adolescents, J. Periodontol. **47**:320, 1976.

Safavi, H., Ruben, M. P., Mafla, E. R., and Bloom, A. A.: Periodontal traumatism produced by sustained increase in occlusal vertical dimension: a histopathologic study, J. Periodontol. **45**:207, 1974.

Saglie, R., Johansen, J. R., and Flötra, L.: Scanning electron microscopic study of tooth surfaces in pathologic pockets, Scand. J. Dent. Res. **82**:579, 1974.

Sangnes, G.: Traumatization of teeth and gingiva related to habitual tooth cleaning procedures, J. Clin. Periodontol. **3**:94, 1976.

Saxton, C. A.: The effects of dentifrices on the appearance of the tooth surface observed with the scanning electron microscope, J. Periodont. Res. **11**:74, 1976.

Schüle, H., and Betzhold, T.: Experimental investigations on the effect of x-ray irradiation on marginal periodontal tissues, Dtsch. Zahnaerztl. Z. **24**:140, 1969.

Schneider, A. R., and Zaki, A. E.: Gingival wound healing following experimental electrosurgery: an electron microscopic study, J. Periodontol. **45**:685, 1974.

Schroeder, H. E.: Formation and inhibition of dental calculus, Berne, 1969, H. H. Huber Verlag.

Schroeder, H. E., and Bambauer, H. U.: Stages of calcium phosphate crystallization during calculus formation, Arch. Oral Biol. **11**:1, 1966.

Schwartz, R., and Massler, M.: Gingival reaction to different types of tooth accumulated materials, J. Periodontol. **42**:144, 1971.

Sconyers, J. R., Crawford, J. J., and Moriarty, J. D.: Relationship of bacteremia to toothbrushing in patients with periodontitis, J. Am. Dent. Assoc. **87**:616, 1973.

Screebny, N. M.: Food consistency and periodontal disease. In Hazen, S. P., editor: Diet, nutrition and periodontal disease, Chicago, 1975, American Society of Preventive Dentistry.

Seltzer, S., and Bender, I. B.: The dental pulp, Philadelphia, 1965, J. B. Lippincott Co., p. 207.

Seltzer, S., Bender, I. B., and Ziontz, M.: The interrelationship of the pulp and periodontal disease, Oral Surg. **16**:1474, 1963.

Selvig, K. A.: The fine structure of human cementum, Acta Odontol. Scand. **23**:423, 1965.

Selvig, K. A.: Ultrastructural changes in cementum and adjacent connective tissues in periodontal disease, Acta Odontol. Scand. **22**:459, 1966.

Seyle, H.: General adaptation syndrome, Montreal Acta, 1951.

Sheiham, A.: Periodontal disease and oral cleanliness in tobacco smokers, J. Periodontol. **42**:254, 1971.

Silness, J.: Periodontal conditions in patients treated with dental bridges, J. Periodont. Res. **9**:50, 1974.

Silness, J.: Periodontal conditions in patients treated with full dental bridges. II. The influence of full and partial crowns on plaque accumulation, development of gingivitis and pocket formation, J. Periodont. Res. **5**:219, 1970.

Silness, J., and Ohm, E.: Periodontal conditions in patients treated with dental bridges. V. Effects of splinting adjacent abutment teeth, J. Periodont. Res. **9**:121, 1974.

Simon, J. H., Glick, D. H., and Frank, A. L.: The relationship of endodontic-periodontic lesions, J. Periodontol. **43**:102, 1972.

Simon, J. H., Glick, D. H., and Frank, A. L.: Predictable failures as a result of radicular anomalies, Oral Surg. **31**:823, 1971.

Simon, B. I., Schuback, P., Deasy, M. J., and Kelner, R. M.: The destructive potential of electrosurgery on the periodontium, J. Periodontol. **47**:342, 1976.

Sinai, I. H., and Soltanoff, W.: The transmission of pathologic changes between the pulp and the periodontal tissues, Oral Surg. **36**:558, 1973.

Solomon, H., Prione, R., and Bross, I.: Cigarette smoking and periodontal disease, J. Am. Dent. Assoc. **77**:1081, 1968.

Sotres, L. S., Van Huysen, G., and Gilmore, H. W.: A histologic study of gingival tissue response to amalgam, silicate and resin restorations, J. Periodontol. **40**:543, 1969.

Stahl, S. S.: The nature of health and diseased roots, J. Periodontol. **46**:156, 1975.

Stewart, D. J.: Minor self-inflicted injuries to the gingival. Gingivitis artefacta minor, J. Clin. Periodontol. **3**:128, 1976.

Stewart, D. J., and Kernohan, D. C.: Traumatic gingival recession in infants. The results of dummy sucking habit, Br. Dent. J. **135**:157, 1973.

Stewart, D. J., and Kernohan, D. C.: Self-inflicted gingival injuries, Dent. Pract. **22**:418, 1972.

Stewart, R. T., and Radcliff, P. A.: The source of components of subgingival plaque and calculus, Periodont. Abstr. **14**:102, 1966.

Stillman, P. R.: Early clinical evidences of disease in the gingiva and pericementum, J. Dent. Res. **3**:25, 1921.

Straub, W. J.: Malfunction of the tongue, Am. J. Orthod. **47**:596, 1961.

Sumner, C. F., III: The water pressure cleansing device, an evaluation. Fifty-first Meeting of the American Academy of Periodontology, Las Vegas, November, 1965.

Sumners, C. J., and Oberman, O.: Association of oral disease with twelve selected variables: I. Periodontal disease, J. Dent. Res. **47**:457, 1968.

Swartz, M., and Philips, R.: Comparison of bacterial accumulations on rough and smooth enamel surfaces, J. Periodontol. **28**:304, 1957.

Taylor, A. C., and Campbell, M. M.: Reattachment of gingival epithelium to the tooth, J. Periodontol. **43**:281, 1972.

Thaller, J. L., Rosen, G., and Saltzman, S.: A study of the relationship of frustration and anxiety to bruxism, J. Periodontol. **38**:193, 1976.

Theilade, J., Fitzgerald, R. J., Scott, D. B., and Nylen, M. U.: Electron microscopic observations of dental calculus in germfree and conventional rats, Arch. Oral Biol. **9**:97, 1964.

Tibbetts, L. S., and Kashiwa, H. K.: A Histochemical Study of Early Plaque Mineralization. I.A.D.R. Abstract no. 616, p. 202, 1970.

Toller, J. R.: The gingival sulcus and the epithelial attachment, Br. Dent. J. **85**:1, 1948.

Toto, P. D., Evans, C. L., and Sawinski, V. J.: Effects of water jet rinse and toothbrushing on oral hygiene, J. Periodontol. **40:**296, 1969.

Townsend, J. D.: Coronal forms. A panel discussion to the American Academy of Periodontists sixty-second annual meeting, San Francisco, November, 1976.

Trachtenberg, D. I.: Allergic response to copper — its possible gingival implications, J. Periodontol. **43:**705, 1972.

Tsatsas, B., Mandi, F., and Kerani, S.: Cervical enamel projections in molar teeth, J. Periodontol. **44:**212, 1973.

Turesky, S., and Glickmen, I.: Histologic and histochemical observations regarding early calculus formation in children and adults, J. Periodontol. **32:**7, 1961.

Vandersall, D. C.: Localized periodontitis induced by rubber elastic: report of case, J. Am. Dent. Assoc. **83:**1326, 1971.

van Valkenburg, J. W., Green, E., and Armitage, G. C.: The nature of root surfaces after curette, cavitron and alpha-sonic instrumentation, J. Periodont. Res. **11:**374, 1976.

Waerhaug, J.: Effect of rough surfaces upon gingival tissues, J. Dent. Res. **35:**323, 1956.

Wasserman, B. H., Mandel, I. D., and Levy, B. M.: In vitro calcification of calculus, J. Periodontol. **29:**145, 1958.

Weintraub, G. S., and Goual, B. K.: Tertiary prevention: a goal of removable partial dentures, J. Prev. Dent. **3:**30, 1976.

Williams, C. H. M.: Present status of knowledge concerning etiology of periodontal disease, Oral Surg. **2:**729, 1949.

Winders, R. V.: Forces exerted on the dentition by the perioral and lingual musculature during swallowing, Angle Orthod. **28:**226, 1958.

Wolfram, K., Egelberg, J., Hornbuckle, C., Oliver, R., and Rathbun, E.: Effect of tooth cleaning procedures on gingival sulcus depth, J. Periodont. Res. **9:**44, 1974.

Zachrisson, B. U.: Gingival condition associated with orthodontic treatment. II. Histologic findings, Angle Orthod. **42:**352, 1972.

Zachrisson, B. U., and Alnaes, L.: Periodontal condition in orthodontically treated and untreated individuals. II. Alveolar bone loss; radiographic findings, Angle Orthod. **44:**48, 1974.

Zachrisson, B. U., and Alnaes, L.: Periodontal condition in orthodontically treated and untreated individuals. I. Loss of attachment, gingival pocket depth and clinical crown height, Angle Orthod. **43:**402, 1973.

Zachrisson, B. U., and Zachrisson, S.: Gingival condition associated with partial orthodontic treatment, Acta Odontol. Scand. **30:**127, 1972a.

Zachrisson, S., and Zachrisson, B. U.: Gingival condition associated with orthodontic treatment, Angle Orthod. **42:**26, 1972b.

Zager, N. I., and Barnett, M. L.: Severe bone loss in a child initiated by multiple orthodontic rubber bands: case report, J. Periodontol. **45:**701, 1974.

Zander, H. A.: The attachment of calculus to root surfaces, J. Periodontol. **24:**16, 1954.

Zander, H. A., Hazen, S. P., and Scott, D. B.: Mineralization of dental calculus, Proc. Soc. Exp. Biol. Med. **103:**257, 1960.

5 Occlusal neuroses

Recognition and elimination of a habit detrimental to periodontal health are of utmost importance in the treatment of the periodontal manifestation. Unless the dentist understands the damage that can or does occur due to a deleterious habit and the need for eliminating or obviating it, he will find himself hindered in periodontal therapy. *In many instances it may be the difference between success and failure.*

In every organ and tissue in the body nature provides a wide margin of safety to take care of demands made on that organ or tissue well beyond what is required by physiologic function. The teeth and their supporting tissues are no exception. There are many instances of breakdown of teeth and of supporting tissues that, although formerly attributed to failure in function, are now clearly recognized to be instances of excessive use and even of abuse far beyond any margin of safety. This breakdown occurs because under certain circumstances the use of part or all of the dentition becomes a repetitive unremitting one, with little or no recovery period to allow for repair. There are oral habits and compulsions in which the use of the teeth creates just such a situation.

These forces have been divided into two broad, general classes: habits and occlusal neuroses. The division is in the main an artificial one because habits are frequently generated by the promptings of inner compulsions; but since habits are practiced in a higher level of consciousness, some logical division may be made. In addition, many occupational practices and general abuses of the teeth have been commonly listed as habits that are, strictly speaking, habits only because they are repetitive. Habits are discussed in Chapter 4.

DEFINITION OF OCCLUSAL NEUROSES

Occlusal neuroses are acts repeated many times by the patient on a subconscious level. A good example of this is nocturnal bruxism. It is a common occurrence for a patient vehemently to deny that he grinds his teeth even though it is explained to him that he may be unaware of the act, and the demonstration of occlusal wear in excess of what would normally be found is indicated to him. It is only when we alert the mate, husband or wife, as the case may be, and go over signs with the patient, for example, morning fatigue in the masticatory muscles, that we can elicit a positive tooth grinding or clenching history from the patient at a later date.

The tenacity of these neuroses of clenching and grinding the teeth is formidable. Before it was realized that they were an extremely difficult compulsion to eradicate, they were regarded as just another habit. Control of these practices was easy under such circumstances. All that one had to do was to admonish the patient to cease and desist and to substitute some other harmless habit to take their place, and the problem was met. Or at least so it was thought. Further study revealed that we were dealing with one of the most deep-seated compulsions; the eradication of this compulsion was found to be an extremely difficult matter that resisted even the most expert psychiatric treatment.

Like all other deviations both psychic and somatic there are various degrees of involvement. It must not be inferred that every patient who grinds or clenches his teeth is similarly involved. There are patients who grind or clench their teeth intermittently as well as those who do so constantly. *It has even been suggested that some grinding and clenching is generated by occlusal imbalances in initial occlusal contact and that the bruxism is generated by unconscious efforts of the patient to reduce the discrepancy. This may very well be true.* It has been claimed that correction of the occlusal discrepancy will eliminate the bruxism. This also is very likely true.

For the most part, however, bruxism and clenching are deep-seated compulsions that have their origin in childhood. Psychiatrists regard bruxism and clenching as the oral outlet for subconscious aggressions. In any case they are difficult to eliminate once they have become well established.*

Bruxism

The effects of bruxism on the dentition are (1) abnormal occlusal wear, (2) thickening of the periodontal ligament space, and (3) occasional concomitant increase of mobility of some or all of the teeth.

In a discussion of occlusal wear notice must be taken of the type of wear as well as the amount. The pattern of wear, no matter what the extent, is facetal. In other words, an even, overall wear pattern is *not* the sign of bruxism. A flattened, highly wear-glazed facet definitely *is* a sign of bruxism. Of course, if the wear facets are large, frequently covering the entire occlusal table or what is left of it, then the bruxism is prominent, all other things being equal. These findings should be checked against the age of the patient. Naturally the older the patient, the longer the grinding has been in effect, and allowance must be made for this in assaying the severity of the case.

To return to the clinical findings, a widened periodontal space usually means increased mobility. This is another sign that the patient is a grinder or a clencher. *Mobility without bone loss or excessive mobility considering the slight amount of bone loss should make the diagnostician suspicious of bruxism or clenching regardless of the subjective response of the patient.*

In many cases the teeth are worn completely flat occlusally. Excessive wear tends to establish the occlusal surface at the widest buccolingual diameter of the tooth. This exerts heavy cantilevering forces upon the tooth because the force on the tooth is not contained within the root range—hence the mobility. If this seems to be a slight imbalance to the reader, let him consider the massive forces exerted upon these teeth in bruxism, uncushioned by an intervening bolus of food, and the unremitting nature of these forces. Functional forces may operate a total of possibly 2 hours per day in widely separated segments. In bruxism the forces exerted are many times as heavy and are continuous. In fact, even the character of wear is

_____

*A study by Thaller et al. has shown that bruxistic patients tend to be more anxious than do nonbruxistic patients. The bruxistic patient tends to use hostility turned inward to remove frustration, whereas the nonbruxistic patient tends to manifest his frustration via punitive action against an object or person; or he glosses over the frustrating situation and is not affected by the situation either externally or internally.

due to the rubbing of tooth on tooth in unrelieved friction.

The treatment for bruxism is palliative. It has been found that bruxism is an extremely deep-seated compulsion that is rarely, if ever, reached by even the most searching psychiatric therapy. Even if the condition cannot be treated and cured successfully, we must mitigate and minimize its most harmful effects. To that end the very first order of procedure is the narrowing of the occlusal table by grinding. It is comparatively easy to reduce the occlusal table buccolingually to almost half its previous width. It must be kept in mind that the reduction is accomplished in grinding the buccal and lingual surfaces near the occlusal surface. The cut surfaces are dressed properly so that the contour is a smooth curve and not interrupted by angular planes. Care must be taken to dress in the occlusal embrasures so that physiologic form is maintained. If these occlusal embrasures are not shaped properly, gingival changes in the papillary region will occur. The ground surfaces must be polished with sandpaper disks and fine polishing wheels. To allow the rough surfaces to remain in a tensional patient is to invite exacerbation of the patient's focus on the oral tissues.

The buccolingual narrowing of the occlusal tables solves the cantilevering problems, but it can be seen that this solution is a temporary one, since the bruxism will continue and rewear wide occlusal tables unless something is done to prevent it. It is at this point that the acrylic night guard assumes considerable value. This appliance has several uses in periodontal therapy but none more critical than the present one. Used by the patient at night it permits any compulsive grinding but effectively splints the teeth that it covers. Further it prevents occlusal wear on the teeth, even on those of the opposing jaw when only a single guard is made.

The bite guard is an acrylic shoe that fits over the occlusal portion of the teeth. The surface occluding with the opposing jaw is made to conform with the occlusal plane of the teeth occluding with it, but the surface is free from indentations for cusp eminences of the occluding teeth. On the buccal aspect half the tooth is invested in the acrylic guard. The lingual or palatal aspects of the teeth are covered completely, and sufficient lingual mucosa or palate is also covered. In fabrication all undercuts are eliminated; no clasps are required for retention. These appliances are worn only at night. The acrylic from which it is made can be highly polished, thus reducing traction in grinding. Also the acrylic is so much softer than the enamel or exposed dentin of the teeth occluding with it that the material wears before damaging the teeth.

The question as to which arch to cover, if only a single guard is to be made, can be answered easily. The guard is made for the jaw in which the teeth have the greatest mobility accompanied by destruction of the supporting tissues. Fixation and coverage for this arch are indicated.

The question of whether to provide the patient with one bite guard or two involves several factors. These appliances naturally invade the interocclusal distance, and two guards will double the intermaxillary opening while they are being worn. Of course, the occlusal thickness of the guards is made as thin as possible, but sometimes it is impossible to avoid invasion of the interocclusal distance. This is especially true in the patient with bruxism. The constant use of the elevator muscles of the jaw creates a hypertonicity of these muscles that tends to shorten them. Whether this is a true shortening or a temporary one is beside the point. The clinical fact is that frequently these patients show no interocclusal distance at all in our methods of assay. Nevertheless the use of the bite guard is helpful in reducing the mobility and saving the teeth. Where both arches are equally involved and the involvement is extensive, two guards should be made. Despite the fact that the interocclusal distance may be intruded upon, the patient is comfortable.

Clenching

Closely related to bruxism, clenching, or clamping, is a similar tensional manifestation. Frequently the clencher suffers from a locked bite and cannot grind his teeth. For this reason examination will show small, highly polished facets where the patient wedges the teeth laterally in an unsuccessful attempt to grind them. There will not be the excessive occlusal flat wear so typical of the grinder. However, the periodontal destruction will be greater, since most of the clenching forces are expended in torquing pressures upon the teeth. Occlusally the interdigitation will be tight and grasping, but the mobility will be more extensive than that found in bruxism. Of the two compulsions, clenching is far more destructive of the periodontium and more difficult to palliate. There is an adage frequently used in these tensional habits which holds that "either the teeth are worn or the periodontium is destroyed." The simple logic of this can be perceived. In a free-wheeling lateral

grinding action there is far less torque than in clamping and wedging.

The very first procedure in therapy is the adjustment of the occlusion so that it is unlocked and lateral movements are possible and freely made. This adjustment necessitates reduction of the long grasping cusps and concomitant narrowing of the occlusal table.

The second aspect of therapy is the construction of a bite guard. It may be argued that the bite guard is less valuable with a clencher than it is with a grinder. This may be true, but the splinting action of the guard is even more valuable in the clenching patient.

BIOFEEDBACK IN TREATMENT OF OCCLUSAL NEUROSES

The habitual clamping and grinding of the teeth are manifestations of stress and tension. Recently biofeedback has been utilized to overcome this problem. Biofeedback is a method of "feeding back" information to persons to make them aware of their physiologic responses. This is accomplished via electronic instruments. Biofeedback with a more highly sophisticated and sensitive electromyographic instrument can make involuntary processes like electromuscular tension perceptible to the senses by way of easily understood audiovisual signals. With an objective indication of normally subconscious behavior patients can begin to learn what thoughts and feelings are for them regularly associated with different tension levels. Thus they progressively develop their own personal electromyographic monitoring capacity. As muscle tension increases, so does electromyographic activity, whereas the opposite occurs with relaxation. When the patient is using the instrument, the muscle activity is translated into an increased or decreased-to-silent beeper tone while at the same time a needle on the instrument panel moves. In this way the patient can recognize objectively excessive muscle activity.

In the case of bruxism the patient wears a headband in which there are electrodes; the headband goes over the frontalis muscles. These are excellent barometers of the patient's relaxation level. The patient hears the beeper via headphones and learns to lower the beeper tone by relaxing. Biofeedback combined with this relaxation therapy program trains patients to relieve and control their habitually increased muscular activity, and as a result bruxism is alleviated. It is said that most patients exhibit useful muscular control skill after ten 60-minute training sessions. Between sessions the patient practices 1 hour per day the techniques, which are recorded on tape.

REFERENCES

Bell, D.: Bruxism, J. Periodontol. **18:**46, 1947.

Benson, H.: The relaxation response, New York, 1975, William Morrow & Co., Inc.

Hirt, H. A., and Mühlemann, H. R.: Diagnosis of bruxism by means of tooth mobility measurements, Parodontologie **9:** 47, 1955.

Ingle, J.: Occupational bruxism and its relation to periodontal disease, J. Periodontol. **23:**7, 1952.

Jensen, M. B.: Muscular tension, J. Prosthet. Dent. **2:**604, 1952.

Klein, E. T.: Abnormal pressure habits, Dent. Surv. **26:**1081, 1950.

Leof, M.: Clamping and grinding habits; their relation to periodontal disease, J. Am. Dent. Assoc. **31:**184, 1944.

Lipke, D., and Posselt, U.: Parafunctions of the masticatory system (bruxism), Periodont. Abstr. **8:**133, 1960.

Massler, M.: Oral habits; origin, evolution, and current concepts in management, Alpha Omegan **56:**127, 1963.

McKenzie, J. S.: Teeth-rocking and teeth-clenching; an important factor in periodontal diseases, J. Fla. Dent. Soc. **19:**9, 1948.

Miller, S. C., and Firestone, J. M.: Psychosomatic factors in the etiology of periodontal disease, Am. J. Orthod. **33:**675, 1947.

Ramfjord, S.: Bruxism, a clinical and electromyographic study, J. Am. Dent. Assoc. **62:**21, 1961.

Roth, H.: Biting habit as a cause of periodontal disease, N.Y. Dent. J. **21:**30, 1955.

Ryan, B. S.: Psycho-biologic foundations in dentistry, Springfield, Ill., 1946, Charles C Thomas, Publisher.

Thaller, J. L.: Bruxism, a factor in periodontal disease, N.Y. Dent. J. **31:**17, 1965.

Thaller, J. L.: The use of the Cornell Index to determine the correlation between bruxism and the anxiety state, J. Periodontol. **31:**138, 1960.

Thaller, J. L., Miller, S. C., and Soberman, A.: The use of the Minnesota Multiphasic Personality Inventory in periodontal disease, J. Periodontol. **27:**44, 1956.

Thaller, J. L., Rosen, G., and Saltzman, S.: Study of the relationship of frustration and anxiety to bruxism, J. Periodontol. **38:**193, 1967.

Tishler, B.: Force as a contributing factor in periodontal pathosis, Dent. Cosmos **76:**638, 1934.

Tishler, B.: Occlusal habit neuroses, Dent. Cosmos **70:**690, 1928.

Wallace, R. K., and Benson, H.: The physiology of meditation, Sci. Am. **226**(2):84, 1977.

6 General health status: effect on periodontal disease and therapeutic response

Although the relationship of general health status and systemic disorders to periodontal disease has been studied extensively, there is no conclusive evidence that they are primary etiologic factors in periodontal disease. It is more accurate to consider systemic diseases as contributing factors in the pathogenesis of periodontal disease. Furthermore, periodontal pathology in patients experiencing an alteration in general health status is indistinguishable from that found in healthy patients. There are no oral signs or symptoms that can be considered pathognomonic of any systemic disorder. Therefore, clinical observations alone are not sufficient to identify the systemic disease that may be contributing to the periodontal manifestations. If an alteration in general health is suspected as a factor in the etiology of periodontal disease, it can only be confirmed by supplementing clinical observations and dental history with a comprehensive medical history and, if indicated, a consultation with a physician.

EVALUATION OF HEALTH STATUS

The rapid advances in medical science and the increasing number of patients (especially older patients) taking one or more drugs have increased the importance of the physical evaluation as a factor in providing comprehensive dental care. Patients taking medications such as steroids, anticoagulants, various cardiac drugs, or immunosuppressant agents require special consideration when undergoing periodontal therapy. The periodontist must be aware of how such medications and the medical problems for which they are used may require alteration in routine periodontal procedures. Thus one of the most important aspects of physical evaluation is the medical history.

The objective of history taking is to elicit information in a logical manner so as to indicate the physical and emotional status of the patient. The medical history will aid in —

1. Identifying patients with undetected systemic diseases that either could be life threatening or complicate dental therapy
2. Identifying what drugs or medications patients may be taking that could interact with drugs the dentist may prescribe or that serve as a clue to a systemic disease the patient has failed to mention
3. Allowing the dentist to modify the treatment plan in light of any systemic disease or drugs being taken
4. Protecting the patient and the dentist from committing malpractice (or allegations thereof)
5. Enabling the dentist to select and communicate with a medical consultant concerning a patient's possible systemic problems
6. Establishing a good doctor-patient relationship (Rose, 1977).

A comprehensive medical history should include the present health status of the patient, major

NAME	TEL. HOME	DATE
ADDRESS	TEL.BUS.	DATE OF BIRTH
REFERRED BY		

DENTAL HISTORY:

Dentist   Telephone #   Last Visit

CHIEF COMPLAINT:

HISTORY OF PRESENT ILLNESS:

PAST DENTAL HISTORY:

MEDICAL HISTORY:

Physician   Telephone #   Last Visit

PRESENT HEALTH STATUS

HOSPITALIZATIONS

ILLNESSES

ALLERGIES   A.S.A.   L.A.   PCN

MEDS.   O.C.

REVIEW OF SYSTEMS

Skin

EENT

Respiratory

Cardiac   RhF   RhHD   M

Gastrointestinal

Genitourinary

Menstrual Hx.   Pregnancy   Children

Endocrine   Diabetes

Extremities

Nervous   Psychiatric

Hematopoietic

FAMILY HISTORY

Diabetes   Hypertension   Cardiac

Epilepsy   Other

SOCIAL HISTORY

Occupation   Smoking   Alcohol   Other

REGIONAL EXAMINATION

1. Face   5. Floor   9. Gingiva
2. Lips   6. Palate-Hard
3. Buccal Mucosa   7. Palate-Soft   10. Lymph nodes
4. Tongue   8. Pharynx   **Vital Signs**   B.P.   P.

MEDICAL SUMMARY: **RECOMMENDATIONS:**

Fig. 6-1. A comprehensive physical evaluation form used to elicit information.

hospitalizations, childhood and adult illnesses, allergies, medications the patient may be taking, pertinent familial and social history, and a review of body systems. The review of systems provides information regarding the signs and symptoms of each organ system in the body (Fig. 6-1). The information elicited from a comprehensive medical history aids in establishing whether the patient's health status is a contributing factor in the etiology of periodontal disease and whether it will therefore dictate the type of periodontal treatment indicated (Rose, 1977).

The remainder of this chapter is devoted to the more common systemic disorders and their influence on the initiation or progression of periodontal disease.

DIABETES MELLITUS

Diabetes mellitus is a major health problem that affects approximately 10 million Americans. The prolonged life span made possible by insulin revealed new complications for the diabetic patient such as kidney disease, gangrene leading to amputation, blindness, and heart disease. In addition diabetes affects certain segments of the population more than others: women, nonwhites, and poverty groups. The chances of becoming diabetic double for every decade of life and more than double for every 20% of excess weight. Life expectancy among people with diabetes is approximately one third less than the general population (Diabetes Forecast, 1975).

Definition. Diabetes has metabolic and vascular components that are probably interrelated. The metabolic syndrome is characterized by an inappropriate elevation of blood glucose associated with alterations in carbohydrate, lipid, and protein metabolism caused by a relative or absolute lack of insulin. The vascular syndrome consists of accelerated nonspecific atherosclerosis and a more specific microangiopathy, particularly affecting the eye and kidney.

Diabetes mellitus ordinarily appears as one of two recognized clinical pictures: the juvenile (ketosis-prone) type or the more common maturity onset (ketosis-resistant) type. The essential abnormalities in the juvenile type are related to absolute insulin deficiency, whereas those of maturity onset diabetes are more often the result of delayed release of endogenous insulin in relation to carbohydrate levels.

Stages of diabetes mellitus. The *overt or clinical diabetic* is known as the frank diabetic, either of the ketosis-prone (juvenile) or ketosis-resistant (adult) type, in which the fasting and random blood glucose levels are definitely elevated. The symptoms related to hypoglycemia and hyperglycemia can usually be elicited.

The *chemical or asymptomatic diabetic* displays a fasting blood glucose level that is usually normal, but the postprandial level is frequently elevated. An oral glucose tolerance test performed in the absence of stress is clearly abnormal. There are no diabetic symptoms. Despite this, diabetic angiopathy may be present.

The *latent or stress diabetic* is a patient who has a normal glucose tolerance test but who is known to have been a diabetic at some previous time, for example, during pregnancy, infection, obesity, or periods of stress.

The *prediabetic* is a conceptual term: a retrospective diagnosis is applied to the time preceding any glucose intolerance. By definition it cannot be diagnosed with certainty except in the nondiabetic twin of a diabetic patient and possibly in the offspring of two diabetic parents (Harrison, 1976).

Relationship of diabetes and periodontal disease

Seiffert (1862) described an association between diabetes mellitus and pathologic changes in the oral cavity. There is, however, no unanimity about the exact relationship between diabetes mellitus and the occurrence of oral disease. Williams (1928) was among the first to conclude that there are certain oral characteristics in diabetes that may themselves lead to a diagnosis. He observed that ''diabetic periodontoclasia'' and ''diabetic stomatitis'' are distinct clinical entities characterized by loose teeth and hypertrophied gingiva.

Two clinical entities that have been described as either being caused by or at least intimately associated with diabetes are the acute gingival abscess and the sessile or predunculated proliferation. The proliferations are polyps that protrude from under the margin of gingiva and tend to push the gum away from the neck of the tooth, producing marked, bright red gingival hypertrophy (Fig. 6-2). These abscesses and polyps are also seen in nondiabetics, but with less frequency (Hirshfeld, 1934).

An experimental animal study utilizing alloxan to produce hyperglycemia, pancreatic disturbances, and symptoms comparable to those in human beings revealed no unique form of gingival disease as a specific oral manifestation of diabetes,

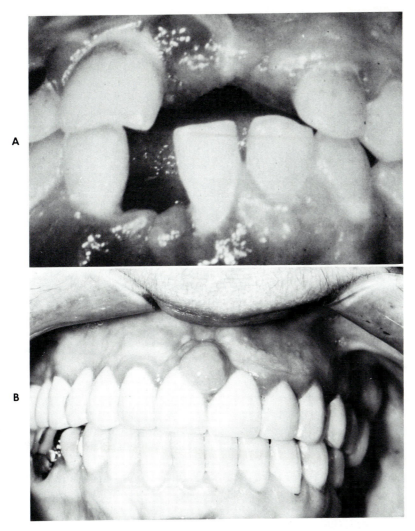

Fig. 6-2. A, Periodontal disease in a 13-year-old diabetic patient. **B,** A 38-year-old diabetic patient who has experienced multiple recurrent gingival abscesses.

nor is the existence of diabetes of itself the precursor of subsequent, inevitable gingivitis (Glickman, 1946).

It has been suggested that the periodontium may react differently in the controlled and uncontrolled diabetic. In the uncontrolled diabetic, the response is characterized by gingival inflammation ranging from marginal gingivitis to acute suppurative periodontitis, mobility of teeth, pain on percussion of teeth, rapid loss of alveolar bone, gradual subgingival proliferations, and multiple gingival abscesses. With control of the diabetes, this group of symptoms may be expected to decrease in severity and occasionally subside. The controlled diabetic exhibits a more gradual resorption of the alveolar bone. This is more chronic and degenerative in nature and seems to be related to the duration of diabetes. The dependence on

the duration of diabetes for development of bone resorption is similar to the other complications of diabetes, for example, angiopathy and neuropathy (Gottsegen, 1962).

Others have observed a dry burning mouth, gingival tenderness, and pain on tooth percussion in patients with a decreased glucose tolerance curve. Also lip dryness, loss of gingival stippling, spontaneous gingival bleeding, pocket formation, tooth mobility, and alveolar bone resorption are found with greater frequency in patients showing evidence of a decreased tolerance to glucose (Cheraskin and Ringsdorf, 1965).

The severity of periodontal disease apparently persists even when such variables as the degree of local irritants and brushing are held fixed. As the degree of local irritants increases, the severity of periodontal disease increases. As brushing fre-

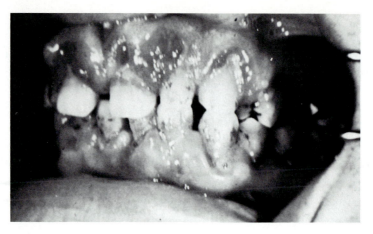

Fig. 6-3. Exaggerated response of gingival deterioration to local irritants in diabetic patient.

quency increases, the severity of periodontal disease decreases. It appears that the severity of periodontal disease found among diabetic patients may be related to other factors. There is mounting evidence to consider vascular alteration as a possible major factor (Belting et al., 1964).

The association of periodontal changes with the duration of diabetes, retinal changes, and insulin dosage has been evaluated. The results suggest that patients suffering overt diabetes for more than 10 years show greater loss of periodontal structure than those with a history of less than 10 years. Insulin dosage does not seem to be related to the degree of periodontal destruction, and diabetics with retinal changes have greater loss of attached periodontium than other diabetics. The modestly increased rate of periodontal destruction seen in patients with long-standing diabetes and retinal changes may reflect some unknown deficiency in the resistance of the diabetic periodontium (Glavind et al., 1968).

A longitudinal study to determine the quantitative differences in the progression of periodontal disease in diabetic and nondiabetic females revealed that both groups experienced an overall increase in tooth mobility and gingival index score at each examination, but that the diabetic group had consistently higher scores. Conversely, soft deposits were consistently lower in the diabetic group. Therefore the diabetic group had a higher gingival index score and a lower soft deposit than the nondiabetic group. Also a significantly higher periodontal index score was noted in the diabetics as compared to the nondiabetics in every examination. This was indicative of more widespread detachment of the attachment apparatus. The increased gingival deterioration and the presence of

a systemic disease in the diabetic group are the only two parameters measured that may account for the advanced destruction of the attachment apparatus. This investigation also suggests that the response of the periodontal tissue reflects a decreased resistance in the diabetic patient (Cohen et al., 1970) (Fig. 6-3).

Vascular changes. Although there is general agreement that gingival disease is initiated by plaque deposition, there is evidence that systemic disease may either have gingival manifestations or influence the local environmental disease processes. Evidence suggests that abnormality of the small blood vessels (microangiopathy) is independent of the diminished carbohydrate tolerance and that the prediabetic may show vascular alterations many years before altered carbohydrate metabolism is detected (McMullen et al., 1967).

Controversy exists as to whether the width of the basement membrane of the small vessels of the gingival tissues of the diabetic is significantly different from that of the nondiabetic. This actually results from different criteria being used in measuring the width of the lamina. Biopsy specimens were taken so that the lamina could be studied under the electron microscope. The basement membrane was found to be larger in the small vessels of the diabetic patient. In addition the membrane appears to widen with increased duration of diabetes (Campbell, 1974). Other investigators report a considerable basal overlap in width and morphologic variation in the gingival capillaries of diabetic patients, but they do not believe that the inflammatory condition of the gingiva is related to basal lamina thickness (Listgarten et al., 1974).

The thickening of the basal lamina may impede

oxygen diffusion and metabolic waste elimination. This may precipitate a physiologic imbalance, thereby increasing the susceptibility of the periodontal tissues to disease (Frantzis et al., 1971; Kitcham et al., 1975).

Treatment. Patients with diabetes have altered resistance to infection. Periodontal disease can cause rapid destruction in these patients, unless they receive proper medical management. If the systemic disease is adequately controlled and the patient is cooperative, periodontal treatment need not be modified and the prognosis is favorable.

Diabetic patients who are difficult to control and are subject to repeated episodes of ketoacidosis may have their glucose metabolism and acid base balance upset by seemingly minor episodes. Emotional upset alone in the absence of any infection may serve to shift the diabetic patient into ketoacidosis. It is not surprising that chronic oral disease in general and periodontal disease in particular have been responsible on occasion for the physician's inability to control the patient's diabetes. It is imperative that the periodontium of diabetic patients be maintained at an optimum state of health. It is therefore the responsibility of the periodontist to stress the importance of good oral health care to both the patient and the physician.

Periodontal treatment may lower the insulin requirement and may reduce fluctuating, uncontrollable sugar levels to a more manageable state. Therefore the treatment of periodontal disease may facilitate the practical regulation of the diabetic patient. Under good medical control and enlightened dental care diabetic patients show no greater tendency toward postdental surgical complications than their nondiabetic counterparts. Dental appointments should be scheduled approximately 1½ hours after breakfast and administration of the morning insulin. Those patients on intermediate- and long-lasting insulin may be treated safely in the afternoon. Every effort should be made to allay apprehension and minimize pain. The administration of analgesics preoperatively is recommended (Campbell, 1967; Gottsegen, 1962).

Summary. The role of diabetes mellitus as an etiologic factor in periodontal disease is not completely understood. Since 1862 many investigators have maintained that a definite relationship exists. It has been proposed that diabetes mellitus lowers the resistance of the periodontal tissues to local irritation or in some manner modifies the response of the gingiva and the underlying supporting structures of the teeth to the local factors.

FEMALE SEX HORMONAL FACTORS

Presently there are insufficient data to define an irrefutable and definitive relationship between pregnancy and periodontal disease. The levels of circulating female sex hormones during pregnancy, puberty, menopause, and the ingestion of oral contraceptives have been implicated, however, as factors in the pathogenesis of periodontal disease by altering the response of the periodontium to local etiologic factors. This discussion concentrates primarily on the response of the periodontium during pregnancy.

There are three primary female sex hormones: gonadotropins, secreted from the pituitary gland, and estrogen and progesterone, produced by the ovaries and the adrenals at puberty. The amount of gonadotropins increases rapidly to a maximum during the first 2 or 3 months of gestation and then decreases to a low level for the remainder of the gestation period. Estrogen and progesterone increase steadily as pregnancy progresses, tending to peak at the beginning of the third trimester and decreasing rather abruptly before parturition. Relaxine is another hormone produced by the ovaries during pregnancy; it rises steadily and reaches its peak toward the end of the third trimester (Löe, 1968).

Periodontal changes in pregnancy

Gingival changes during pregnancy were reported as early as 1877 (Pinard and Pinard, 1877). Observations differ on the incidence of "pregnancy gingivitis," its course during pregnancy, and the role that local and hormonal factors play in the etiology. Some investigators report a variable increase in the incidence of gingivitis during pregnancy (Hilming, 1950; Löe and Silness, 1963), while others believe such a phenomenon is lacking (Glickman, 1969; Maier and Orban, 1949; Ringsdorf, et al., 1962). There seems to be a strong correlation between the severity of gingival inflammation and the rise of gonadotropin production during the first trimester.

During the second and third trimester the gingival response corresponds to an increase in the concentration of estrogen, progesterone, and relaxine. Shortly prior to parturition there is a marked decrease in gingival inflammation and in the excretion of hormones (Löe and Silness, 1963).

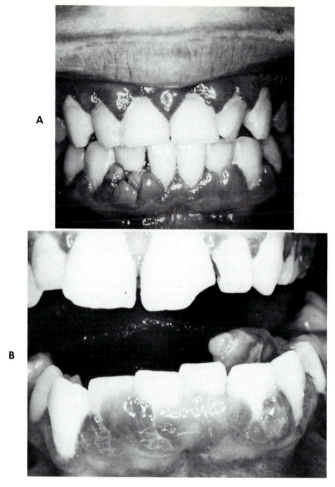

Fig. 6-4. Appearance and severity of gingival changes during pregnancy may vary. **A,** Generalized gingival inflammation. Tissue is edematous, dark red, smooth, and shiny. **B,** Inflammation of gingival tissues is most severe interdentally, producing lobulated hyperplastic tissue.

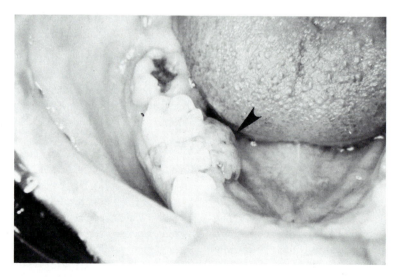

Fig. 6-5. "Pregnancy tumor." Isolated interdental lesion may form between any two teeth, although it is most frequently found between cuspid and bicuspid. Usually adjacent tissues appear clinically normal.

Clinical manifestations. Clinically the gingiva of pregnant women is characterized by inflammatory changes. The gingiva may be edematous, hyperplastic, and dark red. The surface is often shiny, and there is a tendency toward bleeding when brushing teeth or chewing food. The degree of severity may change from patient to patient as well as within the individual dentition (Glickman, 1969; Goldman and Cohen, 1968) (Fig. 6-4). In addition to gingival changes investigators have noted an increase in pocket depth, minimal loss of the attachment apparatus, and increased tooth mobility (Cohen et al., 1969; Hugoson, 1971; Rateitschak, 1967). These changes usually decrease in severity after birth (Cohen et al., 1971). During the course of pregnancy a tumorlike mass may form interproximally between the cuspid and bicuspid; this has been termed the "pregnancy tumor" (Brown et al., 1970). The tissue is red, edematous, and bleeds rather easily. This lesion frequently appears around the second month of pregnancy and gradually increases in size. Histologically it is very similar to a pyogenic granuloma (Kerr, 1961; Shafer et al., 1974). It has been suggested that some form of trauma initiates the lesion and that the hormonal alterations occurring during pregnancy exaggerate the tissue reaction. It may regress after birth, but rarely is eliminated completely (Hatziotis, 1972; Shafer et al., 1974). In most instances surgical excision is necessary (Fig. 6-5).

There are no signs or symptoms that are pathognomonic of gingivitis during pregnancy. It is the medical history that forms the basis for a diagnosis of "pregnancy gingivitis."

Pathophysiology. Some authors feel that the gingivitis occurring during pregnancy relates primarily to an alteration in physiology and that local irritants are secondary factors (Hilming, 1950; Stroh, 1934; Ziskin et al., 1933). Others believe the accentuated inflammatory response to bacterial irritants is related to altered tissue metabolism of the gingiva during pregnancy (Cohen et al., 1969; Löe, 1965; Maier and Orban, 1949; Silness and Löe, 1964). At present the latter concept is more widely accepted. There have been numerous studies in both humans and animals in order to demonstrate the effect of female sex hormones on the periodontium. Experimental investigations in dogs have shown a pronounced effect of exogeneous estrogen and progesterone on gingival tissue exudation, the migration of polymorphonuclear leukocytes within the cervicular epithelium, and the appearance of the dentogingival vessels (Hugoson, 1971; Hugoson and Lindhe, 1971; Hugoson et al., 1972). The increased gingival exudation, demonstrated in humans as well as in animals, has been ascribed to an effect of the hormones on the vascularity and vascular function of the granulation tissue that occurs in chronic gingival inflammation (Lindhe and Branemark, 1968; Lindhe et al., 1968). Although it has been found that both progesterone and estrogen are actively converted in the gingiva and that the inflamed tissue is more efficient in metabolizing these hormones than normal tissue, it is believed that progesterone has a more pronounced effect on the vasculature than estrogen. The amount of gingival exudation correlates with the severity of gingival inflammation during pregnancy as well as with the circulating levels of estrogen and progesterone; it increases during the last months of pregnancy and decreases gradually after parturition (Hugoson, 1970; Hugoson and Lindhe, 1971; Lindhe et al., 1969).

Löe and Silness studied pregnant and nonpregnant women and found that both invariably had gingivitis, although the correlation between plaque and gingivitis was greater in the nonpregnant group. They also demonstrated that teeth kept free of plaque result in resolution of existing gingival inflammation during pregnancy, when gingival inflammation and hormonal activity are likely to be increased. Following prophylaxis and instruction in oral hygiene, soft deposits were reduced and a corresponding improvement occurred in the gingival situation (Löe and Silness, 1963; Silness and Löe, 1966; Silness and Löe, 1964). Other investigators have corroborated these findings.

Cohen et al. reported a strong association between gingival inflammation during pregnancy and the presence of hard irritants and to a lesser extent soft deposits. After birth, there seems to be a greater correlation to soft deposits rather than to hard irritants. On the other hand, Löe considers soft deposits to be the primary factor in the initiation of gingival inflammation both during and after pregnancy. Although there are differences of opinion with regard to the etiology of gingival tissue changes during pregnancy, the majority of research data seems to support the theory that local irritants are the initiating factors in precipitating gingival inflammation and that the accentuation of the inflammatory response is due to the altered tissue metabolism of pregnancy.

From these studies it may be surmised that gingival inflammation during pregnancy is initiated by the same local factors as marginal gingivitis, responds positively to routine local treatment, and can even be prevented (Cohen et al., 1971, 1969).

Treatment of the pregnant patient. Normal pregnancy does not necessarily contraindicate dental treatment if one is cognizant of the stage of gestation and the involvement of the dental procedure to be performed. The first trimester is the period of organogenesis. Approximately 75% to 80% of spontaneous abortions occur before the sixteenth week of gestation. It is best to postpone any procedure during this critical period.

Based on the findings of numerous investigative studies that emphasize the role of local irritants in the initiation of periodontal disease during pregnancy, it is prudent to educate the pregnant woman in good oral hygiene techniques early in pregnancy. All local irritants should be removed as soon as possible before the effects of pregnancy are manifested in the gingival tissues. No elective procedures such as definitive periodontal surgery should be performed during the first trimester. These procedures should be postponed until 8 to 12 weeks postpartum to obtain a maximum state of periodontal health. During pregnancy there are significant increases in the circulating blood volume, cardiac rate, and cardiac output to meet the demands and the requirements of both the fetus and the mother. The cardiac output and blood volume reach their highest level during the third trimester. As is the case in the first 3 months of pregnancy the last 3 months are extremely critical. This is not the time to cause stress to the fetus and mother with involved periodontal procedures. The safest time to perform these procedures is during the second trimester. During this period of gestation organogenesis is essentially complete, and the cardiovascular changes such as cardiac output and blood volume will not reach their maximum level until the end of the seventh month of pregnancy. On the other hand, if emergency treatment is indicated it should be performed at any time during gestation to eliminate the physical and emotional stress caused by the problem. The pain and anxiety precipitated by dental emergencies may be more detrimental to the fetus than the treatment itself. Radiographs should not be taken unless absolutely necessary, and proper precautions should be observed (i.e., lead apron).

All medication should be evaluated to determine whether the drug will pass the placental barrier and what effect it may have on the fetus. The dentist must weigh carefully the indications and contraindications of drug usage. Problems in the pregnant woman are obviously more complex than in the nonpregnant woman because of the presence of the fetus. Prior to the administration of any drugs, whether anesthetics, analgesics, or antibiotics, consultation with the patient's obstetrician is in order.

If a "pregnancy tumor" develops that upsets the patient, is uncomfortable, disturbs the alignment of teeth, and bleeds easily upon mastication, it should be excised. Pregnancy tumors excised before term may reoccur. Therefore, it should be emphasized to the patient that revision of the surgical procedure may have to be performed after birth. It is misleading to advise pregnant patients that their gingival disease is a transitory condition that will disappear after birth. The severity of gingival disease is reduced after childbirth, but the gingiva does not necessarily return to normal. Patients with untreated gingival disease during pregnancy will most likely have gingival disease after pregnancy, although it may decrease in severity (Lyon and Wishan, 1965).

Oral contraceptives

Oral contraceptives alter the circulating levels of estrogen and progesterone. There is much controversy as to what effect oral contraceptives have on the periodontium. Lindhe and Björn (1967) evaluated tissue changes during the use of contraceptives over a 12-month period. They observed that individuals who had almost perfect gingiva at the start of hormonal therapy showed a gradual and significant increase in gingival fluid during the experiment. The length of time that oral contraceptives are used apparently has a bearing on how they affect the gingiva. Gingival changes are greater during the first 1½ years of contraceptive use (Knight and Wade, 1974).

A study in which rats received large dosages of oral contraceptives over 91 days found no overt signs of gingivitis or inflammation although a slight amount of alveolar bone loss was demonstrated (Roth, 1972). Many case reports have described hyperplastic gingivitis and pregnancy tumors following the administration of oral contraceptives, with the inflammation being reversed when the dosage is reduced or stopped (Kaufman, 1969; Lynn, 1967; Sperber, 1969). The divergence of opinion by many investigators could be due to differences in drug composition, dosage, duration of treatment, and species differences.

Menopause

Menopause per se does not seem to be associated with gingival disease. Estrogen deficiencies

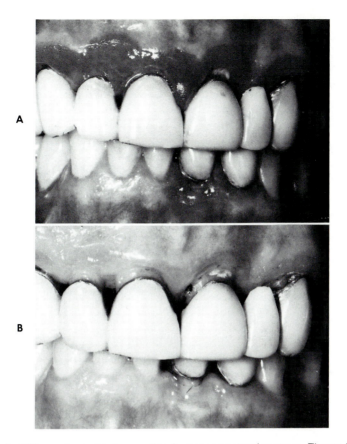

Fig. 6-6. A, Diffuse gingival inflammation in a menopausal woman. Tissue bleeds easily and is quite painful. **B,** Response of tissues to plaque control, root planing and scaling in addition to estrogen supplement.

have been related to desquamative gingivitis, and this disease is seen most frequently in women of middle age and older. It is a disease of the superficial tissues characterized by diffuse areas of inflammation of the gingiva and alveolar mucosa. There is a deficiency in the keratinization of the epithelium, which can easily be removed from the underlying lamina propria (Fig. 6-6). Menopause may so disturb the patient that palliative measures are indicated until adjustment has been made to this period of hormonal change (Glickman, 1969; Ramfjord et al., 1966).

BLOOD DYSCRASIAS

Periodontal disease has been described in association with blood dyscrasias such as leukemia, agranulocytic anemia, neutropenia, and pancytopenia. As is the case with other systemic diseases the blood dyscrasias apparently modify the response of the periodontium to local etiologic factors. Oral findings may suggest the presence of disease but a medical history, physical examination, and appropriate laboratory studies are required before a definitive diagnosis can be made.

Leukemia

Host resistance and the potential for repair appear to be impaired in leukemia patients. This may be due to the alteration of the systemic immunologic mechanisms, as well as a cellular dysfunction, which cause a decrease in phagocytic activity. Both have been associated with leukemia (Dupuy et al., 1971; Lehrer et al., 1972).

Acute leukemia, particularly acute granulocytic leukemia, causes a massive infiltration of leukemic cells into the gingival tissues, producing hyperplastic gingivitis, which at times may be so marked as to cover portions of the teeth (Burket, 1944; Glickman, 1964; Thoma, 1944; Wentz et al., 1949). The gingiva appears to have lost its normal contour and texture. It is hyperplastic, edematous, and bluish red with blunting of the interdental papilla. Varying degrees of gingival inflammation, ulceration, and necrosis have been described (Fig. 6-7). The clinical and histologic appearance of the gingiva is indicative of degenerative changes that have occurred. The tissue is therefore more susceptible to bacterial infection, and the severity of such an infec-

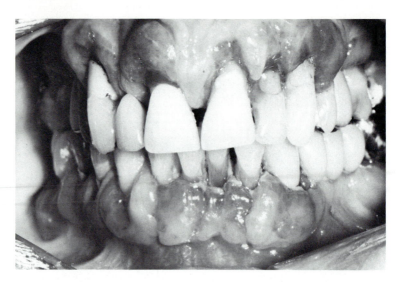

Fig. 6-7. Acute granulocytic leukemia in a 19-year-old young woman. Note dramatic changes in gingival color, contour, and texture.

tion may exacerbate the leukemia (Glickman, 1964).

In chronic leukemia there are very few oral manifestations. Histologically the tissue appears similar to chronic inflammatory disease. Patients who have been treated and are in a state of remission demonstrate gingival tissue that is essentially normal both clinically and histologically (Diehl, 1967; Wentz et al., 1949).

Treatment. The oral complications that occur during leukemia may cause much difficulty for the patient. Toxemia, septicemia, gingival hemorrhage, marked discomfort and pain, and loss of appetite are a few of the complications that may arise. During the acute phase of the disease only those procedures that are necessary to alleviate the discomfort and hemorrhaging should be performed. On the other hand, during a period of remission an attempt should be made to achieve a state of periodontal health. The treatment should be conservative, consisting of the removal of all local irritants, and instruction in good oral hygiene techniques should be emphasized. Treatment procedures involving long periods of time should be avoided.

Agranulocytosis

Agranulocytosis encompasses such diseases as neutropenia and granulocytopenia. These blood dyscrasias are characterized by a decrease or elimination of the granular leukocytes and a reduction in the toal white blood cell count. The etiology of agranulocytosis is essentially unknown although the ingestion of certain drugs such as

aminopyrines, barbiturates, and chloramphenicol has been implicated as a possible cause.

Patients with a decrease in the number of neutrophils are more susceptible to infection, especially where resistance is decreased or where microorganisms are most readily available. Consequently, manifestations often are seen first in the oral cavity and are more severe when in the presence of existing disease such as periodontal disease.

Functioning neutrophils are necessary for the defense of an organism against bacteria. Ulcerations of the marginal gingiva are common findings in patients with abnormal neutrophils. It has been postulated that these lesions are a consequence of bacterial invasion into the tissue (Davey and Konchak, 1969; Swenson et al., 1965). Controversy exists as regards the role of neutrophils. Some investigators are unable to identify any ulcerations of the marginal gingiva or gross bacterial invasion in the gingival tissues (Rylander, 1974).

Cyclic neutropenia. Cyclic neutropenia is a rare form of agranulocytosis. It is characterized by the periodic decrease or disappearance of neutrophils, which occurs approximately every 3 weeks. After 5 to 8 days the neutrophils begin to increase to a level that usually is not higher than 50% of the complete white cell count. Involvement of the periodontal tissues is a manifestation of this disease. Inflammation of the gingival tissues has been noted as well as extensive resorption of alveolar bone about deciduous and permanent teeth (Fig. 6-8). The most significant destruction

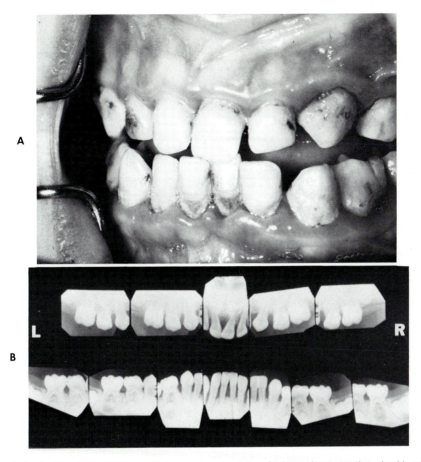

Fig. 6-8. A, Significant accumulation of hard and soft deposits associated with gingival inflammation in a 4-year-old boy with cyclic neutropenia. **B,** Radiographs reveal generalized resorption of alveolar process about primary teeth.

of bone appears to be in the mandibular incisor area (Cohen and Morris, 1961).

Periodontal therapy in patients who have agranulocytic disorders should be performed during a state of remission. At this time conservative therapy is recommended, including scaling, root planing, and oral hygiene instruction. Treatment should be dictated by the limitations created by the systemic disease.

Thrombocytopenic purpura

Thrombocytopenic purpura is a blood dyscrasia associated with a decrease in the circulating platelets. The most common manifestation of thrombocytopenic purpura is spontaneous hemorrhage into the skin and mucous membranes. The disease is also characterized by prolonged bleeding.

Two major forms of thrombocytopenic purpura have been described. Primary (or idiopathic) thrombocytopenic purpura is of unknown etiology. This is a relatively common form of the disease

and is seen more frequently in children and young adults, although it may be seen at any age. Secondary thrombocytopenia is due to a known etiologic factor such as chemicals or drugs (Harrison, 1976). The intraoral signs and symptoms consist of gingival bleeding, intramucosal hemorrhages, and prolonged bleeding with trauma. In addition gingival hypertrophy has been reported.

The severity of the disease and the ability to control the blood dyscrasia and its complications will determine the periodontal treatment that should be initiated. Once the platelet count has stabilized and is within normal limits comprehensive periodontal therapy can be performed.

COLLAGEN-VASCULAR DISEASES: SCLERODERMA

Rhein in 1894 suggested that both acute and chronic rheumatism were contributing factors in periodontal disease. This thought prompted investigators to study the possibility of such a relationship. Some subscribe to the opinion that collagen-vascular disease is an etiologic factor in periodontal disease, while others feel that common factors may account for a predispositon to both illnesses. In addition it has been suggested that the connective tissue junction at which the teeth are lodged in the periodontium (periodontal ligament) should be regarded as a joint, similar to any other joints susceptible to rheumatoid inflammation (Malstrom, 1975).

The data from recent studies have failed to show any positive correlation between rheumatoid and periodontal disease. For instance, Helminen-Pakkala and Laine (1973) found that women of a certain age group who suffered from rheumatoid disease had less calculus, a lower degree of gingivitis, and less tooth mobility than healthy controlled subjects of corresponding age.

Because connective tissue disease syndromes are multisystem disorders and have protean manifestations in many kinds of tissues and because these tissues are well represented and easily accessible in the mouth, it is not surprising to find that many oral structures are affected by collagen-vascular diseases. This group of diseases, however, rarely affects the periodontal tissues.

• • •

When considering all the collagen-vascular diseases, scleroderma is probably the one disease that can affect the periodontium. Periapical radiographs may reveal a widened periodontal ligament space with loss of lamina dura. Hypertrophied periodontal ligament may occur with disorganization of the collagen fibers and thickening of the blood vessel walls. In addition there is pressure resorption and consequent enlargement of the ligament space. The posterior teeth are most frequently involved (Gores, 1957; Stafne and Austin, 1944). Tooth mobility does not seem to be associated with this radiographic observation (Biachi et al., 1966; Christian, 1969; Cummings, 1973) (Fig. 6-9).

The treatment of a scleroderma patient is complicated by rigidity of the lips and difficulty in retracting them. Pseudoankylosis may be caused by the restrictive mouth opening and involvement of the muscles of mastication. Poor oral hygiene and its sequelae can result. If there is sufficient crippling of the hands toothbrushing and other means of oral hygiene may be impossible. Therefore dental procedures for these patients will often present problems. The periodontist should attempt to provide supportive therapy including scaling, root planing, and prophylaxis to maintain good oral hygiene.

STRESS

The emotional status of an individual has been identified as a possible cause of periodontal disease. Acute necrotizing ulcerative gingivitis (ANUG) is the periodontal disease most frequently investigated as having a relationship to stress. A number of studies have reported a positive correlation between stress and ANUG (Kardachi and Clarke, 1974; Moulton et al., 1952). It appears that ANUG is most prevalent in groups of people who are in an environment conducive to stress, for example, military service or college (Kerr, 1945; Schluger, 1949). Psychologic stimuli influence the endocrine and autonomic nervous systems and therefore may be considered possible mechanisms for creating pathologic changes in the periodontium (Giddon, 1963). Manhold hypothesized in 1956 that the constriction of blood vessels that results from continual severe emotional upset could be a complicating or causative factor in the pathogenesis of periodontal disease. Constant vasoconstriction would result in lack of oxygen and nutrients to the periodontal tissues (Gupta, 1966). A variety of stress stimuli have been used in experimental animals to alter emotional stability. Both histologic and clinical observations demonstrate that stress is capable of altering the physiologic state of the periodontium.

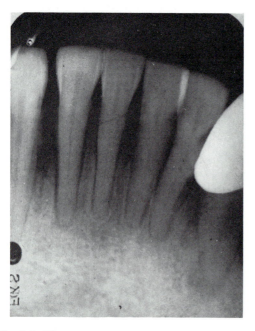

Fig. 6-9. Widened periodontal ligament space with loss of lamina dura in patient with scleroderma.

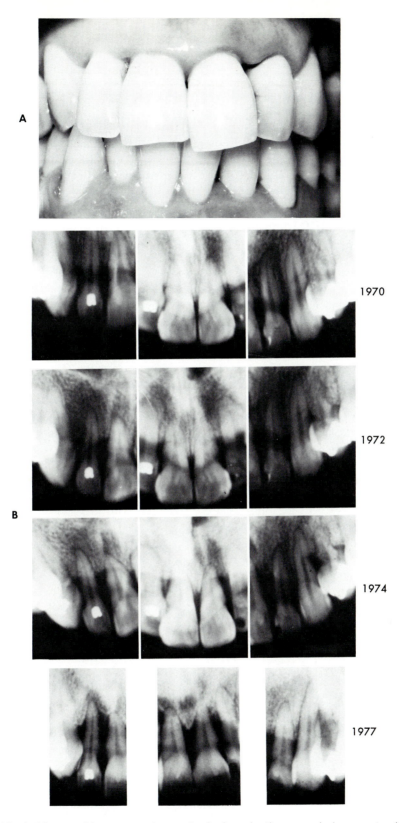

Fig. 6-10. A 29-year-old woman whose physical evaluation revealed no systemic disorders, although she had been experiencing severe emotional instability since 1969. She had had several episodes of acute necrotizing ulcerative gingivitis and had noted increased mobility and migration of her teeth. **A,** Acute symptoms of ANUG have been eliminated, and interproximal cratering is evident, especially about maxillary anterior teeth. **B,** Radiographs demonstrate a rapid destruction of alveolar process.

(Manhold, 1956; Manhold et al., 1971) (Fig. 6-10). However, conclusive evidence to support this theory is lacking. The severity of periodontal disease depends on the type, duration, and extent of the stress and on the host resistance of the periodontal tissues to disease. The mechanisms through which psychic factors may affect the periodontal tissues are discussed as follows.

Oral hygiene. Inadequate oral hygiene is occasionally seen in people who have emotional or psychologic disorders.

Saliva. There may be a decrease in the flow of saliva, which is controlled by the sympathetic and parasympathetic nervous system, in patients suffering from psychologic problems. There is also an alteration in the chemical composition and pH. Acidic saliva and xerostomia may alter the quantity and quality of the microbial flora and contribute to pool oral hygiene.

Diet. An alteration in diet has been observed in people experiencing emotional instability. Frequently the diet consists of excessive carbohydrates, foods with minimal nutritional value, and alcohol. Regressive eating habits may develop, resulting in a soft diet. On the other hand, anorexia may be a consequence of stress.

Oral habits. Many oral habits are psychogenically initiated and practiced unconsciously. Such habits include biting various objects or tissues, clenching and grinding, and tongue thrusting. They usually cause trauma to the oral tissues.

Vasculature. The capilliaries are controlled by the autonomic nervous system. Constriction and dilation of the vasculature in the oral tissues may be precipitated by emotional disturbances. This may result in a decrease in oxygen and inadequate nutrient supply, thereby lowering the tissue resistance.

Endocrine dysfunction. Emotional stimuli may affect pituitary and adrenal function through the autonomic nervous system. The hormones produced by these glands interact with other glands in the body and consequently lead to hormonal imbalance. This imbalance may be a factor in the initiation and progression of periodontal disease.

• • •

All the psychic mechanisms mentioned apparently play a role in host susceptibility and resistance. It is possible that psychic disorders alter the immunologic system, thereby depressing the defense against infection (Epstein et al., 1972; Gupta, 1966).

Treatment. The periodontal treatment of the patient whose emotional stability may be compromised is dictated by the dentist's ability to communicate and motivate his patient (Ringsdorf et al., 1969). A comprehensive medical history and consultation with the patient's physician, if required, will help in evaluating the patient's psychologic status.

DILANTIN HYPERPLASIA

Dilantin hyperplasia was first reported by Kimball in 1939. It has been reported to occur in approximately 40% of patients receiving the drug and is more prevalent in younger patients, with no predilection for either sex or race. Gingival hyperplasia appears approximately 2 to 3 months after the initial administration of the drug and reaches a maximum in 9 to 12 months. Its severity is said to be unrelated to either Dilantin dosage or blood levels. Others have suggested that the degree of hyperplasia is related to the dose of Dilantin (Livingston and Livingston, 1969).

Clinical features. The initial manifestation of gingival hyperplasia is an enlargement of the interdental papilla with the marginal gingiva less commonly involved. Gradually the gingival changes become more diffuse, and the enlargement takes the form of a painless, discrete mass of gingival tissue that is somewhat lobulated, firm, and pale pink. The hyperplastic gingiva gradually encroaches on the anatomic crowns of the teeth with reduction of the clinical crown. It is most prevalent in the anterior regions with the facial gingiva most frequently affected (Fig. 6-11). Edentulous areas are rarely involved.

Inflammation secondary to local irritants alters the appearance of the hyperplastic gingiva. The tissue appears dark pink to red, is edematous, bleeds rather easily, and may be somewhat painful (Livingston and Livingston, 1969). The histopathologic changes involve the connective tissue rather than the epithelium and are by no means pathognomonic. Gingival biopsies routinely reveal inflammatory infiltration of the connective tissue (Angelopoulos, 1975).

Treatment. The inflammatory changes associated with Dilantin hyperplasia can usually be decreased by eliminating the local irritants with good oral hygiene procedures. Surgical removal of the hyperplastic tissue either by gingivectomy or internal bevel procedures is the most common and effective method to treat the hyperplasia. Although the patient should be informed that the hyperplasia will most likely recur, it will be less severe if good oral hygiene is maintained postoperatively.

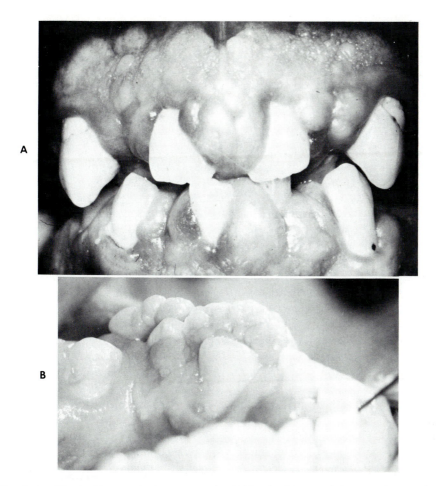

Fig. 6-11. Gingival hyperplasia as a result of Dilantin therapy. It is most frequently seen in children, and its appearance varies from individual to individual. **A,** Tissue is usually firm and pale pink. **B,** At times it may be granular and somewhat lobulated. In presence of local irritants gingiva will appear edematous and bleed rather easily.

NUTRITION

Nutritional disorders are not only a result of inadequate dietary intake, but also may be due to disturbances in absorption and utilization. Dietary deficiencies may be due to economic and educational limitations, self-imposed dietary restrictions, and geographic isolation from an adequate food supply. Alteration in absorption and utilization are usually associated with medical problems (Stahl, 1971).

Diet

The consistency of a diet can affect the health of the periodontal tissues (O'Leary et al., 1966). Gingival inflammation, as well as apical migration of the epithelial attachment and resorption of the alveolar crest, was noted in experimental animals that were placed on a soft diet or given food causing impactions between the teeth (Baer, 1956; Burwasser and Hill, 1939; Egelberg, 1965; Ivy et al., 1931; Klingsberg and Butcher, 1959;

Krasse and Brill, 1960; Mitchell, 1954; Person, 1961; Ruben et al., 1962; Stahl et al., 1958). Thymidine was utilized to quantitate the proliferative cellular activity in the periodontal tissues of experimental animals who were fed either a powder or pellet diet (food-impacting diet). The activity was much greater in the crestal epithelium and in the fibroblast at the interradicular septum of the pellet-fed animals as compared to the animals on the powder diet. This may be due to the abrasive consistency of the pellet diet, thereby relating the proliferative response to functional demands (Weiss et al., 1969).

Nutritional deficiencies

Epidemiologic studies were conducted to evaluate both the periodontal and nutritional status of people in eight different geographic areas: Alaska, Ethiopia, Equador, South Vietnam, Chile, Colombia, Thailand, and Lebanon. Oral examinations were performed utilizing a technique designed specifically for epidemologic studies to determine the incidence and severity of periodontal disease. In order to analyze the nutritional status of the population biochemical tests on blood and urine were used. The survey revealed that most of the variance in periodontal disease was related to poor oral hygiene as well as age. Populations with high scores for periodontal disease tended to be deficient in vitamin A, and there was no correlation with levels of vitamin C (Russell, 1963).

Periodontal disease and the status of oral hygiene had a positive correlation in a study performed in India, although when the people in India were evaluated with people in Atlanta, Georgia, who had similar oral hygiene status, there were significantly higher periodontal disease scores among the Indian group. This may suggest that either the inflammatory response to the local irritants was greater in the people of India than among those from Atlanta or that there were additional factors such as nutritional deficiency present in the Indian group (Greene, 1960).

An evaluation of periodontal disease and nutrition in the people of South Vietnam revealed that although the incidence and severity of periodontal disease was greater where diet was low in total calories, protein, carbohydrate, riboflavin, and iron and relatively high in niacin and calcium, the primary relationship was the oral hygiene and age of the individual. (Russell et al., 1965).

Epidemiologic surveys conducted in Nigeria (Sheiham, 1966) and Gambia (Malberger, 1967) in western Africa have noted the prevalence of acute necrotizing ulcerative gingivitis and the subsequent development of cancrum oris among children. The occurrence of such necrotizing diseases may be due to a relationship between systemic stresses caused by generalized infectious diseases and malnutrition (Emslie, 1963). The evidence to support a relationship between nutritional deficiencies and periodontal disease is at best circumstantial; therefore the remainder of this section will concentrate on two nutritional deficiencies that have been of considerable interest to dentists.

Vitamin C deficiency. "Scorbutic gingivitis" was noted as early as the Crusades when Jacques DeVitry, the Bishop of Acra, described crusaders as having their "teeth and gums so tainted with a kind of gangrene, and the sick could no longer eat." Also sailors who were on extended voyages were said to have loss of teeth and gums that became swollen and hemorrhaged (Van Wersch, 1954).

Studies have demonstrated a significant decrease in the severity of gingivitis and sulcular depth in individuals who have supplemental vitamin C in addition to a prophylaxis as compared to those for whom a prophylaxis was the only treatment (Coven, 1965; El-Ashiry et al., 1964 a and b; Keller et al., 1963). To the contrary, many investigators have been unable to correlate ascorbic acid levels to the status of the periodontal tissues (Dachi et al., 1966; Glickman and Dines, 1963; Shannon and Gibson, 1965). Also there is controversy as regards the effect of vitamin C levels on the mobility of teeth. One series of studies noted a positive correlation (Cheraskin et al., 1968), whereas other studies were unable to demonstrate a decrease in tooth mobility with the administration of vitamin C supplements (O'Leary et al., 1968). Although edema, hemorrhage, resorption of alveolar bone, tooth mobility, and alterations in the periodontal fibers have been reported to occur in the presence of vitamin C deficiency (Waerhaug, 1958), experimental investigations in animals noted that acute vitamin C did not cause gingivitis unless local irritants were present (Dreizen and Stone, 1961; Glickman, 1948a and b). It appears that the periodontium responds to vitamin C in a similar fashion as the connective tissue in other parts of the body.

Protein deficiencies. Protein deficiency has been reported to cause osteoporosis of alveolar bone and a narrowing of the periodontal fibers. It does not appear to affect the epithelial attachment nor does it initiate any local inflammatory reaction (Chawla and Glickman, 1951; Person et al., 1958). In addition protein deprivation has been known to retard the healing of wounds as well as the repair of local tissue irritation (Dunphy, 1960; Levenson et al., 1950; Stahl et al., 1965). South Indian children with severe protein deficiencies (kwashiorkor) were examined for oral mucosal lesions and periodontal disease. The children with kwashiorkor had a greater incidence of acute necrotizing ulcerative gingivitis and higher periodontal disease index scores than were observed in the healthy children (Pindborg et al., 1967). Cheraskin et al., (1968, 1967) evaluated the effects of prophylaxis and protein supplementation on gingival tissues and tooth mobility. They concluded that the effect of local therapy alone, or protein supplementation alone, was not as effective as combined therapy (protein and prophylaxis). This combined approach to therapy is thought to increase host resistance and decrease local irritants.

Protein deprivation in the presence of periodontal tissue injury will decrease the rate of connective tissue and bone repair and frequently cause a breakdown of the healing wound (Stahl, 1966, 1965, 1962). When Stahl et al. (1970) evaluated the effects of low protein feeding in young adult rats utilizing audioradiographic analysis of the gingival response to injury they noted that animals fed a low-protein diet demonstrated less proliferative activity in noninjured periodontal sites than animals on an adequate dietary regimen, although the healing response to injury over 30 days was similar irrespective of diet. It is believed that the stimulus created by inflicting a wound in the animals fed a low-protein diet resulted in tissue compensation for the reduction in proliferative activity.

Russell has stated that:

It seems logical to assume as clinicians have believed for years, that adequate nutrition might be a beneficial factor. This may be true despite our inability to demonstrate any consistent relation, in the epidemiologic surveys that attempted to evaluate disease levels and inadequate intake or body fluid concentrations of such items as vitamin A or ascorbic acid, thiamine, riboflavin, niacin, calcium, protein, iron or total calories. Our findings establish a high probability that periodontal disease is not a manifestation of a specific nutritional deficiency (similar to beri-beri or pellagra); they do not rule out the possibility that non-specific depletion in a combination of factors may hasten the process of deterioration, although not necessarily the same from time to time or place to place. [Russell, 1963]

Deficiencies in nutrition appear to modify the severity and extent of periodontal disease by altering the host resistance and the potential for repair of the affected tissues. To date, evidence is lacking to support nutritional disorders as a factor in the initiation of periodontal disease.

SUMMARY

This chapter has attempted to present interaction of systemic disorders and general health status with periodontal disease. The results of numerous studies evaluating the role that systemic disorders play in the etiology of periodontal diseases seem to support the theory that compromised health status is a modifying factor in the response of the periodontal tissues to bacterial plaque.

REFERENCES

Angelopoulos, A. P.: Diphenylhydantoin gingival hyperplasia, a clinicopathological review, J. Can. Dent. Assoc. **41:**103, 1975.

Baer, P.: The relation of the physical character of the diet to the periodontium and periodontal disease, Oral Surg. **9:**839-844, 1956.

Belting, C. M., Hiniker, J. J. and Dummett, C.O.: Influence of diabetes mellitus on the severity of periodontal disease, J. Periodontol. **35:**476, 1964.

Bianchi, F. A., Bistue, A. R., Wendt, V. E., Puro, H. E., and Keech, M. K.: Analysis of 27 cases of progressive systemic sclerosis including two with combined systemic lupus erythematosus and a review of the literature, J. Chron. Dis. **19:**953-977, 1966.

Brown, G. M., et al.: Pituitary-adrenal function in the squirrel monkey, Endocrinology **86:**519, 1970.

Burket, L. W.: Histopathologic explanation for the oral lesion in the acute leukemias, Am. J. Orthod. Oral Surg. **30:**516-523, 1944.

Burwasser, P., and Hill, T. J.: The effect of hard and soft diets on the gingival tissues of dogs, J. Dent. Res. **18:**389-393, 1939.

Campbell, M. J. A.: The effect of age and the duration of diabetes mellitus on the width of the basement membrane of small vessels, Aust. Dent. J. **19**(6):414-419, 1974.

Campbell, M. J. A.: Periodontal disease in the diabetic patient and its treatment, Aust. Dent. J. **12:**117, 1967.

Chawla, T. N., and Glickman, I.: Protein deprivation and the periodontal structures of the albino rat, Oral Surg. **4:**578-602, 1951.

Cheraskin, E., and Ringsdorf, M., Jr.: Gingival state and carbohydrate metabolism, J. Dent. Res. **44**(3):480, 1965.

Cheraskin, E., Ringsdorf, W. M., Aspray, D. W., Michael, D., and Preskitt, D.: A lingual vitamin C test. X. Relationship to tooth mobility, Int. J. Vitam. Res. **38:**434-437, 1968.

Cheraskin, E., Ringsdorf, W. M., Steyaadmadja, A. T. S. H., and Barrett, R. A.: An ecologic analysis of gingiva state; effect of prophylaxis and protein supplementation, J. Periodontol. **39:**316-321, 1968.

Cheraskin, W. M., Steyaadmadja, A. T .S. H., and Ray, D. W.: An ecologic analysis of tooth mobility; effect of prophylaxis and protein supplementation, J. Periodontol. **38:**227-237, 1967.

Christian, C. L.: In Zegarelli and Kutscher, editors: Human diagnosis of disease of the Mouth and Jaws, Rheumatology, An Annual Review, vol. 4, pp. 451-452, 1969.

Cohen, D. W., Friedman, L. A., Shapiro, J., and Kyle, G. C.: A longitudinal investigation of the periodontal changes during pregnancy, J. Periodontol. **40:**563-570, 1969.

Cohen, D. W., Friedman, L. A., Shapiro, J., Kyle, G. C., and Franklin, S.: A longitudinal investigation of the periodontal changes during pregnancy and 15 months post partum. II. J. Periodontol. **42:**653, 1971.

Cohen, D. W., Friedman, L. A., Shapiro, J., Kyle, G. C., and Franklin, S.: Diabetes mellitus and periodontal disease: two-year longitudinal observations. I. J. Periodontol. **41:**709, 1970.

Cohen, D. W., and Morris, A. L.: Periodontal manifestations of cyclic neutropenia, J. Periodontol. **32:**159, 1961.

Coven, E. M.: Effect of prophylaxis and vitamin supplementation upon periodontal index in children, J. Periodontol. **36:**494-500, 1965.

Cummings, N. A.: The oral mucosal manifestations of rheumatic diseases, Rheumatology, An Annual Review, vol. 4, pp. 60-97, 1973.

Dachi, S. F., Saxe, S. R., and Bohannann, H. M.: The failure of short term vitamin supplementation to reduce sulcus depth, J. Periodontol. **37:**221-223, 1966.

Davey, K. W., and Konchak, P. A.: Agranulocytosis, Oral Surg. **28**(2):166-171, 1969.

Diabetes Forecast: vol. 28, suppl. 1, December, 1975.

Diehl, D. L.: Oral manifestations of acute monocytic leukemia treated with 6-mercaptopurine, Periodontics **5**(3):142-145, 1967.

Dreizen, S., and Stone, R. E.: Nutritional deficiency stomatitis, Pract. Dent. Monogr., Chicago, 1961, Year Book Medical Publishers, Inc.

Dunphy, J. E.: On the nature and care of wounds, Ann. R. Coll. Surg. Engl. **26**:69-87, 1960.

Dupuy, J. M., Kourilsky, F. M., Fradelizzi, D., Feingold, N., Jacquillat, C., Bernard, J., and Dausset, J.: Depression of immunologic reactivity of patients with acute leukemia, Cancer **27**:323, 1971.

Egelberg, J.: Local effect of diet on plaque formation and development of gingivitis in dogs, Odontol. Revy **16**:31-41, 1965.

El-Ashiry, B. M., Ringsdorf, W. M., and Cheraskin, E.: Local and systemic influences in periodontal disease. III. Effect of prophylaxis and natural versus synthetic vitamin C upon sulcus depth, N.Y.J. Dent. **34**:254-262, 1964a.

El-Ashiry, G. M., Ringsdorf, W. M., and Cheraskin, E.: Local and systemic influences in periodontal disease. II. Effect of prophylaxis and natural versus synthetic vitamin C upon gingivitis, J. Periodontol. **35**:250-259, 1964b.

Emslie, R. D.: Cancrum oris, Dent. Pract. **13**:481-494, 1963.

Epstein, R. S., Archard, H. O., Griffin, J. W., et al.: Psychiatric and histologic findings in an unusual type of chronic gingivitis, report of 7 cases, J. Periodontol. **43**(2):101-104, 1972.

Frantzis, T. G., Reeve, C. M., and Brown, A. L., Jr.: The ultrastructure of capillary basement membrane in the attached gingiva of diabetic and non-diabetic patients with periodontal disease, J. Periodontol. **42**(7):406, 1971.

Giddon, D. B., Goldhaber, P., and Dunning, J. M.: Prevalence of reported cases of acute necrotizing ulcerative gingivitis in a university population, J. Periodontol. **34**:366, 1963.

Glavind, L., Lund, B., and Löe, H.: The relationship between periodontal state and diabetes duration, insulin dosage and retinal changes, J. Periodontol. **39**:341, 1968.

Glickman, I.: Clinical periodontology, ed. 3, Philadelphia and London, 1969, W. B. Saunders Co.

Glickman, I.: Acute vitamin C deficiency and periodontal disease. I. The periodontal tissues of the guinea pig in acute vitamin C deficiency, J. Dent. Res. **27**:9-23, 1948a.

Glickman, I.: Acute vitamin C deficiency and periodontal disease. II. The effect of acute vitamin C deficiency upon the response of the periodontal tissues of the guinea pig to artificially induced inflammation, J. Dent. Res. **27**:201-210, 1948b.

Glickman, I.: The periodontal structures in experimental diabetes, N.Y. J. Dent. **16**:226, 1946.

Glickman, I., and Dines, M. M.: Effect of increased ascorbic acid blood levels on the ascorbic acid level in treated and non-treated gingiva, J. Dent. Res. **42**:1152-1158, 1963.

Goldman, H. M., and Cohen, D. W.: Periodontal therapy, ed. 5, St. Louis, 1973, The C. V. Mosby Co.

Gores, R. J.: Dental characteristics associated with acrosclerosis and diffuse scleroderma, J. Am. Dent. Assoc. **54**:755, 1957.

Gorlin, R. J., and Goldman, H. M., editors: Thoma's oral pathology, ed. 6, St. Louis, 1970, The C. V. Mosby Co.

Gottsegen, R.: Dental and oral considerations in diabetes mellitus, N.Y. J. Dent. **62**:389, 1962.

Greene, J. C.: Periodontal disease in India, report of an epidemiological study, J. Dent. Res. **39**:302-312, 1960.

Gupta, O. P.: Psychosomatic factors in periodontal disease, Dent. Clin. North Am., pp. 11-19, March, 1966.

Harrison, T.: Principles of internal medicine, ed. 8, New York, 1976, McGraw-Hill Book Company.

Hatziotis, J. C.: The incidence of pregnancy tumors and their probable relation to the embryo's sex, J. Periodontol. **43**: 447-448, 1972.

Helminen-Pakkala, E., and Laine, V.: The relationship between periodontal findings and articular involvement in a group of subjects suffering from rheumatoid arthritis, Proc. Finn. Dent. Soc. **69**:52-55, 1973.

Hilming, F.: Gingivitis gravidarum, dissertation. Royal Dental College, Copenhagen, 1950.

Hirshfeld, I.: Periodontal symptoms associated with diabetes, J. Periodontol. **5**:37, 1934.

Hugoson, A.: Gingivitis in pregnant women. A longitudinal clinical study, Odontol. Revy **22**:65-84, 1971.

Hugoson, A.: Gingivitis in pregnant women, Odontol. Revy **21**:1, 1970.

Hugoson, A., and Lindhe, J.: Gingival tissue regeneration in non-pregnant female dogs treated with sex hormones, clinical observations, Odontol. Revy **22**:237-249, 1971.

Hugoson, A., Lindhe, J., and Branemark, P. I.: Revascularization of regenerating gingiva in female dogs treated with progesterone. A microangiographic study, Odontol. Revy **23**: 9-20, 1972.

Ivy, A. C., Morgan, J. F., and Farrell, S. L.: The effects of total gastrectomy, Surg. Gynecol. Obstet. **53**:612-616, 1931.

Kardachi, B. J. R., and Clarke, N. G.: Etiology of acute necrotizing ulcerative gingivitis: a hypothetical explanation, J. Periodontol. **45**(11):830-832, 1974.

Kaufman, A. Y.: An oral contraceptive as an etiologic factor in producing hyperplastic gingivitis and a neoplasm of the pregnancy tumor type, Oral Surg. **28**(5):666-670, 1969.

Keller, S. E., Ringsdorf, W. M., and Cheraskin, E.: Interplay of local and systemic influences in the periodontal diseases. I. Effect of prophylaxis and multivitamin therapy on gingivitis score, J. Periodontol. **34**:259-280, 1963.

Kerr, D. A.: Granuloma pyogenicum, Oral Surg. **4**:158-176, 1961.

Kerr, D. A.: Gingival and periodontal disease, J. Am. Dent. Assoc. **32**:31, 1945.

Ketcham, B. S., Cobb, C. M., and Denys, F. R.: Comparison of the capillary basal lamina width in marginal gingiva of diabetic and non-diabetic patients, Ala. J. Med. Sci. **12**: 295, 1975.

Kimball, O. P.: The treatment of epilepsy with sodium diphenyl hydantoinate, J.A.M.A. **112**:1244, 1939.

Klingsberg, J., and Butcher, E. O.: Aging, diet and periodontal lesions in the hamster, J. Dent. Res. **38**:421, 1959.

Knight, G. M., and Wade, A. B.: The effects of hormonal contraceptives on the human periodontium, J. Periodont. Res. **9**:18-22, 1974.

Krasse, B., and Brill, N.: Effect of consistency of diet on bacteria in gingival pockets in dogs, Odontol. Revy **11**:152-164, 1960.

Lehrer, R., et al.: Refractory megaloblastic anemia with myeloperoxidase-deficient neutrophils, Ann. Intern. Med. **76**: 447, 1972.

Levenson, S. M., Burkhill, F. R., and Waterman, D. F.: The healing of soft tissue wounds, the effects of nutrition, anemia and age, Surgery **28**:905-935, 1950.

Lindhe, J., and Björn, A. L.: Influence of hormonal contraceptives on the gingiva of women, J. Periodont. Res. **2:**185-193, 1967.

Lindhe, J., and Branemark, P. I.: The effect of sex hormones on vascularization of a granulation tissue, J. Periodont. Res. **3:**6, 1968.

Lindhe, J., Attstrom, R., and Björn, A. L.: Influence of sex hormones on gingival exudation in gingivitis-free female dogs, J. Periodont. Res. **3:**273, 1968.

Lindhe, J., and Hugoson, A.: Gingival tissue regeneration and gingival exudation in female dogs treated with estrogen and progesterone, J. Periodont. Res. **4**(suppl. 4):26, 1969.

Listgarten, M. A., Ricker, F. H., Jr., Laster, L., Shapiro, J., and Cohen, D. W.: Vascular basement lamina thickness in the normal and inflamed gingiva of diabetics and non-diabetics, J. Periodontol. **45**(9):676, 1974.

Livingston, S., and Livingston, H. L.: Diphenylhydantoin: gingival hyperplasia, Am. J. Dis. Child. **117:**265, 1969.

Löe, H.: Endocrinologic influences on periodontal disease pregnancy and diabetes mellitus, J. Med. Sci. **5**(37):336-348, 1968.

Löe, H.: Periodontal changes in pregnancy, J. Periodontol. **36:** 37-47, 1965.

Löe, H., and Silness, J.: Periodontal disease in pregnancy. I. Prevelance and severity, Acta Odontol. Scand. **21:**533, 1963.

Lynn, B. D.: "The pill" as an etiologic agent in hypertrophic gingivitis, Oral Surg. **24**(3):333-334, 1967.

Lyon, L. Z., and Wishan, M. S.: Management of pregnant dental patients, Dent. Clin. North Am., pp. 623-634, November, 1965.

McKelvy, B., Satinover, F., and Sanders, B.: Idiopathic thrombocytopenia purpura manifesting as gingival hypertrophy: case report, J. Periodontol. **47**(11):661-663, 1976.

McMullen, J. A., Legg, M., Gottsegen, R., and Camerini-Davalos, R.: Microangiopathy within the gingival tissues of diabetic subjects with special reference to the prediabetic state, Periodontics **5**(2):61, 1967.

Maier, A. W., and Orban, B.: Gingivitis in pregnancy, Oral Surg. **2:**334-373, 1949.

Malberger, E.: Acute infectious oral necrosis among young children in the Bambia, West Africa, J. Periodont. Res. **2:** 154-162, 1967.

Malstrom, M.: The nature of the inflammatory process in teeth-supporting tissue of patients with rheumatoid disease. A roentgenologic, histologic and immunologic study, Scand. J. Rheumatol. (suppl.)6:1-18, 1975.

Manhold, J. H.: Introductory psychosomatic dentistry, New York, 1956, Appleton-Century Crofts, Inc.

Manhold, J. H., Doyle, J. L., and Weisinger, E. H.: Effects of social stress on oral and other bodily tissues, J. Periodontol. **42:**109, 1971.

Mitchell, D. F.: Periodontal disease in the Syrian hamster, J. Am. Dent. Assoc. **49:**177-183, 1954.

Moulton, R., Ewen, S., and Thieman, W.: Emotional factors in periodontal disease, Oral Surg. **5:**833, 1952.

O'Leary, T., Rudd, K. D., Crump, P. P., and Krause, R. E.: The effect of ascorbic acid supplementation on tooth mobility, SAM-TR-68-**112:**1-4, 1968.

O'Leary, T., Stumpf, A. J., and Sundberg, P. V.: Oral hygiene procedures in the presence of a tube-type diet, SAM-TR-66-**44:**1-7, 1966.

Person, P.: Diet consistency and periodontal disease in old albino rats, J. Periodontol. **32:**308-311, 1961.

Person, P., Wannamacher, R., and Fine, A.: The response of adult rat oral tissues to protein depletion; histologic observations and nitrogen analysis, J. Dent. Res. **37:**292-300, 1958.

Pinard, A., and Pinard, D.: Treatment of the gingivitis of puerperal women, Dent. Cosmos **19:**327, 1877.

Pindborg, J. J., Bhat, M., and Roed-Petersen, B.: Oral changes in South Indian children with severe protein deficiency, J. Periodontol. **38:**218-221, 1967.

Ramfjord, S. P., Kerr, D. A., and Ash, M. M., editors: Proceedings of the World Workshop in Periodontics, Ann Arbor, 1966, University of Michigan Press.

Rateitschak, K. H.: Tooth mobility changes in pregnancy, J. Periodont. Res. **2:**199-206, 1967.

Rhein, M. L.: An etiological classification of pyorrhea alveolaris, Dent. Cosmos **36:**779, 1894.

Ringsdorf, W. M., Powell, B. J., Knight, L. A., and Cheraskin, E.: Periodontal status and pregnancy, Am. J. Gynecol. **83:**258-263, 1962.

Ringsdorf, W. M., and Cheraskin, E.: Emotional status and the periodontium, J. Tenn. Dent. Assoc. **49:**5, 1969.

Rose, L. F.: Medical history taking is a dental procedure, Dent. Dimens. **1**(1):13-18, 1977.

Roth, G. D., et al.: Effect of contraceptive on the periodontal tissue of rats, J. Periodont. Res. **7:**315-322, 1972.

Ruben, M. P., McCoy, J., Person, P., and Cohen, D. W.: Effects of soft dietary consistency and protein deprivation on the periodontium of the dog, Oral Surg. **15:**1061-1070, 1962.

Russell, A. L.: International nutrition surveys; a summary of preliminary dental findings, J. Dent. Res. **42:**233-244, 1963.

Russell, A. L., Leatherwood, E. C., Consolazio, C. F., and Van Reen, R.: Periodontal disease and nutrition in South Vietnam, J. Dent. Res. **44:**775-782, 1965.

Rylander, H.: Acute inflammation and granulation tissue formation in neutropenic rats, Odontol. Revy **25:**147-156, 1974.

Schluger, S.: Necrotizing ulcerative gingivitis in the army, J. Am. Dent. Assoc. **38:**174, 1949.

Seiffert, A.: Der Zahnaszt als Diagnostiker, Dtsch. Wehn. F. Zahnheil **3:**153, 1862.

Shafer, W. G., Hine, M. K., and Levy, B. M.: Oral pathology, Philadelphia and London, 1974, W. B. Saunders Co.

Shannon, I. L., and Gibson, W. A.: Intravenous ascorbic acid loading in subjects classified as to periodontal status, J. Dent. Res. **44:**335-361, 1965.

Sheiham, A.: An epidemiological survey of acute ulcerative gingivitis in Nigerians, Arch. Oral Biol. **11:**937-942, 1966.

Silness, J., and Löe, H.: Periodontal disease in pregnancy. III. Response to local treatment, Acta Odontol. Scand. **22:** 747-759, 1966.

Silness, J., and Löe, H.: Periodontal disease in pregnancy. II. Correlation between oral hygiene and periodontal condition, Acta Odontol. Scand. **22:**122-135, 1964.

Stafne, E. C., and Austin, L. T.: Characteristic dental findings in atherosclerosis and diffuse scleroderma, Am. J. Orthod. and Oral Surg. **30:**25-29, 1944.

Stahl, S. S.: Nutritional influences on periodontal disease, World Review of Nutrition and Dietetics, vol. 13, pp. 277-297, 1971.

Stahl, S. S.: Influence of prolonged low-protein feedings on eipthelized gingival wounds on adult rats, J. Dent. Res. **45:** 1448-1452, 1966.

Stahl, S. S.: The healing of experimentally induced gingival wounds in rats on prolonged nutritional deprivations, J. Periodontal. **36:**283-287, 1965.

Stahl, S. S.: The effect of a protein-free diet on the healing of gingival wounds in rats, Arch. Oral Biol. **7:**551-556, 1962.

Stahl, S. S., Miller, S. C., and Goldsmith, E. D.: Effects of various diets on the periodontal structures of hamsters, J. Periodontol. **29:**7-14, 1958.

Stahl, S. S., Sandler, H. C., and Cahn, L. R.: The effects upon the oral tissues of the rat and particularly upon periodontal structures under irritation, Oral Surg. **8:**760-768, 1965.

Stahl, S. S., Tonna, E. A., and Weiss, R.: Autoradiographic evaluation of gingival response to injury. IV. Surgical trauma in low-protein fed young adult rats, J. Dent. Res. **49:**531-545, 1970.

Sperber, G. H.: Oral contraceptive hypertrophic gingivitis, J. Dent. Assoc. S. Afr. **24**(2):37-40, 1969.

Stroh, R. E.: Klinische Beobachtungen uber, gingivitis gravidarum, Zahnaertzl. Rdsch. **43:**1749-1755, 1934.

Swenson, H. M., Redish, C. H., and Manne, M.: Agranulocytosis: two case reports, J. Periodontol. **36:**466, 1965.

Van Wersch, J. J.: Scurvey, as a skeletal disease, Nijmegen, The Netherlands, 1954, Dekker and Van De Vegt.

Waerhaug, J.: Effect of C-avitaminosis on the supporting structures of the teeth, J. Periodontol. **29:**87-97, 1958.

Weiss, R., Stahl, S. S., and Tonna, E. A.: The effects of diet on different physical consistencies on the periodontal proliferative activity in young adult rats, J. Periodont. Res. **4:** 296-299, 1969.

Wentz, F. M., Anday, G., and Orban, B.: Histopathologic changes in the gingiva in leukemia, J. Periodontol. **20:**119-128, 1949.

Williams, J. B.: Diabetic periodontoclasia, J. Am. Dent. Assoc. pp. 523-529, March, 1928.

Ziskin, D. E., Blackberg, S. M., and Stout, A. P.: The gingivae during pregnancy, Surg. Gynecol. Obstet. **57:**719, 1933.

7 Gingivitis and periodontitis

GINGIVITIS

The disease process involving the gingival tissue is termed "gingivitis." It is either an acute or a chronic process, the chronic process being the more common. The acute lesion may be found at times of direct injury or acute infections. For example, the acute phase is seen in necrotizing ulcerative gingivitis.

There are many causes for gingival inflammation. Recent investigations suggest that microorganisms and their products play a most significant role in the initiation of the inflammatory lesion while a variety of metabolic factors determine host resistance to the irritants. The specific mechanisms by which the microorganisms induce destruction of the periodontal tissues, however, are still unknown. The following two pathways have been considered: (1) direct initiation of the inflammatory response by injurious microbial metabolites and (2) in the light of recent research, initiation of periodontal inflammation by antigens of oral organisms setting immunopathologic processes into action (Genco, 1970). In addition endotoxins have been shown to adhere to cementum exposed to the oral environment, which may be toxic to cells,

thus limiting or preventing cell attachment at these sites. A symposium dealing with the implications of immune reactions in the pathogenesis of periodontal disease (University of Pennsylvania, 1969) has reviewed the current data in this area and suggested that in the light of recent advances in the field of immunology a potentially great significance can be attached to immune reactions in periodontal tissues (Berglund, 1970). The resultant pathology represents a dynamic and fluctuating interrelation that, once established, is ruled by the changing equilibrium between defensive mechanisms of the host, aggressive mechanisms of the irritant, and many factors influencing both. Recognition of such a dynamic interplay is of extreme clinical importance, since the therapist is often faced with unexpected responses that cannot be explained if only static concepts are employed.

Gingivitis comprises an inflammation of the gingival corium and a change in the sulcular wall. The change in the wall consists of ulceration and proliferation of the epithelium concomitant with destruction of the collagen fibers of the corium. The chronic form is by far the most common. It must be remembered, however, that clinical and histologic diagnoses of periodontal pathology are usually based on primary but not all-inclusive findings of tissue destruction, for evidence of repair activity can usually be found at these sites. This evidence of a dynamic behavior of tissues has led some investigators to consider the marginal lesion as a wound in some stage of breakdown or repair and further to suggest that factors operating in the general repair of wounds may be of significance to the pathology of the marginal lesion (Fig. 7-1).

Clinical features. The very earliest change in the gingival attachment is usually the symptom of bleeding. The form may not be altered, and the interdental tissues may appear intact. However, when probed, the gingival tissue will retract.

The next changes in the gingival tissue comprise alterations in form and color. There is the slightest amount of enlargement of the crestal portion of the gingivae with a tendency for disengagement of the margin, retracting the tissue from the tooth surface. The interdental tissues show evidence of deepening of the col area with slight enlargement of the peaks. Usually the buccal peak is involved rather than the lingual peak. Later the very tip of the buccal peak may be blunted, and the examiner may look directly into the col area after a blast of warm air has cleansed the area of any debris or moisture. Probing will elicit bleeding (Fig. 7-2).

Alterations in color do not occur until the gin-

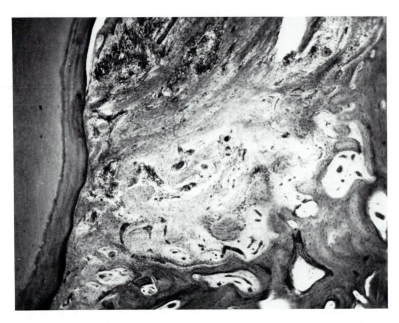

Fig. 7-1. Marginal periodontitis in interdental tissues. Osteogenesis can be seen at crest in fairly close proximity to inflammatory infiltrate. Such biologic adaptations demonstrate multiple host responses to gingival inflammation that take place without specific therapy, thus underscoring tissue's capabilities for repair.

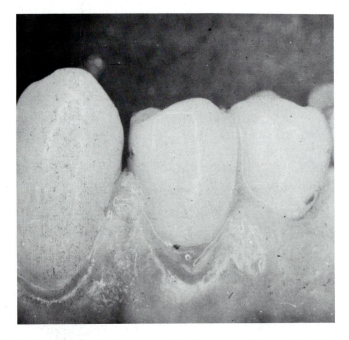

Fig. 7-2. Marginal gingivitis showing some blunting of papillae, particularly between cuspid and bicuspid. Bleeding is present following slight probing.

gival lesion is well established. It is most difficult to appraise this change because gingival complexion varies from individual to individual. One clue, however, is the change of color from area to area in the dentition. The lack of uniformity, with a tendency toward the deeper shades, allows the diagnostician to suspect the deeper inflammatory changes in the gingivae.

The changes in architecture progress with the retraction and enlargement of the gingivae. A distinct collaring irregularity of the gingival margin at this time is a prominent symptom. Interdentally, with deepening of the col, a craterlike lesion develops. Sometimes one or both peaks become broken down, leveling the interdental tissues. On the other hand, the peaks may become considerably enlarged, emphasizing the depth of the crater.

With these changes in the interdental tissues the topographic relation between the marginal gingivae and the interdental papillae may be exaggerated, the normal contour becoming disrupted (Fig. 7-3, *A*).

Upon close inspection with air blast and explorer one often finds plaque or calculus adherent to the tooth surface in the area of gingival destruction. These accretions vary in intensity of color from yellowish to dark brown. They occupy the space down to the area of gingival adherence and can be seen only when the gingival tissue is drawn away from the tooth surface. At times a purulent exudate may be elicited during this procedure. In these instances milking the gingival tissue will also express the exudate. As the disease process involves the tissue more severely, the color change

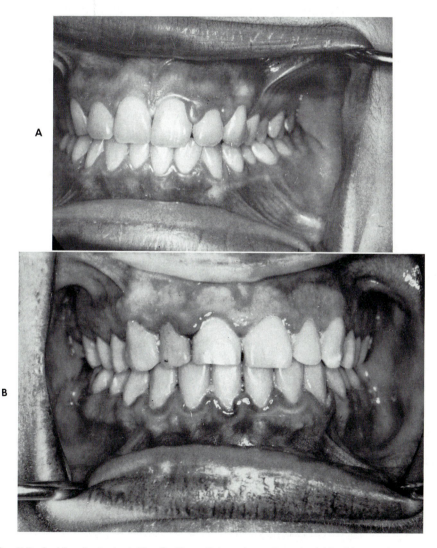

Fig. 7-3. A, Marginal gingivitis. **B,** Necrotizing ulcerative gingivitis. Note enlargement of tissue with blunting and necrosis of interdental gingival margins.

may become even more pronounced. Associated with this deviation may be gross swelling, another sign of the degree of the inflammation. This reaction is extremely variable and differs from individual to individual and also at different times of life. However, in childhood or in young adult life hyperplasia associated with inflammation is pronounced, whereas in late adult life it is seemingly less exaggerated.

Once a gingival inflammation exists, no longer is there a normal gingival sulcus. There is an ulceration of the sulcular epithelium and an accompanying proliferation into the corium as well. A marked inflammatory infiltrate is present in the gingival corium. Associated with these tissue changes is the increased vascularity of the tissue. These changes account for the symptom of bleeding encountered in gingivitis. With the least disturbance of the gingival tissue, blood will exude from it through the ulcerated sulcular epithelium into the pocket and to the surface of the tooth. The inflammation with destruction of the gingival fibers and edema seemingly accounts for the loss in stippling of the tissue that is commonly seen, but no exact correlation can be made.

Occasionally an acute gingivitis is encountered, and this is usually associated with direct injury. Abrasions, cuts, and similar manifestations may cause an acute inflammation. These will subside and heal. However, in some instances a deformity may persist that will allow for a change in gingival pattern and in turn may change into a chronic gingivitis. Acute gingivitis may also occur concomitantly with systemic disease and general infections. It has been noted that an acute gingivitis may arise during a respiratory infection or during childhood disease (smallpox, measles, and so on). Although these gingival disturbances usually heal during convalescence a chronic gingivitis in some instances may persist.

Another acute inflammation of common occurrence is necrotizing ulcerative gingivitis (Fig. 7-3, B). Evidence points to the fact that although spirochetal organisms are probably the exciting cause of this characteristic gingivitis, a predisposing etiologic factor is necessary for the production of the disease. It is probably also necessary to recognize not only the acute form of this disease process but also a subacute one.

Etiology. There are numerous etiologic factors that may produce gingival inflammation. These may be divided into local and systemic causative agents. However, every local injury that constitutes a cause for gingival inflammation is combated by the patient's resistive and reparative powers. Although the local injury initiates the gin-

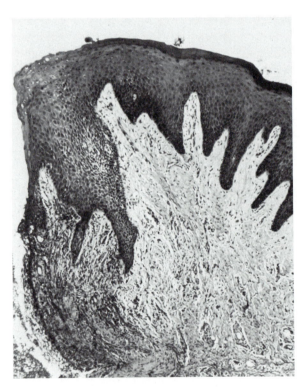

Fig. 7-4. Histologic appearance of marginal gingivitis showing significant inflammatory infiltrate adjacent to sulcular epithelium (left). This is associated with lysis of gingival fibers.

givitis, modified by the intensity of and possible immune response to the causative factor and also by the repetition of the injury, the severity of the lesion and the clinical appearance will be governed and modified by the patient's ability to resist and repair the injury produced. Thus the severity of the lesion is dependent on causative agent, time, age of patient, and resistive and reparative powers of the patient.

The association of oral debris, bacterial plaques, calculus, and gingival pathology has been demonstrated in innumerable investigations, and, con-

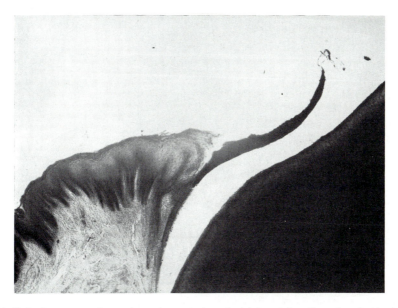

Fig. 7-5. Calculus occupying sulcus, boundaries of which are junction of oral odontogenic epithelium as a base, with enamel surface on one side and oral epithelium on other. A slight reaction in gingival corium is seen adjacent to calculus. This is the early periodontal lesion.

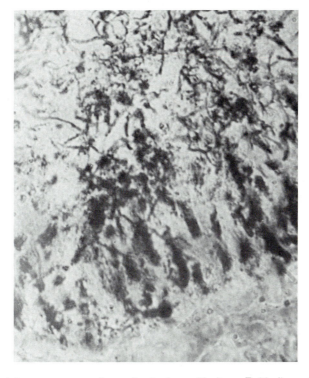

Fig. 7-6. Bacterial masses on surface of sulcular epithelium. Epithelium shows some degenerative changes.

versely, the removal of these materials and the improvement of local hygiene have led to the resolution of the gingival inflammation. What is still to be determined is the exact role of oral accretions in the initiation of gingival disease. However, once the accretions are established they contribute to further injury.

The gingivitis produced by food impaction and other irritants, for example, overhanging filling margins, is similar in character to that associated

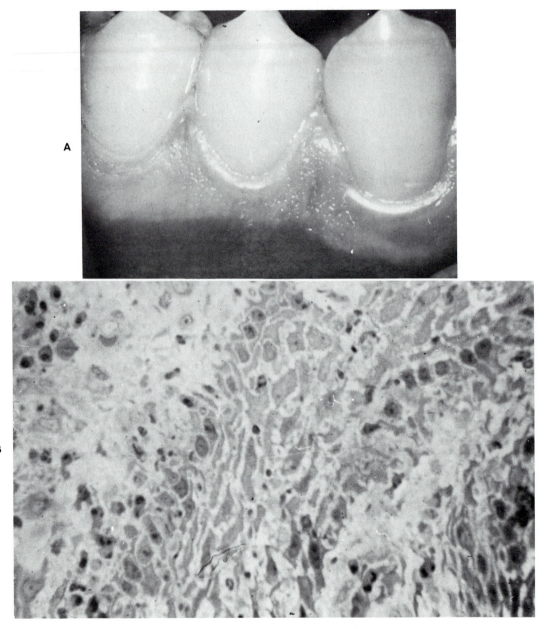

Fig. 7-7. A, Clinically normal gingival margins. First bicuspid in this 14-year-old individual had to be extracted for orthodontic reasons. Sulcus depth at this site was about 1 mm. **B,** Thin section (epon-embedded) of bicuspid facial marginal gingiva shown in **A.** Note reduction of cellular attachment within sulcular epithelium and migration of leukocytes through this layer, even though clinically tissue appeared healthy. **C** and **D,** Corollary to **A** and **B.** Electron micrographs of crevicular epithelium in a 78-week-old mouse exhibiting presence of a granulocyte, **C,** and a polymorphonuclear leukocyte, **D.** (×27,300.) (Courtesy Dr. E. Tonna.)

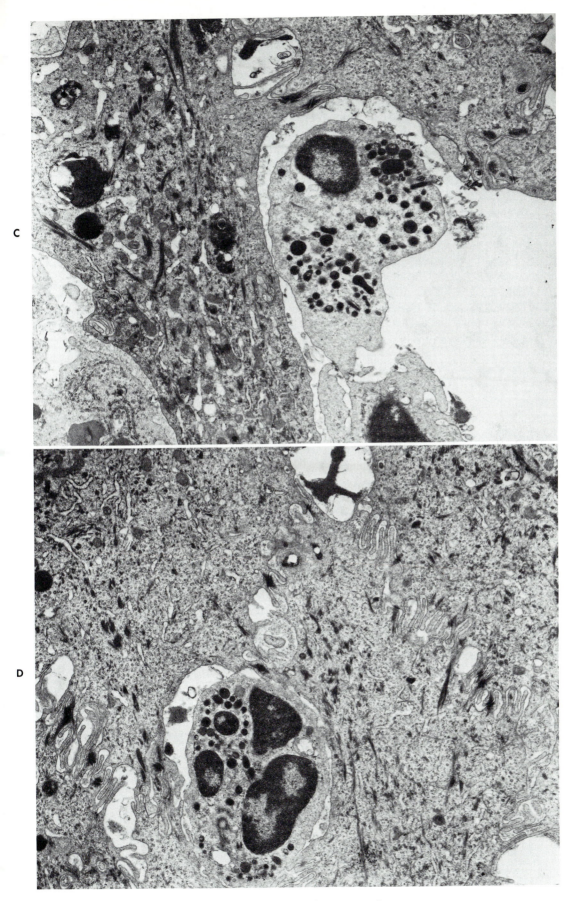

Fig. 7-7, cont'd. For legend see opposite page.

with calculus, probably since microbial components are also present in association with these irritants. Mouth breathing, lack of stimulation of the gingival tissue from soft diets, and mucin accumulation to the teeth at the gingival margins are considered as other causative agents for gingival inflammation. Irregularity in the position of the teeth, improper tilting of the teeth, and abnormal tooth contour allow for food impingement against the gingival margin during mastication, and this irritation causes a gingivitis.

The mentioning of the gingival involvement in many instances of systemic background may be in order. The changes seen in pregnancy, those of hormonal background, those associated in some cases of diabetes, those of Dilantin therapy, and those of nutritional background, although not specifically diagnostic from their clinical picture, are diagnosed after careful evaluation of data obtained from clinical examination, history, and laboratory examination.

Histopathology. The inflammatory process involving the gingiva concerns the sulcular epithelium, the col area, the gingival corium, and later the junctional epithelium and the outer epithelial covering. Early findings reveal a disruption of the oral epithelium at the junction of the odontogenic epithelium, with calculus often occupying the space between the tooth and the gingival wall up to the junction of the oral and odontogenic epithelia. B. Cohen has illustrated the initial lesion in the col site. A subjacent accumulation of inflammatory cells is seen in the gingival corium. These inflammatory cells are chiefly lymphocytes and plasma cells, with some histiocytes and polymorphonuclear leukocytes, the latter adjacent to the sulcular epithelium. Soon the lesion shows ulceration of the sulcular epithelium, with some downward growth of the rete pegs into the corium. The gingival fiber apparatus is disrupted, with collagen fibers being separated by inflammatory cells and finally being destroyed. Concomitantly the junctional epithelium progresses apically onto the cementum, the barrier of the gingival fiber attachment into the cementum having been lost (Fig. 7-4).

At the ultrastructural level the first epithelial changes noted were a widening of the intercellular spaces. When the widening was of moderate degree, intermediate junctions, tight junctions, and desmosomes were still observed. With increased widening the intermediate junctions disappeared first, then the tight junctions, and as a subsequent change there was a reduction in the number of desmosomes. Leukocytes of different types were often present between epithelial cells. In some areas the lamina densa was diffuse or completely absent. In chronically inflamed gingiva widened intercellular spaces were also evident in the sulcular epithelium. Yet despite this widening recognizable bacteria remained confined to the most superficial layers of the epithelium. Such spaces, however, contained a variety of migrating cells, debris, and lysosomes. Lysosomes were also seen in the adjacent connective tissues and were released from disrupting neutrophils. In the connective tissue many types of cells, cellular fragments, and fibrillar elements were encountered immediately adjacent to the crevicular epithelium. Venules showed breaks in the endothelium. Bacterial cells, however, were not seen within the connective tissue (Figs. 7-5 and 7-6).

As the disease process progresses the sulcular wall discloses the proliferation of epithelial rete pegs into the corium. Progressive disintegration of the gingival fiber apparatus is found. Varying degrees of repair may be seen (Fig. 7-7). In some instances the entire gingival corium is replaced by inflammatory cells, whereas in others fibrous tissue, the bundles of which are haphazardly arranged, can be distinguished. The inflammatory process extends deeply up to and often into the transseptal fibers. In the buccolingual aspect the inflammatory infiltrate extends through the gingival wall, reaching into the alveolar mucosa. The degree of inflammatory infiltrate in the gingival wall to a large measure determines the clinical values of color, consistency of tissue, and surface texture. The periodontal ligament, however, is spared, although many sections reveal accumulations of inflammatory cells lying in between the principal fiber groups in the crestal region. These are considered lateral infiltrations via the marrow spaces of the supporting bone. Essentially the extension of the inflammatory cells occurs via the path of lymph drainage (Fig. 7-8).

As clinically denoted, often the peaks of the interdental tissues become hyperplastic either because of the edema associated with the inflammatory process or because of the increase of bulk due to collagen deposition. Chiefly, therefore the enlargement is due to changes in the corium, the reaction varying from local to systemic etiologic agents (Fig. 7-9).

The reaction in the col area in gingivitis discloses ulceration of the epithelium, some degree of downward growth of the rete pegs, and similar response in the corium, as described previously. With breakdown a crater defect occurs. This can be described by loss of tissue, with accompanying tissue reaction, and downward penetration of the rete pegs, with anastomosing of these clawlike epithelial columns. The reaction in the col area is an important phase of gingival disease (Fig. 7-9).

Two gingival reactions may be especially cited: (1) enlargement due to the drug Dilantin sodium and (2) necrotizing ulcerative gingivitis. Patients using Dilantin sodium are likely to react by displaying a distinct gingival enlargement. Histologic examination reveals a marked increase in the bulk of the gingival tissue. The covering epithelium is hyperplastic, exhibiting elongated rete pegs that proliferate into the subepithelial tissue. There is usually an increased width of the malpighian layer and some parakeratosis. The fibrous tissue of the gingival corium is markedly increased in size. Large bundles of collagen fibers may be noted. Subepithelially and interspersed in the connective tissue one finds a chronic inflammatory exudate, chiefly plasma cells and lymphocytes. The blood vessels may be dilated and irregular, and a perivascular infiltrate may be noted. The degree of inflammatory infiltrate varies; in some sections a minimal amount is seen, whereas in others a considerable amount may be noted.

Necrotizing ulcerative gingivitis may be used as an illustration of the changes that occur in local gingival disease, except for the acute and rapid character of the disease process. In this lesion the buccal peaks may become enlarged or completely

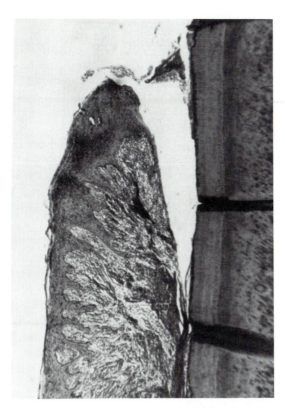

Fig. 7-8. Inflammatory infiltrate has almost completely replaced gingival connective tissue.

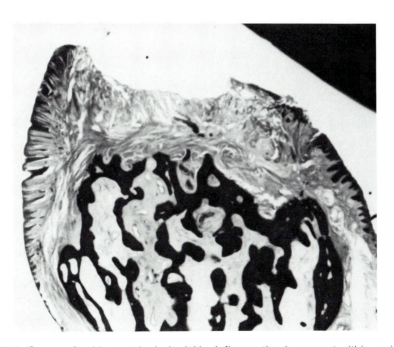

Fig. 7-9. Center of col in marginal gingivitis. Inflammation is present within corium.

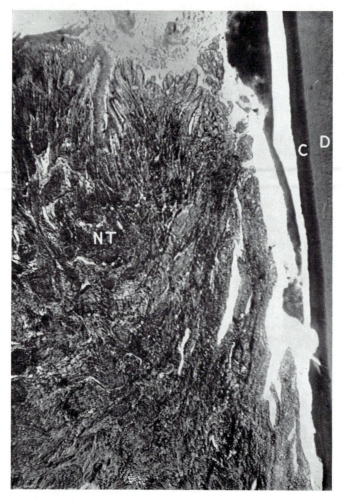

Fig. 7-10. Gingiva in necrotizing ulcerative gingivitis. *NT,* Necrotic tissue; *C,* cementum; *D,* dentin.

destroyed, displaying a blunted and in the acute form a necrotic membrane surface. A necrotic ulcerative process develops in the col area at the same time, resulting in crater defects interdentally. When the peaks remain partially intact, the defects are somewhat hidden. They are more apparent when the peak of the interdental tissue has been completely destroyed. Histologically the covering epithelium is destroyed, with the gingival corium completely occupied by inflammatory cells and polymorphonuclear leukocytes at the surface. This process extends deeply into the subjacent tissue. The surface is covered by a necrotic membrane (Fig. 7-10). Listgarten, using the electron microscope, states that under the necrotic membrane one finds a zone of spirochetal infiltration in which intermediate- and large-sized spirochetes invade the otherwise well-preserved tissues. No other microorganisms are found in this tissue. The more chronic form may be seen in Fig. 7-11, where the surface epithelium remains but displays the influence of an inflammatory response. Some collagen fibers are still present.

MARGINAL PERIODONTITIS

Once the alveolus becomes affected by the inflammatory process occurring in the gingival tissue, the term "marginal periodontitis" is used. It denotes that the lesion no longer resides solely in the gingiva but has extended to involve the marginal area of the bony housing of the tooth. Thus the marginal type of periodontitis develops as a sequel to a persistent chronic gingivitis and hence has the identical etiology. The controlling influences lie within the resistive and reparative factors of the host or within the severity or character of the irritant so as to initiate a more progressive problem. Observations seemingly point to the latter as the responsible agents involved.

Soames et al. (1974) presented the pathway of

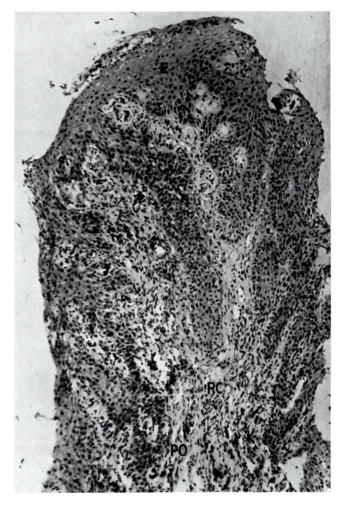

Fig. 7-11. Gingival papilla in necrotizing ulcerative gingivitis. *RC,* Round cell infiltration; *PO,* polymorphonuclear leukocytes.

the spread of the inflammatory infiltrate in the progression of gingivitis to early periodontitis in the beagle dog. Bone resorption in the buccolingual sections progressed from the periosteal surface toward the tooth and interdentally along the crest of the septum into the marrow spaces, similar to that reported in humans. Goldman had also demonstrated this as well as resorption on the periosteal aspect of the interdental septum. This resorptive pattern results in the horizontal bone loss that is seen in marginal periodontitis. Soames et al. also pointed out that the anatomic relationship of the teeth to each other and the original morphology of the alveolar bone may influence the pattern of bone loss in periodontitis.

Clinical features. Marginal periodontitis comprises an inflammation of the soft tissue of the marginal periodontium with resorption of the crest of the alveolus. The tissues affected are the gingiva, the crest of the alveolus, and that portion of the

periodontal ligament above and adjacent to the alveolar crest. Although the marginal periodontium is usually affected, in certain instances the disease may be localized to one or two areas, depending on the causative factors; for example, should the contact area between two teeth be faulty, with resultant food impaction, a single interdental area would be involved.

The signs and symptoms are those of a gingivitis, except perhaps more exaggerated. One major symptom not seen in gingivitis is recession, a process that results from crestal bone loss and accompanying apical shifting of the gingival tissue. Pocket depth varies considerably depending on local environment and secondary factors. Large quantities of calculus, both supragingival and subgingival, are usually noted. Topography of the gingivae (contour), retractability, tissue consistency, surface texture, bleeding, purulent exudate, and status of recession are variable. The amount of repair that has gone on concomitant to the continuous injury determines the clinical expression of the disease process. Also important is the time element involved.

Figs. 7-12 and 7-13 illustrate the typical changes in this disease. The differences in gingival form, loss of interdental tissue, retractability, color value, exudate, and supragingival calculus deposits portray the clinical expressions of marginal periodontitis.

In some instances the peaks of the interdental tissue may tend to become bulbous and purplish red. Calculus and food detritus may fill the interdental spaces. On the other hand, deep interdental

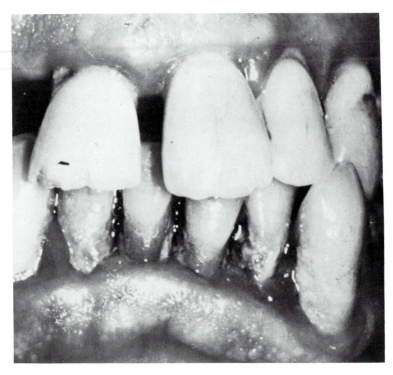

Fig. 7-12. Marginal periodontitis showing gingival enlargement, recession, and exudate associated with marked gingival accretions. Probing demonstrated significant pocketing.

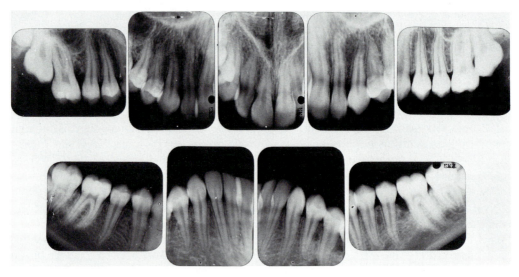

Fig. 7-13. Roentgenograms of a patient with periodontitis. Note evidence of vertical bone resorption around some molar teeth.

cratering may be found, especially in the molar regions. In other instances the gingival tissues return to pink and become dense though hyperplastic; when this happens a fibrosis has occurred. The teeth may either be slightly loose or quite loose depending on (1) the degree of destruction of the gingival fiber apparatus, especially the circular fiber group, in the early stages and (2) the amount of remaining root surface tied to the alveolus by the periodontal ligament.

Once the clinical crown is greater than the clinical root, occlusal relations may cause traumatism and further loosen the tooth.

Roentgenographic study of this disease discloses that alveolar crestal resorption proceeds apically from the alveolar margin of the jaws and progresses slowly and gradually in a horizontal direction without enlargement of the periodontal ligament space. In the early stages a craterlike break is seen in the bony crest. This is minimal, appearing as a central translucency in the alveolar crest portion. Later a characteristic finding is a cuplike resorption of the interdental crest, which serves to differentiate the disease from gingivitis. Fig. 7-14 shows roentgenograms of a patient with advanced marginal periodontitis. Note the resorptive process of the alveolar crest. Thus the cortical layer of the alveolar crest is first attacked, and later the supporting bone, the alveolar bone, or the lamina dura is resorbed.

An explanation of the roentgenographic signs of marginal periodontitis is in order. Roentgenographic interpretation is based on those tissue changes demonstrable on a composite density recording, the roentgenogram. Thus it is important to understand the locations of the osseous destruction. Histologic examination of specimens reveals that the early changes are seen in the interdental crest adjacent to the interdental blood and lymph supply and on the periosteal aspect of the interdental process, as well as on the periosteal side of the buccal and lingual alveolar plates. Two points of information must be stressed: (1) sufficient bone loss must take place before it can be recorded and (2) the lesions on the buccal and lingual plates cannot be seen, since the tooth obliterates these alveolar processes in the roentgenogram. Thus the marginal lesions as seen in the roentgenogram are an expression of the status of the lesion in the interdental region.

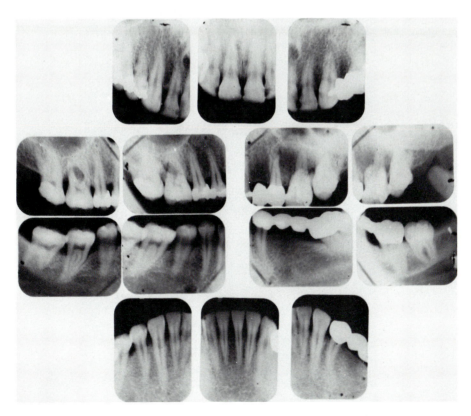

Fig. 7-14. Roentgenograms of a patient with moderate periodontitis. Note significant vertical and horizontal bone resorption in this case.

Since bone resorption may occur both centrally and peripherally in the interdental septum, the roentgenographic appearance may be cuplike in character as denoted by loss of the septum centrally, by translucency of the crestal area blending into the more opaque subjacent portion, or by evidence of loss of tissue on the periosteal side. Varying combinations from interdental area to interdental area in a given case are possible.

Since the clinical characteristics of marginal periodontitis are essentially the same as those of gingivitis, they are different stages of the same disease. Should a gingivitis persist for a long period of time it will terminate as a marginal periodontitis. However, the fact must be explained why in certain instances a gingivitis will remain for a long time whereas cases of early gingival inflammation may be accompanied by loss of the alveolar crest. *Correlation of clinical and roentgenographic findings shows that the severity of the gingival inflammation is not always an index of the degree of bone resorption or pocket depth.*

Microscopic examination. The gingival changes are those seen in a gingivitis. In the gingiva both the epithelium and the gingival corium show evidence of inflammatory changes. The epithelium proliferates into the submucosa in finger-like projections that frequently anastomose and enclose bits of inflamed connective tissue. Inflammatory cells are found in the epithelium. The epithelial lining of the pocket is ulcerated, allowing either a purulent or a serous exudate to be discharged from the inflamed connective tissue of the corium. Often the entire pocket may be filled with this discharge. The type of exudate is dependent on whether the serous or the cellular elements predominate and in turn probably on the character of the microbiology involved. The junctional epithelium is usually intact.

In recent years Waerhaug and Steen have again focused our attention on the fluid that flows from all pockets but is present in only minute quantities in a normal sulcus. Different plasma protein components of the fluid have been identified. Wein-

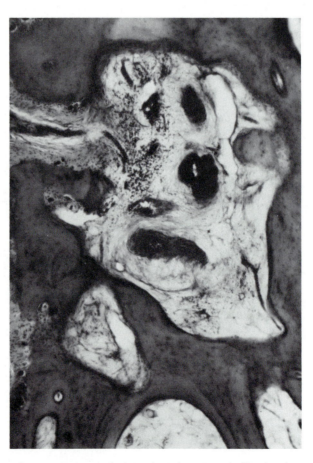

Fig. 7-15. Infiltrate in marrow space in interdental septum, indicating how deeply inflammatory infiltrate has penetrated.

stein and Mandel have suggested that the flushing action, the antimicrobial function, and the fibrinolytic activity of the fluid are among the beneficial aspects of this mechanism. At the same time they point out that enhancement of bacterial growth by nutrients from fluid components and its possible relation to calculus formation may be among the detrimental aspects. Löe and Holm-Pedersen claim that sulci of normal human gingivae do not exhibit flow of fluid. Egelberg essentially concurs with these findings. He states that within minor variations, abnormal permeability of the dentogingival blood vessels does not occur in healthy gingiva. However, a comparison between degree of gingival inflammation as determined by histology and sulcular fluid flow measurements from the same site indicates that as a single measurement on a patient, sulcular fluid recordings may have little diagnostic value. Nevertheless, as Brandtzaeg has pointed out, gingival pocket fluid and saliva may be of significance in local resistance both through mechanical rinsing effects and the presence of antibacterial substances such as lysozymes, and thus play a significant role in the local host resistance mechanism.

Becks has pointed out that the bottom of the gingival sulcus represents an area of lessened resistance to infection when the sulcular epithelium is affected by the accumulated debris at the zone of junction of the oral and junctional epithelium. This had also been pointed out by Box. The epithelial lining of the pocket in marginal periodontitis is destroyed at many places—whether through bacteria from outside or by inflammation in the tissue itself. These breaks allow irritants to enter the subepithelial tissue and cause further inflammation. It is also through the ulcerated sulcular epithelium that the discharge which one finds clinically coming from the periodontal pockets drains. In this connection it should be noted that remodeling of connective tissue during amphibian metamorphosis involves the formation of a collagenolytic enzyme by the epithelial cells and a release of hyaluronidase by the mesenchyma. Furthermore, it has been shown that diseased gingival tissues produce a heat-labile collagenolytic factor that may be of importance in the destruction of gingival collagen observed in periodontal disease, and, most recently, collagenase has also been demonstrated in alveolar bone.

Fig. 7-15 is a photomicrograph of the interdental gingiva in a case of advanced marginal periodontitis. The pockets are moderately deep and are filled with calculus and a purulent discharge. The

entire gingival fiber apparatus and the original transseptal fibers have been destroyed. The crestal portions of the alveolar processes in this section have been destroyed as well.

In the changes in the gingival corium the outstanding feature is an inflammatory cell infiltrate that is so dense at times that very little stroma is evident. Numerous lymphocytes, plasma cells, and histiocytes are found (Fig. 7-16). This infiltrate extends deeply into the marginal periodontium, following along the course of the vessels and separating the connective tissue bundles of the transseptal fibers. These fibers, which pass just above the crest of the bone, are seen in all stages of the disease. Goldman reported that often several sets are present, with new ones being formed as those incisally are destroyed. Inflammatory cells are found adjacent to the alveolar crest and in many instances in the marrow spaces of the interdental bone.

Although in some instances the inflammatory infiltrate occupies the entire gingiva, in others it

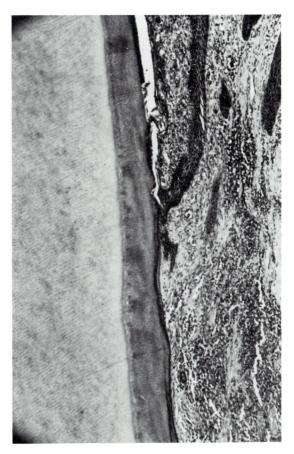

Fig. 7-16. Note marked apical migration of junctional epithelium and significant inflammatory infiltrate associated with lysis of gingival fibers.

may be rather scanty and found interspersed between the dense collagen fiber bundles that are produced as a repair mechanism. When inflammation occurs as a reaction to the irritant, which is the causative agent for the disease initiation, repair of the tissue is seen. In fact inflammation and repair are the agents for the counteraction against injury. Thus in the later stages the repair aspect tends to cause a fibrosis of the tissue, and microscopically a dense collagen is present. Inflammatory cells may be spread diffusely or may be localized to focal accumulations. There is always a dense infiltrate seen adjacent to the ulcerated sulcular epithelium and adjacent to the junctional epithelium.

In the early stages of gingival disease the inflammation is localized to the sulcular area of the gingival tissue. Goldman, studying the problem from a three-dimensional point of view, reported that as the disease progresses this inflammatory process spreads to the subjacent structures. The pathway extends into the interdental septum from the gingiva along the interdental vessels and into the buccal and lingual gingivae. It was also demonstrated that the pattern of osseous resorption followed this spread, that is, the buccal radicular bone and the interdental septum on their periosteal aspects. Also the crestal septum resorbs, causing a hollowing of the otherwise flat or dome-shaped surface.

Weinmann (1941) summarizes his article on the progress of gingival inflammation as follows:

The histological studies revealed the following findings: chronic inflammation of the gingiva progresses, following the course of the blood vessels, into the bone marrow spaces and on the periosteal side of the alveolar bone; only in exceptional instances does it penetrate into the periodontal membrane. Resorption of the alveolar crest from the gingival side leads to destruction, first, of the supporting alveolar bone and then to the lamina dura. The fatty marrow is replaced by fibrous marrow.

Akiyoshi and Mori have reported that in human incipient marginal periodontitis they have noted inflammation of the gingiva spreading into the marginal portion of the periodontal ligament by means of the adjacent canals of the interdental septa. This observation reveals that the spread of gingival inflammation into the underlying tissues may vary in marginal periodontitis.

Fig. 7-17 illustrates the spread of the inflammatory process into the periodontium in the interdental septum. Focal accumulation of inflammatory cells may be seen above the bone crest and lower between the two bone segments. Interestingly the periodontal ligaments have not been infiltrated.

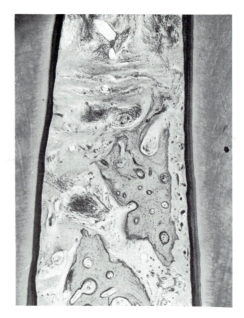

Fig. 7-17. Deep penetration of inflammatory cells in interdental structures. Dense accumulation of these cells may be seen in channel in alveolar process.

Fig. 7-18 shows the inflammatory cells in the buccal gingival tissue extending from the sulcular areas to the alveolar mucosa. Fig. 7-19 shows the pathway of the infiltrate between transseptal fiber bundles. Note that the infiltrate is in gingival tissue per se and has not penetrated the periodontal ligament. Thus one may account for the color changes seen in gingival disease and in marginal periodontitis by the inflammatory process present in the gingival tissue. One often encounters an inflammatory spread into the alveolar mucosa, in which instance the entire gingival wall color is changed, and the demarcating zone between the attached gingiva and the alveolar mucosa is obliterated.

Fig. 7-20 is a photomicrograph of the interdental tissues between the mandibular right premolars, showing the pathologic processes seen in marginal periodontitis. The pockets are very shallow, although there is marked inflammation of the gingival corium. Two sets of transseptal fibers are present; inflammatory cells are seen between the bundles. Resorption of the bone of the alveolar crest is evident. Thus, although the pockets are shallow, resorption of the crestal bone is seen. This demonstrates that the depth of the pocket does not influence the condition of the alveolar crest.

Fig. 7-21 shows the various changes seen in marginal periodontitis in the interdental area. Note

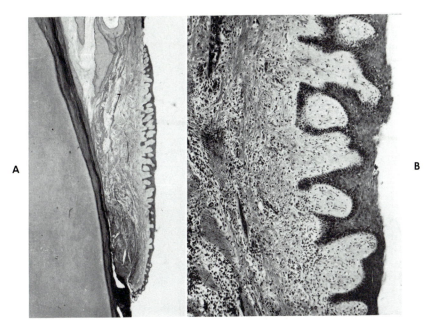

Fig. 7-18. Pathway of inflammation (labial section). **A,** Labial gingiva is situated on root surface of tooth, and calculus adherent to tooth surface is adjacent to gingival tissues. Note dense, inflammatory infiltrate at gingival margin infiltrating apically, extending on outer aspect of alveolar process. **B,** Accumulation of inflammatory cells subjacent to epithelium.

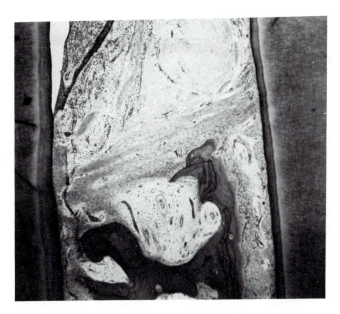

Fig. 7-19. Marginal periodontitis. Note inflammatory infiltrate between transseptal fiber bundles and crestal remodeling.

the course of the inflammation into the deep portions of the periodontium.

Goldman has reported that the inflammatory infiltrate is usually present in proximity to the junctional epithelium and in between the adjacent bundles of connective tissue of the transseptal fibers. The inflammatory cells are chiefly lymphocytes and plasma cells. However, the periodontal ligament is generally spared. In some instances an infiltrate may be seen in the marginal region between fiber groups around the vessels in the periodontal ligament. Their entrance into the periodontal ligament probably occurs through the marrow spaces of the adjacent alveolus. In instances of

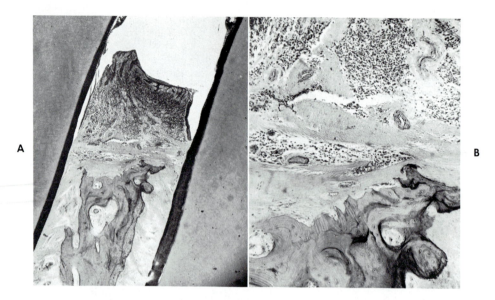

Fig. 7-20. Marginal periodontitis in interdental tissues. **A,** Gingival margin is receded and is now situated on root surfaces of teeth. Note dense inflammatory infiltrate and thinned epithelial covering of gingiva. **B,** Crestal area of alveolar process is undergoing resorption, as noted in lower photomicrograph. Note set of transseptal fibers above alveolar crest. Inflammatory infiltrate is interspersed between bundles of transseptal fiber group.

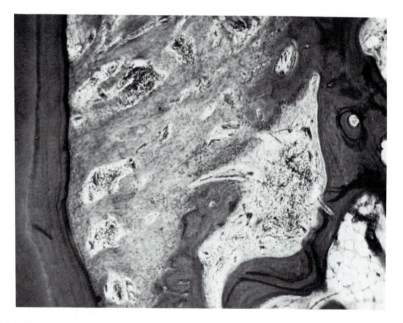

Fig. 7-21. Presence of inflammation throughout transseptal fiber bundles spreading into crestal bone. At periodontal surfaces of this alveolar septum active remodeling takes place, including osteogenesis.

infrabony pockets, however, the infiltrate is seen extending deeper into the periodontal ligament area.

The transseptal fibers comprise groups of collagen fibers in a ligamentlike fashion, extending from one tooth to another. In lesions in which the marginal periodontium has been destroyed, collagen fibers arranged in a similar fashion are seen above the alveolar crest. In some instances more than one set is present. In infrabony pocket areas

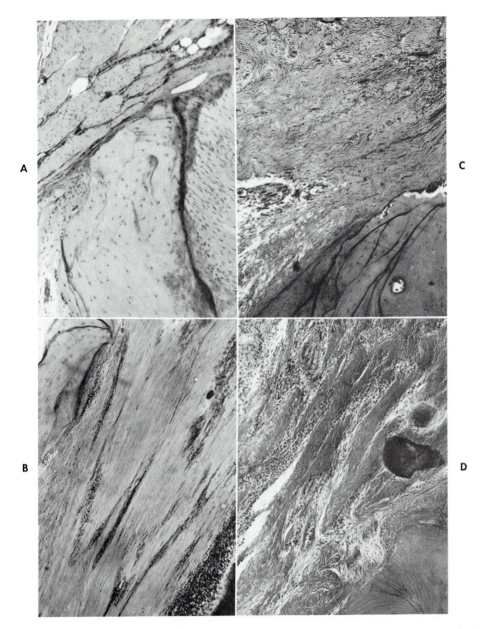

Fig. 7-22. Crestal region in marginal periodontitis. **A,** Alveolar crest in center, surrounded on right by periodontal ligament and on left and above by collagen fibers of gingival fiber group. Note a few inflammatory cells lying between collagen fibers. **B,** Alveolar crest may be noted in upper left portion of photomicrograph, and epithelial covering may be noted in lower right portion. Dense accumulation of inflammatory cells is seen in lower right side subjacent to epithelium. Between collagen fibers, streaks of inflammatory cells may be seen. **C,** Alveolar crest on right, with osteoclastic resorption at tip of this bone. Note inflammatory infiltration between bundles of collagen fibers. **D,** Alveolar crest in lower right. Note heavy infiltration of inflammatory cells between collagen fibers and disrupted gingival fiber apparatus.

the fibers arising between the tooth and the bone can be seen running alongside the bone and passing over the crest to the adjacent tooth. In edentulous areas between two teeth there is a formation of collagen fibers functioning as a transseptal group. Histologic study reveals that these groups are not new formations but are a uniting of previously existing periodontal ligament fibers (Goldman).

The main feature in marginal periodontitis is a

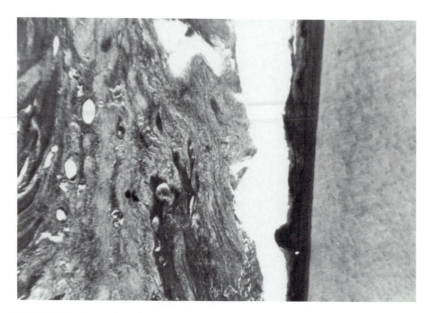

Fig. 7-23. Histologic section demonstrating accumulations of plaque and calculus associated with pocket formation.

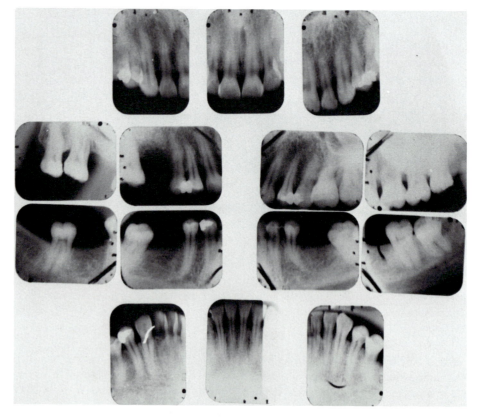

Fig. 7-24. Roentgenogram of marginal periodontitis case. Note crestal resorption patterns.

resorption of the crestal portion of the alveolar process (Figs. 7-22 and 7-23). This resorption goes on in a characteristic fashion, with the bone being resorbed essentially in two sites. The first site is on the periosteal side of the alveolus at the crestal portion, and the second site is interdentally in the crest of the alveolus. In the latter instance the cortical plate of bone of the interdental septum centrally at the area where the blood and lymph vessels emerge is first involved. Once the breakthrough has occurred the supporting bone is destroyed. The process works laterally involving the alveolar bone (lamina dura). This results in a cuplike notch in the alveolar crest, a finding that can be correlated in the roentgenographic examination of the disease process. Osteoclasts in Howship's lacunae along the bone may be demonstrated (Fig. 7-24).

An understanding of the effect of the changes in the gingival tissue on the alveolar crest is essential to comprehend the behavior of this disease process. Bone normally is subject to a coincident tissue growth and absorption that is finely coordinated and comprises a balanced process of anabolism and catabolism. It is not surprising, therefore, that this balance can be upset by many influences. Infection, mechanical factors, metabolic disturbances, growth, and senility all influence the physical properties and architecture of the bone. In the pure state the inflammatory process existing in the gingiva and extending deeper into the periodontium near the alveolar crest causes a disturbance in the balance of bone metabolism. Tendency toward resorption ensues, and bone destruction becomes evident. However, bone apposition also is seen.

The mechanism of bone resorption is still a matter of speculation. However, it is generally considered that bone is dissolved and removed by osteoclastic activity, which is related to the proteolytic capacity of osteoclasts. It is also known that inflammation often accompanies bone resorption, although the mechanism of this action is not clearly understood. It may be related to the participation of lysosomal enzymes, to an increase in either lactic acid or carbon dioxide production, to an increase in blood supply, and to curvatures in bone surface related to differences in electrical potential at these sites.

The effect of the gingival changes on the alveolar crest thus may be controlled by the intensity of the inflammatory process, the extent of the soft tissue repair, and the rate of formation of bone while the bone is undergoing resorption. Goldman demonstrated that the depth of the pocket cannot be correlated to the resorptive process seen in the bone. Thus it can be seen that many variables are present. Microscopic examination of the crest of the alveolus in cases of marginal periodontitis shows evidence of resorption on one surface, whereas on an adjacent surface bone apposition may be evident. Adjacent to such areas the surface of the bone may exhibit evidence of inac-

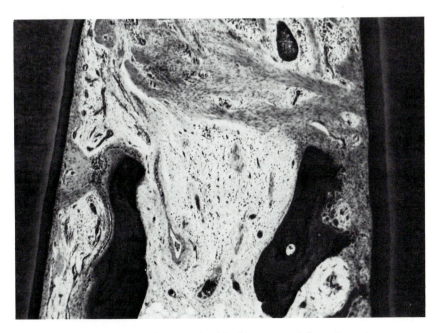

Fig. 7-25. Marginal periodontitis. Note remodeling at crest.

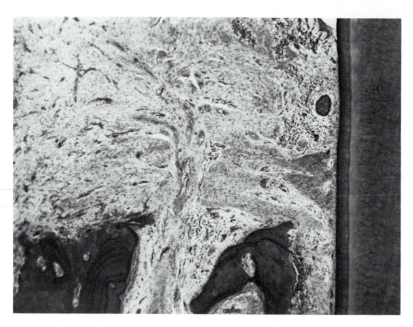

Fig. 7-26. Early marginal periodontitis in which inflammatory infiltrate is essentially above transseptal fiber level although crestal resorption is evident.

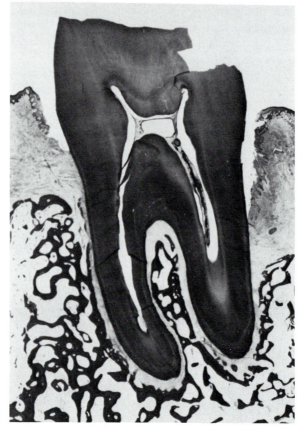

Fig. 7-27. More advanced crestal resorption is evident in this specimen. Note also widened periodontal ligament associated with trauma from occlusion.

tivity. Massler et al. have come to the conclusion that no relationship can be established between the degree of inflammation of the gingival papilla and the level of the roentgenographic appearance of the underlying alveolar crest (Figs. 7-25 to 7-27).

Since the etiologic factors of marginal periodontitis are presistent and chronic in nature, the tissue damage is slow but accumulative in the individual whose repair is normal. Clinically the alveolar crest is slowly resorbed, with the early manifestation of the notchlike resorption extending wider and deeper (Figs. 7-28 to 7-32).

Given the etiologic factors that produce inflammatory changes in the marginal periodontium in an individual whose alveolar and supporting bone is changing because of mechanical factors or metabolic disturbances, the resultant process is more active and destructive. Mikola and Bauer have studied four cases of periodontal involvement in young individuals. The microscopic findings of jaws removed at autopsy from four children 10, 14, 17, and 18 years of age who succumbed to systemic diseases were reported and compared with similar changes in jaws of adults. In all cases inflammatory processes of the subepithelium of in-

terdental papillae were seen to proceed apically, penetrating and loosening the transseptal fibers of the periodontal ligament. The influx of inflammatory cells into the alveolar crest region stimulates the differentiation of osteoclasts, resulting in a resorption of the crest and in many instances perforation through the crest into the underlying bone marrow spaces. They believe that it is the advancing inflammation which separates the Sharpey's bundles from the cementum and alveolar plate and causes the cell of the epithelial attachment to proliferate along the cementum. The apical progression of the inflammatory process stimulates the downward fingerlike proliferation of the surface epithelium and junctional epithelium. Although severe juvenile periodontitis has been observed in other children free of systemic disease (not reported herein) they feel it likely that various systemic involvements, as a predisposing factor for periodontitis, play a more important role in juveniles than in adults. Accordingly diseases of long standing render the tooth-supporting structures more susceptible and less resistant to inflammatory processes. Similar conclusions have been reached in animal studies where gingival healing was impaired when the host animals were fed low-protein

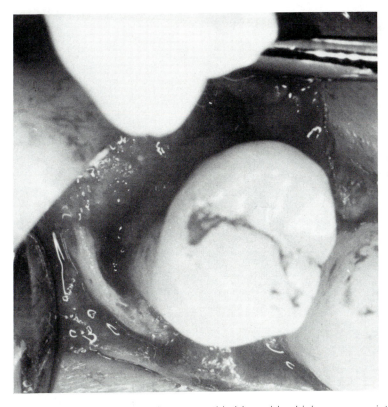

Fig. 7-28. Severe resorption of bone is seen at this bicuspid, which was associated with inflammation within this site (infrabony lesion).

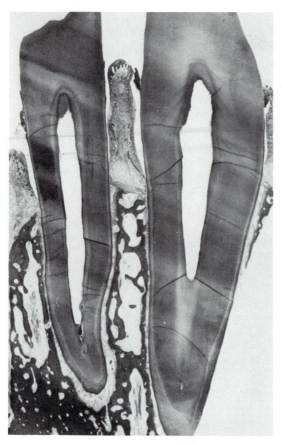

Fig. 7-29. Resorption of crestal bone and significant pocket formation. Calculus accumulations are seen along much of root surfaces.

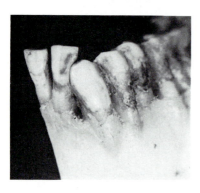

Fig. 7-30. Area of central and lateral incisors, cuspid, and first premolar affected by marginal periodontitis (dried mandible). Note recession of crestal margin, whereas between lateral and central incisors a crater is apparent. Local environmental factors causing this change are discussed in Chapter 4.

diets or received severe metabolic injuries. These findings have been related to a possibly altered immunoresponse of the host and a delay in connective tissue repair due to the metabolic stressors induced in these animals.

Stanley investigated the distance from the bottom of calculus deposits to the alveolar crest and found the measurement to be a mean of 1.97 mm with a coefficient of variation of 33.16%. The length of the junctional epithelium varied between 0.1 and 1.4 mm (mean, 0.57). The means of the distances from (1) the bottom of the calculus to the epithelial attachment, (2) the bottom of the calculus to the alveolar crest, and (3) the bottom of the calculus to the deepest level of inflammatory cells were greater when the subgingival calculus was of the scaly rather than the nodular type.

Limited histochemical and biochemical determinations have also been carried out in inflamed gingiva. An increase in acid mucopolysaccharides, possibly a result of the splitting by proteolytic enzymes of carbohydrate-protein chains, thereby releasing the acid mucopolysaccharides, has been described. A collagenaselike enzyme has also been

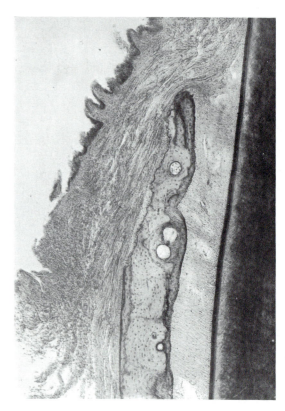

Fig. 7-31. Destruction of buccal alveolus on periosteal side in marginal periodontitis. Note that periodontal ligament is devoid of any inflammatory infiltrate.

demonstrated in inflamed gingiva. Altered activity of enzymes, for example, alkaline phosphatase, aminopeptidase, succinic dehydrogenase, and cytochrome oxidase, have been described. Fluctuations of glycogen in gingival epithelium have been reported, and the frequently seen accumulation of glycogen in epithelial cells has been related to cell injury, thus furthering the concept that this tissue exists in some phase of continuous wound healing.

BIFURCATION OR TRIFURCATION INVOLVEMENT

The extension of pocket formation into the interradicular area of multirooted teeth has been termed "bifurcation or trifurcation involvement." The reason for this terminology is based on clin-

ical experience in problems arising in therapy of pockets having this topography. Fig. 7-33 is a photomicrograph of a maxillary molar cut in the buccopalatal plane. Pocket extension between the two buccal roots into the interradicular area can be observed. All the essential features of pocket formation are present, that is, ulceration of the pocket epithelium as well as inflammatory infiltrate in the gingival corium. Fig. 7-34 shows the bifurcation involvement of a mandibular molar. The interradicular space above the gingival crest, now receded, is partially filled with calculus; the alveolar crest has been resorbed.

PERIODONTAL ABSCESS

A periodontal abscess may form in pockets above the bony crest in the gingival corium or in

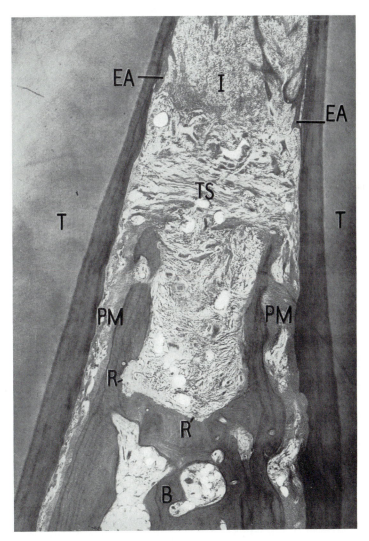

Fig. 7-32. Resorption of interdental bone in marginal periodontitis. Note cuplike notch of alveolar crest, resulting from bone resorption. *T,* Tooth; *EA,* epithelial attachment; *I,* inflammatory cells; *TS,* transseptal fibers; *PM,* periodontal ligament; *B,* bone; *R,* resorption.

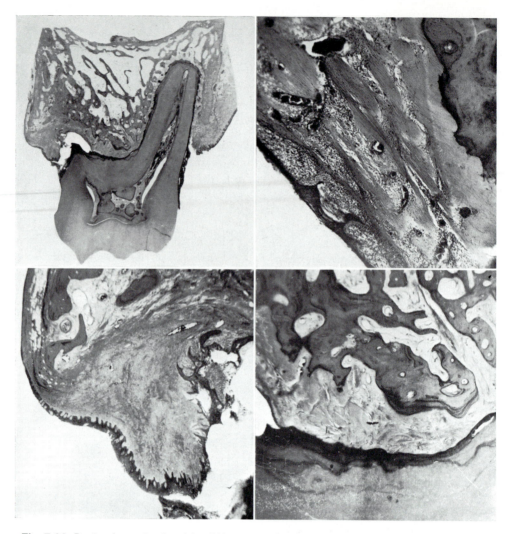

Fig. 7-33. Pocket formation involving bifurcation of buccal roots of maxillary molar. Involvement extends just beyond buccal roots but otherwise leaves interradicular area intact. Note how a ledge of bone on buccal aspect has remained (lower left illustration).

infrabony pockets, at which time it may point through the bone; or it may form in the periodontal ligament not near the gingiva, as occasionally seen in occlusal traumatism. The interradicular area in multirooted teeth is also a site for periodontal abscess formation.

Microscopic examination of these abscesses reveals the same pathology as is usually seen in periapical abscesses. A predominance of round cell infiltration is seen in the chronic type, whereas polymorphonuclear leukocytes are the principal cells seen in the acute type. A connective tissue capsule may be seen if it is of long standing, whereas if the disease is acute the reaction is diffuse. If the abscess is located in the gingival corium the inflammatory reaction is usually surrounded by epithelium that has proliferated into

the gingival corium and has anastomosed (Figs. 7-35 to 7-37).

PERIODONTAL POCKET

Once the clinical signs and symptoms of gingival disease can be recognized, it is evident that a deep-seated lesion has already become established. Clinically speaking the lesion should be termed a ''diseased gingival attachment.'' The term ''pocket'' is used in the dental literature.

Gingival disease is characterized by changes in color, bleeding, exudation, retraction of the gingival margin, loss of form, and later by a possible loss of stippling. These are also signs of pocket formation. Depth of separation of the gingiva from the tooth surface is not solely a reliable index, since a diseased gingiva may not be too retracted,

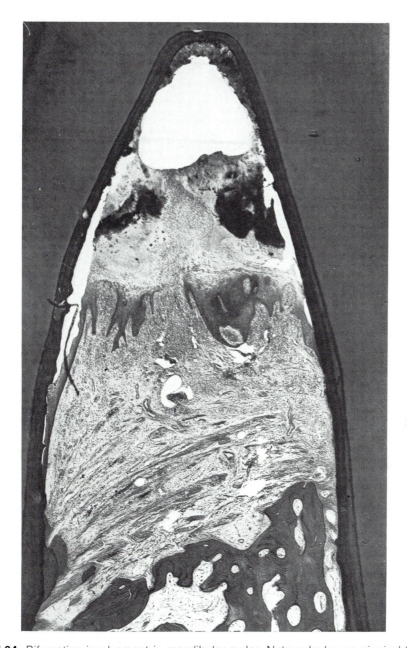

Fig. 7-34. Bifurcation involvement in mandibular molar. Note calculus on gingival tissue and adherent to tooth surface. Gingival inflammation is evident.

nor may the depth of separation be too great. In fact, as seen in necrotizing ulcerative gingivitis, pocket depth may be extremely minimal or negligible.

One must differentiate between the gingival sulcus of 1 or 2 mm in depth, but without clinical or histopathologic manifestations of inflammatory disease, and periodontal pockets. Sulci up to 2 mm in depth occasionally may be seen in mouths that must be considered healthy from a clinical point of view. Therefore it must be recognized that al-

though a gingival sulcus of zero is ideal, a deepened gingival sulcus may exist in a healthy state. Differentiation, therefore, is based on the clinical signs present (Table 14 and Fig. 7-38).

Differentiation between healthy sulcus and pocket

Clinically the loss of stippling of the gingiva can be an indication of an underlying inflammation, although the color and form of the gingiva may not vary from what is considered the range of the

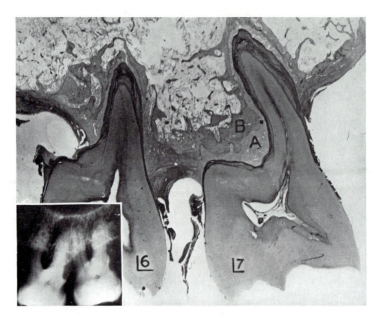

Fig. 7-35. Interradicular abscess or periodontal abscess in upper first and second premolar. *B*, Bone; *A*, abscess.

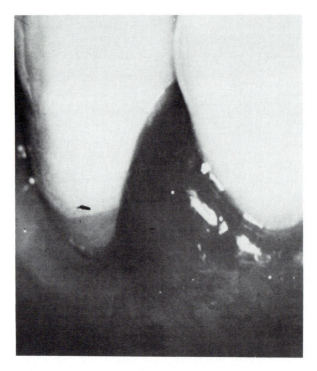

Fig. 7-36. Clinical appearance of gingival abscess.

norm. Stippling has been described as a series of small depressions (by King) and as a network of low ridges (by Orban). It is frequently associated with fully keratinized tissue. This change may be considered one of the first signs of gingival inflammation from the clinical point of view.

In the study of the clinically healthy gingiva one finds lymphocytes, plasma cells, and occasional histiocytes. This finding has led to considerable debate by numerous workers concerning the role of these cells and the interpretation to be made clinically therefrom. Schroeder has recently specu-

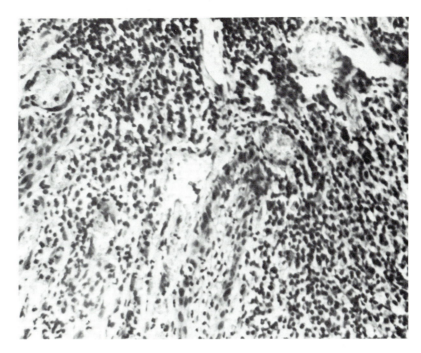

Fig. 7-37. Biopsy of gingival abscess showing typical leukocytic infiltration.

lated that the early inflammatory reactions in the gingiva may be the result of two unrelated cytologic phenomena:

1. The chemotactic migration of leukocytes through the attached epithelium in response to specific factors released by the microbial plaque. As microorganisms elaborating such factors are almost always present, this process, in contradistinction to the conventional inflammatory process, does not cease.

2. The migratory accumulation and mitotic turnover of mononuclear cells, predominantly plasma cells, responding to immunologic factors also released by the microbial plaque or occurring with the general host response.

Changes in corium

A microscopic study of changes in the gingival fibers in cases of gingival inflammation discloses a chronic progressive inflammatory process destroying the gingival fiber apparatus. The inflammatory infiltrate is seen interspersed between fiber groups and later fiber bundles. The early manifestations in the gingival fiber apparatus due to chronic gingival inflammation are characterized by the destruction in the middle sector of those fibers originating directly subjacent to the junctional epithelium. Later changes are evidenced by a dense inflammatory infiltration of the gingival corium, progressively replacing the connective tissue gin-

gival fibers. It is this process that results in the loss of stippling. Thus loss of stippling, while not evidencing in all instances the earliest signs of gingival inflammation, still can be regarded as an important clinical finding of an early inflammatory change, since as a rule neither the form nor the color of the gingiva may have been affected. Therefore histologically the differentiation between a healthy sulcus and a periodontal pocket may be made by the condition of the epithelial lining and the status of the gingival fiber apparatus. Normally the epithelial lining in intact. The greater its thickness, the better protection the subepithelial tissues have and the less likely is inflammation to occur. In periodontal pockets partial destruction of the sulcular epithelium is seen, with the subepithelial tissues exposed. Although a round cell infiltration occurs in the subepithelial tissues, even in healthy gingivae, there is usually more infiltration in periodontal pockets. Also a periodontal pocket shows ulcerations in the sulcular epithelium.

In addition recent studies at both light and electron microscopic levels have demonstrated lysis of the still attached collagen fibrils immediately below the most apical position of the junctional epithelium. Such connective tissue changes associated with those in the adjacent cementum may well be the prodrome for further apical migration of the junctional epithelium. The disruption of the attached gingival fibers is related to gingival inflam-

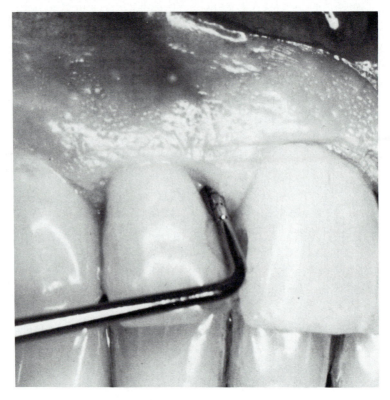

Fig. 7-38. Clinical appearance of periodontitis. Note limited gingival inflammation and marked pocket formation.

Table 14. Correlation of clinical and histopathologic findings of periodontal pocket

Clinical features	Histologic findings
Discoloration—various shades of pink to bluish red	Discoloration—result of inflammatory process occurring in gingival tissue
Loss of stippling	Loss of stippling—result of destruction of gingival tissue because of inflammation and accompanying edema
Retraction—gingival tissue easily reflected from tooth surface	Retraction—result of destruction of gingival fibers because of inflammatory process
Bleeding	Occurrence of bleeding—result of ulceration of sulcular epithelium and new capillary formation in inflammatory process; with occurrence of repair in long-standing gingival inflammations; occurrence of fibrosis and lessening of bleeding are symptoms
Exudate—gentle application of pressure to outer wall of pocket possibly causing exudate to be expressed	Occurrence of exudation in pockets—result of ulceration of sulcular epithelium and inflammatory process in gingiva
Loss of architectural form	Hyperplasia of gingiva—result of inflammatory process and repair going on in various degrees; possible occurrence of recession subsequent to long-standing gingival inflammations

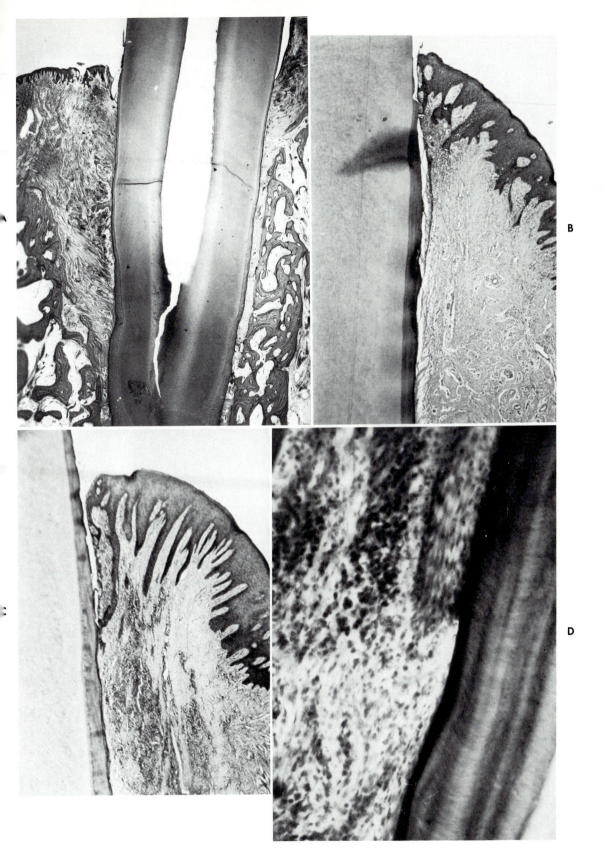

Fig. 7-39. A, Pocket formation is seen along root surfaces associated with significant inflammation and vertical bone resorption (left). **B** and **C,** Apical migration of junctional epithelium. Note enlarged epithelial layer in **C. D,** Note light-appearing area (lysed collagen fibers) immediately below most apical position of junctional epithelium in this section from a case of moderate periodontitis. Also note significant inflammation in area.

mation. Whether or not these still inserted fragments may continue to act as an epithelial barrier once inflammation is reduced is a vital clinical question, for they may in some fashion link with repairing collagen and thus maintain their level of attachment or be lysed completely, thereby enhancing further epithelial downgrowth (Fig. 7-39).

In areas where the epithelium is missing the highly inflamed subepithelial connective tissue is exposed to the contents of the pocket. The connective tissue is usually markedly infiltrated with round cells and, in cases of acute gingivitis, with polymorphonuclear leukocytes. These cells with fluid exude into the pocket and appear as a purulent exudate. The root surface usually shows an accumulation of plaque and calculus, and often food and debris are found in the pockets. Changes in vascularity have also been reported in periodon-titis, consisting primarily of dilation and multiplication of capillaries as well as disappearance of coiled capillaries near the epithelial attachment. These changes have been associated with alterations in blood flow into this area.

Plaque and calculus

Plaque and calculus may be seen occupying the entire pocket, and the relationship of these factors to the adjacent tissue is of interest. Fig. 7-40 shows the interdental tissue between two mandibular central incisors. The epithelial attachment is still on the enamel. The tip of the gingiva is bulbous and seems choked off by calculus. Clinically this gingiva was red, swollen, and bulbous in appearance, with calculus seen on the crowns of the teeth.

Fig. 7-41 shows a low-power photomicrograph

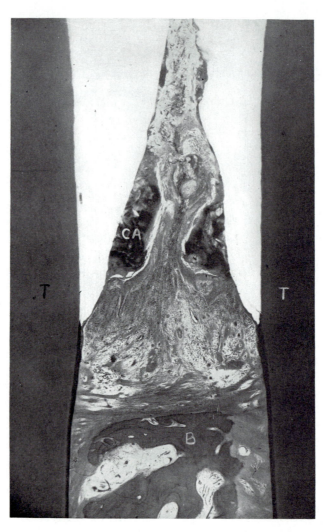

Fig. 7-40. Interdental tissue between mandibular central incisors. Junctional epithelium is still on enamel. Calculus is adherent to teeth. *T,* Tooth; *CA,* calculus; *B,* bone.

of the interdental tissue between two mandibular molars. Clinically there was obvious recession. The gingiva was inflamed, and a heavy calculus deposit was present. Calculus can be seen occupying the entire pocket at *CA;* sulcular epithelium is seen at *CE,* and above the junctional epithelium. Fig. 7-42 is a high-power photomicrograph of the same section. The character of the calculus and the inflammatory condition of the subepithelial tissue are evident. The inflammatory proliferation of the sulcular epithelium into the gingival corium and the ulceration of the sulcular epithelium can be seen. In this relation it must be remembered that the microbial envelope, more than the calcified mass, is the important agent in causing the inflammation.

In these sections the relationship of calculus to the pocket is interesting in that the sulcular epithelium lies adjacent to the calculus. In most sections studied a space appears in this region. We are of the opinion that this occurs in the preparation of the specimen and that in reality the true relationship is as shown in Fig. 7-43. Therefore in the removal of calculus the instrument must be inserted between the calculus and the sulcular epithelium and below the calculus so that it may be removed.

Of interest to the pathologist and the clinician is the manner in which calculus attaches itself to the cementum. Zander has pointed out that the removal of calculus from root surfaces is sometimes easy and sometimes very difficult, with many vari-

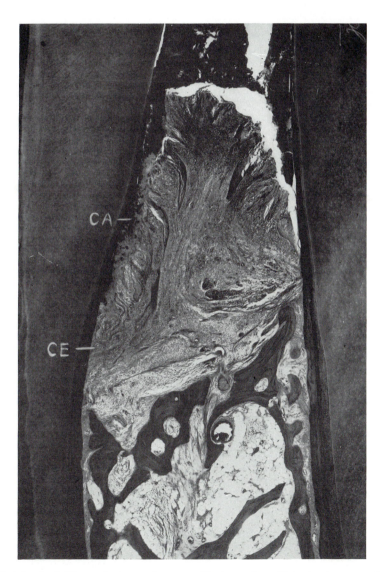

Fig. 7-41. Interdental tissue between two mandibular molars. Calculus is occupying entire pocket at *CA.* Junctional epithelium is at *CE.*

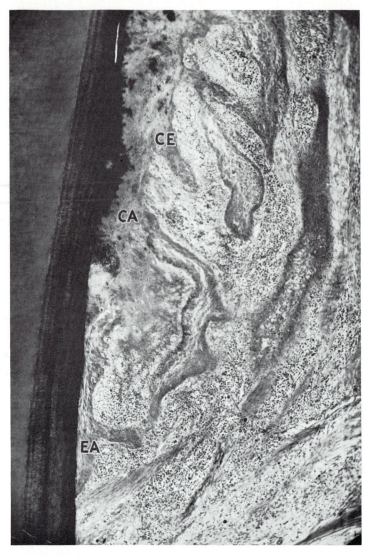

Fig. 7-42. Section shown in Fig. 7-41. Relationship of calculus to sulcular epithelium is seen. *CA,* Calculus; *CE,* sulcular epithelium; *EA,* epithelial attachment (junctional epithelium).

ations between these two extremes. To investigate this subject he studied decalcified and ground sections prepared and stained from autopsy specimens and from freshly extracted teeth. Four variations in modes of attachment were demonstrated: (1) the organic matrix of calculus was attached to the secondary cuticle; (2) the cuticle was absent, and the calculus matrix was attached to minute irregularities in the cemental surface; (3) organisms had penetrated into the cementum and were continuous with the organisms in the calculus matrix; and (4) calculus was locked mechanically in undercut areas of cement resorption.

It has been suggested that these differences in attachment may account for differences in the dif-ficulty or ease with which calculus is removed and may point toward reasons why calculus recurs faster on some teeth in some mouths than on others. Fig. 7-44 shows calculus locked into the cementum as described in the fourth variation.

Purulent discharge

Purulent discharge has long been known as a symptom of periodontal disease. This exudate is due to a discharge from the subepithelial tissue through the ulcerations in the epithelial lining. The amount of purulent discharge from a pocket depends on the degree of destruction of the sulcular epithelium and the amount of cellular infiltration of the subepithelial tissues. Sometimes in very

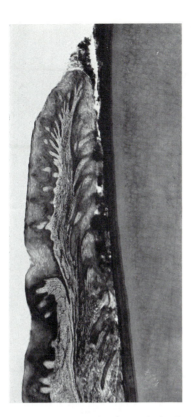

Fig. 7-43. Relationships of tooth, subgingival calculus, sulcular epithelium, and outer epithelial covering. Note that there is no space between calculus and sulcular epithelium.

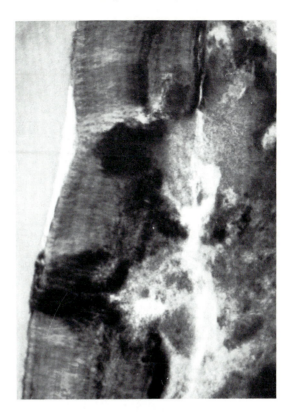

Fig. 7-44. Manner in which calculus may be locked into defect in cementum.

deep pockets there is little discharge. An example is given in Fig. 7-45, which shows a pocket of considerable depth. Little debris or calculus is seen. The epithelial lining is intact in one area about halfway down the pocket. Very little cellular infiltration is seen. The subepithelial tissue is composed of dense connective tissue. Papillary projections of epithelium into the connective tissue are seen; they anastomose. Such a pocket would clinically show but little suppuration.

On the other hand, Fig. 7-46 shows a mesiodistal section of the gingiva between two teeth. The pockets are shallow. Debris can be seen lying on both teeth. The epithelium shows ulcerations in many areas, and the subepithelial tissue is markedly infiltrated with round cells. Only little connective tissue can be noted. The transseptal fibers can be seen running above the alveolar crest. Clinically such pockets may show much suppuration.

Figs. 7-45 and 7-46 demonstrate that the depth of the pocket does not designate the amount of purulent discharge but that there must be an ulceration of the sulcular epithelium and an inflammatory infiltration of the subepithelial tissue.

Gingival bleeding

Bleeding of the gingiva is one of the more prominent symptoms of periodontal disease. Clinically it may be the only complaint of the patient. Fig. 7-47 shows clearly how bleeding occurs from the gingiva. The ulcerated sulcular epithelium, which is the cardinal finding of a pocket, allows for exposure of the subepithelial tissue. Since this tissue shows signs of inflammation, there are numerous capillaries present. Whenever any type of pressure is applied, blood can pass from the exposed connective tissue because the epithelial covering is missing. Often rather large blood vessels can be seen near the surface of the gingiva adjacent to the pocket, and in these cases marked bleeding upon pressure is experienced.

Abscess formation

Occasionally abscess formation occurs in the wall of the periodontal pocket. The abscesses are localized and consist of clusters of lymphocytes and plasma cells, heavily interspersed with leukocytes. At times they consist only of them, especially in acute stages. The abscess formation is seen

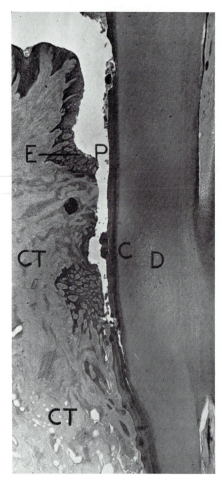

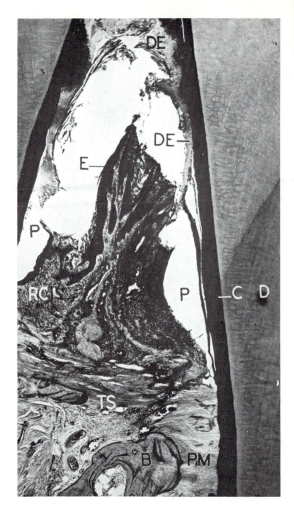

Fig. 7-45. Deep periodontal pocket. Very little cellular infiltration can be seen. *D*, Dentin; *C*, cementum; *E*, epithelium; *P*, pocket; *CT*, connective tissue.

Fig. 7-46. Marked cellular infiltration of subepithelial tissue between two teeth (mesiodistal section). *D*, Dentin; *C*, cementum; *DE*, debris; *E*, epithelium; *P*, pockets; *TS*, transseptal fibers; *B*, bone; *PM*, periodontal ligament; *RC*, round cell infiltration.

beneath the epithelial lining and tends to be situated at the base of the pocket.

Deepening of pocket

The deepening of the pocket is dependent on the apical proliferation of the junctional epithelium alongside the cementum with subsequent separation or hyperplasia of the gingiva resulting from inflammation. Goldman showed that the apical proliferation of the junctional epithelium was hindered by the maintenance of the insertion of principal fibers of the periodontal ligament that lie in apposition to the epithelium. As soon as destruction of these fibers took place the epithelium proliferated to the area of connective tissue attachment (Fig. 7-48). Fig. 7-49 shows a section stained with Wilder's silver stain and illustrates the junctional

epithelium at *EA*, adjacent to which are a few bundle remnants of principal fibers. Apically, at *A*, the fibers are degenerated and widely spaced. The connective tissue appears blotchy, a result of the disintegration of previously intact collagen fibers. At *B* the fibers are closely packed and are of normal thickness and appearance. Epithelial proliferation, stimulated by the inflammatory process in the vicinity, can take place as soon as those few remnant fibers adjacent to the epithelium degenerate. Melcher has described the early changes involved in the spread of inflammation in detail. He reports that initially there is an accumulation of fluid around and then within the fiber bundles. This is followed by fibroblastic nuclear changes. The degeneration of the fibroblasts is followed by degeneration of the fibers, leaving an amorphous once the fibers have become detached, the inflammatory process then acts, leading to the complete destruction of the connective tissue in the area. One must emphasize, however, that whether the apical migration of the epithelium is the result of an initial breakdown of periodontal connective tissue fibers or an initial proliferation of the epithelium it is the inflammatory process that sets off the reaction.

Gottlieb has stated that the barrier against the apical proliferation of the junctional epithelium is the continuous productivity of the cementum. That this is true is evident, since if the principal fiber apparatus of the periodontal ligament remains intact, a cementoblastic layer producing cementum is always seen. Whether the cementum can cease production despite a normal periodontal ligament is the main point in question. At the ultrastructural level an increased occurrence of nonbanded collagen fibrils was observed near the root surface adjacent to marginal areas of chronic inflammation. These changes indicated that they represented partially decomposed collagen fibrils. When destruction of these fibrils became complete the periodontal fibers would loose their attachment. This has been demonstrated by the presence of granular debris and bundles of nonstriated filaments without evidence of typical collagen fibrils in the area immediately below the junctional epithelium. At some of these sites alterations in cementum were also observed. These alterations consisted of removal of the mineral crystals as well as a modification and removal of the matrix collagen in an up to 18 μm wide zone beneath the cementum surface. The localization of the cementum lesions relative to the bottom of the periodontal pocket and to the region of inflammation suggests that the alteration of the organic matrix is caused by the agents responsible for the breakdown of the periodontal fibers, whereas the mineral crystals are removed by a decalcification process (Selvig, 1967). In this relation it should be pointed out that changes in cementum of periodontally involved teeth, for example, an increased mineral content at the cervical cementum and a granular surface at the exposed cementum, have been reported by chemical, microradiographic, and electron microscopic studies. However, the full significance of these changes as related to the apical migration of the junctional epithelium or the detachment of gingival fibers is not yet understood.

Most recently Slavkin and Boyle (1974) have suggested that acellular cementum may be derived from epithelium, with the collagen found in the

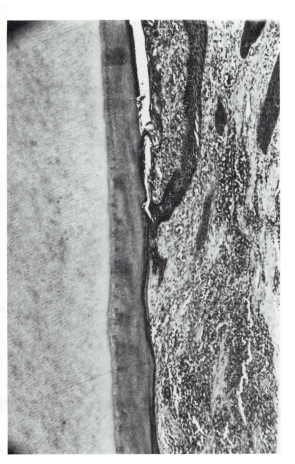

Fig. 7-47. Note ulceration of this crevicular epithelium. Obviously bleeding would occur freely if site were probed.

necrotic mass. With continuing irritation this process proceeds into depth, destroying the adjoining tissues.

Another point of view as to the nature of the epithelial migration apically has been presented by some investigators, notably Wassermann. They indicate that the inflammatory processes and irritation stimulate the epithelium to proliferate rootwise, destroying the subjacent attachment fibers. Two theories have been presented. The first, suggested by Wassermann, is that the proliferating epithelium has some lysing effect on the fibers. This suggestion must be coupled with the recent findings of collagenolytic activity in healing wounds. The second one is that the degeneration of the fibers is caused by pressure atrophy of the epithelial proliferation. It is further explained that

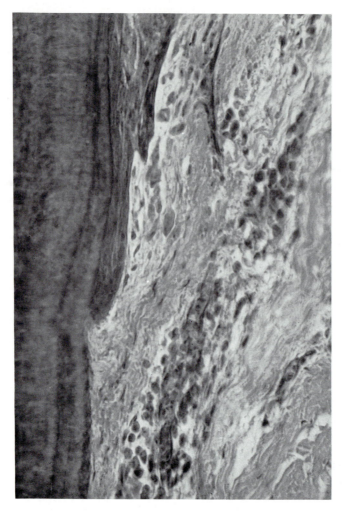

Fig. 7-48. Dense inflammatory infiltrate subjacent to junctional epithelium. Collagen fibers are apparent between base of epithelial attachment and inflammatory cells.

older cementum representing the subsequent influx of fibrils from the periodontal ligament. Since recent evidence suggests that the same proteins involved with amelogenesis may be involved with acellular cementogenesis, the epithelial-specific extracellular proteins in cementum might serve as antigens when this tissue becomes accessible to the immune system in gingival inflammation. This concept presents another vista focusing on the important role of acellular cementum as a component possibly contributing to the inflammatory lesion. To further the above-outlined speculation one should then also consider the type of cementum laid down on previously exposed and subsequently root-planed surfaces following periodontal treatment of, for example, infrabony lesions. Particularly with the use of osseous autografts a new ''scar'' cementum has been shown to deposit on the previously treated root surfaces into which col-

lagen fibers may insert. If the original acellular cementum laid down on the tooth surface during development is epithelial in origin, is the ''scar'' cementum laid down after therapy of a similar nature or is this material mesenchymal in origin? And if indeed it is different in composition does it serve the anchoring need of the periodontal fibers as well as original acellular cementum? Here too one must say that the full significance of our data to clinical therapy awaits future experiments.

Resorption of cementum at the border of the junctional epithelium, if no intervening principal fibers are present, should allow for immediate epithelial proliferation. Fig. 7-50 is a photomicrograph of the mesial junctional epithelium of a maxillary central incisor of a 52-year-old man. Epithelial proliferation over unrepaired areas of cemental resorption is seen at *R*. Repaired cemental defects at the borderline of the junctional epi-

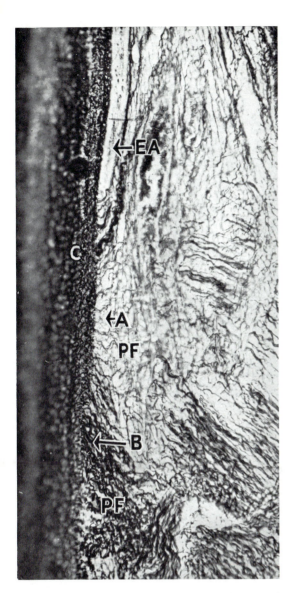

Fig. 7-49. Relation of junctional epithelium and principal fibers of periodontal ligament. At *A* fibers are degenerated and widely spaced. At *B* they are thick and of normal appearance. (Section stained with Wilder's stain.) *EA,* Epithelial attachment; *C,* cementum; *PF,* principal fibers.

thelium are also seen frequently. This is interpreted as follows: if resorption of the cementum occurs at the border of the junctional epithelium, either cemental repair can take place or epithelium can proliferate over the area.

Occasionally a section may show apical epithelial proliferation with intact principal fibers situated in it, as in Fig. 7-50. We interpret these as lateral ingrowths of epithelium along areas where there are no principal fibers present, believing that they do not represent the central area of pocket for-

mation. It is probable that in this manner the pocket progresses laterally.

The pocket depth may also be altered by means of hyperplasia of the gingiva. Inflammation of this tissue, with accompanying edema and increased vascularity, increases the bulk of the tissue. If the bottom of the pocket is either progressing apically or remaining static, the swelling causes greater depth of the pocket. A cycle may develop; the deeper the pocket becomes because of inflammation, the more it can lodge debris and calculus, causing further inflammation and swelling and increasing the depth of the pocket.

Proliferation of sulcular epithelium

Not only does the sulcular epithelium show evidence of ulceration, but papillary projections of epithelium are also given off into the gingival corium. This process varies. In some cases very few offshoots are seen, whereas in others deep anastomosing retia are observed. The epithelium is squamous, and inflammatory cells can be seen in it. Fig. 7-51 shows calculus in a pocket. The sulcular epithelium is ulcerated at several areas, and proliferating epithelium into the gingival corium is marked.

Gingival clefts

The gingival tissues are frequently the location of clefts or fissures in the marginal area; rarely do they occur in the papilla. These clefts have been described as being caused by numerous factors. Clinical evidence of cleft formation discloses that this finding is usually associated with pocket formation. It has also been noticed that clefts may form only to disappear. However, resultant recession is always found. Microscopic examination of cleft formation reveals that it is associated with the proliferation and anastomosing of the epithelium into the gingival corium. When proliferation extends to the outer wall of the gingiva, and final destruction of this tissue results, a cleft can be traced to the inner wall of the pocket. Since the marginal area is thinner than the papillary area, clefts will occur more quickly in this area. Thus spontaneous disappearance of a cleft is the resultant loss of tissue of the marginal area due to pocket formation. In essence, therefore, cleft formation is the result of the fundamental pathologic process of marginal periodontal disease—pocket formation and recession of the gingival margin. A cleft may also start from the outer surface, as is seen in the case of a cleft caused by incorrect brushing of the teeth (Fig. 7-52).

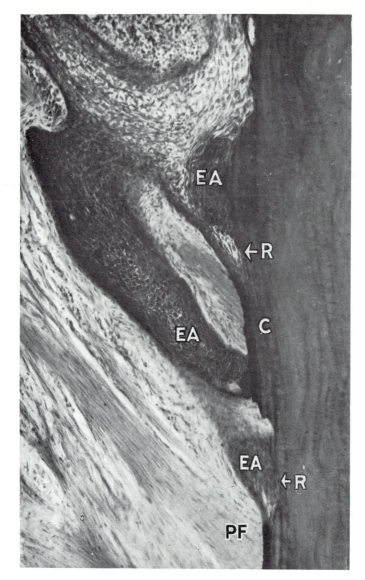

Fig. 7-50. Junctional epithelium proliferating over resorptive areas of cementum. An area of principal fibers of periodontal ligament can be seen at *C*. These bundles are bypassed by lateral ingrowths of epithelial attachment where there are no principal fibers present. *C, Cementum; EA, epithelial attachment; PF, principal fibers; R, resorption.*

Effect of faulty fillings and crowns on gingival sulcus

Faulty margins and faulty crowns may act as irritants to the gingiva. If the margin of the crown is inserted deeply enough into the crevice, ulceration of the tissue occurs. In this event an acute inflammation results, with a purulent discharge evident that will later turn chronic. Histologic sections of teeth that have borne faulty crowns usually show food and calculus accumulated in the crevices. Ulceration of the epithelium is generally seen, with inflammation in the connective tissue of the gingival corium. Resorption of the alveolar bone may be evident.

Classification of pockets

Pockets may be classified as suprabony or infrabony osseous defects (Table 15). However, from a therapeutic point of view the classification of importance is dependent on the osseous contour, that is, whether a defect is present or not. In the suprabony pocket the base of the pocket is coronal to the alveolar crest. The suprabony pocket may be further classified as gingival or periodontal. The former, sometimes called a pseudopocket, may be defined as a gingival inflammation and ulceration of the sulcular epithelium but without apical proliferation of the junctional epithelium. There may or may not be an increase in depth of the gingival

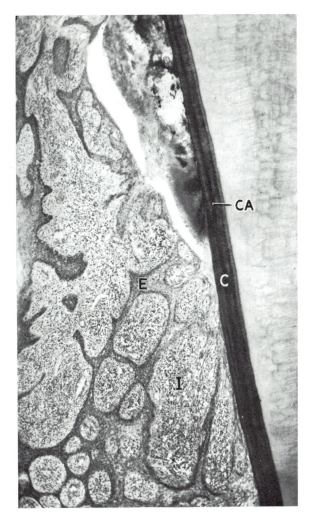

Fig. 7-51. Anastomosing rete proliferating from sulcular epithelium. *C,* Cementum; *CA,* calculus; *I,* inflammatory infiltrate; *E,* epithelium.

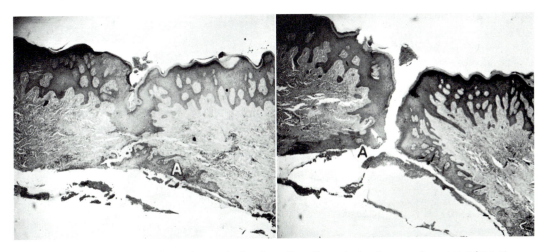

Fig. 7-52. Gingival cleft cut in mesiodistal section. Two photomicrographs were taken at different levels of the cleft. Note sulcular epithelium at *A.*

sulcus. A periodontal pocket may be described as a pathologic deepening of the gingival sulcus produced by destruction of the supporting tissued and apical proliferation of the junctional epithelium. An infrabony pocket is one in which the base of the pocket is apical to the crest of the bone. *The important aspect, however, is the topography of the osseous defect.*

In relation to the classification of pockets, bone in periodontal manifestations may be classified as well. The bone may be unaffected as seen in instances of gingivitis; it may be affected and resorbed but remain in a topography similar to the norm; or it may show signs of irregularity with ridges forming at the buccal-crestal regions. Osseous defects of various contours may be found.

Fig. 7-53 shows the changes in the interdental gingiva in disease. Calculus deposits are present. The junctional epithelia on both teeth have migrated apically, and the gingival margin has receded. The characteristic changes in the corium may be noted. These changes are consistent with pocket formation and are classified as suprabony pockets (periodontal pockets) (Fig. 7-54).

The important aspect of the infrabony pocket is the osseous defect present, the contour of which may be quite varied. Fig. 7-55 shows a deep infrabony pocket (osseous defect) that is relatively narrow on the distal aspect of a lower premolar. Another example is seen in Fig. 7-56. Fig. 7-57 shows a broad defect. Osseous defects in Figs. 7-58 and 7-59 should be compared to the appearance of the crest in Fig. 7-54. Therapy must take into account the topography of the crest. Thus it is important for the diagnostician to differentiate the various bony topographies found in periodontal disease.

There are varied causes for the development of osseous defects. Gottlieb explains that an infrabony pocket is not an intra-alveolar pocket. The alveolar housing of the affected tooth is always gone in the area of pocket formation. An infrabony pocket is impossible on the labial side of an upper

Table 15. Pockets (diseased gingival attachment)

Suprabony (supracrestal)	Infrabony (infracrestal)
Gingival	Three osseous walls
Periodontal	Two osseous walls
	One osseous wall
	Combinations of above

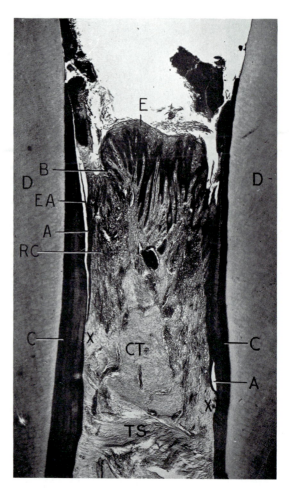

Fig. 7-53. Periodontal pockets. *D,* Dentin; *C,* cementum; *E,* epithelium; *B,* break in epithelium; *RC,* round cell infiltration; *EA,* junctional epithelium; *A,* artifact; *CT,* connective tissue; *TS,* transseptal fibers; *X,* connective tissue attachment to cementum.

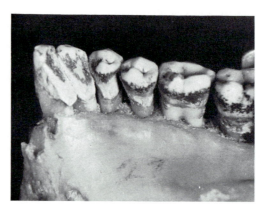

Fig. 7-54. Resorptive lesion in marginal periodontitis (dried mandible). This is so-called horizontal resorptive process.

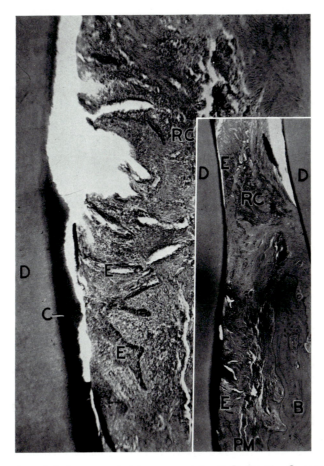

Fig. 7-55. Very deep infrabony pocket (osseous defect). *D,* Dentin; *C,* cementum; *E,* epithelium; *RC,* round cell infiltration; *PM,* periodontal ligament; *B,* bone.

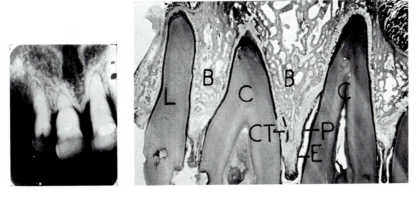

Fig. 7-56. Infrabony pocket on mesial aspect of left central incisor. *L,* Lateral incisor; *C,* central incisor; *B,* bone; *CT,* cemental tear; *P,* pocket; *E,* epithelium.

anterior tooth. If the alveolar bone is gone here, no bone is left, but on the palatal side of the same tooth bone of the hard palate backs the alveolar bone proper. If the alveolar bone disappears from such an area, the palatal bone remains, causing the infrabony pocket. Gingival recession cannot develop here because the palatal bone prevents the gingival margin from following the base of the sulcus and prevents gingival recession. The same applies to any approximal surface when the alveolar bone of one tooth has disappeared and the alveolar bone of the neighboring tooth is intact. This alveolar bone of the neighboring tooth is higher than the level of the base of the pocket of the affected tooth and so produces an osseous defect.

Another explanation for the formation of an osseous defect takes into account the changes that occur in occlusal traumatism and pocket formation in general. Factors responsible for both must be present. Should the attachment apparatus be affected in the crestal region by occlusal traumatism, and should all the factors responsible for pocket formation be present, an infrabony pocket may form.

If one takes into account the indented proximal form of the cervical portion of the root and buccolingual movement of the tooth due to occlusal traumatism, it will be found that the tooth will occlude against the alveolar wall with the least movement. Thus vertical bone resorption will result. Coupled with a gingival involvement of local environmental origin an infrabony pocket may result. An infrabony pocket may also form interproximally in a fashion similar to pocket formation and alveolar crest loss that occur in marginal periodontitis, except that under certain local environmental factors (tooth positions and so on) an osseous defect will form.

Pulpal periodontal interaction

Clinical interest has focused again on the possible relation between pulpal and periodontal pathology. It has long been known that extension of apical lesions into the adjoining periodontium may lead to periodontal pathology. Degeneration of the pulp due to bacteria entering the pulp from an area of periodontal pathosis via lateral canals has also been documented. Recent clinical experience demonstrates that endodontic treatment often leads to the healing of a previously untreatable periodontal lesion and thus clinically supports the contention that lateral canals may act as a passageway for irritants. Further observations have intimated that periodontal pathology may cause secondary

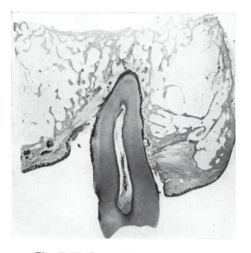

Fig. 7-57. Broad infrabony pocket.

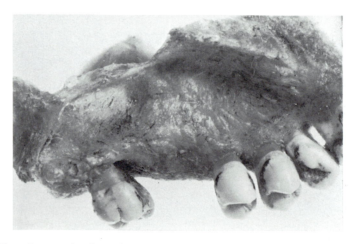

Fig. 7-58. Broad resorptive bone lesion associated with infrabony pocket (dried maxilla). This is so-called vertical resorptive process with only one osseous wall (mesial) remaining.

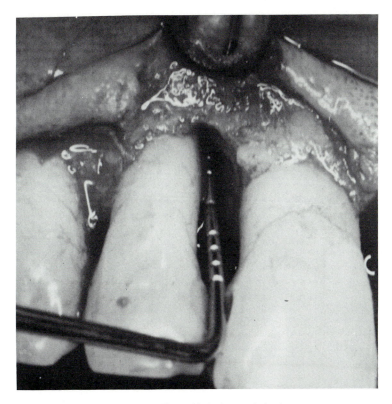

Fig. 7-59. Broad infrabony defect.

dentin formation on the pulpal wall opposite the periodontal lesion in the absence of lateral canals, thus suggesting that noxious agents may pass through the intact tooth wall and produce pulpal irritation. Further study is needed to more clearly define this interaction and its biologic and clinical significance.

REFERENCES

Akiyoshi, M., and Mori, K.: Marginal periodontitis; a histologic study of the incipient stage, J. Periodontol. **38:**45, 1967.

Alleo, J. J., DeRenzis, F. A., Farber, P. A., and Varboncoeur, A. P.: The presence and biologic activity of cementum-bound endotoxins, J. Periodontol. **45:**672, 1974.

Bass, C. C.: A previously undescribed demonstrable pathologic condition in exposed cementum and in underlying dentine, Oral Surg. **4:**641, 1951.

Bass, C. C., and Fulmer, H. M.: The location of the zone of disintegrating epithelial attachment cuticle in relation to the cemento-enamel junction and to the outer border of the periodontal fibers on some tooth specimens, J. Dent. Res. **27:**623, 1948.

Bassett, C. A. L.: The effect of electrical currents on bone structure, J. Dent. Res. **44:**1112, 1965.

Becks, H.: Normal and pathologic pocket formation, J. Am. Dent. Assoc. **16:**2167, 1929.

Benson, L. A.: Study of a pathologic condition in exposed cementum, Oral Surg. **16:**1137, 1961.

Berglund, S. E.: Introduction to conference on the implications of immune reactions in the pathogenesis of periodontal disease, J. Periodontol. **41:**195, 1970.

Berke, J. D.: Etiology and histology of dental tartars, Dent. Cosmos **77:**134, 1935.

Bernier, J. L.: Histologic changes of the gingival tissues in health and periodontal disease, Oral Surg. **3:**1194, 1950.

Black, G. V.: Special dental pathology, Chicago, 1915, Medico-Dental Publishing Co.

Box, H. K.: Gingival clefts and associated tracts, N.Y. Dent. J. **16:**3, 1950.

Box, H. K.: Twelve periodontal studies, Toronto, 1940, University of Toronto Press.

Box, H. K.: Necrotic gingivitis, Toronto, 1930, Canadian Dental Research Foundation.

Box, H. K.: Evolution of periodontal pus pocket, Toronto, 1921, Canadian Dental Research Foundation.

Boyle, P. E.: Periodontal workshop, J. Am. Dent. Assoc. **45:**3, 1952.

Brandtzaeg, P.: Local factors of resistance in the gingival area, J. Periodont. Res. **1:**19, 1966.

Brandtzaeg, P.: Immunochemical comparison of proteins in human gingival pocket fluid, Arch. Oral Biol. **10:**795, 1965.

Brill, N.: Gingival pocket fluid, Acta Odontol. Scand. **20:** Supp., 1962.

Burstone, M. S.: Histochemical study of cytochrome oxidase in normal and inflamed gingiva, Oral Surg. **13:**1501, 1964.

Cantor, M. T., and Stahl, S. S.: The effects of various interdental stimulators upon the keratinization of the interdental col, Periodontics **3:**243, 1965.

Carranza, F. A., Jr., and Cabrini, R. L.: Histochemical reactions of periodontal tissues; a review of the literature, J. Am. Dent. Assoc. **60:**464, 1960.

Cohen, B.: Comparative studies in periodontal disease, Proc. R. Soc. Med. **53:**275, 1960.

Cohen, B.: Morphological factors in the pathogenesis of periodontal disease, Br. Dent. J. **10:**31, 1959.

Cohen, B.: Pathology of interdental tissues, Dent. Pract. Dent. Rec. **9:**167, 1959.

Cohen, D. W.: Pathology of periodontal disease. In Tiecke, R., editor: Oral pathology, New York, 1965, McGraw-Hill, Inc.

Cohen, D. W., Friedman, L. A., Shapiro, J., Kyle, G. C., and Franklin, S.: A longitutional investigation of the periodontal changes during pregnancy and fifteen months postpartum, J. Periodontol. **42:**653, 1971.

Cohen, D. W., Friedman, L. A., Shapiro, J., Kyle, G. C., and Franklin, S.: Diabetes mellitus and periodontal disease: two year longitutional observations, J. Periodontol. **41:**709, 1970.

Cohen, M. M., Winer, R. A., and Shklar, G.: Oral aspects of mongolism, Oral Surg. **14:**92, 1961.

Conference on The Implications of Immune Reactions in the Pathogenesis of Periodontal Disease, J. Periodontol. **41:**195, 1970.

Coolidge, E. D.: Inflammatory changes in the gingival tissue due to local irritation, J. Am. Dent. Assoc. **18:**2255, 1931.

Dragoo, M. R., and Sullivan, H. C.: A clinical and histologic evaluation of autogenous iliac bone grafts in humans. I. Wound healing 2 to 8 months, J. Periodontol. **44:**599, 1973.

Egelberg, J.: Permeability of the dento-gingival blood vessels. II. Clinically healthy gingiva, J. Periodont. Res. **1:**276, 1966.

Eichel, B.: Oxidative enzymes of the gingiva, Ann. N.Y. Acad. Sci. **85:**479, 1960.

Eisen, A. Z., and Gross, J.: The role of epithelium and mesenchyme in the production of a collagenolytic enzyme and a hyaluronidase in the anuran tadpole, Dev. Biol. **12:**408, 1965.

Engel, M. B., Joseph, N. R., Laskin, D. M., and Catchpole, H. R.: A theory of connective tissue behavior, its implications in periodontal disease, Ann. N.Y. Acad. Sci. **85:**399, 1960.

Epker, B. N., and Frost, H. M.: Correlation of bone resorption and formation with the physical behavior of loaded bone, J. Dent. Res. **44:**33, 1965.

Everhart, D. L., and Stahl, S. S.: A possible source of antigen(s) in periodontal disease, J. Dent. Res. **56:**536, 1977.

Felton, J., Person, P., and Stahl, S. S.: Biochemical and histochemical studies of aerobic oxidative metabolism of oral tissues. IV. Additional observations on histochemical oxidase reactions in gingiva, J. Dent. Res. **44:**1238, 1965.

Fish, E. W.: Etiology and prevention of periodontal breakdown, Dent. Prog. **1:**234, 1960.

Fish, E. W.: Surgical pathology of the mouth, London, 1948, Isaac Pitman & Sons Ltd.

Freedman, H. L., Listgarten, M. A., and Taichman, N. S.: Electron microscopic features of chronically inflamed human gingiva, J. Periodont. Res. **3:**313, 1968.

Froum, S. J., Thaler, R., Scopp, I. W., and Stahl, S. S.: Osseous autografts. II. Histologic responses to osseous coagulum-bone blend grafts, J. Periodontol. **46:**656, 1975.

Fullmer, H. M.: A histochemical study of periodontal disease in the maxillary alveolar processes of 135 autopsies, J. Periodontol. **32:**206, 1961.

Fullmer, H. M., and Gibson, W.: Collagenolytic activity in gingivae of man, Nature (London) **209:**728, 1966.

Fullmer, H. M., and Lazarus, G. S.: Collagenase in the bone of man, J. Histochem. Cytochem. **17:**793, 1969.

Garant, P. R., and Mulvihill, J. E.: The fine structure of gingivitis in the beagle. III. Plasma cell infiltration of the subepithelial connective tissue, J. Periodont. Res. **7:**161, 1971.

Genco, R. J.: Immunoglobulins and periodontal disease, J. Periodontol. **41:**196, 1970.

Glickman, I.: Acute vitamin C deficiency and periodontal disease. II. The effect of acute vitamin C deficiency upon the response of the periodontal tissues to artificially induced inflammation, J. Dent. Res. **27:**201, 1948.

Glickman, I.: The bone factor in peridontoclasia, Massachusetts Dent. Bull. **20:**14, 1944.

Glickman, I., and Smulow, J. B.: Alteratons in the pathway of gingival inflammation into the underlying tissues induced by excessive occlusal force, J. Periodontol. **33:**7, 1962.

Glickman, I., and Wood, H.: Bone histology in periodontal disease, J. Dent. Res. **21:**35, 1942.

Goldhaber, P.: Heparin enhancement of factors stimulating bone resorption in tissue culture, Science **147:**407, 1965.

Goldhaber, P.: Collagen and bone, J. Am. Dent. Assoc. **68:**825, 1964.

Goldman, H. M.: Behavior of transseptal fibers in periodontal disease, J. Dent. Res. **36:**249, 1957a.

Goldman, H. M.: Extension of exudate into supporting structures of teeth in marginal periodontitis, J. Periodontol. **28:**175, 1957b.

Goldman, H. M., and Cohen, D. W.: Periodontia, ed. 4, St. Louis, 1957, The C. V. Mosby Co.

Goldman, H. M.: Histologic topographic changes of inflammatory origin in the gingival fibers, J. Periodontol. **23:**104, 1952.

Goldman, H. M.: The topography and role of the gingival fibers, J. Dent. Res. **30:**331, 1951.

Goldman, H. M.: Periodontosis in the spider monkey—a preliminary report, J. Periodontol. **18:**34, 1948.

Goldman, H. M.: A similar condition to periodontosis found in two spider monkeys, Am. J. Orthod. **33:**749, 1947.

Goldman, H. M.: Marginal periodontitis, Am. J. Orthod. **31:**93, 1945.

Goldman, H. M.: The relationship of the epithelial attachment to the adjacent fibers of the periodontal membrane, J. Dent. Res. **23:**177, 1944.

Goldman, H. M., and Cohen, D. W.: The infrabony pocket; classification and treatment, J. Periodontol. **29:**272, 1958.

Gorlin, R. J., and Goldman, H. M., editors: Thoma's Oral pathology, ed. 6, St. Louis, 1970, The C. V. Mosby Co.

Gottlieb, B.: The new concept of periodontoclasia, J. Periodontol. **17:**7, 1946.

Gottlieb, B.: Continuous deposition of cementum, J. Am. Dent. Assoc. **30:**842, 1943.

Gottlieb, B.: The present status of the paradontoclasia problem, J. Periodontol. **2:**99, 1931.

Gottlieb, B.: Formation of the pocket; diffuse atrophy of the alveolar bone, J. Am. Dent. Assoc. **15:**462, 1928.

Gottlieb, B.: Paradental pyorrhea and alveolar atrophy, J. Am. Dent. Assoc. **15:**2196, 1928.

Gottlieb, B.: Tissue changes in pyorrhea, J. Am. Dent. Assoc. **4:**2178, 1927.

Gottlieb, B.: Etiology and therapy of alveolar pyorrhea, Z. Stomat. **18:**59, 1920.

Gottlieb, B., and Orban, B.: Biology and pathology of the tooth and its supporting mechanism, New York, 1938, The Macmillan Co.

Grant, D., and Bernick, S.: The periodontium of aging humans, J. Periodontol. **43:**660, 1972.

Greig, D. M.: Clinical observations on the surgical pathology of bone, Edinburgh, 1931, Oliver & Boyd, Ltd.

Gross, J.: Studies on the biology of connective tissues: remodeling of collagen metamorphosis, Medicine (Balt.) **43:**291, 1964.

Hiatt, W. H.: Periodontal pocket elimination by combined endodontic-periodontic therapy, Periodontics **1:**152, 1963.

Hirschfeld, I.: The dynamic relationship between pathologically migrating teeth and inflammatory tissue in periodontal pockets, J. Periodontol. **4:**35, 1933.

Horton, J. E., Oppenheim, J. J., and Mergenhagen, S. E.: A role for cell-mediated immunity in the pathogenesis of periodontal disease, J. Periodontol. **45**(suppl. 2):351, 1974.

James, W., and Counsell, A.: A histological investigation into "so-called pyorrhea alveolaris," Br. Dent. J. **48:**1237, 1927.

Jordan, H. V., and Keyes, P. H.: Periodontal lesions in the Syrian hamster. III. Findings related to an infectious and transmissible component, Arch. Oral Biol. **9:**372, 1964.

Kelstrup, J., and Theilade, E.: Microbes and periodontal disease, J. Clin. Periodontol. **1:**15, 1974.

Kindlova, M.: Changes in the vascular bed of the marginal periodontium in periodontitis, J. Dent. Res. **44:**456, 1965.

King, J. D.: Gingival disease in Dundee, Dent. Rec. **65:**9, 32, 55, 1945.

Koch, J. D.: Laws of bone architecture, Am. J. Anat. **21:**177, 1917.

Kohl, J. T., and Zander, H. A.: Morphology of interdental gingival tissues, Oral Surg. **14:**287, 1961.

Kramer, I. H.: Alveolar bone in health and disease with special reference to local factors, Dent. Pract. Dent. Rec. **12:**327, 1962.

Kronfeld, R.: Clinical pathology of the periodontal pocket, J. Am. Dent. Assoc. **27:**449, 1940.

Kronfeld, R.: Histopathology of the teeth and their surrounding structures, ed. 2, Philadelphia, 1939, Lea & Febiger.

Levy, B. M., Robertson, P. B., Dreizen, S., Mackler, B. F., and Bernick, S.: Adjuvant induced destructive periodontitis in nonhuman primates. A comparative study, J. Periodont. Res. **11:**54, 1976.

Linde, J. Hamp, S. E., and Löe, H.: Experimental periodontitis in the beagle dog, J. Periodont. Res. **8:**1, 1973.

Linde, J., and Svanberg, G.: Influence of trauma from occlusion on progression of experimental periodontitis in the beagle dog, J. Clin. Periodontol. **1:**3, 1974.

Listgarten, M. A.: Electron microscopic observations on the bacterial flora of acute necrotizing ulcerative gingivitis, J. Periodontol. **36:**328, 1965.

Löe, H., and Holm-Pedersen, P.: Absence and presence of fluid from normal and inflamed gingivae, Periodontics **3:**171, 1965.

Löe, H., Theilade, E., and Jensen, S. B.: Experimental gingivitis in man, J. Periodontol. **36:**177, 1965.

Lövdal, A., Arno, A., and Waerhaug, J.: Incidence of clinical manifestations of periodontal disease in light of oral hygiene and calculus formation, J. Am. Dent. Assoc. **56:**21, 1958.

Macdonald, J. B., Gibbons, R. J., and Socransky, S. S.: Bacterial mechanisms in periodontal disease, Ann. N.Y. Acad. Sci. **85:**467, 1960.

Mandel, I. D.: Calculus formation, Dent. Clin. North Am., p. 731, Nov. 1960.

Mann, W. V.: The correlation of gingivitis, pocket depth and exudate from the gingival crevice, J. Periodontol. **34:**379, 1963.

Mann, W. V., and Stoffer, H. R.: The identification of protein components in fluid from gingival pockets, Periodontics **2:**263, 1964.

Massler, M., Mühlemann, H. R., and Schour, I.: Relation of gingival inflammation to alveolar crest resorption, J. Dent. Res. **32:**704, 1953.

McLean, F. C., and Bloom, W.: Calcification and ossification calcification in normal growing bone, Anat. Rec. **78:**333, 1940.

Melcher, A. H.: Pathogenesis of chronic gingivitis. II. The effect of inflammatory changes in the corium on the overlying epithelium, Dent. Pract. **3:**50, 1962.

Melcher, A. H.: Pathogenesis of chronic gingivitis. I. The spread of the inflammatory process, Dent. Pract. Dent. Rec. **13:**2, 1962.

Mergenhagen, S. E., Tempel, T. R., and Snyderman, R.: Immunologic reactions and periodontal inflammation, J. Dent. Res. **49:**256, 1970.

Mergenhagen, S. E., Wahl, S. M., Wahl, L. M., Horton, J. E., and Raisz, L. G.: The role of lymphocytes and macrophages in the destruction of bone and collagen, Ann. N.Y. Acad. Sci. **256:**136, 1975.

Mikola, O. J., and Bauer, W. H.: Juvenile paradentitis, J. Dent. Res. **28:**650, 1949.

Mueller, E.: Histologic study of a case of extensive resorption in a human being, J. Am. Dent. Assoc. **18:**684, 1931.

Mueller, E., and Rony, H. R.: Laboratory studies of an unusual case of resorption, J. Am. Dent. Assoc. **17:**326, 1930.

Müller, G., and Zander, H. A.: Cementum of periodontally diseased teeth from India, J. Dent. Res. **39:**385, 1960.

Nuckolls, J., Dienstein, B., Bell, D. G., and Rule, R. W., Jr.: The periodontal lesion, J. Periodontol. **21:**7, 1950.

Oliver, R. C., Holm-Pedersen, P., and Löe, H.: The correlation between clinical scoring, exudate measurements and microscopic evaluation of inflammation of gingiva, J Periodontol. **40:**201, 1969.

Orban, B.: Oral histology and embryology, ed. 5, St. Louis, 1962, The C. V. Mosby Co. (Quoting Wasserman, F.)

Orban, B.: Clinical and histologic study of the surface characteristics of the gingiva, Oral Surg. **1:**827, 1948.

Orban, B.: Histopathology of periodontal disease, Am. J. Orthod. **33:**637, 1947.

Orban, B.: Diffuse atrophy of the alveolar bone (periodontosis), J. Periodontol. **13:**31, 1942.

Orban, B., and Mueller, E.: The gingival crevice, J. Am. Dent. Assoc. **16:**1206, 1929.

Orban, B., and Ray, H.: Deep necrotic foci and the gingiva, J. Periodontol. **19:**91, 1948.

Orban, B., and Weinmann, J. P.: Diffuse atrophy of the alveolar bone (periodontosis), J. Periodontol. **13:**31, 1942.

Orban, J. E., and Stallard, R. E.: Gingival crevicular fluid: a reliable predictor of gingival health, J. Periodontol. **40:**43, 1969.

Owings, J. R.: A clinical investigation between stippling and surface keratinization of the attached gingiva, J. Periodontol. **40:**30, 1969.

Page, R. C., and Schroeder, H. E.: Pathogenesis of inflammatory periodontal disease. A summary of current work, Lab. Invest. **33:**235, 1976.

Payne, W. A., Page, R. C., Ogilvie, A. L., et al.: Histopathologic features of the initial and early stages of experimental gingivitis in man, J. Periodont. Res. **10:**51, 1975.

Pevillie, P. E., Nolan, J. P., and Fuch, S. C.: Studies of the resistance to infection in diabetes mellitus; local exudative cellular response, J. Lab. Clin. Med. **59:**1008, 1962.

Quintarelli, G.: Histochemistry of the gingiva. IV. Preliminary investigations on the mucopolysaccharides of connective tissue, Arch. Oral Biol. **2:**277, 1960.

Ramfjord, S.: Local factors in periodontal disease, J. Am. Dent. Assoc. **44:**647, 1952a.

Ramfjord, S.: Tuberculosis and periodontal disease with special references to collagen fibers, J. Dent. Res. **31:**5, 1952b.

Reichborn-Kjennerud, I.: Dento-alveolar resorption in periodontal disorders. In Sognnaes, R. F., editor: Mechanisms of hard tissue destruction, Washington, D.C., 1963, American Academy of the Advancement of Science.

Robertson, P. B., Grupe, H. E., Jr., Taylor, R. E., Shyu, K. W., and Fullmer, H. M.: The effect of collagenase-inhibitor complexes on collagenolytic activity of normal and inflamed gingival tissue, J. Oral Pathol. **2:**28, 1973.

Roper, R., Knerr, G. W., Gocka, E. F., and Stahl, S. S.: Periodontal disease in aged individuals, J. Periodontol. **43:**304, 1972.

Schoenfeld, S. E.: Demonstration of an alloimonune response to embryonic enamel matrix proteins, J. Dent. Res. **54:**72, 1975.

Schroeder, H. E.: Quantitative parameters of early human gingival inflammation, Arch. Oral Biol. **15:**383, 1970.

Schroeder, H. H., and Listgarten, M. A.: Fine structure of the developing epithelial attachment of human teeth, Basel, 1971, S. Karger.

Schultz-Haudt, S. D.: Anatomy and physiology of the periodontal structures. In Ramfjord, S., Kerr, D., and Ash, M., editors: Proceedings of the World Workshop in Periodontics, Ann Arbor, 1966, University of Michigan Press.

Schultz-Haudt, S. D., and Aas, E.: Dynamics of periodontal tissues. II. The connective tissues, Odont. Tskr. **70:**397, 1962.

Schultz-Haudt, S. D., and From, S.: Dynamics of periodontal tissues. I. The epithelium, Odont. Tskr. **69:**431, 1961.

Seltzer, S., Bender, I. B., and Ziontz, M.: The interrelationship of pulp and periodontal disease, Oral Surg. **16:**1474, 1963.

Selvig, K. A.: Biologic changes at the tooth-saliva interface in periodontal disease, J. Dent. Res. **48:**846, 1969.

Selvig, K. A.: Nonbanded fibrils of collagenous nature in human periodontal connective tissue, J. Periodont. Res. **3:**169, 1968.

Selvig, K. A.: Ultrastructural changes in periodontal membrane and cementum in periodontal disease, J. Periodont. Res. **1:**75, 1967.

Selvig, K. A., and Zander, H. A.: Chemical analysis and microradiography of cementum and dentine from periodontally diseased human teeth, J. Periodontol. **33:**303, 1962.

Shaffer, E. M.: Biopsy studies of necrotizing ulcerative gingivitis, J. Periodontol. **24:**22, 1953.

Sheridan, R. C., Jr., Cheraskin, E., Flynn, F. H., and Hutto, A. C.: Epidemiology of diabetes mellitus. I. Review of the dental literature, J. Periodontol. **30:**242, 1959.

Sherp, H. W.: Discussion of bacterial factors in periodontal disease, J. Dent. Res. **41:**327, 1962.

Shimamine, F.: Das sekendare Zement, Z. Stomat. **8:**28, 1910.

Shklar, G., Cohen, M. M., and Yergenian, G.: Histopathologic study of periodontal disease in the Chinese hamster with hereditary diabetes, J. Periodontol. **33:**14, 1962.

Sicher, H.: Ueber Pulpaerkrankungen als Folge von Paradentose, Z. Stomat. **34:**819, 1936.

Sillness, J.: Periodontal conditions in patients treated with dental bridges. II. The influence of full and partial crowns on plaque accumulation development of gingivitis and pocket formation, J. Periodont. Res. **5:**219, 1970.

Simon, J. H. S., Glick, D. H., and Frank, A. L.: The relationship of endodontic-periodontic lesions, J. Periodontol. **43:**202, 1972.

Simpson, D. M., and Avery, B. E.: Histopathologic and ultrastructural features of inflamed gingiva in the baboon, J. Periodontol. **45:**500, 1974.

Simring, M., and Goldberg, M.: The pulpal pocket approach, retrograde periodontitis, J. Periodontol. **35:**22, 1964.

Skillen, W. G.: Normal anatomic and physiologic gingiva and its relation to pathologic processes, J. Am. Dent. Assoc. **18:**600, 1931.

Skillen, W. G.: Normal characteristics of the gingiva and their relation to pathology, J. Am. Dent. Assoc. **17:**1088, 1930.

Slavkin, H. C., and Boyde, A.: Cementum: an epithelial secretory product? J. Dent. Res. **53:**157, 1974.

Snyderman, R.: Immunomechanisms of periodontal destruction, J. Am. Dent. Assoc. **87:**1020, 1973.

Soames, J. V., and Davies, R. M.: The structure of subgingival plaque in a beagle dog, J. Periodont. Res. **9:**333, 1974.

Soames, J. V., Entwisle, D. N., and Davies, R. M.: The progression of gingivitis to periodontitis in the beagle dog: a histologic and morphometric investigation, J. Periodontol. **47:**435, 1975.

Socransky, S. S.: Relationship of bacteria to the etiology of periodontal disease, J. Dent. Res. **49:**203, 1970.

Stahl, S. S.: The nature of healthy and diseased root surfaces, J. Periodontol. **46:**156, 1975.

Stahl, S. S.: The responses of the periodontium to combined gingival inflammation and occluso-functional stresses in four human surgical specimens, Periodontics **6:**14, 1968.

Stahl, S. S.: The effect of hepatic injury on gingival healing in rats, Oral Surg. **19:**188, 1965.

Stahl, S. S.: Influence of antibiotics on the healing of gingival wounds in rats. I. Reattachment potential of soft and calcified tissues, J. Periodontol. **34:**166, 1963a.

Stahl, S. S.: Pulpal response to gingival injury in adult rats, Oral Surg. **16:**1116, 1963b.

Stahl, S. S., Joly, O., and Goldsmith, E. D.: Adaptation of periodontal tissue to combined insults, Dent. Prog. **1:**51, 1961.

Stahl, S. S., Sandler, H. C., and Suben, E.: Histochemical changes in inflammatory periodontal disease, J. Periodontol. **29:**183, 1958.

Stahl, S. S., and Slavkin, H. C.: Development of gingival crevicular epithelium and periodontal disease. In Slavkin, H. C., and Bavetta, L. A., editors: Developmental aspects of oral biology, New York, 1972, Academic Press.

Stahl, S. S., Tonna, E. A., and Weiss, R.: Autoradiographic evaluation of gingival response to injury. V. Surgical trauma in low-protein-fed mature rats, J. Dent. Res. **49:**537, 1970.

Stahl, S. S., Witkin, G. J., DiCeasare, A., and Brown, R.: Gingival healing. I. Description of the gingivectomy sample, J. Periodontol. **39:**106, 1968.

Stahl, S. S., Witkin, G., and Scopp, I. W.: Degenerative vascular changes observed in selected gingival specimens, Oral Surg. **15:**1495, 1962.

Stanley, H. R.: The cyclic phenomenon of periodontitis, Oral Surg. **8**:598, 1955.

Swenson, O., and Claff, L. C.: Changes in the hydrogen ion concentration of healing fractures, Proc. Soc. Exp. Biol. Med. **61**:151, 1946.

Taichman, N. S.: Some perspectives on the pathogenesis of periodontal disease. J. Periodontol., **45**(II):361, 1974.

Theilade, J.: An evaluation of the reliability of radiographs in the measurement of bone loss in periodontal disease, J. Periodontol. **31**:143, 1960.

Thilander, H.: Epithelial changes in gingivitis, J. Periodont. Res. **3**:303, 1968.

Thilander, H.: Effect of leucocytic enzyme activity on the structure of the gingival pocket epithelium in man, Acta Odontol. Scand. **21**:431, 1963.

Thoma, K. H., and Goldman, H. M.: Wandering and elongation of the teeth and pocket formation in parodontosis, J. Am. Dent. Assoc. **27**:335, 1940.

Thoma, K. H., and Goldman, H. M.: Correlation of clinical and pathologic phases of parodontal diseases, Dent. Items Interest **61**:103, 212, 309, 452, 1939a.

Thoma, K. H., and Goldman, H. M.: The pathology of dental cementum, J. Am. Dent. Assoc. **26**:1943, 1939b.

Thoma, K. H., and Goldman, H. M.: Types of resorption of alveolar bone found in parodontal disease, Am. J. Orthod. **24**:62, 1938.

Thoma, K. H., and Goldman, H. M.: Classification and histopathology of parodontal disease, J. Am. Dent. Assoc. **24**:1915, 1937.

Thonard, J. C., and Sherp, H. W.: Histochemical demonstrations of acid mucopolysaccharides in human gingival intercellular spaces, Arch. Oral Biol. **7**:125, 1962.

Toller, J. R.: Studies of the epithelial attachment on young dogs, Northwestern Univ. Bull. **11**:13, 1940.

Toto, P. D., Pollock, R. J., and Gargiulo, A. W.: Pathogenesis of periodontitis, Periodontics **2**:197, 1964.

Turesky, S. S., and Glickman, I.: Histochemical distribution of experimental animals on adequate and vitamin C deficient diets, J. Dent. Res. **33**:273, 1954.

Waerhaug, J.: Subgingival plaque and loss of attachment in periodontoses as observed in autopsy material, J. Periodontal. **47**:636, 1976.

Waerhaug, J.: Presence or absence of plaque on subgingival restoration, Scand. J. Dent. Res. **83**:193, 1975.

Waerhaug, J.: Microscopic demonstrations of tissue reaction incident to removal of subgingival calculus, J. Periodontol. **26**:26, 1955.

Waerhaug, J.: Gingival pocket; anatomy, pathology, deepening, and elimination, Odont. Tskr. **60**:Supp., 1952.

Waerhaug, J., and Steen, E.: Presence or absence of bacteria in gingival pockets and the reaction in healthy pockets to certain pure cultures, Odont. Tskr. **60**:1, 1952.

Wassermann, F.: In Bhaskar, S., editor: Orban's oral histology and embryology, ed. 8, St. Louis, 1976, The C. V. Mosby Co.

Weinmann, J.: Progress of gingival inflammation into the supporting structures of the teeth, J. Periodontol. **12**:71, 1941.

Weinstein, E., and Mandel, I. D.: The fluid of the gingival sulcus, Periodontics **2**:147, 1964.

Weinstein, E., Mandel, I. D., Salkind, A., Oshrain, H. I., and Pappas, G. P.: Studies in gingival fluid, Periodontics **5**:161, 1967.

Weski, O.: Chronic marginal inflammation of the alveolar process, with special regard to alveolar pyorrhea, Vschr. Zahnheilk. **37**:1, 1921.

Wilkinson, F. C.: A patho-histological study of the tissue tooth attachment, Aust. J. Dent. **55**:105, 1935.

Williams, C. H. M.: Rationalization of periodontal pocket therapy, J. Periodontol. **14**:66, 1943.

Zander, H. A.: Attachment of calculus to root surfaces, J. Periodontol. **24**:16, 1953.

Zander, H. A., and Hürzeler, B.: Continuous cementum apposition, J. Dent. Res. **37**:1035, 1958.

8 Acute necrotizing ulcerative gingivitis

Clinical signs and symptoms
Prevalence
Role of bacteria
Communicability
Possible predisposing factors
Treatment

Acute necrotizing ulcerative gingivitis (ANUG) is a distinct, recurrable, periodontal disease, the etiology of which is complex and about which not all factors are understood. It is readily differentiated clinically from marginal gingivitis or periodontitis and responds to therapy.

CLINICAL SIGNS AND SYMPTOMS

The two most significant criteria used in the diagnosis of ANUG are (1) interproximal necrosis and ulceration and (2) history of soreness and bleeding resulting from pressure on the involved area by eating or toothbrushing. The extent and degree of involvement may vary considerably, affecting only a single isolated papilla or practically all the papillae and marginal gingivae throughout the dentition. The different degrees of papillary destruction that are possible in the lower anterior region may be seen clearly in Fig. 8-1, *A*. The adherent grayish slough represents the so-called pseudomembrane, and its presence is indicative of the acute phase of the disease. The typical truncated papillae may be seen in Fig. 8-1, *B*. An example of widespread papillary and marginal gingival necrosis is evident in Fig. 8-1, *C*, whereas in Fig. 8-1, *D*, the destructive process in the lower anterior region has progressed apically, destroying the attached gingiva and partially exposing the root of one of the incisors.

Other clinical signs or symptoms said to be associated with this disease include lymphadenopathy, a characteristic fetor oris, fever, and malaise. Submaxillary lymphadenopathy may be noted in the more advanced cases. Similarly the degree of fetor oris present may be correlated with the amount of destruction present and the state of oral hygiene extant during the period prior to examination. However, it should be noted that some mild cases exhibit no obvious fetor oris. Furthermore the practice of diagnosing ANUG because of a so-called characteristic fetor oris should be condemned, since other oral diseases may manifest a very similar odor.

Perhaps the most confusing and controversial diagnostic criteria are those of fever and malaise. Wilson has stated that there may be an elevation of temperature to 103° F. and that general malaise is common. On the other hand, Stammers maintains that the highest temperature recorded in his study of over 1,000 cases was only 100.1° F. and that in the most severe case seen the temperature was only 98.8° F. Grupe and Wilder have reported that the occurrence of fever is unusual and when present is rarely elevated more than 1° F. above normal. Similar observations have been made in an unpublished article by Goldhaber, who studied 47 acute cases of ANUG in the U.S. Army and found that the oral temperature ranged from 97.4° to 99.7° F., with an average and median temperature of 98.5° and 98.6° F., respectively. In other words, there was just as great a chance of a slight *decrease* in temperature as there was of a slight increase. One of the severest cases observed in this latter series was a Vincent's angina. The patient, despite extensive necrosis of the gingivae and tonsil (Fig. 8-1, *E*), exhibited a temperature rise of only 1° F. Subsequent examinations of numerous civilian patients with ANUG have supported the contention that a moderate to high elevation of temperature is *not* a symptom of this disease and that generalized malaise is rare. It should be stressed that except for their oral discomfiture, patients with ANUG are for the most part in good physical condition.

Contrariwise, the presence of a significantly elevated temperature (102° F. or higher) and generalized malaise should immediately suggest the presence of some disease other than ANUG. Most

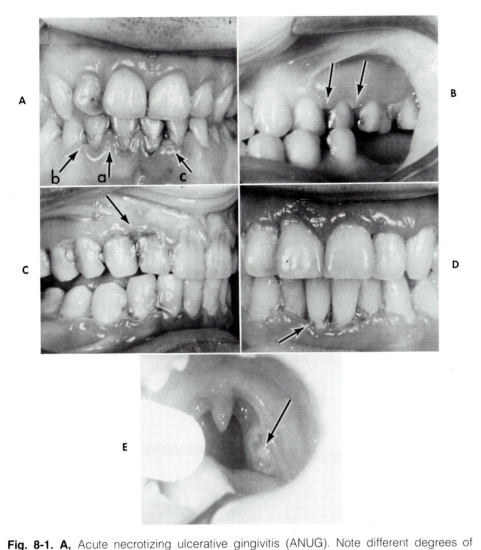

Fig. 8-1. A, Acute necrotizing ulcerative gingivitis (ANUG). Note different degrees of necrosis and ulceration in lower incisor area, demonstrating necrosis of tip, *a,* necrosis and ulceration of one half of a papilla, *b,* and necrosis and ulceration of an entire papilla, *c.* Adherent grayish slough represents so-called pseudomembrane, and its presence is a good indicator of acute phase of disease. **B,** Acute necrotizing ulcerative gingivitis demonstrating "truncated papillae" *(arrows).* **C,** Acute necrotizing ulcerative gingivitis demonstrating widespread papillary and marginal gingival necrosis and ulceration *(arrows).* Note spontaneous bleeding in upper lateral incisor-cuspid area *(arrow).* **D,** Acute necrotizing ulcerative gingivitis demonstrating apical progression of necrosis in lower anterior region that has destroyed attached gingivae and partially exposed root of lower right central incisor *(arrow).* **E,** Vincent's angina, demonstrating a necrotic and ulcerated tonsil *(arrow)* in addition to gingival destruction. (From Goldhaber, P., and Giddon, D. B.: Int. Dent. J. **14:**468, 1964.)

frequently these two symptoms are part of a syndrome related to acute primary herpetic gingivostomatitis (APHG), a viral disease that may be accompanied by bleeding and tender gingivae, marked fetor oris, and lymphadenopathy. Other differentiating features of APHG include the presence of filled or ruptured mucosal vesicles as well as the fact that gingival papillae and margins are not necrotic or ulcerated as in ANUG. Although it is possible to have both diseases simultaneously, there is no need to complicate the problem of diagnosis and nomenclature further by classifying the combination of these two diseases, complex necrotizing gingivitis as opposed to pure simplex necrotizing gingivitis, as has been suggested by Grupe and Wilder.

PREVALENCE

Since acute necrotizing ulcerative gingivitis occurs primarily in young adults between the ages of 18 and 30 years, it is not surprising that most studies of ANUG have involved populations of young men who are serving in the Armed Forces or are in college. Grupe and Wilder have found that 2.2% of 870 U.S. Army inductees had ANUG, whereas Pindborg has reported a prevalence of 4.4% in 8,177 newly conscripted soldiers and sailors in the Danish Armed Forces. Giddon et al. examined 326 entering college freshmen and found that eight (2.5%) had ANUG while four others had histories compatible with ANUG prior to entering college. Follow-up questionnaires indicated that an additional ten students developed ANUG during the following year, making a total of 22 (6.7%) of the entering students with the disease prior to entering college, at the time of entrance, or during their freshman year. It would have been of interest to determine how many additional members of the same class developed ANUG during the remaining 3 years of their college careers. No data are available along this line, but it seems reasonable to assume that approximately 10% of the class would have experienced ANUG by that time and that an even higher percentage would be affected by the age of 30 years.

Although ANUG rarely if ever develops in otherwise healthy children in the western part of the world, Pindborg et al. report that necrotizing gingivitis occurs with surprising frequency (2.4%) among children in South India, and Emslie has found a high frequency of cancrum oris in Nigerian children. He concludes that this condition is an extension of ANUG, which also occurs commonly in these children. Although it has not been possible to correlate these findings with protein malnutrition, it is likely that other factors are operating in these children to make them susceptible to necrotizing gingivitis and cancrum oris.

In a recent study of records of over 800 children and adults residing in a hospital for the mentally retarded for up to 10 years, Brown found that 35% of patients with Down's syndrome (53 of 149) had experienced one or more episodes of necrotizing ulcerative gingivitis as compared with 4% for the other patients (27 of 657).The mean age at the time of the first episode was between 9 and 10 years of age for each group, with some cases occurring as early as 2 to 4 years of age in the Down's syndrome group. Although the diet was considered nutritionally satisfactory it was thought that the lowered resistance to infection in Down's syndrome might be related to the metabolic abnormalities associated with this condition.

ROLE OF BACTERIA

The fact that the acute signs and symptoms of ANUG respond dramatically to penicillin or broad-spectrum antibodies leaves little doubt that bacteria are involved in the production of these signs and symptoms. However, it is not clear whether the bacteria actually *initiate* the disease or are merely secondary invaders. As pointed out by Rosebury and Sonnenwirth fusospirochetal disease always appears to be superimposed on tissue damage induced by other agents, including nutritional disturbances, agranulocytosis, radiation injury, or viral infections. In addition Burnett and Scherp state that overgrowth of a particular bacterial species indigenous to an area does not necessarily indicate responsibility for that disease.

According to Rosebury et al. most investigations concerning the pathogenicity and transmissibility of the so-called fusospirochetal complex have utilized as an experimental model the subcutaneous injection into the guinea pig groin of various oral organisms, singly or in combination. It was found by Macdonald et al. (1956) that the typical experimental fusospirochetal lesion could be produced by a combination of four organisms—two *Bacteroides,* a motile gram-negative anaerobe, and a facultative diphtheroid. Paradoxically none of these was a spirochete or a fusiform bacillus. Further work with this group of organisms by Macdonald et al., writing in 1960 and 1963, has indicated that the primary pathogen is *Bacteroides melaninogenicus,* which produces a collagenolytic enzyme capable of attacking native gingival collagen. However, Hampp and Mergenhagen in 1961 insisted that neither the spirochetes nor the fusobacteria could unequivocally be dismissed as the etiologic agents of ulcerative oral lesions. This conclusion was based on findings by these investigators that localized infections terminating in abscess formation could be produced routinely, following intracutaneous inoculation into the rabbit or guinea pig of 6×10^7 cells of either of the small oral treponemes *Borrelia vincentii* or *Borrelia buccalis.* More recently these same investigators have produced intracutaneous abscesses in rabbits with pure strains of oral fusobacteria injected separately or in combination with strains of oral spirochetes. With regard to the findings of Macdonald et al. in 1956, indicating that spirochetes play no part in the natural and experimental disease in which they occur, Rosebury suggested in 1962 that these workers might have confused fusospirochetal disease with other similar but probably not identical mixed anaerobic infections.

Electron microscopic observations by Listgarten of affected interdental papillae from eight pa-tients with acute necrotizing ulcerative gingivitis revealed the presence of four zones containing spirochetes: (1) the bacterial zone, (2) the neu-trophil-rich zone, (3) the necrotic zone, and (4) the zone of spirochetal infiltration. Most of the microorganisms in the bacterial layer could not be identified, but spirochetes of various sizes could

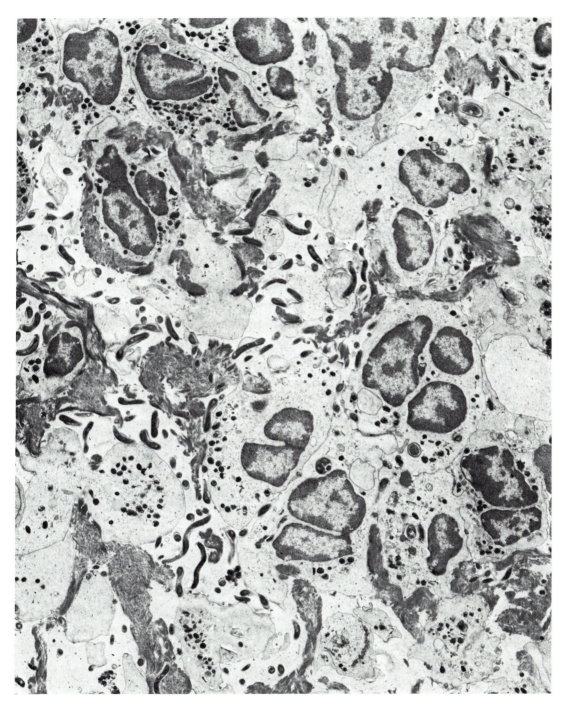

Fig. 8-2. Electron photomicrograph illustrating spirochetal infiltration beneath surface of ulcerated tissue.

be distinguished. Beneath this layer was the closely packed neutrophil layer, occasionally demonstrating phagocytosed bacteria and spirochetes within the neutrophils. The necrotic zone contained necrotic debris, large numbers of spirochetes, and leukocytes. The zone of spirochetal infiltration, about 250 μm beneath the surface of the ulcerated tissue, contained only spirochetes (of the large and intermediate variety), which were found in well-preserved tissues in advance of other bacteria and appeared morphologically different from cultivated strains of *Borrelia vincentii* (Figs. 8-2 and 8-3).

The presence of spirochetes in viable tissue in ANUG should be contrasted with other periodontal diseases wherein the bacteria remain on the

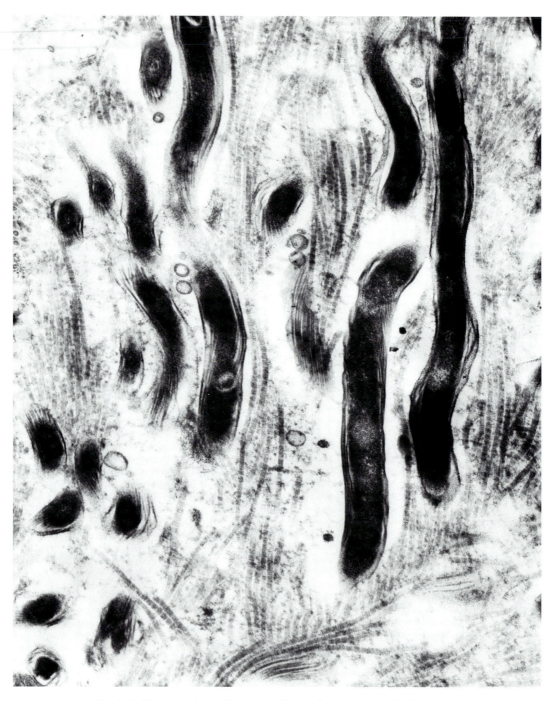

Fig. 8-3. Electron photomicrograph illustrating spirochetal infiltration.

surface of the inflamed tissues. As for the tissue necrosis, it could be brought about by the release of endotoxin from the masses of spirochetes and the subsequent activation of the complement system. Alternatively the spirochetes might provide the chemotactic stimuli necessary to attract the large numbers of neutrophils, which can function in the absence of oxygen to control bacterial proliferation and help clean up debris by releasing their granules, which contain proteases (including cathepsin and collagenase), carbohydrases, lipases, and other enzymes.

COMMUNICABILITY

Since World War II the consensus among clinicians concerning the communicability of ANUG has been that this disease represents an endogenous infection rather than a communicable one. Scattered reports of epidemics of ANUG (particularly in children) probably represent examples of misdiagnosis. Based on his study of over 1,000 cases of ANUG during World War II, Stammers concludes that there is a "most astonishing lack of evidence of the epidemic origin of the disease." The U.S. Army study by Schluger in 1949, in which normal contact by patients with known cases of ANUG failed to influence the development of new ANUG cases, also suggests that the disease is not transmitted by contact or by any of the usual means of transmission of infection. The pattern of distribution of cases in the Army study of Goldhaber similarly fails to support the idea of communicability of this disease. On the other hand, Pindborg in three articles written in 1951 and 1956 has indicated that he believes the disease is communicable, since there was an increased incidence of ANUG in Danish sailors and soldiers after they had finished their preliminary training. This conclusion appears unwarranted, however, since it is possible that the increased incidence was brought about by a change in various predisposing factors. As pointed out by Roseburg in 1938, the mere occurrence of outbreaks of ANUG within populations living under relatively uniform conditions is not sufficient evidence of contagion since other factors affecting the group may be responsible.

The finding by Courant et al. that there is no marked difference in the relative infectivity of bacterial debris (injected subcutaneously into experimental animals) from the normal gingival sulcus area, the periodontal pocket, or the areas of papillary necrosis associated with ANUG suggests that decreased host resistance rather than

increased bacterial virulence is responsible for the development of ANUG.

POSSIBLE PREDISPOSING FACTORS

Although numerous predisposing factors have been suggested for ANUG, there is little agreement as to which are most important primarily because many of the studies have not obtained adequate data along this line. Stammers considers that local predisposing causes, for example, gross neglect, food stagnation, calculus, overcrowding, mouth breathing, smoking, and recent extractions, are of paramount importance in the inception of the disease. Systemic factors such as frequent colds, possible vitamin deficiencies, recent illnesses, operations, pregnancy, overwork, and lack of exercise are considered merely contributory to the local factors. Stammers notes also that the increased prevalence of ANUG coincided with air raids over England in 1940 and 1941 and suggests that the chronically disturbed nights "were definitely responsible not only for lowered general vitality but also for great neglect of oral hygiene" and "very considerable increase in the smoking habit." The fusospirochetal infection, although primarily responsible for the ulceration, was considered of secondary importance. In his 1949 Army study Schluger stressed the role of *fatigue* and *local trauma* (severe beatings about the mouth). Apparently field conditions favored improper food rations, poor oral hygiene, and fatigue brought about by more strenuous work. The importance of *physical debility* and *lowered resistance* was suggested in view of the surprising finding that 7.5% of the cases occurred in patients who were hospitalized for long periods after operations, fractures, or other nonoral problems. Ten years later in a study of ANUG at Camp Chaffee, Ark., Goldhaber found no relationship between the onset of the disease and bivouac. However, of the 61 cases in the study, 21 occurred about the time that the patients entered the Army, and 22 occurred about the time that they went on leave, making a significant total of 43 cases (70%) related to these two periods.

Pindborg considers a *preexisting gingivitis* to be an important predisposing factor, since out of 91 new cases of ANUG, 87 developed from a preexisting, chronic, simple marginal gingivitis, whereas only 4 cases developed from a healthy gingiva. *Tobacco smoking* appears to be another predisposing factor, since only 1 out of 57 patients with ANUG was a nonsmoker as compared to the 12% nonsmokers found in the entire study. These findings with respect to tobacco smoking have been confirmed by Goldhaber, who found that out of 61 patients with ANUG all but 2 were smokers and 41% smoked more than one package of 20 cigarettes per day. In a control group of 185 routine dental patients, however, 25% were non-smokers, and only 5% smoked over one package of cigarettes per day. The percentage of non-smokers in the control group was approximately twice that of Pindborg's study (25% versus 12%). This finding may reflect a difference in the extent of smoking among young men in the United States as compared to those in Denmark. An earlier report of Ludwick and Massler states that 25% of almost 4,000 enlistees at the Great Lakes Naval Station were nonsmokers. Similarly, of the 20 mild ANUG cases in their study, only one patient was a nonsmoker. It should be noted that in Goldhaber's study the two ANUG patients who were nonsmokers had undergone recent extractions a few days prior to the onset of the disease, which appeared to spread from the extraction site. This finding supports the idea of Stammers in 1944 and Schluger in 1949 that local trauma may be an important predisposing or precipitating factor. Of further interest is the clinical impression that the severity of ANUG may be directly correlated with the amount of smoking. Relatively mild cases of ANUG tend to be associated with slight to moderate smoking, whereas severe cases of ANUG tend to be associated with heavy smoking.

The possible relationship of *emotional stress* and ANUG was first introduced into the dental literature by means of scattered case reports, including those of Miller and Firestone in 1947, Roth in 1951, Roth and Weiss in 1951, and Jones in 1951. The study by Moulton et al. in 1952 supports this concept and is particularly significant since the senior author was a psychiatrist. Although the ANUG group comprised only six cases, they stood out clearly from the chronic periodontitis and the periodontosis groups. The most outstanding feature of the ANUG group was the apparent precipitation of the infection "by acute anxiety arising from a life situation of conflict about dependency and/or sexual needs." Local factors and oral habits were found to be at a minimum. The relationship between emotional factors and ANUG is further substantiated by other investigators. Goldberg et al. have reported that 22 patients out of 54 who suffered from ANUG (or 40%) "volunteered some stressful incidents which might be related to the onset of the disease." However, no personality differences

between the ANUG patients and other periodontal disease patients could be determined by means of the Minnesota Personality Inventory and the Word Association Test.

Goldhaber reported in 1957 that a history of acute anxiety could be elicited from the great majority of ANUG patients. The emotional problem usually started 1 to 2 weeks prior to the onset of the disease. In most instances these problems came on about the time that the patient entered the Army or while he was on leave, which probably explains in part why 70% of the cases occurred during these two periods. Although the relationship between acute anxiety and the onset of ANUG is most striking, it should be noted that no attempt has been made to obtain similar histories from a control group of subjects. The study by Moulton et al., however, does include both a periodontitis and a periodontosis group, neither of which had histories of acute anxiety as did the ANUG patients.

A more recent observation by Giddon et al. in 1962 concerning ANUG in a university population, indicated that approximately three times as many students with ANUG as without it had sought psychiatric help; that is, a randomly selected group of dental patients made no greater utilization of the psychiatric services than did the university population as a whole. A subsequent study of college freshmen by Giddon et al. in 1964 revealed that those who by clinical examination or definitive history had developed ANUG by the end of their first year had a significantly higher proportion of withdrawals from school.

It would appear, therefore, that the most conspicuous predisposing factors in ANUG include tobacco smoking and gingivitis or local trauma in association with an acute psychologic disturbance that apparently precipitates the disease in susceptible individuals. As a working hypothesis it is assumed that under proper conditions these predisposing factors may contribute to a decreased general or local resistance, leading to proliferation of the fusospirochetal flora with necrosis and ulceration of the gingiva. The possible mechanisms of action of these predisposing factors have been discussed in detail by Goldhaber and Giddon.

TREATMENT

Although the introduction of this chapter implies that ANUG responds readily to proper and adequate treatment, there has been little agreement as to what constitutes proper and adequate treatment. This point is clearly demonstrated by Miller and Greene, who report that "literally over one hundred medicaments have been advocated."

Treatment of the acute phase of the disease usually consists of repeated gentle scalings and dilute hydrogen peroxide mouth rinses plus the establishment of good oral hygiene for mild to moderate cases. Where possible according to Schluger, deep, immediate, and thorough curettage may be effective. In more advanced cases, or where the response to scaling is slow, oral penicillin (1 million units daily for 4 days) may be used, provided that there is no previous history of sensitivity to the antibiotic. The most usual failing in the treatment of ANUG is the premature discontinuation of therapy after the acute symptoms have been alleviated. Although repeated curettage and the establishment of good oral physiotherapy may result in the regrowth of destroyed papillae, sur-

gical recontouring (gingivoplasty) of the interproximal craters should be carried out where the defect is marked or where papillary regrowth is delayed (Fig. 8-4). Recurrent attacks of ANUG tend to focus about such craters. Various investigators, including Manson and Rand, have noted the relation of recurrences of ANUG to the persisting gingival deformity and have emphasized the importance of eliminating all local predisposing factors.

Therapy of necrotizing ulcerating gingivitis has had just as checkered a career as has its etiology. Early workers warned against the use of curets and debriding instruments on the acute case, lest the infection be spread into the bloodstream and the deeper tissues. This has been found to be without foundation. Immediate subgingival curettage in the acute phase has only a salutary effect on the affected gingivae. This has been seen so many

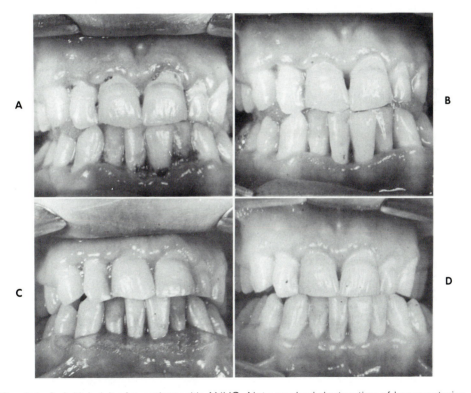

Fig. 8-4. A, Initial visit of a patient with ANUG. Note marked destruction of lower anterior gingiva and large amounts of calculus. Immediate deep scaling was carried out, and patient was put on hot saline rinses. **B,** Same patient 1 week later. Acute symptoms are gone, but note interproximal craters, particularly in lower anterior region. Further scaling was done, and patient was instructed in home care. **C,** Immediately after surgical recontouring (gingivoplasty) of lower anterior gingiva approximately 4 weeks after initial visit. **D,** One month after gingivoplasty. Note reestablishment of proper gingival contour in lower anterior region. Some recontouring of upper anteriors has occurred "naturally," but contour in this region is not satisfactory. (From Goldhaber, P., and Giddon, D. B.: Int. Dent. J. **14:**468, 1964.)

times that it has become a standard response. The more meticulous and complete the subgingival curettage, the more complete will be the response. The usual approach has been to perform some coronal scaling, attempting to avoid the gingival tissues. The exact reverse, however, is the most effective method. The subgingival debridement and curettage are carefully performed as completely as possible in the affected zones, although the coronal scaling is done with no specific attempt at completeness. Stain and fine residual supragingival deposits may be left for a later sitting.

The question frequently arises as to the possibility of performing subgingival curettage on gingivae that are painful and tender. Although this is a minor problem in management it is by no means the barrier to procedure that we have been led to believe it is. Clinical experience has shown that the careful use of curets, with a conscious effort toward minimizing tissue displacement, makes it possible to proceed with no difficulty. In addition it has been noted many times that, as the curettage proceeds, the pain if any becomes less and less acute with the progress of debridement, hemorrhagic lavage, and water flushings. Hot water rinses aid in overcoming the acute symptoms and should be recommended for home care. These should be done for about 10 minutes out of every hour for several hours.

The response to this therapy is dramatic. On the second visit the gingivae will be found to have been comfortable almost immediately after the completion of the first treatment. Also the violent

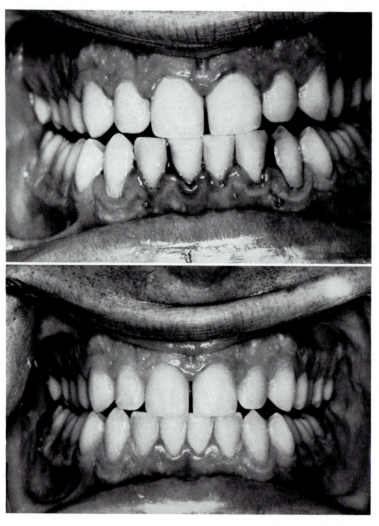

Fig. 8-5. Before and after initial therapy phase of a case of necrotizing ulcerative gingivitis. After photograph was taken 2 weeks later. Periodontal therapy should be continued to obtain gingival health and form.

hyperemia will have subsided. For the most part necrosis will no longer be evident, and on the whole the case assumes a different appearance entirely. Although complete remission of the acute phase usually requires supplementary curettings and home lavage, the gingival tissues are distinctly on the mend at this point (Figs. 8-5 to 8-7).

Further therapy consists of completing the curettage and supervising the home care of the

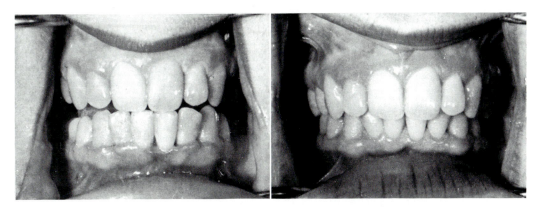

Fig. 8-6. Necrotizing ulcerative gingivitis before and after treatment. Gingivoplasty was performed.

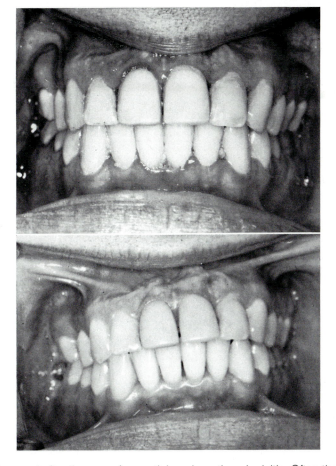

Fig. 8-7. Before and after therapy of necrotizing ulcerative gingivitis. Often there is a problem in therapy of this condition around restorative dentistry, margins of which are not exact. In this instance jacket crowns had overhanging margins; a potential recurrent flare-up can often be expected in such areas. A recommendation for replacement of these jacket crowns was made.

patient. Usually three to four sittings are ample to assure the operator that the episode has been terminated. It will be found that energetic and vigorous therapy carried out early enough will yield a minimum of disfigurement of the gingivae and will avoid crater formation with all its attendant problems. The gingivae will be found to have returned to their previous form and their previous texture.

Antibiotics. Considerable work has been done with the antibiotics, and these agents are widely used in therapy by many operators. Enough time has elapsed to evaluate properly their usefulness and the possible dangers in their use. As has been mentioned before, the response to penicillin, tetracycline, and allied drugs is immediate, although temporary, unless debridement and home physiotherapy are carried out. A case can be made for their use in acute fulminating cases in conjunction with local therapy, but the administration must be carried out with caution and close supervision. If, for example, it is decided to use penicillin, a careful history of previous reactions to this drug must be taken. If this is negative then the drug may be used, but in a standard manner, either by injection of the usual 300,000 unit suspension into the deltoid or gluteal muscles or by mouth in about five times the parenteral dose. Eight 200,000 unit tablets per day may be taken by mouth, in divided doses, for 2 or 3 days. Troches of penicillin should be avoided at all costs, since they constitute a very dangerous sensitizing mechanism.

Home care. The home care of the patient with ANUG consists of frequent flushings, particularly interproximally, with any warm nonirritating solution. A 50% dilution of the common 3% hydrogen peroxide is useful but not indispensable by any means. The use of oxidizing agents has been for the most part of little or no value. Of much more use is the effervescent property of hydrogen peroxide in contact with the tissues in interproximal flushings. However, ordinary warm tap water will serve very well. More important is the method of application. A single mouthful of solution forced between the teeth vigorously for a full minute is more valuable than tall tumblers of solution applied in a perfunctory manner. The patient is instructed in methods of gentle brushing with a soft nylon brush in addition to careful interdental cleansing with a soft balsa wood toothpick.

Regimen of therapy. The following regimen of therapy should be utilized to treat ANUG.

First visit
1. History and work-up
2. Supragingival scaling to remove gross deposits and debris blocking entry into the gingival sulci and craters
3. Careful subgingival curettage of the affected areas with frequent flushing with warm water
4. Instruction in home care: mouth rinses every hour with water or diluted hydrogen peroxide solution, gentle brushing with a soft nylon brush, careful interdental stimulation, and cleansing with balsa wood toothpicks
5. Proper antibiotic administration if it is deemed desirable

Second visit
1. Completion of history and work-up
2. Completion of coronal scaling
3. Reentry into the gingival sulci and craters to check on prior performance
4. Check on home care and test performance

Third visit
1. Polishing of teeth
2. Recuretting subgingivally
3. Instituting more vigorous brushing and interdental stimulation
4. Frequency of mouth rinses reduced

Fourth visit
1. Surveying the tissues for crater formation and setting up a treatment plan for correction if needed

This regimen is of course for the theoretical average case. The routine is merely an organizational aid. The number of visits and the frequency of instrumentation depend upon individual tissue response.

Evaluation of therapy. After the acute episode has been thoroughly and completely treated a careful evaluation of the gingival tissues must be made. If treatment has been sought early enough and if it has been prompt and thorough the chances are that no deformities in the gingivae will result. If delay or repeated exacerbations have been the case, then some crater formation will probably result. There is no hard and fast rule in this direction. *In any event any residual scarring, interproximal craters, or deviation from normal form must be corrected.* To allow these deformities to exist is to invite eventual breakdown of the supporting tissues, with serious consequences to the survival of the dentition. These deformities have often been referred to in the past as chronic necrotizing ulcerative gingivitis, since they are characterized by frequent acute exacerbations. We can no longer support the view that this is a different form of the acute attack. It is merely the sequel of it. The fact that these areas break down again merely labels them as recurrent acute cases. This is obvious since the architectural aberrations invite local breakdown if other factors operate.

The methods for the correction of these deformities will be discussed in Chapter 27.

Despite the most heroic efforts recurrences occur in some cases. It is best to warn the patient during the first or second visit that recurrent acute episodes may take place during the course of treatment or within 6 months to a year following cessation of treatment, particularly if the craters have not been eliminated and the home care instructions have been ignored.

REFERENCES

Brown, R. H.: Necrotizing ulcerative gingivitis in mongoloid and non-mongoloid retarded individuals, J. Periodont. Res. **8:**290, 1973.

Burnett, G. W., and Scherp, H. W.: Oral microbiology and infectious disease, Baltimore, 1962, The Williams & Wilkins Company.

Courant, P. R., Paunio, I., and Gibbons, R. J.: Infectivity and hyaluronidase activity of debris from healthy and diseased gingiva, Arch. Oral Biol. **10:**119, 1965.

Emslie, R. D.: Cancrum oris, Dent. Pract. Dent. Rec. **13:**481, 1963.

Giddon, D. B., Goldhaber, P., and Dunning, J. M.: Prevalence of reported cases of acute necrotizing ulcerative gingivitis in a university population, Abstract no. 40, I.A.D.R. Program and abstract of papers, 1962.

Giddon, D. B., Zackin, S. J., and Goldhaber, P.: Acute necrotizing ulcerative gingivitis in college students, J. Am. Dent. Assoc. **68:**381, 1964.

Goldberg, H., Ambinder, W. J., Cooper, I., and Abrams, A. L.: Emotional status of patients with acute gingivitis, N.Y. Dent. J. **22:**308, 1956.

Goldhaber, P.: A study of acute necrotizing ulcerative gingivitis, Abstract no. 35, I.A.D.R. Program and abstract of papers, 1957.

Goldhaber, P., and Giddon, D. B.: Present concepts concerning the etiology and treatment of acute necrotizing ulcerative gingivitis, Int. Dent. J. **14:**468, 1964.

Goldman, H. M.: Report of the histopathologic study of the jaws of a diet-deficient monkey and its relation to Vincent's infection, Am. J. Orthod. **29:**480, 1943.

Grupe, H. E., and Wilder, L. S.: Observations of necrotizing gingivitis in 870 military trainees, J. Periodontol. **27:**255, 1956.

Hampp, E. G., and Mergenhagen, S. E.: Experimental intracutaneous fusobacterial and fusospirochetal infections, J. Infect. Dis. **112:**84, 1963.

Hampp, E. G., and Mergenhagen, S. E.: Experimental infections with oral spirochetes, J. Infect. Dis. **109:**43, 1961.

Hirsch, J. G.: Neutrophil leukocytes. In Zweifach, B. W., Grant, L., and McCluskey, R. T., editors: The inflammatory process, vol. 1, New York, 1974, Academic Press, Inc.

Jones, H. S.: Emotional stress and gingivitis, Oral Hyg. **41:**657, 1951.

Kelstrup, J., and Theilade, E.: Microbes and periodontal disease, J. Clin. Periodontol. **1:**15, 1974.

Kraal, J. H., and Kenney, E. B.: Polymorphonuclear leukocyte chemotaxis in the absence of oxygen, J. Periodont. Res. **10:**288, 1975.

Lindhe, J., and Helldén, L.: Neutrophil chemotactic activity elaborated by human dental plaque, J. Periodont. Res. **7:**297, 1972.

Listgarten, M. A.: Electron microscopic observations on the bacterial flora of acute necrotizing ulcerative gingivitis, J. Periodontol. **36:**328, 1965.

Listgarten, M. A., and Socransky, S. S.: Ultrastructural characteristics of a spirochete in the lesion of acute necrotizing ulcerative gingivostomatitis (Vincent's infection), Arch. Oral Biol. **9:**95, 1964.

Ludwick, W., and Massler, M.: Relation of dental caries experience and gingivitis to cigarette smoking in males 17-21 years old (at the Great Lakes Naval Training Center), J. Dent. Res. **31:**319, 1952.

Macdonald, J. B., Gibbons, R. J., and Socransky, S. S.: Bacterial mechanisms in periodontal disease, Ann. N.Y. Acad. Sci. **85:**467, 1960.

Macdonald, J. B., Socransky, S. S., and Gibbons, R. J.: Aspects of the pathogenesis of mixed anaerobic infections of mucous membranes, J. Dent. Res. **42:**529, 1963.

Macdonald, J. B., Sutton, P. M., Knoll, M. L., Madlener, E. M., and Grainger, R. M.: Pathogenic components of an experimental fusospirochetal infection, J. Infect. Dis. **98:**15, 1956.

Mackler, B. F.: Plaque dialysate effects on human lymphocyte blastogenesis and inflammatory responses, Arch. Oral Biol. **20:**423, 1975.

Manson, J. D., and Rand, H.: Recurrent Vincent's disease: a survey of 61 cases, Br. Dent. J. **110:**386, 1961.

Mergenhagen, S. E., and Scherp, H. W.: Comparative immunology of the oral cavity, DHEW pub. no. (NIH) 73-438, Bethesda, Md., 1973, U.S. Government Printing Office.

Miller, S. C., and Firestone, J. M.: Psychosomatic factors in periodontal disease, Am. J. Orthod. **33:**675, 1947.

Miller, S. C., and Greene, H. I.: A world-wide survey of acute necrotizing ulcerative gingivitis: a preliminary report, J. Dent. Med. **13:**66, 1958.

Moulton, R., Ewen, S., and Thieman, W.: Emotional factors in periodontal disease, Oral Surg. **5:**833, 1952.

Pindborg, J. J.: The epidemiology of ulceromembranous gingivitis showing the influence of service in the Armed Forces, Parodontologie **10:**114, 1956.

Pindborg, J. J.: Gingivitis in military personnel with special reference to ulceromembranous gingivitis, Odontol. Tidskr. **59:**407, 1951.

Pindborg, J. J.: Influence of service in Armed Forces on incidence of gingivitis, J. Am. Dent. Assoc. **42:**517, 1951.

Pindborg, J. J., Bhat, M., Devanath, K. R., Narayana, H. R., and Ramachandra, S.: Occurrence of acute necrotizing gingivitis in South Indian children, J. Periodontol. **37:**14, 1966.

Robertson, P. B., Cobb, C. M., Taylor, R. E., and Fullmer, H.: Activation of latent collagenase by microbial plaque, J. Periodont. Res. **9:**81, 1974.

Rosebury, T.: Microorganisms indigenous to man, New York, 1962, McGraw-Hill Book Company.

Rosebury, T.: The etiology of Vincent's infection. In Gordon, S. N., editor: Dental science and dental art, Philadelphia, 1938, Lea & Febiger.

Rosebury, T., Clark, A. R., Engel, S. G., and Tergis, F.: Studies of fusospirochetal infection. I. Pathogenicity for guinea pigs of individual and combined cultures of spirochetes and other anaerobic bacteria derived from the human mouth, J. Infect. Dis. **87:**217, 1950.

Rosebury, T., Clark, A. R., Macdonald, J. B., and O'Connell,

D. C.: Studies of fusospirochetal infection. III. Further studies of a guinea pig passage strain of fusospirochetal infection, including the infectivity of sterile exudate filtrates, of mixed cultures through ten transfers, and of recombined pure cultures, J. Infect. Dis. **87:**234, 1950.

Rosebury, T., Clark, A. R., Tergis, F., and Engel, S. G.: Studies of fusospirochetal infection. II. Analysis and attempted quantitative recombination of the flora of fusospirochetal infection after repeated guinea pig passage, J. Infect. Dis. **87:**226, 1950.

Rosebury, T., and Sonnenwirth, A. C.: Bacteria indigenous to man. In Dubos, R. J., editor: Bacterial and mycotic infection of man, Philadelphia, 1958, J. B. Lippincott Co.

Roth, H.: Psychosomatic and nutritional factors related to recurrent necrotizing ulcerative gingivitis, J. Am. Dent. Assoc. **42:**474, 1951.

Roth, H., and Weiss, M.: Recurrent acute necrotizing ulcerative gingivitis, N.Y. Dent. J. **17:**89, 1951.

Schluger, S.: Necrotizing ulcerative gingivitis in the Army; incidence, communicability and treatment, J. Am. Dent. Assoc. **38:**174, 1949.

Snyderman, R.: The role of the immune response in the development of periodontal disease, Int. Dent. J. **23:**310, 1973.

Stammers, A. F.: Vincent's infection; observations and conclusions regarding the aetiology and treatment of 1,017 civilian cases, Br. Dent. J. **76:**147, 171, 205, 1944.

Wilson, J. R. Etiology and diagnosis of bacterial gingivitis including Vincent's disease, J. Am. Dent. Assoc. **44:**671, 1952.

9 Lesions of the attachment apparatus

One of the important manifestations included in the group of lesions termed "periodontal diseases" is that which is produced by changes of function on the tooth. To have a more complete understanding of this manifestation it is best to review the biology of the tooth-supporting mechanism.

CHANGES OF FUNCTION: PHYSIOLOGIC EFFECT

The periodontal tissue reaction to variations in stress via the tooth has been described in numerous reports in the literature. *Yet there is no clear understanding as to how the supporting tissues sustain the effects of the physiologic stress placed on the teeth during mastication, speech, and so on.* The connecting link between tooth and alveolar bone is the periodontal ligament. For many years the thought has been that this connection transmits stress placed on the tooth to the bone, where it is finally assimilated into the supporting bone. Investigations have suggested, however, that the periodontal ligament alone is perhaps not sufficiently oriented for this function and that it does serve as a retention mechanism but only partially as a sustaining one. If this is true, then it becomes necessary for force placed on the tooth to be transmitted into the supporting tissues via another approach.

Turning to the rodent incisor, where there is constant eruption of the tooth, one seemingly can visualize an intermediate plexus. Yet the tooth can withstand a great deal of pressure. One notes also in examining the supporting tissues of this tooth that there is a well-organized arrangement of blood vessels in the bone side of the periodontal ligament. It might be assumed that force placed on the tooth is assimilated in great measure by the milking effect on these blood vessels. Also there is a great deal of fluid in the periodontal ligament space, and the exchange level between fluid in this space and the adjacent marrow spaces can serve as a balancing reservoir for the transmission of force from the tooth to the supporting bone. Thus during physiologic function, when force is placed on the tooth, the periodontal ligament serves passively, allowing for the fluid exchange and the milking of the blood vessels to assimilate the stress. More research is necessary to illustrate and identify the fluid and the exchange mechanism.

Picton has reported that force to a tooth causes compression and tension in the periodontal ligament. Transducers of movement were used to detect the direction and amount of displacement of the alveolar margins of 15 teeth in two adult monkeys. Controlled horizontal and intrusive thrusts were applied manually. Bone displacement started in response to forces less than 100 g and occurred in a linear manner with forces up to 1 kg. Horizontal forces of more than about 50 g tended to cause the labial and lingual alveolar plates to be displaced in the same direction as the applied force. The distance that the bone was displaced and subsequently recoiled was less than the displacement and recoil of the root in the linear phase of movement. This was interpreted by Picton as an increasing tissue compression on the side to which the tooth was moved and a decreasing pressure in the ligament on the other side, with elastic deformation of the socket. Intrusive force resulted in dilatation of the socket. Thus the ligament as a compressive membrane with bone displacement may be considered the mechanism whereby force is dissipated when placed on a tooth.

Function is an important influence. The bony cortex and trabeculae are formed along engineering principles to meet mechanical requirements and to resist the forces brought to bear upon them. Therefore a projecting bone like the mandible, which has to transmit the force, is of an entirely different architectural construction from the completely supported maxilla, although they both have the same purpose, that is, to invest and support the teeth.

Functional stimuli are transmitted through the attachment apparatus to the alveolar and supporting bone, which reacts according to the type, intensity, and duration of the stimulus. Normal function results in a well-arranged structural pattern of the periodontal ligament. The alveolar bone itself is thin and compact and is adjacent to the periodontal ligament. A latticework of cancellous bone connects and reinforces the individual alveoli.

This arrangement may be disrupted for various reasons. Any change of function will result in a change in architecture. If function is greatly decreased over a long period of time, as around teeth having lost their antagonists, the supporting cancellous bone of the alveolar process undergoes atrophy of disuse. Thus one may find only the thin alveolar wall proper, and this may be broken and less compact than normal. The supporting bone may be entirely missing so that only fatty marrow is present. The periodontal ligament is thin and consists principally of indifferent fibers, most of the principal fibers having been lost (Fig. 9-1).

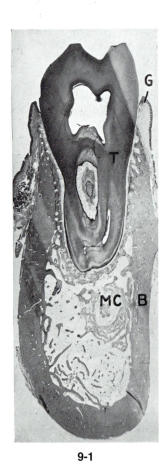

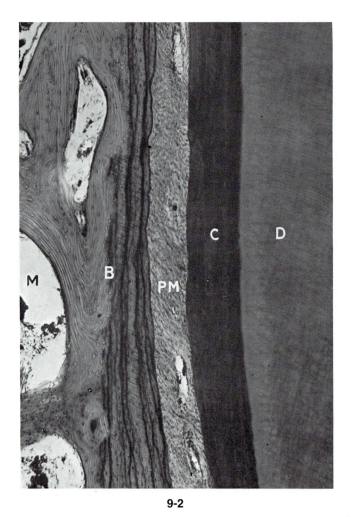

9-1   9-2

Fig. 9-1. Adaptation to heavy function in mandibular first molar (buccolingual section). *T,* Tooth; *B,* bone; *G,* gingiva; *MC,* mandibular canal.

Fig. 9-2. Strong principal fibers of periodontal ligament in heavy function. *PM,* Periodontal ligament; *B,* bone; *C,* cementum; *D,* dentin; *M,* marrow.

On the other hand, an increase in function may result in an adjustment of the periodontium in such a manner that it will withstand the increased stress without damage. Histologically there is a strong periodontal ligament, with a reinforcement of the supporting bone. Similarly, whenever a tooth tips or drifts, owing to missing adjacent teeth, the normal arrangement of the supporting bone changes so as to be able to accommodate the change in the direction of the stress (Fig. 9-2).

Hypofunction

Atrophic changes are quantitative rather than qualitative in nature and are caused by diminished function of a part or by senile or presenile alterations. These alterations can come about by a lack of function of the jaws and indirectly by a lack of function of the teeth or by the loss of antagonists to the teeth. Also lack of jaw function may be the result of malformations (for example, open bite).

In the dental apparatus the root of the tooth is connected to the alveolar bone by the periodontal ligament, the Sharpey's fibers of which are embedded in the cementum and in the bone. Mastication expresses itself in force placed on the tooth and is dissipated in the supporting structures. By this means the attachment apparatus remains in health. When function ceases or is diminished, changes occur in the periodontal ligament and supporting bone. The principal fibers are either less in number or in some instances entirely disappear (when the tooth is entirely nonfunctional), and the supporting bone undergoes atrophic changes. Kronfeld has shown that teeth which evidence changes of atrophy of disuse have a thinner periodontal ligament than normal. The marrow spaces are enlarged, and the bone trabeculae become fewer in number and are smaller in size (Fig. 9-3).

In the instances of hypofunction due to loss of antagonists the continuous eruptive force of teeth is accelerated so that extrusion of the teeth occurs. It has been noticed that maxillary molars extrude more quickly than other teeth although they all move occlusally once the opposing occlusal force is removed. This tendency for continuous eruption usually increases the length of the clinical crown, and in the molars often the bifurcation of the teeth becomes exposed. Thus in cases of missing teeth many patterns of derangement can be seen, depending on the location and number of teeth that are lost, their position in the arch, and the type of occlusion present (Fig. 9-4).

Changes due to hypofunction are generally complex; for example, if the mandibular first and second molars are lost there is a gradual change in the position of the maxillary first molar and possibly of the second molar, depending on whether this tooth becomes locked by the mandibular third molar that tilts mesially. Once the maxillary first molar extrudes a change in contact occurs between it and the second premolar and possibly the second molar (Fig. 9-5). Food impaction occurs, and a gingivitis and subsequently a marginal periodontitis result. Also, when a part is afunctional, the necessary stimulation to the part is not present. It has been noticed that gingival inflammations are prone to occur, especially in areas where plaque tends to collect and the patient does not cleanse the area by brushing.

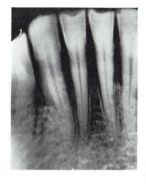

Fig. 9-3. Interdental translucencies between lower incisors associated with diminished use.

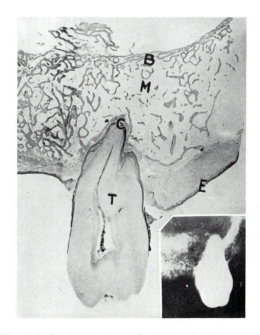

Fig. 9-4. Diminished use. Tooth has lost its antagonist, and disappearance of supporting bone is evident. *T*, Tooth; *E*, epithelium; *B*, bone; *M*, marrow; *C*, cementum.

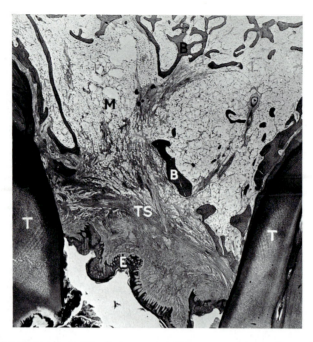

Fig. 9-5. Diminished use in section between maxillary second premolar and second molar. Supporting trabeculae have disappeared, and fatty marrow can be seen. *T,* Tooth; *TS,* transseptal fibers; *B,* bone; *M,* marrow; *E,* epithelium.

On the other hand, cases of open bite in which the anterior teeth do not occlude in any position do not necessarily behave in the foregoing fashion. In these instances stimulation is derived from lip and tongue action, since no occlusal force can be produced. A tongue thrust habit is usually found. These teeth do not tend to extrude, and there is no change in the relationship of clinical crown and root. Microscopic examination discloses that the periodontal ligament consists of only a moderate amount of principal fibers and that the supporting bone is architecturally so arranged and composed of few and small trabeculae. The marrow spaces are large in size and fatty in nature. These changes are variable depending on the functional aspects present. The enlarged marrow spaces are seen roentgenographically and constitute one of the most important methods of diagnosing atrophy of disuse in the periodontium. There is a tendency for gingival inflammations in these cases if the lip and tongue action is not sufficient to cleanse the teeth. Also, because of the positioning of the teeth, plaque accumulates and with food accumulation at the gingival margins, especially on the labial aspects, gingival inflammation is seen.

Microscopic findings. All functional stimuli exerted on a tooth are transmitted to the periodontium as a whole, and the tissues are so adapted to assimilate these stimuli. This adaptation is in re-

ality a reaction to the environment, and if the stimuli should change, the tissues will alter in response to functional demands. In atrophy of disuse, clinical and microscopic examination reveals structural changes in the attachment apparatus and the supporting bone.

Changes in the attachment apparatus in atrophy of disuse center on the change in the periodontal ligament, with varying amounts of principal fiber groups present, depending on the degree of stimulation exerted on the part. Associated with this the periodontal ligament space is thinner. The alveolar bone housing loses its thick cortical appearance, and there are many gaps because of loss of bone. Where the alveolar bone is lost, in many instances the periodontal attachment apparatus is replaced by fatty tissue of the adjacent marrow space that has opened. These findings are especially evident in embedded teeth, where no functional stimuli are possible (Fig. 9-6).

Usually the cementum of nonfunctioning teeth is thicker than that of functioning teeth in the same jaw. Teeth without antagonists have a tendency to move occlusally. This holds true for embedded teeth that also tend to move in the jaw. Such movement tends to cause a widening of the periodontal ligament space, especially at the apex and in the interradicular area of multirooted teeth. To react against this widening, cementum is deposited so

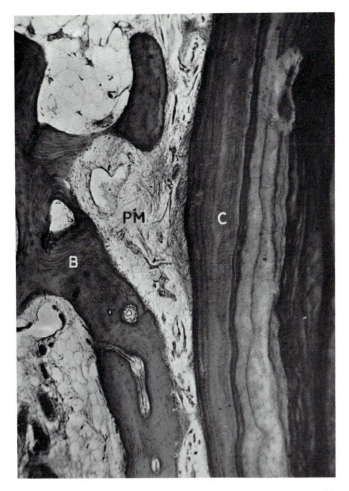

Fig. 9-6. Periodontal ligament of a tooth without function. Loss of principal fibers is evident. Periodontal ligament is composed of indifferent connective tissue. *B,* Bone; *PM,* periodontal ligament; *C,* cementum.

that the periodontal ligament space tends to be of physiologic width. The cementum is deposited evenly on the root surface.

A major change in atrophy of disuse is found in the supporting bone. In some instances the trabeculae of bone comprising the supporting mechanism for the cortical bone of the alveolus disappear. This of course is dependent on the degree of stimulation received. The marrow spaces become larger or even open completely with but few trabeculae evident. The tooth becomes contiguous with the adjacent teeth, and the marrow in many areas has no cortical bone of the alveolar plate remaining. Inspecting the illustrations of atrophy of disuse shows the varying patterns that the remaining trabeculae assume.

It is of importance that the reader be able to correlate these microscopic findings to the roentgenographic signs. Large areas of translucency, with loss of lamina dura integrity or thickness, and the clinical findings are diagnostic signs.

Hyperfunction

At the opposite end of the physiologic range from hypofunction is hyperfunction. In this entity the periodontium adapts itself to heavy forces applied to the teeth. These changes manifest themselves in the attachment apparatus and affect the cementum, periodontal ligament, and alveolar process. Occasionally spike formations of cementum are found on the root surfaces of some teeth on both the apical and the coronal portions. The spikes consist of outgrowths along the principal fibers of the periodontal ligament and are due to heavy function, as demonstrated by Gottlieb in the case of an elderly man who used to carry a heavy pipe hanging on the two lower incisors. But such overburdening is not necessary for the spikes to

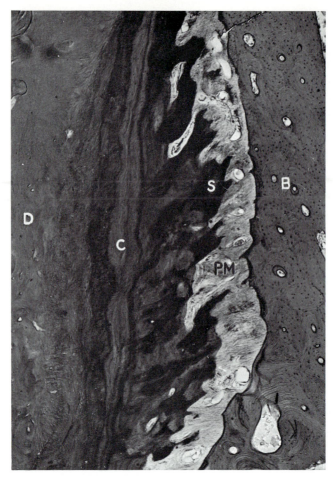

Fig. 9-7. Spike formation. *D,* Dentin; *C,* cementum; *S,* spike; *PM,* periodontal ligament; *B,* bone.

form, for they are found in many cases in which the teeth are involved in heavy occlusal function only. It is impossible to diagnose spike formation clinically, nor can it be ascertained by roentgenographic examination. Necropsy material, however, gives an opportunity for extensive study of this subject. It demonstrates that spike formation, although not common, is frequent in cases of hyperfunction. That it is not constantly encountered under such conditions is due to different reactions to hyperfunction. It can be demonstrated that when stress becomes very great the principal fibers of the periodontal ligament increase in number to give a better attachment to the tooth, and these fibers are found running from the cementum to the alveolar bone. Later, cementum may form along the principal fibers, giving the appearance of a spike (Fig. 9-7).

The periodontal ligament about a tooth in hyperfunction is thicker than normal. Measurements have shown that this dimension may increase to three times normal width. The principal fibers are well defined and on microscopic observation demonstrate the characteristic pattern of the various fiber bundles.

Deposition of the trabeculae of supporting bone is seen in the marrow spaces of teeth under heavy function. Just as the supporting bone is resorbed and not replaced about teeth with hypofunction, so are they actively deposited as a result of the stimulation of heavy forces. The roentgenographic appearance exhibits a fine trabecular pattern, with reduced radiolucent spaces in the supporting bone under heavy function. The roentgenograph plays an important role in diagnosing hypofunction as well as hyperfunction.

OCCLUSAL TRAUMATISM (PARAFUNCTION): PATHOLOGIC EFFECT

The importance of occlusal trauma as an etiologic factor in periodontal disease cannot be overemphasized, and an understanding of its mechanism in producing tissue damage is essential. These changes may be found around a single tooth, or they may be present throughout the jaws; however, in these latter instances the severity will vary. Occlusal traumatism (periodontal traumatism) may be defined as the tissue injury caused by occlusal forces.

At rest position the teeth are apart, and no force is applied to them. During mastication the forces applied to the teeth are relatively small, as has been shown by Manly and Braley. Also the small time element of mastication and the fact that teeth may touch but a minimum during mastication cannot account for the production of traumatism. Therefore occlusal trauma can result only if the teeth are occluded at times other than during chewing. Habits of clenching, bruxism, and so on are agents in producing the traumatic force. The stress generated by these habits is relatively great and sustained and exceeds the adaptive capacity of the attachment apparatus.

Although it is generally agreed that occlusal force against the teeth in its dynamic sense can produce damage to the periodontal tissues, another type of force is not usually recognized. This is the force of the musculature of the lips and cheeks against the teeth as well as the force of the tongue from within the oral cavity. Breitner has brought out this point most clearly. If balance between these forces is not present, damage may result.

The supporting structures of the teeth are subjected not only to influences due to changes in local environment but also to influences of general metabolic conditions, hereditary factors, and conditions generally expressed as systemic factors. As in any other disease process or injury the injuries of the periodontium are combated by the healing process of the individual. Thus as in a wound elsewhere in the body, when there is an interreaction between injury and repair, inflammation and repair are considered to be the same process. The injuries due to occlusal trauma are constantly being repaired. If the injury consists of a single occurrence, then repair will probably be complete, although dependent on the reparative ability of the individual. However, occlusal trauma is a repeated injury, the frequency of which, while variable, is great, since occlusal traumatism is the result of percussions of an afunctional nature (habits of clenching, bruxism, and so on).

It should be kept in mind that the recognizable lesions of occlusal traumatism are the result of the magnitude, severity, and frequency of the applied force *modified by* the repair ability of the host (Figs. 9-8 to 9-10).

We must view occlusal trauma not by the extent of the force being placed on a tooth but by its frequency and the repair process of the individual. If the frequency and the repair ability are satisfactory, an adaptive process will occur that produces changes in the periodontium, enabling it to withstand the forces applied to the teeth. If conditions are not satisfactory, destructive changes in the periodontium are encountered.

Occlusal trauma may be primary in nature, resulting from the factors discussed previously, or it may be secondary in nature, since any tooth that has lost a portion of its supporting tissues is subjected to greater stresses that require these tissues to adapt themselves to the altered relationship. The factors discussed previously still hold true as to whether a destructive lesion will result.

Habits detrimental to periodontal health are common findings when one is taking the dental history of a patient. The importance of suspecting and of determining the presence of a habit may be a deciding factor in the therapy of a case of periodontal breakdown. Each patient must be questioned carefully, since in many instances the habit is an unconscious act. Even if no positive information is gained at the first history taking the patient should be questioned at a later time. Often patients become aware of a habit once they are informed of the possibility that a habit may be operating to the detriment of the health of the periodontium. Although clamping and grinding may be described generally, and although there are certain groups and types of habits, it must be remembered that actually such habits are as multiple and varied as are the individuals who indulge in them.

Forceable clenching of the teeth places tremendous pressure on them, which in turn is transferred to the attachment apparatus. This constant pressure may cause necrosis of the periodontal ligament and other sequelae. Patients may often be aware of this habit, and if it is practiced at night, it may awaken them. The masseter muscle may show evidence of soreness, and the teeth may feel numb and "wooden" when percussed. The patient continues the habit unaware of the damage that it inflicts.

Histopathologic changes

The importance of a knowledge of tissue changes occurring in occlusal traumatism cannot be overemphasized. *If a tooth is subjected to an increased stress of injurious quality that is repetitious in nature, the periodontal tissues may show*

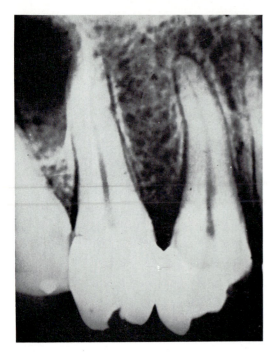

Fig. 9-8. Changes observed in occlusal traumatism, that is, widening of periodontal ligament space and changes in lamina dura. Clinically teeth were mobile.

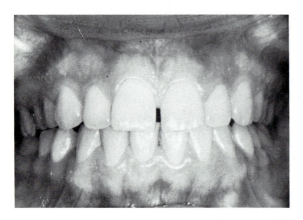

Fig. 9-9. Periodontal traumatism in a young patient. Note that gingival tissue is healthy throughout. Examination revealed intact attachments. Distinct mobility of teeth was present.

evidence of a state of damage, the extent of which is dependent on the reparative ability of the tissue of the individual. The microscopic picture varies with the tissue element, the more recent injuries presenting features without any element of repair. Roentgenographic and histologic correlation of the occlusal traumatic lesion aids the dentist not only in detecting the disturbances caused by occlusal trauma but also in its therapy.

Pressure atrophy is commonly the result of prolonged or continuous pressure upon a local area or group of cells. Pressure apparently affects cells by interfering with their vascular and lymphatic supply, thus preventing proper nutriment from reaching and being absorbed by the cells. This type of change is seen in occlusal traumatism in which a stress of sufficient intensity and duration is placed under heavy pressure. Should an area of the periodontal ligament be subjected to sufficient pressure so as to interfere with cell metabolism completely, tissue death, or necrosis, may result. This is termed "ischemic necrosis."

In studying human autopsy material one finds evidence of occlusal traumatism much more often than might be supposed. It may manifest itself in the following ways: tooth abrasion, cemental tears, fracture of teeth, resorption of the root, injuries to the periodontal ligament, and resorption of alveolar bone.

A frequently observed lesion is the cemental tear—a partial or complete detachment of small portions of the cementum of the tooth. Such lesions are repaired, with the tooth surface being covered by new layers of cementum. Often cemental fragments previously torn away from the tooth become incorporated as layers of new cementum are produced. Root resorption, as the result of occlusal traumatism, can often be detected roentgenographically and histologically. Small areas of cemental and sometimes dentinal resorption are frequent occurrences. In fact when one examines extracted teeth or autopsy material, re-

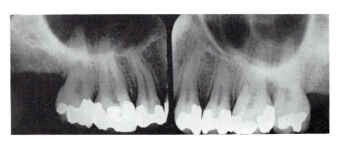

Fig. 9-10. Characteristic signs of occlusal traumatism in attachment of patient in Fig. 9-9. Note widening of periodontal ligament, fraying of lamina dura, and resorption of alveolar housing.

sorptive and reparative areas are extremely common. Fresh injuries in the periodontal ligament and those in the process of repair are also found. Hemorrhage, thrombosis of blood vessels, necrosis, and hyalinization of the connective tissue of the periodontal ligament have been demonstrated. The mechanism of loss of bone tissue as the result of occlusal traumatism has been described in numerous presentations. Minute to large resorptive areas on the bony wall of the alveolus in which osteoclasts may be seen are found. Repair of these defects is constantly encountered.

Abrasion. Tooth abrasion may come either from physiologic wear or from abrasion due to friction. It varies in different persons, since habits and diet play a large role. Abrasion, however, is increased in bruxism owing to grinding of the teeth. In cases of closed bite, abrasion may be marked; often the supporting structure is not affected. However, study of autopsy material reveals that these teeth frequently show evidence of root resorptions and cemental tears.

Cemental tears. Fragments of cementum may tear off, owing to an acute occlusal blow or from intermittent episodes of sustained pressure. These are called "cemental tears." If the fragments are torn away completely, the tears are complete; otherwise they are incomplete. Bauer is one of the first to have shown fracture of a sliver of cementum from an adult tooth, and Coolidge has described a section of an incisor tooth with a cemental tear. These tears are not uncommon and are seen in cases in which many teeth have been lost. Small areas of cementum tear away probably because the attachment of the cementum to the periodontal ligament is stronger than the union at the dentinocemental junction. Often these spicules wander away from the teeth. The defect caused by the tearing away of the cementum is repaired by the ingrowth of connective tissue (Fig. 9-11).

Damage to the periodontal ligament by lateral compression has been recognized, and the changes in the attachment apparatus have been described. Changes in the tension side are generally charac-

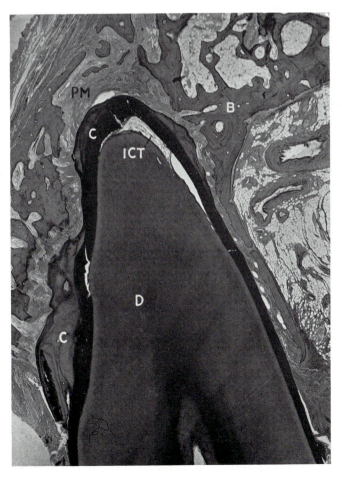

Fig. 9-11. Incomplete cemental tear. *B,* Bone; *PM,* periodontal ligament; *C,* cementum; *ICT,* incomplete cemental tear; *D,* dentin.

terized by apposition of bone; however, damage on this side has also been noted. In areas of tension, cemental tears can occur when the pull of the fibers of the periodontal ligament incorporated in the cementum is stronger than the cementoenamel junction. On the side of pressure these tears cannot take place.

Fig. 9-12 shows a section cut in a labial palatal plane. Two cemental tears can be seen. Repair has already begun.

Tooth repair may be accomplished either by lamellar cementum or by osteocementum, or both. The cervical portion of the tooth may be repaired by either type, whereas in the apical portion osteocementum is more commonly found. Injury to the cementum of the roots is common. It may result when an increased force is placed on the tooth, causing resorption. This resorption is usually repaired by the activity of the cementoblasts in that vicinity, the laying down of new cementum on the original structure. As this repair goes on, new Sharpey's fibers are embedded (Fig. 9-12).

Fracture. Another injury that is repaired by cementum is fracture of the root of a tooth due to

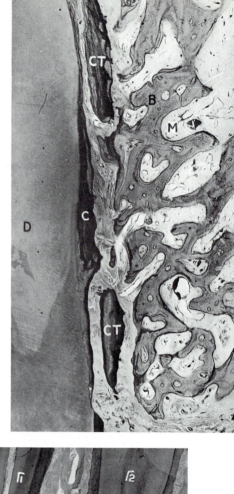

Fig. 9-12. Cemental tears. *D*, Dentin; *C*, cementum; *CT*, cemental tear; *B*, bone; *M*, marrow.

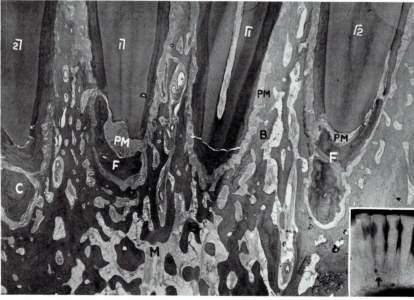

Fig. 9-13. Apical and periapical region of four incisors that were affected by abnormal occlusal trauma. Central incisors show fracture of roots. Lower right lateral incisor presents a fractured end that is not found attached to root in any serial section. Lower left lateral incisor has a complete and an incomplete cemental tear. Repair of these tears has begun, connective tissue from periodontal ligament has invaded tear, and ostocementum is being laid down. *B*, Bone; *M*, marrow; *F*, fracture; *PM*, repaired periodontal ligament; *C*, cementum.

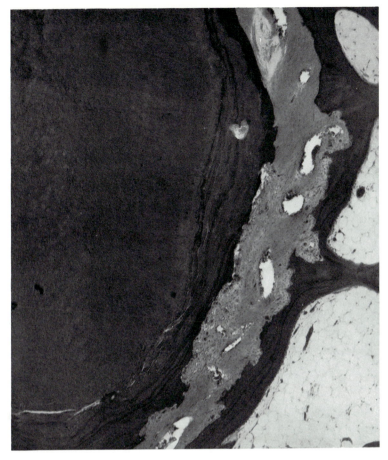

Fig. 9-14. Resorption of tooth and alveolar bone (apex of tooth). Numerous osteoclasts are evident.

occlusal trauma. Fig. 9-13 shows a roentgenogram and a photomicrograph of the mandibular central and lateral incisors in which all four roots have been fractured at the tips from occlusal trauma. The apical fragments have been surrounded by cementum as have the ends of the roots.

Root resorption. Resorption of the tooth root may be found in cases of occlusal trauma. In such cases the surface shows indentations, and large osteoclasts situated in baylike lacunae sometimes extend through the cementum into the dentin (Fig. 9-14).

The tooth, however, resists resorption much more than bone, and when it is forced against the bone, relief is generally brought about by resorption of the bone rather than by resorption of the tooth. Marshall has pointed out that there is a relationship between blood supply and resorption of the tooth, just as there is between blood supply and resorption of the bone. When hyperemia is produced in the periodontal ligament by pressure on the roots, resorptive processes result.

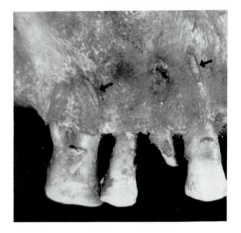

Fig. 9-15. Maxillary right posterior area (human material). Mesiobuccal root of first molar and cuspid root have penetrated alveolus on buccal side. These root fenestrations (*arrows*) are covered by alveolar mucosa. They are commonly observed in occlusal traumatism in necropsy material.

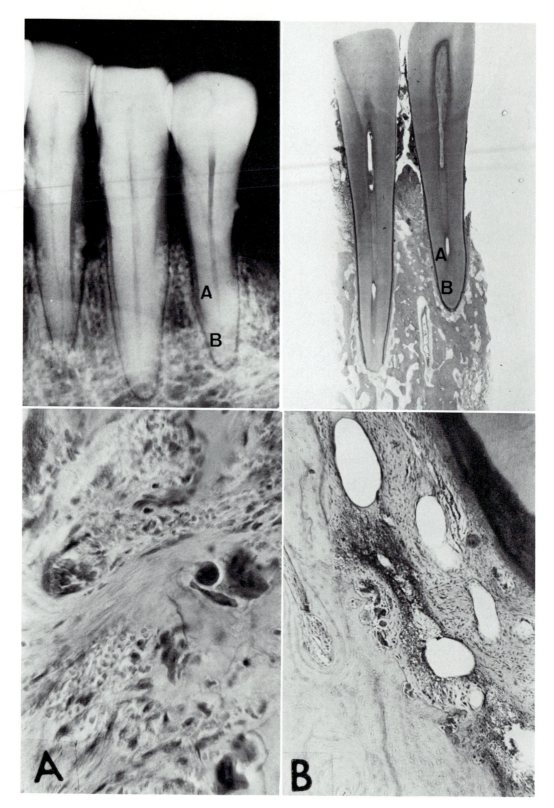

Fig. 9-16. Radiograph and photomicrographs illustrating changes in periodontal ligament histologically. Widening of periodontal ligament (*A* and *B*) is radiographically diagnostic of occlusal trauma. Upper right photomicrograph can be used to orient higher power photomicrographs, **A** and **B. A,** Osteoclasts can be seen in Howship's lacunae. **B,** Hemorrhage in periodontal ligament can be seen. Frontal resorption of bone is also prominent.

Extracted teeth often show records of resorption that has been repaired by apposition of new cementum laid down in the resorptive area. The cementoblasts deposit the matrix around the connective tissue fibers, and as the cementum is laid down, Sharpey's fibers are embedded. This effects reattachment of the tooth (Fig. 9-15).

Injuries to periodontal ligament. Manifestations of occlusal traumatism in the periodontal ligament consist of hemorrhage, thrombosis, and necrosis. Hyalinization of the connective tissue of the periodontal ligament and even cartilage formation have also been noted. Microscopic examination may show minute hemorrhages in the periodontal ligament as well as degeneration of the injured tissue. Necrosis of the small foci of cells may be seen. In more acute trauma the apical fibers of the periodontal ligament may be more severely injured, causing tissue necrosis and finally resorption of the alveolar bone. Coolidge has shown that in long continued trauma of the periodontal ligament degeneration in the form of hyalinization of the fibers may occur. If we remember that stress on the tooth has the effect of a two-armed lever, it is easy to see that the greatest damage occurs at places where there is the greatest pressure. Thus at these areas the periodontal ligament is seen to undergo hemorrhage and even necrosis as well as

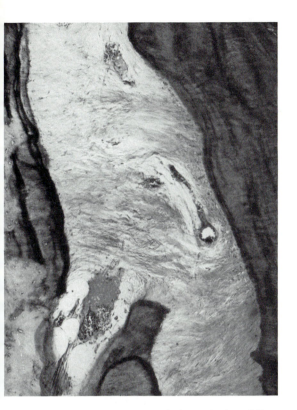

Fig. 9-17. Thrombotic vessels in periodontal ligament.

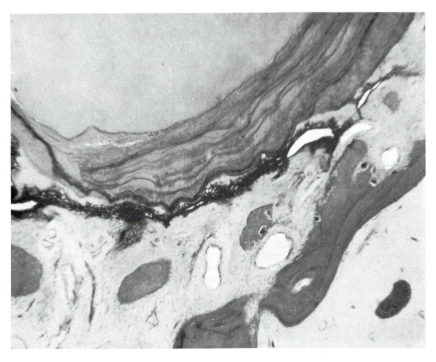

Fig. 9-18. Necrotic area of periodontal ligament in periodontal traumatism. Note active resorption of bone.

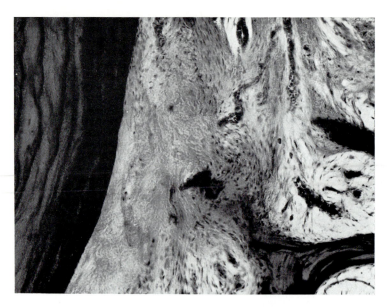

Fig. 9-19. Hyaline degeneration of periodontal ligament.

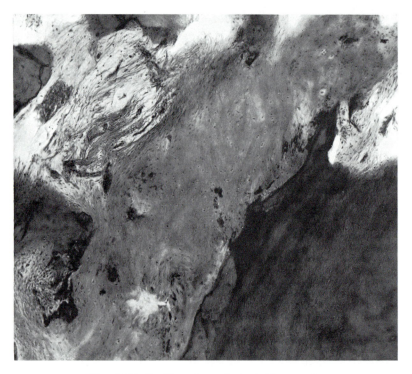

Fig. 9-20. Cartilage in periodontal ligament.

bone resorption. At the opposite area bone building is evident.

Kronfeld has described the traumatic injury to the periodontal tissues in cases of excessive stress, especially in the lateral direction, as a compression and crushing of the soft tissues between the tooth and bone and resorption of the bone and perhaps of the root. These lesions, he points out, have a tendency to be repaired when the stress subsides. If the trauma persists or if the tissue resistance is unusually low, the tooth becomes loosened. Thus the periodontal ligament in such teeth can be completely crushed between the root surface and the bone and transformed into a structureless hemorrhagic mass (Fig. 9-16).

Cartilage may be found in the periodontal liga-

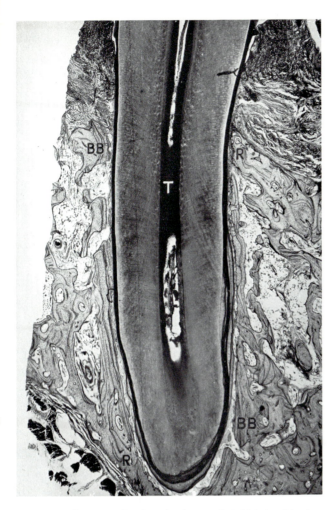

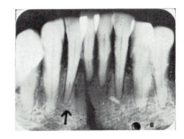

Fig. 9-21. Changes in alveolar bone of right lateral incisor under abnormal occlusal stress. *T*, Tooth; *BB*, bundle bone; *R*, resorption.

Fig. 9-22. Roentgenogram of tooth *(arrow)* in Fig. 9-21.

ment in cases of occlusal trauma. In many instances the connective tissue between the tooth and the alveolar bone may be found to be replaced by cartilage. It is well known that cartilage forms where bone continually rubs against bone. This is seen when the ends of fractured bones repeatedly move against one another, and healing cannot occur. The same process occurs in the periodontal ligament, when the tooth, by pressure against the bone, destroys the ligament and continually exerts force against it. This is shown in Fig. 9-17.

Resorption of alveolar bone. Not only are the tooth and the periodontal ligament affected in occlusal traumatism, but the bone housing the tooth also is affected. Resorptive areas of varying size can be observed, and resorption of the bone occurs around the adjacent marrow spaces. In the early phase osteoclasts may be seen lining a nutritional channel. These widen out, causing openings into the adjacent marrow spaces, the bone margins of which show evidence of a resorptive process. The alveolar bone also becomes destroyed in selective sites. The former is termed "rear resorption"; the latter is termed "frontal resorption." Fig. 9-18 shows a darkened necrotic area in the periodontal ligament subjacent to the root apex. A resorptive process has already removed a portion of the alveolar bone, and at present active resorption can be seen on the right side of the photomicrograph. From these findings one can conclude that the pressure against the tooth must have been in an axial direction.

Vertical bone resorptive defects may be seen interdentally. These resorptive lesions can be described as V-like troughs where bone has been destroyed. The base of the gingival attachment (epithelial attachment) may or may not lie in the troughlike defect. These lesions may or may not be present adjacent to teeth with proximal contacting teeth. If teeth have good proximal contacts there can be no mesiodistal tilting. This defect may be explained by a buccolingual movement of the tooth. Since the root anatomy on the proximal aspect of a tooth usually shows a concavity, the bone housing is under pressure by any buccolingual movement. Thus the alveolar bone of the interdental septum can be affected by traumatic influences, for example, a grasping contact in the buccolingual direction (Figs. 9-19 and 9-20).

The effect of lateral pressure, causing a tilting of the tooth, can be seen in Fig. 9-21, which is a low-power photomicrograph of a mandibular lateral incisor. A roentgenogram of the same tooth is shown in Fig. 9-22. Examination reveals that the tooth is occluded on the incisal edge and rotated on its fulcrum. The alveolar crest on the upper right shows marked osteoclastic resorption,

whereas the alveolar crest on the upper left shows the building up of bone (bundle bone). In the apical region the left surface shows resorption, whereas the right surface shows bone being deposited.

Where does the fulcrum of the tooth lie? As seen in the previous illustrations it is somewhere between the apex and the middle of the root. This has already been shown by Johnson et al. in their experiments on young monkeys. The resorption of the alveolar bone in the apical region was found on the opposite side from that toward which the crown of the tooth was moving, proving that the apex moves in the direction opposite to that in which the crown moves.

Buccolingual stress may resorb the thin crests of the alveolar bone, and thus a lasting injury will result. This lowering of the height of the crest causes an increase in the size of the clinical crown, which results in an increased load on the support-

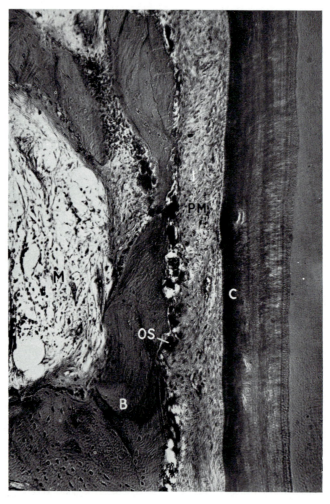

Fig. 9-23. Resorption of alveolar bone in periodontal traumatism. *B*, Bone; *OS*, osteoclast; *PM*, periodontal ligament; *C*, cementum. Note osteoclastic resorption of bone on marrow space side opposite *PM*.

ing tissues. If, however, the rate of apposition of bone is equal to the rate of resorption, the height of the alveolar bone is not lowered.

A common finding is the fenestration of the alveolar plate over the root surface. These defects are found on the buccal aspect where the alveolus is thin (Fig. 9-15).

The alveolar bone undergoes pressure resorption in the areas where force is exerted, unless the injury is of short duration, when the destroyed tis-

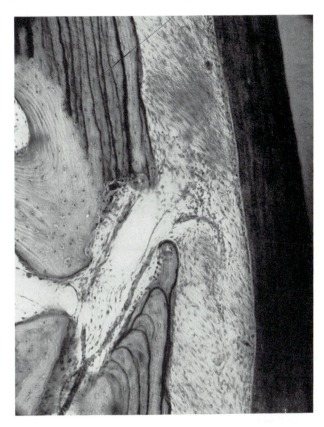

Fig. 9-24. Resorption of bone alongside vascular channel.

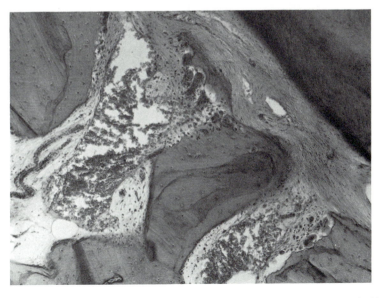

Fig. 9-25. Rear resorption. Note enlarged vessel and multinuclear osteoclasts in Howship's lacunae in marrow alongside bone.

sue will be repaired. Should the stress be intense and its occurrence often, damage will result, since the repair cannot keep up with the damage caused. The longer the time element, the more destruction may be expected. Thus the frequency of the injury is of most importance, but the reparative ability of the individual is also a vital factor. Therefore one finds many variables according to conditions; for example, in slight stress of relatively short duration and in young and healthy patients slight bone resorption may serve only to move the tooth in another position (Figs. 9-23 to 9-25).

On the other hand, a healthy individual who has a clenching habit may exert so much stress on the teeth so often that repair cannot keep pace with the destruction. In this individual severe lesions may be anticipated.

Relationship of pocket formation and occlusal trauma

An understanding of the relationship between pocket formation and occlusal trauma is important because there are two viewpoints expressed in the literature. One viewpoint states the idea that occlusal trauma causes pocket formation, whereas another states that the two processes are not related. Based on the study of animal and human jaws microscopically our belief is that pocket formation is not caused by occlusal trauma. In the study of pocket formation it is found that the epithelial attachment cannot proliferate apically without the destruction of the subjacent connective tissue fibers of the gingival fiber group. The occlusal traumatic lesion, on the other hand, is localized in the attachment apparatus and does not influence the gingival fiber apparatus. These findings are further substantiated by animal experimentation when stress is increased on a tooth or when orthodontic movement is performed.

A study was undertaken (Goldman, 1956) to determine the relationships of the blood supply of the gingiva in occlusal traumatism. The vascular system to the gingivae of the dog has disclosed that the major blood supply arises from vessels on the outer surface of the periosteum although there is a blood vessel route through the periodontal ligament running parallel to the tooth and alveolar housing extending into the gingiva. It was surmised that any gross involvement of the tooth could occlude these latter blood vessels and obliterate a portion of the vascular blood supply to the gingivae. To ascertain whether the gingival blood supply would be sufficient should the periodontal ligament supply to the gingiva be occluded, the following experiment was designed.

Silver crowns were fabricated so that they were in traumatic relationship, wedging the premolars laterally and lingually. They were cemented to the right and left mandibular first premolars. The crowns were left in place for 5 days, after which time 10% gelatin mercury mass was injected into the common carotid artery with the jaws tightly locked. After injection the animals were decapitated, and the heads were fixed in 40% formaldehyde for 1 week. Similar perfusion was performed with India ink. The jaws were removed, and block sections of the crowned teeth were cut. Roentgenograms and sections were made.

The findings showed that although the periodontal ligament on the lingual side was entirely obliterated, with complete occlusion of any possible blood supply, the blood supply of the marginal gingiva was sufficient. The India ink was shown to have perfused from the gingival blood vessels running on the outer surface of the periosteum. Fig. 9-26 illustrates the silver crown in position after cementation. Fig. 9-27, *A,* shows a low-power photomicrograph of the mandibular premolar seen in Fig. 9-26. The section was prepared in the buccolingual plane. The tooth can be seen moved lingually, obliterating the periodontal ligament, the tooth and alveolar bone being almost in contact (Fig. 9-27, *B*). The gingival blood supply may be seen extending from the vessels through the attached gingiva toward the gingival margin. The branches to the papillary area subjacent to the gingival epithelium are evident. The capillary loops of the gingiva are characteristic (Fig. 9-27, *C*). The high-power photomicrograph seen in Fig. 9-27, *B,* shows the obliteration of the periodontal ligament. There is vertical contact between the tooth and the bone. The capillary supply to the gingiva directly above the alveolar crest is seen in Fig. 9-27, *C,* despite the occlusion of the blood supply through the periodontal ligament.

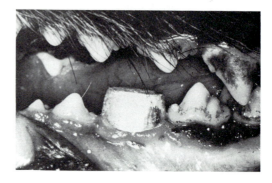

Fig. 9-26. Dentition of a dog in which a silver crown has been placed on one premolar, causing occlusal traumatism.

Some of the defects resulting from traumatic forces are related to the morphology of the alveolar process. When the alveolar process over the root surface is thin, tipping of the tooth may result in resorption of the plate of bone, covering the tooth and permitting the root to pierce the alveolar process. This is called a root fenestration and is frequently found on the mesiobuccal root of the max-

illary first molar, the maxillary canine, and the mesial root of the mandibular first molar. It may not be possible to identify clinically the presence of a root fenestration, since the fenestration may exist under alveolar mucosa in areas where no inflammation or pocket formation is present. If the clinician reflects a flap the fenestration may be viewed. If gingival inflammation extends apically

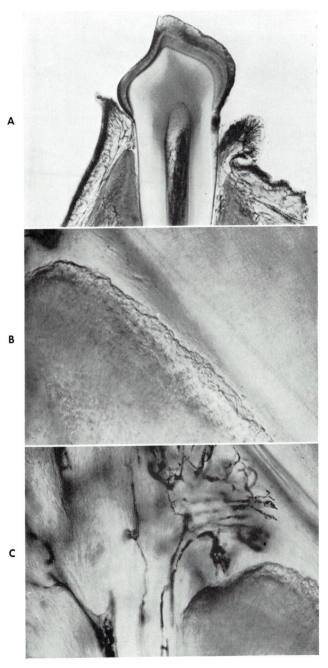

Fig. 9-27. Tooth in Fig. 9-26 has been moved so that it lies directly in apposition to lingual process. **A,** Perfusion of animal illustrated that gingival blood supply remained intact. **B,** Tooth is lying adjacent to bone, whereas in **C** blood supply of gingival tissue above crest can be seen intact.

in an area where a fenestration was present, resorption of the coronal isthmus of bone may result in the formation of a cleft in the gingival tissue and subsequent denudation of the root surface. When such fenestrations are found on the buccal surfaces of maxillary molars, a premature contact in the nonworking or balancing side is frequently observed as one of the etiologic factors (Fig. 9-15).

The entity of primary occlusal traumatism as just described may be seen clinically and is felt to be reversible if the force is relieved. The term "reversible" here is used to imply almost complete repair of the damaged tissues.

Epidemiologic studies indicate that occlusal traumatism frequently occurs about a tooth that has a concomitant gingivitis or periodontitis. The combined lesion of occlusal traumatism and periodontitis has been referred to as occlusal periodontitis. This nomenclature is used for brevity and should not imply that the occlusal factors were responsible for the periodontitis.

Although experimental data have documented in detail the lesion of occlusal traumatism, there still exists some confusion relevant to the interactions of the combined problem of the inflammatory marginal lesion and the degenerative changes of trauma. Some experimental evidence has been offered that excessive occlusal forces may alter the pathways of gingival inflammation into the underlying periodontal tissues and also cause angular remodeling of the alveolar process. Studies of Akiyoshi and Mori on incipient periodontitis in human material have demonstrated that inflammation of the gingiva can spread directly to the marginal portion of the periodontal ligament by means of the adjacent canals of the interdental septa. This occurs more often than has been thought by others and has been observed in material in which there is no evidence of occlusal traumatism. These observations reveal that the pathways of gingival inflammation into the underlying tissues may vary in periodontitis.

Wentz et al. designed an experiment in monkeys in which a jiggling-type trauma was produced. A tooth was subjected to excessive occlusal stress in a buccal direction when it came into contact in centric occlusion and right lateral excision and then pulled back when opening occurred by an orthodontic arch device. Thus the effects of both pressure and tension were recorded in the buccal as well as the palatal periodontal ligament. Examination of the tissue showed thrombosis of blood vessels and hemorrhage, destruction of periodontal

ligament fibers, and bone and cemental resorption. A gradual widening of the buccal and palatal periodontal ligaments occurred until no further resorption took place, and the changes in the attachment apparatus remained the same. It is extremely interesting that the jiggling type of trauma produced angular osseous defects but the supra-alveolar fiber apparatus was unaffected; hence there was no apical proliferation of the epithelial attachment. Wentz et al. questioned whether pocket formation would have occurred if a concomitant gingival inflammation were present. Svanberg and Lindhe also induced occlusal trauma in dogs and found that trauma from occlusion did not cause periodontal pocket formation in dogs with normal gingiva or with overt gingivitis. In other experiments the same investigators induced progressive periodontal destruction around predetermined teeth in ten beagle dogs. Shallow infrabony pockets (around 1 mm deep) were prepared. The experiment illustrated that it is possible in beagle dogs to produce periodontal breakdown around teeth with a rather high degree of reproducibility.

On the other hand, Glickman and Smulow reported that excessive force damaged the periodontal ligament and allowed direct infiltration of the inflammatory process into the ligament area. They noted the following: (1) alteration of the periodontal fiber orientation, opening up a direct pathway for inflammation to enter into the ligament, (2) increased pressure at the crestal areas of the periodontal ligament causing resorption of the alveolar bone, and (3) formation of a funnel-shaped trough at the crestal margins (vertical bone loss). These authors subsequently described two disease zones, the area of irritation and the area of codestruction. The area of codestruction included the coronal portion of the periodontal attachment apparatus. The periodontal ligament fibers in this area became disrupted, allowing the inflammatory process to spread directly into the periodontal ligament. This pattern of the pathway of inflammatory infiltrate, they believed, led to vertical resorption osseous defects.

Comar, Kollar, and Gargiulo in an attempt to ascertain any relation between marginal gingival disease and occlusal trauma in monkeys placed gold crowns on teeth with gross marginal overhangs in such a manner as to allow for food impaction from open contacts. They failed to find a modifying effect of the occlusal trauma produced on the gingival inflammation; however, they commented that the degree of gingival inflammation was not great and may have been insufficient to result in a spread of the inflammatory infiltrate.

While there is no conclusive data confirming the possible modifying role of occlusal trauma on marginal gingival disease, these two conditions do exist together in many and perhaps in most advanced cases of periodontal disease. Thus the therapist must take into account their etiologies, and therapy must be directed toward management of both.

REFERENCES

Akiyoshi, M., and Mori, K.: Marginal periodontitis; a histological study of the incipient stage, J. Periodontol. **38:**45, 1967.

Baer, P. N., Kakehashi, S., Littleton, N. W., White, C. L., and Lieberman, J. E.: Alveolar bone loss and occlusal wear, Periodontics **1:**19, 1963.

Bauer, W.: Ueber traumatische Schädigungen des Zementmantels der Zähne mit einen Beitrag zur Biologie des Zementes, Deutsch. Mschr. Zahnheilk. **45:**769, 1927.

Becks, H.: General aspects in pyorrhea research, Pacific Dent. Gaz. **37:**259, 1929.

Beyron, H.: Characteristics of functionally optimal occlusion and principles of occlusal rehabilitation, J.A.M.A. **48:**648, 1954.

Beyron, H.: Occlusal changes in adult dentition, J. Am. Dent. Assoc. **48:**674, 1954.

Box, H. K.: Twelve periodontal studies, Toronto, 1940, University of Toronto Press.

Box, H. K.: Experimental traumatogenic occlusion in sheep, Oral Health **25:**9, 1935.

Box, H. K.: The pericementum as influenced by physical functional modifications, Trans. Am. Soc. Orthod., p. 154, 1932; Int. J. Orthod. **19:**574, 1933.

Box, H. K.: Traumatic occlusion and traumatogenic occlusion, Oral Health **20:**642, 1930.

Box, H. K.: Necrotic gingivitis, Toronto, 1930, University of Toronto Press.

Box, H. K.: Studies in periodontal pathology, Bull. 7, 1924, Canadian Dental Research Foundation.

Boyle, P. E.: Tooth suspension, J. Dent. Res. **17:**37, 1938.

Breitner, C.: Tooth supporting apparatus under occlusal changes, J. Periodontol. **13:**72, 1942.

Burns, C. G., Orten, A. W., and Smith, A. H.: Development of tumors in incisors of rats on diet low in vitamin A, J. Dent. Res. **16:**317, 1937.

Cohen, D. W.: Changes in the attachment apparatus in occlusal trauma, Alpha Omegan **45:**20, 1951.

Cohen, D. W., and Goldman, H. M.: Clinical observations on the modification of human oral tissue metabolism by local intraoral factors, Ann. N.Y. Acad. Sci. **85:**68, 1960.

Cohen, D. W., and Goldman, H. M.: Oral disease in primates, Ann. N.Y. Acad. Sci. **85:**889, 1960.

Cohen, D. W., Keller, G., Feder, M., and Livingston, E.: Effects of excessive occlusal forces in the gingival blood supply (abstract), J. Dent. Res. **39:**677, 1960.

Comar, M. D., Kollar, J. A., and Gargiulo, A. W.: Local irritation and occlusal trauma as co-factors in the periodontal disease process, J. Periodontol. **40:**193, 1969.

Coolidge, E. D.: Traumatic and functional injuries occurring in the supporting tissues of human teeth, J. Am. Dent. Assoc. **25:**343, 1938.

Coolidge, E. D.: The thickness of the human periodontal membrane, J. Am. Dent. Assoc. **24:**1260, 1937.

Coolidge, E. D.: Evidence of excessive occlusal stress in periodontal tissues of human teeth, J. Dent. Res. **15:**159, 1935.

Coolidge, E. D.: The reaction of cementum in the presence of injury and infection, J. Am. Dent. Assoc. **18:**499, 1931.

Dewey, K. W.: Normal and pathologic cementum formation, Dent. Cosmos **68:**560, 1926.

Ericsson, I., and Lindhe, J.: Lack of effect of trauma from occlusion on the recurrence of experimental periodontitis, J. Clin. Periodontol. **4:**115, 1977.

Feldman, S.: Oral disease of medico-dental interest, Am. J. Orthod. **23:**287, 1937.

Feldman, S.: Diseases of the oral cavity, J. Am. Dent. Assoc. **21:**1401, 1934.

Figi, F. A.: Diseases of the soft tissues of the mouth, J. Am. Dent. Assoc. **22:**1919, 1935.

Fish, E. W.: Parodontal disease, London, 1944, Eyre & Spottiswoode, Ltd.

Glickman, I.: Effect of excessive occlusal forces upon the pathway of gingival inflammation in humans, J. Periodontol. **36:** 141, 1965.

Glickman, J., and Smulow, J. B.: Effect of excessive occlusal forces upon the pathway of gingival inflammation in humans, J. Periodontol. **36:**51, 1965.

Glickman, J., and Smulow, J. B.: Alterations in the pathway of gingival inflammation into the underlying tissues induced by excessive occlusal forces, J. Periodontol. **33:**7, 1962.

Glickman, I., Stein, R. S., and Smulow, J. B.: The effect of increased functional forces upon the periodontium of splinted and nonsplinted teeth, J. Periodontol. **32:**290, 1961.

Goldman, H. M.: Gingival vascular supply in induced occlusal traumatism, Oral Surg. **9:**939, 1956.

Gottlieb, B.: Orthodontic treatment of wandering teeth in cases of diffuse atrophy, Dent. Outlook **28:**551, 1941.

Gottlieb, B.: The formation of the pocket; diffuse atrophy of alveolar bone, J. Am. Dent. Assoc. **15:**462, 1928.

Gottlieb, B.: Traumatic occlusion, J. Am. Dent. Assoc. **14:** 1276, 1927.

Gottlieb, B.: Paradentalpyorrhoë und Alveolaratrophie, Deutsch. Mschr. Zahnheilk. **2:**363, 1926.

Gottlieb, B.: Schmutzpyorrhoe, Paradentalpyorrhoe und Alveolaratrophie, Munich, 1925, Urban & Schwarzenberg.

Gottlieb, B.: Die diffuse Atrophie des Alveolarknochens, Z. Stomat. **31:**195, 1923.

Gottlieb, B., and Orban, B.: Biology and pathology of the tooth and its supporting mechanism, New York, 1938, The Macmillan Co.

Gottlieb, B., and Orban, B.: Tissue changes by experimental overstress, Leipzig, 1931, Georg Thieme.

Granger, E.: Functional relations of the stomatognathic system, J. Am. Dent. Assoc. **48:**638, 1954.

Grohs, R.: Changes in the human periodontal membrane due to overstress, Z. Stomat. **29:**386, 1931.

Haley, P.: Useful procedure in periodontia, Dent. Cosmos **75:**868, 1933.

Haupl, K.: Ueber traumatische verrursachte Gewebsveränderungen im Paradentium, Z. Stomat. **25:**307, 1927.

Haupl, K., and Lang, F. J.: Die marginale Paradentitis, Berlin, 1927, Hermann Meusser.

Hirschfeld, I.: Some types of periodontoclasia and the diagnosis of their incipient symptoms, Dent. Items Interest **48:** 823, 1926.

Johnson, A. L., Appleton, J. L., and Rittershofer, L. S.: Tissue changes involved in tooth movement, Int. J. Orthod. **12:**889, 1926.

Kellner, E.: Das Verhältnis der Zement und Periodontal-breiten zur funktionellen Beanspruchung der Zähne, Z. Stomat. **29:**44, 1931.

Kellner, E.: Histologische Befunde an antagonistenlosen Zähnen, Z. Stomat. **26:**271, 1928.

Kronfeld, R.: Histopathology of the teeth and surrouunding structures, ed. 2, Philadelphia, 1939, Lea & Febiger.

Kronfeld, R.: The physiology of the human periodontal tissues under normal and abnormal occlusal conditions, Illinois Dent. J. **8:**13, 1939.

Kronfeld, R.: Biology of cementum, J. Am. Dent. Assoc. **25:**1451, 1938a.

Kronfeld, R.: Histologic analyses of the jaws of a child with malocclusion, Angle Orthod. **8:**21, 1938b.

Kronfeld, R.: Structure, function, and pathology of human periodontal membrane, N.Y. Dent. J. **6:**23, 1936.

Kronfeld, R.: Influence of function on periodontal membrane, J. Am. Dent. Assoc. **18:**1242, 1931.

Kronfeld, R., and Weinmann, J.: Traumatic changes in the periodontal tissues of deciduous teeth, J. Dent. Res. **19:**441, 1940.

Leonard, H. J.: Research in periodontology, J. Am. Dent. Assoc. **19:**302, 1932.

Leonard, H. J.: Diagnosis in periodontoclasia, Dent. Cosmos **68:**246, 1926.

Leonard, H. J.: Present concepts of periodontoclasia, Dent. Cosmos **68:**145, 1926.

Lindblom, G.: The value of bite analysis, J. Am. Dent. Assoc. **48:**657, 1954.

Lindhe, J., and Ericsson, I.: The influence of trauma from occlusion on reduced but healthy periodontal tissues in dogs, J. Clin. Periodontol. **3:**110, 1976.

Lindhe, J., and Nyman, S.: The role of occlusion in periodontal disease and the biological rationale for splinting in the treatment of periodontitis, Oral Sci. Rev. **10:**11, 1977.

Lindhe, J., and Svanberg, G.: Influences of trauma from occlusion on progression of experimental periodontitis in the beagle dog, J. Clin. Periodontol. **1:**3, 1974.

Looby, J. P., and Burket, L. W.: Scleroderma of the face with involvement of the alveolar process, Am. J. Orthod. **28:**493, 1942.

Lukonsky, E. H.: Fluorine therapy for exposed alveolar atrophy, J. Dent. Res. **20:**649, 1941.

Macapanpan, L. C., and Weinmann, J. P.: The influence of injury to the periodontal membrane on the spread of gingival inflammation, J. Dent. Res. **32:**665, 1953; **33:**263, 1954.

MacMillan, H. W.: Non-use in the development and resistance of the alveolar process, J. Am. Dent. Assoc. **15:**511, 1928.

MacMillan, H. W.: Radiographic and histologic evidence of the functional adaptation of the alveolar process, J. Am. Dent. Assoc. **15:**316, 1928.

MacMillan, H. W.: The clinical significance of disuse atrophy of the alveolar process, J. Am. Dent. Assoc. **14:**697, 1927.

Manly, R. S., and Braley, L. C.: Masticatory performance and efficiency, J. Dent. Res. **29:**448, 1950.

Manson, J. D., and Nicholson, K.: The distribution of bone defects in chronic periodontitis, J. Periodontol. **45:**88, 1974.

Marshall, J. A.: Physiologic and traumatic apical resorption, J. Am. Dent. Assoc. **22:**1545, 1935.

Mertner, S.: Co-destructive factors of marginal periodontitis and repetitive mechanical injury, Thesis. Eastman Dental Center and University of Rochester, Rochester, N.Y., 1975.

Mertner, S.: Co-destructive factors of marginal periodontitis and repetitive mechanical injury, J. Dent. Res. **54C:**78, 1975.

Mühlemann, H. R., and Herzog, H.: Tooth mobility and microscopic tissue changes produced by experimental occlusal trauma, Helv. Odontol. Acta **5:**33, 1961.

Müller, O.: Pathohistologie der Zahne, Basel, 1948, Benno Schwabe.

Orban, B.: Traumatic occlusion and gum inflammation, J. Periodontol. **10:**39, 1939.

Orban, B.: Knorpel im Periodontium, Z. Stomat. **35:**532, 1937.

Orban, B.: Tissue changes in traumatic occlusion, J. Am. Dent. Assoc. **15:**2090, 1928.

Orban, B., and Weinmann, J.: Signs of traumatic occlusion in average human jaws, J. Dent. Res. **13:**216, 1933.

Papillon, M. M., and Lefevre, D.: Deux cas de kératodermie palmaire et plantaire symétrique familiale chez le frère et la soeur; coexistence dans les deux cas d'alterations dentaires graves, Bull. Soc. Franc. Derm. Syph. **31:**82, 1924.

Picton, D. C. A.: On the part played by the socket in tooth support, Arch. Oral Biol. **10:**945, 1965.

Ramfjord, S.: Effects of acute febrile diseases on the periodontium of rhesus monkeys with reference to poliomyelitis, J. Dent. Res. **30:**615, 1951.

Ritchey, B., and Orban, B.: The crests of the interdental alveolar septa, J. Periodontol. **24:**75, 1953.

Rosenthal, S. L.: Periodontosis in a child resulting in exfoliation of the teeth, J. Periodontol. **22:**101, 1951.

Schwarz, A. M.: Movement of teeth under traumatic stress, Dent. Items Interest **52:**96, 1930.

Sicher, H.: Positions and movements of the mandible, J. Am. Dent. Assoc. **48:**620, 1954.

Siegmund, H.: Les recherches scientifiques sur les paradentoses, Parodontologie **12:**1, 1937.

Simonton, F. V.: Pyorrhea, definition and classification, Dent. Cosmos **68:**158, 1926.

Stahl, S.: The responses of the periodontium to combined gingival inflammation and occluso-functional stresses in four human surgical specimens, Periodontics **6:**14, 1968.

Stillman, P. R.: What is traumatic occlusion and how can it be diagnosed and corrected? J. Am. Dent. Assoc. **12:**1330, 1926.

Stillman, P. R., and McCall, J. O.: Clinical periodontia, ed. 2, New York, 1937, The Macmillan Co.

Stuteville, O. H.: Injuries to teeth and supporting structures caused by various orthodontic appliances, and methods of preventing injuries, J. Am. Dent. Assoc. **24:**1494, 1937.

Svanberg, G., and Lindhe, J.: Experimental tooth hypermobility in the dog—a methodological study, Odontol. Revy **24:**269, 1973.

Thoma, K. H.: Cementoblastoma, Int. J. Orthod. **23:**1127, 1937.

Thoma, K. H., and Goldman, H. M.: Correlation of clinical and pathologic phases of periodontal diseases, Dent. Items Interest **61:**103, 212, 309, 452, 1939.

Thoma, K. H., and Goldman, H. M.: The pathology of dental cementum, J. Am. Dent. Assoc. **26:**1943, 1939.

Thoma, K. H., and Goldman, H. M.: Diagnosis of periodontal diseases, Am. J. Orthod. **24:**1071, 1938.

Thompson, J. R.: Rest position of the mandible and its significance to dental science, J. Am. Dent. Assoc. **33:**151, 1946.

Thompson, J. R.: The constancy of the position of the mandible and its influence on prosthetic restorations, Illinois Dent. J. **12**:242, 1943.

Thompson, J. R.: A cephalometric study of the movements of the mandible, J. Am. Dent. Assoc. **28**:750, 1941.

Thompson, J. R., and Brodie, A. G.: Factors in the position of the mandible, J. Am. Dent. Assoc. **29**:925, 1942.

Wentz, F. M., Jarabak, Jr., and Orban, B.: Experimental occlusal trauma imitating cuspal interferences, J. Periodontol. **29**:117, 1958.

Wickham, N. E.: Gingival and periodontal lesions in children, N.Z. Dent. J. **48**:132, 1952.

Williams, C. H. W.: Correction of abnormalities of occlusion, J. Am. Dent. Assoc. **44**:748, 1952.

Woods, E. C., and Wallace, W. R. J.: A case of alveolar atrophy of unknown origin in a child, Am. J. Orthod. **27**:676, 1941.

Znamensky, N. N.: Alveolar pyorrhea—its pathological anatomy and its radical treatment, Br. Dent. J. **23**:585, 1902.

10 Periodontal disease in children

Periodontium: gingival unit
Gingival inflammatory lesions: gingivitis
Gingivosis
Lesions affecting alveolar process and periodontal
ligament

During the past 15 years various epidemiologic studies of the occurrence of periodontal disease in different age groups have focused attention on the susceptibility of the child to periodontopathies. *These studies point out that it is erroneous to consider periodontal disease as primarily a disturbance in adult life.* Surveys of the incidence of gingivitis in children in various parts of this country between the ages of 6 and 17 years reveal that between 28% and 64% (depending on the study) were affected with some form of gingival inflammation. *If untreated many of these lesions will progress, with further destruction in adulthood, and it becomes apparent that to be successful any preventive program to control periodontal disease will first have to eliminate pathologic conditions of the periodontium in children.*

McCall reported in studies conducted at the Guggenheim Dental Clinic in 1938 that gingival lesions were observed in children at 4 to 5 years of age. Development of these gingival alterations occurred in patients with untreated dental caries; however, it is important to note that no correlation between gingivitis and dental caries has been reported. A review of the literature substantiates the universal prevalence of periodontal disease in children; gingival disease has been documented in England, Wales, the Virgin Islands, India, Canada, Israel, Italy, and the United States by numerous investigators. Recent data compiled from the Head Start program has confirmed that the incidence of periodontal disease in children, particularly from the lower socioeconomic level, may approach 75%. Earlier studies would seem to confirm the interrelationship of availability of dental care as a result of socioeconomic status and the

presence or absence of gingivitis in school children. Stahl and Goldman reported 26.9% incidence in Brookline, Massachusetts, that had an active oral hygiene program, whereas Massler and Schour reported a 60% to 70% incidence in Chicago schoolchildren, where no such program existed. In addition the incidence of gingivitis in white children has been shown to be lower than in black children. Socioeconomic factors are probably the primary cause in this difference rather than racial characteristics. Socioeconomic levels have also been shown to be an important variable by King, whose investigations in Dundee, Scotland, of children between the ages 12 and 18 demonstrated a lower incidence in more affluent groups. Additional findings of the study included the following: girls had a lower percentage of gingivitis than did boys (however, this occurrence was implied to be the result of the girls' increasing awareness of oral hygiene) and girls revealed a greater incidence of gingivitis at an earlier age, which was judged to be related to earlier eruption. Baer states that periodontitis may be initiated at the time of puberty and suggests that this situation may be an explanation for the advanced destruction evidenced in young adults.

Stallard maintains that although destructive periodontal disease is most often diagnosed in the third decade of life, its initiation most frequently occurs in childhood. In addition other investigators have postulated that the transition from gingivitis to periodontitis is evidenced generally at age 15.

The purpose of this chapter is not to imply that periodontal disease in children differs entirely in pathology, etiology, and therapy from that in the adult. However, it has been noted that certain forms of the disease process have a predilection for childhood, and trends in experimental studies demonstrate the differences in reaction by the young and old of the species to various stimuli. Many of the variations in response by young and old are attributed to general metabolic differences at the various age levels. It is unfortunate that as yet we

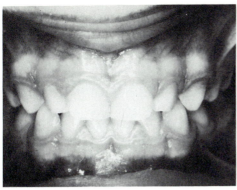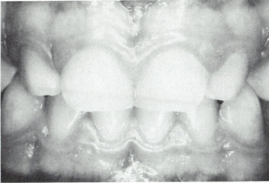

Fig. 10-1. Gingival tissues and dentition of two children 3½ years old. Note prominence of gingival grooves.

cannot pinpoint more of these differences in explaining the peculiarities of the patterns of reaction in the child and the adult to the same etiologic factors. This chapter will be concerned with a description of the normal periodontium of the child as well as with those forms of periodontal disease that have a predilection for childhood. It will not include a discussion of the various diseases that manifest themselves only on the other mucous membrane surfaces of the child's oral cavity, nor will there be any detailed coverage of therapeutic procedures.

PERIODONTIUM: GINGIVAL UNIT

The periodontium consists of the mucous membrane covering (the gingival unit) and the attachment apparatus (the cementum of the root, the alveolar process, and the periodontal ligament).

Gingiva has been demonstrated as a pink, stippled tissue present over the edentulous ridges at birth and separated from the alveolar mucosa by the mucogingival junction, which is located near the vestibular fornix during the first 6 months of life. It has been shown histologically that gingiva begins to differentiate from mucosa at about 8 to 9 weeks in utero and keratinization and epithelial peg formation appear prior to the eruption of the primary teeth. With the eruption of the teeth and the growth of the jaws there seems to be an increase in alveolar mucosa, with the gingiva remaining at approximately the same height, measuring from the margin to the mucogingival junction.

The marginal and papillary gingivae consist of the soft tissue that encircles and approximates the teeth. The marginal area is that small band of gingival tissue that lies on the portion known as the sulcus. The shape of the interdental papilla is pyramidal in a mesiodistal direction, but buccolin-

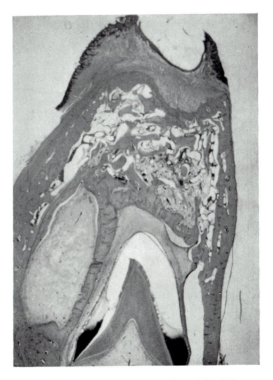

Fig. 10-2. Interdental tissues of a child 2½ years old (labiolingual section). Note presence of col in papilla as well as concavity in alveolar crest. (From Cohen, D. W., and Goldman, H. M.: P. D. M., p. 3, 1962.)

gually its morphology will vary according to the shape of the crowns of the teeth as well as the dimensions of the contact area and the embrasure form. Recent work has demonstrated that the interdental papilla may take the form of a concavity in its mid area in a labiolingual dimension and this col may be a site of early gingival inflammation. When the primary teeth are exfoliated, the col disappears as the papilla rounds over, and a new col may reappear when the permanent teeth begin to erupt. The attached gingiva consists of the stippled, dense tissue bordered by the gingival groove that separates it from the marginal gingiva and the mucogingival junction that limits its apical extent. In some instances the gingival groove is quite distinct, whereas in others it cannot be distinguished at all. Clinically the attached gingiva is keratinized, and its epithelium is a great deal thicker than the alveolar mucosa (Figs. 10-1 and 10-2).

Alveolar mucosa is the continuation of tissue from the attached gingiva to the vestibular fornix. It is rather thin and soft, not keratinized, and of a deeper red than the attached gingiva.

During the period of the primary, mixed, and immature permanent dentitions the gingiva of the child exhibits incomplete passive eruption. Characteristically the epithelial adherence to the enamel surface is great, resulting in a gingival wall that is somewhat flaccid from the gingival crest to the base of the epithelial attachment. Rigidity and retractability are subsequently lessened, which may be the result of a lesser degree of collagen to ground substance in the corium of the marginal gingiva. Recent investigations have demonstrated that the extensively hydrated connective tissues of the young are richer in protein-polysaccharide matrices, whereas with aging the sulfated protein-polysaccharides increase. Concurrently the more soluble collagen present in the young will with age become more insoluble, its polypeptide chains more tightly linked, and its fibrous component exhibiting more tensile strength.

The marginal gingiva of the child presents histologically an extensively delicate reticular and collagen fiber network unlike the dense organized collagen fiber bundles observed in the adult. The absence of incompletely differentiated circular and groups A and B fiber complexes may play a role in the strength of approximation of the gingiva to the enamel. However, the transseptal and group C fibers are dense and well organized with demonstrable attachments to the underlying bony septa and cervical cementum. Arnim and Hagerman have speculated that the circular fiber complex's arrangement supports the free gingiva and aids in its adherence to the tooth surface. More information is necessary to determine accurately the degree of development of the circular fiber complex in children, particularly since Löe suggests that these fibers are extremely abundant constituents of the free gingiva and therefore probably essential to development and maintenance of the dentogingival relationship. Other factors that probably contribute to the stability of this relationship include

the secretion of glycoprotein modalities from epithelial cells, the ionic bonding of cells to dental surface, the effect of hemidesmosomes, and the presence of a plasma filtrate.

The gingiva of the young may also exhibit a very extensive and patent vascularization at the marginal zone; this is made possible by a reduction in containment of vascular patency, the extent of which is inversely proportionate to the degree of collagination and matrical maturation of a tissue. This prominent vascularization may promote transudation of the connective tissue proper, increasing its turgidity, enhancing its hydration, and altering its constitution. Increased passage of the transudate may also occur into the sulcular area or into a more active venular and lymphatic drain. This fluid presence in the connective tissue, together with the augmented fluid transfer from the corium into the sulcus and dentogingival interface, could play a significant role in the diminished adherence of the gingival wall to the tooth surface. These phenomena may be the factors that allowed Waerhaug to insert cellulose strips and extremely fine blades to the cementoenamel junction of newly erupting teeth of dogs. He also reported this finding when examining the gingival sulci of children. In summary we may postulate that the degree of adherence of the gingival wall to the tooth is governed by—

1. Tissue composition, primarily the ratio of ground substance to collagen and the viscosity of the matrical gel
2. The degree of structural rigidity, specifically the arrangement or the organization of the gingival fiber system
3. The state of passive eruption, contributing to the length of adherent gingival wall
4. The vascularity of the gingiva, including tissue hydration, sulcular fluid, and amount of vascular transudate

GINGIVAL INFLAMMATORY LESIONS: GINGIVITIS

The inflammatory lesion of the child is primarily confined to the marginal aspects of the gingiva. This process is evidenced in the unattached but adherent gingival wall, which is coronal to the cementoenamel junction and more specifically separated from the rest of the gingiva. This division is manifested by that part of its corium that is not only attached to the tooth by cementum, but which comprises a well-oriented matt of connective tissue topping and attached to the crest of the bone interdentally and marginally. Clinically, normal childhood gingiva is more flaccid marginally with a tendency toward fullness and rounding of the gingival margin. When affected by the inflammatory process the tissue exhibits not only an accentuation of these features but also a sharply defined marginal erythema induced by the vasodilatory phase of the disease.

This localization of the inflammatory process, with rare extension into transseptal or periosteal fiber areas and bone, can also be seen in the young and adolescents of other species, including nonhuman primates, rodents, and dogs. In children and animals an expansion of a well-circumscribed marginal process into a state of more severe gingival and osseous involvement appears to depend on major local or systemic insult or both: noted with vitamin deficiency in Italian children, as the grossly manifest necrotizing lesions documented in protein-deprived African children, or the severe periodontitis found in Down's syndrome. The periodontal literature is replete with these documentations of severe manifestations in the young, human and animal. However, only minor recognition or cognizance is given to the ubiquitous, contained marginal inflammatory state, and why clinically and histopathologically it is and continues to be so, possibly for a protracted period. An extensive review of the pedodontic and periodontal literature

reveals neither a single, complete histologic analysis of the juvenile marginal lesion nor any explanation of why it should be so, except on a temporal basis, with youth, a mild lesion slowly progressing with age into a more extensive and severe one. Nor does the literature contain a consideration of anatomic influences on the localization of the inflammatory state.

There are other structural attributes that could be related to the nature of the juvenile lesion. The barrier of gingival attachment to tooth and bone is well developed at the time of tooth eruption. In the child, beginning in the edentulous infant, the zone of attached gingiva is firm, stippled, well bound down to bone, and appears inordinately wide. The tooth erupts through the crestal aspect of this tissue with fibers of its dental sac merging with preexisting gingival collagen to form the transseptal and group three fiber complexes. This tooth emergence from the crypt and blending of dental sac with gingival collagen begins prior to the dental entry into the oral cavity and may continue, along with further development of the osseous phase, until the tooth reaches a functional occlusion. The collagenation of the basal aspect of the gingiva, its maturity and insolubility, and the tenacity of gingival attachment to bone and cementum may serve to limit the inroads of inflamma-

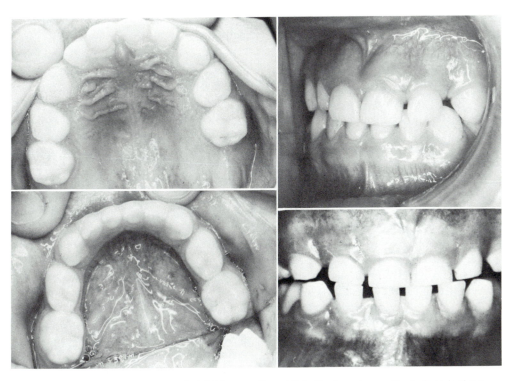

Fig. 10-3. Interdental tissues of child frequently exhibit diastemata, particularly in incisor-cuspid areas.

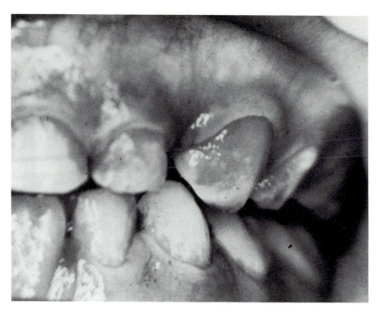

Fig. 10-4. Plaque deposits on deciduous teeth.

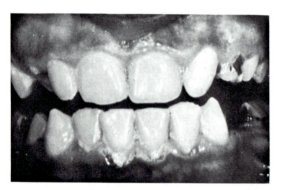

Fig. 10-5. Marked gingival inflammation and retraction in a young individual. Note accumulation of heavy plaque around mandibular incisor teeth.

tory disease into these areas. The marginal connective tissue is formed last and would appear to be less defined until active and passive eruptions are completed. We cannot exclude, however, the consideration of reactive fibroplasia as a response to inflammation in the periosteal zone.

Clinical examination of the interdental tissues with the child, particularly in the incisor-cuspid zones, very often exhibit diastemata. These interdental tissues are in reality structurally comparable to saddle areas, and except in very close association with the tooth these tissues exhibit freedom from inflammatory disease. Examination of the primary molar or primary molar–first permanent molar areas reveals replacement of these areas by coliforms produced by and conforming to the proximal contacts of posterior teeth. Observation has revealed that the inflammatory lesion is more often evidenced in these posterior segments and in anterior zones where proximal dental contacts are present; the character of the interdental tissues concomitantly changes. Consequently the fundamental structure may dictate the onset, presence, continuance, and degree of inflammation (Figs. 10-3 to 10-5).

Histologic evaluation of these diastema areas indicates a surface keratinizing effect, either parakeratinization or orthokeratinization, surmounting stratified squamous epithelium with regular rete peg extension into the underlying corium. There is a continuation of attached gingiva interdentally evolving a potential protection against insult offered by the keratinizing effect of its epithelium. Initial experimental efforts relative to the permeability of these epithelia to labeled tissue fluids and intravascularly administered carbon suspensions suggest that the keratinizing effect limits transudation through such epithelium, thereby containing hydrating and nutritive substances to the epithelium and by inference to the connective tissue. Studies substantiate the inward-outward impermeability of such epithelium and the perviousness of sulcular epithelia. The surface keratinizing quality of an intraepithelial zone of imperviousness (the barrier area at the junction between granular cells and the keratinizing layers) may also act to limit the action and penetration of exogenous irritants and thus protect the gingival corium.

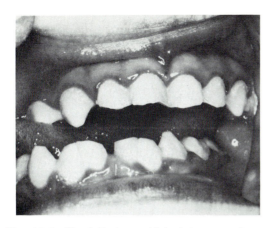

Fig. 10-6. Gingivitis in a child of 4 years of age. Heavy plaque accumulation can be noted. Child did not brush teeth.

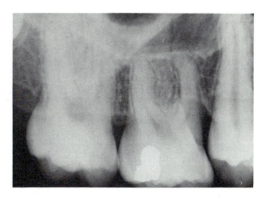

Fig. 10-7. Crestal bone resorption on mesial and distal aspects of maxillary first permanent molar in adolescent 13 years old.

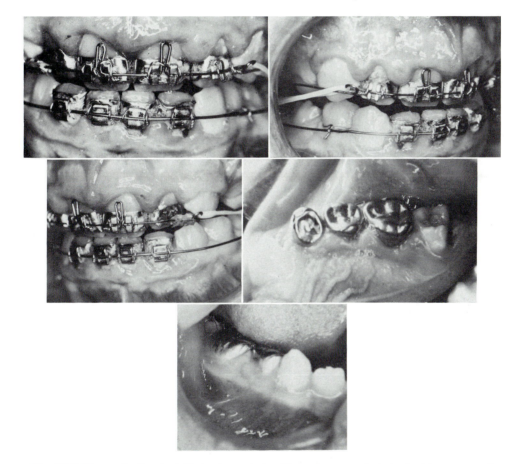

Fig. 10-8. Hyperplastic gingivitis is characterized by enlargement of gingival tissues resulting in pseudopocket formation. Local irritants, that is, orthodontic appliances and stainless steel crowns, are frequently etiologic agents producing this response.

In addition to the epithelial qualities the observations that interdental connective tissues are structurally well organized, better endowed with collagen, and as a complex firmly bound to underlying bone and adjacent gingiva may support the hypothesis that interdental tissues of a saddle nature are more resistant or less affected by inflammatory disease than are interdental tissues topped by ''col'' configurations and the markedly different epithelial nature attending this morphology.

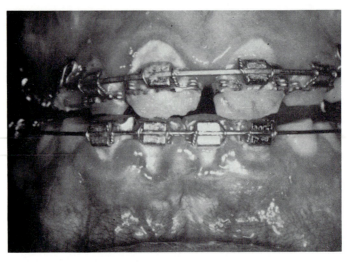

Fig. 10-9. Gingivitis in a child wearing orthodontic appliances. Note collection of materia alba on teeth. (From Cohen, D. W., and Goldman, H. M.: P. D. M., p. 3, 1962.)

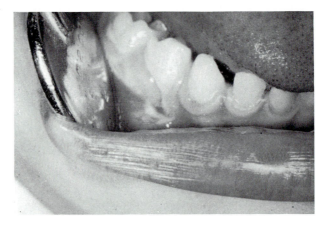

Fig. 10-10. Gingival cleft on mesial root of mandibular first primary molar in a 3-year-old child. Patient had a habit of scratching tissues with his finger. (Courtesy James Dannenberg, Philadelphia; from Cohen, D. W., and Goldman, H. M.: P. D. M., p. 3, 1962.)

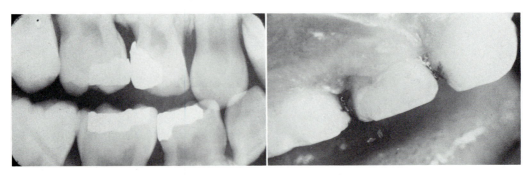

Fig. 10-11. Faulty amalgam restoration in primary molar. Lesion initially occurs in gingiva, progressing from inflammatory infiltrate to osteoclastic activity and resulting in resorption.

Interdental saddle areas may also be shaped convexly, lending itself to the more effective self-cleansing by food abrasion and the detergency of liquids.

Other influences—microbiologic, traumatic, immunologic, inheritable, chemical and enzymatic, cellular, and systemic—are operative in periodontal disease, and their roles individually and in concert with each other may also be tempo-rally variable. Cognizance must also be made of the variance of the vague resistance and reparative abilities that exist at different periods of life and their mediation by the oral, systemic, atmospheric, psychologic, and social ecologies of the individual.

Despite the complexity of influences on the individual and his periodontium, the young, when compared with his elders, manifests a well-de-

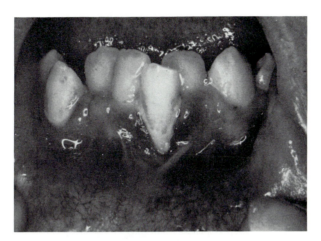

Fig. 10-12. Gingival inflammation in a 12-year-old child. Crowding of mandibular incisors has caused local environmental factors to contribute to periodontal problem. Mandibular labial frenum is perpetuating cleft that developed on labially placed left central incisor. (From Cohen, D. W., and Goldman, H. M.: P. D. M., p. 3, 1962.)

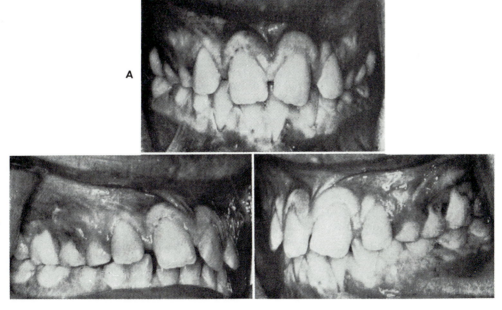

Fig. 10-13. A, Periodontal disease in a young child with mixed dentition. Note recession around lower incisors. **B,** Posterior regions. Note involvement of primary dentition, characterized by recession of gingival margins, gingival inflammation, and loss of interdental structure. Gingivae were irritated by incorrect oral hygiene practices and a tooth-nail habit.

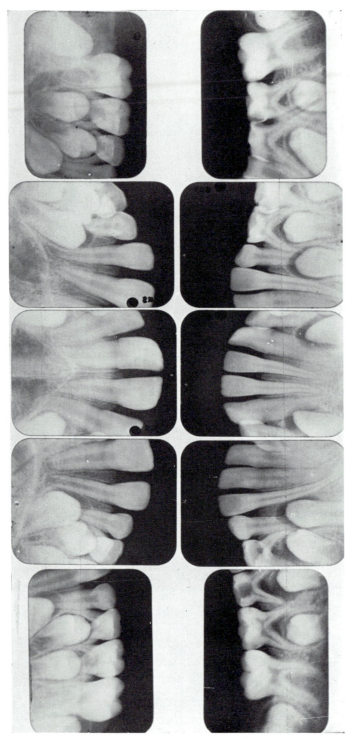

Fig. 10-14. Teeth of patient in Fig. 10-13. Note loss of bone in marginal area around primary teeth.

fined, marginally restricted gingival inflammatory state that remains limited in severity and expanse, often cyclically, until he can no longer structurally, reparatively, or immunologically contain the inflammatory process, whether it remains constant or increases in etiologic or processural intensity.

Gingivitis is the most prevalent periodontal lesion in the child and young adult, and its incidence increases with age. The gingival tissues of the maxillary and mandibular anterior teeth are affected more frequently in this age group than is any other area in the mouth. Studies also point out the high incidence of pockets about the maxillary first permanent molar in children between the ages of 6 and 11 years. Although it has been observed that acute gingival inflammatory disturbances are more common in children than in adults, nevertheless the chronic forms of gingivitis make up the majority of periodontal lesions of childhood. Most of the etiologic factors that are responsible for gingival disturbances in the adult can produce the same changes in childhood. However, there are certain irritating agents that are more prevalent in children (Figs. 10-6 to 10-14).

Studies of the toothbrushing habits and the oral hygiene practices of children between the ages of 6 and 15 years have shown the low frequency of brushing and the minimal time devoted to oral physiotherapy. It is unfortunate that children as well as adults are usually not instructed in proper oral hygiene procedures until some form of periodontal disease has manifested itself.

The irritation of ill-fitting orthodontic appliances may be observed as a cause of gingivitis in the young person (Figs. 10-8, *A* to *C,* and 10-9). Moreover the lack of adequate oral hygiene techniques about properly constructed orthodontic appliances may result in food retention and ensuing gingival inflammation.

Gingivitis associated with herpetic stomatitis, mouth-breathing habits, and hyperplasia noted with Dilantin sodium therapy may be observed in the young patient. However, these conditions are also seen in the adult and are discussed elsewhere in the text.

ERUPTIVE GINGIVITIS

The gingivitis seen in children at the time of eruption of the permanent dentition has been described as eruptive gingivitis. The gingival margin gets no protection from the coronal contours of the tooth during the early stage of active eruption, and the continual impingement of food on the gingivae causes the inflammatory process (Figs. 10-15 and

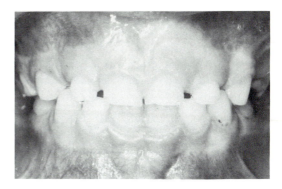

Fig. 10-15. Eruptive gingivitis in a 6-year-old child. Upon full eruption, unprotected gingival margin recedes under coronal contour.

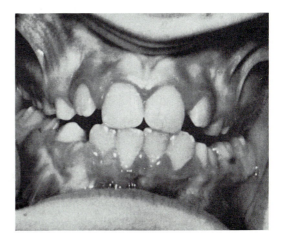

Fig. 10-16. Eruptive gingivitis in a child 10 years of age.

10-16). Plaque has a tendency to collect in these areas and to act as an irritant to the gingival margin.

GINGIVITIS ASSOCIATED WITH PUBERTY

Gingival overgrowth during puberty may occur in both girls and boys; however, it is more prevalent among girls. The gingival enlargement is characterized by a hyperplasia of the marginal gingivae and prominent bulbous interdental papillae. In some instances the gingival tissue is moderately firm and is not unduly discolored, whereas in other cases the hyperplasia presents all clinical features generally associated with an inflammatory process, that is, changes in color and consistency. The gingival tissue may be soft, reddish to reddish blue, and retracted from the tooth surface. Not infrequently are the lingual gingivae free of any change, the labial and buccal portions being solely affected. *Careful examination reveals that local environment factors capable of producing gingival disease cause an increased reaction in the gingiva.* However, in a given instance of puberty change the impression is that the degree of involvement is far greater than one of chronic gingival inflammatory hyperplasia associated with local etiologic agents alone. Although therapy is beneficial, the tendency for recurrence is great. Healing is usually poor with gingival tabs forming and hyperplastic changes following. The slightest local irritation sets off a renewal of gingival enlargement. Once young adult life is reached, there is usually a spontaneous reduction of the gingival tissues; however, complete remission is rare. The sequelae of an untreated case are consistent with the usual inflammatory gingival hyperplasia.

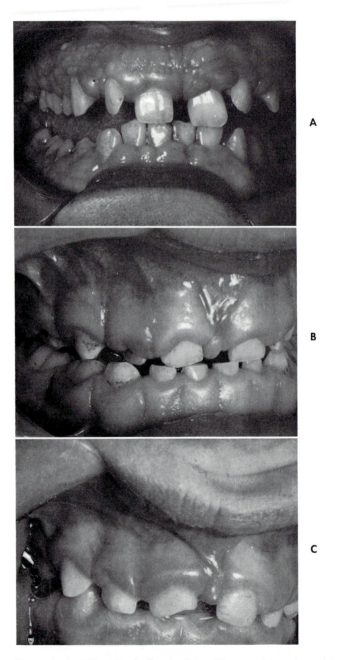

Fig. 10-17. Hereditary gingival fibrosis. **A,** Teeth of the 35-year-old mother of the two children whose photographs are shown in **B** and **C. B,** Teeth of 3-year-old daughter. **C,** Teeth of 5-year-old son. (Courtesy Harry Bohannan and Thompson Lewis, Seattle; from Cohen, D. W., and Goldman, H. M.: P. D. M., p. 3, 1962.)

HEREDITARY DIFFUSE GINGIVAL FIBROSIS

The lesion of hereditary diffuse gingival fibrosis is an uncommon form of severe gingival hyperplasia that may begin with the eruption of the primary teeth or sometimes the eruption of the permanent dentition. This marked gingival enlargement occurs throughout the mouth, and the tissue is firm, dense, pink, and insensitive, with little tendency toward bleeding (Fig. 10-17). Histologic examination of these gingival specimens shows a mild hyperkeratosis of the epithelium. with the production of long rete pegs. The principal cause for the enlargement is the underlying dense connective tissue stroma that consists of well-defined collagen bundles, with some fibroblasts and fibrocytes present. The presence of groups of chronic inflammatory cells is usually in response to the secondary irritation arising from trauma to the hyperplastic gingivae. The etiology of this gingival overgrowth is not known, but most reports point to a genetic factor. Other members of the families of these patients exhibit similar changes, suggesting a hereditary pattern. In some cases systemic defects are observed in addition to the oral changes. The presence of hypertrichosis along with the gingival hyperplasia suggests the possibility of endocrine dysfunction as a possible etiologic factor. The removal of the excessive gingival tissue by gingivectomy procedures seems to be the therapy of choice, although there have been regrowths reported in the literature.

GINGIVAL LESIONS IN CRIPPLED AND HANDICAPPED CHILDREN

One problem of childhood that has been virtually ignored in the dental literature is the high incidence of periodontal diseases in crippled or handicapped children. Clinical observations of children suffering from cerebral palsy, muscular dystrophy, and mental and nervous diseases reveal a high rate of gingival lesions (Figs. 10-18 and 10-19). The paucity of reports on the dental needs of these children points out the tremendous need for future investigations of the oral problems of institutionalized children. In addition to these systemic disturbances the local etiologic factors are multiple and complex. High incidences of mouth breathing, malocclusion, bruxism, caries, and inadequate oral hygiene techniques are common to this group. Because these children are unable to swallow properly, dietary deficiencies are frequent, along with the other physical and emotional problems. With attempts being made by specially trained dentists to treat the carious lesion, it is hoped that in the future consideration will be given to the incidence, etiology, and treatment of periodontal diseases in these children.

GINGIVAL CHANGES ASSOCIATED WITH VITAMIN C DEFICIENCY

Although scorbutic changes in the gingival tissue may be observed throughout life, they are commonly seen in the child under 2 years of age.

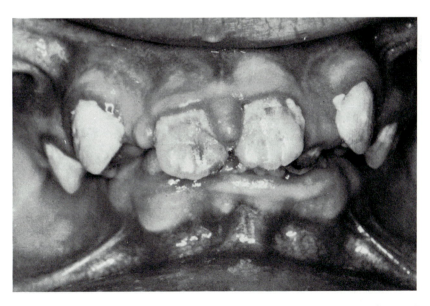

Fig. 10-18. Periodontal disease in a young mentally retarded child. (From Cohen, D. W., and Goldman, H. M.: P. D. M., p. 3, 1962.)

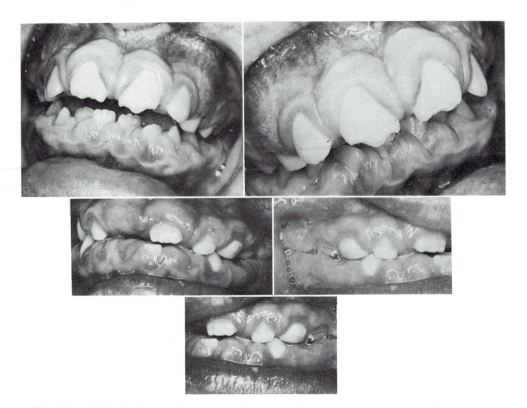

Fig. 10-19. Dilantin therapy for control of grand mal–type seizures may result in gingival hyperplasia. Incidence is highest in children and will vary in its extent. Tissue is generally firm but a superimposed inflammatory infiltrate will result in edema and bleeding.

The gingival lesions may be the first manifestation of vitamin C deficiency in the child. The gingivitis associated with ascorbic acid deficiency is characterized by a marked tendency toward spontaneous hemorrhage and by very painful, swollen, bluish purple gingivae. Ulcerations are present on the spongy gingival tissue, causing acute distress in the child patient. Scorbutic gingivitis may be distinguished from a marginal gingivitis of purely local etiology on the basis of the extreme pain and the tendency for spontaneous hemorrhage. The diagnosis should be supported by blood findings (plasma ascorbic acid levels) and other systemic aspects of scurvy.

GINGIVOSIS

The term "gingivosis" was used by Schour and Massler to describe an unusual and severe type of gingival disease that was observed in malnourished and chronically ailing hospitalized children in postwar Italy. The course of the disease is cyclic and passes through three definite stages. The onset begins insidiously as a low-grade edema of the interdental papilla that spreads to the marginal and attached gingiva. The second stage is characterized by a sudden engorgement of the affected gingivae,

which bleed spontaneously and profusely. This acute stage lasts about 3 to 4 weeks, with complete necrosis of the affected gingivae. There may be desquamation of the alveolar mucosa during this stage. The chronic stage results in necrosis of the gingivae, with recession and denudation of the root. There is little bleeding and no pain in this quiescent phase. The clinical impression is that the disease is of a degenerative rather than an inflammatory nature.

The cases of gingivosis seen in postwar Italy appeared to be related to impetigolike lesions on the skin of the face, and they improved clinically with systemic therapy of niacinamide and pyridoxine.

LESIONS AFFECTING ALVEOLAR PROCESS AND PERIODONTAL LIGAMENT

ERYTHROBLASTIC ANEMIA

Erythroblastic anemia (Cooley's anemia) is a hereditary chronic anemia in children of the Mediterranean groups. This disease is usually fatal and is characterized by leukocytosis, splenomegaly, and generalized skeletal lesions. Patients with this hemolytic anemia are lethargic and appear to be mentally sluggish for their age. The oral mucosa

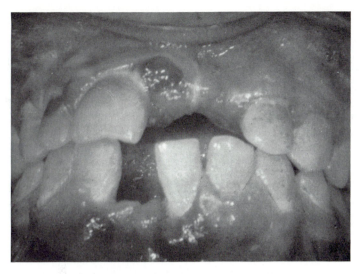

Fig. 10-20. Periodontal disease in a 13-year-old patient with diabetes. Missing anterior teeth were lost as a result of periodontal disease.

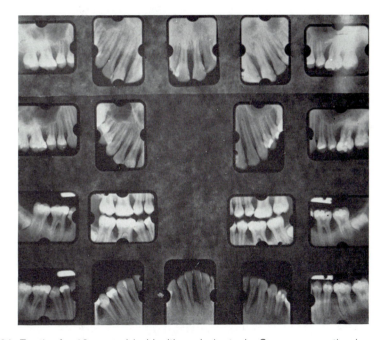

Fig. 10-21. Teeth of a 13-year-old girl with periodontosis. Severe resorption is seen about incisors and first molars. A sister of this child was afflicted by same condition. (Courtesy Edward Jarvis, Cynwyd, Pa.; from Cohen, D. W., and Goldman, H. M.: P. D. M., p. 3, 1962.)

may have a yellowish tint. Strikingly characteristic changes result from a marked overdevelopment of the maxillae and malar bones. These patients develop a mongoloid appearance, and the hyperplasia of the maxillae results in malocclusion, open bite, and diastemata between the maxillary teeth.

JUVENILE DIABETES

Diabetes mellitus in children may be accompanied by gingival inflammation and resorption of the alveolar process. Studies of the periodontal lesions in the uncontrolled juvenile diabetic patient have shown that bone destruction is greater than in children with comparable local etiologic factors without systemic alterations (Fig. 10-20).

PERIODONTOSIS

An interesting periodontal lesion affecting young patients and one that has intrigued clinicians during the past 50 years is the entity known as

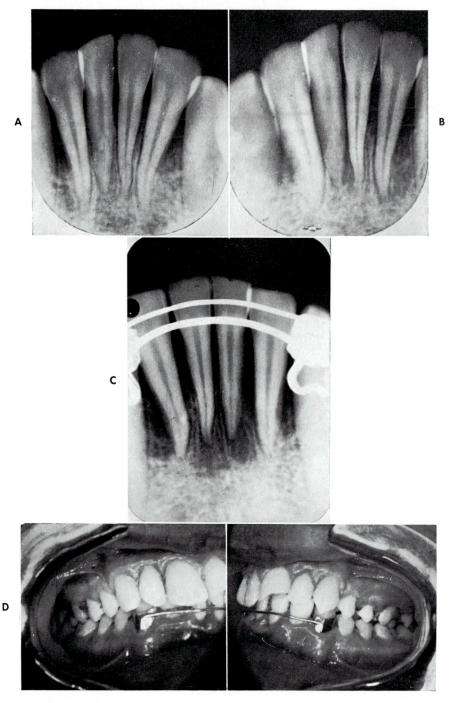

Fig. 10-22. A, Anterior teeth in a 12-year-old boy in November 1938. At this time dentist noticed that anterior teeth were becoming loose. Resorption of alveolar crest is evident. A moth-eaten appearance of bone can also be noticed. **B,** Anterior teeth of patient in **A,** 6 months later. Note further resorption of alveolar bone here as well as widening of periodontal ligament space. Teeth had become much looser in meantime. **C,** Anterior teeth of patient in **A** and **B,** 6 months later. At this time it had become advisable to splint teeth. Further resorption of alveolar bone is evident. Clinically teeth were extremely loose. **D,** Teeth of patient in **A** to **C** January 1940, when splint on anterior teeth was in place. Gingivae around anterior teeth showed marked hyperplasia. Deep pockets could be probed around teeth.

periodontosis. Gottlieb focused attention on a form of periodontal destruction that differed markedly from the inflammatory conditions, and he applied the term ''diffuse atrophy of the alveolar bone'' to this type of periodontopathy. He considered that extraoral or systemic influences played a major role in the etiology of the lesion, and he tried to prove that metabolic alterations affected the biologic state of the cementum. Currently this form of periodontal disease is known as periodontosis, and many attempts have been made to indict a specific systemic factor in its pathogenesis. Although these studies have not been successful in establishing a characteristic systemic alteration, much

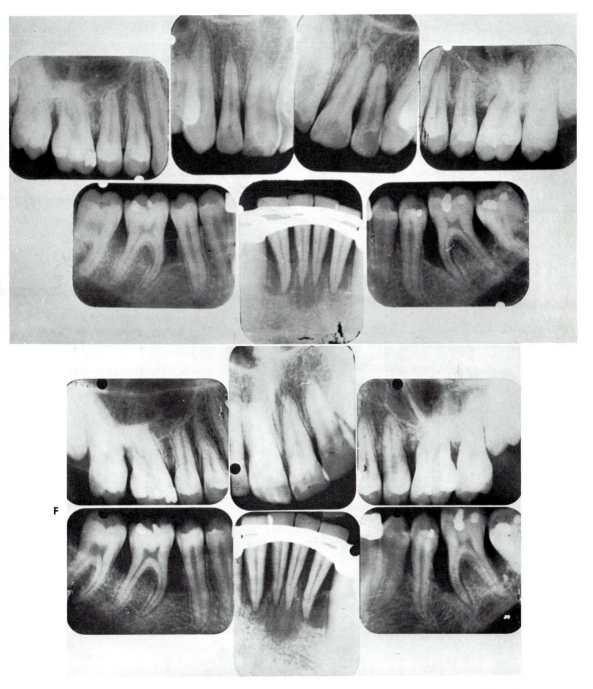

Fig. 10-22, cont'd. E, Teeth of patient in **A** to **D,** 6 months later. Note resorption of alveolar bone around anterior and posterior teeth. **F,** Teeth of patient in **A** to **E,** 6 months later. Note further bone resorption.

Continued.

information has been made available on this condition, which may begin in the first or second decade of life. This rare condition is seen in young patients, and in several studies attempts to localize a common systemic influence have been unsuccessful. Almost all the cases of periodontosis documented in the literature exhibit varying degrees of gingival inflammation.

Clinically, periodontosis, a disease of the alveolar housing essentially, is seen in very young individuals and is characterized by loosening and migration of the teeth. The clinical behavior of this disease is such that bone loss is rapid. The loosening of the teeth is progressive in nature, although cycles of loosening and tightening are noted. The dentist must realize that the incidence of this disease is low, this clinical entity being observed only very infrequently. In its unabated form the prognosis for retention of the teeth is poor (Fig. 10-21).

In some instances a classic picture of "molar-incisor" change can be seen, while in others all the teeth are affected; however, seemingly last to be affected are the premolar teeth. Generally there is minimal plaque accumulation, calculus, or even clinically evident gingivitis. Such individuals have a relatively thin attached bacterial plaque at the gingival attachment orifice (entrance to the sulcus) and little if any plaque attached to the tooth surface in deep subgingival sites. The subgingival accumulations are generally surrounded by polymorphonuclear leukocytes. These organisms are overwhelmingly gram negative. Socransky has described one group of fusiform-shaped organisms that have the ability to glide on agar surfaces. In contrast, organisms from healthy sites in the same patient show gram-positive microorganisms, typical of those seen in individuals free of periodontal disease.

Periodontosis has also been termed "localized juvenile periodontitis." Cianciola et al. have demonstrated defects in white blood cells (polymorphonuclear leukocytes or neutrophils) in these patients. They found that these cells were less efficient both in chemotaxis and in phagocytosis.

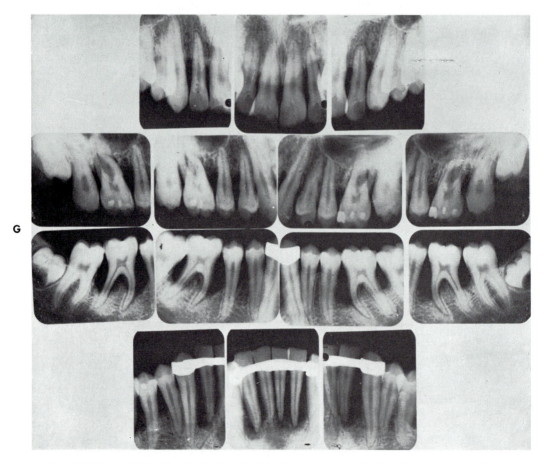

Fig. 10-22, cont'd. G, Teeth of patient in **A** to **F**, 2 years later. Note advanced resorption of bone.

They also found that these patients had no other medical problems and that their other white blood cells responded normally. They suggest that either the causative bacteria release a substance that depresses neutrophils or that the patients have an intrinsic defect in their defense system. The nondiseased siblings also showed neutrophil defects, and because of this these researchers think that the defects are intrinsic characteristics (Fig. 10-22).

Although most cases of periodontosis observed by the dentist are in an advanced stage, since the disease process is not usually recognized in the initial stage, being for the most part asymptomatic to the patient, occasionally the incipient lesion is encountered. In such instances the gingivae may show little involvement, although in a few cases studied gingival abnormalities have been noted. The teeth show a change in alignment as though they were drifting out of position. This is more

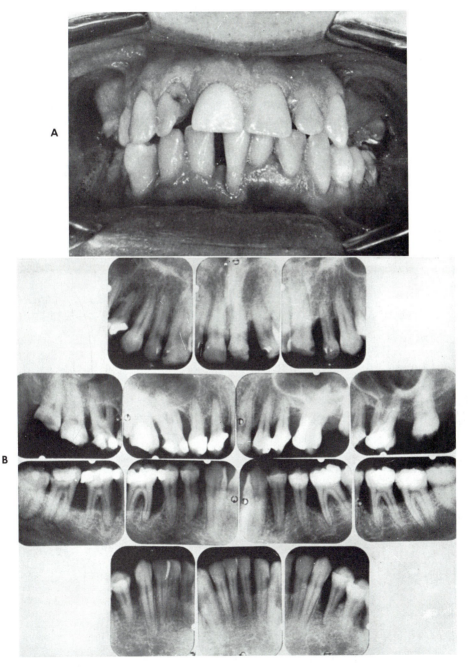

Fig. 10-23. A, Periodontosis in an 18-year-old youth. Note migration of maxillary lateral incisor and mandibular right central incisor. **B,** Teeth of patient in **A.** Note marked resorption of alveolar bone.

noticeable in the anterior portion of the dental arch, where the teeth are freer to move (Fig. 10-23). There is a marked tendency for protrusion and extrusion, with some rotation. This wandering may persist even though the tooth has moved out of occlusion. In the posterior portion the teeth lose contact with one another. Often a space may be found between the second premolar and first molar or between the first and second molars. Loosening of the teeth is an early symptom, and mobility may vary from tooth to tooth. Usually the incisors and first molars are more mobile than the premolars. This finding, however, may vary with the local factors present. Oftentimes the teeth can be depressed into the sockets even though roentgenographically the overall bone loss is not great.

Periodontosis is found in a young age group, the most common age probably being before 20 years. In our experience in some instances only the supporting tissues of the incisors and first molars are affected, whereas in other cases the periodontium throughout has been destroyed. Local factors

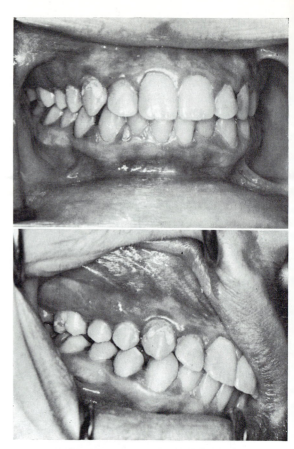

Fig. 10-24. Periodontal disease in a 16-year-old youth showing changes in gingival tissue. This case was diagnosed as periodontosis.

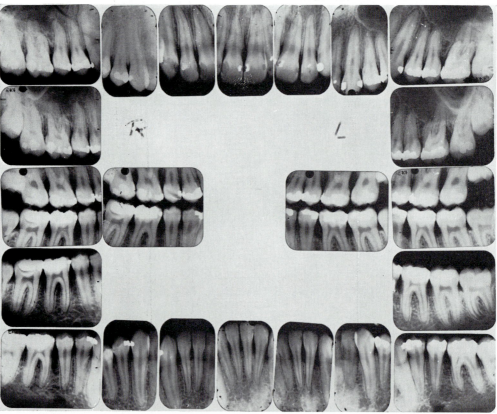

Fig. 10-25. Teeth of patient in Fig. 10-24. Note resorption of interdental bone.

probably play an important role in the course of this disease. Although the disease process may go unabated until all the teeth are lost, many patients lose only a few teeth. The remaining ones may become firm and persist with a functioning attachment apparatus.

In most cases observed, although at first glance the gingival tissue may appear well attached to the tooth surface, long narrow pockets can be found on the side of bone resorption. The tissue immediately surrounding the pockets may show practically no clinical signs of inflammation, but when the pockets are probed the tissue is easily lifted off away from the tooth surface. Bleeding is not a paramount feature as is evident in periodontitis. Late in the disease process marginal changes become prominent, and in this stage the lesion cannot be distinguished from marginal periodontitis (Figs. 10-24 and 10-25).

Roentgenographically the changes are interesting and informative. Bone loss seen roentgenographically in a well-established case is far more advanced than is clinically suspected, and often the

tooth is far looser than is imagined from the roentgenographic findings. Although vertical loss of bone is characteristic, associated advanced horizontal resorption of the alveoli is a consistent finding.

More recently periodontosis has been subdivided on an etiologic basis in which certain common factors seem to play a part in the etiology of the condition. It has been noted that periodontosis may be observed to follow a familial pattern. We have reported on two such families. In the first family all three siblings were affected, whereas in the second group two of five children developed these changes. It was not possible to demonstrate similar findings in the parents. Genetic studies in patients with periodontosis may prove to be fruitful in furthering the understanding of intrinsic factors in the production of this disease.

Periodontosis has been reported as a manifestation of a dermatologic syndrome known as hyperkeratosis palmaris et plantaris or Papillon-Lefevre syndrome. In these cases hyperkeratotic changes may be noted on the hands and feet of children

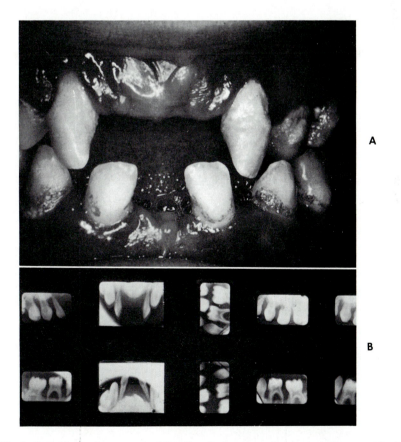

Fig. 10-26. A, Periodontosis as part of Papillon-Lefevre syndrome in a 3-year-old girl. **B,** Teeth of patient in **A.** Note severe resorptive lesion affecting alveolar process. (Courtesy Manuel Album, Philadelphia; from Cohen, D. W., and Goldman, H. M.: P. D. M., p. 3, 1962.)

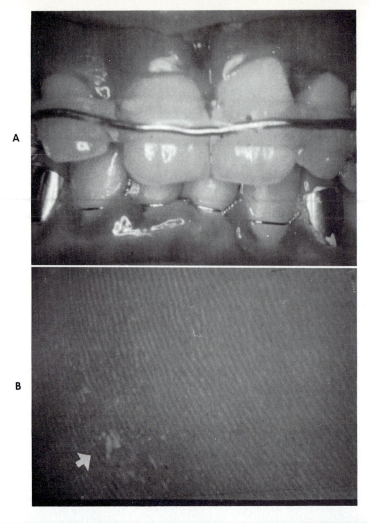

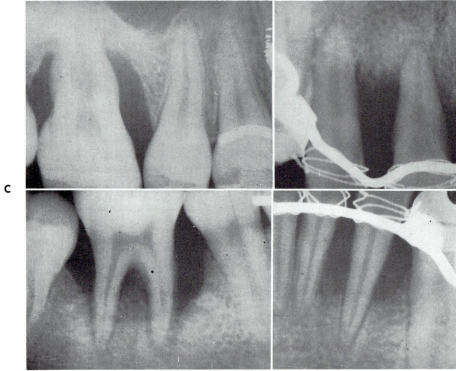

Fig. 10-27. A, Periodontosis associated with hyperkeratosis palmaris et plantaris in a 12-year-old girl. **B,** Hyperkeratotic area on plantar surface of same patient. **C,** Teeth of patient in **A** and **B.**

with severe resorption of the alveolar process about the teeth. This may occur in the primary or the permanent dentitions and may also follow familial patterns. A recent review of the literature by Ingle and a report of a new case demonstrate that hypohidrosis may also be a manifestation of this syndrome. Ingle has discussed as well the possibility of epithelial dysplasia, especially the epithelial rests of Malassez, as part of the pathogenesis of this interesting entity. Two additional cases are reported here. The first is a 3-year-old girl (Fig. 10-26, *A*) with severe destruction of the supporting structures (Fig. 10-26, *B*), causing the premature loss of the primary teeth. Dermatologic studies were shown to be consistent with the hyperkeratotic changes just described. The gingival tissues were red and inflamed. The second is a 12-year-old girl (Fig. 10-27, *A* and *B*) who had the typical vertical resorptive lesion affecting the alveolar process about the maxillary and mandibular incisors as well as the first permanent molars (Fig. 10-27, *C*). The mother mentioned that the child

had extremely dry skin, which she frequently oiled. A hyperkeratotic lesion was noted on one plantar surface (Fig. 10-27, *A* and *B*). In this case the gingival tissues were not markedly inflamed and more closely resembled the case reported by Ingle.

The report by Cohen and Morris of three cases of cyclic neutropenia with concomitant lesions of periodontosis has demonstrated the interplay between this blood dyscrasia and periodontal disease. The youngest patient was a 4-year-old boy (Fig. 10-28, *A*) with resorption of the alveolar process about the primary teeth (Fig. 10-28, *B*). In a 7-year-old girl the periodontal changes involved the mixed dentition, and in a 16-year-old girl (Fig. 10-29, *A*) several permanent teeth were lost because of periodontal disease (Fig. 10-29, *B*). Hematologic studies revealed a pattern of neutrophil count for 3 weeks followed by 1 week of neutropenia and then a return to normal levels. This cyclic pattern of the neutrophil condition was associated with ulcerations of the oral mucosa in two of their

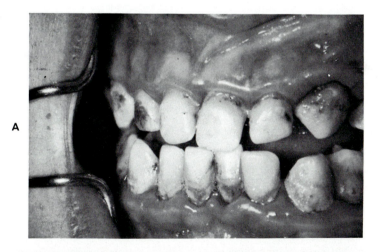

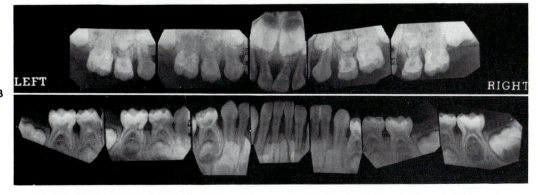

Fig. 10-28. A, Heavy stain, calculus formation, and gingival inflammation in a 4-year-old boy with cyclic neutropenia. **B,** Teeth of patient in **A.** Note horizontal resorption of alveolar and supporting bones throughout mouth.

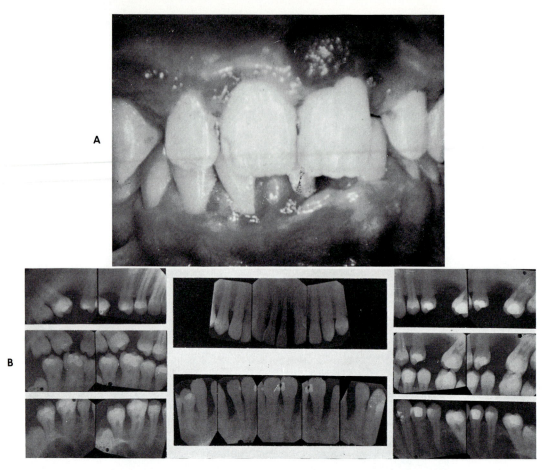

Fig. 10-29. A, Cyclic neutropenia in which red enlarged gingival tissues are observed about maxillary left central incisor and maxillary right cuspid in a 16-year-old girl. **B,** Teeth of patient in **A.** Note advanced resorptive lesion of alveolar process about maxillary and mandibular left central incisors, maxillary right cuspid, and maxillary right posterior teeth.

three cases. Cohen and Morris noted that several other incomplete reports linked periodontosis to this hematologic alteration.

A recent report on the premature loss of primary teeth in three children suffering from hypophosphatasia has linked another systemic alteration with a periodontosislike condition. It is interesting to note that microscopic examination of the exfoliated teeth from these children revealed an absence, hypoplasia, or dysplasia of cementum. It was suggested that the premature loss of teeth in patients with hypophosphatasia was due to aplasia of the cementum and the resultant lack of periodontal fiber attachment. One cannot help recalling the theory of Gottlieb in which he indicted the cementum (cementopathia) as the affected tissue in the pathogenesis of periodontosis. However, it was not obvious in Gottlieb's material that altered cementogenesis had occurred.

Periodontosis has been reported in Down's syndrome children by Cohen et al. They have written that although local factors were present in abundance, the severe alveolar bone loss and the intense inflammatory changes in the gingivae suggested a relationship between systemic factors, brain damage, and the periodontium. Of especial interest was a photomicrograph that disclosed distinct changes in the attachment apparatus, with degeneration of cementoblasts as well as osteoblasts. The arrangement of the collagen fibers was disrupted, and the fibers were almost completely absent on the bone side; remnants of the fiber apparatus were seen on the cemental side. This photomicrograph corresponds to those published for periodontosis.

REFERENCES

Album, M.: Dentistry for the handicapped child, Dent. Radiogr. Photogr. **27:**57, 1954.

Arnim, S. S., and Hagerman, D.: Connective tissue fibers of the marginal gingiva, J. Am. Dent. Assoc. **47:**271, 1953.

Bader, H., and Goldhaber, E.: The passage of intravenously injected tetracycline in the gingival sulcus of dogs, J. Oral Ther. **2:**234, 1965.

Baer, P. N.: Periodontal disease in children and adolescents, a clinical study, J. Am. Dent. Assoc. **55:**629, 1957.

Baer, P. N., Brown, K., Smith, L., Gamble, J., and Swerdlow, H.: Advanced periodontal disease in an adolescent (periodontosis), J. Periodontol. **34:**533, 1963.

Baer, P., and Socransky, S. S.: Periodontosis: case report with long-term follow-up, Periodont. Case Reports **1:**1, 1979.

Bradley, R. D.: Periodontal lesions in children: their recognition and treatment, Dent. Clin. North Am., p. 671, 1961.

Brauer, J. C., Higley, L. B., Massler, M., and Schour, I.: Dentistry for children, ed. 2, Philadelphia, 1947, The Blakiston Co.

Brauer, J. C.: Systemic and local factors in periodontic problems of the child's mouth, J. Am. Dent. Assoc. **30:**45, 1943.

Brauer, J. C.: Periodontal problems in the child patient, J. Periodontol. **11:**7, 1940.

Brill, N., and Krasse, B.: The passage of tissue fluid into the clinically healthy gingival pocket, Acta Odontol. Scand. **16:**233, 1958.

Bruckner, M.: Gingivitis and Vincent's infection in children, J. Dent. Child. **23:**116, 1956.

Bruckner, M.: Studies on the incidence and cause of dental defects in children. III. Gingivitis, J. Dent. Res. **22:**309, 1943.

Butler, J. H.: A familial pattern of juvenile periodontitis (periodontosis), J. Periodontol. **40:**115, 1969.

Carvel, R. J., Halperin, V., and Wallace, J. H.: Immunological studies in chronic severe alveolar resorptive disease: a report of two young female patients, J. Periodontol. **44:**25, 1973.

Cianciola, L. J., Genco, R. J., Patters, M. R., McKenna, J. D., and Van Oss, C. J.: Defective polymorphonuclear leukocytes' function in ahuman periodontal disease, Nature **265:**445, 1977.

Cohen, B.: Morphological factors in the pathogenesis of periodontal disease, Br. Dent. J. **107:**31, 1959.

Cohen, B.: Pathology of the interdental tissues, Dent. Pract. Dent. Rec. **9:**167, 1959.

Cohen, B.: Studies of the interdental epithelial integument, J. Dent. Res. **38:**1219, 1959.

Cohen, D. W., and Goldman, H. M.: Periodontal disease in children, P.D.M., p. 3, July, 1962.

Cohen, D. W., and Goldman, H. M.: Clinical observations on the modification of human oral tissue metabolism by local intraoral factors, Ann. N.Y. Acad. Sci. **85:**68, 1960.

Cohen, D. W., and Goldman, H. M.: Oral disease in primates, Ann. N.Y. Acad. Sci. **85:**889, 1960.

Cohen, D. W., and Morris, A. L.: Periodontal manifestations of cyclic neutropenia, J. Periodontol. **32:**159, 1961.

Cohen, M. M.: Pediatric dentistry, ed. 2, St. Louis, 1961, The C. V. Mosby Co.

Cohen, M. M., and Winer, R. A.: Dental and facial characteristics of Down's syndrome, J. Dent. Res. **44:**197, 1965.

Cohen, M. M., Winer, R. A., Schwartz, S., and Shklar, G.: Oral aspects of mongolism, Oral Surg. **14:**92, 1961.

Corson, E. F.: Keratosis palmaris et plantaris with dental alteration, Arch. Dermatol. **40:**639, 1939.

Dahl, L.: Oral hygiene habits of young children, J. Periodontol. **25:**209, 1954.

Day, C. D. M.: Oral conditions in the famine district of Hissar, J. Am. Dent. Assoc. **31:**52, 1944.

Day, C. D. M., and Shourie, K. L.: Hypertrophic gingivitis in Indian children and adolescents, Indian J. Med. Res. **35:**261, 1947.

Dekker, G., and Jansen, L. H.: Periodontosis in a child with hyperkeratosis palmoplantaris, J. Periodontol. **29:**266, 1958.

Emslie, R. D.: Cancrum oris, Dent. Pract. Dent. Rec. **13:**81, 1963.

Fish, W.: Etiology and prevention of periodontal breakdown, Dent. Prog. **1:**234, 1961.

Gottlieb, B.: Schmatzpyorrhoe, Paradental-pyorrhoe und Alveolaratrophie, Munich, 1925, Urban & Schwarzenberg.

Greene, J. C.: Periodontal disease in India; report of an epidemiological study, J. Dent. Res. **39:**302, 1960.

Greismer, R. D.: Protection against the transfer of matter through the skin. In Rothman, R. S., editor: The human integument, Washington, D. C., 1959, The American Association for the Advancement of Science.

Horton, J. E., Oppenheim, J. J., and Mergenhagen, S. E.: Elaboration of lymphotoxin by cultured human peripheral blood leukocytes stimulated with dental plaque deposits, Clin. Exp. Immunol. **13:**383, 1973.

Ingle, J.: Papillon-Lefevre syndrome; precocious periodontosis with associated epidermal lesions, J. Periodontol. **30:**239, 1959.

Irving, J. T., Newman, M. G., Socransky, S. S., et al.: Histologic changes in experimental periodontal disease in rats non-infected with a gram-negative organism, Arch. Oral Biol. **20:**219, 1975.

Kelsten, L. B.: Periodontal and soft tissue diseases in children, J. Dent. Med. **10:**67, 1955.

Kent, P. W.: Mechanisms of tooth support, Bristol, 1967, John Wright & Sons, Ltd., Medical Publishers.

Kerr, D. A.: Stomatitis and gingivitis in the adolescent and preadolescent, J. Am. Dent. Assoc. **44:**27, 1952.

King, J. D.: Gingival disease in Dundee, Dent. Record **65:**9, 32, 55, 1945.

Kohl, J. T., and Zander, H. A.: Morphology of interdental gingival tissues, Oral Surg. **14:**287, 1961.

Kronfeld, R., and Weinmann, J.: Traumatic changes in the periodontal tissues of deciduous teeth, J. Dent. Res. **19:**441, 1940.

Löe, H.: The dentogingival junction, in miles, structural and chemical organization of the teeth, vol. 2, New York, 1964, Academic Press, Inc.

Massler, M., Cohen, A., and Schour, I.: Epidemiology of gingivitis in children, J. Am. Dent. Assoc. **45:**319, 1952.

Massler, M., and Schour, I.: The P.M.A. index of gingivitis, J. Dent. Res. **28:**634, 1949.

Massler, M., Schour, I., and Chopra, B.: Occurrence of gingivitis in suburban Chicago school children, J. Periodontol. **21:**146, 1950.

McCall, J.: Gingival and periodontal disease in children, J. Periodontol. **9:**7, 1938.

McIntosh, W. G.: Gingival and periodontal disease of children, J. Periodontol. **25:**99, 1954.

Melcher, A. H., and Eastoe, J. E.: Connective tissues. In Melcher, A. H., and Bowen, W. H., editors: Biology of the periodontium, New York, 1969, Academic Press, Inc.

Miller, S. C., and Seidler, B. B.: Periodontoclasia in the young, N.Y. J. Dent. **10:**423, 1940.

Miller, S. C., Wolf, A., and Seidler, B. B.: Generalized rapid alveolar atrophy, J. Dent. Res. **19:**306, 1940.

Newman, M. G., and Socransky, S. S.: Predominant cultivable microbiota in periodontosis, J. Periodont. Res. **12:**120, 1977.

Newman, M. G., Socransky, S. S., and Listgarten, M. A.: Relationship of microorganisms to the etiology of periodontosis, I.A.D.R., Abstract no. 3240, 1974.

Newman, M. G., Socransky, S. S., Savitt, E. D., et al.: Studies of the microbiology of periodontosis, J. Periodontol. **47:**373, 1976.

Novak, A. J.: The oral manifestations of erythroblastic (Cooley's) anemia, Am. J. Orthod. **30:**539, 1944.

Page, R. C., and Schroeder, H. E.: Biochemical aspects of the connective tissue alterations in inflammatory gingival and periodontal disease, Int. Dent. J. **23:**455, 1973.

Papillon, M. M., and Lefevre, D.: Deux cas de keratoderme palmaire et plantaire symetrique familiale chez le frere et la soeur; coexistence dans les deux cas d'alterations dentaires graves, Bull. Soc. Fr. Dermatol. Syphiligr. **31:**82, 1924.

Parfitt, G. J.: Periodontal diseases in children. In Finn, S. B., editor: Clinical pedodontics, Philadelphia, 1963, W. B. Saunders Co.

Ramfjord, S., and Amslie, R.: Epidemiological studies of periodontal disease, Am. J. Public Health **58:**1713, 1968.

Ritz, H. L.: Microbial population shifts in developing human dental plaque, Arch. Oral Biol. **12:**1561, 1967.

Robinson, H. G.: Periodontitis and periodontosis in children and young adolescents, J. Am. Dent. Assoc. **43:**709, 1951.

Rosenthal, S.: Periodontosis in a child resulting in exfoliation of the teeth, J. Periodontol. **22:**101, 1951.

Ruben, M., Frankl, S. N., and Wallace, S.: Periodontal disease in the child, J. Periodontol. **42:**473, 1971.

Russell, A. L., Benjamin, E. M., and Smiley, R. D.: Periodontal disease in rural children of 25 Indiana counties, J. Periodontol. **28:**294, 1957.

Savara, B. S., Sicher, T., Everett, F. G., and Burns, A. G.: Hereditary gingival fibrosis; study of a family, J. Periodontol. **25:**12, 1954.

Schour, I., and Massler, M.: Gingival disease in postwar Italy (1945). I. Prevalence of gingivitis in various age groups: J. Am. Dent. Assoc. **35:**475, 1947.

Schour, I., and Massler, M.: Gingival disease in postwar Italy (1945). II. Gingivosis in hospitalized children in Naples, Am. J. Orthod. **33:**756, 1947.

Sheiham, A.: Epidemiology of chronic periodontal disease in western Nigerian school children, J. Perio. Rev. **3:**257, 1968.

Stahl, D., and Goldman, H. M.: The incidence of gingivitis among a sample of Massachusetts school children, Oral Surg. **6:**707, 1953.

Stallard, R. D.: Current concepts of periodontal disease, J. Dent. Child. **34:**204, 1967.

Sugarman, M. M., and Sugarman, E. F.: Precocious periodontitis; a clinical entity and a treatment responsibility, J. Periodontol. **48:**397, 1977.

Sussman, H. J., and Baer, P. N.: Three generations of periodontosis: case report, Ann. Dent. **37:**8, 1978.

Thomas, B. O. A.: The child patient as a future periodontal problem, J. Am. Dent. Assoc. **35:**763, 1947.

Waerhaug, J.: Plaque control in the treatment of juvenile periodontitis, J. Clin. Periodontol. **4:**29, 1977.

Waerhaug, J.: The gingival pocket, Odontol. Tidskr. **60**(Supp. 1):5, 1964.

Waerhaug, J.: Current concepts concerning gingival anatomy. The dynamic epithelial cuff, Dent. Clin. North Am., p. 715, 1960.

Weinreb, M.: Epithelial attachment, J. Periodontol. **31:**186, 1960.

Zappler, S. E.: Periodontal disease in children, J. Am. Dent. Assoc. **37:**33, 1948.

11 Preventive periodontics

Preventive periodontics encompasses those aspects of dental practice that deal with the establishment and maintenance of an oral environment that is conducive to the preservation of sound, healthy periodontal support to the dentition. The objectives of such practices are to promote optimum health of the periodontium, to prevent departure from the healthy state, to prevent the initial lesion that is most often gingivitis, and to intercept soft and hard tissue lesions already in progress in order to restore health and prevent further damage.

Prevention of the initial lesion is referred to as "primary prevention." Interception of the disease, once initiated, to prevent or limit disability is called "secondary prevention." Primary prevention of periodontal disease is accomplished by the avoidance or the removal of etiologic agents prior to the time when they produce deviations from health. Secondary prevention is largely therapeutic in nature. Early recognition and prompt treatment of gingivitis can prevent extension to deeper structures and loss of bone support. Therapeutic intervention to interrupt and limit bone loss also is secondary prevention, but it is instituted at a more advanced stage of the disease. Delayed recognition and treatment serve to separate these two levels of secondary prevention.

Every case in which the departure from a state of periodontal health has been so extreme that there has been extensive loss of supporting bone represents a failure to prevent or intercept the disease at an early stage. Continued neglect and failure to prevent further loss of bone support result in tooth loss.

Thus all the practices advocated in this text on periodontal therapy have prevention as an objective—the prevention of further extension of the disease and a return to health. The emphasis on prevention of disease has become evident in the legal interpretation of the role of a dentist in the treatment of a patient. A recent court decision found a dentist negligent for failing to indicate a periodontal condition to a patient and for failing to treat this condition, which reached back 15 years. It therefore behooves a dentist to be concerned with the diagnosis of incipient periodontal disease from both a professional and a legal aspect. In fact, preventive periodontics should be the constant concern not only of those providing periodontal therapy but of all dental practitioners working with viable teeth, regardless of their area of special interest. Teeth may be beautiful and carefully preserved but their value and life expectancy are dependent on the health of the structures supporting them.

NEED FOR PREVENTION

With the development and increased application of more effective measures for the prevention of dental caries and the use of improved restorative materials and techniques, more teeth are surviving the childhood years to be exposed to destructive diseases of the supporting tissues in later years. Already more teeth are lost from periodontal disease after the middle of the third decade than are lost from dental caries.

Conservative estimates based on epidemiologic studies using gross diagnostic criteria indicate that destructive periodontal disease is highly prevalent among adult populations throughout the world. A detailed study reported by Marshall-Day et al. using comprehensive diagnostic methods suggests that chronic destructive periodontal disease may affect almost all adults in this country by the age of 40 years (Fig. 11-1). These bone lesions are preceded by inflammatory changes in the gingiva

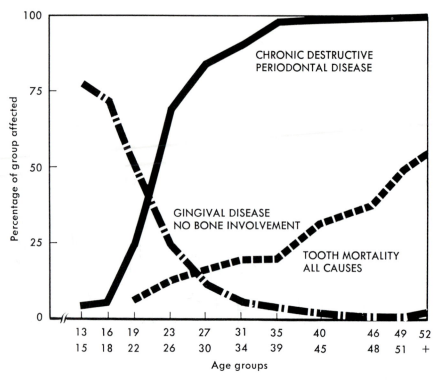

Fig. 11-1. Prevalence of periodontal disease (1187 persons). Percent of persons by age group affected with gingival disease, with no accompanying bone involvement, and percent with chronic destructive periodontal disease. Tooth mortality data are based on percent of persons in study with one or more missing teeth regardless of cause. Edentulous cases were not included. (From Marshall-Day, C. D., Stephens, R. G., and Quigley, L. F.: J. Periodontol. **26:**185, 1955.)

that usually have their inception early in life. In the same study, 77% of the youngest age group (13 to 15 years) had gingivitis. In a study of 602 fourteen-year-old schoolchildren in England using a standard radiographic technique, evidence of chronic periodontitis was found in 51.5% of the children examined.

It is obvious from these data that the periodontal disease problem is of overwhelming proportions. It would be impossible to provide treatment for more than a small fraction of the number already affected. The only possible solution to this major health problem is prevention: primary prevention, or prevention of gingivitis, and early secondary prevention, or prevention of the extension of gingivitis to the deeper structures in order to intercept and reverse the disease before there has been loss of supporting bone. Once destructive disease has begun, therapeutic and maintenance requirements become more extensive, increasing the man-hours needed to prevent further extension.

The great number of persons developing advanced destructive periodontal disease empha-

sizes the need for the dental profession to apply all available measures on as wide a scale as possible for the primary or early secondary prevention of this disease.

Some questions should invariably arise in the mind of the dentist confronted with an advanced periodontal disease case. What circumstances permitted this disease to reach such an advanced stage? What might have been done to interrupt the progress of the disease at an earlier stage? The answers may be accusatory in that they may point to the failure of the dentist or the patient to apply the knowledge at hand; or they may be provocative and create a desire to explore the literature or to conduct research to determine what can be done to prevent or interrupt the disease process at an earlier stage in the next patient.

PREVENTIVE MEASURES: FACTS AND INFERENCES
Population studies

Numerous descriptive epidemiologic studies have identified and compared variations in the prevalence and severity of periodontal disease.

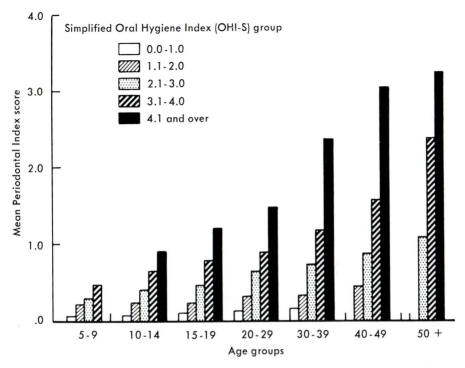

Fig. 11-2. Mean Periodontal Index scores by age group and Simplified Oral Hygiene Index score group for 3,851 civilians examined in Ecuador and Montana. (From Greene, J. C.: Am. J. Public Health **53:**913, 1963.)

They have been made in diverse populations in many parts of the world, with concomitant variations in selected biologic, social, economic, and environmental factors. Such studies have been conducted to describe the magnitude and nature of the periodontal disease problem in various population groups. Another major objective of such descriptive epidemiologic studies has been to identify factors that are associated with variations in the occurrence and severity of the disease. Subsequent investigations of the associated factors may provide the basis for developing effective methods of prevention and control.

When such factors as age, race, sex, socioeconomic status, educational attainment, place of residence, nutritional status, diet, occlusion, and oral hygiene are each compared separately with periodontal disease severity, some highly significant associations can be found. However, when persons with equal oral hygiene status and age are compared the relationships between the other factors and periodontal disease are virtually nonexistent.

The association between oral hygiene and periodontal disease is so strong and so consistent in all populations studied that it may overwhelm associations with other variables. In comparison, associations with any of the other variables except age are weak and inconsistent. The association with age is not completely removed when the effect of the oral hygiene variable is accounted for. Probably the association between disease severity and age in these studies is primarily an expression of the effects of prolonged exposure to local factors included in the oral hygiene assessments rather than to the aging process alone. However, it is possible that with increasing age the ability of the periodontal tissues to ward off harmful effects of the local factors is decreased.

The fact that only age and oral hygiene have been demonstrated to have consistent relationships with periodontal disease does not mean that other factors are not associated with the disease. They may simply be masked by the strong association with oral hygiene. It may be that the study methods available today just are not adequate for identifying other significant associations.

Data from a study conducted in Ecuador and Montana provide a good demonstration of the oral hygiene–periodontal disease relationship seen in descriptive population studies (Fig. 11-2).

In each age group in the Ecuador-Montana study persons with poor oral hygiene status had poor periodontal health. Conversely those with cleaner mouths had healthier periodontal tissues. It appears from these data that if a person were

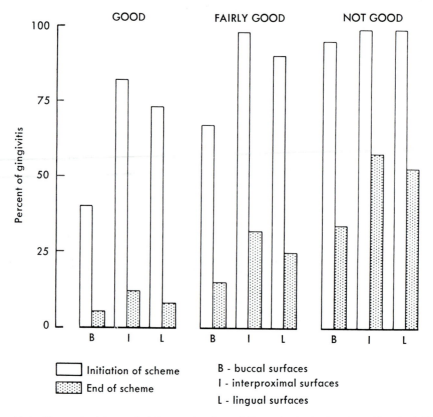

Fig. 11-3. Percent of buccal, interproximal, and lingual gingival units with gingivitis at initiation and at end of a 5-year study according to oral hygiene group. Participants were grouped according to quality of oral hygiene practices at beginning of study. These data are from a study of effects of scaling and controlled oral hygiene conducted on 808 persons. (From Lövdal, A., Arno, A., Schei, O., and Waerhaug, J.: Acta Odontol. Scand. **19:**537, 1961.)

to maintain no better than a fair level of oral cleanliness over a sufficient length of time he would develop serious destructive periodontal disease. On the other hand, the data suggest that if a person were to maintain a good level of oral cleanliness from age 5 to 50 years, he probably would avoid advanced destructive periodontal disease during this major portion of life.

Data from descriptive epidemiologic studies provide pertinent information about the natural history of a disease and its relation to specific variables. However, such data are derived from cross-sectional observations of population groups and do not provide proof of a cause-and-effect relationship. They do not prove that the disease resulted from the accumulation of debris and calculus on the teeth, that persons with poor periodontal health at the age of 50 years had poor oral hygiene at age 10 years, or that persons with poor oral hygiene scores at the age of 10 years will have advanced destructive disease at age 50 years. However, the findings are so consistent and the associations so strong and so compatible with clinical experience that detailed prospective studies have been undertaken to investigate the effects of oral cleanliness on periodontal health in the anticipation that such studies will provide data on which to base preventive practices.

Additional data supporting the assumption that oral hygiene status does play a significant role in periodontal disease are provided from a prospective study conducted by Lövdal et al. This group of investigators attempted to "evaluate the combined effect of subgingival scaling and controlled oral hygiene, i.e., measures which are focused on removal of local irritants in the form of calculus, bacterial plaques, food debris and overhanging margins of restorations." The objective was to evaluate the effects of keeping the mouth essentially free of local irritants throughout the study period. A 5-year study of these factors was conducted on 808 participants. A baseline assessment of percent of gingival units was obtained at the beginning of the study.

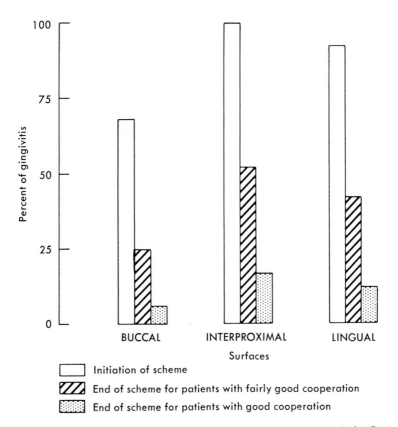

Fig. 11-4. Percent of gingival units with gingivitis at initiation and at end of a 5-year study on effects of oral hygiene according to quality of oral hygiene maintained during study. Levels of oral hygiene maintenance are described in terms of patient cooperation. (From Lövdal, A., Arno, A., Schei, O., and Waerhaug, J.: Acta Odontol. Scand. **19**:537, 1961.)

Each patient received a thorough scaling for removal of all supragingival and subgingival calculus deposits after being instructed in proper toothbrushing and use of toothpicks. Calculus deposits were removed at least every 6 months and every 3 months for those who deposited calculus more rapidly. To avoid introducing more variables, other treatments such as gingivectomy or occlusal adjustments were not given.

The results of the study are depicted in Fig. 11-3. The study population was divided into three groups, based on their oral hygiene practices before the study started without reference to their clinical scores. The figure shows the percent of buccal, interproximal, and lingual areas inflamed at the beginning and at the end of the study. Each of the gingival units in each of the groups had markedly less inflammatory involvement at the end of the study than at the beginning. The improvement was much more makred in the group classified as having good oral hygiene practices before the study started than it was in the other

two groups. The greater response in the group with the best personal oral hygiene practices emphasizes the importance of combined home and professional care.

The significance of good home care is further emphasized by the data shown in Fig. 11-4. The reduction in the percent of gingival units inflamed was far greater in the group practicing good oral hygiene during the study period.

A study reported by Braentzaeg and Jamison has added similar but additional support from a military population. Löe et al. demonstrated that when all oral hygiene measures are withdrawn, healthy persons accumulate soft debris and develop marginal gingivitis in just a few days. The time varied from 10 to 21 days. Reinstatement of oral hygiene measures resulted in a return to healthy gingival conditions and reestablishment of the original bacterial flora. The individual rate of gingivitis development was closely correlated with the rate of plaque accumulation. The gingival inflammation in an area usually disappeared 1 day after the plaque had been removed.

A study by Lindhe et al. reported the effect of regularly repeated professional tooth cleaning on oral hygiene status, gingivitis, and dental caries. Over a 2-year period Swedish schoolchildren were provided with oral prophylaxis performed by a dental nurse every 2 weeks as well as detailed instruction on toothbrushing. During the third year of study the interval between prophylactic sessions was lengthened to 4 weeks in the younger age group and 8 weeks in the older age group. The study indicated that it was possible to maintain a high standard of oral hygiene in the schoolchildren and that marginal gingivitis present at the outset of the study in test children disappeared almost entirely.

Suomi et al. (1971) reported on a 3-year study

to test the hypothesis that the development and progression of gingival inflammation and destructive periodontal disease are retarded in an oral environment in which high levels of hygiene are maintained. After 3 years oral hygiene scores in the control group were four times greater than in the experimental group (Fig. 11-5). Also the gingival inflammation scores were greater in the control group than in the experimental group. The rate of loss of epithelial attachment was more than three times greater in the control group than in the experimental group. Lightner et al. in a study of 470 Air Force Academy recruits divided into test groups with varying frequencies of preventive treatment and varying amounts of toothbrushing instruction found that the groups with the greatest number of preventive appointments (3 to 4 per year) plus toothbrushing instruction at each appointment had the lowest percentage of men affected by loss of epithelial attachment. Groups receiving toothbrushing instruction showed significantly larger decreases in plaque scores than groups that had only prophylaxis without instruction. These findings provide strong evidence to support the importance of good oral hygiene in maintaining periodontal health. These studies also emphasize the importance of patient involvement in the routine maintenance of oral hygiene as well as the necessity of continual professional reinforcement either by dentists or dental auxiliaries.

Laboratory studies

A long-term laboratory study using the beagle hound was conducted to explore further the oral hygiene–periodontal disease relationship. In the study one group of animals had diagonally opposite quadrants of their dentition cleaned every other day. Every 3 months the amount of debris, calculus, and gingival inflammation in the animals were assessed and recorded. Also measurements were made of the distance from notches cut in the teeth to the bottom of adjacent gingival sulci, and roentgenograms were taken every 3 months.

The dogs accumulated large deposits of debris and calculus and developed marked gingival inflammation in the uncleaned areas while there were no significant changes in the cleaned quadrants (Figs. 11-6 and 11-7). The periodontal measurements from the notches to the bottom sulcus increased earlier and more rapidly in the uncleaned quadrants than in the cleaned areas. Marked roentgenographic changes occurred in the un-

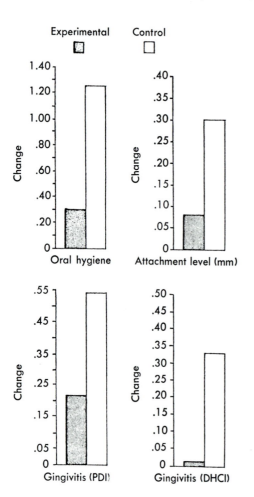

Fig. 11-5. Change in mean oral hygiene, gingivitis, and attachment scores from baseline to 3-year examination for large experimental and control groups. (From Suomi, J. D., Greene, J. C., Vermillion, J. R., Doyle, J., Chang, J. J., and Leatherwood, E. C.: J. Periodontol. **42:**152, 1971.)

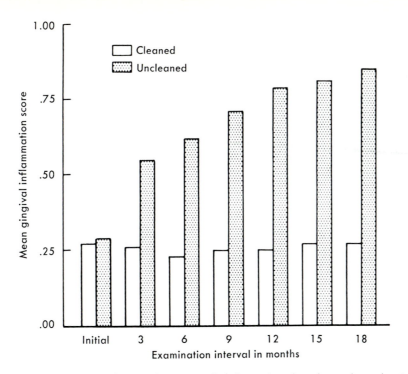

Fig. 11-6. Mean gingival inflammation scores for cleaned and uncleaned quadrants of 39 dogs at 3-month intervals during an 18-month period. Half of each dog's mouth was cleaned every 48 hours. (From Saxe, S. R., Greene, J. C., Bohannan, H. M., and Vermillion, J. R.: Periodontics **5:**217, 1967.)

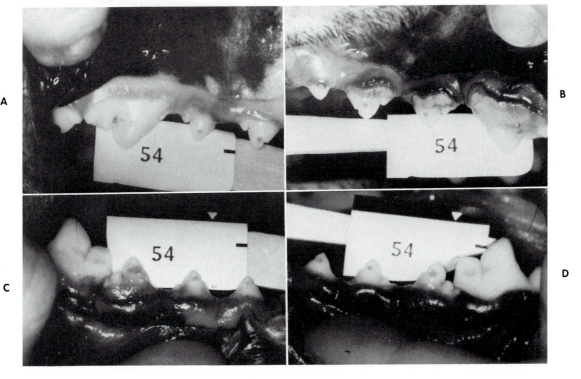

Fig. 11-7. Teeth of one of dogs (no. 54) used in a study of preventive effect of controlled oral hygiene. **A** and **D,** Quadrants cleaned every other day during study period. **B** and **C,** Quadrants not cleaned during study. Note inflammatory changes adjacent to calculus deposits. (From Saxe, S. R., Greene, J. C., Bohannan, H. M., and Vermillion, J. R.: Periodontics **5:**217, 1967.)

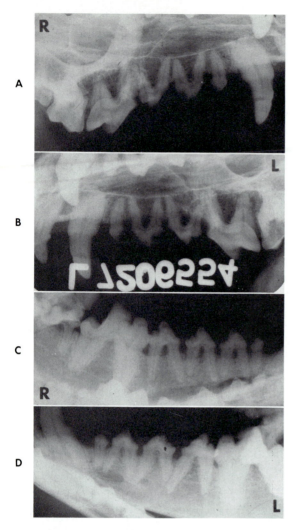

cleaned areas of the majority of the dogs while changes in the cleaned areas were minimal (Fig. 11-8). In another group of dogs, cleaning of previously uncleaned areas in one third of the colony resulted in a dramatic return of the gingivitis scores to approximately the same level as in the opposite quadrants (Fig. 11-9).

These data from a controlled laboratory study provide still more evidence in support of the assumption that keeping debris and calculus deposits off the teeth interferes in the periodontal disease process and that inflammatory changes can be reversed by their removal.

Study inferences

Descriptive epidemiologic and prospective clinical studies in human beings and prospective laboratory studies in dogs have demonstrated that lack of oral cleanliness plays a dominant role in the initiation and progression of periodontal disease. These studies do not rule out the involvement of other factors in the disease process. However, practical application of preventive measures need not await complete knowledge of all causes and effects. Debris or plaque and calculus, which are the factors considered in an assessment of oral hygiene status, may act directly as mechanical irritants to the gingiva. Probably of far greater significance is the bacterial flora that thrives in an unclean mouth and produces substances that may have more direct harmful effects on the periodontal tissue.

These studies also emphasize the need for combined home and professional care to make prevention and control a reality. It is evident that neglect is the chief cause of periodontal disease, that is, neglect on the part of the patient or the dentist or both.

Fig. 11-8. Teeth of same dog (no. 54) in Fig. 11-7. **A** and **D,** Quadrants cleaned every other day during study period. **B** and **C,** Quadrants not cleaned during study. Note difference in bone height in cleaned and uncleaned quadrants. (From Saxe, S. R., Greene, J. C., Bohannan, H. M., and Vermillion, J. R.: Periodontics **5:**217, 1967.)

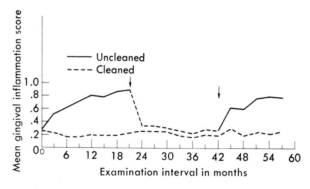

Fig. 11-9. Mean gingival inflammation scores on cleaned and uncleaned sides by examination interval for 12 beagles having changed cleaning regimen. (From Greene, J. C., and Vermillion, J. R.: J. Dent. Res. **50:**188, 1971.)

LOCAL PREVENTIVE MEASURES
The dentist's responsibilities

Early diagnosis. Early diagnosis should be the aim of every practitioner concerned with the health of the periodontium. Every dental problem that brings the patient to the dental office offers an opportunity for examination, early diagnosis, and advice, not only concerning treatment of that problem and prevention of further disability from it but also concerning the remaining dental health potential of the patient. The chronic destructive phase of periodontal disease is almost always preceded by gingivitis. It is important to detect and treat periodontal disease before it reaches the destructive phase, while it is limited to gingival inflammation, and while the pathologic process is reversible. Disease neglected until irreversible changes in the bone have taken place is much more difficult to treat, and because of the altered anatomy the mouth is much more difficult to maintain in a healthy condition, once treated.

In the study reported in Fig. 11-1 it was noted that even in the youngest age groups a very high percentage of the population had gingival inflammation. However, before age 17 to 18 years only a small percentage had developed chronic destructive disease. Although the evidence is unclear as to the actual onset of chronic destructive disease, since in one study (Hull et al.) this condition was demonstrable in 51.5% of a 14-year-old population, it appears that chronic destruction, although present, is still limited in teenagers. Thus it would be well to pay particular attention to patients in their early teens and to diagnose and treat their periodontal lesions while they are completely reversible. All too often both the patient and the dentist permit the disease to progress beyond the early stages until treatment is extensive, probability of success is reduced, and maintenance is made more difficult. Such unfortunate acts of omission result in extensive treatment that is costly to the patient and costly in terms of utilization of already overextended highly trained personnel.

Clinical examination. Prevention begins with the clinical examination. Patients should be given a thorough examination of the entire mouth at least every 12 months. For many people an examination every 6 months is probably necessary. It is important that the examinations include a search for existing or possible contributory factors as well as for periodontal disease. The examination should include an evaluation and charting of gingival status, bone support, oral hygiene, faulty contacts, overhanging margins of restorations, unfilled cavities, and unequal distribution of occlusal stresses. This information should be recorded for treatment planning purposes and for evaluating changes at subsequent dental visits.

Recorded assessments of gingival status should indicate the nature and location of the pathology; for example, the presence or absence of gingivitis may be recorded for each buccal and lingual gingival papilla and margin. The total number of units judged as affected can be used as the patient's score for comparison with subsequent examinations. A similar approach is useful in keeping account of hyperplastic changes in the gingiva.

Bone support may be determined by the use of a probe (to locate the position of the epithelial attachment in relation to a fixed point on the tooth) and by the use of radiographs. Pocket measurements may be made by using a calibrated periodontal probe to measure the distance from the crest of the gingiva to the cementoenamel junction and from the crest of the gingiva to the bottom of the gingival sulcus. The difference between the two measurements is an indication of how far apically the attachment has migrated. The measurements should be made at the mesial and distal interproximal surfaces as well as at the middle of the buccal and lingual surfaces. In areas where extensive pocket formation appears likely continuous probing to distinctly define the contour of the pocket may be useful.

Periapical radiographs provide a permanent record of the bone height and density. However, because of problems of angulation, exposure, and superimposition the radiograph alone is not adequate for evaluation of the bony support. It should not be necessary to repeat the full set of radiographs more frequently than every 12 months. If other parts of the examination reveal no significant changes from the time that the last radiographs were taken the periapical films can be repeated as infrequently as every 24 months unless otherwise indicated.

The status of oral hygiene, on the other hand, should be assessed and recorded at each recall visit. This can best be done with the aid of a disclosing solution or wafer so that the soft deposits are seen easily by both the dentist and the patient. The location and quantity of stained plaques and supragingival and subgingival calculus deposits should be recorded systematically. One way is to apply the scoring criteria of the Simplified Oral Hygiene Index, as reported by Greene and Vermillion in 1964, to each buccal and lingual surface. It is necessary to record the status of oral cleanliness in a systematic way so that it can be repeated in the same way each time that the patient returns. This method provides a way of evaluating the adequacy of the patient's oral hygiene practices and rate of calculus formation.

All interproximal contacts should be examined to determine whether they are sufficiently tight and properly placed to deflect food into the interproximal embrasures as they should. Contacts that are loose or improperly placed should be noted on the chart and corrected, since they encourage wedging of food.

All restorations should be examined for open or overhanging margins because in addition to causing mechanical irritation they provide excellent places for bacterial plaque to form and are almost impossible to keep clean. The radiographs should be examined carefully both for the adequacy of restoration margins and for the proper contour of interproximal restorations. Each tooth should be examined carefully for new or recurrent caries. Open carious lesions not only are a direct threat to the tooth, but they also provide a protected environment for bacterial plaques to thrive and produce substances harmful to the supporting tissues.

Distribution of occlusal forces can be examined by using marking tapes or wax bites. The pattern of occlusal wear should be observed so that clues to premature occlusal contacts, bruxism, or other unusual or harmful bite habits can be obtained.

Use of dental auxiliaries. The dentist is responsible for the examination of the oral cavity and the diagnosis of disease. A definitive treatment plan should be made for every patient after the clinical and radiographic examination including frequency of oral prophylaxis and oral hygiene instruction. Although the dentist manages the total oral care of the patient, most dentists delegate appropriate duties to dental auxiliaries. The increasing availability of dental hygienists has greatly changed the delivery of preventive services. In 1965 there were only 11,600 active hygienists in the United States, or 12 hygienists for each 100 dentists. By 1977 the number almost tripled to 32,200, or 27 hygienists for each 100 active dentists. In addition dental assistants have increased from 87,350 in 1965 to 144,700 in 1977. Dentists now tend to delegate oral prophylaxis to hygienists, and as indicated in a 1974 American Dental Association survey dentists tend to delegate personal oral hygiene education to hygienists and to a lesser extent dental assistants.

The increased use of dental auxiliaries augers well for an increase in preventive procedures available to the public. Responsibility, however, lies with the dentist for total management of the patient even though specific tasks may be delegated.

Oral prophylaxis. Oral prophylaxis is one of the essential elements of a preventive program. The term as generally used in dentistry refers to the process of cleaning the teeth. A thorough prophylaxis should include—

1. Removal of all supragingival and subgingival calculus deposits
2. Planing of all roughened root surfaces
3. Removal of all extrinsic stains and bacterial plaques
4. Correction of overhanging restorations and improperly contoured restorations
5. Polishing of all tooth and restoration surfaces
6. Application of caries-preventive agents
7. Home care instruction

A disclosing solution should be used before the prophylaxis to stain the plaques adherent to the teeth so that the dentist or hygienist can easily see where the soft deposits are located and again after the prophylaxis has been completed to make certain that they have all been removed. The stained material should be removed with a rubber cup and prophylactic paste. All calcified deposits should be completely removed with sharp instruments while care is taken to produce minimum trauma to the gingiva. To adequately complete the task more than one session is often necessary.

After all calculus, stain, and plaque have been removed the surfaces of all teeth and restorations should be smoothed and polished with a rubber cup and polishing paste.

The oral prophylaxis should be repeated at regular intervals. The rate of calculus deposition varies greatly from person to person and with age and will change with significant changes in daily home care. Therefore the time interval between prophylaxes should be varied to suit the needs of the individual. Patients who seldom have new carious lesions and only very slight supragingival calculus deposits after 6 months and who are conscientious about their home care need be seen only every 12 months. Patients with a high caries attack rate should be seen at least every 6 months and given a prophylaxis each time. Patients who have had extensive periodontal therapy and have even moderate supragingival or subgingival calculus deposits after 6 months or who need to be reminded frequently about the importance of good home care probably should be scheduled for recall every 3 or 4 months until the situation is under better control.

No prophylaxis should be considered complete without advising the patient of the proper oral hygiene measures to be used at home. The office appointment is to do only what the patient cannot do himself and then to instruct him how to accomplish his portion of the task of maintaining a healthy mouth.

Treatment. Treatment of diagnosed periodontal pathology should be accomplished as early in the disease process as possible to prevent further damage. Detailed descriptions of the latest methods of treatment are located elsewhere in this text. However, it should be remembered that the objective of all periodontal therapy is to intercept the disease so as to prevent further progression and to return the mouth to a healthy condition that can be maintained. For periodontal therapy to be successful all local irritants must be removed and the mouth placed in such a condition that it is possible for the patient to remove the soft deposits in his daily care.

All carious lesions should be restored and faulty restorations replaced. Properly contoured restorations properly placed contribute significantly to periodontal health. All restoration margins should end either below or well above the gingival margin. The margins should be flush with the tooth surface in order not to create a place for debris to collect. The contour of interproximal restorations should restore firm contact and deflect food into the embrasures and not into the gingival sulcus. Occlusion should be checked, and premature contacts or uneven distribution of occlusal forces should be corrected.

Restorations should reconstitute occlusal dimensions of the teeth so that they are in harmonious contact with the adjacent and opposing teeth. Removable appliances should not place undue lateral or vertical stresses on the teeth or gingiva. Clasps should be kept far enough away from the gingiva to avoid trapping of food at the gingival crest.

Education and motivation of patient. Education and motivation of the patient to take care of his own mouth are essential for effective prevention and control of periodontal disease. Preventive periodontics is a partnership affair. Daily personal care by the patient is perhaps more important than what the dentist does for him. The finest work performed by the dentist or hygienist can be wasted if the patient neglects to take care of his own mouth. The patient must be told and shown that periodontal disease is insidious and usually asymptomatic. The precise status of his own periodontal health should be explained to him. What he personally can do to avoid losing his teeth from this disease should be explained clearly.

Following periodontal therapy it is essential for the patient to maintain good oral hygiene. Lindhe and Nyman in a study of patients with severe destruction of the periodontal tissues who received extensive periodontal therapy found that after a 5-year period no further loss of periodontal support occured. These patients were maintained in a 3- to 6-month recall program that included prophylaxis performed by a dental hygienist and repeated instruction in oral hygiene. Five years after treatment, plaque scores dropped from an average pretreatment level of 1.6 to 0.34.

Patients should be shown areas of gingivitis and stained plaques in their own mouths after disclosing solutions have been applied. They should be shown how to maneuver a toothbrush to clean all areas of the mouth, especially those areas that they have been missing. The technique of showing patients samples of plaque taken from their own mouths under a phase microscope is used to impress on them the need for daily home care. Patient motivation requires frequent reinforcement. Therefore every recall visit should include an evaluation of oral hygiene status and a comparison with the record made at the previous session. The patient should be advised of his progress and told how he can do a better job. The oral hygiene habit should be encouraged and developed by the time the child is 2 or 3 years of age or as young as possible, and it should be reinforced by the dentist at every opportunity.

To motivate patients to perform prescribed oral hygiene practices conscientiously and over a long period of time requires time, patience, and ingenuity. But unless the effort is successfully made, the treatment provided will in large part be rendered ineffective. To be successful in transferring the information to his patients in a convincing way the dentist must be a firm believer in the importance of proper oral hygiene and must practice it conscientiously himself.

Preventive maintenance. After a patient has received periodontal therapy and his mouth has been returned to good health, it is essential that he be placed on a preventive maintenance regimen. The regimen of choice will depend on the extent of destruction caused by the disease and the treatment employed to intercept it. The greater the alteration of the original oral anatomy, the more rigid the regimen should be.

The treated patient has already demonstrated that he is susceptible to the disease. He has neglected his mouth sufficiently to permit the disease to progress until treatment is necessary and the anatomy of his periodontium has been altered. Therefore close surveillance of the patient with treated periodontal disease is essential to prevent deviation from the healthy state that has been restored. Follow-up visits to the dental office should be prescribed according to the needs of each patient. They should be frequent enough to ensure that the patient is keeping the mouth clean and that any new pathologic changes receive prompt attention. The patient's need for care by the dentist does not end with successful treatment; it continues through maintenance of the health that has been restored.

Follow-up visits to the dental office at prescribed intervals are necessary so that the dentist or hygienist can remove accumulated calculus deposits before they cause too much damage. At the follow-up visits the dentist should evaluate the patient's progress, treat any lesions, and remove local irritants that may have developed since the last visit. Previous efforts to motivate the patient to follow conscientiously the prescribed home care regimen should be reinforced at every opportunity.

The patient's responsibilities: daily care

Daily care of the mouth by the patient is the most important phase of preventive periodontics. Techniques for keeping the mouth clean are discussed fully in Chapter 18 so they are only mentioned briefly here. It is incumbent upon the patient to follow the oral hygiene practices prescribed for him by his dentist. Since the objective of the patient's role in prevention of periodontal disease is to keep the teeth and gingiva free of soft deposits, he should make use of all aids available to him. Among the aids to oral health care are toothbrushes, toothpastes, floss interdental stimulators, and dental irrigators. The importance of thorough daily flossing to dislodge interproximal plaque is becoming more generally accepted as the inadequateness of brushing is more fully realized. The effectiveness of dental irrigators in the removal of plaque and loosely attached food debris remains to be documented, but clinically they appear to have considerable promise when used in conjunction with brushes and floss and not instead of them. They are of particular value to some physically handicapped individuals or patients wearing orthodontic appliances.

Disclosing wafers help the patient to evaluate the effectiveness of his cleansing efforts. Their use should be repeated occasionally to make certain that areas are not being habitually overlooked.

The value of gingival massage as a means of prevention is open to question. Although many practitioners believe that this is an essential element of oral physiotherapy, there is little or no evidence to support its use as a preventive measure. However, to the extent that such massage removes or detaches bacterial plaques from the gingiva it should be beneficial. Future research may show that gingival massage in the absence of disease helps to develop positive health of the periodontium and thus helps to prevent the initiation of periodontal disease, but today its use for this purpose is empirical.

Prevention and removal of calculus

Bacterial plaques are precursors of dental calculus. Therefore one of the most effective methods for preventing the deposition of calculus is frequent and thorough cleansing of the teeth by the patient himself. The rate of calculus formation is greater in persons who are heavy pipe or cigarette smokers. Thus in those who smoke the rate of calculus deposition may be decreased by giving up the smoking habit. Removal of rough surfaces to which plaque attaches also helps to decrease calculus formation.

Considerable developmental research is being conducted today to develop calculus inhibiting agents. Mandel states that research efforts to develop methods of plaque control that are not dependent on patient-oriented mechanical removal have focused on five approaches: (1) alteration of the tooth surface to interfere with pellicle or bacterial adhesion, (2) antibacterial or antibiotic agents aimed at preventing proliferation of all or specific bacteria, (3) enzymes to disperse the matrix that holds plaque together, (4) monenzymatic, mucolytic, dispersing denaturing agents that can alter the structure of the plaque, and (5) dietary modification, which can reduce adhesion, prolification, or metabolic activity of plaque bacteria.

To date none of these approaches has provided an acceptable preventive agent suitable for generalized use. The most widely researched agent, utilizing the antibacterial approach, is chlorhexidine gluconate. A 0.2% aqueous solution of chlorhexidine gluconate used as a mouthwash twice daily appears to prevent the formation of plaque. Löe et al. in a 2-year study found that a group using a daily mouth rinse of 10 ml of 0.2% aqueous chlorhexidine gluconate in addition to toothbrushing and interdental cleansing had reduced plaque and gingivitis as compared with a group using a placebo mouthwash, brushing, and interdental cleansing. A significant side effect, however, was staining of the teeth. Other studies reported staining of both teeth and tongue. These stains could be removed by dental prophylaxis. Clorhexidine utilized in dentifrices or in topically applied gels does not appear to have a significant effect in reducing plaque formation. Chlorhexidine is still in the experimental stage, but the concept of a plaque control method that requires relatively little patient effort is worth pursuing.

Investigations of the effect of diet on early plaque formation in animals and in man offer some promise for possible prevention of this precursor of calculus. It appears that the intake of sucrose markedly encourages plaque growth. Perhaps someday removal of certain elements from the diet or addition of others will be used to control plaque formation and thus calculus deposition.

SYSTEMIC PREVENTIVE MEASURES

The evidence available today indicates that local irritants are the major factors that initiate periodontal disease. Control of these local irritants interferes in the disease process and slows or stops its progression. There is no doubt that systemic factors such as metabolism, nutrition, and hormonal balance have an effect on the physiologic actions and reactions of the oral tissues to local irritation. The inflammatory and destructive periodontal changes initiated by local irritants may be accentuated by disturbances of these systemic factors. In some cases to get satisfactory resolution of the periodontal pathology it may be necessary to correct the systemic disturbance as well as to bring the local environment under control.

The systemic approach to primary prevention of periodontal disease by rendering the local tissues more resistant to the local environment has not been developed. However, it stands to reason that all tissues, to function normally, must have proper nutrients, which can be supplied only if there is proper dietary intake and subsequent metabolic preparation. Determining the upper and lower limits of the proper dietary intake for periodontal

health has not been successfully accomplished today. The literature is confusing on the subject of nutrition and periodontal health. Therefore today there is no conclusive evidence on which to base recommendations for the use of specific systemic measures for the prevention and control of periodontal disease.

However, certain systemic disorders do have periodontal manifestations. The blood vessel changes in diabetes and the attachment apparatus changes in scleroderma are examples of these problems. These conditions must be recognized by the examiner. The effects of local irritants certainly become exaggerated under the influences of these underlying systemic conditions such as diabetes, rheumatic heart disease, or leukemia, or on medication such as Dilatin must be admonished to adhere to a rigid oral hygiene regimen.

PRACTICING PREVENTION

Prevention of primary lesions in the periodontium or of secondary damage must be of continuing concern to the dental practitioner if he is to carry out his full responsibility to his consumers. However, working toward the development of a preventive practice offers some difficult challenges initially. Once the practice with major emphasis on prevention has been established, and the majority of patients are returning regularly for evaluation, prophylaxis, and routine preventive maintenance, both the dentist and his clientele are better satisfied. After this type of practice has been in effect for some time, it is seldom necessary to subject patients to major reconstructive procedures that are difficult and taxing for both the patient and the dentist.

The dentist who has entered into an alliance for prevention with his patient has an opportunity to intercept pathologic processes with relatively simple and routine procedures. He seldom is asked to make do or compromise because of delayed diagnoses.

The philosophy of preventive dentistry gives meaning and purpose to the practice of dentistry and guides therapeutic actions, making them a means of reaching the goal of establishing and preserving a healthy mouth for the total well-being of the patient.

Dental practice based on the philosophy of prevention is personally and professionally more rewarding because the dentist can take satisfaction from knowing that he is contributing more to the present and long-term health and well-being of his patients and his community.

SUMMARY

Periodontal disease is so prevalent that the only possible solution to the problem is prevention. According to what is known today the local factors, debris or plaque and calculus, play a major role in the periodontal disease process. Available data suggest that faithful adherence to proper oral hygiene practices should be at least as effective in controlling periodontal disease as fluoridation is in controlling dental caries.

Preventive periodontics requires the active involvement of both dentist and patient. In order to discharge his responsibilities to his patients the dentist must keep the health of the supporting tissues in mind at all times regardless of his special area of practice. Early diagnosis and treatment are essential. The disease should be intercepted in the earliest stage possible to prevent irreversible damage. Local irritants must be removed, and necessary treatment must be given to make it possible for the patient to keep his mouth clean. The patient must be motivated to follow faithfully the oral hygiene practices that have been prescribed and to return for periodic evaluation and prophylaxis. The effectiveness of preventive and control procedures is dependent upon how well the patient follows through with his daily care.

Much more is yet to be learned about the influence of systemic factors such as metabolic disturbances, malnutrition, hormonal disturbances, or systemic diseases on the health of the periodontium. However, application of practical preventive measures need not and should not await complete knowledge of all causes and effects.

REFERENCES

Adams, R. J., and Stanmeyer, W. R.: The effects of a closely supervised oral hygiene program upon oral cleanliness, J. Periodontol. **31:**242, 1960.

Aleece, A. A., and Forscher, B. K.: Calculus reduction with a mucinase dentifrice, J. Periodontol. **25:**122, 1954.

ADA: Legislation and litigation, J. Am. Dent. Assoc. **89:**764, 1974.

ADA Bureau of Economic Research and Statistics: Survey of needs for dental care. II. Dental needs according to age and sex of patients, J. Am. Dent. Assoc. **46:**200, 1953.

Arnim, S. S.: Dental irrigators for oral hygiene, periodontal therapy and prevention of dental disease, J. Tenn. Dent. Assoc. **47:**65, 1967.

Arnim, S. S.: Prevention of dental disease, Pediatr. Clin. North Am. **10:**275, 1963.

Arnim, S. S.: The use of disclosing agents for measuring tooth cleanliness, J. Periodontol. **34:**227, 1963.

Arnim, S. S.: Microcosms of the human mouth, J. Tenn. Dent. Assoc. **39:**3, 1959.

Arno, A., Schei, O., Lövdal, A., and Waerhaug, J.: Alveolar bone loss as a function of tobacco consumption, Acta Odontol. Scand. **17:**3, 1959.

Arno, A., Waerhaug, J., Lövdal, A., and Schei, O.: Incidence of gingivitis as related to sex, occupation, tobacco consumption, toothbrushing and age, Oral Surg. **11:**587, 1958.

Ash, M. M., Gitlin, B. N., and Smith, W. A.: Correlation between plaque and gingivitis, J. Periodontol. **35:**424, 1964.

Astwood, L. A.: Oral irrigating devices; an appraisal of current information, J. Public Health Dent. **35:**2, 1975.

Baer, P. N., Kakehashi, S., Littleton, N. W., White, C. L., and Lieberman, J. E.: Alveolar bone loss and occlusal wear, Periodontics **1:**91, 1963.

Bell, D. G.: Teaching home care to the patient, J. Periodontol. **19:**140, 1948.

Belting, C. M.: A review of the epidemiology of periodontal diseases, J. Periodontol. **28:**37, 1957.

Belting, C. M., and Gordon, D. L.: In vivo effect of a urea containing dentifrice on dental calculus formation, J Periodontol. **37:**26, 1966.

Bernier, J. L., and Muhler, J. C.: Improving dental practice through preventive measures, ed. 2, Saint Louis, 1970, The C. V. Mosby Co.

Blass, J. L.: Motivating patients for more effective dental service, Philadelphia, 1958, J. B. Lippincott Co.

Bohannan, H. M., Ochsenbein, C., and Saxe, S. R.: Preventive periodontics, Dent. Clin. North Am., p. 435, July, 1965.

Brandtzaeg, P., and Jamison, H. C.: A study of periodontal health and oral hygiene in Norwegian Army recruits, J. Periodontol. **35:**302, 1964.

Burket, L. W.: Systemic aspects of periodontal disease, J. Periodontol. **24:**7, 1953.

Carlsson, J., and Egelberg, J.: Effect of diet on early plaque formation in man, Odontol. Revy **16:**112, 1965.

Carter, H. G., Barnes, G. P., and Woolride, E. W.: Effects of using various types of dental floss on sulcus bleeding, Va. Dent. J. **52:**18, 1975.

Castenfelt, T.: Toothbrushing and massage in periodontal disease, Stockholm, 1952, Nordisk Rotogravyr.

Chauncey, H. H.: The comparative efficacy of gum, toothpaste, and mouthwash, J. Dent. Res. **37:**968, 1958.

Crumley, P. J., and Sumner, C. F.: Effectiveness of a water pressure cleansing device, Periodontics **3:**193, 1965.

Cunningham, W. M.: Prevalence of periodontal (paradontal) disease. II. In Australasia, Int. Dent. J. **5:**200, 1955.

Dodds, A. E.: Prevalence of paradontal disease. I. In Africa, Int. Dent. J. **5:**55, 1955.

Dudding, N. J., and Muhler, J. C.: What motivates children to practice good oral hygiene? J. Periodontol. **31:**141, 1960.

Dunning, J. M.: Principles of dental public health, Cambridge, Mass., 1962, Harvard University Press.

Emilson, C. G., Krasse, B., and Westergren, G.: Effect of a fluoride-containing chlorhexidine gel on bacteria in human plaque, Scand. J. Dent. Res. **84:**56, 1976.

Emslie, R. D.: The value of oral hygiene, Br. Dent. J. **117:**373, 1964.

Ennever, J., and Sturzenberger, P.: Inhibition of dental calculus formation using an enzyme chewing gum, J. Periodontol **32:**331, 1961.

Everett, F. G., Tuchler, H., and Lu, K. H.: Occurrence of calculus in grade school children in Portland, Oregon, J. Periodontol. **34:**54, 1963.

Fay, H. D.: The effects of oral prophylaxis and oral health education in reduction of periodontal disease; an epidemiological study, Chin. Med. J. **10:**243, 1963.

Gibson, A. W., and Shannon, I. L.: Microorganisms in human gingival tissues, Periodontics **2:**119, 1964.

Gift, H. C., and Milton, B. B.: Comparison of two national preventive dentistry surveys, J. Prev. Dent. **2:**25, 1975.

Glickman, I.: Nutrition in the prevention and treatment of gingival and periodontal disease, J. Dent. Med. **19:**179, 1964.

Greene, J. C.: Oral hygiene and periodontal disease, Am. J. Public Health **53:**913, 1963.

Greene, J. C.: Periodontal disease in India; report of an epidemiological study, J. Dent. Res. **39:**302, 1960.

Greene, J. C., and Vermillion, J. R.: The oral hygiene index; a method for classifying oral hygiene status, J. Am. Dent. Assoc. **61:**172, 1960.

Greene, J. C., and Vermillion, J. R.: The effect of controlled oral hygiene procedures on the progression of periodontal disease in adults: results after third and final year, J. Dent. Res. **50:**319, 1971.

Greene, J. C., and Vermillion, J. R.: The simplified oral hygiene index, J. Am. Dent. Assoc. **68:**7, 1964.

Gunson, J. J.: Clinical studies on a new calculus-dissolving agent, Dent. Survey **31:**1248, 1955.

Haberman, S.: Inflammatory and non-inflammatory responses to gingival invasion by microorganisms, J. Periodontol. **30:**190, 1959.

Harrisson, J. W. E., Salisbury, G. B., Abbot, D. D., and Packman, E. W.: Effect of enzyme-toothpastes upon oral hygiene, J. Periodontol. **34:**334, 1963.

Hull, P. S., Hillam, D. G., and Beal, J. F.: A radiographic study of the prevalence of chronic periodontitis in 14-year-old English schoolchildren, J. Clin. Periodontol. **2:**203, 1975.

Jensen, A. L.: Use of dehydrated pancreas in oral hygiene, J. Am. Dent. Assoc. **59:**923, 1959.

Johansen, J. R., Gjermo, P., and Eriksen, H. M.: Effect of 2-years' use of chlorhexidine-containing dentifrices on plaque, gingivitis, and caries, Scand. J. Dent. Res. **83:**288, 1975.

Jordan, H. V., and Keyes, P. H.: Aerobic, gram-positive, filamentous bacteria as etiologic agents of experimental periodontal disease in hamsters, Arch. Oral Biol. **9:**401, 1964.

Jordan, H. V., and Keyes, P. H.: Bacteria in periodontal disease, N.Y. Dent. J. **30:**267, 1964.

Krajewski, J. J., Giblin, J., and Gargiulo, A. W.: Evaluation of a water pressure device as an adjunct to periodontal treatment, Periodontics **2:**76, 1964.

Leavell, H. R., and Clark, G. E.: Preventive medicine for the doctor in his community, ed. 3, New York, 1953, McGraw-Hill Book Company.

Lightner, L. M., O'Leary, T. J., Drake, R. B., Crump, P. P., and Allen, M. F.: Preventive periodontic treatment procedures: results over 46 months, J. Periodontol. **42:**555, 1971.

Lindhe, J., Axelsson, P., and Tollskog, G.: Effect of proper oral hygiene on gingivitis and dental caries in Swedish schoolchildren, Community Dent. Oral Epidemiol. **3:**150, 1975.

Lindhe, J., and Nyman, S.: The effect of plaque control and surgical pocket elimination on the establishment and maintenance of periodontal health. A longitudinal study of periodontal therapy in cases of advanced disease, J. Clin. Periodontol. **2:**67, 1975.

Linn, E. L.: Oral hygiene and periodontal disease; implications for dental health programs, J. Am. Dent. Assoc. **71:**38, 1965.

Löe, H.: Present day status and direction for future research on the etiology and prevention of periodontal disease, J. Periodontol. **40:**678, 1969.

Löe, H.: Epidemiology of periodontal disease, Odontol. Tskr. **71:**479, 1963.

Löe, H., Theilade, E., and Jensen, S. B.: Experimental gingivitis in man, J. Periodontol. **36:**177, 1965.

Loos, S.: Prevalence of paradontal (periodontal) disease. III. Europe, Int. Dent. J. **5:**319, 1955.

Lövdal, A., Arno, A., Schei, O., and Waerhaug, J.: Combined effects of subgingival scaling and controlled oral hygiene on the incidence of gingivitis, Acta Odontol. Scand. **19:**537, 1961.

Macdonald, J. B., Gibbons, R. J., and Socransky, S. S.: Bacterial mechanisms in periodontal disease, Ann. N.Y. Acad. Sci. **85:**467, 1960.

Mandel, I.: New approaches to plaque prevention, Dent. Clin. North Am., pp. 663-664, October, 1972.

Marshall-Day, C. D., Stephens, R. G., and Quigley, L. F.: Periodontal disease; prevalence and incidence, J. Periodontol. **26:**185, 1955.

McCauley, H. B., Davis, L. B., and Frazier, T. M.: Effect on oral cleanliness produced by dental health instruction and brushing teeth in the classroom; The 1953-54 Baltimore Toothbrushing Study, J. Sch. Health **25:**250, 1955.

Mehta, F. S., Sanjana, M. K., Schroff, B. C., and Doctor, R. H.: Relative importance of the various causes of tooth loss, J. All India Dent. Assoc. **30:**211, 1958.

Morch, T., and Waerhaug, J.: A quantitative evaluation of the effect of toothbrushing and toothpicking, J. Periodontol. **27:**183, 1956.

Morris, M. L.: Artificial crown contours and gingival health, J. Prosthet. Dent. **12:**1146, 1962.

Muller, E., Schroeder, H. E., and Mühlemann, H. R.: The effect of two oral antiseptics on early calculus formation, Helv. Odontol. Acta **6:**42, 1962.

Ostrander, F. D.: The use of antibiotics in periodontics and endodontics, J. Am. Dent. Assoc. **46:**139, 1953.

Packman, E. W., Abbott, D. D., Salisbury, G. B., and Harrison, J. W. E.: Effect of enzyme–chewing gums upon oral hygiene, J. Periodontol. **34:**255, 1963.

Parfitt, G. J., James, P. M. C., and Davis, H. C.: A controlled study of the effect of dental health education on the gingival structures of school children, Br. Dent. J. **104:**21, 1958.

Peterson, L. N.: Teaching oral hygiene to patients, J. Calif. Dent. Assoc. **28:**6, 1952.

Posselt, U., and Emslie, R. D.: Occlusal disharmonies and their effect on periodontal diseases, Int. Dent. J. **9:**367, 1959.

Poulton, D. R., and Aaronson, S. A.: The relationship between occlusion and periodontal status, Am. J. Orthod. **47:**690, 1961.

Putnam, W. J., O'Shea, R. M., and Cohen, L. V.: Communication and patient motivation in preventive periodontics, Public Health Rep. **82:**779, 1967.

Ramfjord, S. P., Kerr, D. A., and Ash, M. M., editors: Proceedings of the World Workshop in Periodontics, Ann Arbor, 1966, University of Michigan Press.

Ramfjord, S., Nissle, R., and Shick, R.: Subgingival curettage versus surgical elimination of periodontal pockets, J. Periodontol. **39:**45, 1968.

Russell, A. L.: World epidemiology and oral health; environmental variables in oral disease, Washington, D.C., 1966, American Association for the Advancement of Science.

Russell, A. L.: International nutrition surveys; a summary of preliminary dental findings, J. Dent. Res. **42**(suppl.):233, 1963.

Russell, A. L.: Periodontal diseases in well and malnourished populations; a preliminary report, Arch. Environ. Health **5**:153, 1962.

Russell, A. L.: A social factor associated with the severity of periodontal disease, J. Dent. Res. **36**:922, 1957.

Russell, A. L., and Ayers, P.: Periodontal disease and socioeconomic status in Birmingham, Ala., Am. J. Public Health **50**:206, 1960.

Saxe, S. R., Greene, J. C., Bohannan, H. M., and Vermillion, J. R.: Oral debris, calculus, and periodontal disease in the beagle dog, Periodontics **5**:217, 1967.

Schei, O., Waerhaug, J., Lövdal, A., and Arno, A.: Alveolar bone loss as related to oral hygiene and age, J. Periodontol. **30**:7, 1959.

Scherp, H. W.: Current concepts in periodontal disease research; epidemiological contributions, J. Am. Dent. Assoc. **68**:667, 1964.

Schiott, C. R., Briner, W. W., and Löe, H.: Two year oral use of chlorhexidine in man, J. Periodont. Res. **11**:145, 1976.

Stallard, R. E., Volpe, A. R., Orban, J. E., and King, W. J.: The effect of an antimicrobial mouth rinse on dental plaque, calculus and gingivitis, J. Periodontol. **40**:683, 1969.

Stewart, C. G.: Mucinase — a possible means of reducing calculus formation, J. Periodontol. **23**:85, 1952.

Sud, V.: Gingival changes in deficiency states, pregnancy, and lactation period, J. Dent. Res. **30**:19, 1951.

Summers, C. J., and Oberman, A.: Association of oral disease with 12 selected variables. II. Edentulism, J. Dent. Res. **47**:594, 1968.

Suomi, J. D.: Periodontal disease and oral hygiene in an institutionalized population: report of an epidemiological study, J. Periodontol. **40**:5, 1969.

Suomi, J. D., and Barbano, J. P.: Patterns of gingivitis, J. Periodontol. **39**:71, 1968.

Suomi, J. D., Greene, J. C., Vermillion, J. R., Doyle, J., Chang, J. J., and Leatherwood, E. C.: The effect of controlled oral hygiene procedures on the progression of periodontal disease in adults: results after third and final year, J. Periodontol. **42**:152, 1971.

Suomi, J. D., Smith, L. W., McClendon, B. J., Spolsky, V. W., and Horowitz, H. S.: Oral calculus in children, J. Periodontol. **42**:341, 1971.

Theilade, E., Wright, W. H., Jensen, S. B., and Löe, H.: Experimental gingivitis in man. II. A longitudinal clinical and bacteriological investigation, J. Periodont. Res. **1**:1, 1966.

Toto, P. D., Rapp, G., and O'Malley, J.: Clinical evaluation of chewing gum in gingivitis and dental care, J. Dent. Res. **39**:750, 1960.

Waerhaug, J.: Effect of rough surfaces upon gingival tissues, J. Dent. Res. **35**:323, 1956.

Wilcox, C. E., and Everett, F. G.: Friction on the teeth and gingiva during mastication, J. Am. Dent. Assoc. **66**:513, 1963.

W. H. O., Expert Committee on Periodontal Disease: Technical Report Series no. 207, Geneva, 1961, World Health Organization.

Young, W. O., and Striffler, D. F.: The dentist, his practice, and his community, Philadelphia, 1964, W. B. Saunders Co.

12 Examination

Recognition of disease processes is based on a knowledge of healthy tissue appearance and the reactions and deviations that occur when these tissues are affected by disease. Examination is the observation and recording of these changes, and the evaluation of these data constitutes diagnosis.

It is evident that a thorough examination is of the utmost importance in the study of periodontal disease, for only in this manner can a diagnosis be made and the etiologic factors be ascertained. It is necessary to use all the available methods of examination so that as much information as possible may be obtained. The examination must be made methodically with extreme skill and close study. It has been said that the good clinician is one who will spend a sufficient amount of time in examination, for treatment cannot be applied with any degree of success unless a correct diagnosis has been made; a correct diagnosis in turn necessitates the exact collection of data.

The diagnosis and recognition of disease processes of the periodontium and their etiology involve an intimate and complete familiarity with the normal. It is only by deviation from the normal that we can determine the extent and seriousness of disease. It is therefore of great importance to establish the nature of the normal, healthy periodontium. Such a stated objective would seem to imply that there is a single standard of health. But this is not so. Health and normality are not static

concepts. They represent a *range* of variation within which health exists. This range is present in color, texture, and to a certain extent form. The range is modified by factors of age, relationship of the various parts to each other, and even by racial characteristics.

The most effective single method that we possess in diagnosis is *observation*. As in all other methods it must be developed and refined in constant practice. Routine observation will yield only superficial information, and much data of value will remain undiscovered. *Observation must not cease with the arrival at an opinion but must be continued throughout the entire contact with the case. It is in this fashion that problems will be discovered and solutions arrived at that were not apparent at the initial phase of familiarity. Persistent observation is the hallmark of the resourceful, imaginative therapist. For the casual observer there is much that does not appear to exist which is in reality present and waiting to be discovered.*

CLASSIFICATION

For the purposes of clarity, order, and ease in communication a classification of periodontal disease is required. Several of these exist; each based upon one or another of the various approaches to the problem. The following classification is based upon periodontal histopathology and pathogenesis. It is an aid in understanding the disease process with which one is dealing and should in the future promote a more complete comprehension of the underlying factors that create the syndromes one treats.

I. *Inflammation*
  A. Gingivitis—with or without gingival enlargement
    (acute and chronic)
    1. Local etiologic factors
      a. Plaque
      b. Bacterial products
      c. Calculus
      d. Irritating restorations
      e. Food impaction
      f. Other causes
    2. Drug action—allergy

3. Hormonal
4. Systemic
5. Idiopathic

(The severity of a gingival inflammation is dependent on the intensity, frequency, and duration of the local irritant and the resistive factors of the patient. On the other hand, if the causative factor is systemic the severity of the lesion and in some cases its inception may be dependent on a local etiologic agent.)

   B. Periodontitis
     1. Secondary to long-standing gingivitis
     2. Initial lesion: local etiologic factors such as listed under gingivitis
     3. May occur in conjunction with occlusal traumatism

(A marginal periodontitis may evolve after a long-standing gingival inflammation or may occur as a periodontitis in its inception.)

  II. *Dystrophy*
    A. Occlusal traumatism—accentuated or initiated by habits (bruxism, clenching, and so on)
     1. Malfunctional occlusion
       a. Malocclusion
       b. Loss of teeth, drifting, and extrusion
       c. Premature contacts
       d. Faulty centric relationship
     2. Faulty restorations
       a. Incorrect anatomy of occlusal reconstruction
       b. Faulty bridges
       c. Faulty clasps and so on
     3. Secondary to marginal periodontitis where clinical crown becomes greater than clinical root
     4. Secondary to periodontosis
  III. Periodontosis

(A periodontal manifestation seen in young individuals characterized by migration of teeth and rapid bone loss).

PERIODONTAL MANIFESTATIONS OF LOCAL DISTURBANCES

Of importance for the recognition of periodontal manifestations are the signs and symptoms of disturbances of the gingival and periodontal tissues. Some are readily apparent, whereas others are recognized only by a careful clinical examination. They may be listed as follows:

  1. Changes in gingival color
    a. Marginal area
    b. Interdental area—buccal and lingual peaks
    c. Attached gingiva
    d. Alveolar mucosa
  2. Changes in gingival form, position, and surface appearance
    a. Hyperplasia—marginal and peak
    b. Recession
    c. Loss of stippling
    d. Glossy appearance
    e. Clefts
    f. Heavy festooning
  3. Retraction of the gingival tissues
  4. Pocket formation
  5. Bleeding—symptom of incipient disease
  6. Presence of exudate
  7. Topography of the crestal portion of the alveolus
  8. Mobility
  9. Migration
  10. Alterations in occlusion

Gingival color. Changes in gingival color are usually the first sign of periodontal disease noticed upon clinical examination. Although the normal color of the gingivae is coral pink, there is a range of variation in shade. In some individuals the gingivae may be relatively light in color, whereas in others it may be heavily pigmented, as in blacks. All intermediate variations can be found in patients of varying complexions. The color value of the attached gingiva, however, is considerably different from the alveolar mucosa, where it is deep pinkish red. The demarcation between these two zones, called the ''mucogingival junction,'' should be clearly visible. Since the attached gingiva is keratinized its color is uniform from the gingival margin to the alveolar mucosa. Any deviation in color value may be evidence of a pathologic condition. Often the gingival margin itself may be dark red, blending into the normal shade. This is the sign of an early gingival lesion. Frank alterations in gingival color are signs of an active gingival disturbance, although after long-standing gingival inflammation the gingival tissue tends to become fibrotic, at which time there may be a return to the pink color with some deviation in form.

Color changes, diffusely spread through the attached gingiva and blending into the color range of the alveolar mucosa, are indicative of a gingival inflammation not contained but spreading along the blood vessels in the gingiva between the outer periosteum of the buccal alveolar process and the epithelial covering of the gingiva. This observation is not the rule but is of sufficiently frequent occurrence to denote a more severe involvement than that localized to the crestal portion of the gingiva.

Surface texture. The surface texture of the attached gingiva discloses a stippled appearance ranging from a smooth velvet to a decided orange-peel effect. Histologically, examination shows the surface epithelium to have an uneven appearance, ranging from closely spaced to widely separated shallow depressions. The gingival fiber apparatus composes the gingival corium, and fibers can be seen extending into the lamina propria from the cemental surface of the tooth. In inflammatory conditions the gingival fiber apparatus is destroyed, and with the edema and cellular infiltration and concomitant swelling, the surface stippling is lost. Where fibrosis has occurred, stippling may often return. When this finding is encountered, especially where there has been a return to the pink color, the diagnostician must be capable of evaluating these findings and interpreting them correctly. They do not indicate a return to health, but on the contrary represent chronicity and scarring. Thus alterations in stippling must be viewed as an expression of varying degrees of involvement of the attached gingiva in a progressing gingivitis, with history and time factors being important.

Contour and position. Deviations from normal contour and position of the gingival margin should be noted. The position of the gingival margin located on the enamel contour varies in the early age group from the adult group, where the margin is located at the cementoenamel junction slightly apical to the bulge of the enamel contour. Deviations from this position may vary from hyperplasia, covering more of the tooth surface, to recession, denuding part of the root surface. There are numerous etiologic agents capable of causing either of these two findings. In health, contour of the gingival tissue is usually observed as a festooning, with a slightly raised but an adherent, somewhat rounded edge. In an early gingival involvement the margin becomes distinctly rounded and enlarged (Fig. 12-1). These enlargements are known as gingival festoons. In this instance the gingival involvement is usually more localized to the gingival margin area and is the incipient evidence of a progressive gingival hyperplasia, a condition concomitant with gingival inflammation.

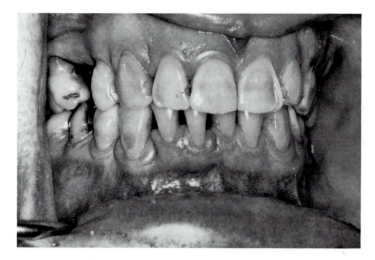

Fig. 12-1. Gingival festoons associated with inflammation and pocket formation.

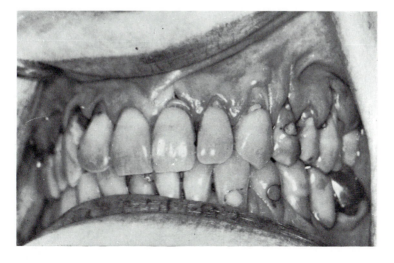

Fig. 12-2. Deep cleft formation in marginal gingiva, extending to vestibular fornix.

With proliferation of the sulcular epithelium and subsequent destruction of the gingival tissue by the inflammation, recession occurs. Thus both processes may occur at the same time. The gingival margins become irregular in contour rather than having the even rounded appearance. In more severe cases the tissue becomes "poxed" and with the color change is diagnostic of a deep-seated inflammatory process (Fig. 12-2).

Clefts. Gingival clefts may be caused by many etiologic factors, ranging from incorrect toothbrushing to a breakthrough to the surface of pocket formation. In the gingiva in which inflammation is present one sees papillary projections of epithelium into the corium. These projections tend to anastomose, isolating areas of tissue with final slough. Since the marginal area is the thinnest the breakthrough is seen in this area. The shapes of the clefts vary since the slough may occur in almost any pattern. When gingival clefts are caused by brushing the teeth incorrectly the clefts originate on the surface and are usually more like V-shaped notches than true clefts. The position of the teeth may also influence the tendency for cleft formation.

Changes in interproximal tissue. The normal interproximal tissue includes a buccal and a lingual peak connected interdentally in a triangular ridge depression termed a "col." It is dependent on the anatomy of the teeth and their position. In some instances the architecture is that of a saddle area. In instances of a col the inner portion of the papilla is triangle shaped as it embraces the proximal surfaces of the teeth and extends through the col to the lingual peak. The interdental tissues conform to the contours of the adjacent teeth. Thus the tissue fills the entire interproximal embrasure. Its for is of utmost importance. It is the prime agency for the interproximal deflection of food debris, and a cone-shaped or pyramidal form is necessary to achieve this function.

Hyperplasia and inflammation are common findings in the peak areas. They are nonspecific inflammatory signs of a wide range of periodontal diseases and are usually associated with ulceration at the depression of the col. This area, unless meticulously cleaned, lends itself to retention of plaque, food debris, calculus, and other forms of gingival irritants that act as etiologic agents of the local inflammation. Often these are not the sole offenders but are the common irritants in concert with other factors such as food impaction (Fig. 12-3).

Some papillary involvements are characterized by destruction and erosion. Gingival craters are the usual result here. In any event surveys reveal that the papillary areas are more often involved in periodontal disease than are any of the other areas of the gingivae.

Pocket. A pocket may be defined as a diseased gingival attachment. It must be emphasized that a pocket exists only because of the pathologic processes in the gingival tissue, initiated by a causative agent for the most part local in origin. Therefore the diagnostician must realize that the diagnosis of a pocket must not be made by measuring the space between the tooth and the gingiva alone but must take into account the condition of the gingival tissue as well. The signs and symptoms of pocket formation are those of gingival inflammation: discoloration, retraction, loss of stippling, bleeding, presence of an exudate, and loss of form in addition to depth of separation. Retraction of the gingival margin from the tooth surface is indicative of an underlying gingival inflammation, the gingival fibers that normally cause the gingiva to hug the tooth having been destroyed. Hence this sign is also evidence of pocket formation.

Of importance in therapy, however, is the extent of detachment of the gingival tissue from the tooth surface. Thus the size, shape, and contour of the pocket must be explored so that a decision can be made as to the method of therapy to be instituted. Pockets, or detachments, may be greater on a single surface of the tooth or may be equal circumferentially. The latter is more often the case. Sometimes the base of the pocket extends apically to the bone crest in the area of a bone defect. This condition is termed an "infrabony pocket." The topography of the pocket is dependent on the degree of hyperplasia resulting from the inflammatory process and the amount of detachment of the gingiva from the tooth surface that has taken place.

Clinical probing with suitable periodontal instruments, for example, the Goldman, Michigan, or Williams calibrated probes, is a prime necessity in delineating the depth, topography, and character of the periodontal pocket. It must be kept in mind that the probe is a searching instrument. The simple insertion of the instrument under the detached gingiva may reveal little or be entirely misleading. The end of the probe may encounter a flake of calculus. If so, it should be lifted away from root contact and gently manipulated in all possible directions to attempt the deepest penetration possible without inflicting tissue damage. It should be angled so that it is not halted by buccal

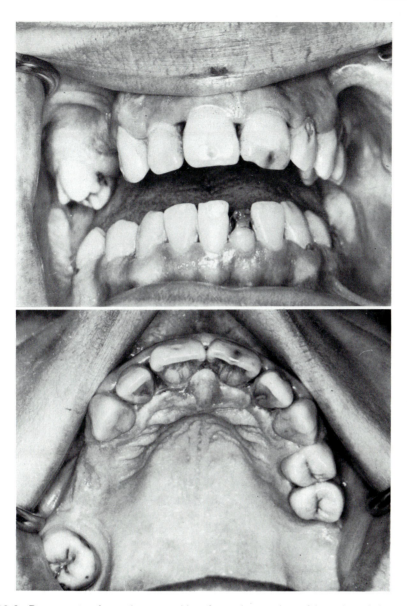

Fig. 12-3. Deep crater formations resulting from destruction of interdental tissues. Examiner must determine whether crater is completely soft tissue or whether there is bone involvement. Example is interdental right central and lateral incisors.

or lingual attachment levels in the interproximal areas. It is not the depth in millimeters that is so important as the location of the base of the detached gingival tissue.

The use of a radiopaque substance to record the actual clinical depth of the pocket roentgenographically is an excellent practice. Gutta-percha points serve well, but the Hirschfeld calibrated silver points are more useful since they establish millimeter markings in addition to locating the gingival margin in the roentgenogram. Thus greater accuracy is possible even with some angulation. Hirchfeld points are easily inserted subgingivally,

and the depth recorded by roentgenographic examination (Fig. 12-4).

Periodontal abscess. The periodontal abscess is an acute exacerbation of a periodontal pocket because of partial or total occlusion of the orifice of the pocket. When drainage is inhibited or stopped we see the typical acute inflammatory situation instead of the chronic process usually encountered.

Roots involved with deep, narrow infrabony pockets usually are prone to periodontal abscess formation because the orifices become blocked. Similarly, teeth with serious interradicular pockets frequently are involved with abscesses even

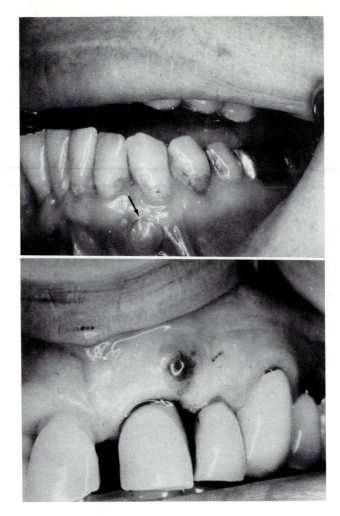

Fig. 12-4. Periodontal abscesses are commonly found. While most patients present complaints, some do not. Examiner must record such incidences.

though the pockets are only partially occluded. On rare occasions no marginal orifice can be demonstrated clinically, which may be due to a fine foreign body such as a toothbrush bristle impinging on the deeper tissues of the periodontium, or there may be deep periodontal infections from another source. Periodontal abscesses are often seen after a scalnig procedure. They result from forcing infectious material into the opened tissues, which leads to further infection and abscess formation. An acute destructive process may be due to occlusal traumatism as a result of an acute pericementitis (not associated with pocket formation).

Some clinicians believe that periodontal abscess formation is more often found in persons with diabetes. Since a glucose tolerance evaluation is not difficult to obtain, this procedure may be indicated if there are multiple acute periodontal abscesses in the mouth.

Interradicular involvement. In multirooted teeth a pocket involving the intraradicular areas is a common finding. Bifurcation and trifurcation involvements in molars and on occasion maxillary first premolars connote a serious lesion of the periodontium. Complication by periodontal abscess formation is a common emergency. Careful exploration of the lesion, however, will reveal many of these pockets to be of the type that may yield to therapy and allow the involved teeth to serve in health for many years.

Interradicular involvements vary in severity. Early involvement is not a particularly serious finding if therapy is instituted promptly. In deeper pockets root form and divergence acquire growing importance. *Even the vitality of the tooth becomes important, since this type of involvement may be periapical via a lateral canal.* The problem of therapy will be dealt with later in the text.

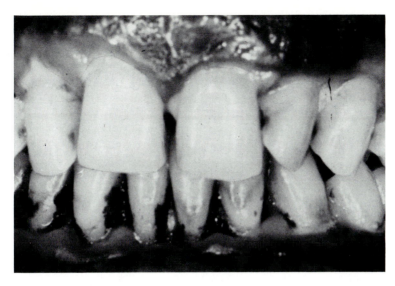

Fig. 12-5. A purulent exudate is an important symptom that must be recognized and recorded. Before scaling, patient must be carefully evaluated, for not infrequently after scaling chills and fever are encountered, denoting a bacteremia. It is wise to prescribe an antibiotic prior to scaling. Also there must be careful manipulation of tissue.

Bleeding and exudation. Bleeding and the presence of an exudate are regarded as signs of a periodontal disease. Both are possible only when the sulcular epithelium is involved, since an intact lining will prohibit the passage of blood and exudate into the sulcus and thence into the oral cavity. The involvement of the sulcular epithelium resulting in ulcer formation and later an inflammatory proliferation of the epithelium is characteristic in gingivitis. Thus any milking of the gingiva allows for blood to pass from the blood vessels of the corium through the broken sulcular epithelium into the space between tooth and gingiva. Probing therefore elicits bleeding. This is also true for the exudate found. However, the amount of suppuration seemingly does not depend on the depth of the pocket but rather on the status of the inflammatory process in the corium. In some areas there is a thick, purulent exudate from a shallow pocket, whereas in others only small quantities or even nonobservable amounts can be found in deep pockets (Fig. 12-5).

Bone involvement. Changes in the alveolus may occur in the crestal region or deeper in the attachment apparatus. It is of extreme importance to recognize the area of involvement, for should only the crestal bone be involved, then the diagnosis rests with the fact that the disease process is limited to the gingiva and the underlying crestal bone. However, should lesions of the deeper attachment apparatus be discerned, then the diagnostician must consider the possibilities of occlusal traumatism, manifestations of systemic diseases affecting bone and connective tissue, or periodontosis. These interpretations of course can be made only roentgenographically, and hence the importance of this type of examination. Roentgenographically the alveolar crest may show evidence of a notchlike defect progressing medially in the alveolar process. Later the crestal portion may be entirely lost, leaving a broad horizontal level to the bone between adjoining teeth. Occasionally the bone level may be slanted interproximally, more pronounced toward one tooth. This finding has usually occurred because of the local environment, for example, the tilt of the tooth, the type of contact between adjacent teeth, or the position of the teeth relative to one another in the jaw itself. In some instances a resorptive lesion may be a vertical one, possibly associated with occlusal traumatism, in which case an infrabony pocket may be present. In the later stages there may be a diffuse resorptive lesion affecting numerous teeth so that the clinical crown–clinical root ratio is markedly disturbed, the end process of a long-standing periodontitis.

Resorptive lesions in the bone may also be detected alongside the periodontal ligament space in the lamina dura. The translucent area may be confined to an isolated spot or may involve an entire side. Sometimes there is a widening of the entire periodontal ligament space, and close inspection of the roentgenogram shows resorptive processes extending from the lamina dura. These changes, together with signs of root resorption, cemental tears, and so on are associated with occlusal traumatism.

Recognition of the topography of the crestal portion of the alveolus is an important factor in the examination and treatment planning today. The therapist treats "regular" bony patterns differently from the way in which he treats altered forms or defects. Since one cannot depend solely on the radiograph in order to recognize the exact topography of the crestal area, clinical observation and examination are necessary to determine the osseous contour.

Mobility. Loosening of a tooth or teeth is an important clinical sign. Mobility may result not only from a decrease in root attachment or changes in the periodontal ligament but also from destruction of the gingival fiber apparatus and transeptal fi-

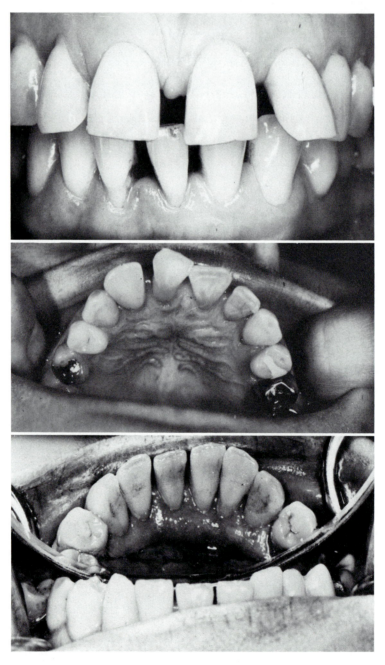

Fig. 12-6. Migration of teeth resulting from loss of periodontal tissues. Examiner must also look for additional factors such as tongue thrusting and a drive from occlusal forces.

bers. These two factors must be distinguished carefully when one is making a diagnosis. Evaluation after therapy may help diagnostically, since there may be a moderation of mobility due to a reduction of the inflammatory process.

In general the more root surface there is for periodontal ligament attachment, the firmer the tooth will be. Thus the square area of the root surface, with respect to the length and circumference of the root, is important; and mobility may be correlated with the degree of loss of attachment by marginal resorption of bone in periodontitis, together with loss of integrity of the gingival fiber apparatus and with changes in the attachment apparatus evident in periodontal traumatism. Both phenomena may be operating concomitantly. In rare cases mobility may be associated with changes in the attachment apparatus occurring in periodontosis.

Migration. Migration of the teeth is one of the characteristic signs of periodontal involvement.

Unfortunately an expression in the literature has given the impression that this sign is diagnostic of an involvement of the periodontium due to a systemic factor. *It must be emphasized that for the most part, migration is associated with various factors such as pocket formation, food impaction, occlusal traumatism, and habits.* In very rare instances, when a case of periodontosis is encountered, wandering of the teeth is found. Here it is a common sign, but it is not specific to that disease (Figs. 12-6 to 12-8).

Characteristically, maxillary incisors tend to migrate labially and then drift either mesially or distally. Usually, however, the latter occurs. This is true of the maxillary lateral incisor and canine. The maxillary premolars tend to wander distally, whereas the molars move mesially. When a tooth loses its antagonist it usually moves into supraclusion. When no disease process or factors that may allow for involvement are present the tooth carries with it the gingiva and alveolar support. In

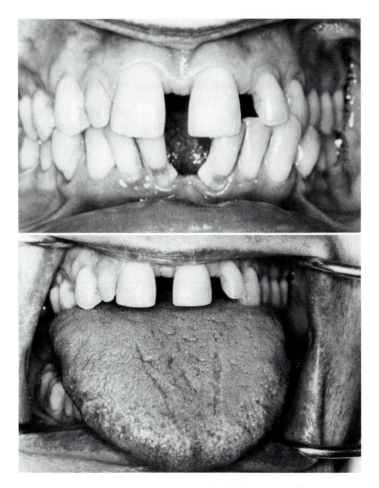

Fig. 12-7. Tongue thrust in association with marked diastemata. There was marked mobility of teeth. Patient was aware of tongue pushing against teeth.

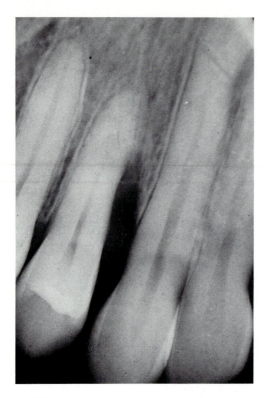

Fig. 12-8. Vertical resorption lesion associated with migration of teeth. Lesion was associated with a premature contact on mesiopalatal surface of first premolar.

the mandible, teeth tend to separate and migrate, losing contact. In cases in which there has been considerable destruction of the periodontium it is not unusual to find one or more teeth wandering from their original positions. Examination of such situations often reveals that a tooth will move away from the area most destroyed by the periodontal involvement.

Disturbances in occlusion. One of the important signs of periodontal involvement is a disturbance of the occlusion, and recognition of the derangement may be the decisive point between success or failure in therapy. However, the fact that individual teeth may be missing from the dentition does not necessarily constitute a disturbance in the periodontium. Adaptation may have occurred, and no periodontal involvement may be present. On the other hand, because a completely intact dentition may be encountered, an involvement cannot be ruled out. A lack of harmony between centric relation and the habitual closing position with a positive habit pattern may be the initiating factors in a disturbance, causing mobility of a tooth or group of teeth, without any in-

volvement of the gingival tissues. Detailed clinical and roentgenographic examination of the dentition in a static and functioning aspect must be performed. Collection of these data and their interpretation constitute a most important aspect of correct therapy.

Thus the examination of the occlusion in cases of periodontal involvement is an important factor in diagnosis and treatment planning. Examination of the patient while he is using his masticatory apparatus will afford a great deal of information as to the patterns of chewing, length of the chewing cycle, and the efficiency of chewing. Examination of study casts for abraded areas and facets is of distinct value. The lingual relationships between the teeth can be better studied in study casts offering a more complete analysis of the occlusal relationships present. Plunger cusps with possible areas for food impaction, the relationship of contact between adjacent teeth, and the overbite and overjet can be observed. Palpation of a mobile tooth during the contact of antagonists in the chewing cycle can be noted by resting lightly the ball of the index finger against two adjacent upper teeth and then against a single tooth. Any movement of the tooth can be detected and is known as fremitus. Another method of study is registration of tooth surfaces in wax after the mandible has been occluded against the maxilla. Detection of a premature contact by the complete displacement of the wax is a valuable method of examination. Many other methods are utilized, the most common being the use of articulating paper markings. Careful examination of facets on the occlusal contacting surfaces is helpful in diagnosis. If only a few teeth exhibit these facets the inference can be made that these are the only teeth to take up the burden. It is to be noted, however, that a tooth may be traumatized without a facet being produced. In these instances the supporting structures have been destroyed, allowing the tooth to move in its socket during the occlusal contact. Excessive mobility of the teeth during function is also a sign of occlusal traumatism. Teeth that on close observation are seen to move in function or those in which the movement can be detected by the placing of a finger over the tooth during the act of occlusion are in traumatism. Soreness of a tooth is usually a late symptom of occlusal traumatism and is related to changes in the periodontium allowing for the tooth to be extruded.

Again it must be emphasized that detailed, careful examination of the occlusion is an essential so that a correct treatment plan can be formulated.

Periodontosis. Periodontosis is seen essentially in very young individuals and is characterized by loosening and migration of the teeth. The clinical progress of this disease is such that bone loss is rapid and the loosening of teeth is progressive in nature, although cycles of loosening and tightening are noted.

Whereas most cases of periodontosis observed by the dentist are in an advanced stage, since the disease process is not usually recognized in the initial stage and since it is for the most part asymptomatic to the patient, occasionally the incipient lesion is encountered. In such instances the gingivae may show but little involvement. There is little or no calculus present, and the architecture of the gingivae is usually within the norm. The teeth show a change in alignment as though they were drifting out of position. This is more noticeable in the anterior portion of the dental arch where the teeth are freer to move. There is a marked tendency for protrusion and extrusion, with some rotation. This wandering may persist even though the tooth has moved out of occlusion. In the posterior region the teeth lose contact with one another. Often a space may be found between the second premolar and the first molar or between the first and second molars. Loosening of the teeth is an early symptom, and mobility may vary from tooth to tooth. Usually the incisors and first molars are more mobile than the premolars. This finding, however, may vary with the local factors present.

Periodontosis is found in a young age group. The most common age probably is before 20 years. In the experience of some observers only the supporting tissues of the incisors and first molars are affected, whereas in other cases the periodontium throughout becomes destroyed. These cases have a distinct plaque ecology (see Chapter 3).

Although at first glance the gingival tissue may appear well attached to the tooth surface, long narrow pockets can be found on the side of bone resorption in many cases. The tissue immediately surrounding the pockets may show practically no clinical signs of inflammation, but when the pockets are probed, the tissue is easily lifted away from the tooth surface. Bleeding is not a prominent feature in periodontosis. In the late stage the lesion cannot be distinguished from advanced marginal periodontitis.

Roentgenographically the changes are interesting and informative. Bone loss seen roentgenographically in a well-established case is far more advanced than is clinically suspected, and often the tooth is far looser than is imagined from roentgenographic findings. Although vertical loss of bone is characteristic, associated advanced horizontal resorption of the alveoli is a consistent finding.

Although the changes of periodontosis can be distinguished from those of periodontitis, it often requires careful consideration to differentiate this condition from one of advanced occlusal traumatism. Vertical bone loss and loosening and wandering of the teeth are characteristic for both conditions. There is a tendency for infrabony pockets to form in these two disease processes under consideration, when the inflammatory process superimposes itself upon the dystrophic lesion. However, in periodontosis the characteristic wandering, the early loosening, the age group, and the grouping of the teeth affected are distinguishing features. A more detailed discussion of periodontosis is found in Chapter 10.

PERIODONTAL MANIFESTATIONS OF SYSTEMIC DISORDERS

All systemic diseases that affect generalized tissues throughout the body may also involve similar tissues within the periodontium. Such responses should be considered as periodontal manifestations of specific systemic diseases (Fig. 12-9). Among these are tumor invasion of periodontal structures by direct extension or metastasis, widening of the periodontal ligament associated with the connective tissue changes that are part of scleroderma, osteoporosis in hyperparathyroidism, and leukemic infiltrations. However, as stated at the outset, such periodontal involvements are part of generalized pathologic states and are not specific for the periodontal tissues. A similar statement can be made about the effect of aging on the periodontium. Although no unanimity exists about the effect of aging per se on the apical migration of the epithelial attachment, bone and soft tissue changes seen in old age also affect similar tissues within the periodontium. It is, however, generally accepted that these altered metabolic states by themselves do not cause gingival inflammation.

The next question to be considered, therefore, must deal with possible modification of periodontal responses to local injury when metabolic stressors are active in the host. Znamensky in 1902 called attention to the interaction of local and systemic factors in the resultant periodontal lesion. Since that time a great deal of experimental and human data has been gathered that suggests that

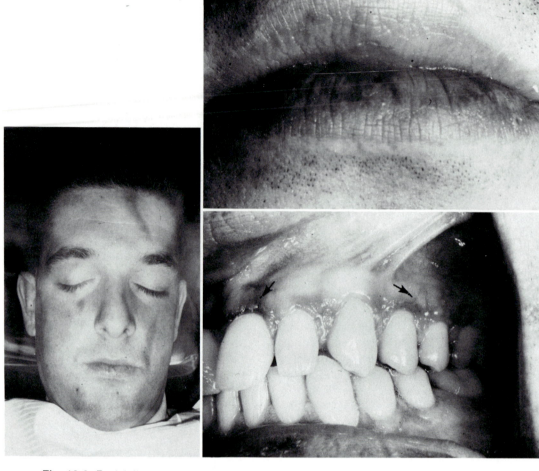

Fig. 12-9. Facial, lip, and gingival lesions in a 30-year-old man whose oral complaint was that of difficulty in chewing. History revealed a systemic condition: lupus erythematosus. Seriousness of disease dictated that only palliative gingival treatment be performed.

the response of the periodontal tissues to local irritants is modified in the presence of some systemic diseases.

Of particular interest to dental investigators have been diabetes, pregnancy, and nutritional disorders (Fig. 12-10).

Recent findings concerning periodontal manifestations in diabetic patients reveal that microangiopathy was discerned in the gingival vasculature. This is true in prediabetic patients as well as in overt diabetics. Microcirculatory impairment was evidenced by disruption of the approximation of endothelial cells, the accumulation of a PAS-positive structureless substance in an area corresponding to the endothelial basement membrane, and the constriction of the vascular lumina. Lipid may also be deposited in the vessel wall. It has also been demonstrated that an endosteal osteoporosis

and a decreased capacity for collagen synthesis may occur. Salivary flow may be decreased. All these factors are important in the etiology of periodontal disease seen in the diabetic patient.

Belting et al. concluded in 1964 that the severity of periodontal disease was significantly greater among persons with diabetes than among those without. Significant differences in severity existed even when such variable factors as degree of calculus, age, and brushing frequency were held fixed in the experimental and control groups. Similar corroborative findings have also been reported by Boorujy and Ship. Belting et al. further noted that as the degree of calculus increased the severity of periodontal disease increased, which focuses on the importance of the local initiating factor.

Recent experimental observations have also demonstrated that gingival disease increases in

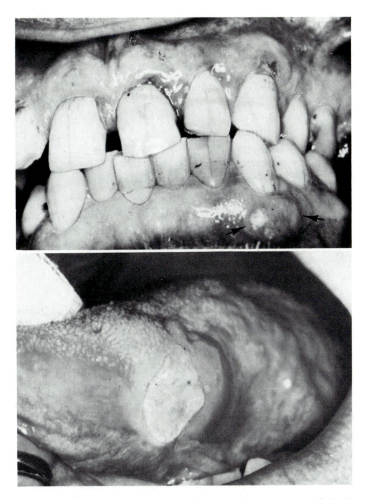

Fig. 12-10. Gingival and tongue lesions in a 60-year-old man who exhibited an advanced periodontal manifestation in addition to an acute periodontal abscess on labial aspect of mandibular left canine and an ulcerous lesion of lateral border of tongue. Tentative diagnosis of tongue lesion was carcinoma, and patient was informed that a biopsy would be done. Patient was hospitalized, and during workup it was found that he was a severe diabetic. Abscess was drained. Patient was placed on a regimen that included insulin injections. In a very short time, tongue lesion healed and gingival condition markedly improved. Patient was subsequently treated periodontally.

hamsters suffering with hereditary diabetes mellitus and that gingival irritants cause greater destruction in alloxan-treated rats than in controls. On the other hand, it is noteworthy that occlusal trauma, which does not affect the marginal gingiva, does not increase marginal gingival pathology in alloxan-treated rats.

Gingival changes associated with pregnancy have been reported as early as 1877. However, it was Ziskin et al. who presented extensive studies relating gingival pathology and the pregnant state. They noted that 40% of the pregnant women in their series had gingivitis and further speculated that the gingival changes were due to hormonal imbalances. Other authors have published a varying incidence of gingivitis in pregnancy, in some studies running as high as 100% of the patients examined. A recently published survey reported gingivitis in all pregnant women in that series which increased from the second month of gestation until the eighth month and then decreased. Of particular interest, however, is Löe's observation that the quantity and character of oral debris do not differ in pregnant and postpartum patients. This finding suggests that in pregnancy some other factor is introduced which, together with the local bacteria, may be responsible for the accentuated inflammation; that is, pregnancy acts as a modifying influence on the gingival response to local irritants.

Cohen et al. in a longitudinal study of the periodontal changes during pregnancy noted that in the presence of similar amounts of both hard and soft irritants, periodontal disease increased with time in both the pregnant and nonpregnant groups. During pregnancy the gingival-periodontal index was significantly higher in the pregnant group. There was also a significant increase in horizontal tooth mobility during pregnancy. An increased level of periodontal disease during pregnancy did not result in increased levels of periodontal disease 15 months postpartum.

Nutritional imbalances and their relation to periodontal lesions have been studied in extensive epidemiologic surveys. Findings have indicated that nutritional imbalances may modify and accentuate the extent of the resultant periodontal lesion but that initiation is probably local in origin. Similar conclusions can also be drawn from experimental studies, particularly from investigations dealing with repair of gingival injuries; for example, gingival wounds in rats have shown delayed repair of connective tissue and bone and reduced resistance to infection when protein deficient diets or hepatic injury were superimposed upon the host either simultaneously or at periods close to the time of gingival injury. Such alteration in repair potential ultimately leads to more severe breakdown of the wound site. However, without local injury local inflammation is usually not present. Further insight into these problems is found in Chapter 4.

With these observations in mind it seems important to contrast the influence of two major factors that do not initiate a periodontal pocket but do affect the severity and extent of the resultant lesion, that is, trauma from occlusion and metabolic stressors. Our present knowledge indicates that occlusal dysfunctions do not affect the repair sequence at the marginal gingiva following injury but may possibly alter the pathway of the resultant inflammation. On the other hand, certain metabolic stressors cause persistent local inflammation and delayed connective tissue and bone repair at the site of gingival injury. It thus seems reasonable to suggest that while both trauma from occlusion and trauma from metabolic stressors act as modifying factors of periodontal disease their mode and site of action are significantly different.

In summary it seems obvious that systemic aberrations do not initiate inflammatory periodontal disease but may modify the extent and severity of the lesion by altering the resistance and repair po-

tential of the affected local tissues. In this manner metabolic shifts that lead to interferences with tissue growth and repair may similarly affect the periodontal tissue response to injury. The resultant accentuation of the local gingival disease might then be thought of as the *specific gingival response* to a variety of *nonspecific metabolic stressors*.

METHODS OF EXAMINATION

Inspection. Observation constitutes the main essential of examination. Minute alterations must be noted, and therefore keen inspection is necessary. In general a routine method may be employed, checking various areas in order. *This may be done first in an overall survey and later in detail*. First the face is studied for contour and swelling or lip lesions. The quality of the breath is noted, and inspection is made of the inside of the mouth: cheeks, palate, fauces, and tongue. Finally occlusion and ability to masticate are studied with the lips raised and the cheeks retracted. Deformities and abnormalities of the dental arch are observed.

The gingivae must be examined carefully in both the upper and the lower jaws. The tone and color should be noted, and small swellings, red spots, ulcers, and fistulous openings should be observed. The gingival margin may be receded or hyperplastic; the interdental papillae may be destroyed or prominent; a pseudopapilla may be present; the gingival sulcus may contain food debris, a purulent exudate, or calculus.

The examiner should determine (1) whether the teeth are high cusped or low cusped, with closed or open contact points; (2) whether they are smooth and well formed; (3) whether they have been well kept and regularly cared for; (4) whether there are few or numerous restorations, of poor quality or skillfully placed; (5) whether any of the teeth are discolored, possibly indicating pulp disease; and (6) whether calculus is present.

A detailed inspection may then be performed. This pertains more particularly to the oral cavity where the tissues are moist and many changes are undistinguishable or indistinct because of moisture coverage. Drying the tissue with gauze or a warm blast of air may reveal tissue changes pertinent to the diagnosis. The examination of the occlusion requires not only the inspection of tooth relationships but also facetal wear and facetal relationships. The matching of facets in centric relation may often be an important clue in the causation of mobility of a tooth.

Thus it may be stated that detailed observation is of utmost importance and that hasty inspection often leads to a misinterpretation of the problem present.

Palpation. Palpation is the use of the sense of touch. Without this type of examination the diagnostician would be unable to gather some data necessary for diagnosis. The ability to feel and touch tissue, testing the consistency, is of utmost importance. Gingival fibrosis, although having certain visual characteristics, certainly can be better diagnosed by palpation of the tissue. The teeth are tested for abnormal mobility while the mouth is open, each tooth being held between two instruments and moved laterally back and forth. They are also tested when articulating during mastication. The patient is asked to chew while a finger is placed lightly over the buccal and labial surfaces of the teeth; first one and then the other side is tested to detect teeth having greater mobility than normal. Gentle pressure applied over the roots may disclose tender places where the alveolar bone has been destroyed by either periapical or periodontal inflammation.

Exploration. Examination of the teeth and the gingivae with the aid of the mirror and explorer is important, since this method shows up small defects of the teeth as well as the condition of the gingival sulci. A good source of light, well directed, is necessary. The examination should be systematic, starting at one side of the mouth. Each tooth, along with its investing gingivae, should be explored in its entirety, and any defect should be carefully denoted. The gingival attachment should be noted, and whether there is any clinical change in color, density, and form should be observed. Retraction of the gingivae should be looked for, since this is one indication of a periodontal pocket. If pockets have formed along the root of a tooth, the size, shape, and contour should be determined. The depth of the pocket is measured by a suitable probe that may be marked off in millimeters. The presence of subgingival calculus and any exudation of a purulent discharge should be noted.

The entire oral cavity should be examined, for valuable information is often brought to light by this procedure. The buccal mucosa, the soft and hard palates, the floor of the mouth, and the tongue should be inspected carefully. Roughness and defects can be examined digitally. A survey of the entire oral cavity is made. *Careful observation is the keynote.*

Percussion. The quality of the percussion may have a marked diagnostic value. A healthy tooth percussed with a metal instrument gives a metallic sound, whereas one embedded in inflamed tissue sounds dull and flat. More often percussion is used to test sensitivity. A tooth with pulp infection or periapical infection may be so affected.

Transillumination. Transillumination is of value chiefly in confirming suspicion of disease. It also aids in the discovery of subgingival calculus. Drying of the area followed by transillumination may show up small deposits that might otherwise be overlooked.

Electrical and thermal tests. The chief purpose of electrical and thermal tests is to determine whether a pulp is vital. Although ethyl chloride may be used to test for cold sensation, and hot gutta-percha may be employed for sensitivity to heat, these thermal tests do not give any indication of the degree of degenerative process encountered. The electrical pulp test gives far more reliable information, but this test also has its limitations concerning degree of pulpal degeneration. Total nonvitality is determined easily.

Chemical tests. Chemical tests are employed especially for the diagnosis of deposits on the teeth. The use of *disclosing solution* is a common procedure to show up mucin plaques as well as materia alba. Often a tooth that looks clean may show deposits under this test.

Radiographic examination. Radiographic examination serves to reveal, confirm, classify, or localize disease. It may establish an early diagnosis by revealing the origin of symptoms and the cause of disease, for example, overhanging fillings causing marginal resorption of the alveolar crest. It also shows the extent of the tissue involved and may be of great value in establishing a differential diagnosis. In all cases the radiographic findings must be correlated with the clinical picture and the results of other laboratory tests. Thus the changes seen in the radiograph must be interpreted carefully from a pathologic point of view with full consideration of the clinical factors.

STEPS IN EXAMINATION

The first step in an examination is the taking of case and dental histories. A certain skill is necessary to accomplish a proper interview; that is, the ability of the examiner to draw out information from the patient comes with experience. This facilitates the interview and also establishes a rapport with the patient. Thus a routine perhaps facilitates the process of history taking. After the necessary information has been elicited clinical and roentgenographic examinations of the periodontium are performed and, if indicated, dietary analysis, laboratory tests, and casts and photographs are undertaken.

Case history

The case history should include age, sex, marital status, nationality, occupation, and former systemic or oral diseases, if any. Observation should be made of weight, height, complexion, physical infirmities, general hygiene, and temperament. The diet should be investigated. If more information is desired concerning the physical condition the patient's physician should be consulted.

The first part of the case history taking is the recording of the medical history. While this may be elicited from direct questioning of the patient concerning organ systems as is performed in medicine, it is convenient and perhaps as rewarding to use a list of questions that the patient can answer before the actual examination. This list is arranged by systems; the patient circles yes or no or don't know. This list should serve as a source for other leading questions that will in turn elicit further information. For example, one question asked is, "Do you have diabetes?" Another asked is, "Is there diabetes in your family?" The answers may be "Yes, I do, and both my parents do." Then, "Are you under treatment?" Yes. "Are you con-

trolled? What does your physician say about you?" "Do you have trouble with your eyes or any numbness?" All these are pertinent questions that must go into the overall evaluation. Another question for elderly patients is "Have you ever had a heart failure?" An affirmative answer certainly would influence the treatment plan concerning the amount of therapy that might be performed at any single time.

The dentist must be aware of any systemic diseases present. He must be familiar with systemic diseases that may produce periodontal manifestations or influence therapy (Fig. 12-11). Complete knowledge of the nature and behavior of these diseases will aid factually in the efficient recording of a medical history.

The dentist must have a fund of information concerning medicine. He need not be *the* physician, but certainly he must be aware of systemic problems in the management of the periodontal patient, as is the otolaryngologist in the surgical management of diseases and disorders for the ear, nose, and throat. All kinds of experiences can be cited to confirm this attitude.

The chart for the patient's physical health status may be seen in the boxed material. Each section relates to a system, and the answers must be care-

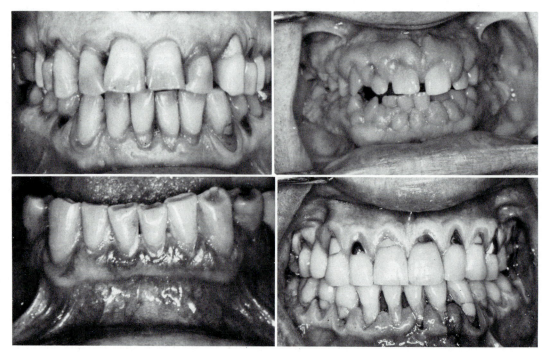

Fig. 12-11. Various health problems that would modify periodontal therapy. Upper left, patient with rheumatic heart disease; upper right, patient with Dilantin hyperplasia; lower left, patient with desquamative gingivitis; lower right, patient with hereditary white sponge nevus.

fully evaluated as to severity, date, relevance, and so on. Each case should have a complete summary as to the possible causal relationship between any medical problem and the dental complaint, and the dentist should tailor therapy to the patient's overall health status. The question of hospitalization may come into consideration. It is wide to consult with the patient's physician to gain an overall evaluation of the health status.

The following questions are often asked: "Should therapy be modified in light of the patient's health problems? Should the therapist seek the ultimate in response and repair? Would it be enough to control bleeding and exudate, stabilize teeth by temporary splinting if necessary, and place the patient on an oral hygiene program?" The answers must come from the dentist; he must be rational and careful to evaluate any problems with medical and dental insight and wisdom.

The detailed systemic history may be of much value in determining the nature, prognosis, and treatment of an oral disease process. It may also dictate the necessity for modifications of treatment, that is, the tailoring of therapy—both primary and adjunctive—to the physical status of the patient (Figs. 12-12 and 12-13). Consider the patient with a history of rheumatic fever; he may certainly require premedication and postmedication with antibiotics to prevent an exacerbation of subacute bacterial endocarditis with is potential grave consequences; or the individual with a history of coronary thrombosis may be on a regimen of anticoagulant therapy. It is evident that precautions should be instituted to prevent bleeding incidents after surgical procedures. When the bleeding time is much prolonged the approach to oral therapeutics may be changed to accommodate to the patient's systemic problem. In general the list should include the following information:

1. Nature of illness—past and present
2. Results of last physical examination
3. Surgical history
4. Gastrointestinal status
5. Cardiovascular history
6. Metabolic and endocrine disturbances
7. Allergic status and drug sensitivities
8. Rheumatic fever
9. Hepatic problems, for example, infectious hepatitis
10. Bleeding tendencies
11. Psychologic problems
12. Past and present medications
13. Dietary regimen

Dental and oral history

The standard beginning of the oral history is the eliciting and recording of the chief complaint. This consists not only of the actual symptom such as pain, swelling, and so on, but also the patient's reason for seeking professional aid. The examiner should listen carefully to the complaint, for often the clue to diagnosis is readily at hand. For example, the patient who describes heat and cold as factors causing pain and tenderness of a tooth may lead the dentist to the diagnosis of pulp involvement. A complaint may consist of more than one finding; often a series of symptoms may be stated. The examiner should not be nonplussed by the pa-

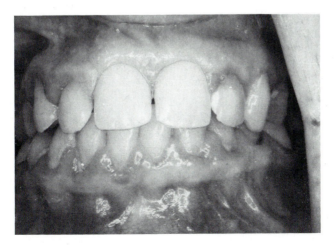

Fig. 12-12. A 35-year-old woman whose history revealed colitis, and who also was on Dilantin medication. Note angular cheilitis. Patient was on a very restricted diet; this fact and effects of Dilantin played a marked role in management of case. Consultation with physician resulted in modification of diet to overcome obvious nutritional deficiency.

No. _____

Health questionnaire

Name _____ Date _____

How old are you? _____ Circle if you are . . Single, Married, Widowed, Separated, Divorced.

Your previous dentist's name _____ Address _____

Your physician's name _____ Address _____

Date of last visit to physician _____

DIRECTIONS TO PATIENTS

Answers to these questions will help the dentist decide how to best treat your dental problem. Try to circle each answer no or yes. If you have no idea of the answer to the question do not circle either answer. Soon after you have completed the questionnaire you will be seen by a dentist in the Admissions Clinic. The questionnaire will then be discussed with you, and you will be examined.

PAST MEDICAL HISTORY

1. Have you ever had hives? No Yes
2. Is there any medicine you cannot take because you are allergic to it or because it makes you sick? No Yes
3. Are you allergic to penicillin? No Yes
4. Has anyone ever told you not to take penicillin or dental anesthesia (novocaine)? No Yes
5. Are you allergic to aspirin or does it make you sick to take it? No Yes
6. Have you ever been a patient in a hospital? No Yes
7. Have you ever had a blood transfusion? No Yes
8. Have you ever been denied permission to give blood to someone (blood donor)? No Yes
9. Have you ever had hepatitis or yellow jaundice? No Yes
10. Have you ever been sick in bed for more than 7 days at a time? No Yes
11. As a child, did you have growing pains or swelling of the joints that required your being put to bed? No Yes
12. Has a doctor ever told you that you had anything wrong with your heart? No Yes
13. Have you ever had a heart attack? No Yes
14. Have you ever had a stroke? No Yes

15. Have you ever had a stomach, duodenal, or peptic ulcer? No Yes
16. Have you ever been treated or taken medication for an emotional problem or for your nerves? No Yes
17. Has a doctor ever told you that you had a heart murmur or an abnormal sound in your heart? No Yes
18. Have you ever had rheumatic fever or St. Vitus' dance? No Yes
19. Have you ever bled too much or for more than 2 days after a tooth extraction or any other dental treatment? No Yes
20. Have you ever had high blood pressure? No Yes
21. Have you ever had anemia, low blood, or thin blood? No Yes
22. Have you ever had tuberculosis? No Yes
23. Have you ever lived with anyone who had tuberculosis? No Yes
24. Have you ever had fits, seizures, convulsions, or epilepsy? No Yes
25. Have you ever fainted? No Yes
26. Have you ever gotten sick because of dental treatment? No Yes
27. Have you ever had syphilis, "bad blood," or a venereal disease? No Yes
28. Have you ever had radiation or x-ray treatments for any disease? No Yes

REVIEW OF SYSTEMS

29. Has there been a change in your general health in the past year? No Yes
30. Have you been treated by a physician in the past year? No Yes
31. Have you lost or gained more than 10 lbs in the past year? No Yes
32. Have you changed the size of your clothes in the past year? No Yes
33. Have you taken off more than a total of 7 days from your job in the past year because of illness? No Yes

34. Have you felt as it you had a fever in the past month? No Yes
35. Do you have anything wrong with your eyes not correctable by glasses? No Yes
36. Do you have nosebleeds as often as once a month? No Yes
37. Do you ever have fever blisters (cold sores) on your lips? No Yes
38. Do you ever have ulcers (sores) in your mouth? No Yes

REVIEW OF SYSTEMS—cont'd

39. Do you have chronic sores or boils of any kind on your skin? No Yes
40. Do you get very short of breath after climbing one flight of stairs? No Yes
41. Do you sleep on two or more pillows at night? No Yes
42. Do your ankles swell during the day? No Yes
43. Do you ever get pains in your chest or over your heart? No Yes
44. Do you ever feel that you heart is beating too fast or irregularly or have palpitations? No Yes
45. Do you have difficulty sleeping? No Yes
46. Are your stools ever black in color? No Yes
47. Do you ever pass blood-stained (red) urine? No Yes
48. Are you now taking or have you taken any medicine in the past 3 weeks? No Yes
49. Have you had any shots (injections) in the past 6 months? No Yes
50. Do you ever have to stop walking because of pain or pressing sensation in your chest? No Yes
51. Do you feel tired or low in energy all day? No Yes
52. Have you taken cortisone treatment in the past year? No Yes
53. Do you seem to be too warm or too cold in a room when everyone else is comfortable?
54. Do you bleed or bruise more easily than other people? No Yes
55. Are there any foods you cannot eat because they make you sick? No Yes
56. Are you troubled by nervousness or tension? No Yes
57. Are you botherd by numbness or "pins and needles" in your legs and feet? No Yes
58. Do you have frequent and severe headaches? No Yes
59. Have you coughed up blood in the past 6 months? No Yes
60. Do you have to pass water (urinate) more than 6 times a day or get up to urinate more than 2 times at night? No Yes
61. Do you have asthma or hay fever? No Yes
62. Do you have sugar diabetes? No Yes
63. Have you lost interest or energy for your job or social life? No Yes
64. Are you frequently sad, depressed, or blue? No Yes
65. Do you take any medicine or pills regularly for allergy, weight control, constipation or do you take aspirin every day? No Yes

FAMILY HISTORY

66. Did anyone in your family (blood related) ever have sugar diabetes? No Yes
67. Did any of your children weigh more than 10 lbs at birth? No Yes
68. Did anyone in your family ever have fits, epilepsy, or mental disease? No Yes
69. How many children do you have? __
70. Have any of your relatives died? (parents, children, or brothers and sisters only) No Yes
71. Are any of your close relatives in poor health? (parents, children, or brothers and sisters only) No Yes

SOCIAL HISTORY

72. Do you smoke more than one package of cigarettes a day? No Yes
73. Do you drink an alcoholic beverage more than six times a week? (six drinks) No Yes
74. Circle the highest grade you reached in school
    Grade 1, 2, 3, 4, 5, 6, 7, 8, High School 9, 10, 11, 12, College, 1, 2, 3, 4, Graduate School 1, 2, 3, 4
75..What is your occupation? _____
76. What is your race? _____

TO BE ANSWERED BY WOMEN ONLY

77. Do you have irregular menstrual periods? No Yes
78. When was your last menstrual period? Date _____
79. Are you taking birth control pills? No Yes
80. Have you had excessive menstrual bleeding in the past 2 years? No Yes
81. Are you pregnant? No Yes
82. How many times have you been pregnant? _____
83. What is your spouse's occupation? _____

Patient's signature _____

Date _____

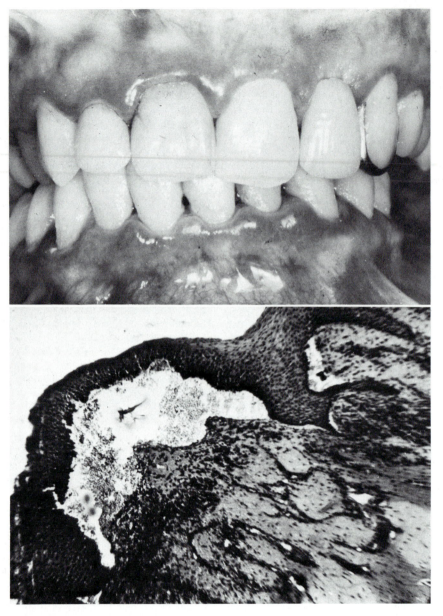

Fig. 12-13. Bullous lichen planus in a woman whose history revealed marked discomfort in chewing. Biopsy showed an interepithelial vesicle. Once diagnosis was made, therapy included local management as well as use of triamcinolone acetonide (Kenalog).

tient's rambling account of a long series of real or imagined ills. Much valuable information may be gleaned from this kind of complaint; in fact the patient's psychologic makeup may be ascertained.

The recording of the complaint should be complete as possible, and the relevant data underlined so that the summary can be utilized as contributing data for evaluation. The complaint should be related to the patient's past history to ascertain whether the problem is a continuation of past symptoms or a new development.

The oral history should review as many of the past dental and oral procedures as possible, including the most recent. The patient who relates that he has had scaling procedures every 3 months for the past 10 years and still has a great deal of subgingival calculus can lead the dentist to conclude that the calculus was never removed or that the accumulation occurred in a most rapid fashion. Reviewing past radiographs could reveal the answer. In any event, such a rapid accumulation of calculus would lead the examiner to ascertain the reason. The patient who relates that herpes infection has occurred every so often in the past and has had a recent episode could have an occurrence after scaling or a surgical procedure. The therapist must be aware of such a problem. If the gingivae are affected by the herpes, then gingival topography may be altered adversely during the infectious phase, even though healing has started.

The dental and oral history may reveal bleeding episodes after scaling or extraction. Again the therapist must be aware of a danger signal. Careful questioning may reveal other data for evaluation. The individual who bleeds for 1 or 2 days after an extraction might bleed after a periodontal operation. It would be wise to do a bleeding and clotting time examination for such a patient.

The history should also include chewing efficiency (how much force sore teeth can provide, chewing efficiency changed because of temporomandibular joint pain, and so on) since such a finding may be the symptom of joint changes—muscular problems as well as advanced periodontal disease where marked mobility of the teeth is present. Chewing efficiency may be altered in the morning because of clenching of the teeth during the night, which makes teeth sore. This finding should lead to questions concerning habits, especially bruxism or clamping.

The history of bruxism or clamping is one that must be elicited from the patient. Often the patient is totally unaware that he or she has such a habit, and it is only when someone in frequent contact confirms that the patient grits his or her teeth that a habitual pattern is ascertained. The recognition of such a habit is of utmost importance in that occlusal trauma is most likely to be present under such circumstances. Wear patterns on the teeth are generally present. This problem is discussed in detail in another chapter, but it is important that it be recognized during the dental and oral examination.

There are other oral habits that should also be recognized such as lip biting, bobby pin opening, tongue placement causing pressure, reverse swallowing, biting on foreign objects, and unrelated chewing. All these may have special influences; soreness and redness of the gingiva on the lingual aspect of the mandibular teeth may be the result of pressing of the tongue against the gingival tissue and alveolar mucosa.

Past acute episodes of necrotizing ulcerative gingivitis or other oral diseases should be covered in the oral history. Recurrent aphthae not only may be painful but may interfere with eating after a surgical procedure has been performed on the other side and the patient has been told not to chew there. Past necrotizing ulcerative gingivitis may account for deep interdental craters.

An important aspect of the examination is the eliciting of information concerning allergies and sensitivity to drugs that may be used in periodontal therapy: anesthetic fluids, antibiotics, aspirin, codeine, tranquilizers, and so on. Drugs or medications currently being taken by the patient also should be known and evaluated in respect to drugs that may have to be prescribed. Any drugs that cannot be used should be marked in large red lettering on the patient's record as well as on the cover as a reminder to the dentist that these drugs cannot be given. Also if a patient must take an antibiotic before treatment, for example, for rheumatic heart disease, it should also be so marked. This reminder allows the dentist to question the patient whether he has taken his medication.

Psychologic considerations should be taken into account during the medical and oral history taking. The patient who reiterates that tooth loss would not be bearable or who is vain about the appearance of his teeth must be recognized. Any change in tooth appearance, sometimes even for the better, may be challenged and set up an emotional problem. On the other hand, the young woman who holds her hand over her mouth when she talks may have a distinct, positive change in personality after dental correction. The dentist must know the patient he or she is treating!

The oral history also may be of considerable importance in attaining the diagnosis and treatment plan; for example, it will explain the patient's interest or lack of attention to his mouth, the possible reasons for excessive tooth wear and the commonly associated occlusal traumatic lesions, and his reactions both psychologically and physiologically to previous dental procedures. It should also elicit the reasons why he seeks the present professional service. Generally, therefore, the oral history will provide the following important information:

1. Chief complaint
2. Recent dental procedures
3. Bleeding history in previous dental operations
4. Habit history, that is, bruxism, clenching, and foreign object chewing
5. Professional and home-care oral hygiene procedures
6. History of acute oral infections, for example, necrotizing ulcerative gingivitis and periapical and pericoronal infections
7. Frequency of dental examinations

Clinical examination of periodontium

The following is a list of the essential points to be checked in a dental and periodontal examination.

- A. Gingival color, form, and texture
  1. Exudate
  2. Bleeding
- B. Deposits
  1. Plaque—amount and distribution
  2. Materia alba—amount and distribution
  3. Supragingival calculus—amount, type, and distribution
  4. Subgingival calculus—amount, type, and distribution
- C. Contour and depth of pockets
- D. Contact relationships of teeth
- E. Food impaction areas, for example, plunger cusps
- F. Marginal ridge, axial, and other anatomic aberrations of teeth
- G. Abnormal frenum insertions
- H. Relationship of pocket base to zone of alveolar mucosa
- I. Areas of gingival recession, for example, clefts
- J. Topography of interdental tissues
- K. Mesiodistal width and height of interdental gingival embrasure, that is, proximity of roots of adjacent teeth
- L. Length of gingival wall, that is, depth of vestibule
- M. Tongue—size, shape, and habits
- N. Occlusal relationships
- O. Signs and symptoms of occlusal traumatism in the following:
  1. Temporomandibular joint and masticatory musculature
  2. Teeth
  3. Attachment apparatus
- P. Wear patterns and facets on teeth
- Q. Occlusal habits, that is, bruxism, clenching, clamping, and percussive habits
- R. Mobility of teeth
- S. Oral habits, that is, tongue thrusting and infantile swallowing
- T. Migration of teeth
- U. Existing restorations and their suitability to conditions that they were designed to correct

In the clinical examination general observations of the oral cavity should be made. The jaws as a whole should be studied. They may be large or small; their relative size and the size of both jaws relative to that of the head may be abnormal.

Examination of arch anatomy. Arch anatomy is an important consideration in the dental examination. The dentist should note the form of the arch, the length of the alveolar process occlusoapically, and the anatomic variations (interferences).

Arch form is especially important. The narrow arch with crowded teeth is conducive to caries and to periodontal disease as a result of nonphysiologic cleansing ability and the obstacles that it presents to home oral physiotherapy; these inadequacies are likely to result in food impaction and plaque and calculus retention.

The *length of the alveolar process* or the length of the gingival wall (gingival margin to vestibular fornix) is variable in different individuals as a consequence of genetic development or the influence of past or present periodontal disease. Therefore the approach to periodontal therapy may require modification to accommodate to the situation at hand. Alveolar length is intimately related to the width of the zone of attached gingiva. Often this zone is narrowed or obliterated in periodontal disease, and therapy must include procedures to broaden this area.

Examination of dentition. The examination of the dentition with respect to the size, contour, and position of the teeth as well as their vitality should be noted. Crown form plays an important role in the protection of the gingival tissues from the traumatizing effects of many foodstuffs. It has been demonstrated that during mastication the bolus of food is deflected away from the gingival margins by the convex axial contours of the tooth crown. Should a tooth surface be flat, there is food impingement against the gingival margin; this is often seen in restorative dentistry when a crown is contoured improperly or when there is wear of an acrylic veneer.

Overly contoured crowns may also be detrimental to gingival health for the opposite reason, that is, trapping of food material cervically to the exaggerated tooth contour.

The inclination of the tooth also must be evaluated, since a lingually tipped tooth, for example, a mandibular incisor, loses its protective capacity for the labial gingiva no matter how well formed its surface may be. Again the gingival tissue on the buccal aspect of a molar tooth retruded in the arch may show signs of a low-grade inflammatory lesion because of the trauma it receives from the pressure of food against it.

Thus crown form and tooth position are important considerations in the etiology of periodontal disease.

Alignment of marginal ridges and loss of contact between approximately teeth, especially with opposing plunger cusps, must be noted in the examination. This loss of approximation is an exceedingly insidious relationship, since food impingement and impaction occur with resultant gingival irritation.

Tooth position should be noted. An example is the buccally positioned maxillary second molar.

When the maxillary second molar is in buccoversion in reference to the first molar, the contact area is located in such a way that it does not adequately protect the interdental tissues. Food impaction commonly occurs in such a situation, with resultant damage to the interproximal gingival tissue and increased likelihood of dental caries. When this occurs the relating mandibular teeth are usually not in proper alignment; here too a similar disease process is often found.

The interproximal area of the maxillary canine and first premolar often presents another special problem because of the turning of these teeth in the arch. The labial surface of the canine may lie in the same plane as the corresponding surfaces of the lateral and central incisors, while the first premolar starts to make the bend so that its buccal surface tends to be in alignment with the buccal surfaces of the remaining posterior teeth. In these instances the buccal portion of the interproximal tissue is wide, but the palatal interdental tissue is extremely narrow and unprotected. Here again the contact areas may not fulfill their protective requirements, with consequent caries and periodontal involvement. A similar situation may also be found in the mandibular canine–first premolar region.

The maxillary lateral incisor in many cases overlaps the central incisor. Here the interdental area is extremely vulnerable to injury, since the positions of the teeth may adversely alter the protective quality of the crown for the gingival tissues. Not infrequently the labial gingival tissue of the central incisor is also traumatized.

The buccal aspect of the mandibular second molar is often involved by cervical caries and by periodontal pocket formation. Such disease is present because the shallow vestibular fornix, the high external oblique ridge of the mandible, and the heavy buccinator musculature combine not only to retain foodstuff in the area, thus detracting from the self-cleansing ability of the part, but also to interfere with oral hygiene measures necessary to cleanse the area.

Individual or collective buckling of the mandibular incisors, when seen, presents a distinct problem. The crown forms do not protect the gingival margins, and as a result a gingival inflammatory lesion is found. Here the examination should entail separate measurements of the distance between the mesial surfaces of the canines and of the combined width of the four incisor teeth. If only three incisor teeth are necessary to fill the intercuspid space, it may be wise to extract one incisor (usually the tooth most involved by periodontal disease) and then by orthodontic means to reposition the remaining incisor teeth in their correct positions to fill the space between the cuspids. The management of the periodontal aspect in these cases must take into consideration not only the repositioning of the gingival margins but also the gingival contours in relationship to crown form. It must also consider the relationship of the mandibular to the maxillary teeth as to their plunger effect.

Root form is ascertained by roentgenographic examination. The length of the root is an important consideration in the evaluation of the tooth for success in periodontal therapy. As a general rule the longer the root, the greater will be the stability of the tooth, and the less costly will be the marginal destruction by periodontal disease.

It should be emphasized here that root anatomy cannot be totally assayed from the roentgenographic examination. The length and buccolingual width of the proximal root surfaces cannot be ascertained; the examiner, however, can determine the anatomy of the apical one third of the root. Since the total square area of the root constitutes the overall surface for binding the tooth by the periodontal ligament to bone, its determination is a prognostic index when the marginal periodontium has been lost. Thus in the case of a tooth with a tapered root, resorption of the cervical third of the supporting bone may constitute a high percentage of square area loss of tooth retention. When half of the periodontium is lost in regard to the length of the root, much more than 50% of the attachment is voided; this is not true when the root form is full. Thus prognosis is directly proportional to the amount of root surface available for attachment of tooth to bone.

The proximity of the roots of adjacent teeth is directly related to crown form. Generally when proximal surfaces of the adjoining crowns are flattened their roots are closer. Because of this there are several factors to be considered, which are as follows:

1. The interproximal tissues of teeth with proximal crown forms that do not allow for a full embrasure space are small and often unprotected.

2. The col form is deep with respect to the buccal and lingual peaks of the interdental papilla. Should an inflammatory change occur in the buccal peak with its attending retractability, the col area will not be protected. Food retention may occur in the col, with resultant crater formation.

3. Since the bulk of interdental tissue is small,

a destructive inflammatory process will tend to produce a deep and narrow defect, thus allowing for further retention of debris. Cause becomes effect, and effect becomes cause.

Examination of the coronal surfaces should include the detection of erosion caries and faulty restorations. All teeth suspected of being pulpless should be indicated and the condition verified by pulp test. These facts should be recorded in relation to the disturbances that they may produce; for example, overhanging fillings not having a proper point of contact with the adjacent tooth may cause not only food impaction but also irritation of the gingiva, resulting in inflammation.

Examination of gingivae. *Color changes* of the gingivae should be observed, since these are the primary visual symptoms of periodontal disease. Normal gingival tissue is pink, varying slightly in shade but uniform throughout for any individual. In some persons it is comparatively light, whereas in others it is almost pink-red. Any deviation from the uniform characteristic color may be evidence of a disease change in that area. It warns that the area is being invaded or encroached upon and that metabolic changes are taking place. The color may be lighter than that of the adjacent tissue (indicative of anemia) or darker (indicative of congestion and inflammation).

Often a color change may be localized in the gingival margin, not extending to the attached gingivae to any extent, whereas in other instances it may involve not only the attached gingiva but also the alveolar mucosa. This is an expression of the extent of the inflammatory infiltrate. Color

changes vary also with the duration of the lesion. A long-standing disease process may not disclose any gingival discoloration but may take on a pink hue and even at times be lighter. This is due to the repair factor present in the course of the disease process. Gingival fibrosis, therefore, may appear lighter in color than a norm but still be the result of disease.

Some cases show a purplish blue line along the gum tissue at about the height of the alveolar crest and extending to the cervical margin. This may indicate chemical poisoning, for example, bismuth; it may also give warning of a systemic involvement. To the critical observer a color change is significant in that it may indicate many different types of disturbances.

Changes in the surface texture are diagnosed on the basis of degree of stippling, loss of stippling, presence of tissue edema, and severity of the inflammatory process. Surface texture is also related to changes in gingival form or topography seen in periodontal disease. Stippling loss in gingival inflammation produces a smooth, often shiny, gingival surface. This change in surface texture and appearance may be localized to the interproximal tissue and the marginal gingivae, or it may be diffusely noted, with variable dimensions, in the zone of attached gingiva. Generally the more severe the inflammatory process, the greater will be the degree and extent of the area of stippling loss, and the more distorted the tissue will be because of edema and hyperplasia. It should be reemphasized that low-grade gingival inflammation, with its accompanying hyperplasia, will often present a

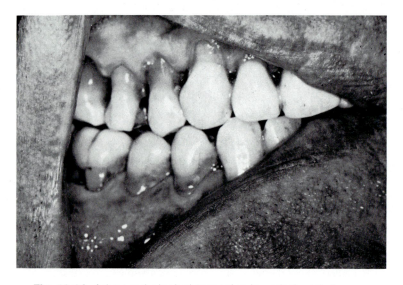

Fig. 12-14. Advanced gingival recession in periodontal disease.

situation in which the tissue is pink, stippled, and variably distorted (Fig. 12-14).

Deviations from normal contour and structure of the gingivae should be noted next. The normal gingiva is festooned around the necks of the teeth with a thin, adherent margin. Thickened, retracted margins may be observed covering the enamel surfaces of the teeth. On the other hand, recession may have occurred, and the gingival margin may be located on the root surface (Fig. 12-15). The location of the gingival margin with respect to the tooth contour is an important relationship,

since a food impaction phenomenon may be present. Recession may be caused by many conditions in addition to the results of a periodontal manifestation, for example, an insufficient contact point of faulty marginal ridges or restorations. These abnormal conditions permit food to lodge between the teeth and on the septal tissue, which is thus gradually forced down from its normal contour into a depression. Food lodging may occur without involving any appreciable recession of the labial, buccal, or lingual gingiva. However, where the interproximal space is deep enough to hold food

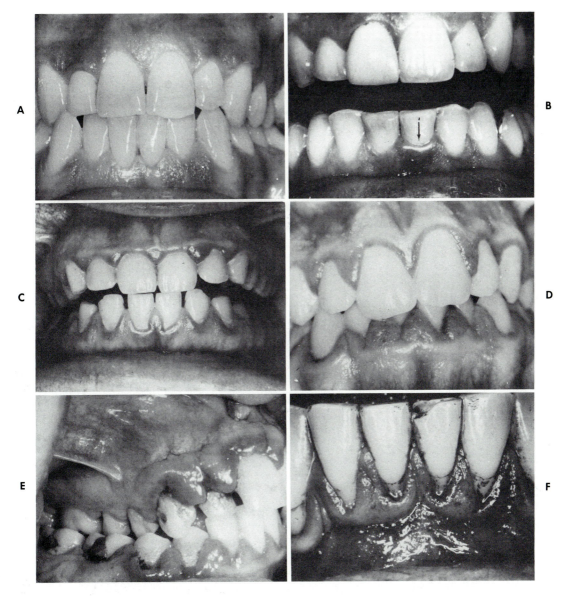

Fig. 12-15. Various gingival conditions that examiner must record. **A,** Fibrotic inflammatory process. **B,** Altered passive eruption. **C,** Gingival hyperplasia. **D,** Marked gingival hyperplasia with some fibrosis. **E,** Extreme gingival inflammatory hyperplasia with a great deal of edema. **F,** Recession and gingival change in topography.

debris, the tissue will soon succumb to disease, and the adjacent tissue will also be gradually invaded.

The irritation of calculus causes a loss of *tissue vitality and tone*. The tissue becomes susceptible to infection, followed by a gradual recession from the normal contour. Faulty brushing of the teeth may cause a recession that is noticeable on the labiobuccal surface, with fairly resistant and firm gingivae and no apparent local irritant. Hypoplasia of the teeth as well as flat enamel labial, buccal, or lingual surfaces are causes of recession inasmuch as food is forced directly from the occlusal

or incisal surfaces onto the gingival margins, thus causing injury; or the gingivae are forced from the cervix of the tooth or teeth, suffering destruction of their normal contour.

Normally the gingival tissue is hard and firm and as a rule highly resistant to injury by brushing of the teeth or by hot, cold, or hard food. The healthy gingiva has a stippled surface. At the first signs of inflammation the structure changes and begins to swell, the gingiva becomes spongy, and there is a loss of tone. Stippling disappears, and the surface of the tissue takes on a glistening appearance.

Abrasions or clefts of the gingivae are to be

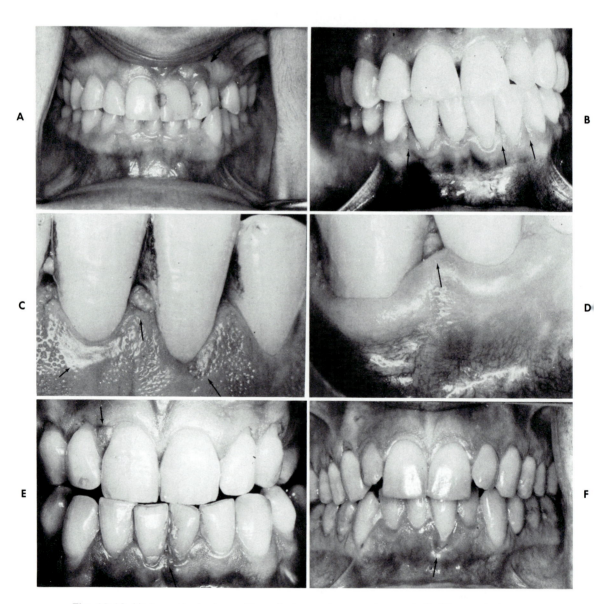

Fig. 12-16. Various gingival conditions that examiner must record. **A,** Change in texture, form, retraction, and color. **B,** Interdental cleft. **C,** Small clefts. **D,** Crater. **E,** Horizontal cleft and interdental loft of tissue *(arrows).* **F,** Recession and frenum.

noted. These may be signs of faulty brushing, which may be caused by a new toothbrush or an improper method of brushing. Clefts may be caused by rotary brushing when the patient uses Fones' technique with a stiff bristle brush.

However, clefts are usually the sign of underlying disease. They may develop on any surface of the gingival margin and are associated with pocket formation. Subgingival deposits may be found and may be an important contributing factor in the etiology. Depressed lines are often seen on the interdental papilla and marginal gingiva. At first glance these lines may indicate a cleft, but on close examination they reveal no separation of tissue. They are *pseudopapillae* such as are often seen in pregnancy and in diabetic gingivitis.

Clefts are apparently due to a breakthrough of the gingiva around the tooth as a result of pocket formation. It was pointed out earlier that in inflammatory conditions such as those seen in marginal periodontitis the crest of the alveolar bone is resorbed. Associated with this condition is a downward growth of the epithelium along the cementum. In the gingiva, where inflammation is present, one sees papillary projections of epithelium that have grown down into the subepithelial tissue and anastomosed; areas of tissue isolated by this anastomosis are sloughed off. An uneven rate of sloughing of the gingiva around the tooth will cause clefts to form (Figs. 12-16 to 12-17).

Examinations of the *interproximal tissues* may show them to be inflamed, hyperplastic, atrophied, or even destroyed; all these are signs of periodontal manifestation. The interproximal gingivae may be destroyed through a necrotizing ulcerative gingivitis, or the buccal peaks may be enlarged because of an inflammatory gingival hyperplasia. Normally the architecture of the interproximal tissue is dependent on the relationship of adjacent teeth. Crown form and root proximations will determine the shape of the papilla. Roots close together allow for diminutive buccal and lingual peaks, whereas should the teeth be separated, a saddle-type area will be present. Overlapping of

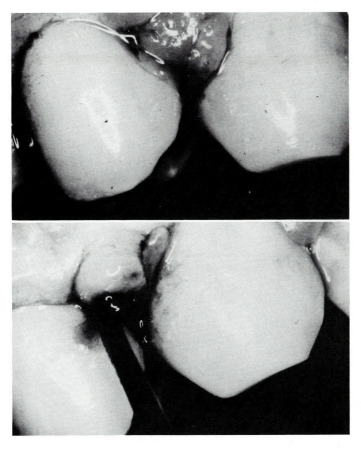

Fig. 12-17. Breakdown of interdental tissue. Note how whole buccal peak can be retracted. Examiner must explore for crater formation.

a tooth alters the shape of the interproximal tissue as well. Thus any changes in tooth relationship due to periodontal disease influence the interdental tissues (Fig. 12-18).

Tooth relationships must therefore be closely inspected for spillways, contact, and lodgment of calculus and food debris as causations for disease. Crowded teeth with closely proximating roots or with roots inclined at poor angulations are often responsible for gingival disease. These relationships must be familiar to the diagnostician for recognition of the problem.

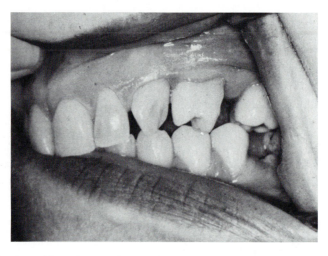

Fig. 12-18. Tooth position plays an important role in periodontal therapy. Note difference in gingival topography between canine and first premolar. Because of close approximation of roots, this may be a difficult area to manage.

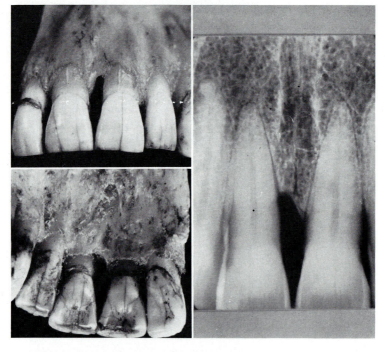

Fig. 12-19. Maxillary incisor section (dried specimen). A vertical resorptive lesion may be seen from both labial and lingual aspects. Here, however, there is no labial or lingual plate. This type of infrabony pocket has only one wall, the septal one. Roentgenographically there is a vertical resorptive lesion. This type of pocket is not amenable to therapy to fill defect. Therapist must ascertain by probing whether one, two, or three walls are present.

The *depth of the pocket* should be ascertained with a probe bearing a millimeter rule (Fig. 12-23). Not only is the depth of the pocket important, but the topography of the pocket is also. Most important, the base of the pocket should be determined; occasionally it may be situated in the alveolar mucosa and present a special problem in therapy. Usually pockets vary in depth around a given tooth, and the differences must be ascertained. Should an infrabony pocket be present, then the examination must disclose whether lateral walls—buccal and lingual— are present. It is im-portant to ascertain the topography of the osseous defect, for therapy will be based upon this.

Examination for crestal topography. In the past roentgenology has been utilized to determine the crestal topography; it has been demonstrated that this procedure has distinct limitations. It is true that vertical resorptive lesions are recognizable; however, the exact topography cannot be visualized. This does not mean that the roentgenogram does not contribute information to the examination but rather that it must be augmented by clinical examination. The clinical examination is

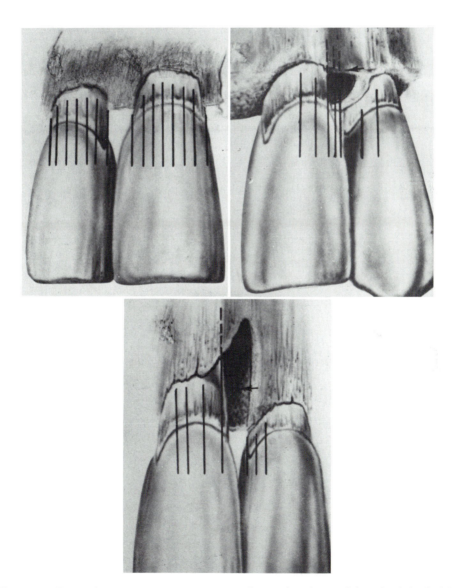

Fig. 12-20. From a fixed point, measurement can be made to base of detached gingival tissue. Band of attachment of collagen fibers covers crestal bone and seems to take on a rather uniform distance. Thus base of detached tissue mimics crestal bone. If examiner records this base around tooth carefully, crestal contour can be ascertained. Note base topographies when horizontal bore loss is seen, in contrast to that found in osseous defects.

directed to ascertain the location of the base of the detached gingival tissue in respect to the bone crest. Thus, these depth recordings locating the bases simulate the base of the osseous loss and to-

gether with probing by needle, the topography can be uncovered. It has long been noted that there is a width of connective tissue between the epithelial attachment of the gingiva and the bone crest. This

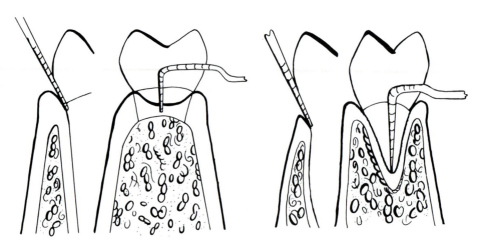

Fig. 12-21. Probing to base of detached gingival tissue must be carefully executed. Buccal and proximal exploration are being performed. An important point is that probe on proximal aspect must be parallel to long axis of tooth. This therefore requires a bend in probe to allow for correct placement. Note relation of base of detached tissue on buccal aspect, in contrast to proximal aspect. In this way a crater can be recognized.

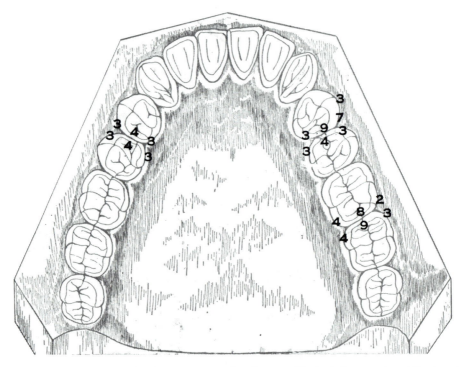

Fig. 12-22. Readings to show bone topography. On mandibular left, crestal architecture is regular; on right, there is a crater between first and second molars and a two-walled osseous defect affecting first premolar. Note that in osseous defect bone rises sharply and covers buccal aspect of tooth (reading of 3). If reading from cementoenamel junction were 7, for example, then examiner would know that root was denuded of bone to same level as interproximal aspect.

width tends to be rather uniform. Thus a shallower recording in respect to a deeper one denotes a tilt, whereas similar recordings denote a straight line (Figs. 12-19 to 12-22).

One important caution is the placement of the probe interdentially so that it is parallel to the long axis of the tooth. The probe must be fine enough to traverse the space between the gingiva and tooth

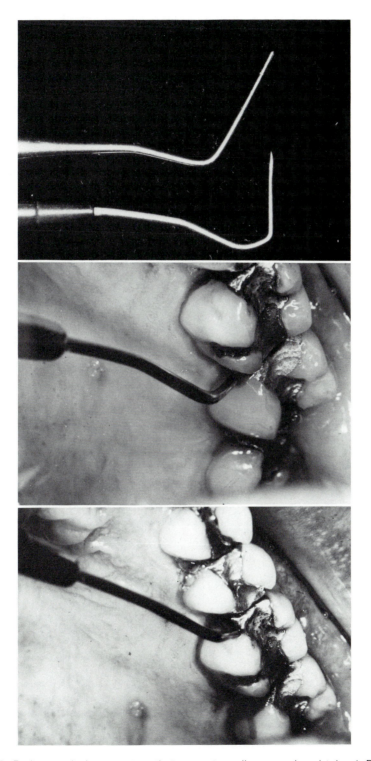

Fig. 12-23. Probes and placement so that correct readings can be obtained. Readings are made from the cementoenamel junction and are recorded on "block system."

without hindrance and should allow for easy reading in millimeters. If calculus interfers with the passage of the probe the examiner must be conscious of this. The calculus should be removed to ascertain a correct reading. Also it is important that the probe be shaped to allow interproximal placement without hindrance by the contact point of the teeth (Figs. 12-23 to 12-26).

In addition, needling, that is, passing a needle into the gingival tissue, allows for determination of tissue thickness and the presence of bone underneath. Hyperplasia may be due to either soft tissue or bone enlargement. It is easily determined by needling. Needling the buccal aspect of a roentgenographic vertical osseous resorptive defect will determine whether there is a bony wall present on

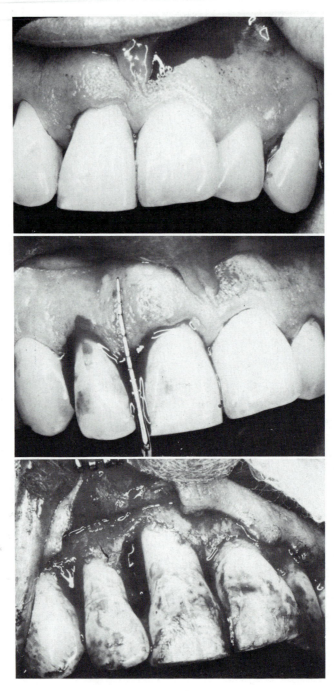

Fig. 12-24. Probing and visualization of a two-walled osseous defect. Recognition prior to therapy is essential so that dentist can decide how to manage problem.

the buccal surface. If penetration is not possible it must be assumed that bone is present. The same is true of the lingual surface.

Recognition of furca involvement is a key issue in the examination. While the roentgenogram offers evidence of such involvement it does not allow for interpretation as to whether the lesion is incipient, is of cul-de-sac topography, or is a through-and-through involvement. The very beginning of loss of tissue in the furca is not recognizable in the x-ray film. Because of this, clinical exploration is necessary. Careful probing allows for entrance into the interradicular space once tissue loss has taken place. In fact a fine wire can be threaded onto the area and directed according to the anatomy of the tooth to the opposite side of the

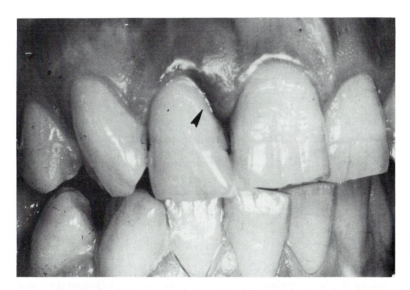

Fig. 12-25. Exploration is a vital aspect of examination. Examiner must not only recognize disease state but must also be capable of exploring detached gingival tissue and interpreting its osseous counterpart. Examiner must relate findings to what is to be done therapeutically. Note lesion on mesial aspect of lateral incisor. Examiner must determine whether an osseous defect is present, and if so, its topography.

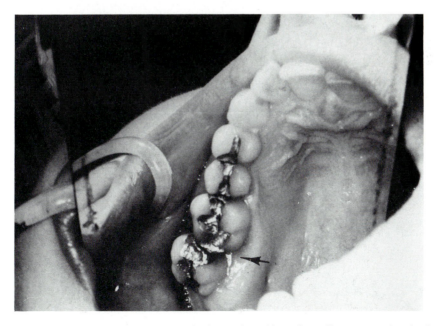

Fig. 12-26. A common problem—namely, buccal position of maxillary second molar in respect to first molar. Defect is usually found in interproximal area; examiner must recognize extent of defect.

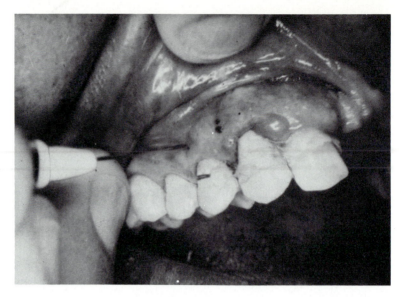

Fig. 12-27. Needling is an extremely helpful diagnostic procedure. Exploration can determine whether a buccal or lingual osseous wall is present; it can determine thickness of soft tissue; and it can locate crestal bone.

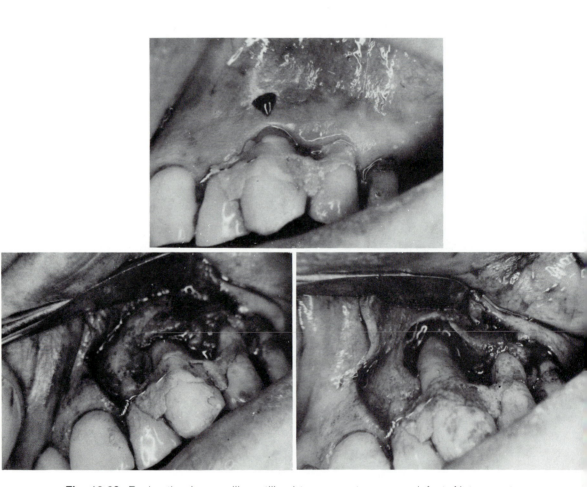

Fig. 12-28. Exploration by needling utilized to map out osseous defect. Note puncture marks that were made. When a flap was raised, defect corresponded to outline visualized by operator.

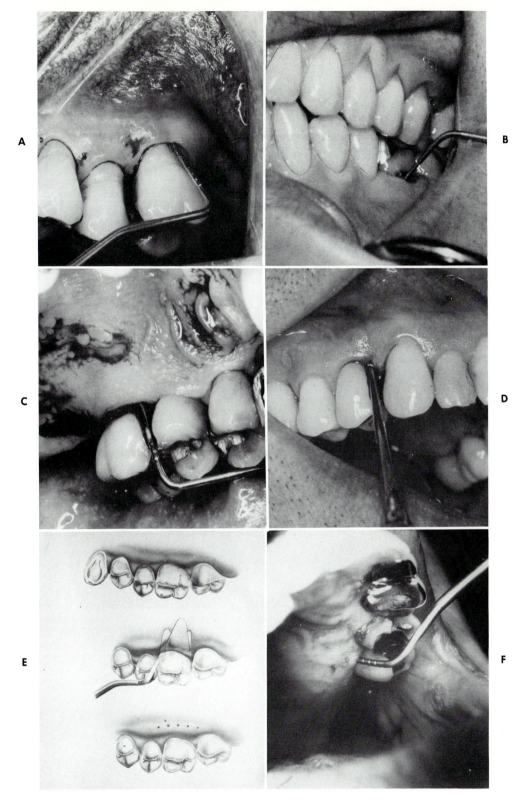

Fig. 12-29. Probing allows for not only pocket depth but also gives information concerning bone topography. **A,** Probe entering buccal furcal entrance. **B,** Entrance being made into furca of mandibular first molar. **C,** Probe sliding along mesial aspect of maxillary first molar. **D,** Entrance on mesial aspect of maxillary first premolar. **E,** Probe exploring mesial aspect of first molar. Outline of base of detached tissue is noted by dotted line. **F,** Examiner exploring base of detached gingival tissue in respect to rather flat palate form.

interradicular area. One of the most important aspects of the examination of maxillary molars (those whose roots are not fused and those in which interradicular involvement has taken place) is the determination as to whether there is bone on the facial aspect of the palatal root. For that matter, should endodontics and root removal be contemplated, the therapist must ascertain how much

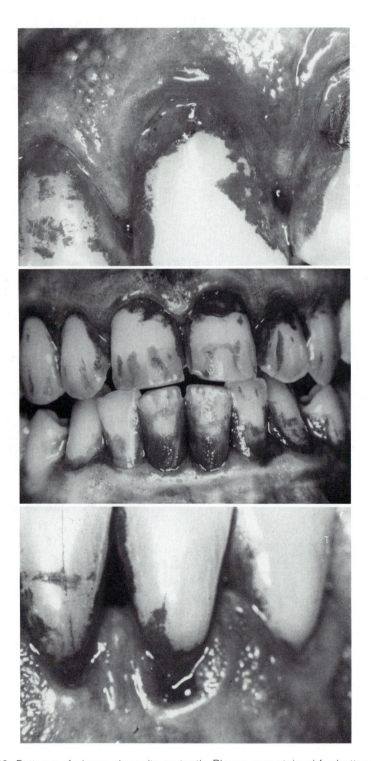

Fig. 12-30. Patterns of plaque deposits on teeth. Plaque was stained for better visualization. Thickness of plaque reveals length of accumulation.

bone remains about each root as well as the potential for repair of the bone after surgical intervention.

Examination for accretions. Accretions both soft and hard have been demonstrated as important etiologic factors in periodontal disease. These include plaque, materia alba (Fig. 12-30), and supragingival and subgingival calculus. The location and extent of their accumulation should be noted. It is important to recognize whether they are spread diffusely or are localized and whether they are placed primarily subgingivally or supragingivally. The time required for the buildup of these accretions deserves careful investigation, since it is well known that the time for deposition varies with different individuals.

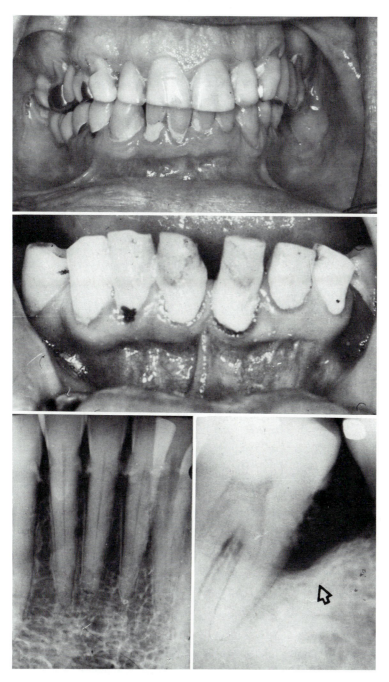

Fig. 12-31. Patterns of calculus deposits—supragingival and subgingival. Note that calculus can easily be recognized in radiographs.

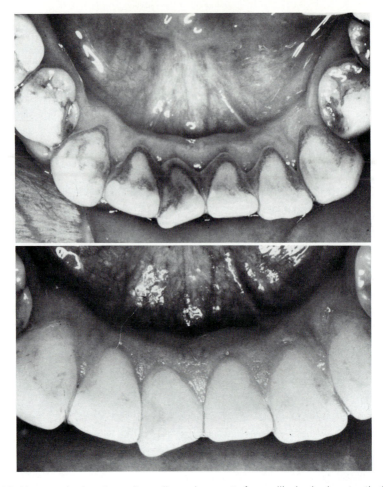

Fig. 12-32. Heavy calculus deposits on lingual aspect of mandibular incisor teeth. Calculus was removed, and patient was taught oral hygiene program. Bottom photograph was taken 1 month later. Note that patient was learning how to prevent formation of calculus. A slight plaque rim can be seen. This was pointed out to patient.

The clearance factor and the formation of plaque upon teeth are interrelated. It has been reported by numerous investigators that these two factors are major etiologic agents in periodontal disease; that is, if they can be controlled there is betterment of gingival health. It is a well-established fact that the better the oral hygiene program practiced by the individual, the less will be the occurrence of periodontal disease. Therefore in the examination one should review in detail not only the severity of accretional deposit but also the control by the patient—*both in attempt and in accomplishment*.

Calculus is a mass with varying degrees of calcification that forms on a tooth surface and adheres to it. The deposit lodges in the gingival margin occlusally (supragingival) and in the sulcular area (subgingival). It varies a great deal in color and hardness, depending on the age of the material and extrinsic factors, for example, dietary consistency and use of tobacco. Supragingival calculus is

easily seen, the greatest accumulations being located on the lingual surfaces of the mandibular anterior teeth and the buccal aspects of the maxillary molars. Subgingival calculus is not readily visible but must be found by careful probing with an explorer; at times it can be seen if a persistent stream of compressed air is directed to retract the gingival margins. It is dense, hard, and firmly adherent to the tooth surface. Its color is dark brown or green black.

The variability of amounts and types of accumulations in different individuals is marked. Recognition of the heavy and rapid calculus producer is important; with such knowledge prophylaxis and calculus removal may be performed at shorter recall intervals, and stringent measures of home oral physiotherapy may be taught and directed.

Examination for anatomic interferences. Anatomic interferences such as frena, high muscle attachments, the low-lying malar process, external oblique and mylohyoid ridges of the mandible, the mental protuberance, and mandibular tori must be checked to determine their possible influences on the production of periodontal disease and the approach to periodontal therapy. If a deformity, for example, deep periodontal pocket formation, narrow zone of attached gingiva, or frenum interferences, is found during examination, its presence and extent will certainly require careful evaluation to assure the successful planning and execution of therapy. In such an instance the dentist should be cognizant of the part that mucogingival surgery can play in the correction of this deformity. The flat palate with deep interdental or palatal pocket formation, again, represents an acute and severe therapeutic problem. Here the approach to therapy is based on (1) the knowledge of the various etiologic factors operating to induce the disease, (2) the actual topography and extent of the periodontal defects on *both* the palatal and buccal aspects of the teeth, and (3) the operative technique that is most likely to produce rapid and effective healing and a dentoperiodontal environment conducive to the maintenance of health.

Examination for mobility. The mobility of each tooth should be tested as directed previously and may be classified into four groups. They are as follows: (1) in some patients only single teeth are affected, whereas in others all the teeth are involved; (2) in early periodontosis, where there are no gingival symptoms, increased mobility and wandering may be the only signs of disease; (3) teeth that have restorations which are slightly high may show an increased mobility for a short time and then become firm; (4) teeth that can be depressed into the socket show roentgenographically a markedly increased width of the periodontal ligament and a loss of the alveolar bone.

Examination of occlusion. In many respects occlusion is the common denominator of *all phases* of dentistry and therefore represents an important aspect of the examination. Examination of occlusion should minimally include observation and notation of the following:

1. Degree of the curve of Spee
2. Measurements of amounts of overbite and overjet and their interrelationship
3. Discrepancy between habitual closure pattern and the terminal hinge position
4. Location, degree, and influence of occlusal prematurities in the terminal hinge position and various mandibular movements
5. Topography of marginal ridges of the teeth
6. Proximal contacts and embrasure areas of the teeth
7. Missing, tilted, rotated, and extruded teeth
8. Abnormal occlusal or proximal wear patterns of the teeth
9. Estimation of adequacy of free-way space
10. Occlusal habit patterns, such as bruxism, clenching, clamping, and so on
11. Measurement of amount of tooth mobility
12. Temporomandibular joint and mandibular musculature symptomatology

From the periodontal point of view the health of the attachment apparatus is directly related to the amount of stress placed on the teeth; this force is transmitted to the supporting structures. Overstress or occlusal traumatism is a direct result of parafunctional tooth contacts brought about by dentally or emotionally induced habits. Therefore it is necessary for the examination to include and record the habitual or convenience occlusal relationship, the terminal hinge position, and the maxillomandibular relationships during the lateral, protrusive, and lateroprotrusive mandibular movements with the teeth in contact. It is important to recognize and record discrepancies between the habitual closure pattern and terminal hinge position, the articular interferences on nonworking (balancing) and working sides during lateral mandibular excursions (to their functional limits), the anterior and posterior tooth contacts during mandibular protrusion, and the role that inadequate group function may play in inducing vertical hyperstress in the incisive position.

There are many causes of malfunctional occlusion—missing teeth, tilting of teeth, and drifting of teeth, to mention three. Missing contact points, resulting in food impaction, are the cause of marginal periodontitis in many instances. Occlusal habits (e.g., bruxism, fingernail biting, and pipe smoking) as well as occupational trauma (e.g., that sustained by needleworkers and upholsterers) should be noted. The type of damage, the teeth used, and the cause of the habit are essential points in the history.

In the examination of occlusion the dentist must be careful that he ascertains the centric relationship of the jaws. In many instances of periodontal disease the patient may open and close his jaws in a constant position, and this may be taken for his centric relationship. However, upon careful examination it will be noted that when the patient places his tongue posteriorly to the roof of the mouth and closes his jaws the mandible is in a more retrusive position than noted previously. This latter position must be taken as the centric relationship, the previous position being one of convenience.

In many cases it will be noted that the damage

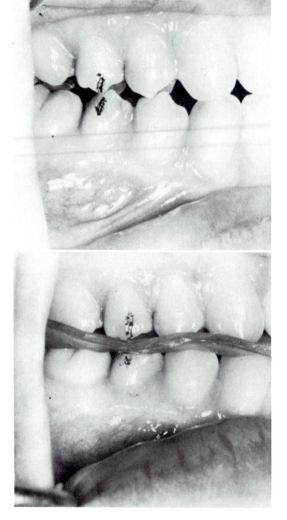

Fig. 12-33. Examination for centric relation is an important phase of determination of occlusal condition. Centric relation has been located and is being recorded in a wax wafer to determine tooth contacts.

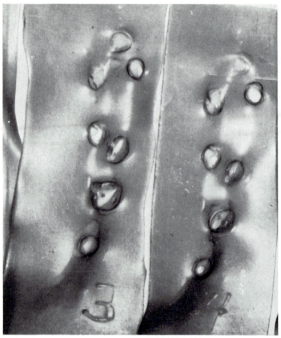

Fig. 12-34. Wax templates denoting occlusal relationship of teeth.

to the supporting structures is located in areas where there is a premature contact in the centric relationship. There may be but few teeth occluding in this position, and these are usually the ones whose periodontium has been damaged.

Thus the examination of the occlusion in cases of periodontal involvement is an important factor in diagnosis and treatment planning. Examination of the patient while he is using his masticatory apparatus will afford a great deal of information as to the habits of chewing, the length of the chewing cycle, and the efficiency of chewing. Examination of study casts for abraded areas or facets is of distinct value. The lingual relationships between the teeth can be studied better, offering a more com-

plete analysis of the occlusal relationships present. Plunger cusps with possible areas for food impaction, relationship of contact between adjacent teeth, and overbite and overjet can be observed. Palpation of movement of a tooth during the contact of antagonists in the chewing cycle can be noted by resting lightly the ball of the index finger against two adjacent upper teeth and then against a single tooth. Any movement of the tooth can be detected. Another method of study is registration of the tooth surfaces in wax after the mandible has been occluded against the maxilla. Detection of a premature contact by the complete displacement of the wax is a valuable method of examination. Many other methods are utilized, the most common being the use of articulating paper markings. Careful examination of facets on the occlusal contacting surfaces is helpful in diagnosis. If only a few teeth exhibit these facets, the inference can be made that these are the only teeth taking up the burden. It is to be noted, however, that a tooth may be traumatized without a facet being produced. In these instances the supporting structures have been destroyed, allowing the tooth to move in its socket during the occlusal contact. Excessive mobility of the teeth during function is also a sign of occlusal traumatism. Teeth that on close observation are seen to move in function or those in which the movement can be detected by the placing of a fin-

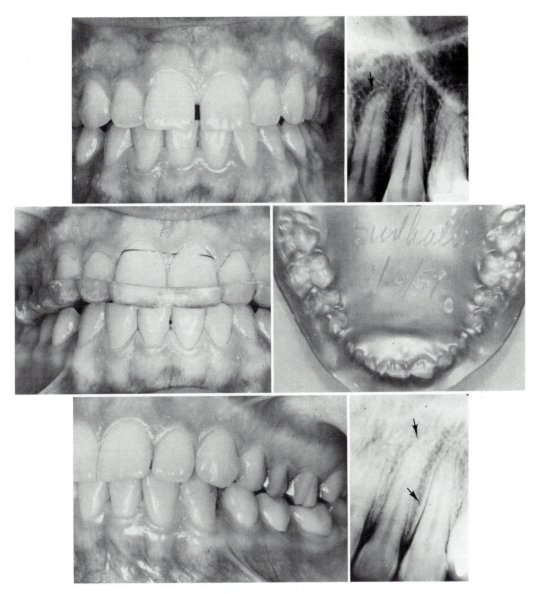

Fig. 12-35. Dentition of a 38-year-old woman who exhibited mobility of teeth. Radiographic findings revealed widening of periodontal ligament space and changes in lamina dura and supporting bone. Centric relation was located, and initial occlusal adjustment performed. Maxillary anterior teeth were retruded orthodontically, and a bite guard was made to stabilize teeth. Mandibular first molars had been lost, and these were replaced by fixed bridges. Occlusal relationships were defined by definitive occlusal adjustment. A wax recording of tooth contacts can be seen. Radiographically, periodontal ligament spaces thinned out, and a distinct lamina dura could be seen. Clinically, teeth became firm. Thus examination is important, for it forms the basis of management.

ger over the tooth during the act of occlusion are in traumatism. Another sign is the blanching of the gingival margin as is at times seen over the maxillary incisors and premolars. This is due to a stretching of the gingiva suspended firmly by the adjacent teeth. Soreness of a tooth is usually a late symptom of occlusal traumatism and is related to changes in the periodontium allowing for the tooth to be extruded (Figs. 12-34 and 12-35).

The occlusal relationship, even though it may appear clinically adverse, may not induce changes in the attachment apparatus. The extent of involvement of the supporting structures in an apparent traumatic situation is dependent on the interplay of the direction, duration, and frequency of the applied force and the ability of the supporting tissues to resist and repair in the presence of the force. When present the occlusal traumatic lesion is characterized by facet wear on the teeth, tooth mobility and migration, and radiographic evidence of root resorption, that is, widening of the periodontal ligament space, fraying of the lamina dura, and resorption induced radiolucencies of supporting bone. All these destructive changes make up the loss of attachment apparatus necessary for the stability of the tooth; this loss of support results in tooth mobility and migration. On the other hand, the occlusal relationship may be such that it represents in the attachment apparatus a condition of *underuse* or *disuse*. During the oral examination the dentist may notice that a tooth has lost its articulating counterpart in the opposite dental arch; this tooth may appear extruded in relation to its neighbors. Roentgenographic examinations may reveal distinct changes in the lamina dura and supporting bone. This disuse, a situation in which

very little stress is placed on the tooth and its attachment apparatus, may reflect roentgenographically a thinning, fragmentation, or fuzziness of the lamina dura and some loss of supporting bone. It should be emphasized at this point that although a tooth may not have occlusal contact, some force is placed on the tooth by the pressure of a bolus of food and by tongue manipulation during speech and deglutition. Hence it is extremely unlikely that a condition of absolute disuse would be found; a partial state of underuse (hypofunction) is the customary finding. Since both the attachment apparatus and the gingival tissue serve as stabilizing tissues, in disuse, if the gingival attachment remains healthy, the tooth does not necessarily exhibit mobility. When there is gingival disease, however, the reverse is true (Figs. 12-36 and 12-37).

Examination of the temporomandibular joint. Examination of the temporomandibular articulation requires not only a knowledge of the anatomy but also of the mechanism by which the joint operates. The physiologic activity of this articulation

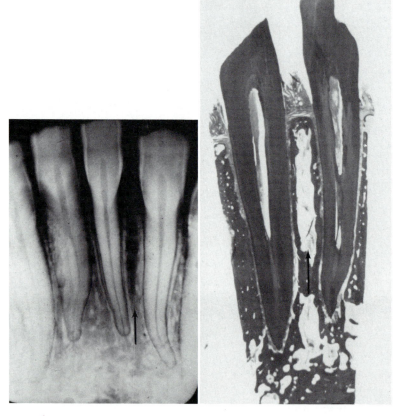

Fig. 12-36. Radiologic and histologic correlation of an instance of atrophy of diminished use. Radiograph is of a mandibular anterior area of an open bite case. Note translucency in interdental septum in both radiograph and histologic photomicrograph.

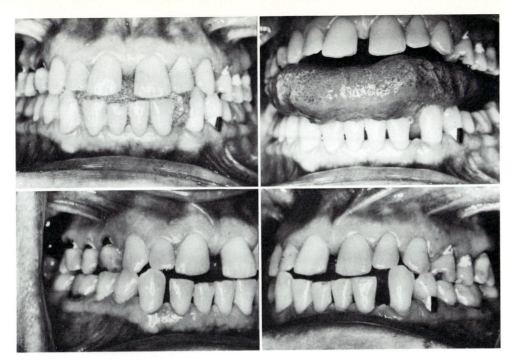

Fig. 12-37. Occlusal trauma not only results from tooth contacts, but also from pressure exerted by tongue, as in this instance. Not only did migration occur, but also mobility was a distinct symptom.

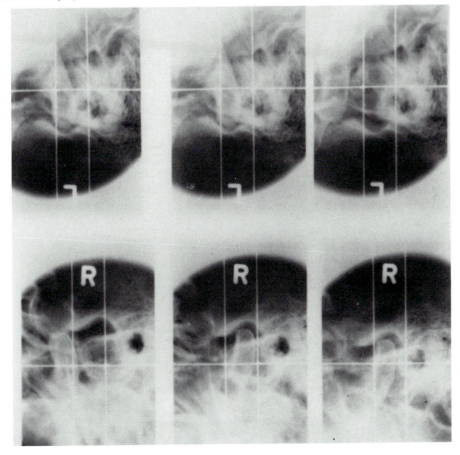

Fig. 12-38. Radiographs of temporomandibular joints in closed, protrusive, and open positions. Examination is performed in instances where there is a complaint of joint pain or cracking to rule out possibility of disease.

is complex, but once it is understood, examination becomes a matter of differential diagnosis. The history is an important facet of the examination; pain, difficulty in opening the mouth, tenderness in front of the ear, and generalized soreness are some of the descriptions that may be offered as a complaint (Fig. 12-38).

The first step in examination is the determination of whether the head of the condyle is moving smoothly. This can be ascertained by placing the index fingers in the patient's ears from behind the patient and having him open and close his mouth. Another method consists of placing a stethoscope in front of the ear and determining whether any gritting is heard. A smooth glide can easily be distinguished from an irregular movement. The next step comprises checking for tenderness of the pterygoid muscles. The patient should open the mouth as wide as possible. The index finger is carried down along the anterior border of the ascending ramus and then brought medially across the anterior border of the muscle. If the muscle is tender or in spasm, the patient will react to the pressure of the fingers. Also the examiner will feel a "bunching" of the muscle. This step is followed by manipulation of the mandible to ascertain whether it will retrude in respect to the habitual relationship of the mandible to the maxilla. The lower jaw is jiggled against the maxilla. This must be done gently, since if any force is placed on the mandible the patient will react and become tense and the examiner then will not be able to jiggle the mandible.

While there is no radiographic technique to determine any deviation of the mechanism of the temporomandibular articulation, the radiograph is important in determining the anatomy of the joint and any disease entity such as arthritis, tumors, and so on.

Examination for habits. Habits of lip or cheek biting and fingernail or foreign object biting are often the cause of overstress on the teeth. Clenching of teeth to control the emotions, bruxism, and occupational habits also may be prominent etiologic factors in the production of periodontal disease. In the examination of the patient these factors must be borne in mind, and the patient must be questioned carefully regarding them.

The use of a habit history chart is of benefit. The patient is questioned, and the answers are recorded. However, these answers must not be taken as absolute, since oftentimes a patient will return on a subsequent visit and relate an entirely different accounting made possible by his becoming ac-

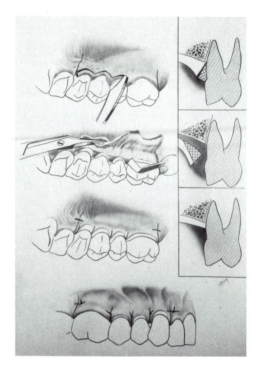

Fig. 12-39. Management of a flat palate represents one special problem with which therapist must cope. Presence of a flat palate has been determined, and operative procedure is pictured. Note how palatal mucosa has been thinned to achieve apical repositioning of flap.

quainted with the problem. A married person may sometimes ask his mate about grinding habits. Therefore a second period of questioning is important.

Special considerations. The following is a list of special considerations in the periodontal examination of individual areas:

A. Maxillary second molar area
  1. Topography of retromolar area, that is, tuberosity height, depth of hamular notch, angle of mesiodistal slope
  2. Depth of distal involvement
  3. Buccal or palatal interradicular involvement
  4. Depth of palatal vault; angle of slope of palatal aspect of alveolar process
  5. Buccal vestibular depth
  6. Malar process
  7. Angle of flare of palatal root
  8. Root fusion
  9. Infrabony defect—with or without interradicular involvements
B. Interdental area of the maxillary second and first molars
  1. Relative position of the proximal contact
    a. Mesiodistal width of gingival embrasure; height of gingival embrasure
    b. Contact of teeth along linguoproximal line angles; width of buccal embrasure

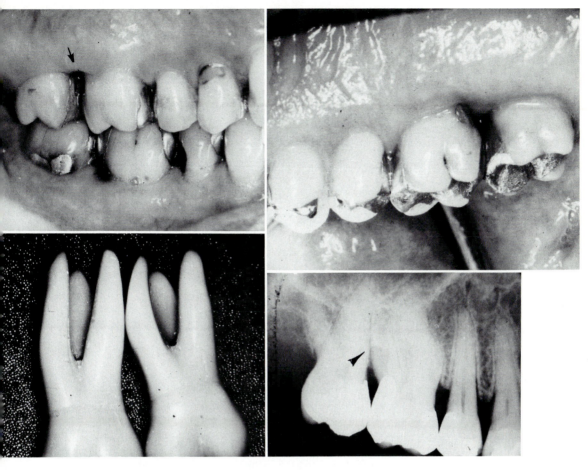

Fig. 12-40. Crater formation and root approximation of maxillary molars. Root approximation plays an important role in therapy in that the only manner interdental space can be widened is to remove one buccal approximating root. This would require endodontics, although vital root resection is being actively explored.

2. Interdental soft tissue crater
3. Interdental osseous crater
4. Proximity of roots of second molar to those of first molar; mesiodistal width of interdental septum
C. Maxillary first molar
  1. Buccal bifurcation involvement; proximity of buccal roots; mesiodistal width of interradicular septum; depth of palatally directed penetration of pocket; connection with interradicular (furcation) involvement from palatal aspect
  2. Palatal interradicular involvement; proximity of palatal to buccal roots, width of furcation involvement; distal furcation, mesial furcation, or both; trifurcation involvement
  3. Flare of palatal root
  4. Flatness of palate (not usually so much as next to second molar)
  5. Low dipping malar process
D. Interdental area of maxillary first molar and second premolar
  1. Type of proximal tooth contact; mesiodistal width of interdental septum; proximity of molar

to premolar roots; width and height of gingival embrasure
E. Maxillary premolars
  1. Nature of proximal contact (see D)
  2. Palate form
  3. Interdental cratering—soft tissue and/or osseous
  4. Proximity of roots; width of interdental septum
F. Maxillary first premolar
  1. Interradicular involvement; width of palatal embrasure between premolar and cuspid; proximity of roots; height of palate
G. Maxillary premolar—cuspid area (Fig. 12-41)
  1. Nature of proximal contact
  2. Embrasure form
  3. Width of interdental septum
  4. Interdental soft and/or hard tissue crater
  5. Caries distal to cuspid
  6. Proximity of roots
H. Lateral incisor
  1. Relationship to central incisor; proximity of lateral to central incisor roots; mesiodistal width of interdental septum; size of access to gingi-

val embrasure of lateral and central incisors

2. Shape of crown—bell, peg, normal; protection of axial walls for gingival margin
3. Partial anodontia—missing lateral incisor; relationship of cuspid to central incisor
4. Form of cingulum; relationship of deep overbite; palatal infrabony pocket; slope of anterior palatal wall
5. Palatal gingival grooves

I. Maxillary central incisors
1. Labial frenum
2. Incisive papilla
3. Nature of proximal contact; influence of diastema
4. Position of teeth relative to basal bone; lingually tipped central incisors; form of cingula; deep overbite relationship; class II, division 2 relationship
5. Palatal gingival grooves

J. Mandibular second molar
1. Distal retromolar problems; depth of distal in-

volvement; angle of slope of anterior border of ramus; influence of external oblique ridge; character of retromolar tissue
2. Position of tooth relative to basal bone; lingual tipping with cul-de-sac at lingual gingival margin area; relationship of buccal axial tooth form to buccal gingival margin; width of zone of attached gingiva
3. Bifurcation involvement—buccal, lingual, through and through; proximity of roots; enamel spur into bifurcation zone
4. Zone of attached gingiva; pockets into alveolar mucosa; slope of buccal wall of alveolar process; depth of vestibular fornix; position of external oblique ridge
5. Infrabony pockets—buccal, lingual, distal; with and without third molar
6. Impacted third molar; relationship to second molar and distal pocket
7. Missing first molar; mesial tipping of second molar

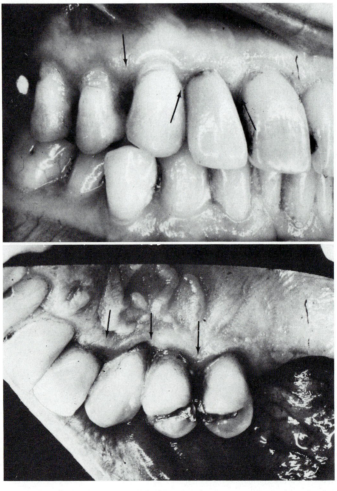

Fig. 12-41. Maxillary canine premolar area is an area that oftentimes presents a special problem because of proximal contact of teeth. In this instance, buccal interdental tissue is wide, but practically nonexistent on palatal aspect. The problem is compounded should palate be flat. There are also problems in adjacent teeth in this instance because of proximal contacts of teeth.

K. Interdental area of mandibular second and first molars (Fig. 12-42)
  1. Nature of proximal contact; embrasure form; mesiodistal and buccolingual dimensions of interdental septum; proximity of roots; interdental crater; soft and/or hard tissue type
  2. Adequacy of zone of attached gingiva—pocket into alveolar mucosa

L. Mandibular first molar
  1. Buccal or lingual bifurcation involvements; communicating buccal and lingual involvements; proximity of roots; width of interradicular septum; enamel spur into bifurcation zone
  2. Proximal infrabony pocket; communication with lingual or buccal infrabony defect; relationship of form to dimensions of interdental septum

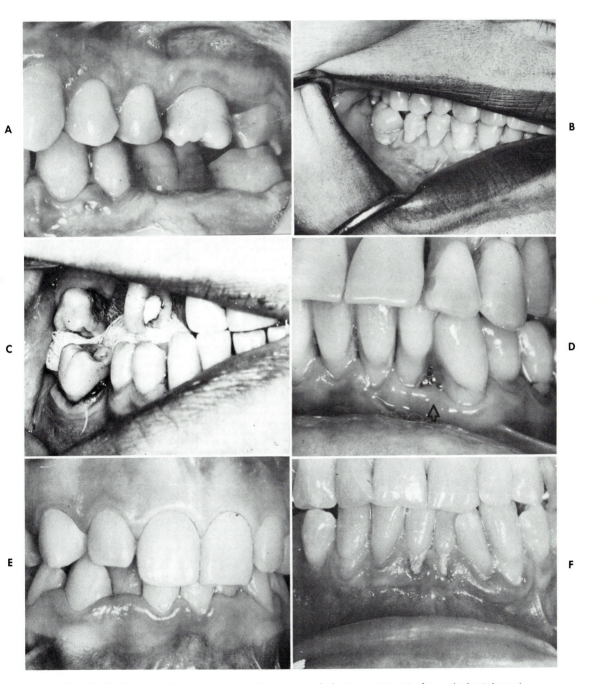

Fig. 12-42. Tooth positioning plays an important role in management of a periodontal manifestation. **A,** Relationship of a mandibular first and second molar. **B,** Tilting of a mandibular second molar due to loss of first molar. **C,** Pocket formation extending into alveolar mucosa. **D** to **F,** Crowding of teeth.

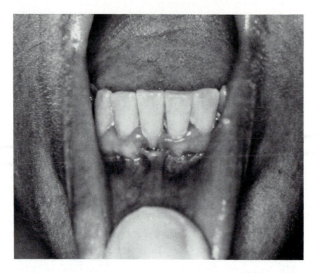

Fig. 12-43. Recognition of abnormal frena attachments is an important aspect of examination. In this case not only is there a heavy frenum present, but vestibule is shallow and gingival wall is short (gingival margin to vestibule).

3. Zone of attached gingiva; depth of vestibular fornix
4. Thickness of buccal osseous wall; position of tooth in basal bone; axial tooth protection to gingival margin; buccal infrabony pocket; communications of buccal infrabony defect with bifurcation or proximal infrabony pocket
5. Thickness of lingual osseous wall; position of tooth in alveolar housing; overprotection of axial wall of tooth to gingiva; lingual cul-de-sac; lingual infrabony pocket communication with furcation or proximal involvements

M. Mandibular first molar–premolar relationship
1. Nature of proximal contact
2. Form of interdental tissues
3. Embrasure form
4. Width of buccal attached gingiva and depth of vestibular fornix

N. Mandibular premolars
1. Proximal form and contact
2. Zone of attached gingiva; vestibular fornix (usually deeper)
3. Buccal frenum
4. Tooth–basal bone relationship
5. Crowded second premolar—effect of linguoversion; altered proximal contacts; protection of buccal tooth surface to gingiva; buccal osseous defects; short lingual wall of alveolar process
6. Lingual tori; lingual bony shelf; lingual infrabony defects
7. Cervical erosions or caries on buccal aspects of teeth; root exposure and sensitivity; gingival recession
8. Thin zone of alveolar mucosa; degree of thickness of buccal osseous wall
9. Buccal osteophytes

O. Mandibular first premolar–cuspid relationship
1. Nature of proximal contact
2. Proximity of roots

P. Mandibular cuspid
1. Relationship to basal alveolar process; lingual tipping; labial axial tooth form relative to gingiva; position of lingual gingival margin
2. Width of zone of attached gingiva
3. Pocket into alveolar mucosa
4. Depth of vestibular fornix
5. Relationship to lateral incisor; interdental gingival embrasure of cuspid and lateral incisor; topography of interdental crest; soft or hard tissue crater
6. Thickness of labial osseous plate

Q. Mandibular incisors (Fig. 12-43)
1. Buckling; crowding
2. Lingual tipping of teeth
3. Frenum
4. Zone of attached gingiva; depth of vestibular fornix; relationship of gingival margin to alveolar mucosa and frenum
5. Type of proximal contacts; dimensions of interdental septa; proximity of roots
6. Ankyloglossia (tongue tie)—frenum to gingiva relationship
7. Deep overbite; labial gingival fibrosis
8. Gingiva-tooth relationships—altered passive eruption
9. Interdental cratering—hard or soft tissue involvement
10. Length of lingual gingival wall and relationship of gingival margin to floor of mouth; attached or movable lingual gingiva

Roentgenographic examination: interpretation and evaluation of periodontal changes

Roentgenographic examination should never be relied upon as a sole diagnostic method. However, examination by roentgenograph is indisputably one of the most valuable means of detecting periodon-

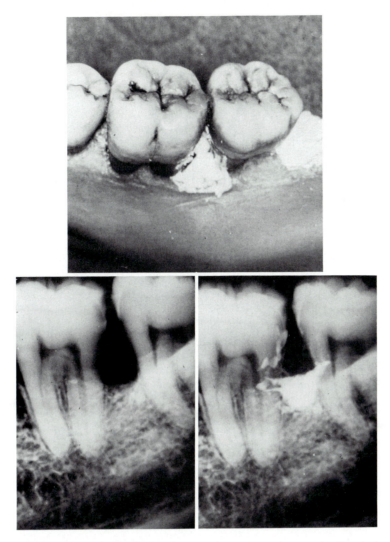

Fig. 12-44. Radiologic examination is of utmost importance in examination, but examiner must not try to read into radiographs that which is not possible. In photograph a radiopaque mass is placed into a crater. Radiograph shows depth of crater, which was not seen in photograph.

tal disease, and any departure from the normal should be noted. To understand pathologic changes one must have an understanding of the relation of histology to roentgenographic appearance (Figs. 12-44 to 12-48).

As a routine a minimum of 14 roentgenograms should be made. A better survey can be made if 22 are used. This number provides at least two views of each dental area, and since they are obtained from different horizontal angles the effect is somewhat stereoscopic. In other words, with the two views it is possible to see more of the approximal surfaces of the roots of the teeth than with a single view. The long cone parallel technique should be utilized. The Updegrave holder is an excellent method for holding the film as well as for lining up

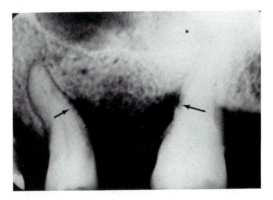

Fig. 12-45. Radiograph showing bone loss in an irregular pattern *(arrows)*; however, exact topography cannot be visualized. This must be done clinically.

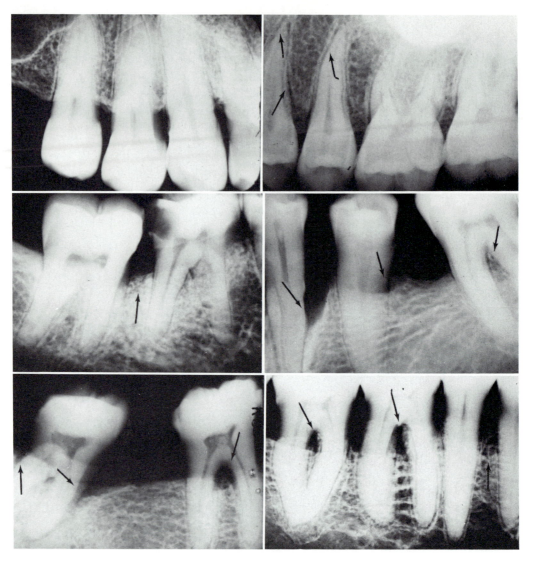

Fig. 12-46. Radiographic findings that are possible to determine: loss of crestal bone, widening of periodontal ligament space, changes in lamina dura, vertical resorptive lesions, and furca involvements.

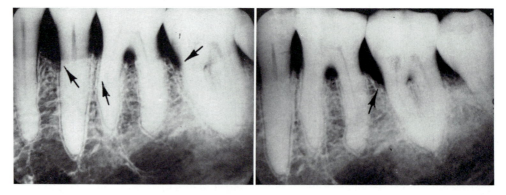

Fig. 12-47. Radiographs showing changes in crestal areas. These can be correlated to changes found on skull. Clinically, however, crestal topography would have to be determined by probing and needling.

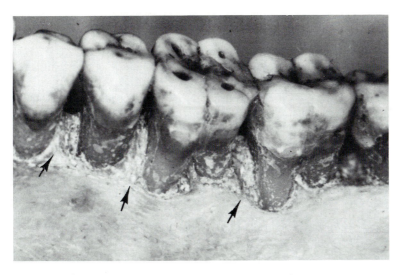

Fig. 12-47, cont'd. For legend see opposite page.

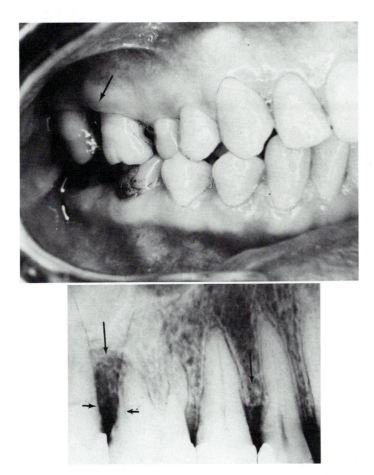

Fig. 12-48. Clinical and radiologic correlation. Loss of bone between first and second molars can be compared to status in premolar region. Clinically, loss of tissue interdentally in molar area conforms to a crater. Examiner must determine buccal and palatal bony walls; also thickness of palatal wall must be ascertained. Thickness of palatal wall is of importance in treatment.

the cone for correct vertical and horizontal angulation.

As has been pointed out, exact knowledge of the changes that have occurred in the bone structure is important. This requires roentgenographic portrayal of the interproximal bony crest, the periodontal ligaments, and the lamina dura for the following purposes:

1. To determine the size of the tooth, its position, and the number of roots—length and shape of root are most important
2. To tabulate abrasion, erosion, caries, and condition of the filling and other restorations
3. To study the condition of the interproximal bony crests–horizontal pattern of resorption, vertical bone resorption
4. To determine clinical crown–clinical root ratio
5. To assist in discovering irritating factors such as lack of approximal contact allowing for food impaction
6. To investigate periapical changes, e.g., widening of the periodontal ligament space, root resorption, or hypercementosis
7. To determine the presence or absence of a complete lamina dura
8. To locate calculus on the roots
9. To determine the character of the bone itself

In many cases it may be well to insert gutta-percha points in the pocket prior to taking roentgenograms. These show the exact depth of the pocket and the relationship of its bottom to the alveolar crest. This relationship is widely misunderstood, and many operators believe that both are on the same level. The bottom of the pocket is much higher up on the tooth than the point opposite the alveolar crest. Roentgenograms taken with gutta-percha points give an accurate record of the case and help to measure its progress under treatment.

Radiopaque material placed into the pocket prior to taking the roentgenogram not only gives information concerning the depth of the pocket perma-

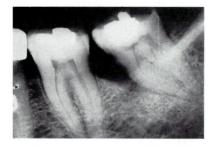

Fig. 12-49. Mandibular molar region. Second molar has been lost, and third molar has drifted forward to take its place. However, there is no contact between teeth. Note interdental resorptive lesion that assumes a vertical character in relation to third molar. This lesion is due to food impaction, resulting in a marginal periodontitis, and it has created an infrabony pocket. Occlusal traumatic lesion has been caused by contact between mandibular and maxillary molars. Osseous defect is present on mesial aspect of last molar. However, exact osseous topography cannot be read from radiographic evidence. Probing and clinical examination are necessary.

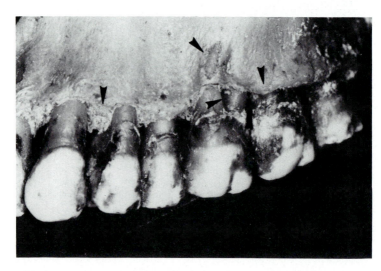

Fig. 12-50. Skull showing hemiseptum, furca involvement, a ledge, and a dehiscence. This topography is unacceptable, and therapist must change bone architecture to achieve an acceptable gingival topography and attachment.

nently recorded, but also illustrates the exact relationship between the bottom of the pocket and the alveolar crest. This information is of extreme importance in treatment. In one type of pocket, the *suprabony pocket,* it will be found that the bottom of the pocket is coronal to the alveolar crest; this is the type most commonly seen. In the other type, the *infrabony pocket,* the bottom of the pocket is apical to the alveolar crest, there being bone in the lateral wall. These lesions are termed osseous defects.

The recognition of osseous defects is perhaps the most important factor for treatment planning.

It is well recognized that although radiographic signs reveal the presence of vertical loss of alveolus, it does not aid in the recognition of interdental craters or the exact topography of the osseous defect that may be present. The recognition of these defects, therefore, is based on clinical examination (Figs. 12-49 to 12-55). The examiner utilizes the probe to relate pocket depth to crestal osseous topography. This system utilizes the fact that there is a distance of fiber apparatus between the base of the pocket and the crestal alveolar bone. Thus the crater is detected by depth of pocket interdentally in comparison to the gingival detachment at

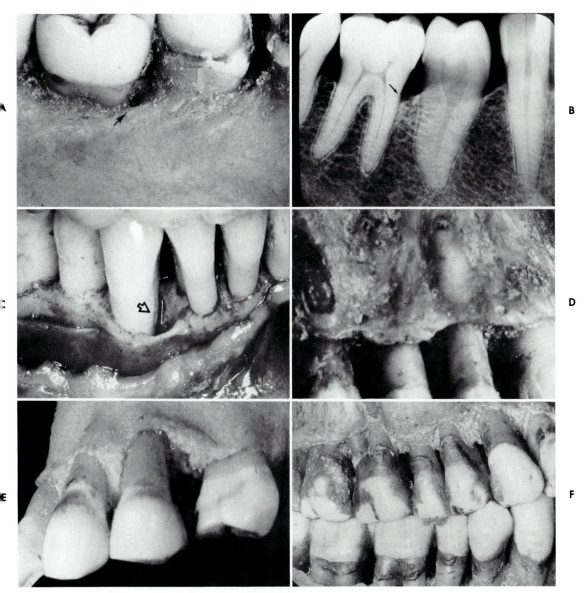

Fig. 12-51. Osseous defects ranging from three walls, **A** and **C**, (**B** is radiograph of **A**) to two walls, **E,** to a variety of bone changes, **F. F** shows hemisection, ledges, furca involvement (maxilla), and craters and furca involvement (mandible). Dentist must be able to visualize defects and select either excisive or reconstructive, reparative procedures on basis of total treatment plan.

the buccal and lingual line angles of the teeth. Thus a typical recording is 3 to 4 mm of depth of gingival detachment at the line angles, but 9 or 10 mm directly in the middle of the proximal aspect of the teeth. Such findings leave no doubt. However, in the circumstances of a shallow crater, the depth recordings are closer in range, giving not as clear-cut an interpretation. The same system is utilized for the detection of the various ''types'' of osseous defects.

In evaluating the changes of bone tissue as they

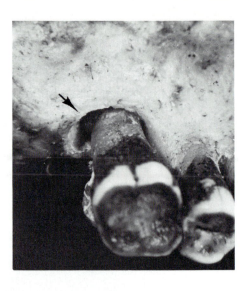

Fig. 12-52. Osseous defect involving palatal root of molar.

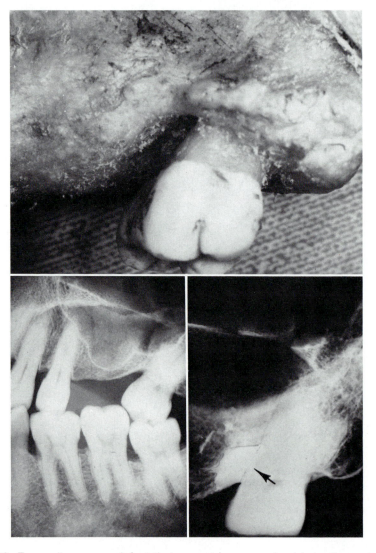

Fig. 12-53. Two-wall osseous defect that cannot be recognized in radiograph. A radiopaque mass was inserted into defect prior to taking of radiograph at lower right. In this way, outline of defect can be discerned.

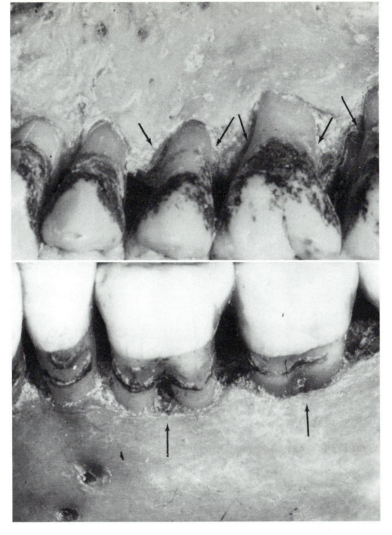

Fig. 12-54. Furca entrance from mesial and distal aspects of maxillary first molar and furca entrances on buccal aspect of mandibular first and second molars (top). These furca involvements may be classified as incomplete or cul-de-sac. It is extremely important to recognize such involvements during examination. Entrance to mandibular furca can be seen in lower photograph. Note difference in bone topography between first and second molars.

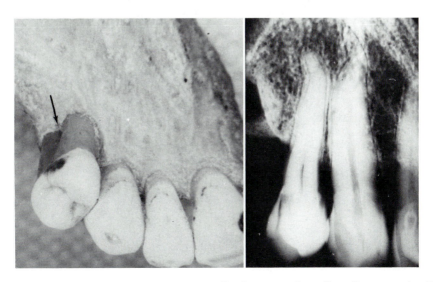

Fig. 12-55. Furca entrance can be seen on distal aspect of maxillary first premolar. Note that involvement is not recognizable in radiograph but must be recognized clinically.

are seen in the roentgenogram, one must realize that the translucencies and opacities are dependent on the different permeabilities of bone and marrow spaces to the roentgen rays. Thus the configuration of bone tissue represents the topography of the bony trabeculae and their arrangement, registering opaque in contrast to the translucency of the marrow spaces.

Structural changes of bone can be recognized only if the normal configuration and distribution of the bone tissue are utilized as a standard for comparison. Thus extreme osteoporotic changes seen, for example, in atrophy of disuse can be recognized for the disappearance of the normal opaque configurations substituted by a translucent registration (Fig. 12-56).

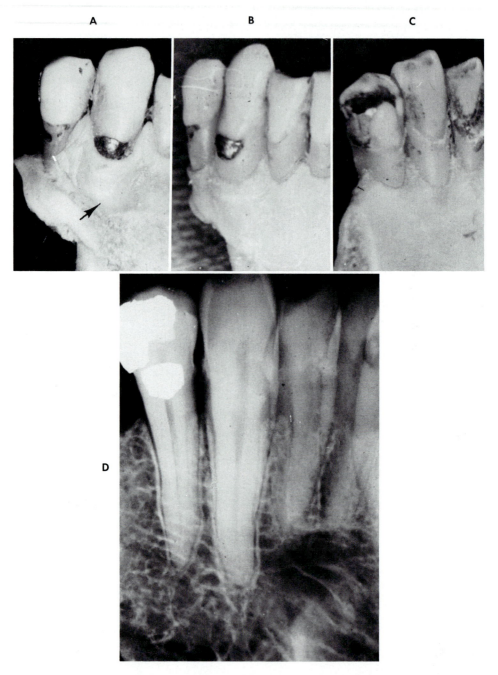

Fig. 12-56. Periodontal therapy is based on bone topography. **A,** Gingival condition. A diagnosis of marginal periodontitis can be made. Gingiva was stripped away, and one can see regularity of bone. This topography is acceptable. **D,** Radiographic findings.

Therefore it is important that roentgenograms be evaluated on the basis of tissue topography and not simply as shadows registered on a film.

The use of the roentgenogram in studying the patterns of morphologic changes in periodontal disease is of infinite value to the clinician. It is not our purpose to evaluate the advantages and disadvantages of the bisecting and paralleling techniques, but it should be understood that the films must clearly show the complete tooth and its attachment apparatus with a minimum of quantitative and qualitative distortions. For correct technique the student is referred to any of the textbooks on oral roentgenology. Utilizing a complete roentgenographic survey consisting of 22 films properly exposed and processed will greatly enhance the diagnosis as well as the prognosis and treatment plan.

Although it is inconceivable that the practitioner would attempt a complete diagnosis without a complete roentgenographic survey, he must be aware that roentgenograms are of limited value in certain respects. One of the limitations of present-day dental roentgenology is that the film will show only the interproximal periodontal structures with any degree of clarity. The roentgen ray penetrates 10 to 14 mm of tissue thickness before reaching the film, and therefore one sees a composite picture on the roentgenogram. Because of the denseness of the tooth structure the buccal and lingual aspects of the periodontium are obscured on the film. For this reason the clinician cannot depend on the roentgenograms alone to determine the presence of a bifurcation involvement. The osseous destruction may extend into the bifurcation on the buccal side, but because of an intact alveolar process on the lingual side this pathologic condition may not be observed clearly on the film. Thorough probing of all pockets must be performed, since the level of the epithelial attachment is not registered on the roentgenogram. Radiopaque objects, for example, periodontal probes, Hirschfeld points, gutta-percha points, or opaque masses, are necessary to demonstrate the bottom of the pocket, but they will not show the length of the epithelial attachment.

Although a calculus deposit, if sufficiently heavy, can be detected on a roentgenogram, this should not mean that sole reliance is placed on the film when deciding on the presence of the deposit or the thoroughness of its removal. Many deposits cannot be observed with present techniques.

Today there has been developed a practical apparatus that will standardize the angulation and exposure of periapical roentgenograms just as the cephalometer enables the dentist repeatedly to obtain accurate profile roentgenograms of the patient (Updegrave).

A thorough knowledge of the roentgenographic appearances of normal structures is necessary before studying pathologic conditions. One of the most accurate means of studying the roentgenographic changes in periodontal disease is to study closely histopathologic serial sections of human material that has been radiographed accurately. In this way the microscope is employed as a diagnostic tool in interpreting aberrations registered on the film. The following observations and findings have been collected in this manner from human necropsy material.

Gingivitis. As the term implies, gingivitis is an inflammatory lesion of the gingiva. Roentgenographically, no changes are observed due to absence of the gingivae from the usual dental film. The roentgenograms can be employed by the clinician in certain cases of hyperplastic gingivitis to measure the length of the anatomic crowns of the teeth. This information is useful when comparing the length of the anatomic crowns with the measurements of the clinical crowns, which have been reduced by the gingival overgrowth.

Marginal periodontitis. As the inflammatory process extends in an apical direction from the gingivae, any of several changes may be observed in the alveolar crests on the roentgenograms (Fig. 12-57).

The most typical change in the crest in marginal periodontitis is a cuplike defect that is due to the resorption of the cortical crest, leaving the alveolar bone that makes up the proximal borders as well as the buccal and lingual cortical plates unaffected. This horizontal pattern of resorption may vary according to which part of the osseous tissue that makes up the interproximal septum is destroyed. If the infiltrate results in resorption of the cortical crest as well as part of the buccal and lingual cortical plate but leaves the adjacent alveolar bones intact, then a notchlike deformity (between first and second molars) is observed. However, the disease process may result in destruction of the cortical crest and also the adjacent alveolar bone, but it does not involve the buccal and lingual plates of bone. This also results in a craterlike defect that has a different appearance on the roentgenogram. Another less frequently encountered situation is the destruction of the cortical crest, the adjacent alveolar bones, and either the buccal or lingual cortical plate of bone. This leaves a ramplike defect between the first and second molars.

As the disease progresses the defect becomes larger, and the translucency extends apically into the interdental supporting bone. This characteristic allows for the exaggeration of the notchlike appearance seen roentgenographically. As the disease progresses the lateral walls of the defected crest become lost, tending either to flatten the alveolar crest or if only one side should be lost to cause an oblique crestal margin. Thus roentgenographically in this stage either a horizontal or oblique loss of the alveolar crest can be seen. Oftentimes, subjacently, a translucency can be traced deeply into the alveolar process following along the interdental vessels. On the other hand, in many instances examination of the roentgenograms reveals a subjacent opacity or sclerosis to the crestal defect, even when quite a bit of the interdental septum has been destroyed. This zone of bone formation varies in thickness and may be interpreted as bone deposition, a reactive phenomenon to halt the progress of the destructive process.

Occasionally, however, this opacity is due to an overlay of cortical bone, ridgelike in topography, which is found on the buccal cortical plate. In some angulations this cortical layer superimposes over the crestal area, and an opacity in the roentgenogram results. The deformities observed roentgenographically in marginal periodontitis should be correlated with the situation encountered clinically in the mouth. The local environmental conditions must be studied closely for tooth shape, tooth-to-tooth position, contours and contacts of restoration, etc. because they will enhance the interpretation of the roentgenograms and also clarify some of the more subtle etiologic factors that are responsible for these changes on the roentgenogram.

Occlusal traumatism. The roentgenogram is of paramount importance in diagnosing occlusal traumatism. However, the therapist must correlate the roentgenographic findings in light of the clinical signs and symptoms: mobility, wear facets, and premature contacts as well as the presence of habit patterns (Figs. 12-58 and 12-59).

One of the cardinal roentgenographic changes in occlusal traumatism is the thickening of the periodontal ligament space. This widening is usually due to resorption of tooth structure as well as alveolar bone. Loss of contiguity of the lamina dura and minor areas of root resorption usually accompany the thickened periodontal ligament space. Widening of the periodontal ligament space at the crestal and apical regions is a sign of a tilting lesion. Here the tooth is being tilted, rotating on its fulcrum, which is located about two thirds apically rootwise.

Careful scrutiny of the roentgenogram may reveal cemental tears or larger areas of root fractures. In the more advanced lesion vertical resorp-

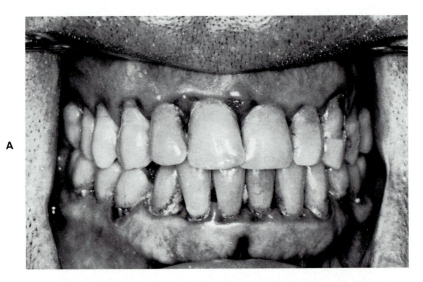

Fig. 12-57. A, Marginal periodontitis of long standing. Deep pocket formation is present associated with heavy calculus deposits. Bases of detached tissues must be located, and osseous topography determined. Radiographs will contribute to ascertaining bone crest locations in a general fashion as well as furca involvements. **B,** Teeth of patient in **A.** Note advanced crestal bone destruction, heavy calculus, some vertical resorptive lesions, and furca involvements.

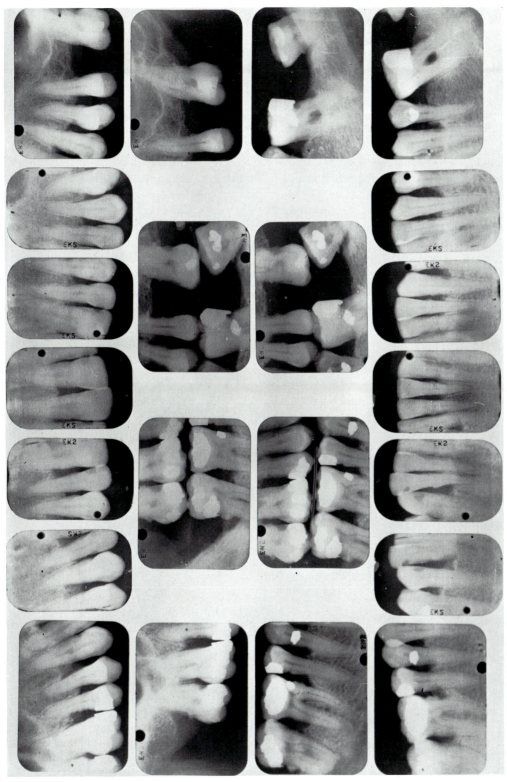

Fig. 12-57, cont'd. For legend see opposite page.

B

tion of the alveolar crest may occur. When a gingival irritant is present, causing inflammatory changes, an infrabony pocket may ensue.

Occasionally in advanced cases of traumatism the buccal and lingual plates of the alveolar process are more prominent on the roentgenogram. The alveolar crest on either the buccal or lingual plates is at a more apical level because of the extensive resorption. They become more clearly seen in the roentgenogram because the root of the tooth is thinner in a buccolingual direction as it tapers apically.

Periodontosis. It is imperative to study carefully the clinical picture in conjunction with the roentgenographic changes. Bone resorption is pronounced, the pattern of which is correlated to the environmental factors to which the teeth are subjected. In the later stages, once the bone resorptive process is advanced and the occlusion has been altered, the gingival changes become more pronounced. Deep pocket formation occurs, and the signs and symptoms are characteristic of those of marginal periodontitis with which occlusal traumatism is associated.

Fig. 10-22, *A* shows a roentgenogram of the anterior teeth in a boy 12 years old. At that time the dentist noticed that the anterior teeth were mobile. Roentgen-ray examination revealed the

alveolar crest to be resorbed and the bone to be osteoporotic in appearance. The patient was told to return in 6 months, at which time roentgen-ray examination showed further loss of bone. Clinical examination showed a well-developed boy who had no systemic complaints. All the laboratory tests were negative, and physical examinations revealed no disease. Roentgenograms taken when the patient was last seen are shown in Fig. 10-22, *G*.

Dietary analysis

In many cases a dietary analysis should be made, since a nutritional deficiency may be a causative factor in the production of the oral disease. One method for evaluating the diet is to have the patient keep a record of all the foods eaten and the approximate quantity for 1 week. The diet is then studied on the basis of caloric intake per day, protein, fat, and carbohydrate proportions, acid-alkali balance, roughage, minerals, and vitamins. Suggestions can then be made to correct any imbalance or deficiency. Although the diet should be made adequate in all respects, often additional elements such as vitamins may be prescribed in order to fortify the diet and to overcome more quickly a deficiency state. However, the dentist must realize that while the diet may be adequate, the absorp-

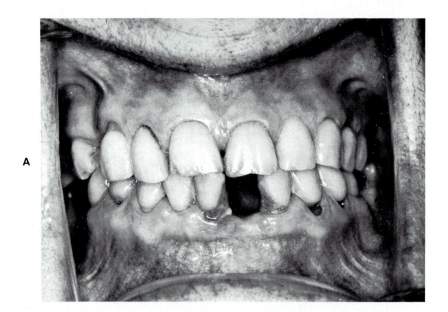

Fig. 12-58. A, Periodontal traumatism. Teeth were excessively mobile. **B,** Teeth of patient in **A.** Note widening of periodontal ligament space almost throughout entire remaining dentition as well as vertical bone loss in several areas. Of special interest are maxillary and mandibular left second premolars. Widening of periodontal ligament space circumferentially can be seen. Maxillary right premolars show typical roentgenographic signs of occlusal traumatism.

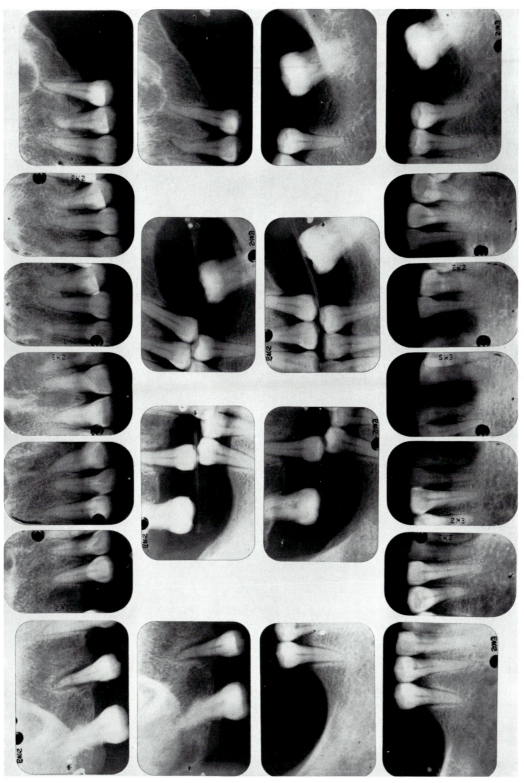

Fig. 12-58, cont'd. For legend see opposite page.

B

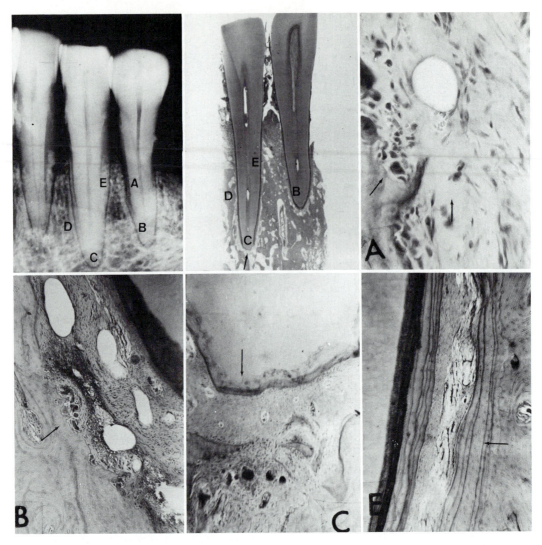

Fig. 12-59. Radiologic and histologic correlation of an instance of occlusal traumatism. Radiologically there is widening of periodontal ligament space, as confirmed in photomicrograph. At *A* there is bone resorption and hyalinization of the connective tissue; at *B*, necrosis of the periodontal ligament and bone resorption; at *C*, previous root resorption with repair; at *E*, bone apposition.

tive power of the body may be lacking. *In prescribing a diet the dentist should take into consideration the general history of the patient, and most often he should consult the patient's physician.* He should not prescribe dietary measures in the presence of a disease such as diabetes, nephrosis, cardiorenal disease, gastrointestinal disorders, and so on but should refer the patient to the physician for dietary correction (boxed material).

Laboratory tests

The literature on the application of laboratory procedures to dentistry is meager, and aside from a few articles no attempt has been made to point out their value in the diagnosis of oral lesions. The importance of differential diagnosis by these methods in certain gingival lesions, for example, hyperplasia and ulceration, is obvious.

Many cases of blood diseases have been mistaken for local infections, and the patients have been treated for such until they became gravely ill. If a laboratory examination had been made the diagnosis would have been determined in the beginning. There are also many generalized systemic diseases having manifestations in the jaws that go unrecognized and are treated as local conditions without avail. An example of this was a case of lipoid histiocytosis seen by us. The patient

---

Nutritional evaluation form (part I)

Patient's name_____ Case number_____

Inclusive dates of study _____

PROCEDURE TO BE FOLLOWED

1. Patient should fill in a separate sheet for each day. The chart will be evaluated weekly. The information should include all foods and beverages (including alcoholic) consumed and the amounts.
2. Since the dietary habits of patients vary widely each daily chart should be broken into six sections: (1) breakfast; (2) midmorning; (3) lunch; (4) midafternoon; (5) dinner; (6) after dinner.
3. From this information, using tables, one can calculate (1) approximate intake of protein (g); (2) fat (g); (3) relative proportion of saturated to unsaturated fats; (4) carbohydrate (g); (5) cholesterol (mg); (6) calcium (mg); (7) iron (mg); (8) vitamin A (IU); (9) vitamin D (IU); (10) thiamine (mg); (11) niacin (mg); (12) riboflavin (mg); and (13) ascorbic acid (mg). The relative proportions of protein to fat to carbohydrate intake should be calculated (g% basis) to determine balance of diet. Also the percent of calories from protein, fat, and carbohydrate should be determined and alcohol calories should be calculated and reported. Particular attention should be paid to the qualitative content of the carbohydrate intake (i.e., attention to excessive intake of refined sugar or products containing refined sugar). The overall evaluation for the week should include the adequacy of the fibrous content of diet provided by grains, legumes, fruits, and vegetables.

AFTER ANALYSIS OF THE WEEKLY CHART THE PATIENT SHOULD BE PROVIDED WITH A VERBAL EVALUATION OF THE FOLLOWING ITEMS   (✓)

1. Adequacy of diet   _____
2. Any evidence of dietary excess   _____
3. Easily understood advice on improving diet   _____
4. Selection of foods to provide adequacy and balance   _____
5. Selection of a quality diet for those on limited incomes   _____

Continued.

---

had been treated as for an advanced case of local periodontal disease. When he was examined a yellowish tinge to the gingivae was noted. A biopsy was performed, and a routine blood examination was made. The biopsy showed a lipoid histiocytosis present, and a later blood test showed high cholesterol.

Many more similar instances can be cited to show why the dentist should avail himself of laboratory tests in all cases for which he can ascribe no etiologic factors after a careful examination (Fig. 12-60).

The reader may be referred to tests on clinical laboratory procedures for this information.

BIOPSY

Biopsy is the removal of a small piece of tissue from the living body for microscopic examination. Although this method of examination is not generally used in the practice of dentistry, when considered in relation to the clinical findings it is of extreme benefit for diagnosis; for example, gingival enlargements may be excised, prepared for sectioning, and viewed under the microscope for the type of tissue present. In cases of periodontosis the presence of large amounts of lymphocytes in the gingiva may offer a clue as to the possibility of lymphokines and the osteoclast-releasing factor (Fig. 12-61).

Biopsy may be used for differential diagnosis. In many gingival enlargements some sections show marked hyperplasia with round cell infiltration and hyperemia of the blood vessels, whereas others show hyperplasia of the connective tissue without much cellular infiltration. This discrepancy gives valuable information regarding treatment, since in the first case subgingival curettage will reduce the inflammation, and the gingiva will shrink, whereas in the second case subgingival curettage will not bring any successful re-

Text continued on p. 372.

Nutritional evaluation form (part II)

Patient's name _____ Case number _____

Does patient select food because of state of dentition?

_____

_____

Does the patient have dentition problems that can affect food selection?

_____

_____

Also comment on patient's masticatory ability.

_____

_____

Is food selected because of convenience?

_____

_____

Is diet restricted because of economics?

_____

_____

Does patient recognize the importance of a balanced diet?

_____

_____

Does patient recognize that dietary excesses may be related to certain chronic disease problems?

_____

_____

Has the importance of a balanced and adequate diet in relation to general health been discussed with patient?

_____

_____

Have the retentive properties of certain foods been adequately discussed with patient?

_____

_____

Which food tables were used for analysis of diet?

_____

_____

Additional comments and overall evaluation of dietary intake

_____

_____

_____
Signature of student

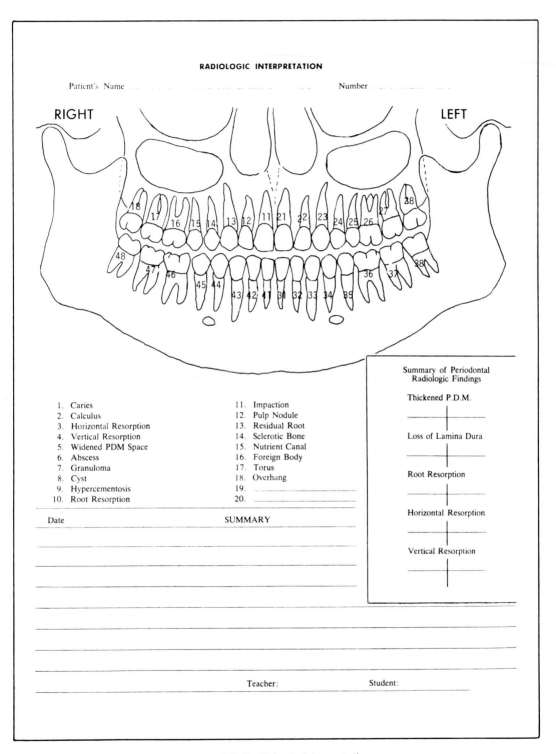

Fig. 12-60. Radiologic interpretation.

CASE NO:

PERIODONTAL DISEASE

STUDENT NAME: DATE:

PERIODONTAL DISEASE FINDINGS

Draw teeth in their position in the dentition and mark location of gingival margin and mucogingival junction and frenae. Also record interradicular involvement and vertical resorption of alveolus as seen in the radiograph. X teeth which have negative prognosis. Draw deficient proximal contacts, drifting, plunger cusps, extruded teeth, root proximity, form, and root resorption. Draw in base of pocket in any area where pocket depth is near or beyond the mucogingival junction.

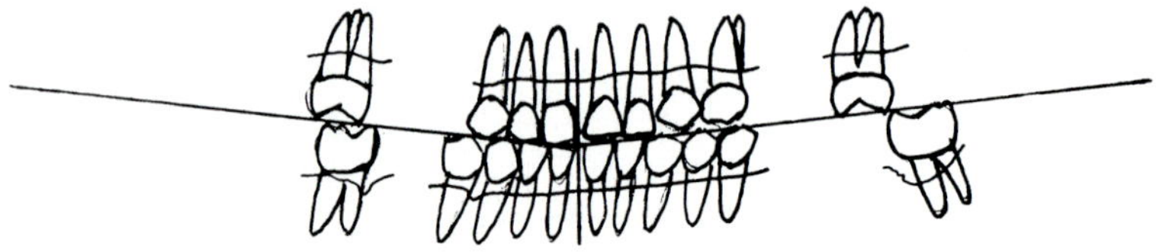

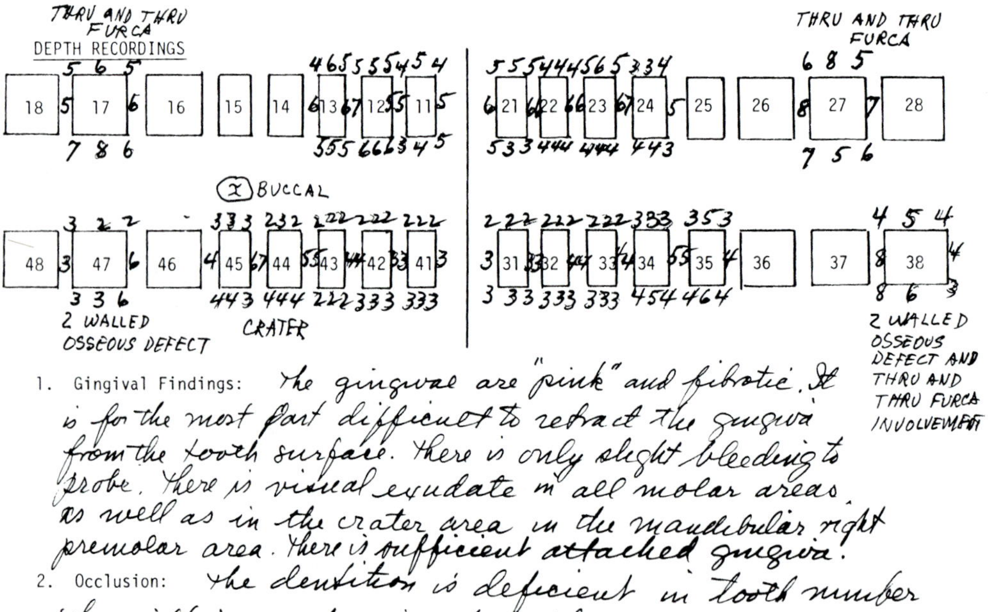

1. Gingival Findings: The gingivae are "pink" and fibrotic. It is for the most part difficult to retract the gingiva from the tooth surface. There is only slight bleeding to probe. There is visual exudate in all molar areas as well as in the crater area in the mandibular right premolar area. There is sufficient attached gingiva.
2. Occlusion: The dentition is deficient in tooth number The midline is not coincident. The mandible retrudes in centric relation. (See occlusion chart)

Fig. 12-61. Periodontal disease chart.

3. Alveolar Crest Findings: Horizontal bone loss except for the mandibular right premolar area and the four molar teeth, all of which have osseous defects. The bony topography in the maxillary anterior region is regular and acceptable; there is a slight ledge of bone on the labial aspect in the mandibular anterior region. This probably, however, will present no interference.

4. Periodontal Ligament and Lamina Dura Findings: Lamina dura intact in the anterior segment. Widening of periodontal ligament space around molar teeth.

5. Mobility: Distinct mobility of the four molar teeth. The teeth in the anterior segment are relatively firm.

SUMMARY OF FINDINGS OF PERIODONTAL DISEASE

This is a case of marginal periodontitis with supra and sub-gingival calculus. There is a great deal of plaque accumulation. The patient does not brush regularly and also has poor manual dexterity. I believe, however, that the patient can be motivated. The anterior segment has a favorable prognosis whereas the molar teeth present problems.

TREATMENT PLAN

1. Initial preparation - scaling and toothbrush instruction
2. Investigation as to the retention of the palatal roots of the maxillary molars $\overline{17}$ and $\overline{127}$ after endodontics and removal of the two buccal roots. The question whether there is sufficient bone on the buccal aspects of the palatal roots (interradicular bone) is critical. The stability of the roots will determine prosthetic treatment.
3. Treatment of the two-walled osseous defect $\overline{47}$
4. Investigation as to the retention of the distal root of $\overline{38}$ after endodontics and removal of mesial root.
5. Elimination of $\overline{45\cdot44}$ crater by osteoectomy - flap procedure.
6. Maxillary and mandibular gingivectomy - sufficient attached gingiva and bony topography presents no interference
7. Determination of prosthetic prescription after evaluation of periodontal therapy

Fig. 12-61, cont'd. Periodontal disease chart.

STUDENT NAME:

CASE NO:
DATE:

OCCLUSAL HISTORY AND EXAMINATION FOR THE DENTULOUS PATIENT

I. Occlusal History:

    A. Patient's own evaluation of:

        1. Esthetics

        2. Function (phonetics, mastication).

        3. Comfort: Locate   a. Tooth sensitivity.   b. Food impaction areas.

           c. Duration of missing teeth and spacing of teeth, etc.

    B. Patient's habit history:

        1. Tooth to tooth contact (clenching, grinding, doodling)

           a. first visit   b. second visit

        2. Oral musculature to tooth contact (adult or infantile tongue thrust, lip biting, cheek biting)

        3. Foreign object to tooth contact (pipe, pencil biting, etc.)

    C. Temporomandibular joint disturbances (pain, clicking, lack of function, traumatic injury, etc.)

II. Examination of Mounted Study Casts

    A. Examination of maxillary and mandibular arches.

	Maxillary cast			Mandibular cast		
	Yes	No	Location	Yes	No	Location
Arch symmetry						
Interarch harmony						
Faulty contact areas						
Faulty marginal ridges						
Malposed teeth						
Wear patterns						
Posterior bite collapse						
Open bite						
Migration of teeth						
Disrupted arch integrity						

    B. Examination of study casts in the maximum intercuspal position (centric occlusion, acquired centric, habitual closure, etc.)

        Articulator settings   Condylar <u>R</u> | <u>L</u>   Bennett <u>R</u> | <u>L</u>   Intercondylar distance

        1. Angle's classification (circle) I, II Div 1, II Div 2, VI

        2. Overbite _ _ _ _ _ _ _ _ _ mm.

        3. Overjet _ _ _ _ _ _ _ _ _ mm.

        4. Incorrect landmarks

           a. Mesio-distal
<u>18 17 16 15 14 13 12 11</u> | <u>21 22 23 24 25 26 27 28</u>
48 47 46 45 44 43 42 41 | 31 32 33 34 35 36 37 38

           b. Bucco-lingual
<u>18 17 16 15 14 13 12 11</u> | <u>21 22 23 24 25 26 27 28</u>
48 47 46 45 44 43 42 41 | 31 32 33 34 35 36 37 38

Fig. 12-62. Occlusal chart.

	Verified by Oral Examination	
	Yes	No

C. Examinations of study casts in the retruded contacting position (centric relation).

1. Angle's classification (circle)   I,   II Div. 1,   II Div. 2,   III

2. Overbite _____ mm.

3. Overjet _____ mm.

4. Initial contact at the retruded contact position (centric relation).

　　a. Tooth numbers of teeth hitting at simultaneous contact _____

5. Mandibular movement from the retruded position (centric relation) to the maximum intercuspal position (centric occlusion).

　　a. Distance of mandibular deflection _____ mm.

　　b. Direction of mandibular deflection _____

6. Locate: incorrect landmark relations

　　a. Mesio-distal

```
18 17 16 15 14 13 12 11 | 21 22 23 24 25 26 27 28
48 47 46 45 44 43 42 41 | 31 32 33 34 35 36 37 38
```

　　b. Bucco-lingual

```
18 17 16 15 14 13 12 11 | 21 22 23 24 25 26 27 28
48 47 46 45 44 43 42 41 | 31 32 33 34 35 36 37 38
```

III. Examinations of Mandibular Function:

A. Unguided (active) function:

1. Estimated free way space in rest (postural) position _____ mm.

2. Swallowing pattern: a. normal,   b. adult tongue thrust,   c. infantile tongue habit

　　d. resulting tooth displacement finding(s):

3. Maximum jaw opening _____ mm. Deviation (circle)   R   L

4. Fremitus (palpable tooth movement) in maximum intercuspal position.

5. Fremitus in horizontal mandibular glides _____ .

6. Excursive interference   Right | Left

　　a. Working

　　b. Non-working

　　c. Protrusive

B. Guided (passive) function: Estimated freeway space in the retruded position _____ .

IV. Diagnosis of Occlusion

A. Healthy physiological occlusion   ☐

B. Primary occlusal traumatism   ☐

C. Secondary occlusal traumatism   ☐

D. Temporomandibular joint disturbances   ☐

E. Posterior bite collapse   ☐

V. Etiology

A. Poor tooth relationship   ☐

B. Parafunctional habits   ☐

C. Orthodontic movement   ☐

D. Poor restorations   ☐

E. Non-replacement of teeth   ☐

F. Other _____   ☐

VI. Treatment Recommendations

A. No treatment needed   ☐

B. Occlusal adjustment needed   ☐

　　1. Selective grinding needed   ☐

　　2. Selected extractions needed   ☐

　　3. Orthodontic treatment needed   ☐

　　4. Restorative treatment needed   ☐

　　　　a. Simple restorations

　　　　b. Fixed

　　　　c. Removable

　　　　d. Splints and night guards

C. Referral to TMJ clinic   ☐

D. Referral to Post-graduate division   ☐

E. Not possible to treat at school   ☐

Student _____Instructor _____Date _____

Fig. 12-62, cont'd. Occlusal chart.

sult. In the second case the gingiva should be excised.

SMEARS

Occasionally it is advisable to make a bacteriologic smear of an oral condition. Gingival inflammations of mixed bacterial origin or fungus infections are not too uncommon. Consultation with a bacteriologist and a mycologist in these instances is advisable. Although a diagnosis of necrotizing ulcerative gingivitis cannot be made from a smear, it is at times advisable to determine the presence and abundance of Vincent's organisms. Investigate plaque ecology when necessary.

Casts and photographs

In the study of a case of periodontal disease, models and photographs have become important adjuncts in examination and diagnosis. The examination of a study model that is true in its reproduction of the original may aid in the detection of occlusal trauma, food impaction, anatomic abnormalities (e.g., malalignment of teeth), and many other conditions.

The study model should be exact and neat. The bases should be carefully contoured as desired by the dentist. The gingival margins and incisal edges must be defined sharply and the contours of the gingivae not obliterated. Facets should be distinct to show the wear of the tooth. The models should be mounted in the true centric relationship of the patient. In this way the occlusion can be studied carefully not only from the buccal aspect but also from the lingual aspect. Faulty cusp relationships, defective contact surfaces, and often premature occlusal contacts can be detected. Study models aid not only in examination but also in planning restorations and in determining the prognosis of questionable teeth. If the occlusion is to be altered it is desirable to have a record of the case at the beginning of treatment.

The condition of the gingivae and other phases cannot be memorized or even exactly recorded; photographs, especially those taken in color, serve excellently in this capacity. They should be taken close up, and if necessary three may be taken, one from each side and one anteriorly.

CHARTING OF PERIODONTAL CASES

The charting of cases in periodontal disease is of extreme importance, since it furnishes a complete record of findings that can be referred to at a later date. Charting is best done in the presence of the patient. Data should be written down as the history is taken and while the examination is being made. The result of laboratory investigations can be entered when such reports are received.

It is good practice to have a standardized procedure of recording symptoms, since one will probably fail to obtain all the possible data when recording in a hit-or-miss fashion. Once the record chart is made it not only serves as an aid in making the diagnosis but also reminds the operator of the conditions needing continuous surveillance during treatment. The technique for charting may in general be as follows, but the requirements of the case presented must determine the type and scope of each inquiry.

Physical and dental history

1. Name, address, telephone number, date of examination, age, occupation, temperament (normal, nervous, phlegmatic), height, weight, recent loss or gain in weight
2. Reason for presentation
3. Past dental conditions with special reference to swelling, exudation of pus, toothache, neuralgia, pain due to thermal changes, pain caused by impact or pressure on the teeth, periodic tenderness or mobility, accidental trauma, bilateral or unilateral masticatory habit, reasons for loss of missing teeth, previous treatment of periodontal disease, mouth hygiene (personal attention and periodical prophylaxis)
4. Characteristic breath odors suggesting neglected oral conditions, digestive disorders, Vincent's disease, diabetes, and so on
5. Present health condition as outlined by patient or reported by physician
6. Dietary data with reference to appetite, food preferences, masticatory habits, regularity of meals, eating between meals; daily diet record to check intake of proteins, carbohydrates, vitamins, and so on with average daily requirements or to compare intake of foods having acid end products with those of alkaline type
7. General appearance—nourishment, carriage and posture, color and texture of skin, color of ears, any enlargement of the thyroid area, protrusion of eyes

Intraoral examination

1. Lips: color, evidence of abnormal conditions, e.g., ulcers, fissures, cysts, herpes, mucous patches, chancres, neoplasms
2. Tongue: size, coating, mucous patches, ulcers, fissures, leukoplakia, neoplasms, typical markings caused by certain diseases

3. Subgingival area: evidence of inflammation, ulcers, cysts, mucous patches, neoplasms
4. Mucous membrane of cheeks: color, evidence of hyperplasia, ulcers, mucous patches, cysts, indurations, neoplasms
5. Hard palate: form, possible presence of neoplasms, fistulas, ulcers, traumas from prosthetic restorations
6. Soft palate: inflammation, ulcers, perforation, clefts, neoplasms; color and appearance in reference to typical manifestations produced by certain systemic diseases

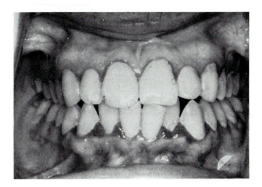

Fig. 12-63. Effects of hormonal imbalance in a young female patient. Vaginal smear and urine examination for estrins, together with clinical history, revealed a hormonal imbalance. Findings in this instance show value of laboratory tests.

7. General hygiene of mouth
8. General condition of gingivae: evidence of gingivitis, hyperplasia, atrophy, metallic poisoning
9. Presence of supragingival calculus
10. Evidence of immunity or susceptibility to caries (DMF)
11. General impression of masticatory efficiency in relation to occlusal contacts of teeth present

Dental and periodontal examination

1. Missing teeth
2. Vitality of teeth
3. Abnormal reactions to percussion on individual teeth
4. Evidence of mobility
5. Evidence of malocclusion in previous operative and prosthetic restorations, obtained by using the different functioning positions of the mandible
6. Restorations, with reference to contours, contact points, marginal ridges, cervical margins
7. All tooth surfaces for caries and erosion, with use of explorers and strong mouth lamp, roentgenograms
8. Presence of hypoplasia and Hutchinson's incisors
9. Gingivitis, hyperplasia, congestion, recession of gingival tissue

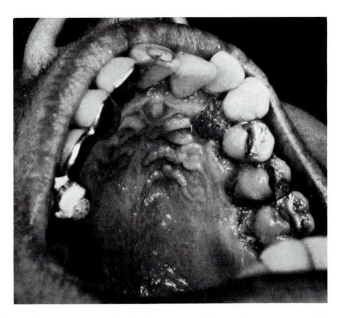

Fig. 12-64. Pyogenic granuloma of gingiva on palatal surface of upper left canine. It appeared as a mulberry mass, soft and blanching under pressure. Examination of this tissue miscroscopically is only method by which character of such a lesions can be revealed. Microscopic examination of tissue, therefore, should be done in many instances.

Minor tooth movement chart

Patient's name _____ Case number _____

Draw in position of teeth to be moved orthodontically. Superimpose desired new position of teeth.

Reason for tooth movement

_____

_____

Methodology

_____

_____

Type of appliance and anchorage

_____

_____

Prognosis

_____

_____

Evaluation of therapy

_____

_____

10. Subgingival tissue: periodontal pockets (shallow or deep) topography, exudation of pus, presence of calculus
11. Tenderness or painful areas, congestion, exudation of pus on palpation of gum tissue over root area
12. Anomalies of tooth form, size, or number (Fig. 12-62).

Roentgenographic examination
1. Any marked deviation from normal in alveolar bone formation
2. Evidence of rarefying or condensing osteitis of alveolar bone
3. Evidence of root surface changes, absence of lamina dura, abnormal thickening of periodontal ligament, periapical rarefaction
4. Presence or absence of root canal filling in pulpless teeth
5. Condition of alveolar crests and any widening of marrow spaces; evidence of alveolar atrophy
6. Indications of caries, abrasion, or erosion

As the examination proceeds, the findings should be recorded on a suitable chart. In Figs. 12-63 and 12-64 the teeth are drawn in position as found: the teeth present, their proximity, their proximal contact, their inclination and position in the arch, and so on. The depth recordings are performed to ascertain the bone and crestal contour. The remainder of the chart is narrative in character and requires the examiner to describe findings in detail. In addition to the recording of the chart, photographs of the patient are exceedingly helpful for an exact recording of the gingival tissue as well as for tooth placement and so on (boxed material). Nine photographs make up a set: three buccal, three palatal, and three lingual. The full dentition set of radiographs also should be taken.

After all the information obtained at the chair has been recorded on the charts, and after roentgenograms, photographs, and impressions have been taken, the patient may be dismissed. At a later date any additional data obtained can be filled in. At that time the data should be analyzed and a differential diagnosis made. The etiologic factors should be listed, after which a diagnosis and prognosis can be made. Once the diagnosis is decided upon, the type of treatment that will best remove the exciting causes and symptoms present can be selected.

REFERENCES

Alldritt, W. A. S.: Radiology in periodontal practice, Dent. Pract. Dent. Rec. **5:**123, 1954.

Arnim, S.: The use of disclosing agents for measuring tooth cleanliness, J. Periodontol. **34:**227, 1963.

Baer, P. N.: The case for periodontosis as a clinical entity, J. Periodontol. **42:**516, 1971.

Baer, P. N., and Bernick, S.: Age changes in the periodontium of the mouse, Oral Surg. **10:**430, 1957.

Baer, P. N., and Kilham, M. D.: Rat virus and periodontal disease. III. The histopathology of the early lesion in the first molar, Oral Surg. **17:**116, 1964.

Barros, L., and Witkop, C. J., Jr.: Oral and genetic study of Chileans, 1960. III. Periodontal disease and nutritional factors, Arch. Oral Biol. **8:**195, 1963.

Beagrie, G. S., and James, G. A.: The association of posterior tooth irregularity and periodontal disease, Br. Dent. J. **113:**239, 1962.

Belting, C. M., Hiniker, J. J., and Dummett, C. O.: Influence of diabetes mellitus on the severity of periodontal disease, J. Periodontol. **35:**476, 1964.

Belting, C. M., Schour, I., Weinmann, J. P., and Shepro, M. J.: Age changes in the periodontal tissues of the rat molar, J. Dent. Res. **32:**332, 1953.

Bernier, J. L.: The role of organ systems and of age in periodontal disease, J. Periodontol. **29:**247, 1958.

Bissada, N. F., and Schaffer, E. M.: Histopathologic changes in the periodontium of alloxan diabetic rats with and without local factors, Abstract no. 63, I. A. D. R. Program and abstract of papers, 1965.

Bjorn, H., Halling, A., and Thyberg, H.: Radiographic assessment of marginal bone loss, Odontol. Revy **20:**165, 1969.

Boorujy, S. R., and Ship, I. I.: An epidemiologic and clinical study of the prevalence of periodontal disease in diabetics, Abstract no. 58, I. A. D. R. Program and abstract of papers, 1965.

Box, H. K.: Experimental traumatogenic occlusion in sheep, Oral Health **25:**9, 1935.

Box, H. K.: Traumatic occlusion and traumatogenic occlusion, Oral Health **20:**642, 1930.

Box, H. K.: Necrotic gingivitis, Toronto, 1930, University of Toronto Press.

Breitner, C.: The tooth supporting apparatus under occlusal changes, J. Periodontol. **13:**72, 1942.

Burket, L. W.: A histopathologic explanation for oral lesions in acute leukemia, Am. J. Orthod. **30:**516, 1944.

Burnette, E. W.: Limitations of roentgenograms in periodontal diagnosis, J. Periodontol. **42:**293, 1971.

Carranza, F. A., Jr., and Glickman, I.: Some observations on the microscopic features of the infrabony pocket, J. Periodontol. **28:**33, 1957.

Carranza, F. A., Jr., Gravina, O., and Cabrini, R. L.: Periodontal and pupal pathosis in leukemic mice, Oral Surg. **20:**374, 1965.

Castelli, W. A., and Dempster, W. T.: The periodontal vasculature and its responses to experimental pressure, J. Am. Dent. Assoc. **70:**890, 1965.

Cawson, R. A.: Periodontosis associated with gingival lesions in a child, J. Periodontol. **30:**95, 1959.

Cohen, D. W., Friedman, L., Shapiro, J., and Kyle, G. C.: A longitudinal investigation of the periodontal changes during pregnancy, J. Periodontol. **40:**563, 1969.

Cohen, D. W., and Goldman, H. M.: Clinical observations on the modification of human oral tissue metabolism by local intraoral factors, Ann. N.Y. Acad. Sci. **85:**68, 1960.

Cohen, D. W., Shapiro, J., Friedman, L., Kyle, G. C., and Franklin, S.: A longitudinal investigation of the periodontal changes during pregnancy and fifteen months post-partum, J. Periodontol. **42:**862, 1971.

Cohen, M. M., Shklar, G., and Yerganian, G.: Pupal and periodontal disease in a strain of Chinese hamsters with hereditary diabetes mellitus, Oral Surg. **16:**104, 1963.

D'Amico, A.: Application of the concept of the functional relation of the canine teeth, J. Calif. Dent. Assoc. **27:**39, 1959.

Dummett, C. O.: Abnormal color changes in gingivae, Oral Surg. **2:**649, 1949.

Easley, J. R.: Methods of determining alveolar osseous form, J. Periodontol. **38:**112, 1967.

Ewen, S. J., and Stahl, S. S.: Response of the periodontium to chronic gingival irritation and long-term tilting forces in adult dogs, Oral Surg. **15:**1426, 1962.

Feldman, S.: Oral disease of medico-dental interest, Am. J. Orthod. **23:**287, 1937.

Fish, E. W.: Etiology and prevention of periodontal breakdown, Dent. Prog. **1:**234, 1961.

Fitzgerald, G. M.: Dental radiography, J. Am. Dent. Assoc. **41:**19, 1950.

Fleming, H. S., and Soni, N. N.: SE polyoma virus and the periodontium, Periodontics **2:**115, 1964.

Gargiulo, A., Wentz, F. M., and Orban, B.: Dimensions and relations of the dentogingival junction in humans, J. Periodontol. **32:**261, 1961.

Glickman, I.: Role of nutritional therapy in the management of periodontal disease, J. Am. Dent. Assoc. **52:**275, 1956.

Glickman, I., and Smulow, J. B.: Effect of excessive occlusal forces upon the pathway of gingival inflammation in humans, J. Periodontol. **36**:51, 1965.

Glickman, I., Smulow, J. B., and Moreau, J.: Effect of alloxan diabetes upon the periodontal response to excessive occlusal forces, J. Periodontol. **37**:146, 1966.

Glickman, I., and Weiss, L. A.: Role of trauma from occlusion in initiation of periodontol pocket formation in experimental animals, J. Periodontol. **26**:14, 1955.

Goldman, H. M.: Extension of exudate into supporting structures of teeth in marginal periodontitis, J. Periodontol. **28**:175, 1957.

Goldman, H. M.: Gingival vascular supply in induced occlusal traumatism, Oral Surg. **9**:939, 1956.

Goldman, H. M.: Marginal periodontitis, Am. J. Orthod. **31**:93, 1945.

Goldman, H. M.: Acute aleukemic leukemia, Am. J. Orthod. **28**:89, 1940.

Goldman, H. M., and Stallard, R. E.: Limitations of the radiograph in diagnosis of osseous defects in periodontal disease, J. Periodontol. **44**:626, 1973.

Gorham, L. W., and Stout, A. P.: Hemangiomatosis and its relation to massive osteolysis, Trans. Assoc. Am. Physicians **67**:302, 1954.

Gottlieb, B.: The formation of the pocket; diffuse atrophy of alveolar bone, J. Am. Dent. Assoc. **15**:462, 1928.

Gottlieb, B.: Paradentalpyorrhoë und Alveolaratrophie, Deutsch. Mschr. Zahnheilk. **2**:363, 1926.

Gottlieb, B.: Schmutzpyorrhoe, Paradentalpyorrhoe und Alveolaratrophie Munich, 1925, Urban & Schwarzenberg.

Gottlieb, B.: Die diffuse Atrophie des Alveolarknochens, Z. Stomat. **31**:195, 1923.

Gottlieb, B., and Orban, B.: Biology and pathology of the tooth and its supporting mechanism, New York, 1938, The Macmillan Co.

Green, J. C.: Periodontal disease in India; report of an epidemiological study, J. Dent. Res. **39**:302, 1960.

Greenberg, J., Haster, L. L., and Listgarten, M. A.: Transgingival probing as a potential estimator of alveolar bone level, J. Periodontol. **47**:514, 1976.

Hassell, T. M., Germann, M. A., and Saxer, U. P.: Periodontal probing: inter-investigator discrepancies and correlations between probing force and recorded depth, Helv. Odontol. Acta **17**:38, 1973.

Haupl, K.: Ueber traumatische verrursachte Gewebzveräderungen im Paradentium, Z. Stomat. **25**:307, 1927.

Haupl, K., and Lang, F. J.: Die marginale Paradentitis, Berlin, 1927, Hermann Meusser.

Hirschfeld, I.: A calibrated silver point for periodontal diagnosis and recording, J. Periodontol. **24**:94, 1953.

Hirschfeld, I.: Periodontal symptoms associated with diabetes, J. Periodontol. **5**:37, 1934.

Hirschfeld, I.: Importance of casts in periodontia practice, J. Am. Dent. Assoc. **20**:1223, 1933.

Hirschfeld, I.: Diagrammatic recording of periodontal disease, J. Am. Dent. Assoc. **18**:1927, 1931.

Hirschfeld, I.: Toothbrush trauma; recession, J. Dent. Res. **11**:61, 1931.

Hirschfeld, I.: Interdental canals, J. Am. Dent. Assoc. **14**:617, 1927.

Hirschfeld, I.: Some types of periodontoclasia and the diagnosis of their incipient symptoms, Dent. Items Interest **48**:823, 1926.

Hugoson, A.: Gingivitis in pregnant women, Odontol. Revy **22**:65, 1971.

Itoiz, M. E., Carranza, F. A., Jr., and Cabrini, R. L.: Histologic and histometric study of experimental occlusal trauma in rats, J. Periodontol. **34**:305, 1963.

James, W. W., and Counsell, A.: The primary lesion in so-called pyorrhoea alveolaris, Br. Dent. J. **49**:1129, 1928.

Kakehashi, S., Baer, P. N., and White, C. L.: Comparative pathology of periodontal disease. I. Gorilla, Oral Surg. **16**:397, 1963.

Kelly, G. P., Cain, R. J., Knowles, J. W., et al.: Radiographs in clinical periodontal trials, J. Periodontol. **46**:381, 1975.

Klinkhamer, J. M.: Quantitative evaluation of gingivitis and periodontal disease. II. The mobile mucus phase of oral secretions, Periodontics **6**:253, 1968.

Klinkhamer, J. M.: Human oral leukocytes, Periodontics **1**:109, 1963.

Klinkhamer, J. M., and Zimmerman, S.: The function and reliability of the orogranulocytic migratory rate as a measure of oral health, J. Dent. Res. **48**:709, 1969.

Lipke, D., and Posselt, U., editors: Functional anatomy of the temporomandibular joint, J. West, Soc. Periodont. **8**:48, 1960.

Löe, H.: The gingival index, the plaque index and the retention index systems, J. Periodontol. **38**:610, 1967.

Löe, H.: Periodontal changes in pregnancy, J. Periodontol. **36**:209, 1965.

Looby, J. P., and Burket, L. W.: Scleroderma of the face with involvement of the alveolar process, Am. J. Orthod. **28**:493, 1942.

MacLeod, K. M., Bety, P. K., and Ratcliff, P. A.: An index of gingival architectural form, J. Periodontol. **36**:413, 1965.

Manly, R. S.: Factors affecting masticatory performance and efficiency among young adults, J. Dent. Res. **30**:874, 1951.

Manson, J. D., and Nicholson, K.: The distribution of bone defects in chronic periodontitis, J. Periodontol. **45**:88, 1974.

McCall, J. O.: The radiogram as an aid in diagnosis and prognosis of periodontal lesions, J. Am. Dent. Assoc. **14**:2073, 1927.

McMullen, J. A., Legg, M., and Gottsegin, R., et al.: Micro-angiopathy within the gingival tissues in diabetic subjects with special reference to the prediabetic state, Periodontics **5**:61, 1967.

Miller, S. C., and Pelzer, R. H.: An original classification of alveolar types in periodontal diseases and its prognostic value; corroboration by plasma phosphatase determination, J. Am. Dent. Assoc. **26**:565, 1939.

Mühlemann, H. R.: Tooth mobility: a review of clinical aspects and research findings, J. Periodontol. **38**:686, 1967.

Mühlemann, H. R.: Tooth mobility, J. Periodontol. **25**:22, 125, 198, 1954.

Nabers, C. L., Spear, G. R., and Beckham, L. C.: Alveolar dehiscence, Texas Dent. J. **78**:4, 1960.

O'Conner, T. W., and Briggs, N. L.: Interproximal bony contours, J. Periodontol. **35**:326, 1964.

O'Leary, T. J.: Tooth mobility, Dent. Clin. North Am. **13**:567, 1969.

Oliver, L. P.: Pain patterns, Aust. Dent. J. **6**:79, 1961.

Orban, B.: Traumatic occlusion and gum inflammation, J. Periodontol. **10**:39, 1939.

Orban, B., and Weinmann, J.: Signs of traumatic occlusion in average human jaws, J. Dent. Res. **13**:216, 1933.

Person, P.: Dynamic equilibria of oral tissues, J. Periodontol. **26**:7, 1955.

Persson, P-A., and Wallenius, K.: Metastatic renal carcinoma (hypernephroma) in the gingiva of the lower jaw, Acta Odontol. Scand. **19:**289, 1961.

Posselt, U.: Bite guards, bite plates, and orthodontic treatment in periodontal disease, Dent. Prod. **11:**126, 1960.

Prichard, J.: Role of the roentgenogram in the diagnosis and prognosis of periodontal disease, Oral Surg. **14:**182, 1961.

Prichard, J., and Goldman, H. M.: Periodontal traumatism, Oral Surg. **15:**404, 1962.

Ramfjord, S.: Effects of acute febrile diseases on the periodontium of Rhesus monkeys with reference to poliomyelitis, J. Dent. Res. **30:**615, 1951.

Ramfjord, S., Kerr, D., and Ash, M., editors: Proceedings of the World Workshop in Periodontics, Ann Arbor, 1966, University of Michigan Press.

Ramfjord, S., and Kohler, C.: Periodontal adaptation to functional occlusal stress, J. Periodontol. **30:**95, 1959.

Reeves, R.: Occlusal traumatism; its pathologic effects and diagnosis, J. Am. Dent. Assoc. **59:**439, 1959.

Ritchey, B., and Orban, B.: The crests of the interdental alveolar septa, J. Periodontol. **24:**75, 1953.

Russell, A. L.: International nutrition surveys; a summary of preliminary dental findings, J. Dent. Res. **42:**233, 1963.

Russell, A. L., Leatherwood, E. C., Consolazio, C. F., and Van Reen, R.: Periodontal disease and nutrition in South Viet Nam, J. Dent. Res. **44:**775, 1965.

Sandler, H. C., and Stahl, S. S.: The influence of generalized diseases on clinical manifestations of periodontal disease, J. Am. Dent. Assoc. **49:**656, 1954.

Sandler, H. C., and Stahl, S. S.: Prevalence of periodontal disease in a hospitalized population, J. Dent. Res. **39:**439, 1960.

Sheridan, R. C., Cheraskin, E., Flynn, F. H., and Hutto, A. C.: Epidemiology of diabetes mellitus. I. Review of the literature, J. Periodontol. **30:**242, 1959.

Stafne, E. C., and Austin, L. T.: A characteristic dental finding in acrosclerosis and diffuse scleroderma, Am. J. Orthod. **30:**25, 1944.

Stahl, S. S.: Healing of gingival tissues following various therapeutic regimens; a review of histologic studies, J. Oral Ther. **2:**145, 1965.

Stahl, S. S., Cantor, M., and Zwig, E.: Fenestrations of the labial alveolar plate in human skulls, Periodontics **1:**99, 1963.

Stahl, S. S., Miller, S. C., and Goldsmith, E. D.: The effects of vertical occlusal trauma on the periodontium of protein deprived young adult rats, J. Periodontol. **28:**87, 1957.

Stallard, R. E.: Occlusion: a factor in periodontal disease, Int. Dent. J. **18:**121, 1968.

Stallard, R. E.: The effect of occlusal alterations on collagen formation within the periodontium, Periodontics **2:**49, 1964.

Strahan, J. D.: The relation of the mucogingival junction to the alveolar bone margin, Dent. Pract. Dent. Rec. **14:**72, 1963.

Suomi, J. D., Palumbo, J., and Barbano, J. P.: Comparative study of radiographs and pocket measurements in periodontal disease evaluation, J. Periodontol. **39:**311, 1968.

Theilade, J.: An evaluation of the reliability of radiographs in the measurement of bone loss in periodontal disease, J. Periodontol. **31:**143, 1960.

Thoma, K. H., and Goldman, H. M.: Correlation of clinical and pathologic phases of periodontal diseases, Dent. Items Interest **61:**103, 212, 309, 452, 1939.

Thoma, K. H., and Goldman, H. M.: Diagnosis of parodontal diseases, Am. J. Orthod. **24:**1071, 1938.

Tibbetts, L. S.: Use of diagnostic probes for detection of periodontal disease, J. Am. Dent. Assoc. **78:**549, 1969.

Waerhaug, J.: Pathogenesis of pocket formation in traumatic occlusion, J. Periodontol. **26:**107, 1955.

Weinberg, L. A.: Technique for temporomandibular joint radiographs, J. Prosthet. Dent. **28:**284, 1972.

Weiner, G. R.: Radiology in prevention, diagnosis, and treatment of periodontoclasia, J. Periodontol. **8:**33, 1937.

Weinmann, J. P.: Progress of gingival inflammation into the supporting structures of the teeth, J. Periodontol. **12:**71, 1941.

Wentz, F. M., Jarabak, J., and Orban, B.: Experimental occlusal trauma initiating cuspal interferences, J. Periodontol. **29:**117, 1958.

Wickham, N. E.: Gingival and periodontal lesions in children, N.Z. Dent. J. **48:**132, 1952.

Williams, C. H. M.: Investigation concerning the dentition of the Eskimos of Canada's Eastern Arctic, J. Periodontol. **14:**34, 1943.

Woods, E. C., and Wallace, W. R. J.: Alveolar atrophy of unknown origin, Am. J. Orthod. **27:**676, 1941.

Young, A. P.: Methods in the production and use of intraoral x-ray film in connection with periodontal conditions, N.Y. J. Dent. **8:**364, 1938.

Zabinska, O.: The use of the iodine text of Schiller as an index of gingival inflammation, Adv. Periodontics **1:**30, 1970, Paradon. Acad. Rev **2:**65, 1968.

Zander, H. A., and Mühlemann, H. R.: The effect of stresses on the periodontal tissues, Oral Surg. **9:**380, 1956.

Ziskin, D. E., Blackberg, S. N., and Stout, A. P.: The gingiva during pregnancy, Surg. Gynecol. Obstet. **57:**719, 1933.

13 Rationale of periodontal therapy

The paradigm of an anatomically desirable healthy periodontium would be a stable virgin tooth in ideal interarch and intra-arch relationships, invested in a well-formed bony housing crested with margins of parabolic form peaking interdentally, and veneered with a sizable mat of firmly adherent keratinized mucosa that filled the embrasure spaces completely. This protective layer of gingiva would have the color of health, a shallow sulcus, a tight seal, be difficult to retract, and upon gentle probing elicit no pain or bleeding. Additionally the dimension and topography of the jaw and its alveolar extensions would create the framework for a deep reflection of the mucosal fornix at a distance from the gingival margin that would provide an adequate zone for attached gingiva. When aberrations or deviations from this ideal are encountered because of congenital development or disease or both the central issue in planning an approach to treatment is the rationale of the therapeutic modalities, conceptualized at this stage in the development of periodontology, that may be utilized to intercept, abort, or reverse a condition that threatens the longevity of the teeth of the dentition.

IS PERIODONTAL THERAPY NECESSARY?

Epidemiologic studies reveal that the predominant cause of tooth mortality after midlife is peri-

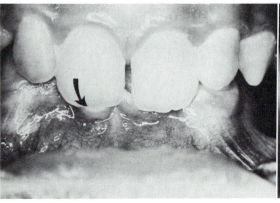
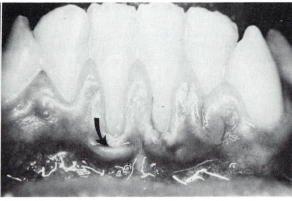

A   B

Fig. 13-1. Periodontal destruction resulting from malocclusion in a 12-year-old child. Deep overbite, **A,** has caused maxillary central incisors to strip attached gingiva from labial surfaces of mandibular central incisors, **B.** Arrows in **A** and **B** indicate position of incisal edge of maxillary right central incisor when mandible is closed. In this instance orthodontics played a key role in treatment of periodontium.

odontal disease but only reflect by inference an earlier disease incipiency. Other studies, however, indicate that periodontal disease among the young can be considered pandemic. It seems *plausible,* therefore, to assume that the disease that begins in childhood (Figs. 13-1 to 13-3) progresses with varying degrees of abatement and subsequently terminates in tooth loss during the middle and later years in a large segment of the world's population.

The principal raison d'être of periodontal therapy is to interrupt this sequence of events. Therefore for all the reasons that teeth are important— mastication, speech, appearance, the psyche, and in general a sense of well-being—periodontal therapy is warranted. Unfortunately, unlike other diseases (the common cold) periodontal disease is not self-limiting. Without an interceptive program

of treatment this ubiquitous, progressively destructive disease will eventuate in loss of the dentition (Fig. 13-4).

PREDICTABILITY OF THERAPEUTIC RESULTS

The heart of periodontal therapy is the question, "Does it work?" Some obvious emergency periodontal treatment measures may be required during the chronology of periodontal disease because of swelling, pain, dysfunction, or infection, but is a well-planned, well-executed treatment program predictably successful? Are the results of present treatment regimens temporal in nature or can tooth mortality be reduced by periodontal therapy? The documentation on answers to these questions is sparse indeed. We are dependent

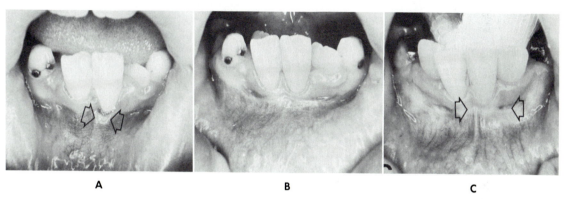

A   **B**   **C**

Fig. 13-2. A, Periodontal problem presented by a 4-year-old child in which mandibular left central incisor erupted slightly labial to a ridge adjacent to a shallow vestibule and a high frenum attachment *(arrows).* In **B,** 2 months after treatment (repositioning), and in **C,** 17 months later, interceptive mucogingival surgery has allowed a healthy development of dentition. Arrows in **C** indicate that new mucogingival junction has remained stable.

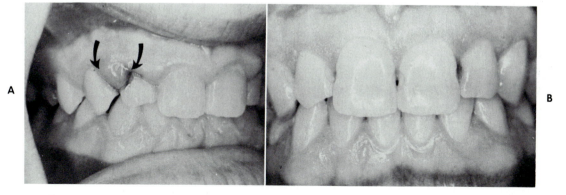

Fig. 13-3. Timely periodontal therapy in developing dentition can have beneficial effect on adult dentition. In **A,** 14-year-old boy demonstrates gingival enlargement and easy bleeding *(arrows)* consistent with diagnosis of gingivitis. In **B,** 7 years later, periodontium is healthy and well formed, indicating a good response to interceptive periodontal therapy. Plaque control, root planing, gingivectomy in the anterior maxilla, and gingival curettage in remaining dentition was treatment carried out.

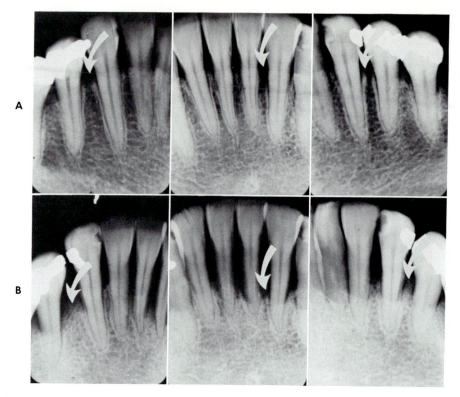

Fig. 13-4. Comparison x-ray films of a patient with a periodontitis in which pockets remained untreated over a 10-year span. Original series, **A,** indicate early crestal resorption *(arrows).* Failure to manage these lesions with definitive therapy at this relatively early stage in progress of disease has resulted in severe loss of bone *(arrows)* seen in **B.** Many similar instances of progressively destructive periodontal disease when no therapy is rendered provide a logical rationale for treatment of the early lesion.

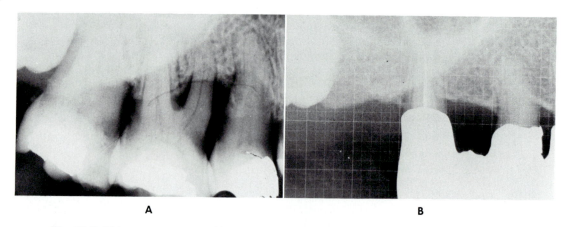

Fig. 13-5. This case was treated by strategic extraction, root sectioning, osseous surgery, and periodontal prosthesis. X-ray film in **B** was taken 19 years after x-ray film in **A.**

primarily on the evidence of long-term results based on the records of treatment over a span of years by various clinicians. Figs. 13-5 to 13-8 illustrate the results over many years of a variety of periodontal treatment procedures in individual cases. These and innumerable similar cases give

credence to the contention that periodontal therapy in its various forms is an effective modality. The logic of periodontal therapy is therefore based on the premise that in the light of some studies validating the usefulness of periodontal therapy, and the apparently successful results of treatment

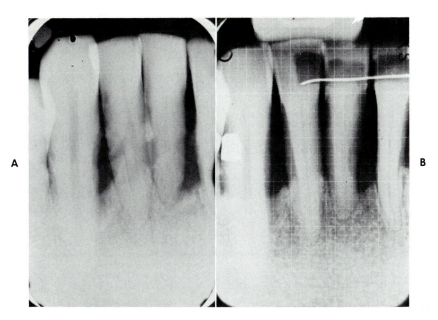

Fig. 13-6. Case treated by open curettage and wire-and-acrylic stabilization. X-ray film in **B** was taken 11 years after x-ray film in **A.**

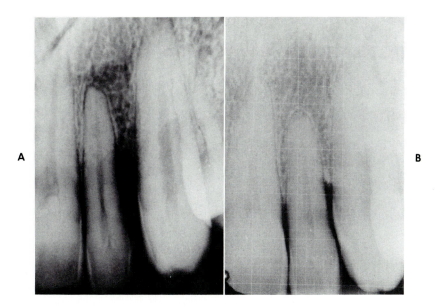

Fig. 13-7. Fifteen-year treatment result, **B,** of periodontal lesion between the maxillary lateral and cuspid in **A,** using orthodontics and osseous surgery.

by individual therapists, periodontal treatment is preferable to the reality of tooth loss when no treatment commitment is made.

BASIC TENETS OF PERIODONTAL THERAPY

When considering treatment of periodontal disease it is easy to be misled. Although this group of diseases may have a common termination, tooth loss, it manifests itself in a variety of ways: acutely or chronically destructive, limited to gingiva or invasive to bone, or confined to a single tooth, group of teeth, or diffuse throughout the dentition. It may appear in apparently healthy individuals or be concomitant with numerous syndromes and diseases. Its symptomatology may vary widely: spontaneous hemorrhage or none, swelling or none, acute pain or painless, mobility with no bone loss or stability with advanced loss, color ranging from shiny red to stippled pink, and

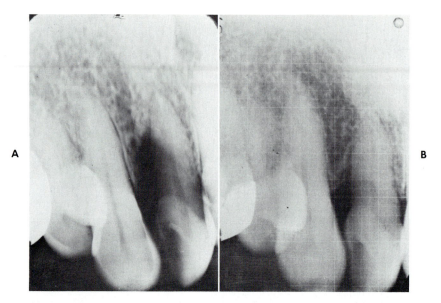

Fig. 13-8. Sixteen-year postoperative x-ray film, **B,** indicates substantial restoration of the septal intraosseous lesion seen in **A.** In this case surgical approach was a "self-fill" procedure because of diagnosis of a periodontal lesion with three osseous walls.

heavy calculus or minimal plaque. Each case has its own history, appearance, and character and is first observed at a time in the individual's life cycle in which constitutional, psychic, or accidental influences may have been, may be, or will be a factor. It is therefore a basic tenet in the rationale of periodontal therapy that we are faced not with a disease in isolation but with a *patient* afflicted with a type of periodontal disease that requires treatment. This discussion, however, will limit itself to the rationale of the *intraoral* treatment of diseased gingival and periodontal attachments, fully cognizant of the critical influences that peripheral factors may exert.

TREATMENT HYPOTHESES

Periodontal therapy is based on the following three propositions:

1. Bacterial plaque is the key etiologic agent in the initiation and perpetuation of periodontal disease; therefore any treatment that eliminates, minimizes, or prevents its accumulation and adherence is beneficial to the periodontium.

2. The periodontal attachment apparatus—cementum, periodontal ligament, and bone—can be damaged by untoward force applied to it; therefore any treatment that intercepts or rearranges forces so they are received within acceptable limits (the physiologic range) is beneficial to the periodontium.

3. The quality, quantity, and topography of the periodontium may preclude or deter the inception, progress, or extent of periodontal disease; therefore any treatment that enhances these structural defense factors is beneficial to the periodontium.

The rationalization of the entire range of periodontal therapy as practiced today is based on the preceding analysis. Each case will of course present great individual variation, and each therapist will justify the reasoning for his treatment regimens on the weight of each factor he places on the scales of his own training, experience, and perception.

Rationale of periodontal therapy based on bacterial etiology: plaque control

We have known that bacteria are living residents of the dental environment and adhere as a potentially harmful mat or plaque on teeth and gingivae for a very long time. It is not within the scope of this chapter to delineate every shred of evidence in support of the bacterial factors in periodontal disease. However, careful scrutiny of the literature will indicate that (1) the bacterial microcosm can initiate periodontal disease; (2) a program of plaque control can decrease the incidence of periodontal disease; and (3) removal of plaque can diminish the inflammatory response in periodontal disease.

The logical conclusion is therefore that plaque prevention and control are rational periodontal therapy. Additionally, *any environment that en-*

courages plaque accumulation or that makes plaque removal more difficult or impossible is not in the best interest of periodontal health and should be changed. This may be termed environmental control, a reference to the influence of tooth position, iatrogenic dentistry, and gingival morphology. Most importantly, however, it refers to the management of the dentogingival space, that is, the sulcus, in health or disease.

PLAQUE AND TOOTH POSITION

Clinicians who carry out an orderly, disciplined program of plaque control find it self-evident that the morphology, position, and contacting relationships of teeth are prime factors not only in food

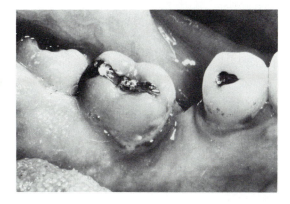

Fig. 13-9. This mandibular second molar drifted mesiolingually after extraction of first molar and is a typical example of plaque retention as a result of faulty tooth position. This situation adds a new dimension of difficulty in an area notoriously a problem in plaque control even under ideal conditions.

impaction and retention but also in the deposition of plaque and calculus. The dentition, moreover, has a poor self-cleansing mechanism, is not *substantially** aided in its hygiene by diet, and therefore requires either chemical or mechanical deplaqueing. Although chemical control of plaque is an exciting idea and is being investigated, we are at this time still dependent on mechanical debridement for effective control. Crowded lower incisors, tipped molars, and short square teeth with broad contacts contribute to the difficulty in plaque removal (Fig. 13-9). When such situations exist, odontoplasty, orthodontics, and strategic extraction are some of the methods employed to intercept or alleviate this problem (Fig. 13-10).

PLAQUE AND RESTORATIVE DENTISTRY

It hardly needs pointing out that gingival inflammation and periodontal disease are frequently attendant to overhanging restorations and large proximal carious lesions. Not only do these dental lesions and restorations act as plaque retainers but they also make plaque removal a complicated if not impossible endeavor. It is often so discouraging for the patient to repeatedly catch or break dental floss on a poor margin (Fig. 13-11) that it reduces his enthusiasm for plaque control in the other parts of his dentition. Therefore a treatment plan that focuses on superior restorative dentistry with its connotation of marginal perfection, ideal

---

*Egelberg's study does indicate a beneficial cleansing effect from a hard diet in dogs, but Arnim's investigation and the work of Lindhe and Wicen appear to be more germane to the cleansing effect of a hard diet in man's dentition, especially in the difficult proximal areas.

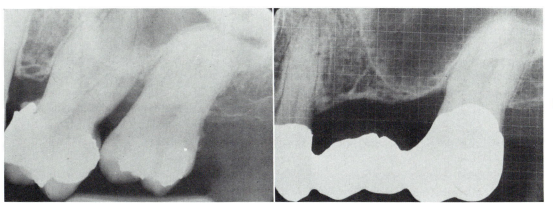

A   **B**

Fig. 13-10. One could anticipate that retention of first molar in **A** would result in an extremely difficult proximal plaque problem after periodontal therapy. X-ray film in **B** illustrates 12-year result of strategic extraction, osseous surgery, using a flap approach, and a fixed bridge. Gingival topography and prosthetic restoration have been designed to minimize plaque accumulation and to facilitate plaque removal.

contour, and proper contact relationships is rational periodontal therapy. This is true for both preventive and corrective periodontics.

PLAQUE CONTROL AND GINGIVAL MORPHOLOGY: POCKET ELIMINATION

There are occasions, however, when tooth position and restorative dentistry are within normal limits, but the contiguous gingival morphology predisposes the area to plaque accumulation. This is particularly true of those cases of altered passive eruption in the posterior segments. The combination of broad contacting surfaces, especially in the molar areas, and coronally positioned gingival margins create soft tissue craters that act as harbors

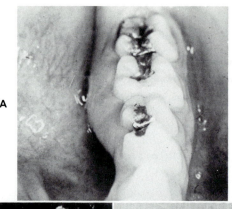

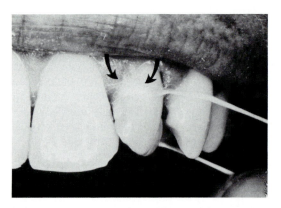

Fig. 13-11. Breaking and shredding of dental floss *(arrows)* as seen here is evidence of importance of ideal restorative dentistry in periodontal health. In this case floss is catching on overhanging margin of proximal synthetic restoration in maxillary lateral. Not only does a poor restorative margin retain plaque, but it hinders its removal as well.

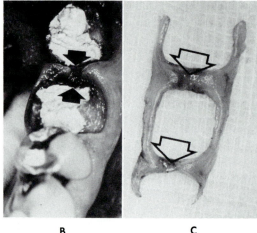

Fig. 13-12. This mandibular molar area, **A,** has all the anatomic conditions conducive to proximal periodontal disease: short square teeth, altered passive eruption, and an uncommonly wide alveolus. These combine to form a proximal topography ideal for plaque retention. **B,** Similar case resulting in cratering *(arrows)* and in diseased gingival attachments *(arrows)* seen in excised gingival tissue in **C.**

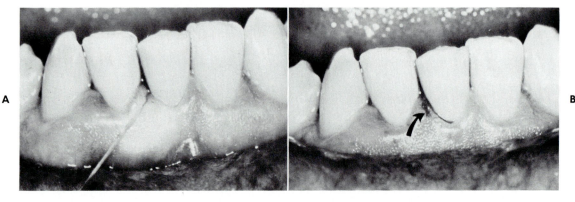

Fig. 13-13. Although use of floss is instrumental in plaque control, improper manipulation of floss, **A,** in attempt to remove plaque from craters can result in the floss lesion *(arrows)* seen in **B.** Ideal gingival topography and good plaque control are complementary.

for the bacterial invaders (Figs. 13-12 and 13-13). This topographic situation is also commonly found in cases of chronic necrotizing gingivitis. It is well nigh impossible to remove the plaque from these depressions without causing injury to the covering gingiva (Fig. 13-13). Excessively rounded, thick, or irregular gingival margins are additional examples of the influence of gingival morphology in plaque control. This is the rationale of gingivoplasty, the surgical removal and shaping of gingival tissue designed to facilitate the prevention and management of bacterial plaque. In surgical periodontics, subsurface healing is temporal if ideal gingival morphology is disregarded.

The most obvious, largest, and safest harbor for bacterial plaque is of course the periodontal pocket. The great variations in the depths, widths, and configurations of pocket morphology make it self-evident that no patient-operated mechanism of plaque control can reach the innermost tortuous labyrinths of many periodontal pockets. In Fig. 13-14 one can observe a probe reaching 10 mm beyond the gingival margin of an upper canine. However, ready access to the canine environment for plaque control is meaningless now because the plaque and calculus are protected by a cover of gingiva and are located subgingivally too distant from the margin for any successful debridement technique by the patient. Knowing, moreover, that plaque can be found on the tooth within the periodontal pocket to a point within 1 to 2 mm of the epithelial attachment, as shown by Hoffman

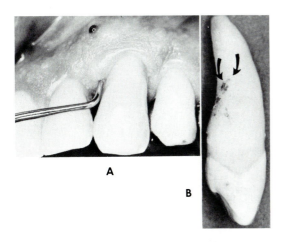

Fig. 13-14. A, Periodontal probe 10 mm into diseased gingival attachment. **B,** Arrows point to the estimated apical residence of root plaque. No patient-operated control program can deplaque this area. It is beyond reach of patient and in reality beyond reach of consistent debridement by therapist as well.

and Gold, and that plaque removal is critical to periodontal health, we are obviously entirely dependent on the therapist for definitive plaque control in the remaining 8 mm of this particular dento-gingival space. To do this effectively as in the case illustrated or in similar topographic protectors of the bacterial microcosm requires not only a highly skilled operator working with exquisitely sharp scalers or curets or both but also a schedule of visits at extremely short intervals. This is necessary because new plaque begins to form almost immediately after its removal. If the potential pathogenicity of the plaque is dependent on its numbers and its aging (a reflection of nonremoval), then pocket elimination is a reasonable methodology in plaque control.

In addition to this analysis one can make a brief for pocket elimination as follows:

1. Generally there is no *acute* loss of the bony alveolus (as in the case of a periodontal abscess) unless a periodontal pocket is present. There are exceptions, of course, such as in instances of sudden alveolar loss associated with pulp pathology.
2. Generally there is no chronic wasting of the bony sockets unless pockets accompany the phenomenon. Gingival atrophy may be an exception to this statement, but, even in these cases, the alveolar loss is commonly only one-sided on the facial aspect.
3. Conversely, when the alveolus does survive from childhood to old age, pockets are generally not present or are of minimal depth and the plaque has a nonvirulent potential (Fig. 13-15).
4. As a sequela of pocket depth, with its accompanying breakdown in the integrity of the sulcular lining, an inflammatory infiltrate can be demonstrated in the gingival corium and, depending on the extent of the lesion, in and contiguous to the alveolus.
5. Bone resorbs in the continued presence of inflammation.
6. Filling in of bony defects caused by or associated with pocketing and cessation of bony resorption does take place after pocket elimination (Figs. 13-16 and 13-17).

It is presumptive then that loss of the alveolar housing is a reflection of breakdown in the sulcular lining followed by inflammation in the subjacent and contiguous tissues and that the pocket is an etiologic factor in periodontal disease: as demonstrated, pocket elimination is a rational approach to the management of periodontal disease.

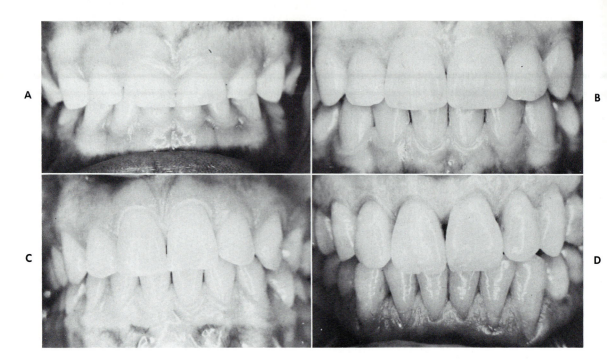

Fig. 13-15. From deciduous dentition, **A,** to 15-year-old adolescent, **B,** young adult, **C,** and elderly, age 76, in **D,** gingival topography remains consistent and covers a similarly shaped osseous foundation if pocketing is prevented. In four cases illustrated, sulcus depth was minimal.

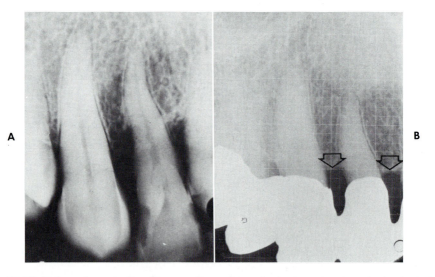

Fig. 13-16. Before, **A,** and after, **B,** x-ray films of a patient whose treatment plan included osseous surgery and periodontal prosthesis as key factors. X-ray film in **B,** taken 19 years postoperatively, illustrates crestal definition and position consistent with healing *(arrows).*

Dentogingival space elimination to zero depth is therefore a desirable goal *even though this objective may be difficult to achieve as well as impossible to maintain.* As almost every clinician will attest, there is usually a "cuffing out" process that occurs postsurgically. As a result some sulcus depth may be observed even after the most successful therapy. This in no way denigrates the value of seeking zero depth as an objective in treatment. *In the absence of contradictions* the attempt at the dentogingival junction to reach the perfection of a zero sulcus that may ultimately mature to a 1 or 2 mm space makes more sense than acceptance of 3+ mm with its obvious man-

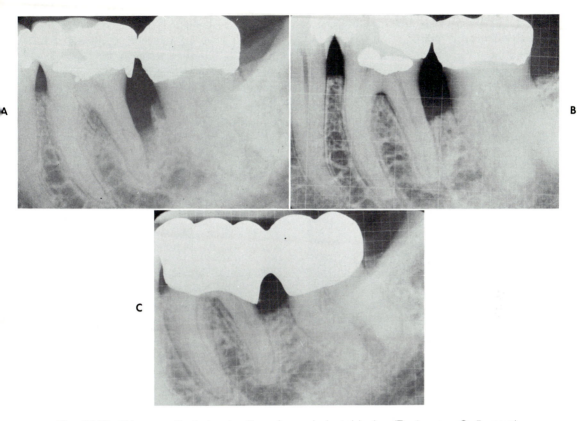

Fig. 13-17. This case illustrates healing of a periodontal lesion (**B**, 4 years; **C**, 5 years). First molar distal intraosseous lesion in **A** was a combination of three and two osseous walls. Treatment involved a mucoperiosteal flap approach, complete debridement of lesion, and placing some autogenous bone chips removed from mesial osseous lesion of second molar into defect. This case lends credence to rationale of treating such osseous lesions with our present therapeutic armamentarium.

agement problems and questionable future dimension. *The twin objectives of minimal sulcus depth and plaque control are therefore complementary and are not only the cornerstone of rational periodontal therapy once disease has occurred, but of preventive periodontics as well.*

Great prudence must be exercised in pocket therapy, however, for it is easy to be beguiled by a concept of zero sulcus. The fact that there is a measurable distance between the gingival margin and the epithelial attachment does not *in itself* justify sulcus or pocket elimination. There are a substantial number of contraindications to committing every deep sulcus to surgery. Any physical health or psychologic deterrent to surgery as well as local environmental anatomy quite often rules out any definitive elimination of pocket depth or makes its maintenance at its corrected level unlikely. Bony exostoses, shallow palatal vaults and the external oblique ridges of the mandible adjacent to the bases of pockets, deep lingual pocketing associated with a shallow mouth floor, roots

in close approximation, or pocketed second molars with an abruptly rising mandibular ramus are but a few examples of situations when acceptance of some sulcus depth may be good clinical judgment. There are additional instances, however, when the dental and jaw anatomy may favor definitive surgery, but the oral anatomy or gag reflex may influence the operator in the direction of a nonsurgical approach. Fig. 13-18 illustrates the oral opening of a woman who presented herself with a periodontitis treated definitively by periodontal surgery under normal circumstances. In this case, however, the combination of an extremely small oral aperture, pendulous cheek pads, and long dental arches prevented pocket elimination distal to the second premolars. Inadequate access and visibility were critical factors in the decision not to operate on the molar segments.

When a probe measures a sulcus to a depth greater than the operator is willing to accept, it is imperative to determine if the depth is in reality a pocket or is normal for the part. Bleeding is a key symptom. Should it occur either by probing or brushing, it is evident that the lining of the gingival attachment has undergone inflammatory change. Proximal measurements, particularly, are influenced by the morphology of the teeth, their contacting relationships, the shape of the embrasures, and the positions of the approximating ce-

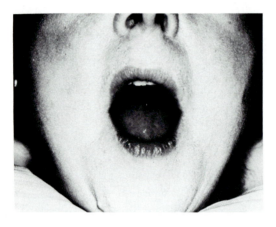

Fig. 13-18. Inadequate visibility and accessibility to molar areas are the result of a restricted oral opening. This is an anatomic variation that may preclude desired result in posterior segments.

mentoenamel junctions. Not only do these junction positions have an influence on the shape of the interdental alveolar crests, as shown by Ritchey and Orban, but these positions can affect the normal sulcus depth (health) as well. Finally, if the achievement of zero sulcus is the operator's only goal and is reached at a cost of eliminating all remaining attached gingiva, creating an impossible plaque control situation because of margin position of sensitivity or producing a frank cosmetic failure, then the price paid was much too high. As in clinical medicine the decision to operate is a judgment based on an assessment of all factors involved and is a reflection of the art as well as the science of the discipline.

Rationale of osseous therapy in pocket elimination

The fact that the bony alveolus is affected by periodontal disease is self-evident and universally accepted. As shown in Fig. 13-4 loss of bone is the normal consequence of untreated periodontal disease and is the rule rather than the exception. *It is destruction of bone, not gingiva, that results in tooth mortality.* The most pertinent question in periodontal therapy is therefore, ''What is the best

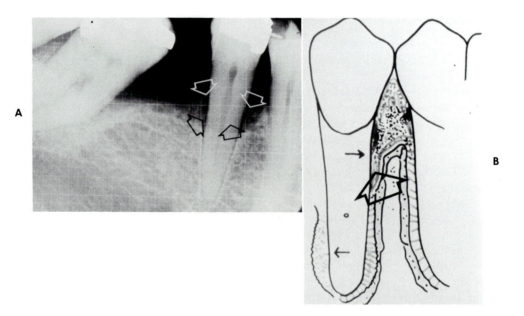

Fig. 13-19. A, X-ray film of a periodontal osseous lesion typical of one in which occlusal forces and inflammation are common overlapping etiologic factors. In this case, A splint between bicuspids is not beneficial in correcting lesion that has been established to depth reached by a probe *(arrows).* However, splinting or occlusal correction or both may intercept new lesions of occlusal trauma that may be occurring apical to arrows. In **B,** a representation of this case indicates that inflammatory infiltrate has entered area previously lysed (softened up) by excessive occlusal force *(open arrow).* This area is no longer amenable to occlusal therapy and now requires pocket elimination techniques.

treatment regimen for preventing additional loss of bone or rebuilding that which has already been lost?''

To answer this, one must be conversant with the various mechanisms of alveolar breakdown, the available treatment modalities in osseous therapy, and the dynamics of wound healing as well as have an appreciation of the soft tissue (gingiva) and hard tissue (bone, tooth) morphologic relationships that enhance maintenance of a treated case in health.

The essential local factors leading to alveolar destruction in periodontal disease are inflammation and excessive force. These allopathic influences may be working separately in any individual case or be operating in consonance (Fig. 13-19, *A*). Regardless of the weight of each factor in the derivation of a particular osseous defect, once a pocket with an osseous component has been established, only treatment of the inflammatory component (the pocket) will arrest the lesion. Although treatment of the occlusion to redirect or alleviate untoward forces on the attachment apparatus may still be indicated in such a case, its role now is one of preventing additional pathology in the region of the cementum–periodontal ligament–bone interface rather than correcting the damage that had previously been incurred at the pocket level. Remodeling of bone within the pocket wall, by redesigning the occlusion, does not occur (Fig. 13-19, *B*). We are therefore completely dependent on the direct therapy of the gingiva or bone or both to intercept additional bony loss *within the inflammatory zone.*

Although aberrant bony levels can be main-tained in some instances by repeated pocket débridement, there is general agreement, as discussed earlier, that pocket elimination is more reliable in aborting further deterioration. Pocket eradication, with its primary goal of minimum sulcus depth, therefore remains the key challenge in the treatment of the bony alveolus jeopardized by periodontal disease. The success of this venture, however, is impeded by the irregular patterns of bone destruction concomitant with the pathogenesis of detachment. The indications for simple excision of the gingival wall (gingivectomy) as a routine technique for treatment of a pocket are uncommon, for *it is successful in total pocket elimination, with good gingival form, only when the base of the pocket is suprabony* (Fig. 13-20).

The pathways of inflammation operating in conjunction with or without the destructive effects of occlusal trauma and superimposed on varying congenital morphologies have a pathoplastic effect on the alveolar housing that results in many bizarre configurations. Bony craters, dehiscences, fenestrations, hemisepta, inconsistent margins, ledging, and lipping as well as one-, two-, or three-wall intraosseous defects can be observed in isolation or combination (Fig. 13-21). In the face of this great variation in the housing topography subgingivally there is a common conceptual denominator in planning treatment of all bony lesions. *The foundation of all osseous therapy is based on the idea that the postsurgical objective of a healthy sulcus with minimum depth is dependent on the parallel and harmonious relationship between gingiva and bone that simulates normal periodontal architecture.* Departures from this concept are cer-

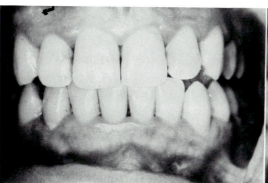
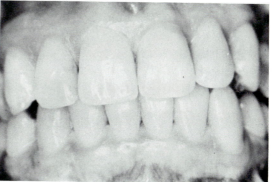

A

B

Fig. 13-20. Example of periodontal surgery successful because of proper procedure selection. In this case, gingivectomy was carried out because cratering in **A** was all supracrestal. In **B**, 7 years later, one can observe ideal gingival topography and considerable ''creeping.'' Such results can be anticipated in gingivectomy technique only if periodontal lesions probe coronal to osseous crests.

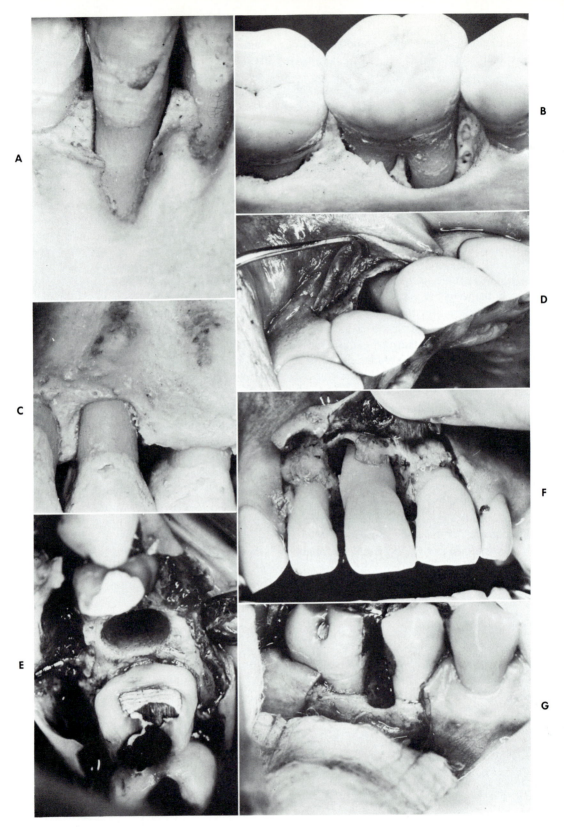

Fig. 13-21. Skull, **A** to **C,** and clinical, **D** to **G,** illustrations of enormous variety of osseous lesions that occur as a result of destructive effects of inflammation, trauma, or both superimposed on different congenital morphologic configurations. Despite these bizarre topographic findings, basic phenomena of destructive processes remain the same.

tainly indicated when peripheral circumstances dictate a different approach; compromise is at times prudent clinical judgment. But instances of contraindication in no way minimize the validity of the basic philosophy of an idealized parabolic form and should be understood for what they represent—exceptions to a fundamental rule.

Fulfillment of the objective of ideal bony form, in the presence of complex structural changes, may be realized by the subtraction of bone (osteoectomy, osteoplasty, osseous resection) or the addition of bone (grafts). Although successful grafting of bone has the advantage of gaining additional attachment and may be the treatment of choice in many instances, removal of bone to achieve physiologic form is a common surgical procedure provided that the loss of bone does not endanger the retention of the tooth or teeth. Simplicity of execution, predictability of results, and no waiting period for determining the success of a "take" are some of the advantages osseous reduction techniques have over osseous grafting procedures. In addition grafting procedures logistically are more complex for they may require a second-stage corrective surgical procedure and frequent deplaqueing visits during the long healing period. Despite these difficulties, grafting techniques have become more widely used as evidence of successful results begin to accumulate (Fig. 13-17). It has been demonstrated that new healthy periodontal ligament and cementum formation occurs in the areas of apparently successful grafts and as a result has become a rational approach to treatment of the periodontal osseous lesion. However, in instances of minimal postoperative loss of bone in subtraction techniques, osseous resection, *sensibly executed* *with modifications when necessary,* remains a standard treatment for a large variety of osseous problems.

Rationale of mucogingival surgery based on fiber barrier principle

It will be remembered that the gingival attachment to the tooth is composed of two parts: the epithelial lining, which can be termed a "barrier," and the gingival fiber apparatus, which accounts for the adherence quality of the attachment. An insufficient zone of attached gingiva will not accommodate sufficient gingival fibers, and thus the adherence quality will be affected. Therefore there should be an adequate zone of attached gingiva.

If inflammation is the basic phenomenon in destructive periodontal disease, then obstruction to or impedance of the spread of inflammation is a rational treatment objective. The most reliable naturally occurring defense structure is the connective tissue complex. Dissolution of this collagen fiber system by epithelial or cell-bound collagenases (and various other lytic mechanisms) elicited in the inflammatory state is considered essential to the apical migration of the epithelial attachment. In the absence of conclusive histologic and statistical evidence it seems logical to assume that dense, closely packed collagen fiber groups found in zones of attached gingiva are better deterrents to the infiltration of inflammatory elements than in the loosely arranged fiber milieu of alveolar musoca (Fig. 13-22). Progression of a periodontal lesion that has traversed the mucogingival junction is often quite rapid and frequently results in loss of a facial bony plate, especially in the presence of congenitally thin structures (Fig. 13-23).

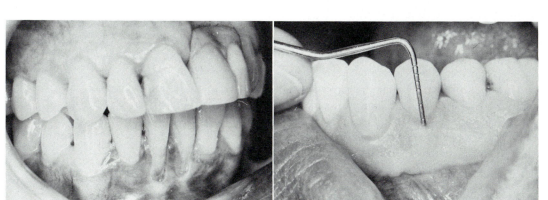

Fig. 13-22. In **A,** one can observe extremely thin mucosa covering prominent root structure in mandible. In presence of inflammation or toothbrush abrasion, one could anticipate premature loss of this tissue and its subjacent thin bony plates, a phenomenon that has already occurred over central incisors. In **B,** however, attached gingival zone is thick, wide, and firmly bound down to underlying bone, all anatomic factors deterring easy inflammatory spread and its destructive sequelae.

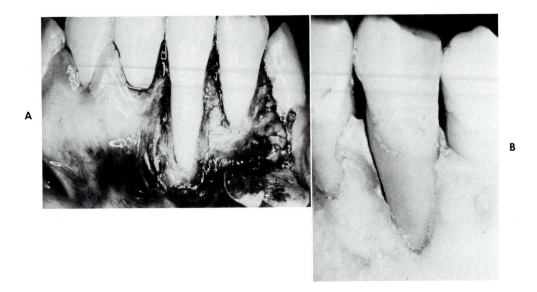

Fig. 13-23. Typical findings can be observed in the clinical case, **A,** and skull specimen, **B,** when one removes thin gingival covering over prominent root formations. Loss of thin, labial bony plates can usually be predicted; surgical plan should anticipate this and proceed accordingly.

The clinical implications are readily drawn. In the absence of solid defense bastions of dense collagen fiber bundles (attached keratinized gingiva), restructuring the vulnerable zones with a new fiber barrier system is a sensible treatment modality. Löe recently has indicated that 2 mm of attached gingiva is sufficient for the maintenance of health. This is an extremely difficult research problem, since the topographic, inflammatory, traumatic, and age factors in each case are found in such varied combinations. In addition the projected postsurgical management of the treated zone may exercise a strong influence on a clinician's attitude in a particular situation. For example, if major extracoronal fixations are planned after periodontal therapy, the operator may deem it prudent to pursue greater gingival dimension than "normal" as insurance against injuries he may unavoidably induce in tooth preparation, impression-taking, and cementation. The clinical knowledge that subgingival crown margins may be responsible for increased plaque accumulation and more severe gingivitis, even when magnificently executed, often leads to an attempt at creating an added safety zone. This is "built-in" preventive dentistry and is akin to the extension-for-prevention concept in restorative dentistry carried out in the periodontal structures. Even in circumstances when no postsurgical iatrogenic injury is contemplated it is reasonable to protect the periodontium by overbuilding its physical defenses (attached keratinized gingiva) in the face of anticipated repeated bacterial attack. Even the most disciplined and enthusiastic patient in the arena of plaque control experiences occasional behavioral changes that may endanger the vulnerable sulcular epithelial wall. It is reassuring to have a strong second line of defense.

As Congdon noted, "In the theory of therapeutic processes there seems to be a theme of substitution or replacement that goes back to earliest man." Periodontology is no exception. Numerous surgical techniques have been devised and proposed to treat mucogingival problems from a tenuous beginning of denudation to the current era of repositionings, pedicles, and free gingival grafts. The development of improved conversion procedures in the mucogingival field has been steady, well intentioned, and imaginative. Its prime objective, since the earliest wound-healing studies evidencing the possibilities of postsurgical loss of bone, has been the creation of an "adequate" dimension of attached gingiva without destruction of fragile facial or lingual bony plates. In pursuit of this goal, various complex flap designs, dissection procedures, suturing techniques, and dressing materials have been developed. Some of these are not considered standard techniques, whereas others have been discarded, but most have contributed some part in the development of mucogingival surgery. The casual finesse with which these techniques are carried out today (Figs. 13-24 and

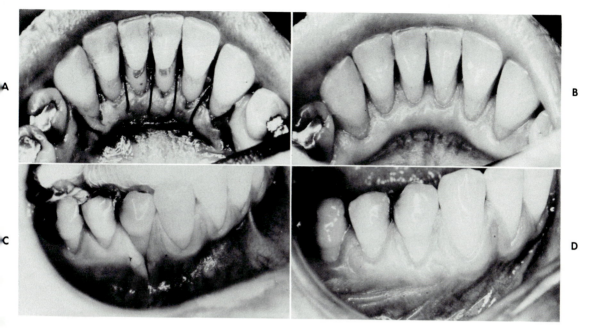

Fig. 13-24. Examples of commonly employed current therapeutic modalities. **A,** Partial-thickness flap repositioned and designed to eliminate lingual pocketing and gain attached gingival dimension, **B.** In **C,** cleft in mandibular first bicuspid area is treated by laterally repositioning proximal papillary gingiva to eliminate defect and create a healthy zone, **D.**

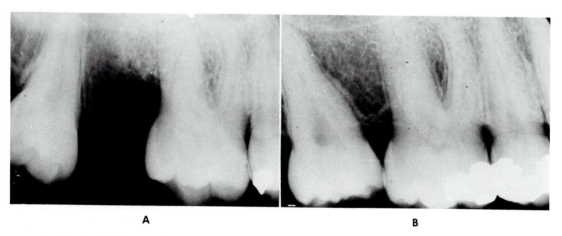

Fig. 13-25. This case illustrates what can be expected from a rational biologic approach to periodontal therapy. In **A,** x-ray film reveals a deep intraosseous lesion distal to maxillary first molar involving edentulous second molar site. Using orthodontic techniques, third molar was repositioned to second molar contact. Subsequently, an intraosseous "self-fill" surgical procedure was carried out because examination of the lesion with patient under anesthesia indicated it had three osseous walls. Ten years later, **B,** osseous septum approximates normality for existing tooth positions, teeth are firm and functioning, and sulci probe to minimal depths.

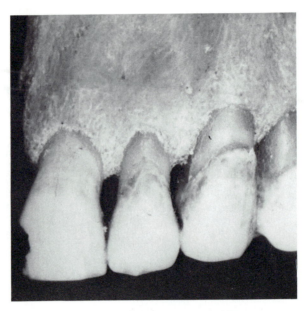

Fig. 13-26. Skull showing regular, parabolic form of alveolar housing, although bone margins are more apical than their original locations.

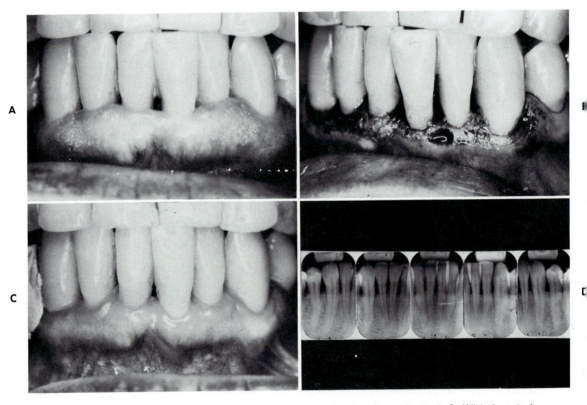

Fig. 13-27. Case in which excisional therapy (gingivectomy) is indicated. **A,** Wide band of keratinized gingiva with blunting and soft tissue cratering. **B,** Gingiva has been removed to base of craters in an attempt to create normal gingival architecture in incisional design. **C,** Two months later, healing has occurred; however, new calculus is being formed. Oral hygiene is being taught as treatment progresses. **D,** X-ray studies of this area show relatively flat mesiodistal profiles of osseous crests since bone has been resorbed evenly.

13-25) owes its sophistication to the men who pioneered, often with great anxiety, the procedures of yesterday.

SURGICAL APPROACHES IN PERIODONTAL THERAPY: RESECTIVE AND RECONSTRUCTIVE TECHNIQUES

As one examines the numerous and various surgical approaches previously and currently employed to treat periodontal disease it becomes apparent that they fall into two major categories: those involving soft tissue (gingiva, mucosa) and those involving bone. It is important to recognize, however, that even in those instances in which only soft tissue is being treated bone may (Figs. 13-26 and 13-27) or may not (Figs. 13-28 and 13-29) be involved by the disease process or by developmental factors.

The preponderance of soft tissue therapy (gin-gival curettage, gingivectomy) is excisional and designed to obtain healing of the disease process by elimination of damaged tissues. This is accomplished by the healing of the surgical wound: a healthy soft tissue complex is formed to seal the dentogingival junction. The pedicle and free mucosal autografts may be considered reconstructive techniques. In these cases not only are diseased tissues removed but a greater quantity and improved *quality* of gingiva is created by the surgical technique (Figs. 13-30 and 13-31). The intentional "reconstruction" of soft tissue is generally limited to these instances. Occasionally a new and increased amount of gingiva forms following excisional therapy by "creep" (Fig. 13-20).

When the normal configuration of the alveolar process has been altered due to periodontal disease (Fig. 13-21) the conceptual approach to the

Text continued on p. 400.

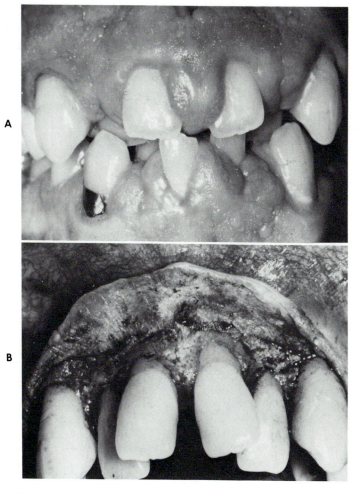

Fig. 13-28. Case of Dilantin gingival hyperplasia in which excisional therapy of gingiva is indicated. **A,** Gingival enlargement is observed prior to surgery. **B,** Excision of gingiva is being accomplished by a flap approach. One can observe normal osseous architecture.

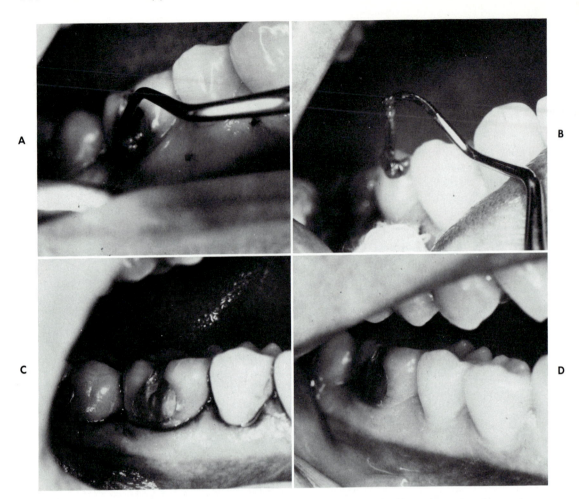

Fig. 13-29. Soft tissue excisional therapy (gingival curettage) with no bone involvement. **A,** Curet moving through sulcus to enucleate wall of pocket. **B,** Sulcular epithelium and subjacent granulomatous tissue are removed. **C,** Appearance of gingival margin immediately after curettage. **D,** Topography of healed case 6 months after surgery.

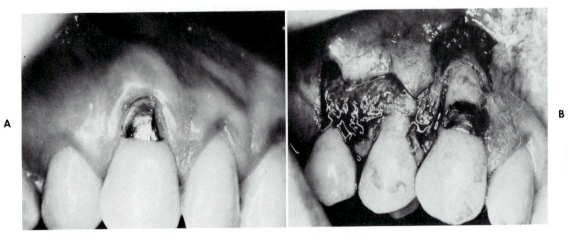

Fig. 13-30. "Reconstruction" of gingiva with underlying bone loss. **A,** Gingival margin of canine can be probed to a depth of 5 mm. **B** and **C,** Combined full- (over first premolar) and partial-thickness (over second premolar) pedicle is being dissected and sutured to denuded, planed root of canine. **D,** Healing 6 months later shows an "attached" gingival margin with a wide zone of keratinized tissue. Little if any injury has occurred at donor sites.

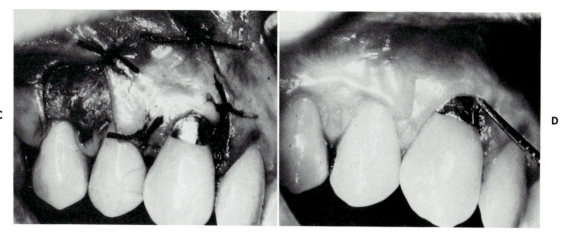

Fig. 13-30, cont'd. For legend see opposite page.

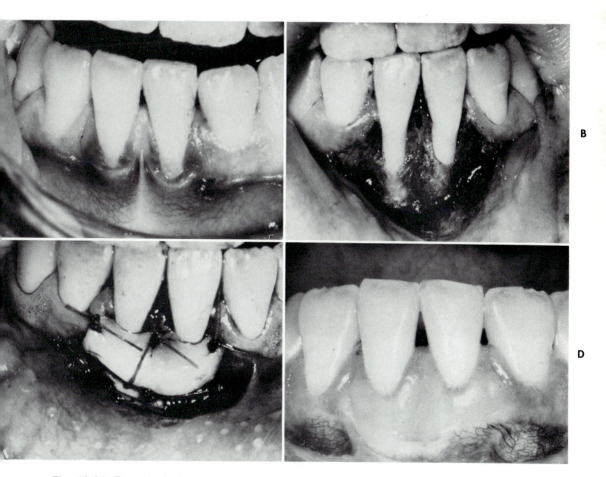

Fig. 13-31. Free gingival autograft. **A,** Inflamed mucosal margins labial to lower central incisors. **B,** Labial plate loss can be observed. This recipient bed has been prepared, and roots planed for placement of graft are seen in **C. D,** "Reconstructed" gingiva over denuded central incisors. Dentogingival junction can be probed 2 mm. Obviously creeping attachment has taken place.

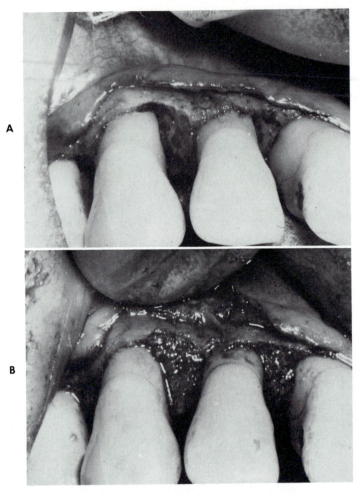

Fig. 13-32. Case of loss of bone from a periodontal disease in which ostectomy is contra-indicated. Depth of osseous lesions, **A,** precludes removal of remaining supporting bone. **B,** Ideal osseous morphology is being "reconstructed" with iliac crest marrow.

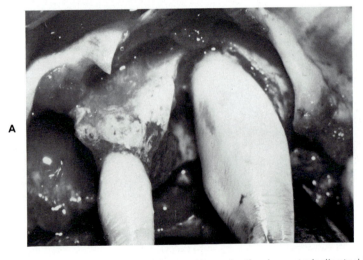

Fig. 13-33. A, Osseous lesions in which osseous reduction is contraindicated because of extent of bone loss.

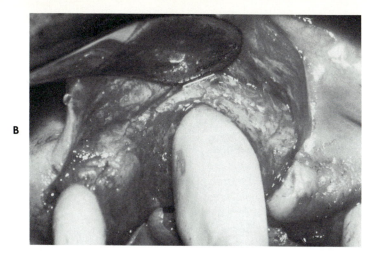

Fig. 13-33, cont'd. B, Osseous morphology is now examined on a reopening procedure for osseous shaping 9 months after bone graft was taken from maxillary tuberosity.

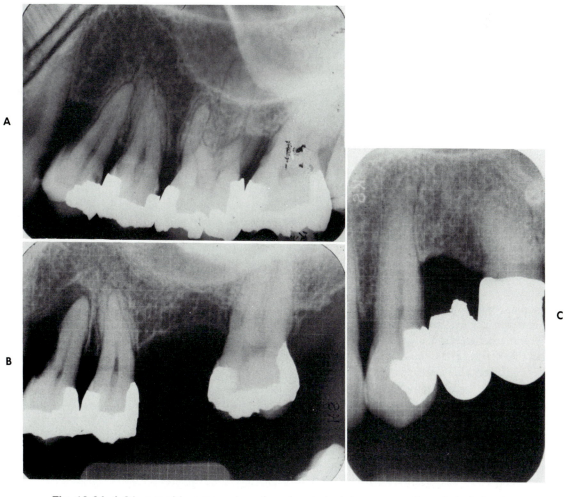

Fig. 13-34. A 34-year-old woman who refused periodontal surgery and pocket elimination procedures. After a program of root planing and closed curettage she was placed on 1-hour recall visits every 3 months. **A,** Original x-ray film with advanced osseous loss mesial to first premolar and between first and second molars. **B,** Ten years later with loss of first molar due to a periodontal abscess (from trifurcation) and advanced loss of bone mesial to first premolar, which has remained vital. **C,** First premolar has now been removed, and osseous reshaping of housing of adjacent teeth has been carried out previous to construction of a fixed bridge. Pocket "maintenance" in such cases more often results in eventual tooth loss, as shown with this patient.

treatment of these bony lesions is ideally derived from the answer to the basic question, "Is this particular lesion amenable to reconstructive therapy or is the optimum approach resective in nature?" As stated earlier, attempts to rebuild alveolar housing destroyed by periodontal disease have in the past been less frequently indicated than resective techniques for a variety of reasons. However, it appears that additional grafting procedures have caught the imagination of and are an intellectual challenge to the profession and will be a steadily increasing option for the sophisticated clinician. There are, moreover, instances in which an osseous graft may be the *only* choice of treatment (Figs. 13-32 and 13-33) short of extraction or a long difficult maintenance program involving deep pockets that are vulnerable to acute exacerbations and eventual loss of osseous support despite meticulous and frequent curettage (Fig. 13-34). The predictability of preserving osseous support in these deep lesions is haphazard and leaves much to be desired. There are, however, numerous cases in which precise pocket elimination therapy may be ruled out by extenuating circumstances and in which repeated curettage may not be the treatment of choice but rather the treatment of necessity.

SUMMARY

Periodontal therapy is based on the understanding that there is a logical and rational methodology in the management of periodontal disease. These treatment regimens have been developed with the biologically sound concept that periodontal disease can be prevented, aborted, and controlled if the apparently causative factors (plaque, occlusal trauma) are understood and properly managed and the defense mechanisms are strengthened by a variety of restructuring techniques. If carried out meticulously with a reasoned and disciplined approached, successful results can be anticipated and will justify the occasionally lengthy and costly treatment. Conversely, periodontal treatment based on empiricism or fadism may terminate unhappily for both patient and dentist. If one practices periodontal therapy with a pragmatic attitude, that is, that the validity of the theories in the etiology, pathogenesis, and correction of periodontal disease should be tested on the anvil of practical application, he is usually impressed with the accuracy of these beliefs and the predictability of his results. Finally, the art and science of periodontology owes its present position of esteem to the rationally thinking men whose enthusiasm for new ideas in therapy was properly tempered by facts and logic but who were also transfixed with the idea that prevention is better than treatment.

REFERENCES

A.D.A. Bureau of Economic Research and Statistics: Survey of needs for dental care. II. Dental needs according to age and sex of patients, J. Am. Dent. Assoc. **46:**200, 1953.

Akiyoshi, M., and Mori, K.: Marginal periodontitis: a histologic study of the incipient stage, J. Periodontol. **38:**45, 1967.

Allen, E. F.: Statistical study of the primary causes of extractions, J. Dent. Res. **23:**453, 1944.

Arnim, S.: Use of disclosing agents for measuring tooth cleanliness, J. Periodontol. **34:**227, 1963.

Bass, C.: Optimum characteristics of dental floss for personal oral hygiene, Dent. Items Interest **70:**921, 1948.

Belting, C. M., Hiniker, J. J., and Dummett, C. O.: Influence of diabetes mellitus on the severity of periodontal disease, J. Periodontol. **35:**476, 1964.

Bjorn, H., and Carlsson, J.: Observations on a dental plaque morphogenesis, Odontol. Revy **15:**23, 1964.

Brautzaeg, P., and Jamison, H.: Effect of controlled cleansing of the teeth on periodontal health and oral hygiene in Norwegian army recruits, J. Periodontol. **35:**302, 1964.

Brekhus, P. J.: Dental disease and its relation to the loss of human teeth, J. Am. Dent. Assoc. **16:**2237, 1929.

Caffesse, R. L., Ramfjord, S. P., and Nasjleti, C. E.: Reverse bevel periodontal flaps in monkeys, J. Periodontol. **39:**219, 1968.

Cohen, D. W., and Morris, A. L.: Periodontal manifestations of cyclic neutropenia, J. Periodontol. **32:**159, 1961.

Congdon, C. C.: Bone marrow transplantation, Science **171:**1116, 1971.

Dobell, C.: Antony van Leeuwenhoek and his little animals, New York, 1960, Dover Publications, Inc.

Dragoo, M. R., and Sullivan, H. C.: A clinical and histologic evaluation of autogenous iliac bone grafts in humans. I. Wound healing, 2-8 months, J. Periodontol. **44:**599, 1973.

Egelberg, J.: Local effect of diet on plaque formation and development of gingivitis in dogs. I. Effect of hard and soft diets, Odontol. Revy **16:**31, 1965.

Fish, E. W.: Surgical pathology of the mouth, London, 1948, Sir Isaac Pitman & Sons, Ltd.

Friedman, N., and Levine, L.: Mucogingival surgery: current status, J. Periodontol. **35:**5, 1964.

Fullmer, H., Gibson, N., Lazarus, G., Bladen, A., and Whedan, K.: The origin of collagenase in periodontal tissues of man, J. Dent. Res. **48:**646, 1969.

Gilmore, N., and Sheiham, A.: Overhanging dental restorations and periodontal disease, J. Periodontol. **42:**8, 1971.

Glickman, I., and Wood, H.: Bone histology in periodontal disease, J. Dent. Res. **21:**35, 1942.

Goldman, H. M.: Extension of exudate into supporting structures of teeth in marginal periodontitis, J. Periodontol. **28:**175, 1957.

Goldman, H. M.: Relationship of the epithelial attachment to the adjacent fibers of the periodontal membrane, J. Dent. Res. **23:**177, 1944.

Groat, J. E., and Bhatnagar, R. S.: Endogenous collagenase in periodontal disease, Periodont. Abstr. **17:**147, 1969.

Halliday, D. G.: The grafting of newly formed autogenous bone in the treatment of osseous defects, J. Periodontol. **40:**511, 1969.

Hiatt, W. H., Stallard, R. E., Kramer, G. M., and Grant, D. A.: Is the simple gingivectomy obsolete? Periodont. Abstr. **8**:64, 1965.

Hoffman, I. D., and Gold, W.: Distances between plaque and remnants of attached periodontal tissues on extracted teeth, J. Periodontol. **42**:29, 1971.

Ingle, J. I.: Papillion-Lefevre syndrome: precocious periodontosis with associated epidermal lesions, J. Periodontol. **30**:230, 1959.

Ivancie, G. P.: Experimental and histological investigation of gingival regeneration in vestibular surgery, J. Periodontol. **28**:259, 1957.

Jenkins, G. N.: Composition and formation of dental plaque, Am. Inst. Oral Biol. Annu. Meet. **25**:99, 1968.

Keyes, P. H., and Shern, R. J.: Chemical adjuvants for control and prevention of dental plaque, J. Am. Soc. Prev. Dent. **1**:18, 1971.

Klingsberg, J.: Periodontal scleral grafts and combined grafts of sclera and bone: two year appraisal, J. Periodontol. **45**:262, 1974.

Lindhe, J., and Wicen, P. O.: The effects on the gingivae of chewing fibrous foods, J. Periodont. Res. **4**:193, 1969.

Löe, H.: The formation and growth of dental plaque on gingival-dental structures. International Conference on Plaque, New York, 1969, Warner-Lambert Pharmaceutical Co.

Löe, H.: Hjemmetandpleje [Home care for the dentition], T. Sygepl. **68**:200, 1968.

Löe, H., and Schiott, C.: The effect of mouthrinses and topical application of chlorhexidine on the development of dental plaque and gingivitis in man, J. Periodont. Res. **5**:79, 1970.

Löe, H., Theilade, E., and Jensen, S.: Experimental gingivitis in man, J. Periodontol. **36**:177, 1965.

Lovdal, A., Arno, A., Shei, O., and Waerhaug, J.: Combined effect of subgingival scaling and controlled oral hygiene on the incidence of gingivitis, Acta Odontol. Scand. **19**:537, 1961.

Lovdal, A., Arno, A., and Waerhaug, J.: Incidence of clinical manifestations of periodontal disease in light of oral hygiene and calculus formation, J. Am. Dent. Assoc. **56**:21, 1958.

MacDonald, J., Gibbons, R., and Socransky, S.: Bacterial mechanism in periodontal disease, Ann. N.Y. Acad. Sci. **85**:467, 1960.

Marshall-Day, C. D., and Shourie, K. L.: Roentgenographic survey of periodontal disease in India, J. Am. Dent. Assoc. **39**:572, 1949.

Matherson, D. G.: An evaluation of healing following periodontal osseous surgery in monkeys, master's thesis. University of Rochester, Rochester, N.Y., 1964.

Matherson, D. G., and Zander, H. A.: Evaluation of osseous surgery in monkeys (abstract), J. I. A. R. **41**:116, 1963.

McDougall, W. A.: Studies on the dental plaque. I. The histology of the dental plaque and its attachment. II. The histology of the developing interproximal plaque, Aust. Dent. J. **8**:261, 398, 1963.

Melcher, A.: Pathogenesis of chronic gingivitis. I. The spread of the inflammatory process, Dent. Pract. Dent. Rec. **13**:2, 1962.

Oliver, R. C.: Tooth loss with and without periodontal therapy, Periodont. Abstr. **17**:8, 1969.

Pennel, B. M., King, K. O., Wilderman, M. B., and Barron, J. M.: Repair of the alveolar process following osseous surgery, J. Periodontol. **38**:70, 1967.

Pfeifer, J. S.: Growth of gingival tissue over denuded bone, J. Periodontol. **34**:10, 1963.

Pritchard, J. F.: The etiology, diagnosis and treatment of the infrabony defect, J. Periodontol. **38**:455, 1967.

Prichard, J.: The infrabony technique as a predictable procedure, J. Periodontol. **28**:202, 1957.

Prichard, J.: Regeneration of bone following periodontal therapy, Oral Surg. **10**:247, 1957.

Ritchey, B., and Orban, B.: Crests of the interdental alveolar septa, J. Periodontol. **24**:75, 1953.

Ritz, H. L.: Microbial population shifts in developing human dental plaque, Arch. Oral Biol. **12**:1561, 1967.

Robinson, R. E.: Osseous coagulum for bone induction, J. Periodontol. **40**:503, 1969.

Rosenberg, M.: Free osseous tissue autografts as a predictable procedure, J. Periodontol. **42**:195, 1971.

Rosenzweig, K. A.: Gingivitis in children of Israel, J. Periodontol. **31**:404, 1960.

Russell, A. L.: Epidemiology of periodontal disease, Int. Dent. J. **17**:282, 1967.

Sandler, H. C., and Stahl, S. S.: Influence of generalized diseases on clinical manifestations of periodontal disease, J. Am. Dent. Assoc. **49**:656, 1954.

Schallhorn, R. G.: The use of autogenous hip marrow biopsy implants for bony crater defects, J. Periodontol. **39**:145, 1968.

Schallhorn, R. G.: Eradication of bifurcation defects utilizing frozen autogenous hip marrow implants, Periodont. Abstr. **15**:101, 1967.

Schallhorn, R. G., Hiatt, W. H., and Boyce, W.: Illiac transplants in periodontal therapy, J. Periodontol. **41**:566, 1970.

Schei, O., Waerhaug, J., Lovdal, A., and Arno, A.: Alveolar bone loss as related to oral hygiene and age, J. Periodontol. **30**:7, 1959.

Scherp, H.: Discussion of bacterial factors in periodontal disease, J. Dent. Res. **41**:327, 1962.

Schluger, S.: Osseous resection—a basic principle in periodontal surgery, Oral Surg. **2**:316, 1949.

Schoen, M. H.: Frequency of tooth loss in relation to the dentist's ability to prevent the necessity of extraction, Dent. Clin. North Am. **13**:741, 1969.

Schour, I., and Massler, M.: Gingival disease in postwar Italy (1945). I. Prevalence of gingivitis in various age groups, J. Am. Dent. Assoc. **35**:475, 1947.

Schultz-Haudt, S., Bruce, M. A., and Bibby, B. G.: Bacterial factors in non-specific gingivitis, J. Dent. Res. **33**:454, 1954.

Seibert, J. S.: Reconstructive periodontal surgery: case report, J. Periodontol. **41**:113, 1970.

Silness, J.: Periodontal conditions in patients treated with dental bridges, J. Periodont. Res. **5**:60, 1970.

Silness, J.: Periodontal conditions in patients treated with dental bridges. II. The influence of full and partial crowns on plaque accumulations, development of gingivitis and pocket formation, J. Periodont. Res. **5**:219, 1970.

Silness, J., and Löe, H.: Periodontal disease in pregnancy, III. Response to local treatment, Acta Odontol. Scand. **24**:747, 1966.

Socransky, S. S., Gibbons, R. J., Dale, A. C., Bortnick, L., Rosenthal, E., and MacDonald, J. B.: Microbiota of the gingival crevice area of man. I. Total microscopic and viable counts and counts of specific organisms, Arch. Oral Biol. **8**:275, 1963.

Theilade, E., Wright, W. H., Jensen, S. B., and Löe, H.: Experimental gingivitis in man. II. A longitudinal clinical and bacteriologic investigation, J. Periodont. Res. **1**:1, 1966.

Weinmann, J. P.: Periodontitis: etiology, pathology, symptomatology, J. Am. Dent. Assoc. **44:**701, 1952.

Weinmann, J. P.: Progress of gingival inflammation into the supporting structures of the teeth, J. Periodontol. **12:**71, 1941.

Wilderman, M. N., Wentz, F. M., and Orban, B. J.: Histogenesis of repair after mucogingival surgery, J. Periodontol. **31:**283, 1960.

Williams, J. L.: A contribution to the study of pathology of enamel, Dent. Cosmos **39:**296, 1897.

14 Prognosis

Concept of cure
Prognosis of dentition
Factors concerning prognosis

Prognosis is an evaluation of the condition, based on the etiologic factors responsible for the disease process and the benefits from therapeutic measures to be instituted, as well as the possibility of maintaining the status of a functionally dynamic reparation. Thus prognosis must be considered at the same time that treatment planning is formulated. Therefore Chapters 14 and 15 should be considered and studied as a unit.

Obviously in the formation of a prognosis there are many intangibles that may be described best as therapeutic judgment. It is just as obvious that in the less than expert operator this is the area of greatest deficiency. He may find teeth that have ample support and are loose and teeth that have little support but are firm; and he must cope with all the perplexing variations in between.

Prognosis depends on a combination of factors; the following are some general considerations:

1. Extent and type of the disease process, for example, suprabony, osseous defects, and zone of attached gingiva
2. Causative factors
   a. Local environmental factors—correctable or noncorrectable
   b. Physical health status of the patient influencing periodontal therapy—correctable or noncorrectable
   c. Habits—correctable or noncorrectable
3. Occlusal factors
4. Number and distribution of teeth remaining
5. Age of patient
6. Cooperation of patient

The question of periodontal prognosis is one that arises in almost every treated case. It is common experience for the patient, after case presentation, to inquire as to survival chances of the teeth and to express the desire for reassurance on the probable success of the case. This presents no great problem in the slightly or moderately involved teeth

and in the hopelessly involved teeth. The periodontist can give a definite unequivocal answer to these, since the outcome is fairly obvious. The borderline cases and those with a doubtful outcome present the real problem. It is with this type of case that this chapter will concern itself.

The problem is compounded by the fact that not only are individual teeth themselves in question but also often a large and complex restorative treatment plan depends on the retention and use of these very teeth as key abutments. This places a rather heavy burden of responsibility on the diagnostician under any circumstances (Figs. 14-1 to 14-3).

In such situations the establishment of a formula is useless. Rules have been expressed in the literature concerning proportional bone loss, for example, one third or one half the supporting bone loss as condemning a tooth for extraction. In practice these rules have been found to be of little value, and they have even been conducive to the sacrifice of teeth that might have been retained in health. The difficulty in establishing a formula or

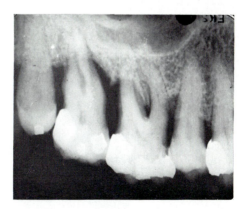

Fig. 14-1. Bone loss resulting in a diminution of approximately two thirds of attachment apparatus of molars. Prognosis for these teeth is poor. Although there is less bone loss around third molar than around other two molars, tapering shape of root is detrimental in that greatest square area of attachment apparatus is situated in marginal area. Because of loss of tissue here, prognosis is poor.

rule is that there are more exceptions than there are conforming cases. The best way to meet the problem is to establish certain basic principles, criteria of judgment, and probable behavior patterns of doubtful teeth under the conditions in which they must function.

CONCEPT OF CURE

The very first consideration is the concept of cure. Any tooth or collection of teeth that has become capable of functioning in health may be considered to be cured of disease. These teeth may be

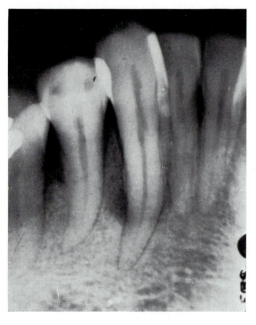

Fig. 14-2. Bone loss around root of cuspid. Clinically an osseous defect on labial aspect burrowed lingually around tooth.

able to function alone, or they may require stabilization and splinting to survive. In other words, if seriously involved teeth have been rendered healthy gingivally and yet do not possess enough investing attachment after the ravages of periodontal disease to support themselves in function, they may still become useful members of a dentition with some help. They must of course make a useful contribution to the splint, but this requirement is far less than that required to stand unaided. There is no point in retaining a useless tooth just for the sake of retaining it. On the other hand, frequently we encounter a situation in which a seriously involved tooth is flanked by others only slightly less involved. This poses problems of weak abutment teeth, and the question arises as to where to stop extracting. In these indications it is quite possible that they may all do better together than they would with one member missing.

PROGNOSIS OF DENTITION

The second consideration is the flexibility to sacrifice the single tooth and still succeed in the case. In all other branches of dentistry the prime consideration is the saving of an individual tooth or of several teeth. In periodontal procedures the prime consideration is the preservation of the dentition as a functioning unit. This means that individual components are not so vital as the overall function of the entire organ. The loss of a single tooth or even of several teeth does not destroy the dentition, provided the dentition can be restored.

The inference is obvious that if a given tooth is involved seriously and the outcome of therapy is in doubt, the tooth may be retained only on a provisional basis. But if response to therapy is not up

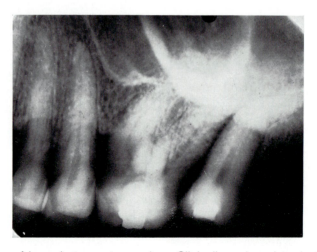

Fig. 14-3. Loss of bone between two molars. Clinically a deep interdental crater was present. Note root proximity.

to hopes or expectations the question must be asked, "How vital is this tooth to the overall plan?"

If the tooth can be dispensed with and enough remaining members can be maintained to ensure adequate support for a fixed prosthesis, then obviously the tooth may be sacrificed. If the same tooth in question is a key tooth in the plan the decision to retain it must be made on several factors other than the degree of involvement only. It is at such a point that diagnostic ability and therapeutic judgment serve one well. The problem of malposed and malaligned teeth often enters into the overall prognosis in a patient with periodontal disease. These conditions must be judged on an individual basis because of the various conditions that have to be considered. A knowledge of prosthesis and of orthodontics may be essential to solve the problem. There are, however, several criteria that we may use.

FACTORS CONCERNING PROGNOSIS

Questions that one might ask in considering a periodontal prognosis include the following:

1. *How long has the tooth been so seriously involved?*

If the degree of involvement has been more or less static for some years without help, it is reasonable to assume that with therapy the tooth should do well. Old roentgenograms are invaluable in determining the rate of bone loss. Sometimes these are surprising. If it is determined that the rate of destruction is rapid, then this particular factor of degree of involvement is a distinctly negative one.

2. *How radically can the environment of the tooth be changed (Figs. 14-4 and 14-5)?*

Local environmental factors have been described and discussed in a previous chapter. These problems may again be reviewed. Obviously the ability to change the local environmental factors for the tooth or teeth in question is a vital one; for example, if a tooth is in heavy trauma and is failing as a single unit in the total occlusion, the question must be answered whether splinting that tooth, cutting down the forces exerted upon it, or having it function in concert with a corrected occlusion will alter appreciably the displacing forces brought to bear upon it. If a given molar with interradicular involvement can be so reconstituted through therapy that all the heretofore inaccessible areas are open to home physiotherapy, will this procedure plus other factors such as occlusal adjustment and stabilization support establish a climate of health so that the tooth can survive? A corollary to this question may very well be, "Can such a tooth bear up under the requirement of occlusion?" To this the periodontist must bring a knowledge of the tensional habits of his patient and his own ability as therapist to mitigate or palliate the effects of those

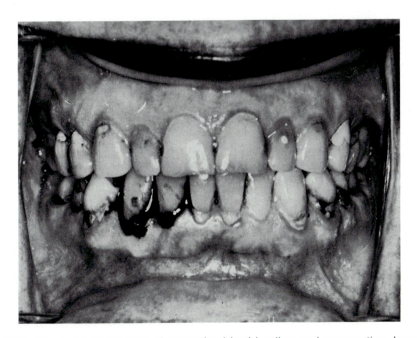

Fig. 14-4. Gingival inflammation characterized by bleeding and suppuration. Local environment can account for disease process, and hence prognosis is favorable.

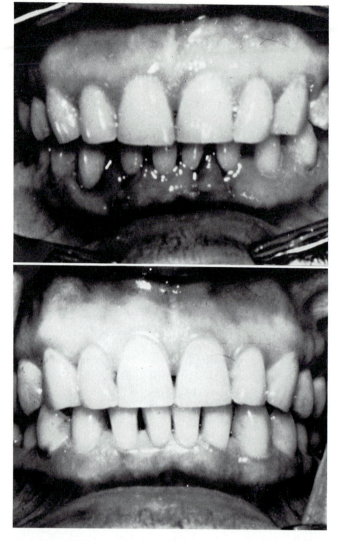

Fig. 14-5. Gingival inflammation associated with calculus deposits. Therapy was success-ful. Note shrinkage obtained and resultant architecture.

habits by secondary appliances such as night guards, and he must assay the reparative properties of his patient. The next question that arises is, "Can part of the tooth be retained?" Removal of one bucal root of a maxillary molar will result in a tooth with two roots that in many instances can be retained in health.

The introduction of the provisional fixed splint and the night guard as adjunctive therapy to peri-odontal treatment has been of tremendous import. The fixed provisional splint, particularly, gives the therapist the opportunity to observe response to therapy without finally committing the patient to a given restorative treatment plan. Only when the tissue response to therapy has been established in the desperately involved case can final procedures be established with confidence. The night guard is

a more conservative expedient because of its low cost and ease of fabrication. It serves to splint the teeth at night during the uninterrupted and most harmful time of tensional movements such as clenching and grinding.

3. *At what point in the proportion of bone loss to retained investing tissue would the tooth be considered hopeless?*

In answer to this question it can be stated that there is no such point. Basically if the tooth and the surrounding tissues can be returned to health and if the tooth can maintain itself in function, then it should be retained even if three fourths of the sup-porting bone has been lost. There are many teeth in this category that have given good service for many years and that continue in health.

On the other hand, there are some teeth with

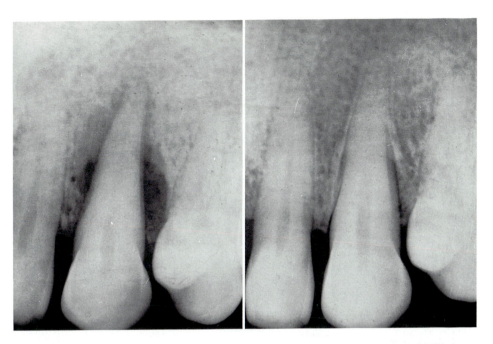

Fig. 14-6. Before and after therapy of infrabony pocket. Note healing of area with bone regeneration.

about one fourth of the supporting bone missing that have a hopeless prognosis because they cannot be returned to health. We have all seen teeth with extensive bone loss that have surprising stability because of a good physiologic response by the remaining investing tissues to the demands made upon them. Not always is it the amount of bone loss that must be considered, but the topography of the loss. Three-walled osseous defects have a relatively favorable prognosis, whereas a deep, one-walled defect may have a poor prognosis. Therefore the therapist must take into consideration the potential for repair as well as reconstruction of the area. Fig. 14-6 illustrates a condition that could be considered hopeless, yet bone fill resulted after therapy.

4. *Of what benefit is the assay of root form to prognosis?*

This factor can be of critical importance. Roots that are conical, even though they be of adequate length and dimension, are not to be relied upon for stability as much as are those that are club shaped. This is part of the secret of the remarkable stability of teeth with little apparent support. In the cone-shaped root a bone level of one third reduced from the crest involves almost two thirds of the total support. On the other hand, much less is lost in the club-shaped root than appears in viewing the roent-genographic profile. Root investment must be thought of in square millimeters of attachment rather than in profile proportions.

Naturally the crown-root ratio figures prominently here also. This is a more obvious factor. Thin, spindly, short roots under a broad, heavy crown constitute an unfavorable prospect in the face of extensive periodontal damage unless the ratio of crown to root support can be altered radically. Here occlusal narrowing and splinting accomplish much. Fixation accomplishes far more than borrowing support from stronger members to support weak ones. The arch form of the jaw lends tremendous mechanical advantage to units tied to each other. This factor often is minimized in case design. The conservative therapist still thinks in terms of individual units acting individually. The whole principle of the keystone in the arch is based on the basic premise of divergent or convergent vectors of force canceling each other out and making for stability. Root form plays an important role in prognosis in yet another aspect. Crown and root form are related to proximity of roots in the jaws when the embrasure area and interdental septum are reduced in size. Crater formation is often seen, and this makes for difficulty in therapy. Widely separated roots because of either size or position also present a problem in therapy (Fig. 14-7).

5. *Does the presence of a large osseous defect necessarily denote a negative prognosis for the tooth?*

Although the presence of an osseous defect presents a serious problem in therapy, for the most part these defects can be managed successfully.

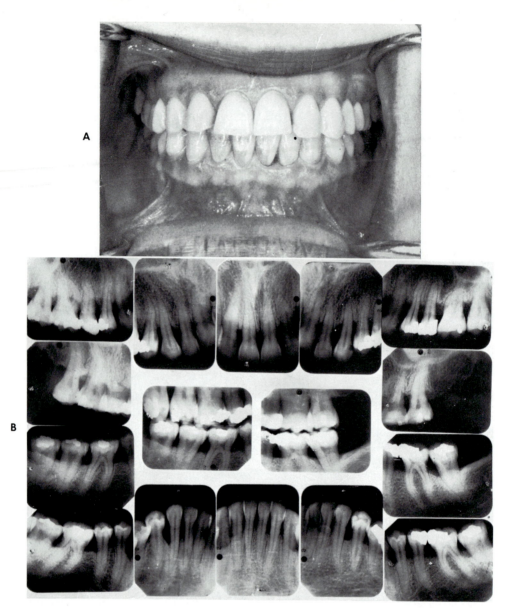

Fig. 14-7. A, Periodontal involvement that could not be attributed to local environmental factors. No habit history could be elicited. Teeth showed marked loosening. **B,** Teeth of patient in **A.** Note advanced bone loss. It is in cases of this nature that prognosis is less favorable than in those cases in which disease process can be attributed to local factors present.

Osseous defects may be classified as craters, totally encompassed, partially encompassed, or non-encompassed defects (three, two, or one osseous walls). The various surgical approaches are directed to allow for repair and fill of the defect or to remodel and contour the bone to eliminate the defect. Treatment planning is directed toward evaluation of the topography of the defect and the surgical approach. This in effect constitutes the relative prognosis. In detail each of the procedures has definitive objectives, and whether a success-

ful operation is possible is based on the general principles of prognosis determination.

6. *Is mobility a serious factor in periodontal prognosis?*

The answer to this basic question lies in several directions. If the mobility is due to extensive loss of support for the tooth, then the answer lies in the possibility for stabilization and for the return of the remaining tissues to health. All the factors discussed previously apply here. If, however, the mobility is due to heavy occlusal trauma without extensive pocket formation but with the usual picture roentgenographically of a widened periodontal space, then the prognosis is distinctly favorable. These teeth respond completely to proper therapy and correction of the occlusal factor.

Another aspect of this question should be mentioned. In the mobile tooth that shows extensive loss of periodontal support, a careful assay must be made of the pattern of loss of support. Often in these cases the deepest areas of loss of support are on the buccal or labial and lingual aspects of the tooth. The buccolingual direction is also the one in which mobility is most easily assayed clinically. These teeth lend themselves very well to therapy, and stabilization through splinting is extremely effective.

7. Is a young patient a better risk than an old one, given a similarly serious involvement?

In general the older the patient, the better is his prognosis in similarly involved cases. This is contrary to popularly held theories on resistance and disease. It is believed generally that the younger the patient, the greater his recuperative powers will be as well as his resistance to all disease. In a sense this confirms the stated opinion because if the younger patient who ordinarily is resistant to periodontal disease succumbs so completely as to constitute an advanced case of periodontal disease, there must be a serious lack of resistance in him, or the factors promoting periodontal disease must be of an overwhelming nature. Whether the response of the older patient to therapy is due to a diminution of inflammation as compared to the younger individual or whether the tissues themselves become inherently resistant to periodontal disease is difficult to determine. Both possibilities may be factors. In any case the clinical fact is apparent; only the explanation is uncertain.

8. Is suppuration from periodontal pockets an unfavorable prognostic sign?

Suppuration from the periodontal pocket indicates that the sulcular epithelium is ulcerated and that minute abscesses are present in the connective tissue. This is of course a sign of a serious periodontal lesion, but it does not affect the prognosis on its presence alone. Since proper therapy is successful in changing the sulcular lining and since the objectives of therapy are directed toward the elimination of as much of the sulcus as possible, it can be seen that suppuration need be only a transitory phenomenon. Of much greater import are such factors as bone loss vis-à-vis remaining support, interradicular involvement, and time interval of involvement.

9. Does the presence of a removable prosthesis affect the general prognosis of a periodontally involved dentition?

Generally speaking, in the periodontally involved mouth the fixed prosthesis is a stabilizing one, whereas the removable prosthesis is a displacing one. Such factors as soft tissue compressibility and rigid or springy retaining devices on the remaining teeth are inconsistencies that cannot be resolved adequately. This assumes that the case is one that can be restored only with a removable prosthesis. A distal extension case is such an example. In this contingency it must be kept in mind that the saddle area and other mucosal surfaces constitute an abutment in the restoration. This type of abutment used in conjunction with natural teeth as additional abutments can only exert torquing forces on the abutment teeth. Of course, a well-designed and carefully fabricated removable prosthesis, utilizing fixed splinting of the abutment teeth, will be less deleterious than will one that is poorly designed and made. The difference may be the key to the prognosis. The fixed restoration, on the other hand, uses abutments of similar quality and texture and will therefore behave as a single unit under stress.

Important considerations concerning the construction of removable partial dentures are as follows:

1. Occlusal disharmonies must be corrected.
2. Abutment teeth should have properly contoured crown form or restorations.
3. Abutment teeth should be stable and many times be utilized in multiples (fixed splinting).
4. Occlusal rests should direct force along the long axis of the tooth. Retention may be achieved by external, internal, or telescopic attachments. The latter two have many advantages over cast clasps.
5. The design of the appliance must be based on biomechanical principles.

Although there may be indications other than the distal extension case in which the removable restoration may be used, it is erroneous to believe that the long span or the space with weakly supported teeth as abutments is sometimes adequately restored by removable appliances. In reality weak teeth need splinting and stabilization rather than displacement, and a long span is just as long if there are clasps or retainers at both ends.

It is not the purpose here to enter into a long discussion of periodontal prosthesis other than to establish certain principles that will aid in the preservation of a dentition with damaged support. The therapist should consider several factors:

1. It is not necessary either for aesthetics or for adequate function to restore a dentition to a complement of 28 teeth. Many function well with a second premolar on one side as the distal tooth. It is far more important to stabilize the remaining teeth for their preservation.

2. Teeth with damaged support require help in stabilization. Removable appliances generally do not by themselves offer this support. Fixed splinting of abutment teeth is necessary.

3. In a situation in which a key tooth is in some jeopardy the considered risk may be taken with provisional appliances, making the possible failure of the tooth part of a plan of procedure.

These are a few of the basic considerations to use as an aid in prognosis where restoration is involved.

10. *Can the forces of occlusion be minimized in a periodontally damaged key tooth?*

Actually the forces of physiologic occlusion, that is, the forces of chewing food, really are well within the tolerance limits of a seriously involved tooth, even if that tooth helps support others. The debilitating stresses to which such a tooth is subjected are inflicted upon it by clenching and bruxism. Usually although not always these are nocturnal compulsions. They can be helped not only by an acrylic night guard but also by the guard's being adjusted so as to bring most of the stresses to bear on teeth that are better able to withstand them. This is done easily by minor adjustments in the occlusal surface of the guard. Stresses can be thrown on either the anterior segment or the posterior segment as desired. In so relieving a weak member the splinting property of the guard is maintained, and even some of the controlled and modified occlusal stresses can be minimized and diverted.

11. *Can the therapist provide for failure of a key tooth or key teeth in a complex restorative treatment plan if the restoration consists of a fixed prosthesis?*

There are situations in which this may be done. Usually, although not necessarily, these key teeth are distal teeth. In the case of distal teeth, however, it must be remembered that a full complement is not necessary for adequate function. We must also remember that we are dealing with crippled, mutilated dentitions that must be salvaged and maintained, so our objectives for an acceptable result must be tempered by minimum requirements in aesthetics and function. Such a result must be compared with the efficiency of full dentures. The primary objective of survival is not paramount. Therefore in many instances we can accept a single first molar of the upper and lower arches in occlusion on one side as adequate, even if the distal teeth on the other side of the arches are an upper and lower second premolar. This will effectively meet the minimum masticatory and aesthetic requirements of the patient. Within this general framework much can be done to preserve the dentition with a fixed prosthesis. Provision can be made to cut off crowns distal to these teeth for the removal of the teeth that they cover if they fail to survive in health. It is of paramount importance to provide for such a contingency in the original treatment plan. Provision should be made whenever possible for failure of a questionable tooth and for convenient retreat without the removal and remaking of the entire appliance.

The importance of this entire question and of the attempts to meet it is that we never become prisoners of an appliance and think in terms of the prosthesis. We must think in terms of the teeth and of the supporting tissues. The rest is just a collection of methods and materials for the preservation of the teeth. The teeth do not exist to support the appliance.

12. *Of what importance is the systemic factor in periodontal prognosis?*

The possibility of the removal of etiologic factors is of utmost importance in determining the prognosis in a given case. Local factors such as missing contact points, overhanding restorations, and so on can be removed easily; however, if the predisposing causes are of systemic origin, correction may not be possible. Therefore the prognosis is dependent upon the conditions present.

The state of health of the patient may determine the outcome of treatment. Health may make the difference between success and failure. In patients with systemic disturbances recognized as detrimental to periodontal health the prognosis for periodontal therapy is poor unless the systemic disease process can be eliminated or controlled.

• • •

Twelve questions in periodontal prognosis have been posed, and an attempt made to answer them. As indicated previously no formula exists that will be useful in seriously involved teeth. The safe formula would condemn many useful teeth to extraction. Those teeth that would fit into a formula prescription usually present no vexing problems in prognosis. Thus there is no point in helping the therapist make easy decisions. It is the difficult decision and situation with inherent danger of failure that must be met if we are to attempt any but the most routine of cases. As is usual in such matters the successful solution to the difficult case brings with it the greatest rewards to the therapist in terms of personal satisfaction and professional fulfillment, and it serves to advance the periodontal horizon.

Finally, prognosis is dependent on the experience of the operator, his ability to examine carefully and interpret his findings, his judgment concerning the healing capacity of the patient, and his technical ability, all combined with the patient's cooperation.

REFERENCES

Cohen, D. W., and Chacker, F. M.: Criteria for selection of one treatment plan over another, Dent. Clin. North Am., p. 3, March, 1964.

Dummett, C. O.: Significant considerations in the prognosis of periodontal disease, J. Periodontol. **22:**77, 1951.

Kantor, M., Polson, A. M., and Zander, H. A.: Alveolar bone regeneration after removal of inflammatory and traumatic factors, J. Periodontol. **47:**12, 1976.

Lindhe, J., and Nyman, S.: The effect of plaque control and surgical pocket elimination on the establishment and maintenance of periodontal health. A longitudinal study of periodontal therapy in cases of advanced disease, J. Clin. Periodontol. **3:**110, 1975.

Miller, S. C., and Pelzer, R.H .: An original classification of alveolar bone types in periodontal disease and its prognostic value, J. Am. Dent. Assoc. **26:**565, 1939.

Morris, M. L.: The diagnosis, prognosis, and treatment of the loose tooth, Oral Surg. **6:**957, 1953.

Moskow, B. S.: Repair potential in combined pulpal and periodontal lesions, N.Y. State Dent. J. **34:**209, 1968.

Pennel, B. M., King, K. O., Wilderman, M. N., et al.: Repair of the alveolar process following osseous surgery, J. Periodontol. **38:**70, 1967.

Rosling, B., Nyman, S., and Lindhe,, J.: The effects of systematic plaque control on bone regeneration in infrabony pockets, J. Clin. Periodontol. **3:**38, 1976.

Rosling, B., Nyman, S., Lindhe, J., et al.: The healing potential of the periodontal tissues following different techniques of periodontal surgery in plaque-free dentitions, J. Clin. Periodontol. **3:**233, 1976.

15 Treatment planning

The chapters on therapeutics that follow describe a number of techniques and methods designed to correct particular periodontal lesions. The choice of methods and the sequence of their use often present a bewildering problem to the therapist. In most cases the success or failure in a given case depends on the correct choice of techniques. Even proper technique, however, gives rise to floundering and haphazard treatment if an orderly approach is not employed. Much time is used needlessly and much more effort is expended when a systematic approach is not used. It is for this reason that treatment planning assumes paramount importance.

Periodontal therapy consists of those procedures, properly planned and applied in light of a detailed examination and exacting differential diagnosis, utilized to induce healing in periodontal tissues and in some instances to restore lost parts of the periodontium. It also aims to create a dentoperiodontal atmosphere that is conducive to the *prevention* of recurring disease. Adequately conceived treatment reflects a consideration of the spatial relationships and interactions, in health and disease, of the many tissues and structures that make up the oral apparatus, for example, the jaws, temporomandibular articulation, tongue, mandibular and facial musculature, the articulation of teeth, the salivary glands and their secretions, the lining oral tissues; it also considers this oral complex in association with the structure, physiologic and biochemical mechanisms, and the pathophysiology of other tissues and organ systems.

OBJECTIVE: PREVENTION OF PERIODONTAL DISEASE

The primary goal of all health professional activity is the prevention of disease and deformity. Although in a limited number of cases the causation of periodontal disease may be elusive and its prevention and cure not attainable, an overwhelming majority may be obviated or inhibited by the routine, systemic, and fastidious removal of bacterial plaque from the dentition and the gingiva. Calcified accretions — the sequelae to the initial or continuing deposit of the mucoid mass — can only be effectively removed or negated through direct professional care. In this context the dentist and his auxiliaries direct their attention not only to the agents that harbor and elaborate the tissue irritants, but also to the perfection of the dentogingival atmosphere. These environmental derangements — whether they be dental hypoplasias, carious lesions, structural defects iatrogenically produced, malpositions of teeth singly or in concert with others, and so on — provide nidi for plaque lodgment and inhibit its removal by the patient and the dentist. Thus integral to the prevention of periodontal disease are the recognition and correction of these ecologic variations.

If we extend the classic definition of periodontal disease, which includes lesions solely of inflammatory derivation, to include manifestations that are the direct or indirect products of such agencies as occlusal discrepancies and psychologic disturbances, we may find that direct prevention may not lie primarily within the scope of the patient. Preventive measures in these instances are the province and the responsibility of the dentist, at times in consultation with those in the applicable allied health professions.

Preventive periodontics includes the following:
1. The accumulation and collation of knowledge obtained through research and expert clinical observation relative to —
   a. Biology of periodontal, dental, oral, and body tissues
   b. Deviations from biologically acceptable norms, and the mechanisms of their development and progress
   c. Singular and collaborative roles of the causative and contributive agents to disease processes
   d. Chronologic variations of normalcy and

of disease (the natural history of the condition)

e. Influence of preventive and therapeutic modalities on the onset, progression, and termination of the lesion, and so on

2. Data transfer at all levels of professional and paraprofessional education performed with scientific conviction, energetic and lucid delivery, provocative discussion, and on a continuous basis

3. Lay education that is simple, direct, forthright, and presented with clarity and a positive approach at the chair, in the schools, and through the press and other media relative to—

    a. Progress in the oral health area

    b. Periodontal disease with its local and extraoral manifestations

    c. Prevention and control of periodontal disease

    d. Relatively simple, inexpensive measures that can be applied by each individual and the profession to improve the oral health status

4. Preventive programs that are broadly applicable as well as regimens tailored to the requirements of the individual's dentition or dentoperiodontal atmosphere (In the latter context not only may prevention consist of customized plaque and accretion control, but also of professional modification or correction of dentition, occlusion, dietary consistency and composition, and so on so as to minimize the accumulation or activity of agents with disease producing potential.)

5. Treatment in all its ramifications, rationally conceived and expertly applied, carried out to erase the lesion and the deformity that the disease has induced

The rationale of periodontal therapy is based on bone topography. The architecture of the osseous tissues is best determined by a combination of careful clinical probing and radiographic examination. It has been demonstrated by numerous investigators that radiographic examination alone is not sufficient to determine accurately the osseous structure configuration. Osseous defects are frequently masked by variations in radiographic technique, particularly angulation, which often create false impressions. However, in most instances careful clinical probing in conjunction with well-angulated radiographs will reveal the osseous topography. A thin, graduated periodontal probe is used as a sounding instrument to determine the walls of an osseous defect. A needle can be passed through the gingiva; this procedure must be performed under local anesthetic, which is not usually needed for routine measurements of periodontal pockets. The presence or absence of buccal or lingual plates of bone may be determined by horizontal insertion of the needle through the gingiva until its progress is halted by the presence of bone. This examination procedure is described in Chapter 12.

Periodontal therapy consists of evaluation of cause and effect and control of these factors to obtain a healthy, secure gingival attachment over an acceptable bony crestal topography. The teeth should be capable of functioning as part of the dentition for chewing and swallowing.

Therapy for disease of the periodontium is based on achievement of these objectives. Control or elimination of etiologic factors translates itself into initial preparation, or the presurgical phase. The concept of pocket elimination or the attainment of a healthy, secure gingival attachment is a fundamental objective of periodontal therapy. It has also been accepted that to eliminate detached gingival tissue, gingival resection or gingivectomy is not indicated in those instances in which attached gingiva is insufficient, in which the underlying osseous contour is either irregular or ledged, or in which osseous defects are present. Procedures practiced today concern the reestablishment of the integrity of the dentogingival junction so that there can be a physiologic relationship between the clinical crown of the tooth and both the attached gingiva and the alveolar mucosa apical to the mucogingival junction. As a result the host is better able to maintain and prevent reestablishment of periodontal disease by proper cleansing methods. It is easily seen that an improper gingival attachment does not allow for plaque removal at the gingival tooth junction (Figs. 15-1 and 15-2).

Although resective methods of therapy have been firmly established in periodontics, it has become obvious that reconstructive and reparative treatment procedures are more favorable and desirable for both gingival and osseous tissue loss. This knowledge has led to techniques in soft tissue and osseous grafting.

Periodontal treatment planning may be influenced by the systemic factors of the patient. The health status may be a contributing factor to the periodontal disease state, and in that case therapy will largely depend on the correction or control of the systemic disease. Also the health status may

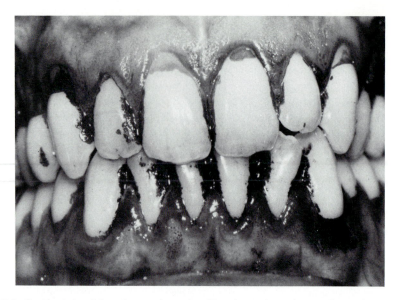

Fig. 15-1. Teeth stained for plaque deposits. Note how deposits are formed on proximal aspect and at cervical portions of teeth, where recession is present. Photograph taken in morning, approximately 2 hours after brushing. Obviously, individual was unable to remove plaque. There is a generalized gingival fibrous hyperplasia throughout. Dentist must be cognizant that not only must patient be carefully taught toothbrushing, but also that there must be no interferences to make cleansing difficult.

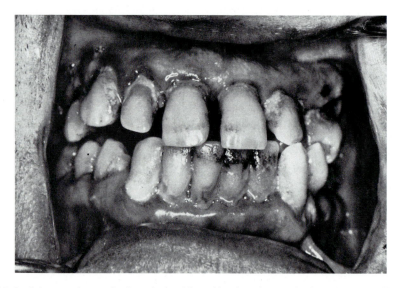

Fig. 15-2. Advanced marginal periodontitis, with abundant calculus deposits. Teeth are markedly deranged as well. In treatment plan one must evaluate question as to whether patient will produce heavy calculus after therapy and how oral hygiene will be able to combat this deposition.

be a factor in the management of the patient, for example, as in a patient who has cardiac disease with angina. Modification of the treatment plan is often required. The patient cannot be overtaxed, and therapy may have to be carried out over a longer period. In addition anesthetic requirements may have to be changed.

The object of periodontal therapy consists of a return of the periodontal tissues from the diseased state to a state of health. In particular its goals are a healthy gingival tissue and gingival attachment to the tooth covering a cortical alveolar crest, the topography of which is acceptable in light of anatomic requirements. In periodontal disease the alveolar bone may not be affected as seen in a gingivitis; the bone may be affected but the topography may remain acceptable as often seen in marginal periodontitis; the bone crest may be irregular, ledged, or ridged and in that case unacceptable; or the crestal bone may be affected with osseous defects and in that case unacceptable. In the first two examples the focus of attention is on the gingival tissue, whereas in the latter two the bone becomes the area of concern. Periodontal therapeutic techniques may be divided into those that are excisive in nature and those that are reparative and reconstructive. Both have indications and contraindications.

Certain posttreatment attributes are considered as essential characteristics of periodontal health and primary to its maintenance; these include the following:

1. Pocket elimination — obviation of the inflammatory lesion
2. Establishment of physiologic tissue contours necessary for self-cleansing and ease of physiotherapeutic management
   a. Thin, parabolically curved gingival margins
   b. Pyramidically shaped interdental papillae that conform architecturally and adapt tightly to tooth contours while permitting the free egress of food and debris from the interproximal areas (Once surgical intervention is dictated because of existing disease, it is appropriate to eliminate the "col" form of gingiva interdentally and to substitute an occlusally convex tissue form shy of the contact areas between adjacent teeth.)
   c. Adequate width and rigidity of the zone of keratinizing attached gingiva (Rigidity implies density as well as firm attachment to tooth and bone.)
3. The placement of teeth and the modification of their morphology in a manner to protect the periodontium from the effects of local environmental insults
4. Eradication of positive occlusal habits and control of their effects
5. Application of measures for tooth stabilization to protect the attaching tissues and to permit their full healing potential
6. The acquisition of patient cooperation and facility in the performance of preventive physiotherapeutic measures

Cure, as a consequence of periodontal therapy, does not imply the salvage of hopelessly involved teeth or those that are marginally capable of contributing to a well-functioning dentition. Cure does not require the complete reconstitution of portions of the periodontium lost because of disease. It has been demonstrated that teeth can function and be stable despite the fact that they have lost a great deal of their investing and supporting tissues. Cure further connotes that adjuncts such as fixed prosthesis can be utilized in the procurement of function and the maintenance of health.

Successful periodontal therapy, and thus cure, is dependent on the expert application of therapeutic regimens that are specifically designed for the elimination of etiology, correction of the local environment, negation of the lesions and its effects, and the attainment of physiologic tissue form and oral relationships. Therapeutic success requires the tailoring of specific operative procedures to specific lesions operating in a specific oral environment. "Rules of thumb" and "panaceas" have no place in treatment planning and execution; it is necessary to establish biologically sound therapeutic precepts to which must be added expanding and scientifically flexible clinical acumen and judgment.

It must never be forgotten that we are treating a patient and not a masticatory organ. Patients require some prediction of time factors, even if the predictions are general in nature. Periodontal therapy may be a rather long and time-consuming procedure at times, and a number of patients will be found to discontinue treatment because of discouragement with the length of time required to demonstrate a result. Some of this is inevitable, even with the most efficient organization of efforts. It is obviously far more common when faulty organization draws the time for therapy out to disproportional dimensions.

INITIAL THERAPY

The critical nature of a rational choice of technique needs no elaboration. In each chapter a rational approach to the potential of each method is stressed. Although there will of necessity be some repetition here, a survey of these factors will be of benefit. It would be of definite value to review this section after the material under each individual method has been covered. The blending of a large amount of material is the hallmark of the skilled therapist, and nowhere is this more useful than in treatment planning.

Hopelessly involved teeth. In many cases there are one or more teeth that are *obviously* hopeless and are destined for sacrifice. It is highly desirable that they be removed at the very outset of therapy. Several reasons for this are as follows:

1. Their presence needlessly complicates therapy of adjacent teeth.
2. They frequently are prone to acute exacerbations that create situations requiring emergency care.
3. Patients routinely forget that these teeth were condemned as hopeless and consider the result a partial failure when they find that the loss of the teeth can be postponed no longer.
4. The presence of these hopelessly involved teeth often encourages the patient to postpone the restorative phase of therapy to the detriment of the entire case.

As in all other general rules there are exceptions to this one. Aesthetic considerations and the availability of adequate provisional restorative skills are two problems that frequently enforce a change in procedure. It will be found, however, that all compromises are followed by complications, and the operator should expect them and be prepared to manage them with as little disruption of orderly procedures as possible.

Caries. Caries are another aspect of a case that must be corrected or arrested before actual periodontal therapy begins. It is unfortunately too common an experience for the operator to be embarrassed at the progress made by a ''harmless'' carious lesion while periodontal therapy is in progress.

If during the initial work-up of a case the periodontist determines on the basis of existing restorations and on the basis of the history that the patient is still subject to rather active caries, he must then consider seriously the effect of root exposure after surgery. Root caries are a difficult complication to manage, and many teeth that have been treated successfully periodontally have been lost because of them. These cases present individual problems in treatment planning.

When caries are treated before periodontal therapy begins it usually is the better part of wisdom to restore the teeth in cement if occlusal and proximal surfaces are involved and if the eventual permanent restoration is to be an inlay or a crown. The reason for this is that during the occlusal phase of therapy teeth generally are altered in form. The presence of an inlay or crown frequently complicates this procedure for obvious reasons. The presence of old restorations is vexing enough without fabricating new ones until the form of the tooth has been established definitely.

Inflammatory involvement. Since in practically every case other than in an emergency the patient suffers from a chronic inflammatory involvement of the periodontium, it would seem logical to begin by the elimination of the cardinal sign of the disease.

It might be helpful at this point to reiterate briefly the broad general principles of therapy in the field. Subgingival scaling and concomitant curettage constitute procedures to reduce and treat the inflammatory lesion. Many therapists perform definitive supragingival and subgingival scaling first to contain the inflammatory process. Once the tooth surface has been cleansed and the area allowed to heal, curettage of the sulcular wall is accomplished (Fig. 15-3).

As might be expected, most cases show only a partial response to root scaling. When properly done there is a resolution of edema and inflammation, but this result is only a partial solution to the problem of pocket elimination.

The objective of scaling is to eliminate gross calculus deposits. Definitive scaling of subgingival deposits must be done most carefully. Recent investigation has disclosed that haphazard instrumentation to remove calculus pushes calculus, cementum, and all sorts of foreign material into the gingiva. Therefore careful instrumentation is paramount in the initial preparation of a given case. This type of therapy can accomplish or control the inflammatory process and is within the tolerance capability of a patient with limited emotional and physical ability.

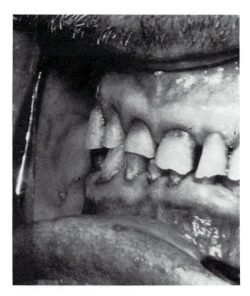

Fig. 15-3. Not only is gingival form an important aspect in treatment planning, but alveolar housing must also be taken into consideration. In this instance osteoplasty will have to be performed to secure a proper gingiva-tooth relationship.

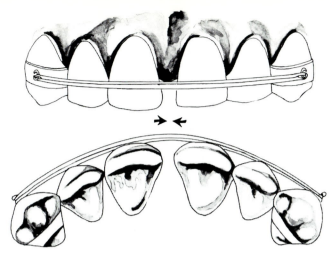

Fig. 15-4. Orthodontics is often performed in initial preparation phase. In this instance, maxillary anterior teeth are being retruded to close anterior diastema. Etiologic factors must be ascertained and either corrected or modified. There may be many reasons for this procedure; for example, there may be osseous defects affecting these teeth, and new alignment may be beneficial for healing process. Occlusal relationship must allow for retrusion of maxillary anterior teeth.

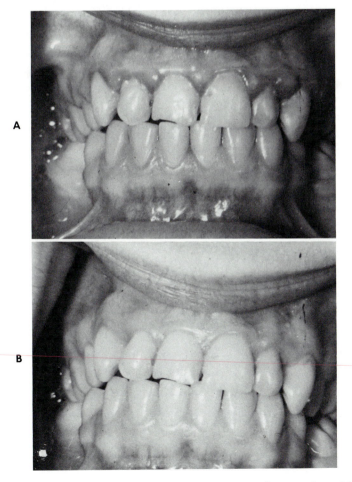

Fig. 15-5. Examiner must be able to determine amount of regression of inflammatory process once etiologic factors are eliminated. **A,** Mandibular teeth were scaled 1 week before. Changes after scaling of maxillary teeth 3 weeks later are shown in **B.** Evaluation should be performed at this time.

In the débridement technique, when properly applied, the result should be a resolution of edema and inflammation and a shrinkage of the gingiva involved. There are times when this shrinkage alone is sufficient to recapture normal form and result in the elimination of the pockets. There are two factors that may prevent this from occurring: (1) the nature, composition, and environment of the soft tissue and (2) the patterns of resorption of the underlying bone.

In most instances, especially in cases of advanced disease, a choice of surgical procedures must be selected. However, before such a course can be pursued there are several considerations that must be taken into account. In the first place it must be determined whether the patient will be treated in a routine manner so that pocket elimina-tion is the objective or whether for some reason excision procedures are contraindicated. There are a number of reasons why the operator may be well advised to eliminate this modality from his treatment plan in the given case. Factors of such a nature are age of the patient and psychologic considerations.

Additional considerations

Age. In aged patients the objectives of therapy often are lowered. The reasons for this are manifold. It may be understood that survival of the dentition despite lack of treatment implies resistance somewhat above average and that maintenance may suffice to retain the teeth in comparative health for the remaining years. In addition there is the physical health status of the patient to consider. Further, with advancing age the inflam-

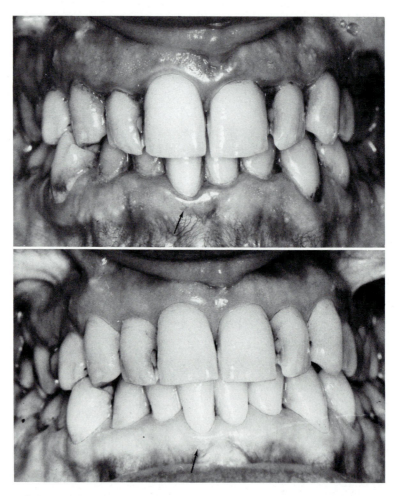

Fig. 15-6. Before and after a scaling procedure showing changes in gingiva. Evaluation at this time will determine definitive therapy. A pocket traversing into alveolar mucosa is seen at *arrow*. Treatment plan must take into consideration elimination of pocket. Should therapist look for recession with a zone of attached gingiva (excisive technique and repair of attached gingiva) or should he attempt an attachment as far coronally as possible with an adequate zone of attached gingiva (pedicle graft and reconstructive repair)?

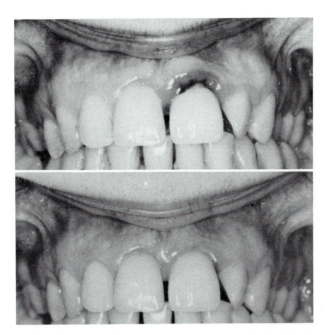

Fig. 15-7. Before and after photographs of a marked gingival inflammation in conjunction with an inadequate margin of a full veneer crown. In treatment plan a decision was made to curet sulcular wall in initial preparation to determine definitive therapy that might be needed.

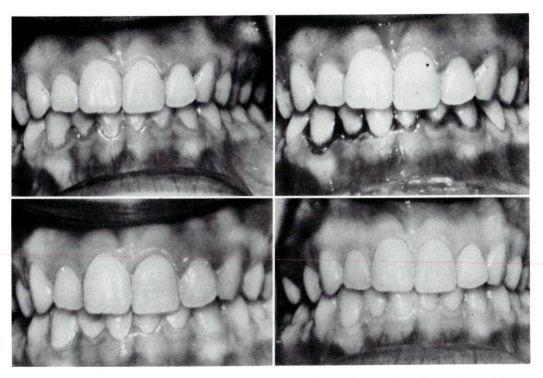

Fig. 15-8. Healing of a gingival inflammation treated by scaling and curettage. Therapist must decide mode of therapy best suited to overcome inflammatory process and result in an intact gingival attachment.

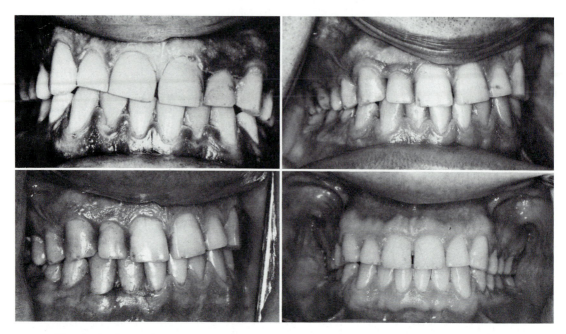

Fig. 15-9. Case of necrotizing ulcerative gingivitis treated initially with débridement to overcome acute phase and followed by resection of gingival tissue to achieve acceptable gingival topography. After photograph taken 23 years postoperatively. Case must be carefully planned; successful therapy is dependent upon an understanding of etiology and behavioral pattern of disease process and of therapy that allows for healing and reconstruction of part.

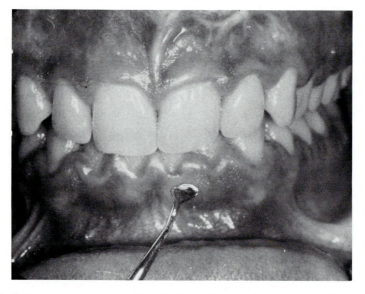

Fig. 15-10. This case represents a fibrotic gingival hyperplasia best treated by resection of gingival tissue, accomplishing gingival form and a healthy gingival attachment. Curettage would not result in regression of tissue. There is an adequate zone of attached gingiva, and alveolar crest seemingly is not affected.

matory reaction to an irritant is somewhat less than is the case in a younger individual.

Psychologic considerations. A considerable number of patients suffer from neuroses of varying severity. Some patients find it impossible to submit to extensive surgical procedures. In these instances, although the major objective is the survival of the dentition, therapy can be carried out over a longer period in less lengthy operations with smaller sites.

Tooth movement. Tooth movement to close contacts to realign migrating teeth or to alter local environment is often a necessary element of peri-

odontal therapy. It has been found that if orthodontic tooth movement is performed prior to definitive therapy, retention is far less a problem. Also if tooth movement is done at this time it may be combined with subsequent management of osseous defects (Fig. 15-4).

Provisional occlusal adjustment. At this point we should be dealing with a patient in whom the active inflammatory lesions have been controlled. If no other factor intervenes, attention should be focused on the occlusal problem both in regard to tooth relationship in a dynamic sense and in regard to mobility factors that qualify function.

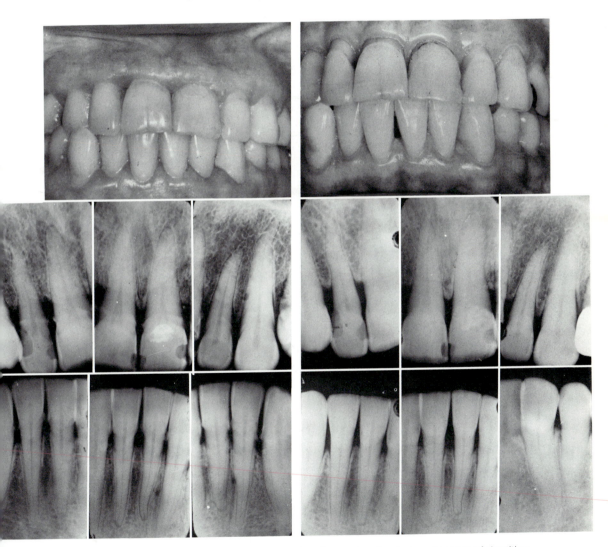

Fig. 15-11. Before and after photographs and radiographs of anterior segment of dentition treated by scaling, oral hygiene instruction, and gingivectomy. After photograph (right) taken 14 years postoperatively. Note crestal changes in before radiographs (left) and cortical crests in after radiographs (right). Gingivectomy technique was selected because of adequacy of attached gingiva and acceptable topography of alveolar bone. Although gingival recession was produced, there was no aesthetic problem because of a low lip line. Also, patient was able to brush adequately.

In many cases some temporary splinting is indicated. This is a logical point in therapy to introduce it. When mobility is a serious factor, occlusal adjustment is complicated by its presence. Teeth that move in function are difficult to adjust properly.

No attempt will be made here to enter into the various methods of temporary splinting, since the subject is covered in Chapter 21. We are merely attempting to give a sequence of procedures in a hypothetic case.

It must be understood that occlusal correction made at this time will be examined and finalized later in therapy. After the initial gross adjustment there are inevitable changes in the occlusal pattern

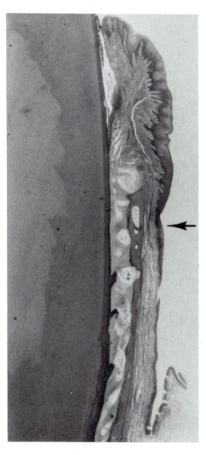

Fig. 15-12. Photomicrograph showing entire gingival wall from gingival margin to vestibule. There is gingival recession onto root, and mucogingival line is seen at *arrow*. If gingival resection were performed, then certainly there would be an insufficient attached gingiva left. Treatment plan in such a case must take into consideration formation of an adequate zone of attached gingiva either by an apically repositioned flap or a gingivectomy together with a free mucosal graft.

that frequently require correction and refinement (Figs. 15-5 to 15-19).

DEFINITIVE THERAPY

The patient is now at a point in treatment when the remaining marginal lesions must be corrected and the environmental problems in the mucosa of adjacent areas must be managed.

The reader must be cognizant of the various methods to be brought to bear on these problems. They present a wide range of surgical approaches and fall into three general classes: (1) reparative techniques, (2) plastic repair of marginal lesions, and (3) environmental or mucogingival procedures.

From the standpoint of treatment planning these methods must be evaluated from two points of view:

1. How do they apply to the lesion and deformities at hand?
2. What is the time factor involved in each?

In answer to the first requirement our basic need is adequate diagnosis. If the lesions have been charted adequately against the tissue complex in which they exist, treatment planning follows as a logical extension of diagnosis; for example, careful probing may reveal the presence of craters, particularly where the process is broad. This means that the simple insertion of the probe to measure pocket depth is not enough to give the operator the information that he requires. There must be a circumferential probing to outline bone topography as well. In addition the depth and extent of the pockets must be plotted against the mucogingival topography, and a survey of the extent of the vestibular trough must be made. It is only in this fashion that a clear picture of operative procedure comes into focus.

The objectives of curettage are débridement of the gingival wound so that epithelization, resolution of inflammation, and repair of the corium can occur. Two factors are important: (1) the extent of the debrided area cannot be too great, or complete wound healing will not result and (2) the technique for débridement must be considered carefully. Too often the col area is completely destroyed, leaving two peaks intact with resultant deformity after healing.

It must be determined at this stage of planning how definitive procedures will be organized. Many operators divide the dentition into quadrants for surgery and administer corrective therapy in this fashion, progressing from one area to the next as healing of the last operative site has advanced to the point where such a course is feasible. A number of periodontists operate on both upper and lower quadrants of a given side at a single sitting. This system has many advantages in that a considerable area of the dentition is completed at each surgical visit. It has, however, one serious disadvantage. The terminal point of each quadrant is in the anterior region, which is awkward when there is mucogingival surgery to be done in this region. To overcome the problem, the operator can extend the quadrants of one side to include the anterior regions and shorten the operative field in the remaining areas.

Another method is to divide the dentition into six operative areas of two posterior sections and one anterior section in each arch. The upper and lower anterior sections are almost always done at a single sitting. There is rarely mucogingival

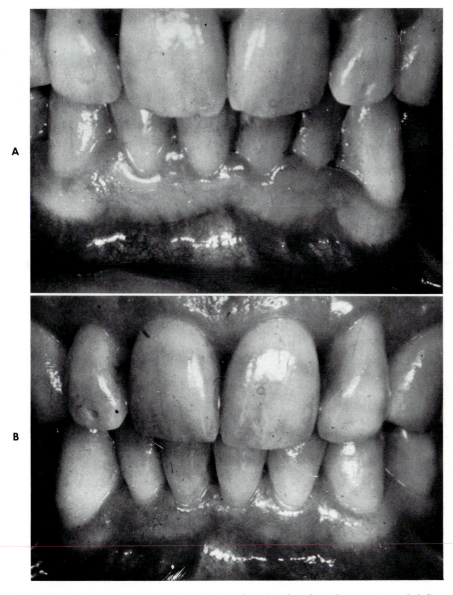

Fig. 15-13. It is essential in treatment planning that local environment, as it influences therapy, be considered. **A,** In this instance retruded lateral incisor, with respect to the canine, is an area that offers a therapeutic problem. Tissue must be contoured with respect to tooth contour in both lateral incisor and canine regions. Tissue topography must conform to accepted physiologic standards. It may be necessary because of insufficient attached gingiva to perform mucogingival surgery. In this instance an apically repositioned flap was performed. **B,** Apically repositioned flap.

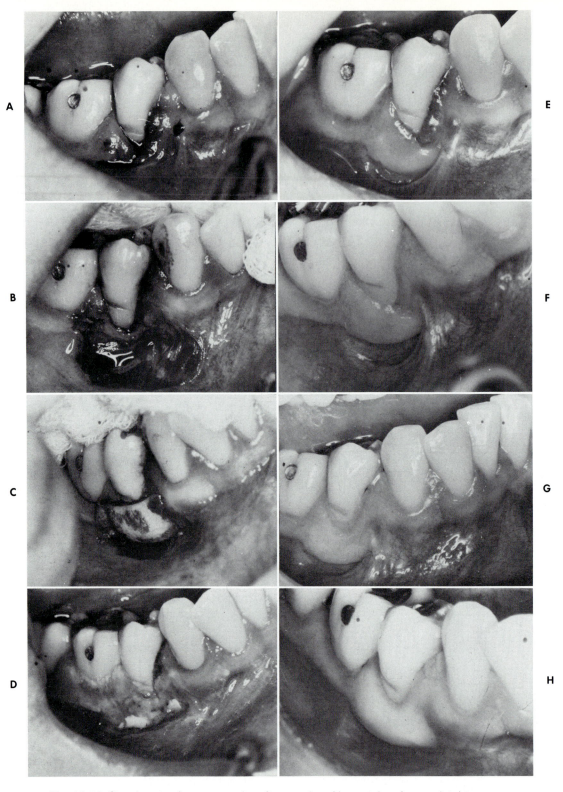

Fig. 15-14. Step-by-step free mucosal graft procedure (tissue taken from palate) to secure an adequate zone of attached gingiva. **A,** A marked gingival inflammation with practically no attached gingiva and a shallow vestibule. **B,** Bed was prepared; note that bed extends to gingival margin. **C,** Inflamed gingival tissue was resected, and graft tissue was placed into position and held by a covering of surgical dressing. **D** and **E,** Site 1 week and 2½ weeks postoperatively, respectively. Area healed completely (**F** and **G**), and gingival attachment and zone of attached gingiva 1 year later are seen in **H.**

surgery to be done on both of these areas, and the advantages of a single course of dressing applications here are obvious.

Exactly the same method of management may be used in posterior sections on a given side.

The point to remember in all these approaches is that proper planning can reduce the time factor in periodontal therapy without compromising the quality of effort. This, in the final analysis, is the only proper time-saving device to be considered.

In answer to the second requirement the osseous defect presents a special problem in treatment planning (Figs. 15-20 to 15-23). If it is determined by diagnostic methods that the osseous defect is a suitable lesion for reparative filling techniques the question becomes one of therapeutic management. With fill methods as with all others consideration is given to other procedures required in the area, and all techniques are blended into a single operative visit. With reattachment methods, however, there often are still additional conditions to be met, for example, temporary splinting and endodontic evaluation, and these too are fitted smoothly into the overall operation of the section or quadrant under therapy.

The reader will note also that fill procedures require a somewhat longer period under dressing than is the usual course in periodontal surgery. This factor should induce the limiting of therapy to the opposing arch on the same side so that time is not spent needlessly in waiting for adequate healing before advancing to other areas. It must be kept in mind that when we move to other operative sites on other sides of the arches the healed area is subjected to rather heavy use in chewing. This is a factor that must be considered before setting up appointments.

Consideration for aesthetics. An important factor in periodontal therapy is the aesthetic problem of the maxillary anterior segment of the dentition. The lip line presents an important aspect; a high lip line shows the entire dentition, whereas a low lip line hides the teeth. Any slight change

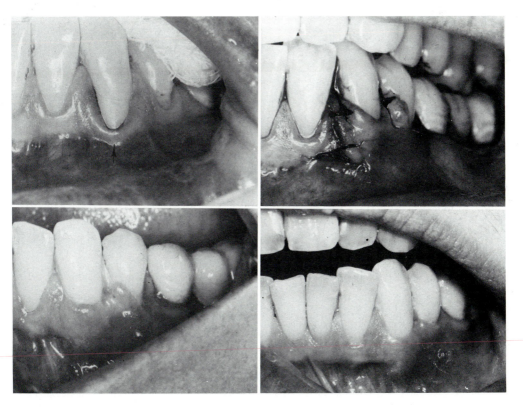

Fig. 15-15. Examination disclosed recession and detachment of gingival tissue to a point at mucogingival line. Vestibule was shallow in this area. A periosteal pedicle graft was performed to not only eliminate pocket, but also to secure an adequate zone of attached gingiva. If therapist accepts recession, then treatment plan must take into consideration elimination of pocket and procurement of a keratinized gingiva. In this case a free graft may be done with resection of gingival pocket.

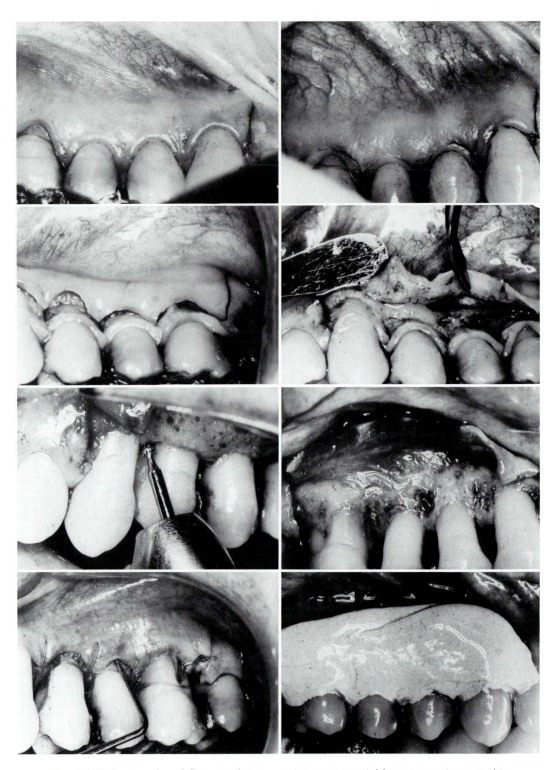

Fig. 15-16. Inverse bevel flap used to correct an unacceptable osseous topography. Osteoplasty was performed to allow gingiva to be tautly stretched over bone so that a healthy gingival attachment would result. At its worst, gingival sulcus can only be as deep as thickness of flap. (Courtesy Dr. Gerald Isenberg.)

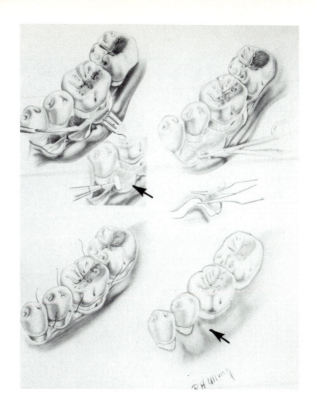

Fig. 15-17. Elimination of interdental osseous craters by flap procedure and osteoectomy. Examination must determine extent of craters, their topography, and best approach for therapy.

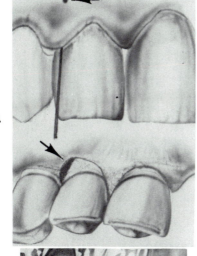

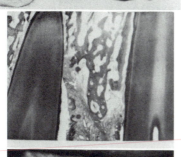

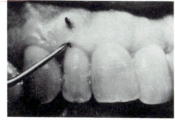

A

B

C

Fig. 15-18. A two-walled osseous defect on distal aspect of a maxillary lateral incisor managed by a collapsed flap. Note changes that occurred radiographically. **A,** Drawing of clinical findings. **B,** Photomicrograph of such a defect. **C,** Instrument in pocket and extending into a labial fistula. **D,** Immediately postoperatively. **E** and **F,** Healing of area.

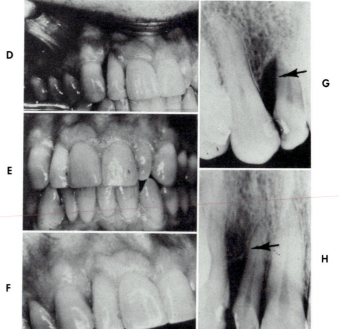

D

E

F

G

H

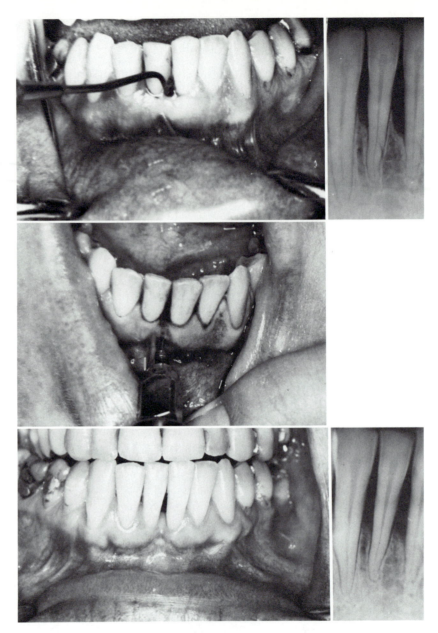

Fig. 15-19. Examination of a one-walled osseous defect diagnosed by probe, needling, and radiology. An osteoectomy was performed via a flap procedure. Note changes radiographically.

such as spacing, zones of exposed labial cementum, and elongation of the clinical crowns causes aesthetic changes and often difficulty in speech as well. In treatment of this area the operator must be aware of the changes that will take place and must evaluate them on the basis of circumstances. The cardinal rule is that the objectives of periodontal therapy cannot be compromised; therefore if an aesthetic problem is present all attempts should be made toward reparative and reconstructive management (Fig. 15-24). The treatment plan should incorporate therapy to enhance aesthetics rather than detract from them. To achieve desired results restorative dentistry may often be required. Above all the patient should be thoroughly informed about the problem. Often it is wise to draw a diagram of the existing situation and show the patient the change that will take place. The reasons for the proposed therapy should be discussed with the patient.

Definitive occlusal adjustment. At the completion of the surgical phase it usually is found con-

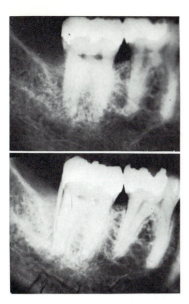

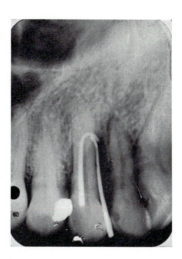

Fig. 15-20. Lower right second molar. In upper roentgenogram resorptive lesion can be seen on distal aspect in a V-shaped manner. Actual depth of pocket cannot be determined. In lower roentgenogram by insertion of a gutta-percha point, base of defect can be determined accurately in relation to root. Examiner must determine topography of osseous defect. Probing on buccal, distal, and lingual will disclose topography. If reading at buccal line angle of tooth reads 4 mm, distal portion 10 mm, and lingual line angle of tooth 4 mm, then diagnosis of a three-walled osseous defect can be made. On the other hand, if readings reveal 4 mm on lingual, 10 mm on distal, and 10 mm on buccal line angle, then two-walled osseous defect is present.

Fig. 15-21. Upper right canine with gutta-percha points placed in pocket before roentgenogram was made. Outline of pocket may be seen as evidenced by location of gutta-percha points. In this instance a two-walled osseous defect is present. This could be treated by a collapsed flap or by an osseous or periosteal implant. While first procedure is predictable, its drawback is a distinct recession. Second procedure is not as predictable but if successful, entities would be good and there would be more housing for tooth.

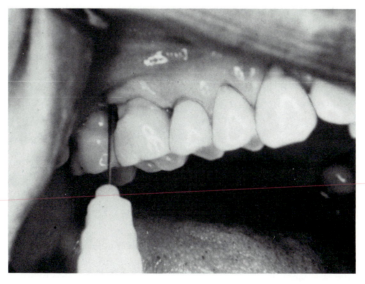

Fig. 15-22. Needling to determine buccal crest of an interdental crater. Once topography of this osseous defect is determined, therapist must decide whether to perform osteoectomy to eliminate crater or try to reconstruct defect.

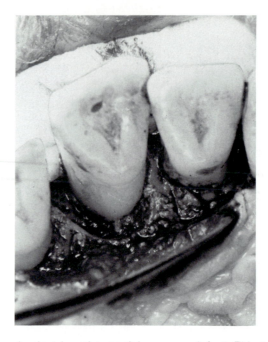

Fig. 15-23. Osseous implant in palatomesial osseous defect. This type of defect has a poor prognosis if implant procedure is not performed.

venient to give the tissues time for complete healing and for the maximum benefit to be derived from home physiotherapy. This is the time to complete the definitive occlusal adjustment. In most cases it will be found that there has been a shifting of the teeth and an altered occlusal relationship from that achieved at the earlier provisional occlusal adjustment. During the surgical phase of therapy the teeth become somewhat more mobile than they were preoperatively. With the minute extrusions and increased mobility during this period it is easy to understand how relationships may be slightly altered in so dynamic an arrangement as the human occlusion, which is at best an unstable complex. It follows logically that this adjustment of the occlusion may not be a more detailed operation than was the initial attempt. Although there is never a really final occlusal adjustment, it must be considered that the one at hand will remain more or less as it is left until the patient is rechecked in the maintenance phase. It is because of this that the teeth that have been reshaped are disked and polished carefully so that all sharp edges have been rounded and all scratches from coarse grinding have been polished.

Maintenance during therapy. It might seem strange to the reader to learn that there is a certain amount of maintenance while active therapy is in progress. It will be found, however, that be-

cause of the presence of dressings, restricted function, curtailed and modified brushing due to surgical procedures and to minor discomforts that follow, and altered chewing, a considerable amount of stain and debris collects about the teeth and roots. Because of this there is a periodic course of maintenance required, consisting of coronal scaling and polishing fortified by whatever subgingival scaling is possible.

Instruction periods in brushing methods and interdental stimulation are repeated constantly, and this phase of maintenance is stressed again and again.

Restorative dentistry. In most patients a periodontal prosthesis is not required for the completion of active periodontal therapy, but restorative dentistry always is a problem to be met under all contingencies. It will be recalled that earlier in the chapter the problem was met on a provisional basis with cement fillings after the carious lesion had been well excavated. It is now propitious to convert to more permanent restorations. The form of the teeth has been established, and occlusal relationships have been adjusted to a level definitive enough to be considered fairly stable. This is a good time to establish proper contact relationships, consistent marginal ridges, adequate spillways, and proper form to teeth so that basic etiologic mechanisms that lead to periodontal disease

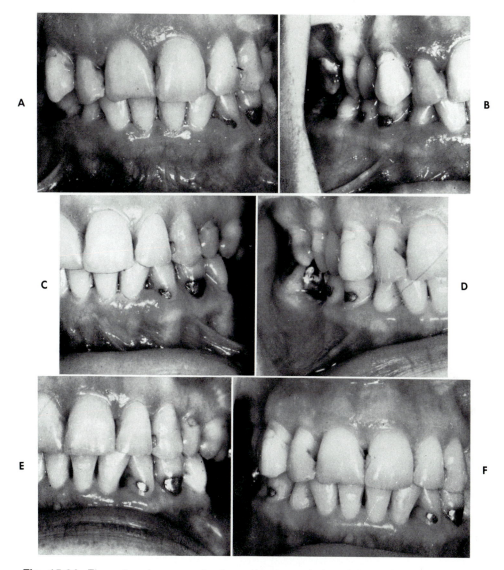

Fig. 15-24. There has been much discussion in periodontal literature concerning advisability of performing gingivectomy in anterior portion of dentition. It is often claimed that postoperative results are disfiguring and unaesthetic. The question therefore arises in the minds of many periodontists whether to allow pockets of fairly considerable depth to exist after periodontal therapy. One method of elimination of any deformity or unaesthetic value is to change the shape of the teeth. It can be noted in the text that integrity of gingival papillae is a key feature in gingivectomy operation advocated. Hence, postoperative papillae resemble the ideal of physiologic interdental tissue seen in health where no recession has occurred. **A** to **C,** Before. **D** to **F,** After. Note that despite the fact that several millimeters of gingival tissue have been resected, postoperative results are pleasing to the eye. Maxillary anterior teeth have been shortened, cementoenamel junctions have been eliminated, and incisal edges have been cut so that it is difficult at first glance to note changes after gingivectomy. For comparison, however, one may use initial carious area in **A** on maxillary right lateral incisor, mesial surface, as a landmark. Note that in postoperative result, **F,** considerable root has been exposed. Still by contouring tooth the periodontist has preserved anatomy, and aesthetic value has not been diminished. Contouring tooth is an important phase in treatment planning of any given case. It is important not only from an aesthetic point of view but also from a functional point of view in that the tooth-gingiva relationship is one important aspect of periodontal therapy.

are eliminated. It is the responsibility of the periodontist to require a level of craftsmanship adequate to the necessities of the case. Damaged periodontal support cannot afford indifferent restorations (Fig. 15-25).

Reevaluation. After we have completed our efforts toward rehabilitation of the tissues, pocket elimination, marginal and environmental corrective procedures, and all the other techniques that we have brought to bear on the case, the time has

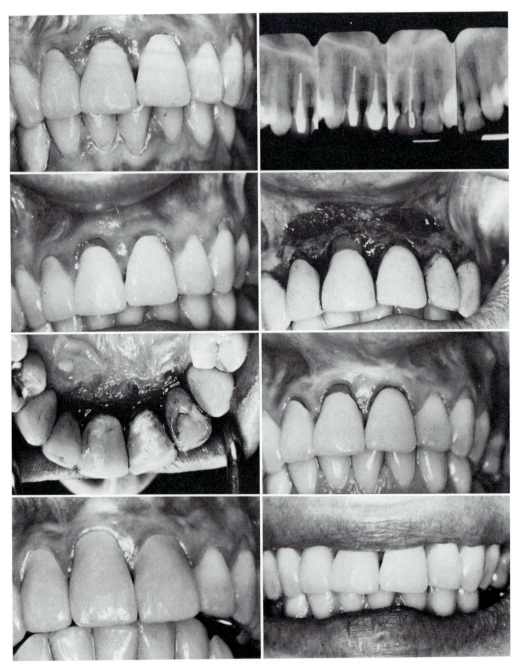

Fig. 15-25. Treatment plan usually must take into consideration the problem of restorative dentistry. There was a marked gingival inflammation associated with full veneer crowns of two central incisor teeth. Gingivae were debrided for initial preparation, followed by gingivectomy. Gingival tissue healed. Note keratinized tissue. Although new crowns were now much longer (because of recession), aesthetic pattern was acceptable since patient only showed about half the maxillary teeth.

arrived when a careful examination of our results is in order. Although the methods may have been well chosen and skillfully applied, it is one of the incontrovertible facts of life that all good techniques are not uniformly successful. There are at times areas that may require redoing or treatment of a different order. Teeth that have been assigned a doubtful or guarded prognosis may not have yielded to treatment and may have to be sacrificed as hopeless.

Objectivity in this regard pays good dividends. Not only does the periodontist protect both the patient and the referring dentist from subsequent disappointment in his efforts and skill, but he also establishes a reputation for therapeutic integrity, without which he cannot discharge his responsibility to his professional colleagues and to his patients.

Those areas in which there remain aberrations in form or residual pocket depth may, if it is deemed rewarding, be retreated on the spot. These usually are minor deficiencies, and no protracted course of treatment is indicated. If on the other hand the operator decides that a second application of the original method with necessary modifications will effect no greater success, then the area in question must be set down as a partial result or compromise and must be carried as such during the maintenance phase of treatment.

Conversion to maintenance phase. The completion of the treatment phase of therapy does not mean that responsibility for the survival of the dentition has been discharged. The fact that there are elements of resistance and repair inherent in the tissues over which neither the periodontist nor the patient has control implies supervision and maintenance over an indefinite period. Exactly the same set of circumstances obtains in all other phases of dentistry. It is for this reason that maintenance must be included in the overall plan for the preservation of the dentition.

Most periodontists find it useful and necessary to establish a second visit for reevaluation of active therapy about 3 months after the completion of treatment. The reasons for this are grasped easily. The operator can examine the tissues after a reasonable interval of time to determine the effect of final healing in many areas of surgical intervention. He also can determine whether there has been a proliferation of gingiva in given areas. Compromise zones can be checked, the rate of calculus deposition can be recorded, and the performance of the patient in home physiotherapy can be evaluated properly.

This information not only aids in the proper handling of any residual disease, but it also is invaluable in setting a recall interval and in supervising home care in the patient. It is not at all uncommon to find a falling off in the performance of this duty by the patient at such a time. The necessity for rigid performance in this phase is obvious.

After a 3-month time lapse the recall interval is set on the basis of some knowledge of the behavior of the case in normal function away from the constant supervision incident to the weekly visit.

SPECIAL PROBLEMS IN TREATMENT PLANNING

Local environmental factors. Success of periodontal therapy is dependent on the collection of data, its evaluation, and the treatment plan proposed for therapy. The realization of the problems at hand is the first step. The therapist cannot initiate an optimal environment for healing unless he is concerned with those environmental causative agents that have allowed the lesion to occur or with those conditions that have secondarily become involved. An example may be cited as follows. The therapist often notes a deep crater-shaped defect in the interdental area of the maxillary first and second molars when the teeth are incorrectly aligned. Often the maxillary second molar is in buccoversion. As a result of this environment a destructive lesion results. If left uncorrected the lesion progresses until a deep crater occurs in the interdental septum; thus buccal and palatal spines are present. Should a flat palate be present, complications in therapy are manifold. The therapist must take into consideration such factors for successful therapy (Figs. 15-26 and 15-27).

Therefore treatment planning must encompass the many and varied local environmental factors influencing periodontal therapy. These involve labial and lingual tooth contour, proximal contour, root proximity, proximal tooth relations in the arch, position of the tooth in the jaw, and many secondary influences, for example, frena, inadequate zone of attached gingiva, pockets extending into the alveolar mucosa, and interference of a flat palate, rugae, oblique ridge, and high mylohyoid ridge.

A list of local environmental problems would include the following:

1. Altered passive eruption and sequelae
2. Incipient soft tissue crater

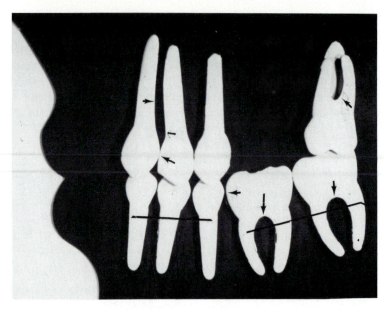

Fig. 15-26. Examiner must be careful to evaluate local environmental problems that may be present. These must be taken into consideration in treatment plan. *Arrows* point to possibilities that may be present: furca involvement of maxillary first premolar, contact deficiency between canine and first premolar, and close approximation between these two roots. Furca involvement may be present on all molar teeth, and contact between mandibular second premolar and first molar is deficient. Lines in mandible denote mucogingival line and signify that there may be insufficient keratinized gingiva.

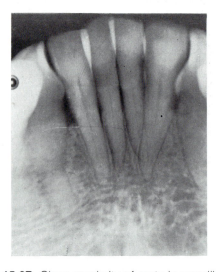

Fig. 15-27. Close proximity of roots in mandibular central incisor region creates a local environmental problem that must be taken into consideration in therapy.

3. Incipient loss of buccal or lingual peaks of interdental tissues
4. Irregularity of gingival margins
5. Incipient buccal recession
6. Cleft formation in attached gingiva
7. Thickened marginal crest
8. Soft tissue crater
9. Interradicular involvement
10. Involvement of mandibular and maxillary retromolar regions
11. Complications of frena, rugae, flat palate, oblique ridge, mylohyoid ridge, mental protuberance
12. Inadequate zone of attached gingiva
13. Invasion of alveolar mucosa by pocket formation
14. Periodontal abscess
15. Saddle areas
16. Interference of thick marginal bony crests
17. Osseous defects, for example, attached gingival zone sufficient, but initial incision at alveolar mucosa line
18. Improper proximal contact seen in maxillary first and second molar region when second molar in buccoversion—other areas: maxillary first premolar and canine,

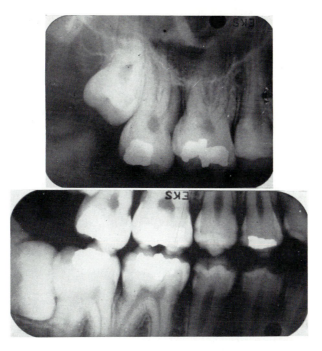

Fig. 15-28. Loss of interdental alveolar process in maxillary first and second molar regions as a result of food impaction. Cause is a faulty contact between first and second molars. There is infraclusion of the mandibular second molar and supraclusion of maxillary second molar. Supraclusion resulted from impaction of mandibular third molar against second molar. In this way maxillary second molar could extrude beyond contact point, allowing for food impaction.

mandibular incisors (buckling), and mandibular lateral incisor and canine (Fig. 15-28)

19. Narrow interdental spaces

The problems listed should be recognized in the examination, and their therapeutic correction should be planned prior to the operative procedure. In this way due consideration may be given to setting up an environment that will be conducive to health maintenance.

Periodontal prosthesis. A number of cases require a periodontal prosthesis for ultimate success in the preservation of the remaining natural dentition. It goes without saying that the necessity for this therapy should be obvious to the diagnostician in the initial workup of the case. It is a matter of considerable importance that the use of a prosthesis be included within the span of periodontal therapy or at least be begun during the active treatment phase.

This will necessitate special considerations in setting up a treatment plan. Since it is obvious that the fabrication of a final periodontal prosthesis is impossible during periodontal treatment a cooperative effort must be made for the use of temporary fixed splints during this period. The advantages are as follows:

1. Hopelessly involved teeth may be sacrified and replaced quickly. This is especially important in the anterior segment.
2. No temporary, poorly designed removable appliances need be used for aesthetics.
3. Teeth undergoing therapy are stabilized and may be treated under optimum conditions.
4. Since many if not all of the teeth are to be reduced for the temporary splint, the occlusal phase may be left to the prosthetist in consultation.
5. Temporary fixed splints obviate a common tendency on the part of patients to postpone periodontal prosthesis at the termination of active treatment.
6. Splints facilitate periodontal therapy because they may be removed for treatment and replaced in temporary cement.

When in the treatment plan is the best time to introduce temporary periodontal prosthesis? The most logical time in the overall treatment plan is after the initial débridement. In lieu of temporary treatment for caries the temporary splint may be used, and care for the carious lesions on teeth not included in the splint may be completed.

From that point forward the case is carried into the surgical phase for the correction of marginal and environmental lesions. At each operative visit the splint or splints may be removed easily to facilitate access to all areas involved. The splint or splints may then be replaced before the wound is dressed.

The patient enjoys maximum comfort, maximum function, and good aesthetics during a therapy, which is about as all inclusive as can be imagined.

After the completion of the active treatment phase, when the gingival margins have been established in their ultimate positions on the roots and are composed of tissue mature enough to be stable, then the temporary periodontal prosthesis may be converted to a permanent appliance. This usually is about the time for the 3-month recall visit for the second reevaluation.

Physical health status of patient. Reference must be made to the particular disease or disability from which the patient is suffering. Obviously the ulcer patient who is on a restricted and nondetergent diet is a problem in hygiene but is not a problem insofar as his ability to withstand a normal treatment regimen is concerned. The same cannot be said for the patient suffering from cardiovascular disease. Here some modification must be made in the extent and duration of the individual treatment. Calling the physician about the patient does not absolve the periodontist from responsibility in the case. It may divide the responsibility somewhat, but it should be remembered that the physician has no concept of periodontal procedures or just how elective they are. These decisions must be made by the periodontist, and a treatment plan must be devised that will enable therapy to be administered in an efficient, straightforward manner. It goes without saying that the treatment time will be somewhat extended.

As far as other physical health problems are concerned, a more complete assay of diseases of interest to periodontists is contained in Chapter 6.

Contingency. There are times in the management of the case when a procedure, usually a surgical procedure, is performed either partially or completely on an exploratory basis. This is particularly true of seriously involved but strategically important teeth. It is in these very areas that the greatest resourcefulness of the operator is called into play. Naturally the more skilled and experienced the diagnostician, the less often is the operator surprised. There are inevitably, however, times when the most experienced operator is confronted with a bizarre pattern of destruction that may change the prognosis and the outcome of the entire case. Although these areas may for the most part be marked, they should be recognized as potential trouble spots in the mouth, and a contingent diagnosis should be made as well as the more standard diagnosis. The patient must of course be apprised of its situation and must be given the alternatives. Commonly these contingent conditions will require periodontal prosthesis where none was deemed necessary before. Simple logic requires that these areas be definitely disposed of early in treatment so that a radical change in treatment method and sequence can be made without disrupting orderly management.

Comprehensive surgical approach. There are periodontists who perform the entire surgical phase in a single operation in a hospital with the patient remaining in the hospital for postoperative care and feeding. The operation may be performed with the patient under either local or general anesthesia. Although this approach makes a rather extensive surgical procedure for a patient who can be treated on an outpatient basis, the periodontists who use it feel that the advantages outweigh the disadvantages.

Some of the disadvantages are as follows: (1) protracted nature of the operation, (2) tendency to compromise on thorough-going procedures, especially if a general anesthesia is used and a general surgical operating room is utilized, and (3) postoperative course. The advantages of course are (1) that time is saved in healing and (2) that the apprehensive patient is treated in a single operation under general anesthesia. If this procedure is to be used it must be planned carefully so that the periodontist is available for bleeding episodes postoperatively, pain control, and usual surgical and anesthetic complications.

CHECKLIST FOR TREATMENT PLANNING PROCEDURES

A good practice to follow is to set down the treatment plan for the patient as an itemized list of procedures in the order in which they are to be used. The list may be used by the operator as a checklist so that when it has been completed the patient is ready for the first reevaluation. This method has been found to be effective in encouraging an orderly progress of case management.

A provisional outline that may serve as a sample

is as follows:

I. Initial preparation
  A. Scaling and root planing
  B. Instruction in oral physiotherapy
  C. Excavation of all caries, treatment of endodontic problems, extraction of hopeless teeth
  D. Orthodontic tooth movement
  E. Temporary stabilization of mobile teeth
  F. Occlusal adjustment by selective grinding
  G. Reevaluation
II. Definitive periodontal procedures
  A. Excisive
    1. Subgingival curettage
    2. Gingivectomy
    3. Apically repositioned flap
    4. Flap procedure with osteoplasty and osteoectomy
    5. Excision of frena
  B. Reparative and reconstructive
    1. Pedicle graft
    2. Free mucosal graft
    3. Flap procedure with débridement of osseous defect—self-fill
    4. Flap procedure with osseous graft
    5. Flap procedure with periosteal graft
    6. Flap procedure with contiguous autograft
    7. Periosteal pedicle graft for two-walled osseous defect with or without free periosteal graft
    8. Periosteal pedicle graft for cul-de-sac furca with or without free periosteal graft
  C. Special problems concerned with pocket elimination and production of physiologic form—tooth positions in arch and opposing tooth relationship influencing periodontal therapy
III. Desensitization of teeth
IV. Reevaluation of periodontal status and corrections, if necessary
V. Fulfillment of anatomic and physiologic requirements
  A. Dental anatomy
  B. Localized splinting of teeth
  C. Occlusal adjustment
  D. Replacement of missing teeth (multiple abutments)
  E. Periodontal prosthesis
VI. Habit preventives and correctives
  A. Maintenance of oral hygiene
  B. Routine prophylaxis
  C. Occlusal adjustment
VII. Recall interval established

It must be emphasized that periodontal therapy is not performed by one type of procedure but that there is a blending of the various techniques to accomplish the desired results. *Thus in a given quadrant a gingivectomy may be performed on the lingual aspect and a repositioned flap on the buccal aspect. An operation for an osseous defect may be included, as is also sometimes a mucobuccal fold extension. Therefore it may easily be seen that the indicated operation is performed for the local area but is combined with other procedures to treat the entire segment.* It must also be stressed that there is no one constant approach to follow in therapy. Often in one patient a procedure may be performed early, whereas in another it may be performed later.

Therapy consists of measures to obtain a healthy gingival attachment and an intact functioning attachment apparatus. It can be considered successful only if both the gingiva and the attachment apparatus are in a healthy state.

REFERENCES

Berdon, J. K.: Blood loss during gingival surgery, J. Periodontol. **36:**102, 1965.

Beube, F.: In our opinion, J. Periodontol. **19:**71, 1948.

Bjorndahl, O.: Reattachment and bone regeneration; report of a case, J. Am. Dent. Assoc. **36:**356, 1948.

Blanquie, R. H.: The rationale of pocket elimination in the treatment of periodontal disease, J. Periodontol. **21:**139, 1950.

Blanquie, R. H.: Periodontal problems, Dent. Surv. **10:**37, 1937.

Boyens, P. J.: A coordinated system for the treatment of paradentosis in its various phases, Dent. Items Interest **60:** 605, 1938.

Chase, R.: Methods and values of tooth planing in periodontal therapy, J. Periodontol. **32:**233, 1961.

Cohen, D. W., and Chacker, F. M.: Criteria for selection of one treatment plan over another, Dent. Clin. North Am., p. 3, March, 1964.

Fleming, W. E.: A clinical and microscopic study of periodontal tissues treated by instrumentation, Pacific Dent. Gaz. **24:**568, 1926.

Friedman, N.: Periodontal osseous surgery; osteoplasty and osteoectomy, J. Periodontol. **26:**257, 1955.

Goldman, H. M.: A summary of the treatment of periodontal diseases, Am. J. Ortho. **29:**183, 1943.

Goldman, H. M.: Diagnosis and treatment of periodontal diseases, Massachusetts Dent. Bull. **17:**14, 1941.

Goldman, H. M.: Periodontal diseases—a summary of examination, diagnosis, and treatment, Harvard Dent. Alumni Bull. **1:**29, 57, 1941.

Leof, M.: Clamping and grinding habits, their relation to periodontal disease, J. Am. Dent. Assoc. **31:**184, 1944.

Leonard, H. J.: Question of reattachment, J. Periodontol. **14:**5, 1943.

Linghorne, W. J., and O'Connell, D. C.: Studies in the regeneration and reattachment of supporting structures of the teeth, J. Dent. Res. **29:**419, 1950.

Lundquist, G. R.: Regeneration of the gingiva following surgical treatment of pyorrhea with special reference to the epithelium, J. Am. Dent. Assoc. **16:**128, 1929.

Lundquist, G. R., and Skillen, W. G.: An experimental study of periodontal membrane reattachment in healthy and pathologic tissues, J. Am. Dent. Assoc. **24:**175, 1937.

Morris, M. L.: Reattachment of human periodontal tissues following surgical detachment; a clinical and histologic study, J. Periodontol. **24:**220, 1953.

Morris, M. L.: Reattachment of periodontal tissue, Oral Surg. **2:**1194, 1949.

O'Leary, T. J.: Tooth mobility, Dent. Clin. North Am. **13:** 567, 1969.

Prichard, J.: The infrabony technique as a predictable procedure, J. Periodontol. **28:**203, 1957.

Ramfjord, S. P.: A rational plan for periodontal therapy, J. Periodontol. **24:**88, 1953.

Ramfjord, S. P.: Experimental periodontal reattachment in rhesus monkeys, J. Periodontol. **22:**67, 1951.

Ramfjord, S. P., Kerr, D. A., and Ash, M. M., editors: Proceedings of the World Workshop in Periodontics, Ann Arbor, 1966, University of Michigan Press.

Skillen, W. G., and Lundquist, G. R.: Experimental gingival injury in dogs, J. Dent. Res. **15:**165, 1935.

Smith, T. S.: The treatment of two periodontal cases, J. Periodontol. **20:**129, 1949.

Smith, T. S.: A summary of periodontal research findings, J. Periodontol. **19:**47, 1948.

Smith, T. S.: Constructive treatment of diseases of the paradental tissues, J. Am. Dent. Assoc. **22:**1477, 1935.

Sorrin, S.: Bone changes induced by periodontic treatment, J. Dent. Res. **9:**359, 1929.

Stones, H. H.: The reaction and regeneration of cementum in various pathological conditions, Proc. R. Soc. Med. **27:** 728, 1934.

Swenson, H. M.: Experimental periodontal pockets in dogs, J. Dent. Res. **26:**273, 1947.

Williams, C. H. M.: In our opinion, J. Periodontol. **19:**76, 1948.

Williams, C. H. M.: Rationalization of periodontal pocket therapy, J. Periodontol. **14:**66, 1943.

16 Initial preparation

Although the term "initial preparation" continues to be used in the literature, its connotation is different for many clinicians. Initial preparation constitutes one of the essential phases of periodontal and restorative therapy. Yet what is meant by initial preparation, and how does one define it?

Since the middle 1940s the term "initial preparation," coined by Goldman, has been utilized to describe those procedures employed to reduce clinical gingival inflammation by elimination of accretions on the teeth (scaling and root planing) and the institution of oral hygiene measures. In addition, reduction in mobility was accomplished by occlusal adjustment or stabilization by temporary splinting or both. In deranged articulations orthodontic tooth movement was performed. A reevaluation period was advocated at the conclusion of these various steps. Previous discussions seemed to be concerned with whether scaling, root planing, and oral hygiene were necessary prior to surgical intervention (Glickman 1961, 1957). The only procedures apparently considered as initial preparation—scaling, root planing, and oral hygiene—were not performed in a number of surgically treated cases. If they were performed their importance was understated. With changing ideas about the clinical treatment of the gingival unit and the attachment apparatus and with the results of a number of wound-healing studies, new procedures were introduced prior to pocket elimination in the so-called initial preparation phase.

In the late 1950s and 1960s initial preparation became firmly entrenched. It included orthodontic therapy and fixed temporary splinting when indicated. Thus the initial preparation phase increased in time and scope. It allowed for longer evaluation of the patient prior to definitive surgical intervention. This extended duration allowed for a better understanding of the patient's response to removal of local factors and therefore helped the clinician to better determine not only prognosis but the best treatment for the patient. The optimal treatment for a particular individual can only be determined by a constant evaluation process over time. Although each seasoned clinician develops a "gut" reaction derived from experience, this feeling must be substantiated by critical evaluation of the patient's response to treatment.

Additional procedures not only increased the time of the initial preparation phase of treatment, but the total time involved for periodontal therapy. One notes that over the past 20 years this phase of treatment has been greatly expanded (Ramfjord et al., 1966). Today, with utilization of Hawley bite plane therapy and more frequent use of orthodontics, a further increase in time is encountered in this phase of therapy. However, the final results justify this increased time as healing has been demonstrated in both the gingival unit and the attachment apparatus (Fig. 16-1). This healing has in many instances diminished the extent of periodontal surgery or has eliminated its need altogether. It appears that debate and controversy over the need for presurgical scaling and root planing have succumbed to a more logical integration of a number of procedures designed to treat the gingival unit and the attachment apparatus (Cohen and Chacker, 1964). The periodontal procedures have become much more closely integrated with the restorative considerations in rendering total patient care (Chacker and Serota, 1966).

The objectives of initial preparation are directed toward obtaining repair. They consist essentially of eliminating all known local etiologic factors and adverse environmental influences prior to

439

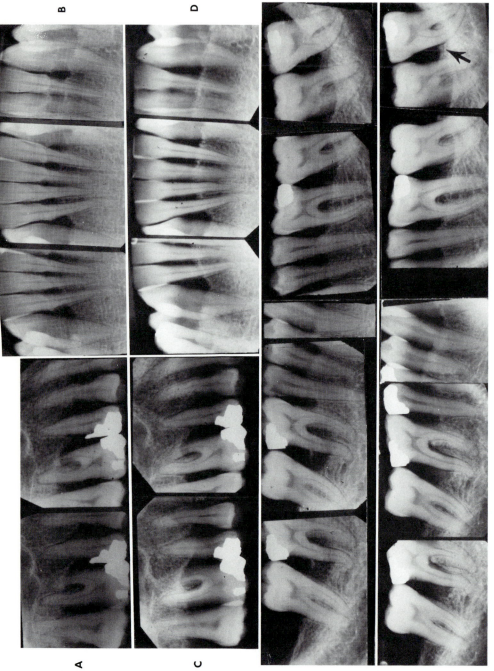

Fig. 16-1. A, Preoperative radiographs of maxillary right quadrant of a 45-year-old white man. **B,** Lower anterior preoperative radiograph. **C,** Note healing in attachment apparatus after 7 months of Hawley bite plane thearpy in conjunction with elimination of inflammation and occlusal adjustment by selective grinding. **D,** After initial preparation note absence of root resorption and lack of stabilization with 60% bone loss functioning against a properly adjusted bite plane. **E,** Lower posterior preoperative radiographs. **F,** Again note healing associated with scaling, root planing, occlusal rest, posterior eruption, and occlusal adjustment. *Arrow* indicates "lipping" of bone associated with posterior eruption. External oblique ridge and

definitive periodontal procedures and prior to the establishment of a sequence of therapy for the restorative phase (if one is needed) (Hine and Swenson, 1952). An attempt should be made to ensure that a minimum of irreversible procedures are accomplished during this phase so that as many options in therapy as possible remain available to the patient. Initial preparation constitutes the most critical part of periodontal therapy, since it is during this period that the decision is made as to what the final solution to the patient's dental problem will be.

The procedures involved in initial preparation are presented as follows: (1) emergency care and documentation, (2) instruction in oral physiotherapy, (3) scaling, root planing, and soft tissue curettage, (4) excavation of all caries, and treatment of endodontic problems, (5) extraction of hopeless teeth or parts of teeth, for example, hemisection or root amputation, (6) tooth movement procedures, for example, modified Hawley bite plane therapy and adjunctive orthodontics, (7) temporary stabilization for mobile teeth or anchorage for tooth movement, (8) occlusal adjustment, and (9) reevaluation. The complexities of each case and the treatment that is to be rendered to each patient determine the components and their sequence in the initial preparation phase (Goldman and Burket, 1959).

In order to understand the value and the need for initial preparation one must consider tissue character, wound-healing processes, and restorative requirements. One can then outline a series of steps on which to begin repair.

Documentation

Documentation of the patient's status upon presentation is essential if one is to subsequently evaluate his response to treatment. A complete data base, models, radiographs, charts, clinical photographs, occlusal documentation, and so on all afford the clinician a reference point for subsequent evaluation of the patient. It would of course be invaluable to obtain all previous dental records on any patient in an attempt to determine what the rate or progression of the disease process had been. This background is critical in determining prognosis.

Scaling, root planing, and soft tissue curettage

The gingival tissue in the marginal periodontal manifestation is constantly being exposed to repeated injury, with continual attempt at repair.

Calculus lying adherent to the tooth and adjacent to the sulcular tissue acts as a constant irritant. The inflammatory response to this irritant is the attempt to overcome the harmful effects. Concomitant with this inflammatory and immunologic response is repair. In some individuals the gingival tissue is almost completely filled with inflammatory cells without any production of collagen fibers (the basic constituent of the repair mechanism), and clinically one sees soft, red, and edematous tissue. In others the connective tissue response is marked, and one sees a dense and fibrotic pink tissue (Ambrose and Detamore, 1960).

The importance of scaling prior to further procedures should be stressed (Chace, 1974; Stone et al., 1966). Removal of calculus deposits prior to surgical techniques has several distinct advantages (Ross et al., 1966). The reduction of inflammation by scaling in many instances changes the quality of the tissue so that it is easier to incise or reflect (Fig. 16-2). Moreover, it may eradicate the pocket and thereby do away with the need for surgery altogether. The reduction in gingival inflammation may also confine the necessary surgical technique to a more limited area. This is frequently seen in cases of gingival clefts. Presurgical scaling may also prove advantageous by giving the operator a wider band of gingiva to utilize than existed prior to the removal of the deposits. This results from the coronal movement of the gingival margin and the current emphasis on conservation of gingiva for certain flap procedures: the more gingiva that is available, the greater will be the possibilities for surgical treatment. Subgingival scaling will also minimize the time that the wound must remain open during surgery (Gottsegen, 1961; Prichard, 1972; Zamet, 1966).

In some instances the inflammatory reaction is not contained at all, and there is an extension of the infiltrate through the attached gingiva into the alveolar mucosa. Clinically the change in color extends throughout the entire gingival wall, and no demarcating lines are visible. The gingivae are soft, edematous, and friable. It has been noted that an incision into this tissue does not heal readily, since granulation tissue tabs result, and complete epithelization of the wound is sometimes delayed. The healing of such soft, friable tissue to any expected architectural form cannot be ensured. Also excision of this type of tissue may result in proliferation of the gingival margin, creating sulci of a depth beyond that which is acceptable. Removal of the irritants in these instances, which allows the tissue to heal prior to surgery, leads not only to a relatively uneventful healing but enables the tissues to heal in the form achieved by the operation.

The scaling and root planing procedure is directed toward the removal of all calculus deposits both on the exposed surfaces of the teeth and sub-

gingivally (Schaffer, 1956). The calculus deposits should be removed thoroughly, and the tooth surfaces should be left smooth and clean (Zander, 1953). It has been shown that calculus formation is accelerated when a nidus of material is present on the tooth. A warm air blast used to dry the tooth often will disclose remnants of supragingi-

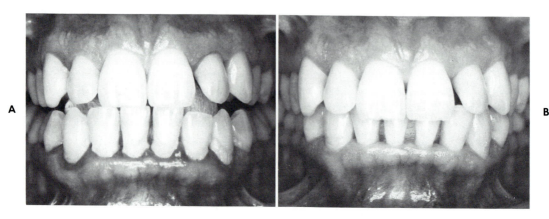

Fig. 16-2. Tissue type is an important factor in selection of a particular therapeutic procedure. **A,** Appearance of tissues at time of initial examination. **B,** Note tissue response after 9-week period of scaling, root planing, curettage, and proper oral physiotherapy.

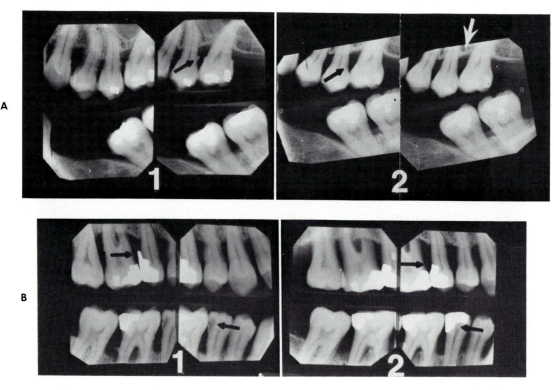

Fig. 16-3. Bite-wing radiographs can be helpful in checking for calculus removal. **A,** Preoperative bite wings in *1*. *2*, After scaling and root planing note improvement in crestal dura. **B,** Preoperative vertical bite wings, *1*, can usually be utilized even in advanced cases. *2*, After scaling, root planing, elimination of caries, removal of overhangs, and selective grinding.

val calculus; if these are allowed to remain a rather large formation will be found within a short time. Calculus deposits themselves can be planed to the point of feeling very smooth. Therefore once all root surfaces feel adequately planed additional radiographs can be very useful. In particular, several bite-wing radiographs will expose remaining subgingival calculus deposits (Fig. 16-3). Too much emphasis cannot be placed on the attainment of well-polished surfaces for the prevention and control of calculus formation (Hirschfeld, 1952). Therefore after the scaling procedure the teeth should be polished. Disclosing solution is of distinct benefit. Although one generally directs the curet against the root surface subgingivally, there usually occurs an inadvertent removal of the epithelium and connective tissue lining the pocket wall (Ramfjord and Kiester, 1954; Zamet, 1966). This occurs when a double-edged curet is used, because the curet's side is usually larger than the pocket dimensions. Although this soft tissue removal or curettage may be inadvertent, it will aid healing and provide for shrinkage of inflamed tissues. This shrinkage will be quite noticeable in the soft, red, and edematous tissue, but less noticeable in the firm and dense tissue (Sternlicht, 1961). Quite often more definitive curettage is performed along with scaling and root planing to better control the gingival inflammation. However, in those instances where deep pockets are present and one is having difficulty controlling the gingival inflammation, it may be necessary in the initial preparation phase to perform an internal beveled incision to remove the granulomatous tissue. This is a definitive removal of the epithelium and connective tissue lining the pocket wall. This procedure can expose osseous tissue and usually requires suturing and a periodontal dressing. Many names have been associated with this type of operation: Widman flap, mini-flap, open-flap, or clean-out procedure. This would not be done prior to control of occlusal etiology (Fig. 16-4). It is frequently necessary in cases requiring orthodontic therapy.

Also during initial therapy overhanging, rough, cervical margins should be removed, caries eliminated, improper contact points corrected where possible, and irregular marginal ridges recorded. Correction of these problems may aid in preventing the retention and accumulation of food and debris, which can act as a source of irritation (Glickman, 1972).

When teeth are filled with restorations having poor anatomic form and flat marginal ridges or ridges that slant toward the contact point, food is forced toward the interproximal area instead of through the spillways of the occlusal surface buccally or lingually. This food is wedged between the teeth, causing an impingement on the papilla and possibly a separation of the teeth. Anatomic features can be carved with a fissure bur, and sulci fissures, cusps, and especially marginal ridges can be formed.

Instruction in oral physiotherapy

The equation for successful periodontal therapy contains one important variable: the patient. After performing intricate therapeutic procedures requiring years of training and experience, the clinician must turn the treated case over for maintenance to the patient, an inexperienced layman. The results of poor oral physiotherapy can be devastating. The risk of failure is great if the patient is not taught oral hygiene techniques until the completion of therapy. He may prove completely incapable of carrying out the proper exercises, thus wasting much in the way of time, effort, and expense and causing himself unnecessary discomfort. It is far more advisable to make the teaching of oral hygiene part of the earlier aspects of therapy (Hirschfeld, 1939). Thus the patient's ability to carry out proper oral physiotherapy can be checked during the reevaluation phase of treatment. This may help the clinician to determine whether further periodontal therapy has a reasonable chance to succeed. Recent clinical investigation has established that some patients may be taught to maintain their mouths in acceptable condition while others may fail to do so despite repeated lessons given by the dentist. The latter are poor risks and are unlikely to benefit from more advanced procedures.

The introduction of oral hygiene procedures in the initial preparation stage of therapy aids in keeping the teeth free of debris and new accretions both soft and hard. Should the patient continue with a poor oral hygiene program after scaling, new deposits will occur that may hinder healing (Lovdal et al., 1961). Of greater benefit, however, is the achievement in a sense of oral cleanliness, should the patient be instructed in an oral physiotherapy technique at this time. It is true that during some of the initial preparation procedures the patient will not be able to carry out brushing in certain areas. However, not only can he keep the remaining portion of the dentition clean, but he can also prevent debris and accretions from accumulating around the dressings by rinsing. A soft, multituft, rounded, bristle-type brush perhaps is the best choice, since during the instruction period the patient is not likely to injure the gingivae with this type. The brushing technique may be the Charters, the modified Stillman-McCall, the Bell, the Bass, or any other that is suited to the case at hand. Interproximal and sulcular cleaning must be stressed. Utilization of dental floss, Super Floss, Stim-U-Dents, Perio-Aids, and so on should be directed toward complete removal of bacterial plaque. The disclosing solutions may become paramount in demonstrating to the patient the presence of plaque. Each patient should be given instruction designed for him individually and not a kit of all the home care aids known to dentistry, which tends to be self-defeat-

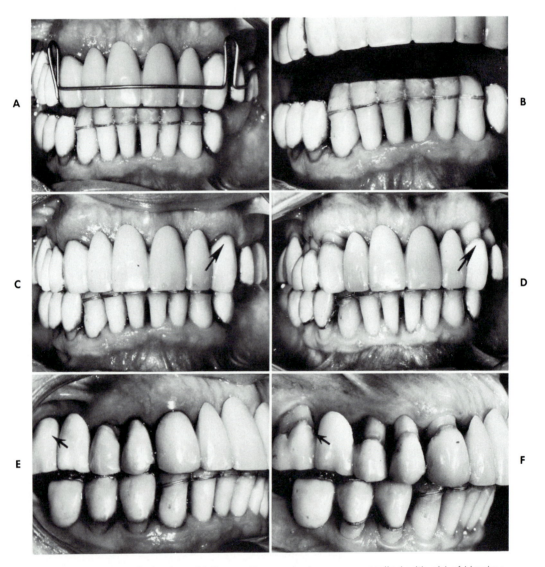

Fig. 16-4. During elimination of inflammation occlusion was controlled with aid of Hawley bite plane. **A,** Early insertion of bite plane for disarticulation to achieve redirection of force, occlusal rest, posterior eruption, and so on. **B,** Wire and orthodontic bond material used to stabilize lower anterior segment. **C,** Note overhanging margin initially. **D,** Removal of overhang and soft tissue shrinkage obtained after several months of root planing. **E,** Preoperative buccal contour. **F,** Removal of marginal overhang and reduction in soft tissue depth. **G,** Maxillary right quadrant initially. **H,** After initial preparation. **I,** Lower right quadrant preoperative radiographs. **J,** Seven months postoperative. **K,** Lower anteriors exhibited class II mobilities initially. **L,** Note return of lamina dura and lack of root resorption after many months of bite plane therapy.

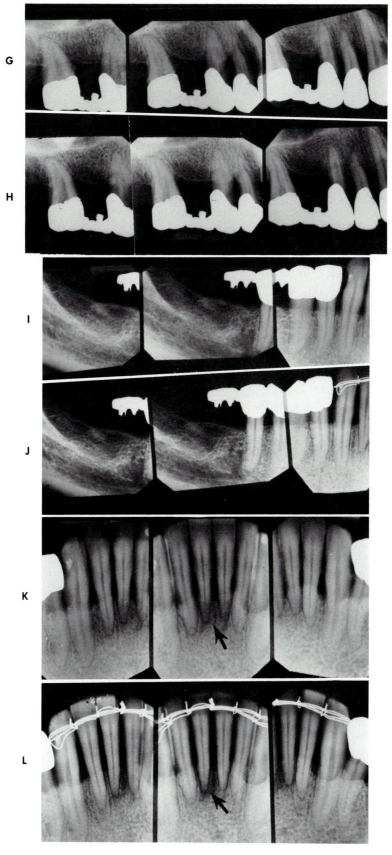

Fig. 16-4, cont'd. For legend see opposite page.

ing by its enormity. After therapy, when the gingivae have healed, the patient should be instructed again in the chosen techniques. These considerations are presented in Chapter 18.

Caries excavation, treatment of endodontic problems, strategic extraction, and hemisection and root amputation

Since periodontal, orthodontic, and restorative therapy can extend over long periods of time, it is advisable to remove all caries early. Caries can cause breakdown of contacts and shifting of teeth, and they can impair the healing process of the gingival tissues by retaining debris and plaque. Also one would want to avoid any pulpal problems and other unnecessary discomforts to the patient during the postoperative healing of a surgical area. Endodontic manipulation could be difficult as well as painful.

To prevent unnecessary complications during the surgical phase an endodontic evaluation of all questionable teeth should be performed and all recommended therapy should be completed in the initial preparation phase. Those teeth that require hemisection or root amputation should be filled, or if the root is in question at least instrumentation of the canals can be performed. Then at the time of an exploratory procedure or peri-

odontal surgery, the root can be removed and postoperative discomfort associated with pulpal origin can be avoided. When a tooth is questionable it may be economically beneficial to the patient to undergo instrumentation of the canals first in the event it is determined that later poor prognosis would indicate extraction.

It is recommended that the selected roots be removed in the initial preparation phase if possible. This would then allow the socket area where the root was removed to heal prior to the reevaluation step. In some cases no further surgery may be indicated, but in the majority of cases these areas have to be reopened because pocket depth with osseous defects are still present. This early root removal allows for optimum osseous regeneration and healing prior to completion of pocket elimination.

One should also be aware of the many combined endodontic-periodontic problems. In the combined lesion the endodontic therapy should be performed first because treatment of the endodontic lesions may either eliminate the need for or add to treatment of the periodontal lesion.

By taking advantage of the healing of extraction sockets and by anticipating the replacement of osseous tissue after extraction, the operator may decide to sacrifice a tooth to save alveolar support around a key abutment (Fig. 16-5) or

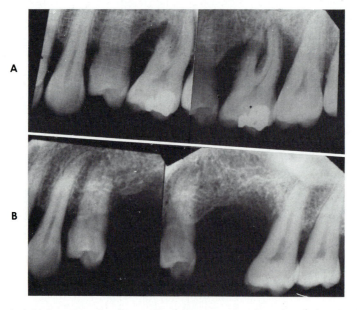

Fig. 16-5. In initial preparation it may be wise to extract hopelessly involved teeth prior to definitive therapy. In this maxillary quadrant, first molar was removed to afford maximum healing on mesial aspect of viable second molar abutment and prevent mesial furcation involvement. **A,** Preoperative radiograph. **B,** After several months of postoperative healing.

adjacent teeth. This may prevent the necessary removal of large amounts of osseous tissue in establishing optimal bony architecture during surgical intervention. This is also an indication for early root removal.

Adjunctive orthodontics: tooth movement

Tooth movement for restorative and periodontal needs may be necessary to correct existing local etiologic factors contributing to the disease process. If favorable osseous and soft tissue changes

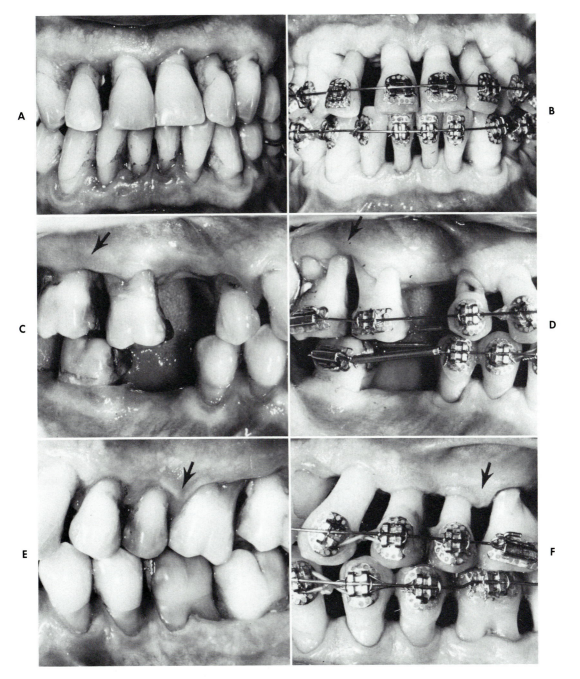

Fig. 16-6. A, Initial examination. **B,** Note soft tissue remodeling and shrinkage associated primarily with elimination of inflammation. **C,** Right posterior area preoperatively. **D,** After resolution of inflammation and axially positioning posterior teeth. **E,** Accentuated mesial drift preoperatively. **F,** Soft tissue change with closed root planing and curettage along with tooth movement.

attributed to proper tooth repositioning are to be obtained, the most critical aspect of this procedure is proper periodontal preparation before initiating tooth movement. Also when utilizing the modified Hawley bite plane for redirection of force, occlusal rest, posterior eruption, to facilitate occlusal adjustment, active tooth movement, and so on the key is proper elimination of inflammation. Eruption of teeth passively or with active appliances where calculus and inflammation are present will render less than optimal results.

If an adult patient is being prepared for extensive orthodontic therapy involving change of arch form or arch-to-arch relationships, treatment time may be in excess of 2 years. It is inconceivable that several visits with the hygienist would suffice to properly prepare this patient for orthodontic banding. Extensive root planing and elimination of all inflammation must precede insertion of the appliance. In addition the patient must be kept free of inflammation by root planing and curettage throughout tooth movement procedures (Fig. 16-6). This is done as frequently as necessary to maintain the patient inflammation-free during orthodontic therapy. If this is not rigidly adhered to, irreversible bone loss will inevitably result in the periodontally susceptible patient. This inflammation-free state is considerably easier to describe than to accomplish clinically. The same meticulous preparation and continuous root planing are necessary to successfully achieve proper tooth movement of local dental malpositions.

In cases with advanced bone loss, furcation involvements, and severe pocket depth it may be necessary to do an open-flap procedure for removal of diseased gingival tissue and proper root planing prior to the orthodontic therapy. Because of better visualization and access more definitive root planing can be performed in these deeper pocket areas and tortuous root configurations. Obviously this procedure would not be done in the advanced case without control of the occlusion prior to the open-flap débridement. Control of the occlusion can readily be accomplished with the aid of the Hawley bite plane.

In the case of occlusal periodontitis a clinician must critically evaluate the patient prior to placement of appliances as to whether prognosis appears favorable or unfavorable. Patients who must undergo advanced periodontic, orthodontic, and restorative dentistry procedures to maintain their natural dentition should (barring unknown or detectable systemic factors) expect a favorable prognosis. In reviewing hundreds of successfully treated advanced cases the one common denominator that these patients demonstrated was early healing in the attachment apparatus. Therefore not only are we looking for favorable soft tissue resolution, but radiographs can be taken early in treatment to check for calculus that remains and to evaluate radiographic evidence (return of lamina dura, normalization of the periodontal ligament spaces, changes in trabecular pattern of bone and so on) of healing in the attachment apparatus (Fig. 16-7). Naturally reduction in mobility patterns and resolution of other clinical occlusal symptoms would also be expected. Upon

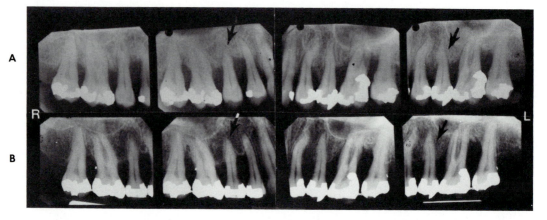

Fig. 16-7. A, Preoperative radiographs of maxillary posterior segments. **B,** Months later note healing in attachment apparatus. *Arrows* indicate normalization of periodontal ligament space and return of lamina dura. (In conjunction with Dr. C. Kvistad, Edmonds, Wash.)

receiving a favorable response the patient could then be advised to continue with the tooth movement phase of initial preparation. The clinician who relies solely on instinctive reaction to a patient upon initial presentation to determine the ultimate treatment plan will more frequently experience disappointing case failures than an operator who allows individual patient response to influence the course of treatment.

Tooth movement is part of initial preparation not only because it may be necessary to establish acceptable occlusal landmarks, optimal axial inclinations of teeth, and proper embrasures and provide an adequate path of insertion for prostheses and so on, but it can also minimize the amount of supporting bone that may have to be sacrificed by definitive osseous surgery. It may eliminate the need for osseous and mucogingival surgery altogether because properly performed tooth movement can favorably change the osseous and soft tissue topography around the teeth (Brown, 1973; Corn, 1968). Forced eruption of teeth via active appliances has been used to salvage teeth fractured off at the gingival margin and to aid in eliminating infrabony defects (Ingber, 1974). The potential for osseous regeneration and recontouring associated with active tooth movement is presented in Chapter 21.

In summary tooth movement from a periodontal point of view can be considered to be preventive, interceptive, and therapeutic. It is *preventive* when proper tooth position allows normal gingival and osseous topography, which is not only more self-cleansing but can allow areas previously inaccessible to cleansing to be adequately cared for. It is *interceptive* where previous inflammation existed. Reestablishment of proper soft and osseous tissue to coronal form relationships may resolve the local factor and stop further progression of the disease process. It is *therapeutic* in the many ways that have been outlined in correction of periodontal deformities. In addition proper tooth position helps to promote a more physiologic distribution of force and stress (critical in the advanced case) by the attachment apparatus. These are all objectives of the initial phase of therapy.

Tooth movement logically precedes definitive periodontal surgery. It would be superfluous to attempt to establish acceptable osseous and gingival forms knowing that tooth movement would change them both. The optimal approach is to place the teeth in their final position, establish a stable occlusion, then wait a minimum of 6 months before opening the case for definitive periodontal procedures.

Temporary stabilization

Teeth that have varying degrees of mobility due to lost support from periodontal disease may require additional aid for their stabilization (Wulff-Cochrane, 1967). Normal stresses in a given dentition with a healthy periodontium become abnormal forces when there is a lessened amount of support for these teeth. In some instances eliminating the disease and adjusting the occlusion to a functional balance are sufficient for these teeth to become firm again (Wust et al., 1961). However, it may be necessary to splint temporarily so that repair can occur (Fig. 16-8).

Temporary stabilization is also utilized in tooth movement procedures to provide anchorage prior to tooth movement and to immobilize teeth for retention and stabilization after movement.

The provisional restoration (Amsterdam and Fox, 1959) may be necessary in mutilated dentitions with many missing teeth or in musculature problem cases. However, following tooth movement the natural tooth structure would usually be preferable for further periodontal therapy for reasons of patient comfort, ease for the restorative dentist, and evaluation of patient response to establishment of a stable posterior occlusion. In many instances once the posterior occlusion has been properly set up, very little attachment apparatus may be necessary to maintain the anterior teeth in health.

In severe cases of secondary occlusal traumatism with excessive mobility it may be necessary to splint the teeth temporarily to provide a fixed position that will allow for an occlusal adjustment without the teeth shifting in all directions during functional movements. Techniques and methods of stabilization are presented in Chapter 21.

Occlusal adjustment

Occlusal adjustment may be made by orthodontics, selective grinding, extraction, restorative dentistry, or some combination of the above. However the sequence of therapy (Chapter 30) for a particular case may involve elimination of inflammation, control or elimination of occlusal etiology, and correction of remaining soft and hard tissue deformities (Amsterdam, 1974). Any case will follow this sequence although each step may not be necessary.

The rationale and technique of occlusal adjustment by selective grinding are presented in Chap-

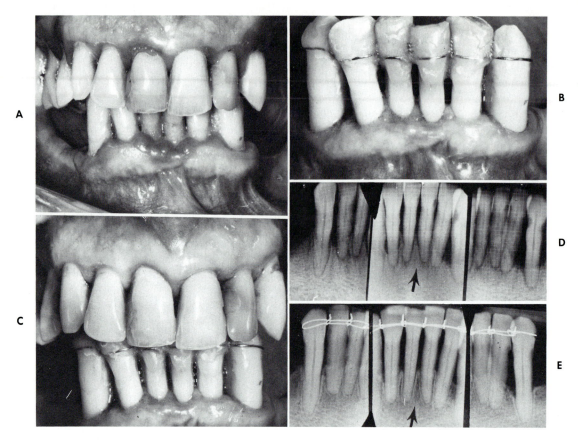

Fig. 16-8. A, Upon initial presentation this 65-year-old white woman exhibited two-plus mobility patterns on lower anterior teeth. **B,** Five years after stabilization by extracoronal wire ligation covered by orthodontic bond material. **C,** Five years after operation. Initial stabilization has not been added to or altered. **D,** Preoperative radiographs exhibiting widened periodontal ligament spaces and loss of lamina dura. **E,** Five years after operation radiographs indicate results of scaling, root planing, oral physiotherapy, and stabilization. Note healing in attachment apparatus as indicated by return of lamina dura, normalization of periodontal ligament spaces, and so on.

ter 30. However, it should be pointed out that this is a definitive procedure, with the objective of decreasing tooth mobility and allowing for healing in the attachment apparatus.

Occlusal adjustment may start at the time of insertion of the Hawley bite plane to eliminate interferences in the periodontally involved patient. Taking advantage of a discrepancy between retruded contact position and the intercuspal position to alleviate excessive trauma on anterior teeth is frequently beneficial (Fig. 16-9).

The response of the patient to occlusal therapy must be critically evaluated. The surgical phase of therapy should not be begun prior to control of occlusal etiology. After a stable occlusion has been established and the inflammatory element has been eliminated, reevaluation should be performed.

Reevaluation

Although constant evaluation of each procedure of initial preparation is performed, a final step to evaluate and coordinate all the procedures is suggested prior to pocket elimination. Reevaluation will help determine the direction, course, and extent of further therapy by assaying the patient's response to all the preceding procedures.

Reevaluation should provide information concerning the patient's motivation, oral hygiene effectiveness, and healing capacity. It should allow the operator to observe the nature and the healing process of the gingival tissues (edema, bleeding, suppuration, fibrosis) as well as the resultant gingival architecture. It should aid in evaluating any changes in pocket depth, gain or loss of attached gingiva, roentgenographic changes of osseous defects, extension of pockets beyond the mucogin-

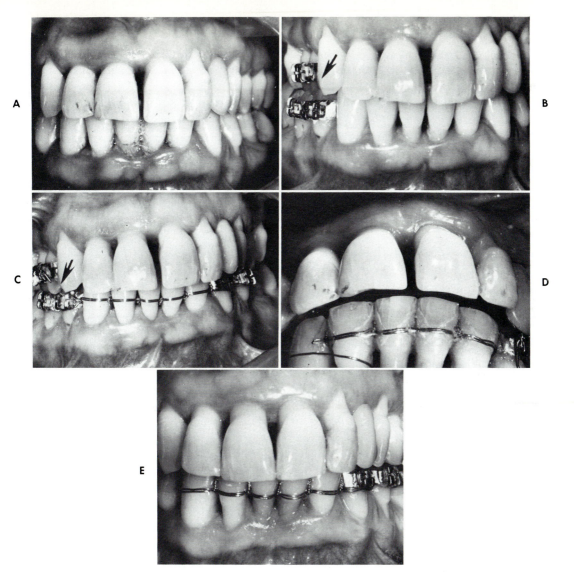

Fig. 16-9. A, Upon presentation this 37-year-old white woman exhibited posterior bite collapse and incisor flaring as indicated by maxillary diastema. **B,** She was placed in a bite plane for disarticulation during tooth movement. Note right premolar cross bite. **C,** Correction of premolar cross bite and establishment of a stable posterior occlusion. **D,** Note overjet that was developed by establishing a stable posterior occlusion in retruded contact position, taking excessive force off maxillary anterior incisors. **E,** With removal of bite plane maxillary incisors moved back from lip pressure alone, closing diastema.

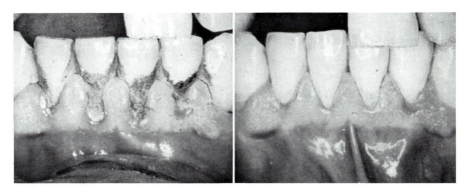

Fig. 16-10. Deposits on mandibular incisors and a narrow band of attached gingiva. If periodontal surgery were performed and calculus removed, it would be most difficult to do any type of mucogingival surgery. However, after initial preparation a broad band of attached gingiva resulted. Thus definitive therapy can only be programmed after local etiology factors have been either eliminated or controlled. (Courtesy Dr. H. Corn.)

gival junction, and frena and muscle attachments related to clefts or interfering with surgical pocket elimination. In the examination of a periodontal manifestation involving major portions of the dentition, marked deformities are seen to be caused by the disease process. Fig. 16-10 presents such an instance. Should pocket elimination be contemplated without initial preparation, the operator must slant the procedure to overcome the existing gingival deformity. In Fig. 16-10, i

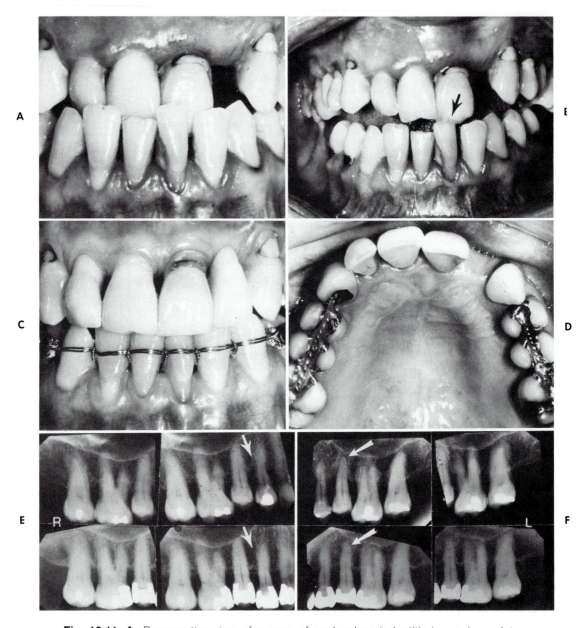

Fig. 16-11. A, Preoperative view of a case of occlusal periodontitis in maximum intercuspation. **B,** Initial contact on retruded arc of closure. **C,** After initial preparation that consisted of scaling, root planing, instruction in oral physiotherapy, adjunctive tooth movement, stabilization utilizing aid splints, and occlusal adjustment by selective grinding. This photograph presents case at time of reevaluation, prior to definitive mucogingival and osseous procedures. **D,** Note stabilization of maxillary posterior segments with aid splints. **E,** Maxillary posterior segments preoperatively. *Arrows* indicate osseous defect on distal aspect of maxillary right first premolar and widened periodontal ligament space and loss of lamina dura on maxillary left second premolar. **F,** Nine months later note radiographic evidence of changes in crestal topography associated with eruption, elimination of inflammation, and evidence of healing in attachment apparatus.

gingivectomy is instituted, where would the initial incision be made? Would it be at the vestibular fold in order to eliminate the pocket on the labial aspect of the mandibular right cuspid? If the procedure were so performed, would not the resulting topography be a greater deformity than that created by the disease process? Initial preparation therefore allows for healing. It will initiate repair; in some instances it will provide complete repair. Not infrequently one sees improvements in topography, so that subsequent management to overcome the deformity is more easily attained.

When occlusal adjustment, tooth movement, temporary stabilization, or a combination is performed the operator should observe changes in mobility and fremitus patterns as well as in intra arch and interarch relationships of the teeth. Radiographic evidence of healing in the attachment apparatus must be evaluated. There should be a favorable response to elimination of occlusal etiology (Fig. 16-11).

Based on the restorative plan selected and the financial capabilities of the patient, teeth with questionable or poor prognosis may be extracted if they have not responded favorably to initial preparation.

Thus reevaluation assays the patient and his initial response to therapy and therefore provides for a more definite course in future periodontal and restorative procedures.

• • •

In essence, initial preparation can provide the clinician with a logical sequence to a sometimes unpredictable and imperceptible healing process. It can protect the patient and the operator as regards time, expense, and effort. It can also ensure success.

REFERENCES

Ambrose, J., and Detamore, R.: Correlation of histologic and clinical findings in periodontal treatment; effect of scaling on the reduction of gingival inflammation prior to surgery, J. Periodontol. **31:**238, 1960.

Amsterdam, M.: Periodontal prosthesis — twenty-five years in retrospect, Alpha Omegan **67:**3, 1974.

Amsterdam, M., and Fox, L.: Provisional splinting principles and techniques, Dent. Clin. North Am., p. 73, March, 1959.

Brown, I. S.: The effect of orthodontic therapy on certain types of periodontal defects. I. Clinical findings, J. Periodontol. **44:**742, 1973.

Chace, R.: Subgingival curettage in periodontal therapy, J. Periodontol. **45:**107, 1974.

Chacker, F. M., and Serota, B. H.: Provisional periodontal prosthesis, Periodontics **4:**265, 1966.

Cohen, D. W., and Chacker, F. M.: Criteria for selection of one treatment plan over another, Dent. Clin. North Am., p. 3, March, 1964.

Corn, H.: Osseous changes and bone fill associated with tooth movement, Hollywood, Florida, 1968, American Academy of Periodontology meeting.

Glickman, I.: Clinical periodontology, ed. 4, Philadelphia, 1972, W. B. Saunders Co.

Glickman, I.: The effect of prescaling upon healing following periodontal surgery — a clinical and histological study, J. Dent. Med. **16:**19, 1961.

Glickman, I.: Is scaling prior to gingival surgery a necessary procedure? Periodont. Abstr. **4:**99, 1957.

Goldman, H. M., and Burket, L. W.: Treatment planning in the practice of dentistry, St. Louis, 1959, The C. V. Mosby Co.

Gottsegen, R.: Should the teeth be scaled prior to surgery? J. Periodontol. **32:**301, 1961.

Hine, M. K., and Swenson, H. M.: Role of prophylactic procedures in the treatment of periodontal disease, J. Am. Dent. Assoc. **45:**301, 1952.

Hirschfeld, I.: The toothbrush — its use and abuse, Brooklyn, N.Y., 1939, Dental Items of Interest Publishing Co., Inc.

Hirschfeld, L.: Subgingival curettage in periodontal therapy, J. Am. Dent. Assoc. **44:**301, 1952.

Ingber, J. S.: Forced eruption. I. A method of treating isolated one and two wall infrabony osseous defects — rationale and case report, J. Periodontol. **45:**199-206, 1974.

Lovdal, A., Arno, A., Schei, O., and Waerhaug, J.: Combined effort of subgingival scaling and controlled oral hygiene on the incidence of gingivitis, Acta Odontol. Scand. **19:**537, 1961.

Moskow, B.: The response of the gingival sulcus to instrumentation — a histologic investigation, J. Periodontol. **33:**282, 1962.

Prichard, J.: Advanced periodontal disease; surgical and prosthetic management, ed. 2, Philadelphia, 1972, W. B. Saunders Co.

Ramfjord, S. P., Kerr, D. A., and Ash, M. M., editors: Proceedings of the World Workshop in Periodontics, Ann Arbor, 1966, University of Michigan Press.

Ramfjord, S. P., and Kiester, G.: The gingival sulcus and the periodontal pocket immediately following scaling of teeth, J. Periodontol. **25:**167, 1954.

Ross, S. E., Malamed, E. H., and Amsterdam, M.: The contiguous autogenous transplant — its rationale, indications and technique, Periodontics **4:**246, 1966.

Schaffer, E. M.: Histological results of root curettage of human teeth, J. Periodontol. **27:**296, 1956.

Sternlicht, H. C.: Curettage, its place in the treatment of periodontal disease, Tex. Dent. J. **79:**4, 1961.

Stone, S., Ramfjord, S. P., and Waldron, J.: Scaling and gingival curettage — a radiographic study, J. Periodontol. **37:**63, 1966.

Wulff-Cochrane, V.: Splints in periodontal treatment, Leeds Dent. J. **6:**55, 1967.

Wust, B. P., Rateitschak, K. R., and Muhleman, H. R.: The influence of local periodontal treatment in tooth mobility and gingival inflammation, Dent. Abstr. **6:**270, 1961.

Zamet, J. S.: Initial preparation of the gingival tissues prior to surgery, Dent. Pract. Dent. Rec. **17:**115, 1966.

Zander, H. A.: The attachment of calculus to root surfaces, J. Periodontol. **24:**16, 1953.

17 Scaling and root planing

Coronal and root surface scaling is a basic technique in periodontal therapy. In actual present-day use there is little question that it is the initial phase of therapy.

Basically, root surface scaling is a technique of root surface cleansing. Its aim is to remove accretions of calculus and debris in large or small quantities in both the supragingival and subgingival uninvested areas of a tooth. Although the objective may be simply stated, it is not easily achieved. Great skill must be developed through constant practice and objective evaluation to master this technique adequately. The difficulty lies in the development of tactile acuity in seeking out and removing deposits that cannot be seen.

However, some aspects of scaling involve the removal of gross deposits that are easily found but difficult to remove without damage to the cemental surface. *This wide range of application makes root surface scaling one of the most demanding of all periodontal techniques* (Fig. 17-1).

The deposition of supragingival and subgingival calculus is one of the most interesting phenomena to be encountered in periodontics. The position of calculus on the root under the gingival mucosa creates a rather anomalous condition. Since the calculus is rough, septic, and irritating to the adjacent tissue, it is not surprising to find the reaction to it by this tissue to be inflammation, epithelial ulceration and degeneration, and edema. On occasion a purulent exudate

---

Fig. 17-1. Root surface curettage or scaling constitutes first phase of periodontal therapy. Removal of all accretions from exposed surfaces of teeth and those located subgingivally demands a technical skill that dentist must develop; however, it is essential that he be familiar with tissues involved. In this illustration four photomicrographs depict supragingival and subgingival calculus deposits and gingival tissues. **A,** Calculus on gingival margin close to tooth. Space seen between tooth and calculus is an artifact due to preparation. In this instance no calculus lies between gingiva and tooth. Gingival corium is densely infiltrated with inflammatory cells. Note that gingival margin is situated on cementum, recession having taken place. **B,** Calculus deposited between gingiva and tooth. Clinically this is termed subgingival calculus. Note that calculus completely occupies pocket space. Inflammatory infiltrate in corium is evident, as is proliferation of sulcular epithelium due to inflammation. **C,** Heavy calculus deposit adherent to tooth surface, occupying pocket space completely. This is another example of subgingival calculus. In this photomicrograph densely inflamed corium of gingiva is evident, as is proliferation of sulcular epithelium. Note apical limitation of epithelial attachment by band of collagen fibers. **D,** Subgingival calculus in a deep labial pocket. All characteristics of pocket formation are evident. From these photomicrographs it is evident that in root surface scaling procedure instrument must be placed between calculus and gingival wall at expense of soft tissue; then it must be brought apically until calculus deposit is engaged. With even smallest instruments it is impossible not to remove sections of soft tissue in the scaling operation. It seems apparent that in most instances both sulcular epithelium and epithelial attachment would be removed in any extensive scaling.

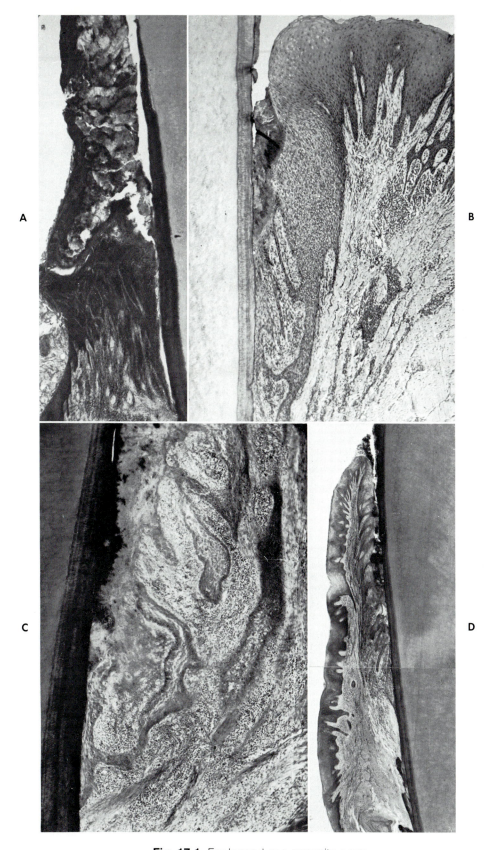

Fig. 17-1. For legend see opposite page.

is formed in the sulcular ulcerations because of microscopic abscess formation in the connective tissue, and droplets may occasionally be elicited by a stroking, milking pressure on the gingiva with the finger.

Coronal scaling connotes the procedure of the removal of gross and fine deposits on a more or less visual basis, with no extensive excursion subgingivally except to engage a heavy ledge of calculus that is discernible supragingivally. Subgingival scaling refers to the removal of calculus and accretions within the periodontal pocket as a precise definitive technique. Subgingival scaling is the more demanding and requires much application to do well.

It is very well known that the slower the deposition of calculus, the denser its structure will be and the smaller its crystals. Also it is attached to the cementum more tenaciously. We know also that subgingival calculus is much denser and more tenacious than is supragingival calculus because it is formed in a protected cryptlike area and is formed slowly and without being disturbed. This fact presents the operator with a difficult problem. Constricted terrain would require a small, delicate instrument, whereas a hard tenacious deposit would require a heavy blade for its delivery. This is a problem that frequently taxes even the most resourceful technician. Files are sometimes useful in initial crushing. Occasionally a push curet will split the flake nicely. In any event these are problems that have no stock solution but

depend on diagnosis of the shape, location, and character of the calculus and pocket with which we are dealing. After the initial break has been made, the removal of the smaller pieces is quite simple (Fig. 17-2).

The skillful use of instruments is a basic requisite of adequate scaling. There are many sets of instruments of various types designed to reach most of the different patterns of periodontal pocket formation. Although these instruments show wide differences in design, they are basically not so different from each other as might be inferred from a casual glance. They fall into broad classes of scalers (chisels, sickles), hoes, files, and curets. Most sets of instruments contain several of these types. Some are composed exclusively of one type and depend on supplementary instruments for complete treatment (Figs. 17-3 to 17-5).

More important than the instrument itself is the development of skill in its use. The therapist must be cognizant of the fact that in the scaling procedure care must be exercised not to push calculus or cemental shavings into the gingival tissue. Many clinicians perform scaling and root planing procedures under a washed field technique to avoid displacing calcified particles into the gingival tissues. A brief description of the various instrument types will be offered, together with the techniques for their use. There is no intention to disparage an instrument because it is limited in its use. Each has its place, and skilled use of it will yield rewards in the results of therapy.

Text continued on p. 461.

Fig. 17-2. Choice of instruments is a matter of taste and experience. As an operator gains skill, he usually learns to employ a fewer number of instruments more efficiently. Instruments should be simply designed and capable of being sharpened easily. The more uses to which an instrument can be put, the greater is its value in the scaling procedure. Last, knowledge of what is to be accomplished, not the particular instrument to be employed, is the all-important factor. It is the operator who accomplishes the task, not the instrument. The chief requisite is that calculus deposits be removed effectively and completely and that enamel and root surfaces and soft tissue not be excessively traumatized in the process. Instruments used to remove calculus in cleaning the teeth are called scalers, curets, hoes, and files. Curet scaler has an elongated pear-shaped blade that terminates in a rounded end. Cutting surfaces of base are approximately parallel. Back of face is convex, allowing for repeated sharpening of instrument. Sickle scaler has a blade with two or four cutting edges; in cross section, blade is triangular or rectangular in shape. It is intended for general work, when instrument need not penetrate deeply between gingiva and tooth surface. Hoe has a single cutting edge that is approximately at right angles to shank. In order for hoe to perform efficiently, angle of blade should be over 88 degrees so that it will dislodge calculus deposits and allow tooth surface to be planed smooth. File is essentially a series of hoes set close together; it is best used as a smoothing instrument. File should be small so that it can penetrate periodontal pocket easily. In this illustration periodontal chisel, curet, file, hoe, and scaler are shown in that order.

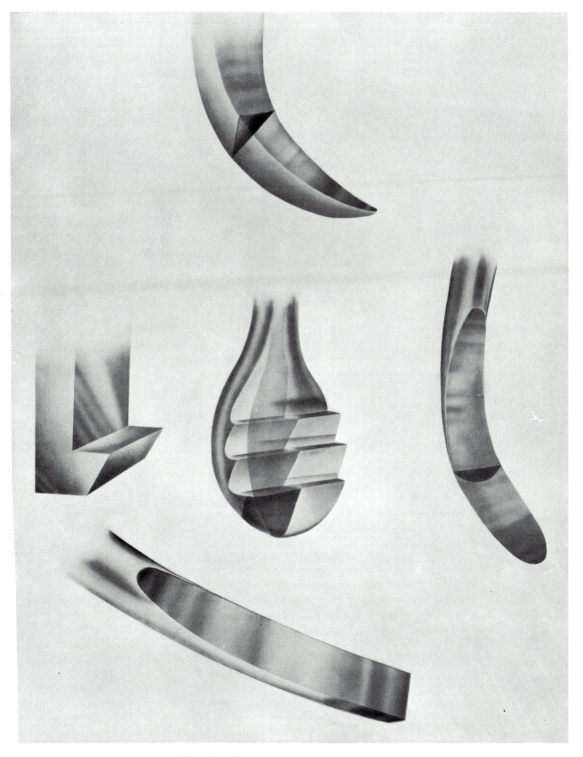

Fig. 17-2. For legend see opposite page.

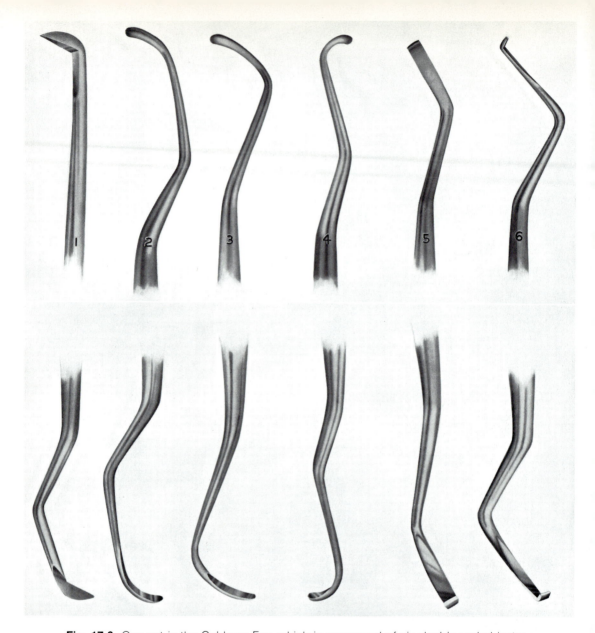

Fig. 17-3. One set is the Goldman-Fox, which is composed of six double-ended instruments: one scaler, three curets, and two hoes. Except for scaler, other instruments compose a right and left angulation. No. 1 has a small, straight blade of scaler type at right angles to shaft, whereas other end has an offset in shank, blade being of same character. This instrument, although universal, can be used most effectively on proximal surfaces and on flat buccal and palatal surfaces. Blades are small enough and shaped so that they penetrate pocket easily. Blades of curets are small and sharp and can easily remove sections of soft tissue. In all instances blade is in direct line with handle so that instruments are well balanced. Hoes also are constructed as are curets and are designed to be able to approach all surfaces of teeth. Thus cutting edge can be brought to any portion of tooth at correct angle. Curets are designed so as to reach the very bottom of pocket without excessive distention of gingival tissue. These instruments can be made very sharp, which facilitates removal of deposits from root surface. Instruments should be applied with a firm downward push of thumb and index finger, the force of which is controlled by firm pressure of shank against third finger. They should be moved in short, quick, even planing strokes, gradually smoothing root surface and dislodging deposits. Forearm and rocking movements will naturally follow to facilitate operation. No. 1 is used as a universal instrument to remove heavy deposits; it is especially useful on proximal surfaces. No. 2 is a curet intended for incisors, cuspids, and premolars, whereas no. 3 is used for premolars and molars. Contra-angle of latter facilitates scaling in instances in which inclination of tooth is such that the no. 2 instrument cannot be placed in same long axis as tooth. No. 4 is utilized for molars in that extra bend of shank allows for better placement of instrument. Nos. 5 and 6 are hoes. No. 5 is primarily for buccal and lingual surfaces of molars and for other surfaces of other teeth. No. 6 is used for molars.

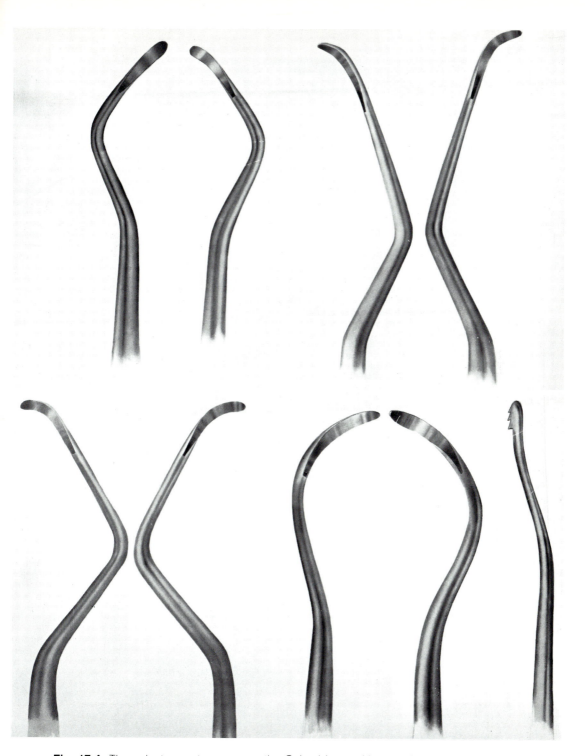

Fig. 17-4. These instruments compose the Columbia set. Upper left pair of instruments are Younger-Good nos. 13 and 14. These are extremely slender fine curets, designed for removal of thin subgingival deposits and exploration of root surfaces. They are used with a pull stroke or a push-pull stroke; and they are very useful in completing the smoothing operation. Pair of instruments on upper right are the 2R and 2L McCall's; these are likewise fine and slender curets, used to dislodge small, thin accretions. They are excellent instruments for final preparation of tooth surface. Lower left pair of instruments are McCall 4R and 4L and are identical to pair on upper right, with exception of a more acute angle to the shank. This allows for easier approach to roots of posterior teeth. In lower center McCall nos. 17 and 18 are illustrated. These are heavy spiral curets for removal of adherent flakes of calculus. They are also extremely useful for circumferential curettage. Instrument shown on lower right is a Hirschfeld-Dunlop file, obtainable in nos. 3, 5, 7, 9, and 11; these have various angulations for approach to different surfaces of teeth.

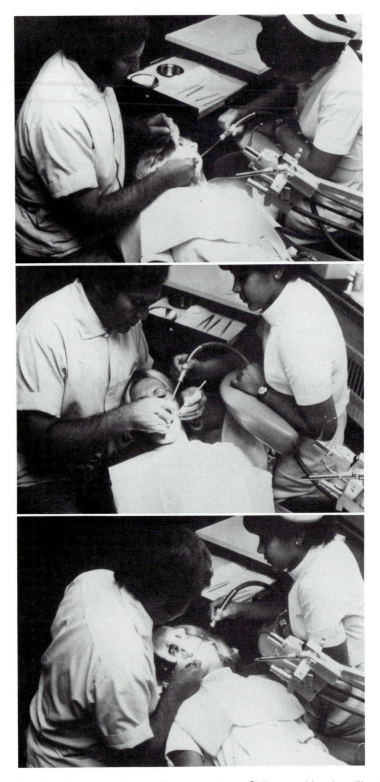

Fig. 17-5. Position of operator for scaling procedure. Sitting position is utilized. In top photograph, operator is on side of patient with patient's head turned to left for scaling buccal aspects of teeth. In lower photograph, dentist is in front of patient. Scaling area is palatal aspect of maxillary right teeth. Note that patient's head is turned to right. By varying operator position and head position of patient, a direct visual approach is possible. Also note assistant's body and hand positions.

In the root planing technique the clinician attempts to establish a root surface that is smooth, hard, and glasslike in consistency. Root planing is a definitive procedure and extends beyond the scaling technique.

INSTRUMENTS

Periodontal chisel. The simplest form of scaler is the periodontal chisel. It is used with a push stroke and depends upon a right-angled edge blade for its action, which consists of scaling or splitting of calculus. It is most useful in the splitting of heavy accretions on the anterior teeth, the mandibular teeth particularly. The instrument is passed interproximally through the embrasure, in tight contact with one of the approximating root surfaces, toward the lingual surface in a labial to lingual direction. In this manner the heavy plate of calculus is either fractured or in some instances completely removed.

A modification of this scaler is used by some operators in an apical direction for root surface scaling. Specially shaped shanks make application of the chisel to posterior areas possible. No particular advantage is derived from this type of instrument, and it is rather destructive to cementum when not perfectly seated. On the whole it is much too coarse and powerful an instrument to be used subgingivally. To avoid this, the blade is made more springy by making it very thin. Even then it is not suitable for subgingival root cleansing.

Sickle. The sickle scaler is a hook-shaped instrument in various sizes and weights. It is an instrument designed to be used supragingivally on deposits of some tenacity. In cross section its blade usually is a rectangle so that there are four edges on this versatile instrument; some sickles are triangular in cross section. It may be used with a pull stroke or a push stroke, depending on the edge employed. The very tip of the blade ends in a sharp point so that it may be used interproximally as well as labially and lingually.

Various forms of the sickle are obtainable. All are basically hook shaped or have right-angled blades. Several are bent so as to be adapted to posterior use interproximally. Of necessity these come in pairs, right and left.

The sickle scaler is used with a short, powerful, dislodging stroke. Because of its design and size it is not adaptable for subgingival use. This is fortunate since extensive root and soft tissue damage may be inflicted by its careless use. It is a useful instrument as a preliminary scaler where the deposits are massive and strongly attached.

Hoe. The action of the hoe is similar to that of the chisel in that its blade is a right angle of steel, but it is designed to be used with a pull stroke. It is a rather heavy instrument, with some of its action due to crushing as well as cutting or scaling. Its pull action makes it suitable for use in a vertical direction within a pocket, since its action is in effect a withdrawal. However, the sharp corners of the hoe are a distinct hazard within a pocket. If the blade of the hoe is not well seated, the corner edge gouges a deep groove on the root surface. It also is a heavy, coarse instrument that is not particularly sensitive, and it has rather sharply limited application in subgingival work. It is not as maneuverable as the fine curet.

File. The file is in reality a miniature series of hoes on a single blade face. Its action is similar to that of the hoe, with the important variation of size. Because it can be made in very small, flat sizes, for example, the Hirschfeld-Dunlop files, it is especially suited to negotiate sharply constricted pocket orifices because it causes a minimum of tissue displacement on entry. It is used solely with a pull motion and is not a sensitive instrument in a tactile sense. Its use is therefore purely adjunctive and never primary. Even in fine sizes it is capable of some crushing of a flake of calculus. This is an important consideration when a deeply placed tenacious flake of calculus is encountered in tight quarters. It is, however, not easily sharpened.

Curet. The curet is a standard instrument for subgingival scaling. It is spoon shaped and has two blades along the edges of the elongated spoon. The working blade is the inner edge in pull curets, and the offset blade is the outer edge. In curets designed to be used with a push stroke the edges are just the reverse. Both push and pull curets are valuable and useful instruments.

Curets are made in various sizes. Generally speaking they should be fairly fine to enable them to negotiate constricted areas. An important consideration is that the shank be fairly rigid. An instrument of this sort that is too springy behaves in the manner of a shock absorber and does not transmit vibrations indicating roughness of the root surface. In addition the instrument gives instead of bites when some force is applied. This is important when a stubborn flake of calculus is encountered.

Grasp. The method in which the curet is grasped for use has often been misunderstood. It is almost always referred to as the pen grasp, but practice will show that such a grasp gives the utmost flexibility in maneuver to the instrument without conveying the controlled force and sensitive acuity to vibration so necessary to successful scaling.

It must be kept in mind that tactile values are foremost in this discipline. It is only through actual tactile sensations that the operator can determine performance level. For this reason the standard pen grasp, with the tips of the thumb and forefinger contacting the shank of the instrument and the middle finger tucked under the shank for complete maneuverability, sacrifices sensitivity for complete freedom of action.

In the correct grasp the tips of the thumb, forefinger, and middle finger are all in direct contact with the shank of the instrument. This position sacrifices some freedom of action in maneuver but retains enough to negotiate the arc necessary to complete the successful curetting stroke. On the other hand, the grasp conveys the sensitivity in tactile values so vital to a correct appraisal of the curetting effort.

Finger rests. The finger rest becomes an important factor in the scaling arc. Most operators use the third finger rest because this allows the widest possible arc of movement consistent with tactile acuity. There are some, however, who prefer the middle finger rest, using the same finger as one of the holding fingertips. This rest permits the use of great power but makes possible only a very short, constricted scaling arc. Another disadvantage is the fact that the rest must of necessity be immediately adjacent to the work area and not, as in the third finger rest, some distance removed if desired. The disadvantage of this constricted range of action is apparent in posterior teeth, where such proximity of rest to working blade is practically impossible in a normal mouth. That is not to say that the powerful stroke possible with the middle finger rest is not useful on isolated tenacious flakes of calculus. It is frequently used to dislodge such a calculus deposit. It is not, however, uniformly useful in the standard procedure of scaling.

Basic strokes. Having considered the grasp of the instrument and the finger rest used, let us turn to a brief review of the various strokes.

There are two basic strokes used with the curet in negotiating subgingival cementum: the exploratory stroke and the working stroke. In the exploratory stroke the instrument (the curet in this case) is held with a modified pen grasp and a feather-light purchase in the fingertips. The blade of the curet is inserted into the pocket, with the edge of the blade engaging the cementum surface. When the term "engage" is used in this sense, what is meant is "bite" of the blade so that a tactile sensation is manifest. This bite is feather light in the case of the exploratory stroke, but it is nonetheless in definite shaving contact with the root surface. The clinical sense of bite or shaving purchase with a sharp instrument is clearly felt and determined. In the exploratory stroke the curet blade is passed into the depth of the pocket and gently withdrawn in contact with the root to determine the topography of subgingival deposits in each arc made by the instrument. This stroke is repeated until the entire outline of the pocket is delineated both vertically and laterally so that the confines of the operative field are delimited. On meeting an apparent end or obstruction to the blade in exploration the dentist should lift the blade slightly from the root and gently attempt further extension. The blade might have been butting against a ledge of calculus and not the attachment as had been thought.

The working stroke is the same as the exploratory stroke except that it is initially a short power stroke, with blade engaging root surface, followed by a smoothing, shaving stroke done with finesse and absolute control. The shaving stroke is somewhat longer than the power stroke, which is designed to split or dislodge calculus from the root surface. The shaving stroke is not, however, so long and sweeping as the exploratory stroke discussed previously.

After the appropriate curet has been selected for the tooth surface being worked on, the instrument is placed against the root with the face of the blade toward the tooth. The angle between the face of the blade and the tooth surface should be closed so that the blade can enter the sulcular area easily. Often the shank of the instrument may interfere from complete closing of the blade; in this case the blade should be closed as much as possible. Once entrance has been made and the accretion bypassed, the blade should be opened to engage the calculus.

Both the power and shaving components of the working stroke are stepped to cover the entire root surface exposed by the pocket. This is best accomplished by the use of a fixed finger rest, with the greater part of the movement performed by a rocking motion of the wrist and forearm about this fulcrum and a comparatively minor but important part of the movement furnished by the contracture of the fingers holding the instrument.

It is possible to perform this operation in a routine fashion and to fail completely. Constant

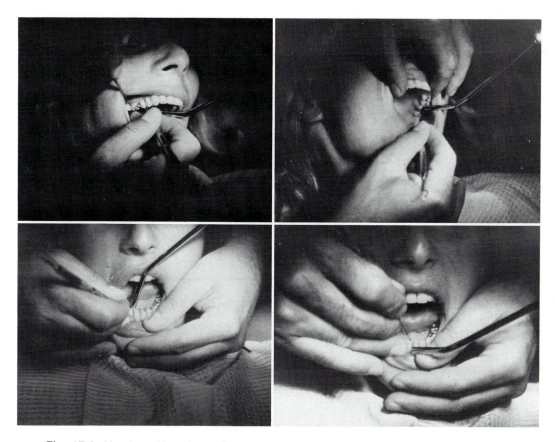

Fig. 17-6. Hand positions in scaling procedure. Note how left hand is retracting while right hand is operating. Finger rests are being employed to steady right hand so that short, precise working strokes are possible. Also note positions of suction tip.

alertness and tactile acuity must be maintained at all times to achieve a creditable performance of successful débridement.

The circumferential stroke is also useful in standard scaling. There are certain problem areas that make curettage in a vertical direction difficult and tedious. Line angles of molar roots are such areas. The circumferential stroke is very well suited to such an area as a finishing stroke, but is not too well adapted as a basic power stroke (Figs. 17-6 to 17-22).

Sharpening of instruments. Sharpening of instruments is essential if the operator is to use them successfully. The prime requisite in the sharpening of any instrument is that it shall maintain a predetermined angle to the stone. Hoes are sharpened with a flat stone, whereas curets are best sharpened with a cylindric or tapered stone used on the face of the instrument, thereby sharpening both cutting edges simultaneously. The instrument must at all times have a definite keen edge so that it may accomplish the task to which it is put.

Curets may be sharpened with a mounted Moyco Ruby stone or a no. 186 Carborundum stone that has two flat surfaces and two rounded edges, each with a different curvature. The smaller curvature is for the smaller curets, and the larger is for the sickle scaler and large curets. The flat surfaces are used to sharpen the hoe scalers, but they also may be used to shave down the outer surfaces of the curet blades. Very small knife-edged Arkansas stones or small jeweler's files are used to sharpen the files. The sharpened instruments may be tested for their sharpness by scraping against the fingernail. If a small stroke is made with light pressure, with the instrument held at the angle usually used against the root surface, a minute bit of the nail should be shaved off. If the instrument glides over the nail surface, it requires more sharpening.

SCALING

In root scaling the objective of removing all irritants from the subgingival operative field has another aspect: to allow for remission from edema

Text continued on p. 485.

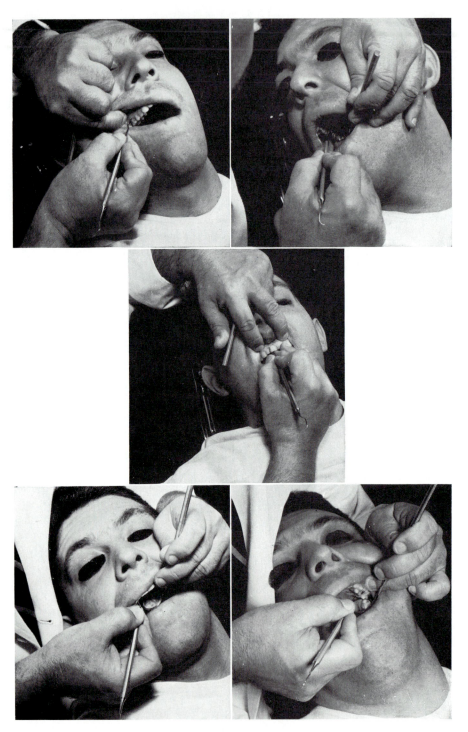

Fig. 17-7. Hand positions and finger rests for scaling maxillary teeth.

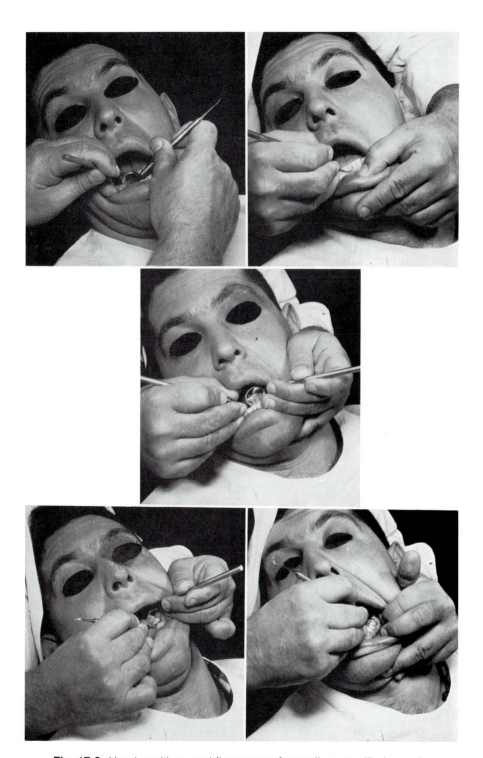

Fig. 17-8. Hand positions and finger rests for scaling mandibular teeth.

Fig. 17-9. Instrument should be held between thumb and the index and third fingers, grasped firmly but not tightly enough to cramp muscles of fingers or to tire them during scaling procedure. A proper grasp allows for easy rolling of instrument by thumb between index and third fingers. This type of grasp is a modification of the hold of a writing instrument. Other two fingers are used for a rest or perch from which movements can be made. Thus instrument can be pivoted on a fulcrum, allowing for necessary wrist movement associated with scaling procedure and permitting instrument to be placed subgingivally and to be moved in and out in a straight line. This grasp also allows for a high degree of sensitivity to touch, an indispensable quality needed to discover and remove calculus. Holding instrument lightly but firmly, with a positive rest either on a tooth or at some position away from operative area, operator introduces instrument into pocket. He should have complete control of instrument, allowing it to transmit sensations that can be translated into topography and contents of pocket. If instrument is grasped tightly, fingertips become less sensitive, thus making it impossible to perform scaling procedure either completely or without pain to the patient. Not only are placement and type of instrument important in scaling procedure, but also positions of fingers are important, that is, those of left hand in retraction and those of right hand assuming proper finger rests to control instrument properly. A rest is obtained for second and third fingers as near as possible to site of operating area. An adjacent tooth, a finger of left hand, or external site on face may serve as a location for rest. In this illustration a curet is being placed on mesial surface of maxillary right second molar. Note that an external site on face is serving as a rest position. Working edge of blade is placed against surface of tooth and will be brought down in a short stroke.

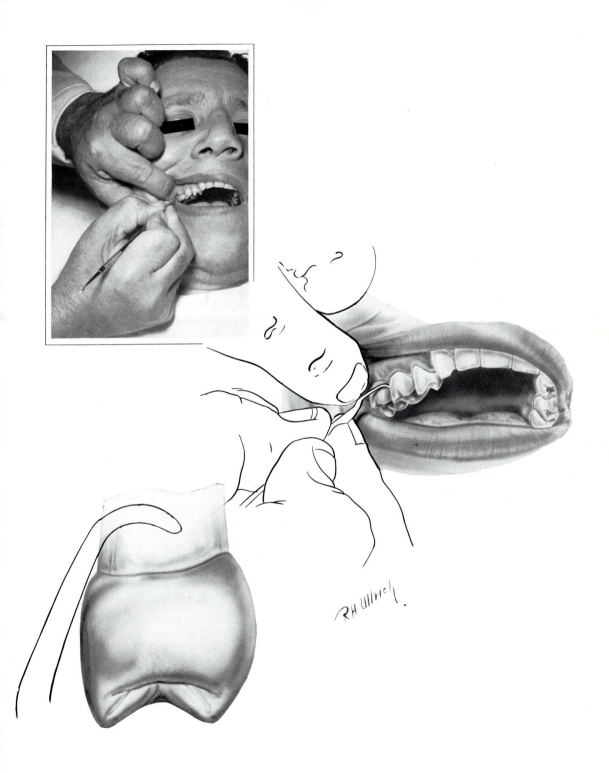

Fig. 17-10. In pull stroke instrument is inserted to base of pocket, traveling along soft tissue side and engaging lower edge of calculus. With a short pull stroke toward mouth of pocket calculus is dislodged. Several short strokes may be necessary. It is best to keep strokes short, generally within pocket. This pull stroke is extremely effective in removal of large subgingival calculus deposits. It can be performed without too much discomfort to patient, especially if care is taken in inserting instrument and in keeping strokes short, thereby not tearing soft tissue. It is improper handling of soft tissue that makes scaling painful to patient. Push-pull stroke is often effective but can be used with only certain instruments. This procedure consists of moving instrument along tooth surface in a continuous to-and-fro movement that will crush or crack any calculus present. It should be employed in removing thin, hard, adherent deposits of calculus that cannot be disengaged by pull motion. This stroke must be executed carefully, with care that all calculus has been removed and not merely rounded over; also soft tissue should not be torn in movement. In this stroke movements should be short, and instruments should convey to operator condition of tooth surface. Push stroke is most difficult to perform correctly because of character of motion. It must be employed with instruments designed for this stroke; however, once mastered, stroke is highly effective. Instrument is placed on tooth surface at mouth of pocket and inserted. Thin, hard pieces of calculus will be removed. Smooth tooth surfaces can be obtained in this fashion. Movement of instrument in pocket should be smooth. This is effected by a coordination of grasp and a movement or rock of hand; coordination is result of wrist action. Thus finger muscles do not quickly become fatigued, which would result in impairment of tactile sense so necessary for proper control and working of instrument. Application of a curet against mesiolingual surface of maxillary molar may be seen in this illustration. Note rest position and retraction of lip.

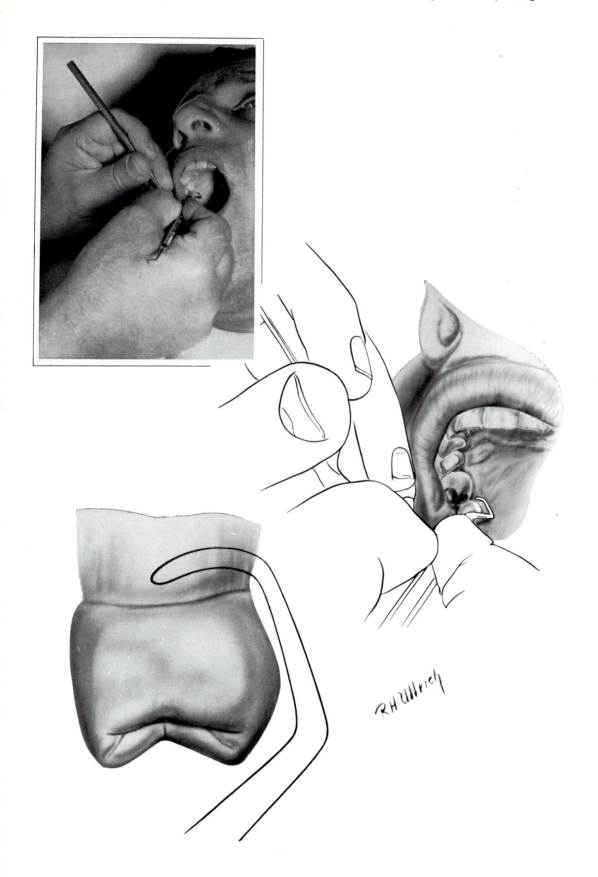

Fig. 17-11. A Goldman-Fox no. 2 instrument is being inserted into pocket on mesial aspect against root of maxillary first premolar, approaching it from buccal side. This is a curet; angulation of blade shaft allows blade to be inserted in the pocket from buccal or mesial side, keeping cutting edge parallel to tooth surface (closed position). In this way very depth of pocket can be reached. Any stroke can be utilized with this instrument. Head of instrument bypasses deposit and engages it (open position). With a pulling motion directed downward and slightly buccally the instrument head moves slowly and deliberately along the tooth surface. Scaler no.1 is also useful. Access with this instrument is easy. Position of head and stance of operator are especially important in working on palatal surfaces. When working on right side, operator turns patient's head away and tilts it upward, allowing for direct vision of this area. Chair should be tilted back so that patient's head can be placed in proper position more easily. When working on left side, operator turns patient's head toward him. Care must be taken that line angles of root are cleansed as well, for often only broad surfaces of tooth are scaled. If operator is uncertain whether all calculus deposits have been removed, he can use a fine explorer to examine tooth surface. Instruments designed for the purpose, for example, Cross probe, can be used effectively. Retracting gingival wall, thereby extending mouth of pocket by use of a warm air blast, is an extremely useful adjunct. A positive check for interproximal surfaces can be made by use of roentgenograms.

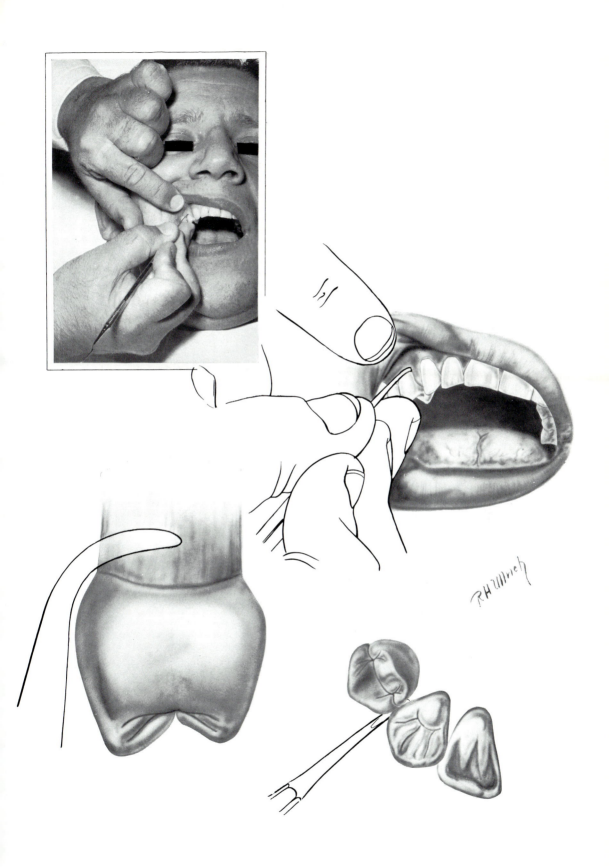

Fig. 17-12. As anterior portion of jaw is reached, access becomes easier, and working view is direct. In this instance a curet is being placed on labial surface of maxillary left central incisor. Retraction of upper lip is being accomplished by thumb and forefinger of left hand, while grasp of instrument and finger rest allow for complete control in placement and movement. It is of utmost importance that all calculus deposits be removed completely. Therefore it is expedient to work within a small field of a few square millimeters at a time, removing calculus completely. Otherwise, as instrumentation continues, deposits may become decreased in size and finer, making them more difficult to remove. Many failures are result of operator's inability to recognize presence of deposits or result of his inability to remove them. This is especially true of subgingival deposits as well as thin coatings of calculus that may remain after large deposits have been eliminated. These fine plaques serve as retention areas for further calculus formation, hastening the process of deposition. Thus calculus should not be shaved off in layers, but rather the entire thickness of the particular section should be removed in toto if possible. Root surface must be freed of all coatings—the smoother the surface, the better will be the chances of its remaining free of further depositions. Operator must develop a sense of feel when applying an instrument to the tooth surface. He must be able to distinguish various sensations, interpreting them so that he may operate effectively. Calculus formations, irregularities of root surface, and other contours must be recognized. Whereas heavy deposits can be made out easily, thinner pieces are felt as grainy substances, in contrast to smooth surface of tooth. Pocket must be explored for deposits prior to the scaling, and exploration must be repeated in detail during and after procedure. Since pockets may have irregular shapes, it is essential to detect to their limits all calculus that may be present. Although scaling procedure consists of operating as effectively as possible in a single sitting, it is not infrequent that some deposits are left behind. Careful examination at a subsequent sitting and repetition of scaling procedure are indicated. Thus, although scaling procedure can be done on a single visit, cleansing all the particular teeth at that time, it is wise and often advantageous to treat mouth in work areas. This allows for more time to be spent on a single location and does not tax patient excessively. Also on subsequent visits, areas previously operated on can be rechecked. Gingival health, as determined by color, tone of tissue, and condition of attachment area, can be evaluated. Testing for suppuration can be done.

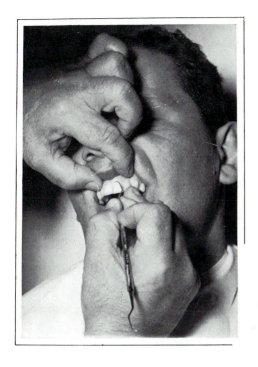

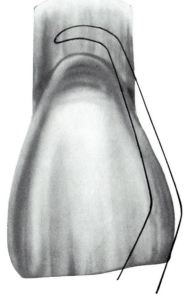

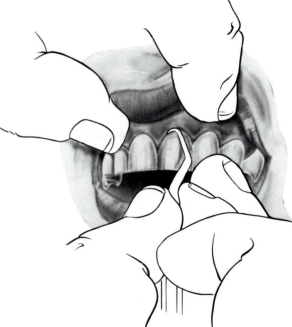

RHUllrich

Fig. 17-13. Palatal aspect of maxillary central incisor is approached via indirect vision. Finger rest is on right premolar area. In description of scaling operation position of head of patient, operator's stance and position (standing or sitting), and placement of hands (left hand for retraction and occasionally even for perch of finger rest and right hand for instrument grasp and finger rest) are important considerations. Depending on these, opposites in angulation of heads of instruments may be employed for identical areas. By changing hand position and stance operator may employ an edge used on mesial surface of a tooth on distal surface. In this instance operator is standing slightly back and to the right of the patient. Note that curvature of blade approximates tooth surface closely. Routine use of topical anesthetics and in some instances local anesthesia is of extreme benefit in keeping patient comfortable and in allowing the operator to work more easily. The operator, however, should be aware that careful handling of soft tissues and good control of the instrument reduce operative pain. When using a topical anesthetic, operator saturates a cotton pledget with solution and applies it to gingivae. He then places a drop of solution in pocket with instrument to be used before instrumentation. When teeth are very sensitive, infiltration anesthesia may be employed.

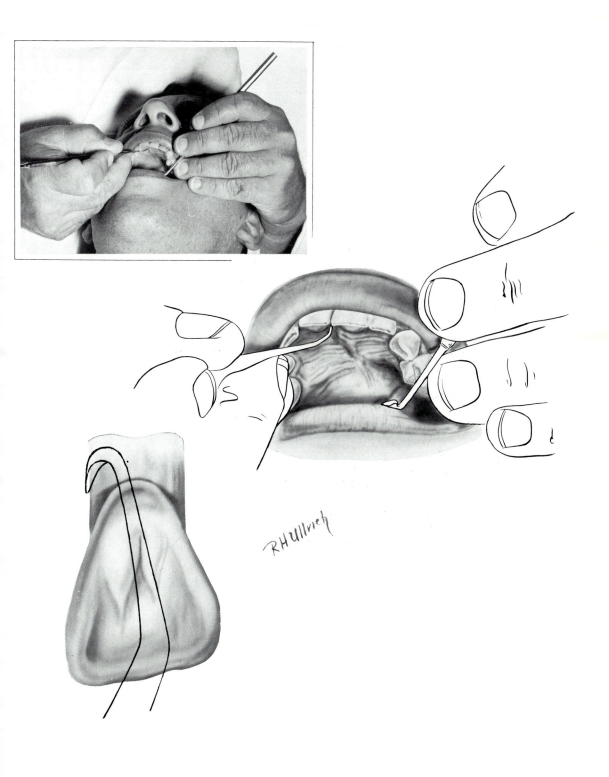

Fig. 17-14. Approach of maxillary left side. Mesiobuccal aspect of first molar is being scaled by a curet. Patient's head is tilted back and slightly to the right. Forefinger of left hand serves as a retractor for access to operative site. Instrument is held in a modified pen grasp and is positioned in such a manner that angulated part of blade is closely adapted to tooth surface. Control of instrument is achieved by placing terminal phalange of third finger against first and second molars while palm of hand cups the chin. This allows for ease of approach and for simple short strokes employed in a deliberate fashion, which requires little in the way of arm motion, and thus added extraoral rest is satisfactory. Operator is standing to left and slightly in front of patient. There are several suggestions for instrumentation that are pertinent. They are as follows:

1. Be sure that instruments are as sharp as possible.
2. Work by direct vision whenever possible.
3. Have control of instrument, employing proper finger rests and grasp.
4. Employ proper strokes and correct relationship of instrument blade to the tooth.
5. Do not traumatize soft tissues unnecessarily.
6. Make sure that all calculus has been removed and that tooth surface is smooth.
7. Make stroke short. It should include only deposit on tooth. Any longer stroke is of no value, since effective portion of the stroke is that part when blade is in contact with tooth and calculus.
8. Use topical anesthesia or in some instances local anesthesia to keep patient comfortable during operative procedure.
9. Realize importance of procedure in overall therapy of periodontal diseases.

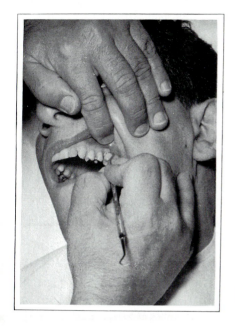

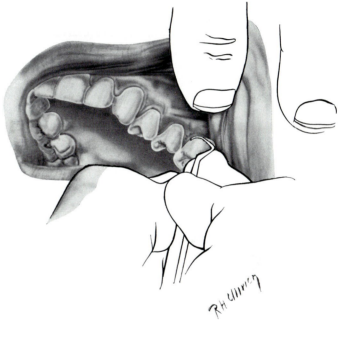

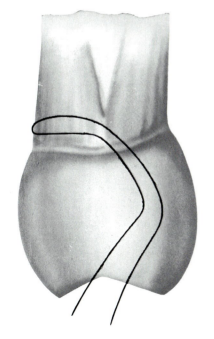

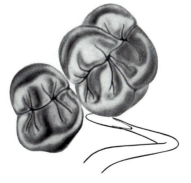

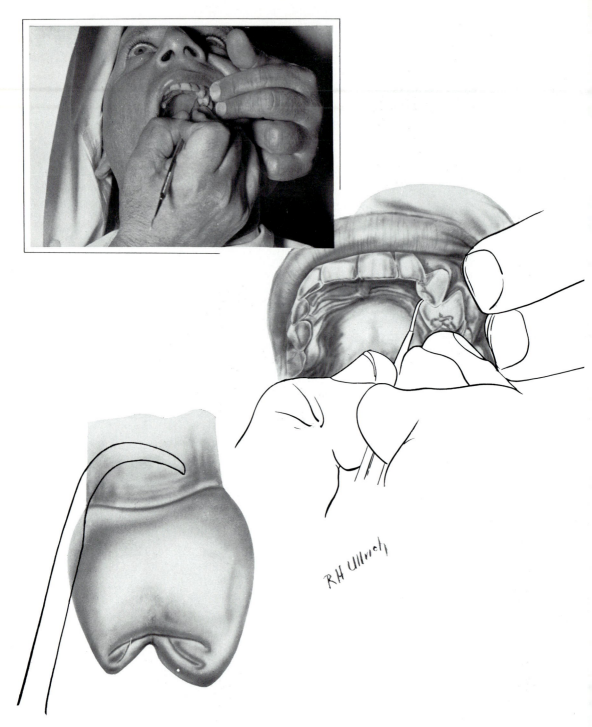

RH Ullrich

Fig. 17-15. Approach to maxillary left side, first premolar area. Instrumentation is being done via direct approach. Patient's head is slightly turned away from operator and is tilted upward. Operator stands in front and to side of patient so that there will be direct access to area. Retraction of upper left lip is accomplished by first and second fingers of left hand. Instrument is held in a modified pen grasp and is placed on mesial aspect of first premolar, with third finger being used as a rest on second premolar. Instrument, while held firmly, is not grasped too tightly lest operator lose sense of feel of instrument. If instrumentation were done via reflection through dental mirror, operator would stand to right of and slightly behind patient. Scaling stroke consists of placing cutting edge of the instrument against tooth surface at closed position and opening it directly apical to and in contact with calculus deposit. With a slight rotary motion of arm from elbow, operator pulls instrument toward occlusal surface with a short forceful stroke.

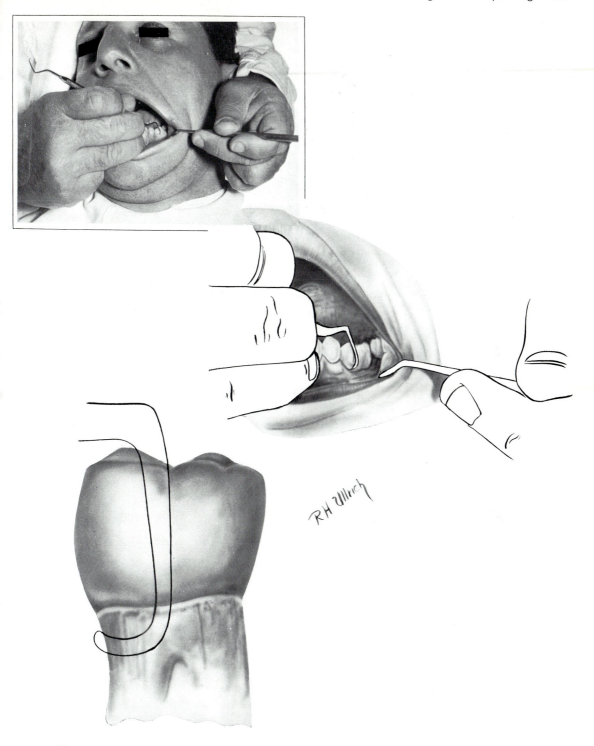

Fig. 17-16. Buccomandibular left side, premolar, and molar regions may be operated on by direct vision. Patient's head is tilted to right and upward. Operator is standing in back and slightly to right of patient. Left arm encircles head, and mirror retracts lip. Finger rest is on labioincisal surface of left anterior teeth. In this instance curet is being placed on mesiobuccal angle, with concave surface against tooth to draw blade onto mesial surface. Lingual surface of mandibular left side may be approached from patient's right, left arm encircling head. Left side is retracted by second and third fingers as dental mirror is utilized to displace tongue. By tilting mirror correctly operator can reflect additional light onto right anterior incisor–cuspid–first premolar area. Necessarily instrument, although held in modified pen grasp, is grasped long. Depending on situation, Goldman-Fox nos. 2, 3, and 4 curets or Younger-Good nos. 13 and 14 curets may be used.

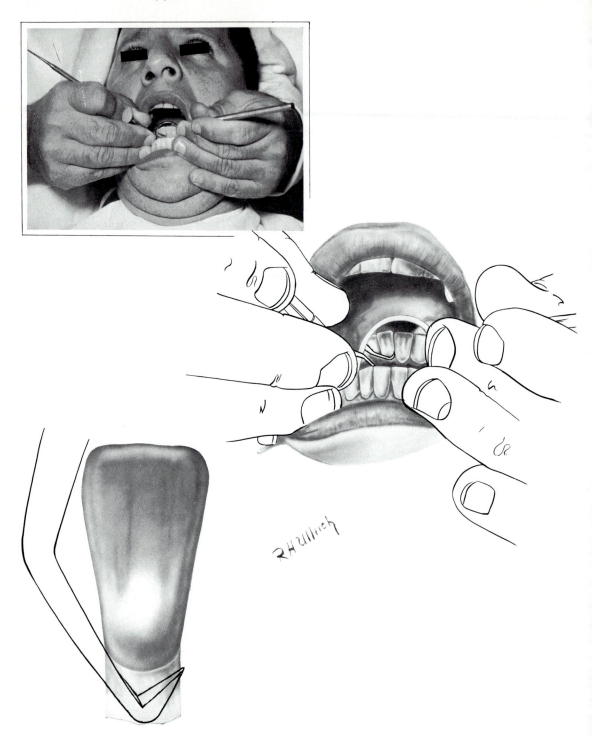

Fig. 17-17. Finger rest, grasp of instrument, and retraction of lower lip for instrumentation of lingual surfaces of mandibular teeth. Operator is standing to right of and almost completely behind patient. Left arm encircles patient's head. Mirror acts as a tongue retractor and also reflects light onto operative site. Actually in this stance operative area can be seen by direct vision. Once scaling procedure has been finished, surfaces of these teeth can be checked by operator standing behind and to the left of patient; with aid of a mirror, he can view teeth easily and in this way can easily approach mesiolingual surfaces of lower incisors.

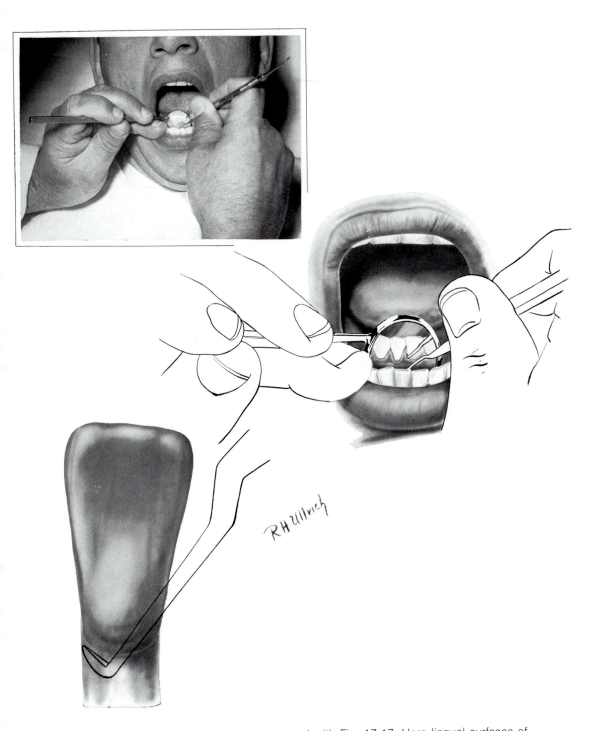

Fig. 17-18. This illustration may be compared with Fig. 17-17. Here lingual surfaces of mandibular incisors are approached from a stance in front of patient. Operator is standing to right and in front of patient, whose head should be tilted downward. Dental mirror is used to retract tongue and to reflect light onto operative area; third finger is used to retract lip. Third finger of right hand is used as a finger rest; it is located on left premolar area. Labial surfaces of mandibular anterior teeth are approached from right, with operator standing slightly behind patient. Left arm encircles head, and thumb acts as a retractor. Left hand holds mandible at same time. Finger rest is on labial surface of adjacent teeth to right.

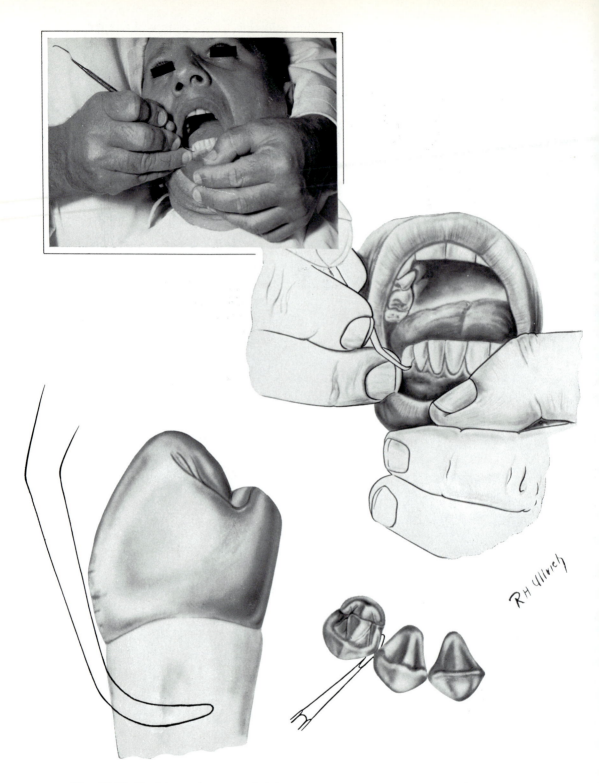

Fig. 17-19. Mesiobuccal aspect of right premolar area is approached from right, with operator standing to right and in back of patient. Left hand supports mandible, and thumb is used as a retractor for lip. Operative area is seen by direct vision. Instrument is held in modified pen grasp, with third finger placed on buccal surfaces of adjacent posterior teeth as a finger rest. First molar may also be approached in a similar fashion, but usually operator must change his stance to move more to side of patient and sometimes to front, changing finger rest to anterior teeth. A change in instruments is necessary when stance of operator is varied. Also, when posterior teeth are scaled, instrument with a longer shank is necessary so that blade can be positioned correctly.

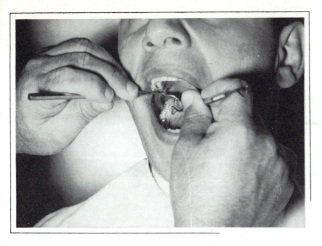

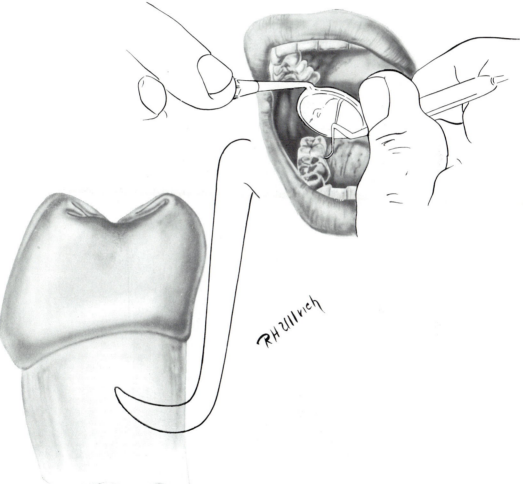

Fig. 17-20. Instrumentation on lingual surface of lower right side. Note instrument grasp with instrument being held long. Note also retraction of lower lip and rest position on left anterior teeth, with reflection of light onto operative area by dental mirror. Operator is standing in front and slightly to left of patient. Patient's head is held slightly to left and down, allowing for direct vision of region to be scaled. Because of long hold of instrument operator must be careful of its use, directing stroking in a precise manner. Oftentimes instrument may be held in normal fashion, short and with finger rest in cuspid area of same side. Operator approaches lingual surface with blade parallel to tooth surface. In many instances he may stand to right of patient and, with reflected image from dental mirror, approach these surfaces with suitable instruments. Head is tilted to right so that lingual surfaces become parallel to operator, thus making for an easier approach.

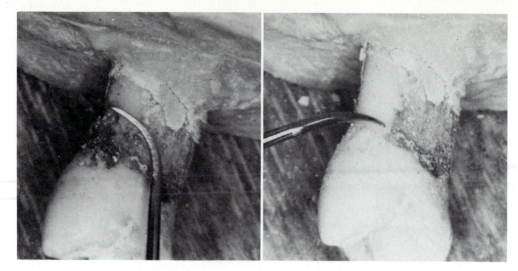

Fig. 17-21. Scaling procedure utilizing curet. Blade is in open position and stroke started at terminus of calculus deposit and continued, breaking up calculus deposit and freeing it from tooth surface. Material brought to orifice will be picked up by suction. Any material remaining on instrument will be removed by suction prior to reentry. Right photograph shows root surface planed and smooth.

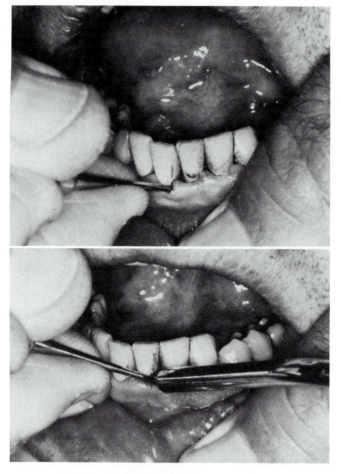

Fig. 17-22. Suctioning accretion at orifice is important. Note how closely suction tip is applied to gingiva. Assistant must be able to move tip as operator moves instrument. Once instrument is out, it must be cleansed by suction. In top photograph, entry beyond calculus deposit has been made. Note retraction of gingiva. In lower photograph scaling stroke has been made; assistant is now suctioning away freed calculus.

and inflammation and to contain the inflammatory process. The dentist performing this aspect of instrumentation may reverse the curet blade so that it engages the soft tissue side. Since it is soft tissue that is now being curetted, the tactile value of the bite of the blade is missing. Soft tissue gives no such response to the instrument. In addition the tissue itself must often be stabilized to the action of the curet so that it is not displaced with each stroke, thus preventing curettage. This stabilization is easily achieved on the buccal and lingual surfaces by the placement of a finger of the left hand on the gingiva to fix it. The blade can then be felt through the thickness of the gingiva as a faint ripple. Only a few strokes are needed to complete sulcular débridement, using the curet in a circumferential stroke throughout the entire confines of the pocket.

Mention has been made several times of the absolute requirements of instrumentation. Lest the absoluteness of these requirements discourage the therapist in the practical development of his skill in this direction, let him be reminded that this is the one aspect of therapy that can be repeated, with no loss of tissue to the patient or any compromise in the final result. What counts most here is not the time factor but the completeness of the effort. Repetition of the method is no barrier to quality.

Instrumentation can be called the basic skill in the practice of periodontics.

Scaling by ultrasonic instrument

Ultrasonic vibrations are mechanical in nature and are the same as sound waves but of a frequency range above that audible to the human ear. The instrument used is an ultrasonic power generator that delivers vibrational mechanical energy with a water supply to specially designed tips. A wide variety of tips is available. They must be so contoured that they can be placed in direct contact with the tooth surface so as to remove any accretion. Some of the tips are blunt; others are sharp. Only blunt tips are recommended for supragingival and subgingival calculus removal. Water is utilized to cool the instrument head as heat is liberated by the sound waves. Cutting down the water supply causes heating of the instrument. In operation the water is pounded against the tooth at a rate of many thousands of times per second. The operator must be aware that unless contact is made by the instrument against the calculus the calculus will not be dislodged. The instrument is useful in the removal of calculus, but root planing is not possible (Fig. 17-23).

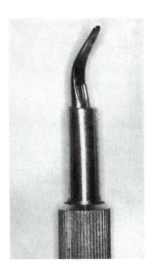

Fig. 17-23. Tip used for scaling in an ultrasonic machine. Note that edges of end are rounded and whole tip is blunt.

In the use of the ultrasonic instrument the therapist must develop a manipulative sense, since there is no tactile ability; also the hanging cord at the end of the instrument is a new sensation for the dentist. The operator must be capable of feeling uneven spots on the tooth surface and of placing the point against this area, thus allowing the instrument to work. Distention of the gingival tissue when approaching subgingival areas is necessary. Because of the water flow the whole sulcular area is flushed. The instrument therefore must be angulated to allow for this flushing effect. All debris and accretions are prone to be washed away, which is a decided advantage, but of course control of the overflow of water into the mouth by an efficient suction apparatus is necessary.

The ease of manipulation and the rapid removal of supragingival calculus make for an advantage of ultrasonic scaling in this respect. Subgingival scaling, however, is more difficult, and the technique must be mastered. The flat surfaces of the tooth are moderately easily reached, but concavities must be covered carefully with the instrument. However, this is also true for hand instrument scaling.

Coronal scaling

Instruments used in coronal scaling are classed as chisels, sickle scalers, hoe scalers, curets, and modifications of each. All of these are obtainable in various sizes from fine to heavy, but they all generally are limited to removal of coarse, gross deposits, and most of them are confined to supragingival use. Some slight subgingival application is possible by compression of the gingiva so that a ledge of calculus may be engaged, but that is about the extent of their subgingival use, except in wide-mouthed pockets. These may be inserted for variable distances, but they are suited only for coarse deposits, and the dangers of root damage are always present in their subgingival use.

For the most part, the coronal deposits to be removed can be fairly well visualized. We will concern ourselves therefore only with the working or power stroke and not with the exploratory techniques. The working stroke is a short powerful, dislodging stroke executed with controlled force. The instrument is held with the modified pen grasp.

In even a superficial examination of the dentition it will be seen that there is an affinity of calculus deposition to certain locations, for example, the lingual surfaces of the lower anterior teeth and the buccal surfaces of the upper molars. As in all generalities there are exceptions to this distribution of calculus, but for the most part it holds true in clinical experience.

In a situation of overlapping, common in crowded anterior teeth, access is particularly difficult in the interproximal areas. For such teeth a chisel of extremely fine caliber or a small thin sickle scaler (Goldman-Fox no. 21) is useful in removing the very thin flakes of calculus interproximally. For stain on the approximating surfaces linen strips with a fine garnet texture are excellent polishing agents. Fine sickle scalers are also useful in removing stain from comparatively inaccessible areas.

Subgingival scaling

Subgingival scaling, as has been mentioned previously, is a technique of root surface cleansing. In those areas in which subgingival calculus is present in large or small quantities, it affects the removal of these accretions. It is also designed to plane and scrape the root surface so that the

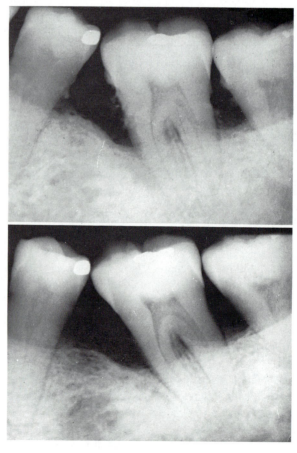

Fig. 17-24. Preoperative and postoperative scaling. Note that calculus has been removed in lower roentgenogram.

surface presents a clean, smooth aspect unmarred by roughness and foreign material. There is, during instrumentation, an added inadvertent side effect. Due to the offset blade of the curets used in subgingival scaling, some gingival lining is removed while the root surface is being treated. In many if not most cases the epithelial attachment is also removed with the same inadvertence. This attendant action is treated more fully in chapter concerning curettage.

An important sequel to subgingival scaling is the unavoidable extravasation of blood that attends any instrumentation of these areas when the gingival tissues are hyperemic and ulcerated. The gingiva not only is hyperemic but also is afflicted with localized circulatory stasis. Some of the actual enlargement is due both to edema and to the entrapped blood. The minor bloodletting relieves this localized stasis more quickly than would be the case, it seems, if the blood were allowed to remain. It is obvious that this gingival bleeding is automatic and unavoidable in instrumentation (Figs. 17-24 to 17-28).

Whether the removal of calculus and the general cleansing of the pocket will prove *completely* effective in attaining the remission from gingival inflammation and other sequelae depends upon the following two factors:

1. In a low-grade chronic inflammation such as is commonly found in periodontal pockets there is a tendency for fibrosis to occur if the process has been in operation for a considerable length of time. This is merely an attempt at healing on the part of the involved tissue and is a

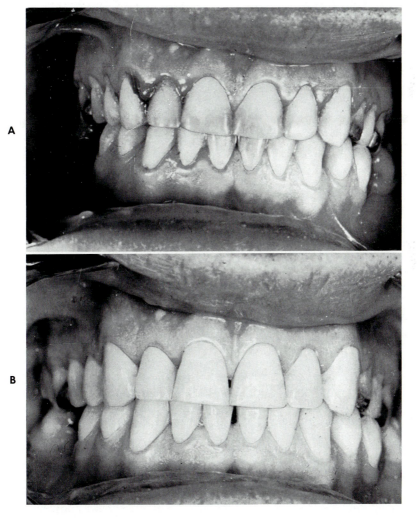

Fig. 17-25. Before, **A,** and after, **B,** a scaling procedure. Note healing that has resulted and changes in gingival form.

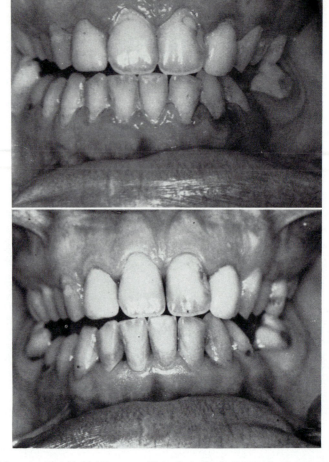

Fig. 17-26. After results of initial therapy. Note that gingival margins have assumed a more physiologic architectural form and that they hug gingivae closely. Evaluation at this time will decide further therapy concerning gingivae.

Fig. 17-27. Results of scaling teeth. Removal of direct irritants, especially calculus, is first phase of initial therapy. This procedure consists of scaling and polishing teeth thoroughly. It is not good practice to apply procedure indiscriminately. Instead each tooth in succession should be thoroughly scaled and polished. Since scaling is best done systematically, one should begin instrumentation as well as polishing at a definite point and continue it in such a way that certain surfaces of teeth will not be overlooked. It matters little what system is adopted so long as it is followed regularly. Treatment should remove all accretions from root surfaces of teeth. Operator should develop a firm yet soft touch, and gentle handling of lips, cheeks, and tongue should be carefully observed. The object of scaling teeth is to eliminate as many irritants of gingiva as possible. Shrinkage of gingival tissue occurs with resolution of inflammation. The amount, however, is dependent on character of tissue. Operator may often be surprised to see how many pockets heal and that gingivae assume a physiologic architecture after thorough scaling. Many operators prefer to scale a group of teeth at one time, using one instrument for same surface of group, then using another instrument for another surface. When all surfaces are completed, next group of teeth may be approached. This procedure reduces number of times that instruments must be picked up and laid down. When large numbers and single-headed instruments are used, this method is especially advantageous. With fewer and double-ended instruments it is not as necessary. Thus in this manner each tooth must be scaled carefully; however, not only must all calculus be removed, but contents of pockets must be removed also. Once scaling has been performed, tissues may be irrigated thoroughly with hot water to remove any adherent debris between teeth. Note resolution of inflammation and shrinkage of tissue in this illustration. After healing, following initial therapy, periodontal status is evaluated for further therapy.

physiologic reaction to injury. If such is the case it may be masked in the generalized enlargement of the gingival tissues due to edema and attendant phenomena. It is only when these are resolved that the residual fibrosis or scarring becomes manifest. This fibrosis does not disappear when the irritant is removed but must be corrected by surgery.

2. When the gingival lining in the pocket degenerates an extensive proliferation of the rete pegs of the pocket epithelium, ulceration, and a general indolent hyperemia of the soft tissue wall of the pocket occur. If allowed to remain long enough this process sets up a dynamics of its own so that the removal of the irritant, the subgingival calculus, does not by itself relieve the soft tissue signs. In these instances curettage is indicated to remove the gingival lining so that the sulcus becomes lined by an intact, healthy epithelium. Shrinkage of the gingival tissue will ensue, depending on the nature of the tissue.

This process is an equivocal one in that the

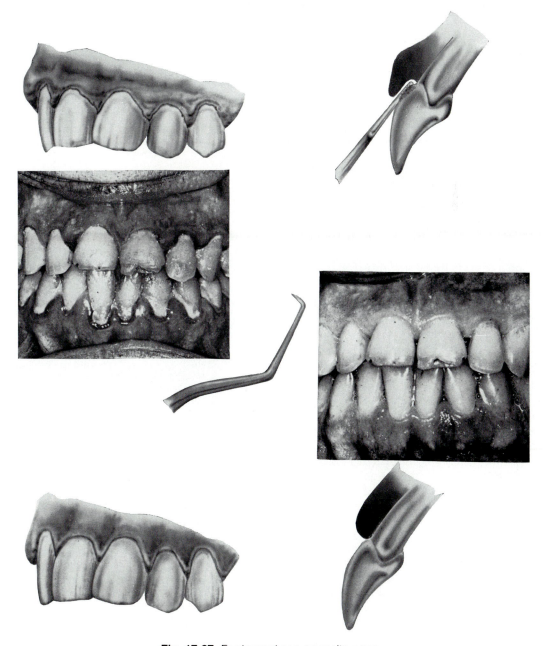

Fig. 17-27. For legend see opposite page.

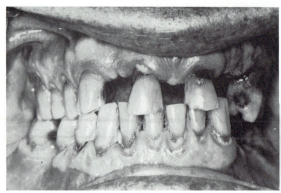

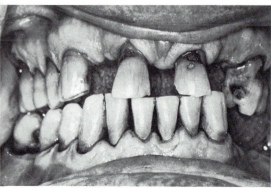

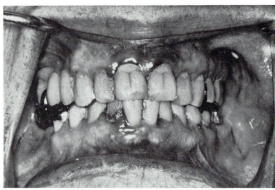

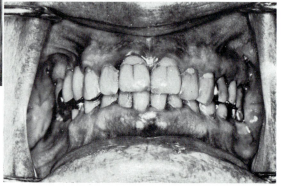

Fig. 17-28. Ideal way to teach instrumentation is to observe student as he removes calculus, making recommendations as he works and illustrating instrument grasp and finger rests for him. Of great benefit, however, is student's participation in preclinical instruction on removal of calculus from Dentoform teeth placed in a mannequin. Roots of teeth are covered with a mixture of plaster of Paris and shellac to simulate calculus. Teeth are placed in the mannequin, and student is taught methods of instrumentation and scaling. Once operation is completed, he can remove teeth from mannequin and inspect them as to effectiveness of his scaling. Student must also be taught principles regarding handling of soft tissue. Tearing and traumatization of tissue only retard healing. Postoperative evaluation of calculus removal and gingival healing should be discussed by student and instructor. In this illustration results of two cases of scaling, essential component of initial therapy, are depicted. Both cases represent severe periodontal involvements characterized by deep pocket formation, retraction of gingival tissue, heavy calculus formation, bleeding, and suppuration. Postscaling evaluation determines remaining therapy.

pocket wall is usually peeled off incident to root surface scaling, as mentioned previously, and many of our successful results are due to both the scaling and débridement plus the accidental curetting of the gingival wall. There are times, however, when this does not occur, and the soft tissue curettage must be performed as a separate operation.

In root surface scaling the requirements in performance level are high. It can be seen that any subtotal removal of accretions will allow the soft tissue wall to continue to remain in contact with rough, septic calculus, which will elicit the same inflammatory response from the tissues. Root planing requires the removal of any soft or necrotic cementum. The passage of a sharp instrument over a thoroughly planed root will cause a screeching sound. The root surface will feel glasslike to the instrument.

Considered in its true light, root surface scaling allows the soft tissues to shrink through the reduction of edema, hyperemia, and stasis. It is in subgingival scaling that both the exploratory stroke and the power stroke of the instrument come into the fullest play. In this technique the instrument becomes the eyes and ears of the operator, since all the sensations are tactile. It is through the instrument that all sensations of roughness or smoothness are realized because the operative field is hidden from the operator. It is for this reason that a few words on the condition of the instrument will not be amiss.

There is an old adage in periodontics to the effect that nothing lies like a dull curet. This is true because a dull curet blade burnishes and does not bite or engage calculus. It sends no vibrations through the shank to warn its user that rough area has been encountered. It must be stressed that this is the only avenue that we have for critical evaluation of subgingival scaling performance.

It is for this reason that experienced operators are constantly sharpening their curets and scalers, and it is for this reason that the curet blades, particularly, wear down rather quickly. Every periodontist has many of these worn-out, or rather "sharpened out," curets ready to be discarded. However, they make ideal instruments for checking on scaling performed with other and more sturdy instruments. Since they are extremely thin and sharp, they are extremely sensitive in exploration and evaluation when used with a light, delicate exploratory stroke. Of course their delicacy makes them useless for a working stroke, but they are ideal for checking.

Moskow has demonstrated that tears in the gingival wall during scaling may account for the presence of much of the foreign material seen in sulcular areas and that bits of calculus embedded in the gingival tissues will elicit severe foreign body reactions. Kohler and Ramfjord have noted pieces of calculus in the gingiva 112 days after operation. Because of these findings the therapist must exercise care in the scaling procedure. The pull stroke, therefore, is most likely to be the safest and most thorough means of irrigating the sulcular area in order to rid the region of any foreign material. The use of adequate suction is recommended.

Hard deposits are usually removed by firm, short strokes of a curet; these are called work strokes. The blade should bypass the calculus in the placement of the instrument and begin the removal at the apical edge of the deposit, trying to break the accretion away from the tooth surface in one piece rather than shaving it off bit by bit. The blade angle to the tooth should be about 75 to 85 degrees, thus allowing the blade edge to catch the calculus; the blade should be placed firmly so that the instrument will not slip over the deposit. At times the calculus may be so adherent that it will be difficult to budge the deposit. Under this circumstance it is often wise to crack the calculus with the blade and then remove the deposit or to reposition the blade laterally and take the edge of the accretion off. This will tend to loosen the deposit from the tooth surface. If the deposit is still resistant it may be wise to use a periodontal hoe; this instrument must be carefully employed, but if correctly placed and engaged, a pull stroke will dislodge the deposit. Once the calculus is thought to be removed the therapist should carefully explore the tooth surface with the instrument to make sure that all the accretion has been removed. If there is still roughness the area should be planed carefully. Oftentimes the instrument blade might be dull; if so it should either be sharpened or another instrument should be used.

Tenacious calculus. The mode of attachment of calculus to the tooth surface has been investigated. So far as can be determined there are various types of attachment: (1) simple apposition, (2) attachment with a cuticle, and (3) projection into the cementum or resorption areas of cementum. The last is so tenacious that a major effort is necessary to remove it. Frequently it cannot be dislodged successfully without removing some of the adjacent cemental surface. Care must be taken when such a situation is encountered subgingivally not merely to smooth over and plane the surface of the calculus. For this reason it is advisable to check on performance with an exploratory stroke of a fine curet when visual examination is not possible. The use of hoes in such an area is indicated, but care must be taken with the corners of the instrument. The objective is a splitting or scaling of the entire flake of calculus and not a shaving or planing action.

ROOT PLANING

Root planing on a tooth is performed after calculus deposits have been removed. Its purpose is to eliminate any roughness of the tooth surface that may occur during the scaling procedure. This roughness may be small, adherent, residual bits of calculus or even be the tooth surface itself; also it may be a slight defect due to instrumentation. Root planing, properly performed, will smooth the surface. The blade must be sharp, and the strokes must be smooth, short, and precise without too much pressure; overlapping strokes are utilized. The operator must make sure that the planing is done evenly and must not allow the blade to skip over the surface. The objective of the root planing technique is to eliminate any roughness, but in no way should it cause any new defect.

CONTROL OF BLEEDING

Bleeding of the gingivae during instrumentation is unavoidable, and the operator should not defer the removal of deposits for this reason. Although he or she should guard against the laceration and destruction of tissue, scaling must be thorough. Bleeding of tissue is caused by the removal of calculus and disturbance of the gingiva. The epithelial lining is ulcerated when calculus is attached to the teeth, and it is through these ulcerated areas that bleeding takes place. The use of suction by an assistant perhaps offers the best aid in the control of bleeding during the scaling procedure. Pressure with sponges against the gingiva during scaling is also a valuable aid.

POLISHING

Many clinicians find it useful to employ a disclosing solution before beginning polishing. This practice is a helpful one to dramatize to the patient the general inefficiency of his efforts if indeed they are inefficient, and to reveal to the operator the extent of calcareous and mucinous deposition on the teeth. Its use is not limited to preoperative application but is an excellent preparation to check on one's efforts after the prophylaxis is completed.

The formula and methods of application are found in Chapter 18.

The object of polishing is to remove plaque as well as soft deposits from the teeth. The polishing of the area at the gingival margin creates an optimum environment for the gingiva in that it presents no source of irritation. The plaque can be discovered easily by the use of disclosing solution. It infiltrates the film or plaque and stains it. In this way plaque that is almost colorless and invisible to the eye is recognized easily, since if the solution is applied to the surfaces of the teeth and washed off with water, all the plaque will stand out against the natural color of the tooth.

Polishing must be executed carefully. It may be done by hand or by the dental engine. A recommended method is to polish the gingival margins by hand and the outer surfaces with a rubber cup run by the engine. Fine pumice in water makes an excellent polishing agent; it should be applied very wet. As in scaling operations, a regular system of polishing should be followed.

After polishing with a porte-polisher and the dental engine the dentist should polish the approximal surfaces as well as the contact points with ribbon floss. If the teeth are close together, ordinary floss may be employed. It should be passed between the teeth with care so that it will not snap past the contact point and injure the papilla, and it should be drawn back and forth on the distal and mesial surfaces of the adjoining teeth. If the ends are wound around the first fingers, the floss can be manipulated easily.

Proximal surfaces may be polished with linen strips. Many periodontists follow the polishing procedure with a supplementary application of stannous fluoride paste or a saturated solution of sodium silicofluoride used with a soft rubber polishing cup. They feel that this procedure imparts some densensitizing properties to the exposed cervical areas. For additional material on desensitizing drugs the reader is referred to Chapter 22.

REMOVAL OR CORRECTION OF MECHANICAL IRRITANTS

Overhanging fillings may be the cause of gingival irritation and resultant inflammation; until this defect is corrected the gingival condition will persist. The same is true of faulty crowns. It may be necessary to remove a bridge that not only has faulty crowns or overhanging inlays but is also overburdening the abutment teeth. Partial dentures whose clasps are injuring the gingiva or causing trauma to the teeth must not be worn. All

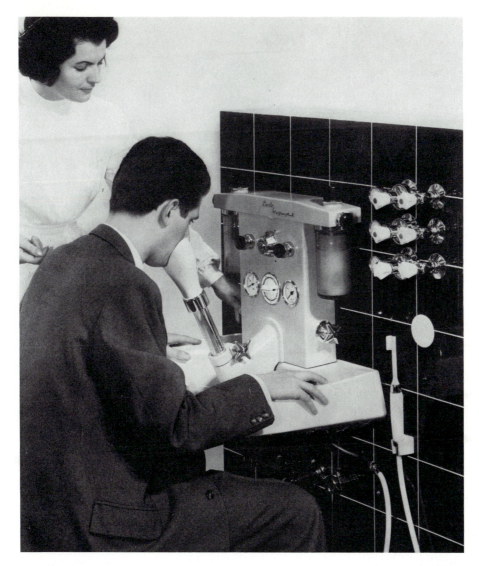

Fig. 17-29. Patient utilizing Weissenfluh mouth irrigation unit after scaling procedure. This instrument controls temperature and pressure of solution and is used for 4 to 5 minutes after treatment. Irrigant helps to flush out particles of loosened debris.

those conditions that have presumably been recorded in the examination chart as etiologic factors must be corrected (Fig. 17-29).

REFERENCES

Allen, D. L., and Kerr, D. A.: Tissue response in the guinea pig to sterile and non-sterile calculus, J. Periodontol. **36:**121, 1965.

Barnes, J. E., and Schaffer, E. M.: Subgingival root planing; a comparison using files, hoes, and curettes, J. Periodontol. **31:**300, 1960.

Björn, H., and Lundke, J.: The influence of periodontal instruments on the tooth surface, Odontol. Revy **13:**355, 1962.

Boedecker, C. F.: The difficulty of completely removing subgingival calculus, J. Am. Dent. Assoc. **30:**703, 1943.

Box, H. K.: Necrotic periodontitis, Oral Health **36:**321, 1945.

Bunting, R. W.: Oral hygiene and preventive dentistry, Philadelphia, 1930, Lea & Febiger.

Cripps, S.: Elimination of the periodontal pocket by pressure packing, Br. Dent. J. **90:**235, 1951.

Cross, W. G.: Scaling, Br. Dent. J. **90:**130, 1951.

Green, E.: Root planing with dull and sharp curettes, J. Periodontol. **39:**348, 1968.

Haley, P. S.: Packing the gingival crevice to eliminate the pyorrhea pocket, Dent. Cosmos **73:**965, 1931.

Hine, M. K., and Swenson, H. M.: Role of prophylactic procedures in the treatment of periodontal disease, J. Am. Dent. Assoc. **45:**301, 1952.

Hirschfeld, I.: Subgingival curettage in periodontal treatment, J. Am. Dent. Assoc. **44:**301, 1952.

Hodge, H. C., and Leung, S. W.: Calculus formation, J. Periodontol. **21:**211, 1950.

Johnson, W. N., and Wilson, J. R.: The application of the ultrasonic dental unit to scaling procedures. I. J. Periodontol. **28:**264, 1957.

Jones, S. J., London, J. and Boyde, A.: Tooth surface treated in situ with periodontal instruments, Br. Dent. J. **132:**57, 1972.

Lovdal, A., Arno, A., Schei, O., and Waerhaug, J.: Combined effect of subgingival scaling and controlled oral hygiene on the incidence of gingivitis, Acta Odontol. Scand. **19:**537, 1961.

McCall, J. O.: The evaluation of the scaler and its influence on the development of periodontia, J. Periodontol. **10:**69, 1939.

Meyer, K., and Lie, T.: Root surface roughness in response to periodontal instrumentation studied by combined use of microroughness measurement and scanning electron microscopy, J. Clin. Periodontol. **4:**77, 1977.

Moscow, B.: Calcification in gingival biopsies, Dent. Prog. **1:**30, 1960.

Pameyer, C. H., Stallard, R. E., and Hrep, N.: Surface characteristics of teeth following periodontal instrumentation; a scanning electron microscope study, J. Periodontol. **43:**628, 1972.

Parr, R. W., et al.: Subgingival scaling and root planing, Section on Instructional System Design. Division of Periodontology, School of Dentistry, University of California, San Francisco, 1976.

Ramjford, S., and Kiester, G.: The gingival sulcus and the periodontal pocket immediately following scaling of teeth, J. Periodontol. **25:**167, 1954.

Rosenberg, R. M., and Ash, M. M., Jr.: The effect of root roughness on plaque accumulation and gingival inflammation, J. Periodontol. **45:**146, 1974.

Schaffer, E. M.: Objective evaluation of ultrasonic versus hand instrumentation in periodontics. Dent. Clin. North Am., p. 165, March, 1964.

Schaffer, E. M.: Histological results of root curettage of human teeth, J. Periodontol. **27:**296, 1956.

Tascher, P. J., and Ewen, S. J.: An ultrasonic method of root scalings, preliminary report, N.Y. Dent. J. **23:**266, 1957.

Theband, J.: Some microscopic aspects of the curetted surface of the cementum after the subgingival curettage, J. Can. Dent. Assoc. **17:**127, 1951.

Waerhaug, J.: Effect of rough surfaces upon gingival tissue, J. Dent. Res. **35:**323, 1956.

Waerhaug, J., Arno, A., and Lovdal, A.: The dimensions of instruments for removal of subgingival calculus, J. Periodontol. **25:**281, 1954.

Zander, H. A.: The attachment of calculus to root surfaces, J. Periodontol. **24:**16, 1953.

18 Oral physiotherapy

The past 2 decades have been marked by significant advances in procedures for eliminating pockets and restoring hard and soft tissues lost as a result of periodontal disease. Despite these impressive gains, however, the long-term success of periodontal treatment depends for the most part on the effectiveness and regularity of the patient's oral hygiene measures. It is disheartening to treat successfully an individual with periodontitis, only to be confronted later with a recurrence and progression of the disease because of the patient's ineffective or irregular oral hygiene habits. *Clinicians agree that motivating and teaching patients to routinely and effectively remove bacterial plaque are essential elements of any treatment plan to arrest inflammatory periodontal disease.*

ORAL HYGIENE STATUS AND PERIODONTAL DISEASE

Epidemiologic studies within the past 20 years have clearly demonstrated the relationship between oral cleanliness and periodontal health status. All these reported investigations show a close association between the two, and additional evidence is available in a classic study by Löe. When all oral hygiene measures were withdrawn from individuals with healthy gingiva, bacterial plaque accumulations on the teeth increased markedly, and clinically evident gingivitis developed in 10 to 21 days. Bacterial counts dropped substantially, and the gingiva returned to health a few days after oral hygiene procedures were resumed. Löe stated that bacterial plaque was unquestionably a prime requisite in the production of gingival inflammation.

Longitudinal studies have further confirmed the relationship between bacterial plaque and periodontal disease. Over a 5-year period the combined effect of subgingival scaling treatments and controlled oral hygiene was evaluated in a group of 1,428 male and female factory workers and office personnel. Over the test period the average incidence of gingivitis dropped to one eighth in individuals who started the project with "good" oral hygiene. The incidence decreased to about one third in the individuals who were originally classified as "fairly good" in oral hygiene, while in the group originally classified as "not good" the incidence dropped to one half.

A United States Public Health Service study showed that individuals receiving intensive preventive periodontal care and oral hygiene instruction over a 3-year period had healthier gingiva and less loss of epithelial attachment than individuals in the control groups. A follow-up study of the participants 32 months after termination of the active phase revealed that although the gingival status had deteriorated somewhat, the experimental group still had significantly healthier gingiva than the control group. A 46-month study of the effect of preventive periodontal care and instruction in oral hygiene has been reported by United States Air Force personnel. Groups that received the most frequent preventive treatment and instruction in toothbrushing had the lowest percentage of individuals experiencing loss of epithelial attachment. There were significantly larger decreases in plaque scores for groups receiving toothbrushing instruction than in the groups not receiving instruction.

In an investigation among Swedish children of the effect of thorough training in use of the toothbrush, the experimental group had significantly better gingival health and less plaque accumulation than the control group. However, a final examination 1 year after the end of the supervised brushing regimen revealed that gingival status had deteriorated in the experimental group to the extent that it did not differ from the control group. Plaque scores at the final examination were almost identical for the two groups. The investigators speculated that failure to achieve a prolonged effect might have been caused by their failure to tell the students why they should use the particular brushing method and to explain that it should also be used at home.

Data from these and many other studies show that training in oral hygiene procedures brings about a reduction in plaque accumulation and a healthier gingival status. Follow-up studies that reveal a deteriorating gingival status after supervision is discontinued point up a problem familiar to periodontists. After active therapy, patients sometimes unconsciously change their hygiene techniques or become preoccupied with other matters, with the result that plaque control becomes ineffective and the disease reappears. The possibility of such occurrences after treatment necessitates preventive maintenance care. Although patient motivation is not dealt with in this chapter, its importance is evident. Without it the patient will not long continue effective oral hygiene procedures.

Our knowledge of bacterial plaque has increased tremendously over the past 10 years. Much less is known concerning variations in how individual patients respond to bacterial irritants. On the other hand, there is indisputable evidence that inflammatory periodontal disease can be prevented by the routine application of effective oral hygiene measures.

ORAL HYGIENE AIDS AND AGENTS
Disclosing agents

Preparations that disclose stainable material on the teeth for patient education have long been available. One such preparation, Bismarck brown disclosing solution, does a good job of plaque detection and does not stain soft tissues, lips, and tongue as vividly as some other compounds and tablets. The formula is as follows:

Bismarck brown (powder)	3 g
Ethyl alcohol	10 ml
Glycerin	120 ml
Anise oil	1 drop

The Bismarck brown powder is available through all major chemical supply companies.

A fluorescent disclosing solution, DC yellow no. 8 fluorescein, has recently been shown to be more effective than erythrosin solution for plaque detection without imparting a red stain to the mucosa and lips. A dichroic filter placed over the dental or bathroom light renders the plaque fluorescent. A special light utilizing this filter is available for patient use (Plate 1).

Of recent development is a two-tone dye test for dental plaque that uses FDC red no. 3 and FDC green no. 3. The solution stains thick accumulations of plaque blue, and thin deposits are stained red. The main advantages cited for the solution are that blue offers a considerable contrast to the teeth and that tissues and plaques of different ages stain differently.

In the past few years disclosing tablets have become available for use in the office and for plaque detection at home. These tablets, containing a water-soluble vegetable dye, FDC red no. 3 (erythrosin), make it easy for a patient to see stainable material on the teeth, and their periodic use should result in better oral hygiene (Fig. 18-1). They are probably of greatest value during the early period when the patient is learning how to

A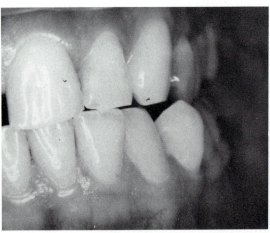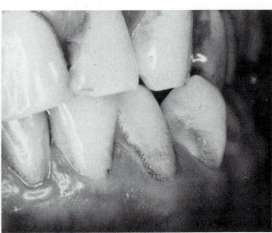

Fig. 18-1. A, Clinical appearance of unstained teeth. Unless bacterial plaque is present in gross amounts, it is difficult for patient to see it. **B,** After use of disclosing tablets, bacterial plaque is readily evident to patient.

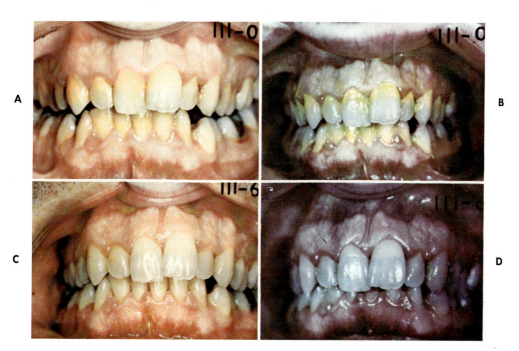

Plate 1. Use of D.C. yellow no. 8 disclosing solution, with Plak-Lite as source of illumination. **A,** Initial visit without disclosing solution. **B,** Initial visit using disclosing solution. Note bacterial plaque glowing yellow. **C,** Six weeks after initial visit without Plak-Lite. No instructions in toothbrushing technique had been given to patient. **D,** Six weeks later with Plak-Lite. Patient had been given instructions to remove all yellow stain from teeth. Note absence of plaque. (From Cohen, D. W., Stoller, N., Chace, R., and Laster, L.: J. Periodontol. **43:**333, 1972; courtesy International Pharmaceutical Corp.)

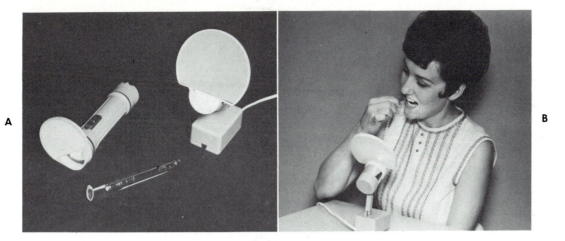

Fig. 18-2. A, Three types of light sources that enhance patient's ability to see various areas of mouth for oral hygiene. **B,** Patient using auxiliary light during plaque control session in dental office.

position the toothbrush and execute brushing strokes or how to use interdental cleaning agents in various areas of the mouth.

Disclosing solutions and tablets have certain limitations. They do not selectively disclose bacterial plaque, but rather stain all soft debris, pellicle, and bacterial plaque on the teeth. When a patient's plaque control is being evaluated in a clinical situation or when a study is being conducted, the stained areas must be probed to determine if the material is soft and comes away on the instrument. Exposed cementum in particular can stain vividly, although it is free of bacterial plaque. In the home, disclosing solutions are limited in their usefulness by the patient's inability to see some areas of the mouth and by inadequate lighting in the average bathroom. Several light sources are now available to eliminate this problem (Fig. 18-2).

Toothbrushes and brushing techniques

The toothbrush in its present form dates back only about 200 years. In earlier times toothpicks and chew sticks of various kinds were the chief oral hygiene aids. The specifications for an acceptable toothbrush, established by the Council on Dental Therapeutics of the American Dental Association, cover physical requirements as to size, shape, texture, maneuverability, and cleansability, along with desirable functional qualities. These are general specifications and permit inclusion of almost any type of brush that can be imagined. The few comparative investigations of the effectiveness of various brush designs, types, or configurations of bristles have not demonstrated a clear-cut advantage of any one type. Results of one study indicate a possible correlation between the number of filaments in a brush and its cleansing effect.

Two hand brushes with radically different bristle angulations have recently been proposed. In both brushes the bristles are offset at angles that it was claimed would make plaque removal more effective. Insufficient data are available to evaluate the plaque-removing efficiency of the brushes. Minor modifications in design such as variations in bristle thicknesses and heights between the outer and middle rows and in the number of tufts in the brush head have been made by individual manufacturers. Data to support claims of increased effectiveness with the new designs are not available.

No single brush size or bristle configuration has been shown to be clearly superior to the rest, but most clinicians favor a soft or medium-firm nylon bristle brush with a reasonably small head and square-cut or rounded bristle ends. A child's brush is often prescribed for the adult patient with a small mouth, malposed teeth, or a limited opening (Fig. 18-3).

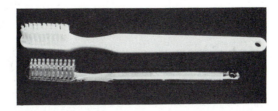

Fig. 18-3. Child and adult size, level trimmed, multi-tufted, soft nylon bristle toothbrushes.

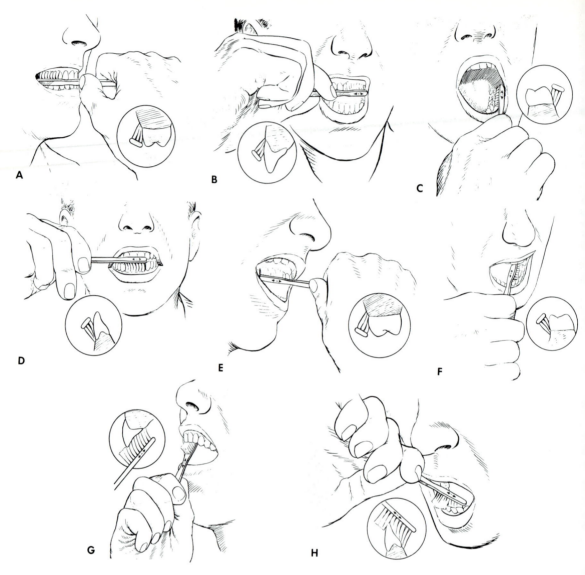

Fig. 18-4. Placement and activation of toothbrush in Bass technique. (From O'Leary, T. J., and Nabers, C. L.: J. Periodontol. **40:**27, 1969.)

The Bass, the roll, the horizontal scrub, and the Charters' technique are the most commonly taught methods. However, each therapist teaches according to his or her concept of the particular technique, and that concept may vary considerably from what the originator of the method had in mind.

In the Bass technique the bristles are applied to the tooth at a 45-degree angle, pointed apically so that the bristle tips enter the gingival sulcus (Fig. 18-4). The brush is then activated with a slight vibratory motion. Those who support the Bass technique consider it the most effective means of cleaning the dentogingival junction, since they feel that the bristle tips actually penetrate into the gingival crevice for a short distance, dislodging plaque from the tooth surfaces. Advocates of the roll technique say that it removes plaque effectively and requires less time to teach and less skill to use than the Bass or Charters' technique (Fig. 18-5). The horizontal scrub method may be viewed as a modification of the Bass technique since the bristles are applied at right angles to the tooth surfaces and activated by back-and-forth horizontal scrubbing strokes (Fig. 18-6). In the Charters' technique the bristles are placed at right angles to the long axis of the tooth, gently forced interproximally, and vibrated

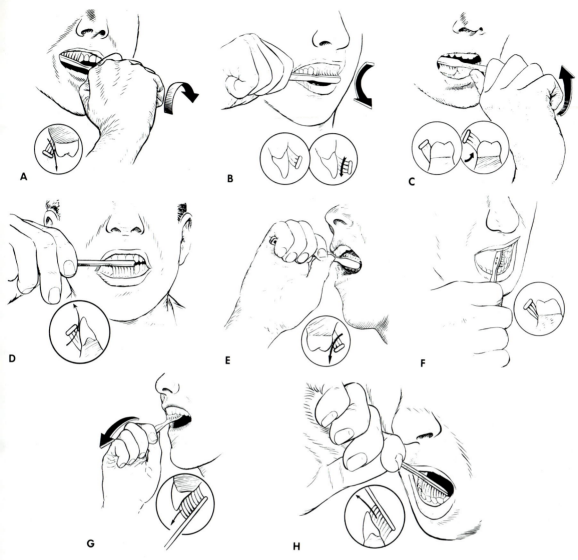

Fig. 18-5. Roll technique. Note in **F** that lingual surfaces of mandibular posterior teeth are cleaned by Bass technique. (From O'Leary, T. J., and Nabers, C. L.: J. Periodontol. **40:** 27, 1969.)

to clean and massage the gingival margin and interproximal areas (Fig. 18-7).

There have been few comparative studies of toothbrushing techniques. In one study comparing two vertical brushing methods the investigators reported no statistically significant differences in regard to the prevention or removal of bacterial plaque accumulation. A study comparing the Charters' and roll techniques of brushing reported no significant differences in reducing gingival inflammation or extrinsic stains on the teeth. In an investigation of preschool children the horizontal scrub method proved to be more effective for deciduous teeth than the roll method. The same result was obtained when either the child or the parent carried out the brushing procedure. A comparative study of the Charters', the roll, the horizontal scrub, and a modified Fones' technique showed that the horizontal scrub method was the most effective in preventing plaque accumulation and the Charters' was least effective. There was no real difference in effectiveness between the roll and modified Fones' methods.

Considerable interest is attached to two recent studies by a group of investigators on the effectiveness of the Charters', scrub, and roll methods of brushing for plaque removal. When a dentist or a hygienist did the brushing, an interaction was

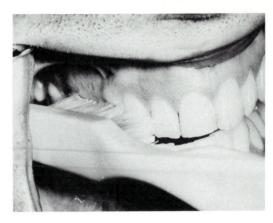

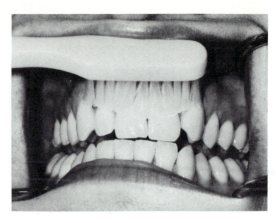

Fig. 18-6. In scrub brush method bristles are applied at right angles to tooth surfaces and activated by short back-and-forth horizontal scrubbing strokes.

Fig. 18-7. Bristles are forced interproximally in Charters method.

observed between the one doing the brushing and the brushing method. In the second study participants brushed their own teeth. Again, an interaction between instructor and toothbrushing method was detected. In both studies the interaction indicated that the effectiveness of any method was partly dependent on the instructor and that no one method was superior to the others in plaque removal. However, both the Charters' and the scrub methods appeared to be superior to the roll technique. None of the brushing methods was effective in removing interproximal plaque deposits.

Any toothbrushing study will have several hard-to-control variables. As in the study results just described the dentist or plaque-control therapist can influence the results of a study. If an individual believes that one technique is superior to another, his enthusiasm in teaching that technique or his lack of enthusiasm in teaching another can influence the patient or the study's results.

If the teacher happens to be more adept at performing and demonstrating one of the test methods, that too may influence the results. Most toothbrushing studies are relatively short term, which means that the Hawthorne, or subject, effect may further influence the reliability of the result. Some variables can be controlled or eliminated in toothbrushing studies, but the results will be of doubtful reliability unless different groups of investigators report the same findings.

In deciding on the toothbrushing technique to be taught, such factors as anatomy of the teeth, position of the teeth in the arch, and manual dexterity of the patient should be taken into account. One of the most important factors to consider is the teacher's conviction as to the most effective method. At present most periodontists appear to favor the Bass or the horizontal scrub method.

Electric toothbrushes are available with various types of brushing motion, head design, and bristles. When they were introduced many viewed them as the answer to plaque control problems. However, short-term studies comparing the effectiveness of hand and electric brushes have not conclusively demonstrated that an electric brush is superior to a manual toothbrush in the hands of a reasonably adept individual. One 2-year study found no evidence that the electric brush was superior to the hand brush in reducing oral debris, calculus, or periodontal disease, nor did the use of one kind of brush result in more gingival recession than the other. On the other hand, reports indicate that the power toothbrush is superior for oral hygiene procedures in the physically and mentally handicapped.

There is a widespread misconception that anyone can brush his teeth acceptably well with little or no instruction. Periodontists generally find that uninstructed patients usually miss entirely or only partially clean several areas of their mouths in toothbrushing.

Interdental cleaning agents

Periodontal disease occurs more commonly and causes more destruction in the interdental areas than on the facial and lingual aspects of the teeth. The toothpick was the first recorded oral hygiene aid and is still probably the most commonly used device for interdental cleaning. Devices for interdental cleaning include various types of toothpicks, interdental brushes, rubber and plastic tips of various sizes and shapes, and waxed and un-

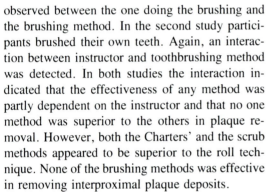

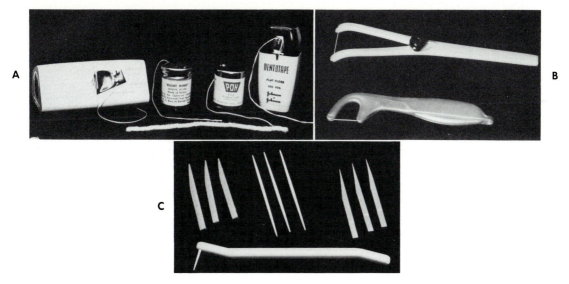

Fig. 18-8. A, Waxed and unwaxed dental floss, waxed dental tape, and yarn for cleaning interproximal tooth surfaces. **B,** Auxiliary aids for flossing interproximal surfaces are useful for handicapped patients and persons with poor manual dexterity. **C,** Wood and plastic interdental cleaning agents. At bottom the tip of a toothpick is inserted in Perio-Aid.

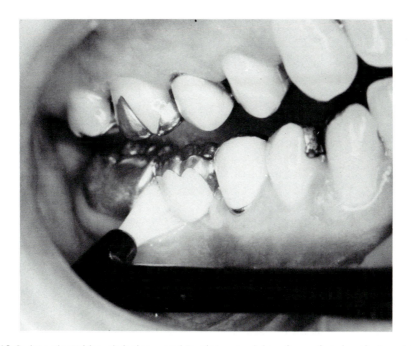

Fig. 18-9. Interdental brush being used to clean mesial surface of molar abutment tooth.

waxed dental floss (Fig. 18-8). Devices such as the interdental brush, rubber tips, and the various types of toothpicks require little instruction, and the patient can use them in almost any environment. A conscientious, motivated patient can clean most of the facial interproximal surfaces quite well with the various types of toothpicks and the interdental brush (Fig. 18-9). It is difficult, however, to remove plaque from the mesial-lingual and distal-lingual line angles of teeth with these devices. The hard wooden toothpick, either by itself or held in the Perio-Aid, is a useful adjunct for cleaning grooved root surfaces where floss cannot reach (Fig. 18-10). The Perio-Aid toothpick holder is one of the most effective aids available for cleaning exposed furcations after periodontal therapy.

Long before the importance of bacterial plaque

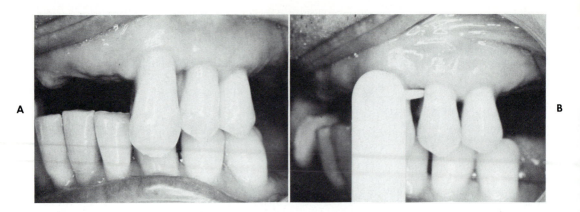

Fig. 18-10. A, Dental floss cannot reach and remove bacterial plaque from grooved root surfaces. **B,** Toothpick held in Perio-Aid allows patient to clean grooved surfaces.

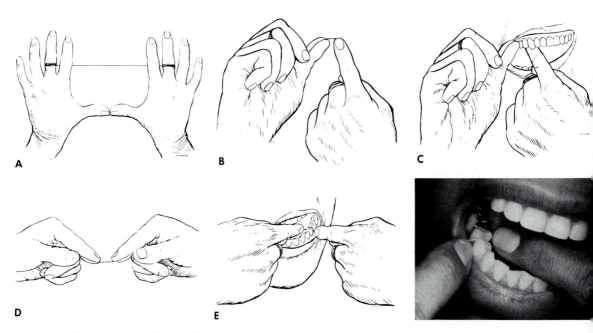

Fig. 18-11. A to **E,** Handling floss for cleaning interproximal tooth surfaces in various areas of mouth. **F,** Patient inserts floss through contact between mandibular right bicuspids. Less than ½ inch of floss is between fingers. Floss is held taut so that it scrapes plaque from teeth with a knifelike action. (**A** to **E** from O'Leary, T. J., and Nabers, C. L.: J. Periodontol. **40:**27, 1969.)

was generally recognized, waxed dental floss was commonly used to remove large particles of food or oral debris from between the teeth. However, it was not generally thought of as a method for removing organized bacterial plaque. Unwaxed dental floss has been generally available only during the last decade. Its smaller diameter means that it can be slipped through interdental contacts more easily than waxed floss. The individual filaments of the unwaxed floss contact the tooth surface and scrape off the organized microbial

colonies (Fig. 18-11). It is essential that any supragingival or subgingival calculus deposits and rough or overextended margins of restorations be removed before the patient begins to use unwaxed floss. If not removed they can cause bleeding and soreness of the gingival tissues, along with catching, fraying, and breakage of the floss (Figs. 18-12 and 18-13). Many restorative dentists recognize the value of unwaxed floss and routinely use it to check the marginal adaptation of castings.

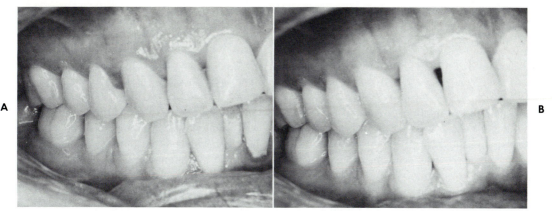

Fig. 18-12. A, Heavy subgingival calculus deposits are present on interproximal tooth surfaces. Unwaxed floss will catch, fray, or break if used in area. Use of either waxed or unwaxed dental floss can result in bleeding and soreness. **B,** Calculus deposits have been removed so that floss can be used effectively and without discomfort.

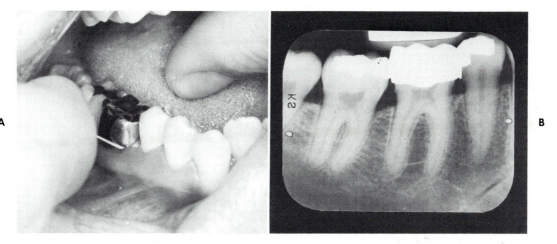

Fig. 18-13. A, Dental floss caught by overhanging margin of casting. **B,** Radiograph showing overhanging mesial margin of casting and calculus on distal surface of root.

When properly used either waxed or unwaxed dental floss will effectively clean all flat or convex interproximal surfaces. More chairside instruction is generally required for a patient to become proficient in flossing, and it is more time consuming for the patient than some other aids; however, the high state of interdental cleanliness and interproximal gingival health attained by patients who use floss attests to its great value in an oral hygiene regimen.

Although the use of supplemental aids for interproximal plaque removal is favored by most periodontists, relatively few studies have compared the effectiveness of the various aids. Recent studies have evaluated the following: (1) a standard toothbrush compared to unwaxed and waxed dental floss, (2) the single-tufted brush compared

to the interdental brush, to toothpicks, and to waxed dental tape, (3) a multitufted nylon brush compared to wooden toothpicks and to unwaxed dental floss, and (4) a soft-bristled toothbrush compared to waxed dental floss and to round, rectangular, and triangular toothpicks. The conflicting results of the various studies may be accounted for by the differing methods of patient selection and by the differences between the various experimental procedures. However, in the presence of wide interdental spaces it appears that the interdental brush, waxed dental tape, and triangular toothpicks all effectively remove proximal plaque deposits. The enthusiasm or lack of it displayed by the individual who teaches the use of the individual interdental cleaning aids could have a significant effect on the outcome of any comparative study. At present most periodontists in the United States seem to recommend the use of unwaxed dental floss for cleaning the interproximal tooth surfaces.

Oral irrigation

Although oral irrigation has been advocated and used as a cleansing aid for over 75 years, there has been a recent upsurge of interest in it, perhaps because several devices have become available that permit the procedure to be carried out quickly and easily. Some of these devices attach directly to the faucet and deliver either a continuous or a pulsating stream of water. Others have a reservoir from which water is delivered in a pulsating stream; water pressure is controlled by a dial regulator. Many studies have investigated the effect of oral irrigation on gingivitis, plaque, calculus, pocket depth, and other variables. In general a reduction in gingival inflammation, both clinical and microscopic, has been reported as well as a reduction in pocket depth and calculus formation, but little reduction in bacterial plaque. One investigator has speculated that irrigation may affect the qualitative composition (pH, bacterial and chemical composition) of the plaque.

A study has been reported of the effect of various solutions delivered in water by pressure irrigation on the bacteriologic content of the periodontal pocket. An oxygenating agent was found to be most effective in reducing the pus content of periodontal pockets, and a quaternary ammonium compound was the next most effective, whereas physiologic saline was ineffective. In a recent short-term study testing the effect of water, 1% hydrogen peroxide, and 0.5% hypochlorite administered through a water irrigation device, both the 1% hydrogen peroxide and the 0.5% hypochlorite resulted in less plaque retention on the test teeth and a smaller fall in mean pH of the plaque after a 20% sucrose rinse. The authors suggested that water-irrigating devices may be useful for delivery of therapeutic agents.

There have been reports of possible harmful effects from the use of water-irrigating devices. One study using three different irrigating devices found that carbon particles frequently penetrated the sulcular epithelium and underlying connective tissue of beagle and human gingival tissues when the areas were irrigated with water containing carbon. Another investigator found that a 1% solution of alcian blue dye penetrated apparently intact gingival tissue of cats when applied through a pulsating irrigator at maximum pressure.

In a clinical study 30 patients with untreated periodontitis used an irrigating device at medium pressure for 1 minute to flush out debris from the gingival crevices. One minute later blood samples were taken and cultured. Microorganisms were obtained from 15 of the 30 postirrigation blood samples. Streptococci and staphylococci were most frequently found, and the authors noted that these were the most prominent organisms mentioned in the etiology of bacterial endocarditis.

Several oral irrigation devices have been classified as acceptable by the Council on Dental Materials and Devices of the American Dental Association. The council regards them as an effective aid to the toothbrush and interdental cleaning agents in promoting oral cleanliness. On the other hand, the council does not consider that these devices can prevent or treat oral diseases.

When one of these devices is prescribed for patient use, the operator should stress that it will not take the place of routine effective brushing and interdental cleaning. Unfortunately patients tend to regard such a device as a substitute for either or both measures. Such a substitution can have a most unfavorable impact on gingival health.

Chemotherapeutic agents

Chemotherapeutic agents that were as effective as brushing and interdental cleaning procedures in controlling bacterial plaque would be of great value in preventing the inception and progress of periodontal disease. Accordingly, several types of agents have been investigated.

The effect of enzymes on calculus or its precursor, bacterial plaque, has been investigated, and marked reductions in plaque, calculus, and gingivitis scores have been reported. However, the objectionable taste, odor, and prolonged contact time needed to make such preparations effective appears to make them unsuitable for general use.

Erythromycin, tetracycline, polymyxin, vancomycin, and the macrolide antibiotic cc 10232 are among the antibiotics that have been studied for their effect on bacterial plaque. Except for vancomycin, which will be discussed separately, they usually caused a reduction of the entire plaque accumulation or of specific types of organisms within the plaque. Vancomycin, produced by *Streptococcus orientalis,* is a true topical because it is not absorbed across the mucous membranes. Incorporated into an ointment it has proved effective in the control of bacterial plaque among retarded institutionalized patients and in the initial

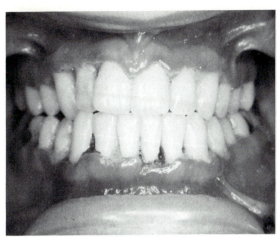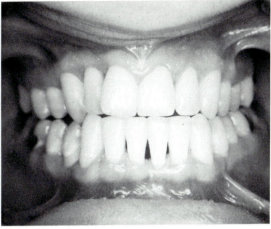

Fig. 18-14. A, Patient with acute necrotizing ulcerative gingivitis. **B,** Same patient 17 days later with complete resolution of inflammation. Acute stage was treated by careful scaling and initiation of oral hygiene procedures. Antiplaque solutions would be useful in treating acute problems of this type.

treatment of acute necrotizing ulcerative gingivitis. In another study six subjects with clinically healthy gingiva at the start used as their only oral hygiene measure a 0.5% solution of vancomycin for 1 minute three times a day. All subjects developed a clinically obvious gingivitis at the same rate as the control group, which rinsed with distilled water. The vehicle used may have been responsible for the difference in results between these studies, since vancomycin in ointment form would remain in contact with the teeth and gingival tissue longer than when used in a water solution and rinsed with for 1 minute.

Although some antibiotics effectively reduce plaque accumulations, their potential usefulness is severely limited because of a number of possible problems, including sensitivity reactions, the emergence of drug-resistant strains of organisms, and undesirable side effects due to changes in the normal flora of the intestinal tract.

Chlorhexidine, an antimicrobial biguanine, has received considerable attention as a possible antiplaque agent. Before it attracted the interest of dental investigators it had been used as an antiseptic in medicine for many years. Through animal toxicity tests and long experience with its use in medicine it is known to have a low level of toxicity when applied orally or topically. In oral use it is absorbed by substances in the mouth from which it is slowly released, thus exerting a prolonged bactericidal effect on both gram-negative and gram-positive organisms. In short-term studies relatively low concentrations of the agent applied topically once a day, used as a rinse once or twice

daily, or used in a toothpaste twice daily have caused significant reduction in plaque accumulations. The plaque-inhibiting action of chlorhexidine in a study using humans was reported to be undiminished after 2 years. However, when the preparation was used on beagle dogs for 1 year it prevented plaque formation and gingivitis for up to 6 months, but during the last 6 months the scores for plaque and gingival health status rose to about half the level found in the control animals. Differences in the oral flora may well have been responsible for the varying results in the two studies.

Several undesirable side effects have been reported, notably an objectionable taste and staining of the tongue, teeth, and silicate restorations. However, no dangerous side effects have been reported in a number of studies with medical and dental students and with handicapped individuals.

Chlorhexidine or some similar agent would appear to have great potential for use as an antiplaque agent in both short- and long-term application (Fig. 18-14).

TEACHING ORAL HYGIENE PROCEDURES

Teaching a patient to carry out oral hygiene procedures appears to be easy, but it is not. One prerequisite for success is that the dentist and his staff believe in and practice meticulous oral hygiene themselves. This personal conviction is extremely important if we expect our patients to follow our advice and teaching. The therapist must also establish the need for the procedures in the patient's mind, motivate him to employ them, and then teach him to carry them out routinely and effectively.

Establishing the need. For many reasons the first, or examination, appointment is the most important session that a practitioner will have with a patient. In the case of the patient with inflammatory periodontal disease it is the appointment at which the need for oral hygiene procedures is first established. This need can be established in several ways. Periodontal pathology can be pointed out in the patient's mouth. He can be shown bone loss on his radiographs. Teeth that have been loosened by bone loss or severe gingival inflammation can be called to his attention.

Motivating the patient. Setting desirable and attainable goals is essential in motivating a patient to carry out oral hygiene procedures (Chapter 19). These goals may vary from one person to another. Younger people in particular can often be motivated by promising them an improved appearance that will impress their contemporaries. Of course many older persons are also vitally concerned with their personal appearance. These individuals can be motivated by appealing to their pride and pointing out how much more attractive they could be with healthy oral tissues.

Many people are health conscious. They are concerned with maintaining an optimum weight, an ideal dietary intake, regular sleeping habits, and physical fitness. Such persons often can be motivated by pointing out the presence of bacteria-containing plaque on the teeth, demonstrating its injurious effects on the periodontium, and noting that transient bacteremias may occur during function. They can be told that a healthy mouth can be attained by eliminating this source of disease.

Another effective motivator is the fear of aging and becoming edentulous. Many people associate edentulousness with aging and are particularly concerned at the thought of growing old. Explaining to these patients that the loss of teeth changes facial contour and appearance is an effective motivational technique.

Older patients are often concerned about the potential loss of chewing efficiency. The periodontal patient who is told that he may face the loss of one or more teeth and who knows from the experiences of others about the problems sometimes encountered with prosthetic appliances is more easily motivated to learn and regularly carry out oral hygiene procedures.

Another type of patient is the person who has a powerful drive to be successful in anything he attempts. Improving his oral hygiene is a challenge to this individual, which he will make every effort to meet successfully.

One question on the health history form that the patient fills out before the periodontal examination can provide useful information as to how the patient regards his teeth and how easily he may be motivated. The question is, "How much would it bother you if you had to lose all of your teeth and wear false teeth?" A response indicating that the patient would be extremely upset usually signifies that he places a high value on his natural dentition and can be readily motivated to carry out the necessary oral hygiene regimen. Conversely, a reply stating that he would not be too concerned or that he has always expected he would lose his teeth by this time raises quite a different problem. If the patient's answer is simply due to a lack of knowledge about the disease and its treatment, the practitioner will have to make sure that the necessary information is provided. However, this type of answer may be the result of the patient's socioeconomic values; that is, his parents, siblings, and acquaintances have become edentulous at an early age and he has come to expect the same thing. In this situation the patient must first be made aware of the fact that barring congenital defects or accidents, any individual should be able to retain his teeth throughout life. Changing one's beliefs is difficult, and the task becomes even more difficult with increasing age. Whenever possible, a simplified treatment plan should be developed for this type of individual, as his prior dental experience is probably limited and he may not be conditioned to accept a long and complicated course of treatment or be motivated to follow through with it. The prescribed oral hygiene procedures should also be kept as simple as possible.

Approach to instruction. The teaching of oral hygiene procedures should be a continuing part of a practice, not something to be carried out only at one or two appointments, but something that requires periodic reinforcement as long as the patient is seen. Many instructional methods have been used, including the use of posters, charts, and stone or plastic models with oversized toothbrushes in the classroom or at the dental chair. These methods have merit but it has become increasingly evident that oral hygiene procedures are demonstrated and taught most effectively in the patient's mouth.

Oral hygiene education logically starts at the

examination appointment. Prior to the clinical examination the patient is given some information about periodontal disease and its treatment by means of audiovisual or written educational material. At the beginning of the clinical examination

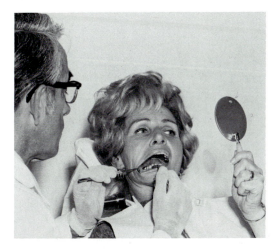

Fig. 18-15. Periodontal pathology is pointed out to patient.

he is given a hand mirror so that he can view the procedure (Fig. 18-15). Areas of obvious gingival inflammation or periodontal pocketing are pointed out to the patient as the examination progresses. When disclosing solution is applied the bacterial plaque present on the teeth in the areas of inflammation and pocketing is shown to the patient. The patient's recognition of disease in his own mouth and of the relationship between the disease and the bacterial plaque accomplishes three things: (1) it makes the disease process a real, not an abstract, entity to the patient; (2) it shows him the major reason for the disease process; and (3) it makes him aware of the need to remove the plaque from the teeth. Many clinicians routinely take plaque samples from the teeth, prepare slides, and demonstrate the bacterial activity of the plaque to the patient under the phase contrast microscope as part of the education process (Fig. 18-16).

Once the relationship between periodontal health and oral hygiene status has been thoroughly explained and demonstrated to the patient, the actual teaching of the cleaning methods can be

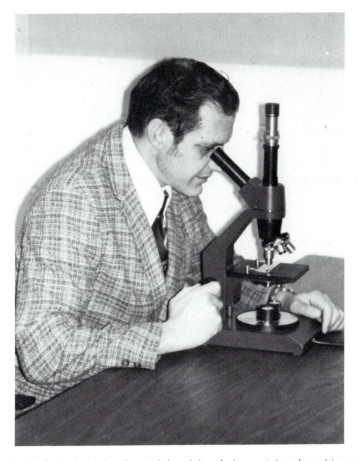

Fig. 18-16. Patient viewing bacterial activity of plaque taken from his mouth.

delegated to a hygienist or other auxiliary personnel. However, it is false economy for the dentist to delegate the responsibility of explaining the periodontal disease–plaque relationship to an auxiliary. When this is done the patient subconsciously feels that oral hygiene cannot be too important or the dentist would have taken time to discuss it. As a result the patient may be negligent both in the frequency and in the effectiveness with which he carries out his cleaning procedures.

Some offices employ a "dental educator" or "plaque-control therapist" whose major function is teaching oral hygiene procedures. Using auxiliary personnel for this phase of periodontal treatment offers advantages in that the patient can be more readily appointed for the necessary number of instructional sessions and the cost of the service can be kept to a minimum. There is some question as to whether all teaching of oral hygiene procedures should be delegated to one auxiliary or whether two or more of the assisting staff should share this important responsibility. Proponents of the single person approach feel that this method assures standardized instruction; the others feel that the sharing of responsibilities lessens the chance that a single designated teacher will become bored and ineffectual.

There is no generally accepted time schedule for teaching oral hygiene techniques. They are probably most frequently scheduled as part of routine treatment appointments, several days to weeks apart. Recently, some clinicians have termed oral hygiene education the "disease control program" or "plaque control program," and teaching sessions have been scheduled daily for 5 or 6 days. There is no conclusive evidence that one schedule of teaching is more effective than the other.

Teaching process. In the first stage of instruction a disclosing agent may again be used to make the plaque and other stainable materials easily visible to the patient. He is then given a toothbrush and asked to clean his teeth. If after brushing his present method appears to be adequate in most areas of the mouth, the basic technique is retained. He is simply shown how to improve his cleaning efficiency in the deficient areas.

When the patient's present method is markedly ineffective a method is prescribed that will allow him to effectively clean his teeth. The technique is first demonstrated in the patient's mouth, and he is given an orderly sequence for brushing so that no tooth surfaces are missed. Patients appreciate definite instructions as to the sequence for brushing the various teeth and the number of

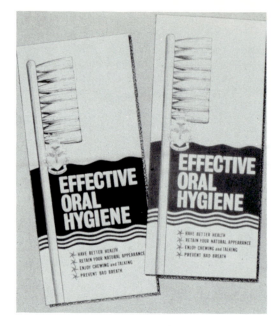

Fig. 18-17. Booklets describing and illustrating roll and Bass techniques of toothbrushing. Both booklets include handling of floss for cleaning interproximal tooth surfaces. (From O'Leary, T. J., and Nabers, C. L.: J. Periodontol. **40:**27, 1969.)

strokes to be used for each area. The patient is then asked to demonstrate the technique and the clinician makes corrections as needed. Interdental cleaning (flossing) may or may not be introduced at this first learning session, depending on the toothbrushing ability of the patient and the condition of the interproximal surfaces of the teeth.

There is a prevalent but erroneous belief that one period of instruction in oral hygiene procedures should result in a marked decrease in plaque levels. This is not true. The patient assimilates only part of the information given at the first teaching appointment and will remember and be able to put into practice at home only a part of what he assimilated. For this reason many clinicians give patients instructional booklets that describe the toothbrushing technique and the type of interdental cleaning that they want the patient to use (Fig. 18-17).

At the beginning of the second instructional appointment a disclosing solution is used to determine the patient's progress in mastering oral hygiene procedures. The degree of improvement depends to some extent on the amount of plaque that was present on the teeth initially. If all or most of the tooth surfaces were covered with plaque at the first instructional session a marked reduction can be expected. If on the other hand

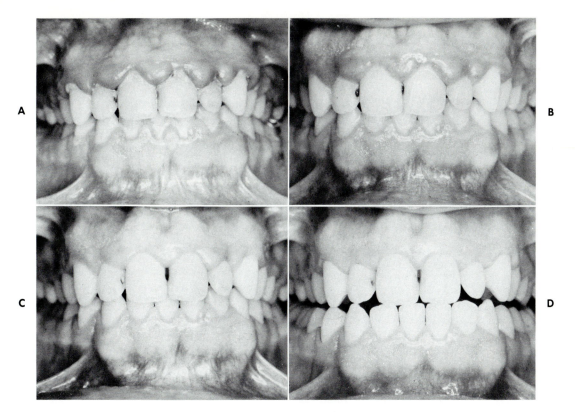

Fig. 18-18. A, This patient presented with marked gingival inflammation and enlargement. Gross calculus deposits were removed and patient was instructed in toothbrushing at this appointment. **B,** Appearance of gingival tissue 7 days later. Toothbrushing instruction was reinforced at this appointment. **C,** Fourteen days after first appointment. Patient was instructed in use of unwaxed dental floss at this time. **D,** Twenty-nine days after first appointment. There has been a marked resolution of gingival inflammation and enlargement. Instrumentation was carried out only at first appointment.

half or less of the surfaces had plaque accumulations before any instruction was given the reduction is usually much smaller. In all types of patients the initial reduction in plaque scores after one session of oral hygiene instruction probably approximates 25%.

The average patient usually requires four periods of instruction to achieve a satisfactory level of plaque control (Figs. 18-18 to 18-20). When correcting a patient's technique errors it is important to see that any criticisms are accompanied by appropriate compliments on the patient's progress. If after the second or third session the patient is not progressing satisfactorily a change in approach may be indicated. It may develop that for a particular area the technique originally prescribed is inappropriate because of the patient's poor manual dexterity, malposed teeth, or some other reason. At this time it may be advantageous to instruct the patient in a new technique for cleaning the problem areas. Ordinarily instructions in

oral hygiene are completed during the initial phase of therapy while the teeth are being scaled and root planed, and hopeless teeth are eliminated from the mouth. Most clinicians feel that it is unwise to proceed further with treatment if the patient has not demonstrated satisfactory proficiency in oral hygiene procedures (Fig. 18-21). Instruction may be continued if the lack of proficiency is traced to the patient's poor manual dexterity. When the lack of proficiency is due to a lack of motivation, the treatment plan is either drastically revised or treatment is terminated.

A number of forms have been devised that permit recording of the patient's progress with cleaning procedures. These charts also appear to have a motivating effect on the patient. Fig. 18-22 shows the plaque control record with each tooth represented by a circle divided into four areas: mesial, facial, distal, and lingual. At the initial appointment when the disclosing solution is used, surfaces having plaque at the gingival margin

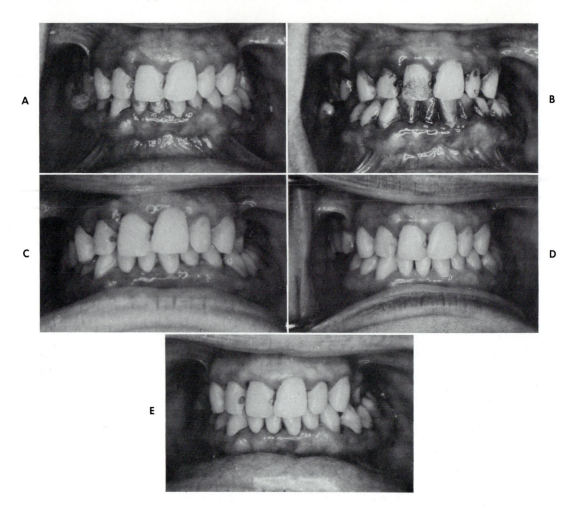

Fig. 18-19. A, This patient presented with marked gingival inflammation and enlargement. **B,** Disclosing solution shows gross amounts of bacterial plaque on teeth. Patient was instructed in Bass method of toothbrushing and use of unwaxed dental floss at this appointment. No instrumentation was carried out. **C,** Appearance of tissues 1 week later. Instruction in oral hygiene procedures was reinforced. **D,** Patient 2 weeks later. Marginal inflammation and enlargement are subsiding. **E,** There has been marked resolution of inflammation and gingival enlargement. Only therapy to date has been instruction in oral hygiene.

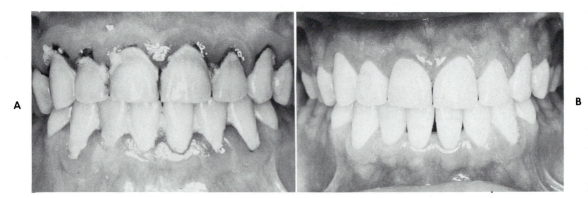

Fig. 18-20. A, This patient presented with gross amounts of uncalcified and calcified marginal irritants. Teeth were scaled and patient was instructed in toothbrushing and use of unwaxed dental floss. **B,** Gingival tissues at next appointment, 10 days later.

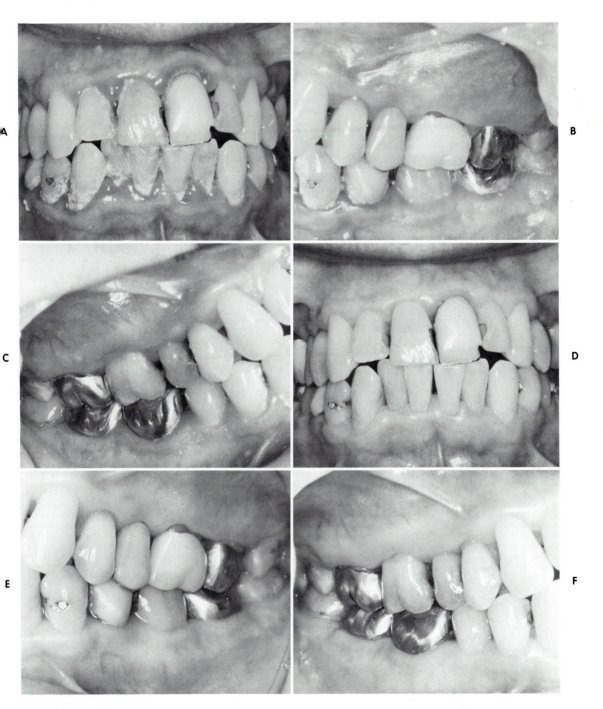

Fig. 18-21. Older patient with generalized severe pocketing and gross accumulations of uncalcified and calcified irritants. Because of patient's past history of indifferent oral care there was some question as to whether he could be motivated to carry out routine, effective oral hygiene procedures. **A** to **C,** Frontal and right and left lateral preoperative views of patient. **D** to **F,** Same areas 3 months after completion of initial therapy with resolution of gingival inflammation. Obviously, patient has been motivated. However, pocket elimination procedures are still necessary in all segments since deep pockets are still present. Extended time between completion of initial therapy and beginning of pocket elimination procedures permits clinician to better evaluate patient's continued motivation. It also permits greatest possible resolution of gingival inflammation.

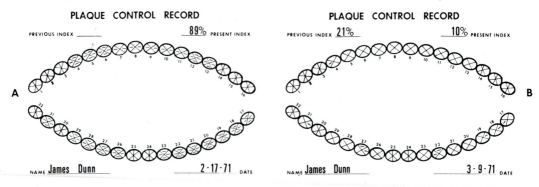

Fig. 18-22. A, Plaque control record filled out at first appointment for teaching plaque control measures. **B,** Plaque control record after four sessions of instruction. Patient's plaque level is such that definitive treatment can begin.

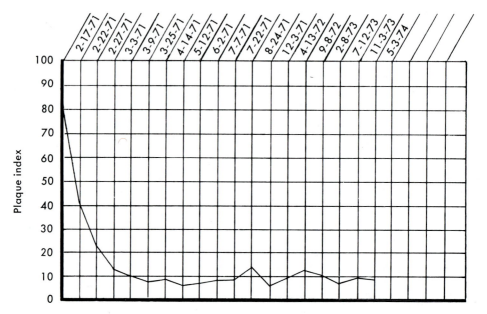

Fig. 18-23. Plaque index scores recorded at initial and all subsequent appointments are plotted on graph so that clinician can easily review long-term effectiveness of patient's oral hygiene.

are scored as "a–." Surfaces with no plaque are left blank. The plaque index is determined by dividing the number of stained surfaces by the number of surfaces available for staining. Recording of this information at instructional sessions takes 3 to 4 minutes. It permits a determination of the improvement that occurs with instruction and it points out the areas where the patient is having continued difficulty in cleaning. The Plaque Index graph (Fig. 18-23) offers a convenient method of maintaining a record of the patient's plaque control during both the active and maintenance phases of therapy.

Other considerations. The objective of oral hygiene procedures is to remove the bacterial plaque without damaging the teeth or gingiva. The minimum procedures needed to accomplish this are prescribed. The patient who has neglected his oral health and hygiene measures over many years can be literally overwhelmed by being immediately introduced to several hygiene techniques. It is usually best to begin by instructing this patient in brushing only. Attempting to introduce all necessary cleaning procedures at one time can invite failure. The patient may listen quietly as techniques are described and demonstrated but may inwardly decide that there is no possibility of learning and successfully performing all these procedures.

Some clinicians tend to overprescribe hygiene

agents and procedures. Again, the patient may appear to accept the added demands on his time, but eventually he may rebel and refrain from even the basic techniques.

Information is not available as to the optimal frequency of carrying out oral hygiene procedures for the prevention of periodontal disease. However, it has been shown that little plaque adheres to the teeth in the first 24 hours after a thorough cleaning. It is probable that effective once-a-day cleaning, including the interdental areas, is adequate for maintaining gingival health. Since many patients tend to do only part of what is asked of them, it may be advantageous to prescribe more than once-a-day cleaning procedures.

The teaching of oral hygiene procedures will not result in every surface being free of plaque from that time on. Realistically these procedures should be taught with the objective of reducing the plaque on the teeth to a level compatible with gingival health. Even a successfully treated patient with clinically healthy gingiva will usually have small discretely scattered areas of retained plaque. Every individual probably has a plaque level that is compatible with clinical gingival health. This level will vary from person to person and in all probability will vary over an individual's lifetime. The goal in teaching oral hygiene is to help the patient reach and maintain that level.

During the pocket elimination phase of periodontal treatment, plaque levels may increase as some patients are reluctant to clean with their customary vigor for fear of dislodging the periodontal surgical dressing. This is a transient period, and after the final dressing is removed the patient's plaque levels should again fall to a satisfactory level.

MAINTENANCE PHASE OF THERAPY: PLAQUE CONTROL

On completion of periodontal and any necessary adjunctive treatment many patients tend to relax their oral hygiene efforts. Therefore it is wise to arrange the first maintenance appointment not later than 3 months after the termination of active therapy. An important part of this appointment is an assessment of the patient's oral hygiene. One of several things may be observed. The patient may be performing the procedures as meticulously as during active therapy, the patient may admit that he has slackened somewhat, or the clinician may find one or more areas where the patient has unconsciously changed his technique and is no longer effectively removing the

bacterial plaque. Remotivation and reinstruction are called for, and if necessary the patient is rescheduled to check his progress.

REFERENCES

ADA: Guide to dental materials and devices 1974-1975, ed. 7, Chicago, 1974, American Dental Association.

ADA: Accepted dental therapeutics 1969-1970, ed. 33, Chicago, 1969, American Dental Association.

ADA Council on dental materials and devices: Irrigating devices, J. Am. Dent. Assoc. **74:**799, 1967.

Amenta, C., Corn, H., Haselnus, D., Mittelman, J., and Reed, O.: Making prevention pay, Dent. Manage. **11:**23, 1971.

Arnim, S. S.: Dental irrigators for oral hygiene, periodontal therapy and prevention of dental disease, J. Tenn. Dent. Assoc. **47:**65, 1967.

Arnim, S. S.: The use of disclosing agents for measuring tooth cleanliness, J. Periodontol. **34:**227, 1963.

Barkley, R. F.: Unshackle your patients, J. Tenn. Dent. Assoc. **49:**25, 1969.

Bass, C. C.: An effective method of personal hygiene. II. J. Louisiana M. Soc. **106:**100, 1954.

Bay, I., Kardel, K. M., and Skougaard, M. R.: Quantitative evaluation of the plaque-removing ability of different types of toothbrushes, J. Periodontol. **38:**527, 1967.

Beeuwkes, H., and de Vries, H. R.: Chlorhexidine in urology, Lancet **2:**913, 1956.

Bergenholtz, A., Bjorne, A., and Vikstrom, B.: The plaque-removing ability of some common interdental aids, an intraindividual study, J. Clin. Periodontol. **1:**160, 1974.

Black, G. V.: Special dental pathology, ed. 3, Chicago, 1924, Medico-Dental Publishing Co.

Block, P. L., Lobene, R. R., and Derdivanis, J. P.: A two-tone dye test for dental plaque, J. Periodontol. **43:**423, 1972.

Bunting, R. W.: Oral hygiene, ed. 2, Philadelphia, 1954, Lea & Febiger.

Charters, W. J.: Immunizing both hard and soft mouth tissue to infection by correct stimulation with the toothbrush, J. Am. Dent. Assoc. **15:**87, 1928.

Cofield, K. R., Ferguson, E. W., and Toye, A. E.: Topical application of penicillin in the treatment of Vincent's infection, J. Am. Dent. Assoc. **34:**406, 1947.

Cohen, D. W., Stoller, N., Chace, R., and Laster, L.: A comparison of bacterial plaque disclosants in periodontal disease, J. Periodontol. **41:**333, 1972.

Cohen, M. M.: A pilot study testing the plaque-removing ability of a newly invented toothbrush, J. Periodontol. **44:**183, 1973.

Collins, J. F., and Hood, H. M.: Sensitivity of oral microorganisms to vancomycin—an in vitro study, J. Oral Ther. **4:**214, 1967.

Curtis, G. H., McCall, C. M., and Overaa, H. I.: A clinical study of the effectiveness of the Roll and Charter's methods of brushing teeth, J. Periodontol. **28:**277, 1957.

Dunkin, R. T.: A new approach to oral physiotherapy with a new index of evaluation, J. Periodontol. **36:**315, 1965.

Ennever, J., and Sturzenberger, O. P.: Inhibition of dental calculus formation by use of enzyme chewing gum, J. Periodontol. **32:**331, 1961.

Felix, J. E., Rosen, S., and App, G. R.: Detection of bacteremia after the use of an oral irrigating device in patients with periodontitis, J. Periodontol. **42:**785, 1971.

Fitzgerald, R. J., Keyes, P. H., Stoudt, T. H., and Spinell, D. M.: The effect of a dextranase preparation on plaque and caries in hamsters, a preliminary report, J. Am. Dent. Assoc. **76:**301, 1968.

Flotra, L., Gjermo, P., Rolla, G., and Waerhaug, J.: Side effects of chlorhexidine mouthwashes, Scand. J. Dent. Res. **79:**119, 1971.

Frandsen, A. M., Barbano, J. P., Suomi, J. D., Chang, J. J., and Burke, A. D.: The effectiveness of the Charters', scrub and roll methods of toothbrushing by professionals in removing plaque, Scand. J. Dent. Res. **78:**459, 1970.

Frandsen, A. M., Barbano, J. P., Suomi, J. D., Chang, J. J., and Houston, R.: A comparison of the effectiveness of the Charters', scrub and roll methods of toothbrushing in removing plaque, Scand. J. Dent. Res. **80:**267, 1972.

Geraci, J. E., Heilman, F. R., Nichols, D. R., Wellman, W. E., and Ross, G. T.: Some laboratory and clinical experiences with a new antibiotic, vancomycin, Mayo Clinic Proc. **31:**564, 1956.

Geraci, J. E., Nichols, D. R., and Wellman, W. E.: Vancomycin: its use in serious staphylococcal infections, Arch. Intern. Med. **109:**507, 1962.

Giesecke, M.: History of the toothbrush, Oral Health **48:**554, 1958.

Gjermo, P.: Chlorhexidine in dental practice, J. Clin. Periodontol. **1:**143, 1974.

Gjermo, P., Baastad, K. C., and Rolla, G.: The plaque-inhibiting capacity of 11 antibacterial compounds, J. Periodont. Res. **5:**102, 1970.

Gjermo, P., and Eriksen, H. M.: Unchanged plaque-inhibiting effect of chlorhexidine in human subjects after two years of continuous use, Arch. Oral Biol. **19:**317, 1974.

Gjermo, P., and Flotra, L.: The effect of different methods of interdental cleaning, J. Periodont. Res. **5:**230, 1970.

Gjermo, P., and Rolla, G.: The plaque-inhibiting effect of chlorhexidine containing dentifrices, Scand. J. Dent. Res. **79:**126, 1971.

Glickman, I.: The use of penicillin lozenges in the treatment of Vincent's Infection and other acute gingival inflammations, J. Am. Dent. Assoc. **34:**406, 1947.

Goldman, H. M., and Bloom, J.: The topical application of Aureomycin for the treatment of the acute phase of necrotizing ulcerative gingivitis (Vincent's Infection), Oral Surg. **3:**1148, 1950.

Grant, J. C., and Findlay, J. C.: Local treatment of burns and scalds using chlorhexidine, Lancet **2:**862, 1957.

Greene, J. C.: Oral hygiene and periodontal disease, Am. J. Public Health **53:**913, 1963.

Hamp, S-E., Lindhe, J., and Löe, H.: Long term effect of chlorhexidine on developing gingivitis in the beagle dog, J. Periodont. Res. **8:**63, 1973.

Hill, H. C., Levi, P. A., and Glickman, I.: The effects of waxed and unwaxed dental floss on interdental plaque accumulation and interdental gingival health, J. Periodontol. **44:**411, 1973.

Hiniker, J. J., and Forscher, B. K.: The effect of toothbrush type on gingival health, J. Periodontol. **32:**346, 1961.

Hoover, D. R., and Robinson, H. B. G.: The comparative effectiveness of the Water Pik in a noninstructed population, J. Periodontol. **39:**43, 1968.

Horowitz, A. M., and Suomi, J. D.: A comparison of plaque removal with a standard or an unconventional toothbrush used by youngsters, J. Periodontol. **45:**760, 1974.

Hugo, W. B., and Longworth, A. R.: The effect of chlorhexidine on the electrophoretic mobility, cytoplasmic con-

stituents, dehydrogenase activity and cell walls of *Escherichia coli* and *Staphylococcus aureus,* J. Pharm. Pharmacol. **18:**569, 1966.

Hugo, W. B., and Longworth, A. R.: Some aspects of the mode of action of chlorhexidine, J. Pharm. Pharmacol. **16:**655, 1964.

Jensen, A. L.: Use of dehydrated pancreas in oral hygiene, J. Am. Dent. Assoc. **50:**923, 1959.

Jensen, S. B., Löe, H., Schiott, C. R., and Theilade, E.: Experimental gingivitis in man. IV. Vancomycin induced changes in bacterial plaque composition as related to development of gingival inflammation, J. Periodont. Res. **3:** 284, 1968.

Kelner, M.: Comparative analysis of the effects of automatic and conventional toothbrushing in mental retardates, Penn. Dent. J. **30:**102, 1963.

Konig, K. G., and Guggenheim, B.: In-vivo effects of dextranase on plaque and caries, Helv. Odontol. Acta **12:**48, 1968.

Krajewski, J. J., Giblin, J., and Gargiulo, A. W.: Evaluation of a water pressure cleansing device as an adjunct to periodontal treatment, Periodontics **2:**76, 1964.

Krajewski, J. J., Rubach, W. C., and Pope, J. W.: The effect of water pressure cleansing on the clinically normal gingival crevice, J. South. Calif. Dent. Assoc. **43:**452, 1967.

Lainson, P. A., Bergquist, J. J., and Fraleigh, C. M.: Clinical evaluation of pulsar, a new pulsating water pressure cleansing device, J. Periodontol. **41:**401, 1970.

Langley, K. B., and O'Bannon, J. Y.: The plaque index graph, Presented at the Periodontic Section, annual meeting of the American Dental Association, Washington, D.C., November 11, 1974.

Lightner, L. M., O'Leary, T. J., Drake, R. B., Crump, P. P., and Allen, M. F.: Preventive periodontic treatment procedures: results over 46 months, J. Periodontol. **42:**555, 1971.

Lindhe, J., and Koch, G.: The effect of supervised oral hygiene on the gingivae of children. Lack of prolonged effect of supervision, J. Periodont. Res. **2:**215, 1967.

Lindhe, J., and Koch, G.: The effect of supervised oral hygiene on the gingiva of children. Progression and inhibition of gingivitis, J. Periodont. Res. **1:**260, 1966.

Lobene, R. R.: The effect of a pulsed water pressure cleansing device on oral health, J. Periodontol. **40:**667, 1969.

Lobene, R. R., Brian, M., and Socransky, S. S.: Effect of erythromycin on dental plaque and plaque-forming microorganisms, J. Periodontol. **40:**287, 1969.

Lobene, R. R., Soparkar, P. M., Hein, J. W., and Quigley, G. A.: Evaluation of an irrigating device for delivering oral therapeutic agents, Abstract No. 277, I. A. D. R. Program and abstract of papers, 1971.

Löe, H.: Formation and growth of plaque on gingival-dental structures, oral presentation given at the International Conference on Dental Plaque, New York, Oct. 8, 1969.

Löe, H., and Schiott, C. R.: The effect of mouthrinses and topical application of chlorhexidine on the development of dental plaque and gingivitis in man, J. Periodont. Res. **5:** 79, 1970.

Löe, H., Theilade, E., and Jensen, S. B.: Experimental gingivitis in man, J. Periodontol. **36:**177, 1965.

Löe, H., Theilade, E., Jensen, S. B., and Schiott, C. R.: Experimental gingivitis in man. III. Influence of antibiotics on gingival plaque development, J. Periodont. Res. **2:**282, 1967.

Lovdal, A., Arno, A., Schei, O., and Waerhaug, J.: Combined effects of subgingival scaling and controlled oral hygiene on the incidence of gingivitis, Acta Odontol. Scand. **19:**537, 1961.

Lowbury, E. J., Lilly, H. A., and Bull, J. P.: Methods for disinfection of hands and operation sites, Br. Med. J. **5408:** 531, 1964.

McClure, D. B.: A comparison of toothbrushing technics for the preschool child, J. Dent. Child. **33:**205, 1966.

McKendrick, A. J. W., Barbenel, L. M. H., and McHugh, W. D.: A two-year comparison of hand and electric toothbrushes, J. Periodont. Res. **3:**224, 1968.

Mitchell, D. F., and Baker, R. B.: Topical antibiotic control of necrotizing gingivitis, J. Periodontol. **39:**81, 1968.

Mitchell, D. F., and Holmes, L. A.: Topical antibiotic control of dentogingival plaque, J. Periodontol. **36:**202, 1965.

Mobley, E., and Smith, S. H.: Some social and economic factors relating to periodontal disease among young Negroes, J. Am. Dent. Assoc. **66:**486, 1963.

O'Leary, T. J., Drake, R. B., and Naylor, J. E.: The plaque control record, J. Periodontol. **43:**38, 1972.

O'Leary, T. J., Shafer, W. G., Swenson, H. M., Nesler, D. C., and Van Dorn, P. R.: Possible penetration of crevicular tissue from oral hygiene procedures. I. Use of oral irrigating devices, J. Periodontol. **41:**158, 1970.

Packer, M., and Smith, T.: Massed versus spaced appointments in teaching oral hygiene, Abstract no. 278, I. A. D. R. Program and abstract of papers, 1971.

Parsons, J. C.: Chemotherapy of dental plaque — a review, J. Periodontol. **45:**177, 1974.

Raybin, M.: Disclosing solutions, their importance and uses, Dent. Outlook **30:**159, 1943.

Rodda, J. C.: A comparison of four methods of toothbrushing, N. Z. Dent. J. **64:**162, 1968.

Roethlisberger, F. J., and Dickson, W. J.: Management and the worker, Cambridge, Mass., 1939, Harvard University Press.

Rolla, G., Löe, H., and Schiott, C. R.: The affinity of chlorhexidine for hydroxyapatite and salivary mucins, J. Periodont. Res. **5:**90, 1970.

Russell, A. L.: International nutrition surveys: a survey of preliminary findings, J. Dent. Res. **42:**232, 1963.

Sanjana, M. K., Mehta, F. S., and Shroff, B. C.: The effect of irrigation treatment on the bacteriological contents of the periodontal pocket, J. All India Dent. Assoc. **34:**74, 1962.

Schei, O., Waerhaug, J., Lovdal, A., and Arno, A.: Alveolar bone loss as related to oral hygiene and age, J. Periodontol. **30:**7, 1959.

Schmid, M. O., Balmelli, O. P., and Saxer, V. P.: Plaque-removing effect of a toothbrush, dental floss, and a toothpick, J. Clin. Periodont. **3:**157, 1976.

Seliger, W. O.: A technique for measuring the penetration of pulsating-jet oral irrigators, Arch. Oral Biol. **14:**435, 1969.

Shick, R. A., and Ash, M. M.: Evaluation of the vertical method of toothbrushing, J. Periodontol. **32:**346, 1961.

Skinner, F. H.: The prevention of pyorrhea and dental caries by oral prophylaxis, Dent. Cosmos **56:**299, 1914.

Smith, J. F., and Blankenship, J.: Improving oral hygiene in handicapped children by the use of an electric toothbrush, J. Dent. Child. **31:**198, 1964.

Stallard, R., Volpe, A. R., Orban, J. E., and King, W. J.: The effect of an antimicrobial mouthrinse on dental plaque, calculus, and gingivitis, J. Periodontol. **40:**683, 1969.

Suomi, J. D., Greene, J. C., Vermillion, J. R., Doyle, J., Chang, J. J., and Leatherwood, E. C.: The effect of controlled oral hygiene procedures on the progression of periodontal disease in adults: results after third and final year, J. Periodontol. **42:**152, 1971.

Suomi, J. D., Leatherwood, E. C., and Chang, J. J.: A follow-up study of former participants in a controlled oral hygiene study, J. Periodontol. **44:**662, 1973.

Toto, P. D., Evans, C. L., and Sawinski, V. J.: Effects of water jet rinse and toothbrushing on oral hygiene, J. Periodontol. **40:**296, 1969.

Vowles, J. K.: Assessment of an automatic action toothbrush (Broxodent) in spastic children, Br. Dent. J. **115:**327, 1963.

Wolfe, G. N.: An evaluation of proximal surface cleansing agents, J. Clin. Periodont. **3:**148, 1976.

19 Motivation of patients

It is important to study motivation as it relates to the treatment of human periodontal disease because motivation is closely involved with the patient and his role in the actual therapy. Our techniques and armamentaria are completely under our control, but the patient's mind is his own, and only he can make and maintain his dentition in a healthy state indefinitely (Derbyshire, 1970, 1968, 1964). "Remember that it is not enough to have the method, and the art, and the power, nor even that which is touch, but you shall also have the conviction that nails the work to the wall."

Stress, as well as motivation, is important as an etiologic factor in oral disease. In a study utilizing naval aviation cadets (Formicola et al., 1970) it was established that certain personality traits correlated with the occurrence of ANUG in this group. Treatment for periodontal disease must partly address itself to a change of life-style by the patient, which requires a positive motivation to reduce stress. Bruxism is also thought to be linked to emotional stress in most cases. Even a patient's oral hygiene performance has been linked to socioeconomic status, age, and sex (Awwa

and Stallard, 1970). Manhold found that neglect of oral as well as of general health was characteristic of the nonauthoritarian personality (Manhold, 1972, 1961). Therefore as an etiologic factor that affects patient motivation the relationship between psychology and dental disease is an important one, and one that demands a well-motivated patient for successful change in the course of the disease process.

Motivation is a powerful force that dictates whether and how a person will act in a given situation and as such must be comprehended so that we can aid the patient in making a decision to treat his periodontal disease or understand why many persons, even when informed, will not act to save their teeth by dental therapy. Greene (1966) has stated this concept in the following manner: "Perhaps the most important and difficult problem that remains to be solved before much progress can be made in the prevention of periodontal disease is how to motivate the individual to follow a prescribed-effective oral health care program throughout his life." Reed (1970) has stated, "Treating without preventing is like chasing without catching." Barclay (1971, 1970) phrases it somewhat differently when he says that before he instituted his dental disease control program "I treated a diseased mouth much like a carpenter working on a burning building."

There are many factors capable of influencing motivation. However, one specific point requires emphasis. Specifically, both dentist and patient must regard themselves as cotherapists, partners, or equals in therapy. The patient's basic role must be clearly defined early in therapy. Briefly stated, it is one of keeping his dental disease under control by his personal dental disease control (PDDC) program. The dentist's equally important role is then to make it possible for the patient to practice his PDDC program. This is accomplished by good operative dentistry.

Katcher (1964) has stated that the traditional role of the physician or dentist has been to dispense "health" in small periodic doses to a totally passive, "good" patient. All too frequently the dosage was not so much health, but treatment of the symptoms or deformities caused by the disease. To practice preventively the physician must relinquish some of his unchallengeable, superior, conciliatory attitudes and make the patient a full partner in treatment. This means a fully informed partner who is to be given credit for success and responsibility for failure as it pertains to his task. The patient must clearly recognize that the physician cannot and should not be expected to perform the patient's task, and, as well, the patient should not expect the physician or dentist to do anything for the patient that he cannot do for himself.

Before leaving the discussion of the doctor-patient relationship we should explore each of the two principal characters, the dentist and the patient, in greater detail.

THE DENTIST
Personality

Like most professionals, the dentist tends to be a compulsive personality type with a well-developed ego and superego that combat the instinctual id drives. He therefore may manifest many of the following attributes: (1) he pays attention to details and is somewhat of a perfectionist; (2) he demonstrates a devotion to duty and responsibility; (3) he is capable of a long-sustained work effort; (4) he is capable of postponing his instinctual pleasure, or id drives, because of his well-developed ego and superego; and (5) he tends to conform to moral and social codes of society.

With these personality traits the dentist is further influenced by the nature and location of his work. Some of its characteristics are as follows: (1) he works in a confined area, (2) he has little or no opportunity for release of tension through motor activity, (3) he has a rather constant preoccupation with pain or prevention of pain, and (4) he is in contact with patients who are consciously or subconsciously hostile toward him and his work.

Therefore, given these personality traits and conditions of work, it is not surprising that the dentist is somewhat prone to anxiety and tension that are manifested in the high rate of cardiovascular disease, ulcers, headaches, lower back problems, and suicide.

Self-image. Sociologic studies of various service occupations indicate that most workers in a given occupation believe the public at large does not have as favorable an image of that occupation as the workers believe they should have. This is true of dental students, many of whom believe that the public thinks of dentists as sadistic mechanics who charge too much (Quarantelli, 1961). This negative attitude is then built into a dentist's self-concept. The negative self-concept then will heavily influence the social relationship that exists between a dentist and his patient.

It is of utmost importance that the dentist handle patient hostility in the proper manner for his own sake and so that he may properly influence the patient to make the proper decision for treatment and to take the proper responsibility for oral hygiene through plaque control.

Role in society

It is also important to outline the basic role of the dentist in our society. Depending on the person consulted on this topic, the answer to the question, "What is the dentist's role?" (Amsterdam, 1963-1964) would probably include the following duties: (1) to prevent dental and oral disease, (2) to maintain a functioning dental apparatus for mastication, speech, and aesthetics, (3) to allow for mastication of a wide variety of foods necessary for a balanced diet, (4) to detect and treat local disease processes found in the oral cavity, (5) to make sure that there are no irritative factors that may lead to tissue alterations, and (6) to detect incipient oral tumors and to initiate their therapy. Although all these answers are true, none of them represents the *basic* reason why the dental profession exists today in our society.

Consider the following statements.

1. Periodontal disease may occasionally have serious consequences relative to the general health of the patient, but periodontal disease is rarely a life-and-death situation.

2. Unlike animals, which soon die without teeth, and primitive man, who was greatly dependent on good teeth, modern man in our Western society no longer needs teeth to maintain proper nutrition. The advent of refined, nutritious, solid, and liquid foods and dietary supplements makes chewing for dietary reasons unnecessary.

3. The emotional significance of teeth and the integrity of the oral cavity make teeth most important from an aesthetic and psychologic standpoint.

Therefore the basic role of the dentist in our society seems to be one of helping to maintain the psychologic well-being of our patients. This is accomplished by dental techniques that may maintain, restore, or even destroy the patient's natural teeth. Acceptance of this basic role for our profession does not necessarily change the specific techniques that we utilize, but it certainly does affect the reasons for which we perform these techniques. It demands a change in philosophy of dental practice (Chaves and Frichofer, 1966) that takes into account the varying degrees of importance that patients place upon their teeth and the reasons for this variance. Acceptance of such a philosophy in no way reduces the goals of the profession. Indeed it forces these goals to a higher plane where we may actually minister as a true physician to the patient's mind and body. Recognition of our true task in life requires understanding the patient's needs and values. A well-motivated patient is absolutely essential if we are to prevent dental disease and preserve the natural teeth.

THE PATIENT

Having briefly profiled the dentist let us now examine the patient. The following anecdote provides a good starting point. A small boy came to the office of a dentist and very aptly stated, "I hope you know what you're doing because it's me, and I don't want anything to happen to me" (Dunlap, 1977). In the opinion of many patients, dentists, and psychiatrists (Firestein, 1976; Hammerman, 1954) all dental patients are anxious. Hammerman states that this is correct "regardless of whether or not the anxiety is evident overtly, whether the patient admits this anxiety or whether he is completely unaware of the existence of anxiety." Anxiety is related to dread of situations that symbolize unconscious conflict and may be considered as a subjective warning of such danger. Fear, on the other hand, is related to more specific objective dangers. Stunkard (1956) states that a patient never comes to a doctor unless he is anxious. This has been referred to by Meares (1957) as disquiet of mind. In other words a person feels uncomfortable and seeks out the dentist for treatment to reduce his anxiety.

However, many patients have conflicting anxieties that counteract the one previously mentioned. Some of these latter anxieties, which would prevent a patient from following through with his original intentions, stem from unconscious conflicts that center around the oral cavity. These conflicts manifest themselves as hostility toward the dentist, the dependent situation in which the patient finds himself, and the possible loss of teeth or tooth structure with all of its psychologic implications. To understand these conflicts better, the unique emotional significance surrounding the oral cavity should be reviewed.

Emotional significance of oral cavity: anxiety related to dental visits

Freudian viewpoint. One of the main bases for anxiety in the dental patient is connected with unconscious conflicts that center around the oral cavity, which is the special province of the dentist. In the development of personality, according to Freud, one of the earliest stages is called the oral stage of development. This lasts from birth to the age of about 12 months and is the period when the infant utilizes his mouth almost exclusively to maintain contact with his environment. The mouth is not only the site of food ingestion but also an organ of exploration with which the child samples everything from his fingers and toes to any object with which he comes in contact. With his mouth he feeds, deriving considerable pleasure from this act itself and also from being held, cuddled, and talked to while feeding. In this parent-child relationship vast amounts of learning take place in an emotionally charged setting.

The oral stage of personality development is followed by a so-called anal phase and a genital phase, in which these respective areas become the center of the child's attention and interest and therefore become important in his emotional development. All children pass through these stages of personality development. Normally we pass through the early stage into the next and more advanced stage of emotional growth. It is to be expected that traces of each stage remain.

As previously stated the child from birth to about 1 year of age utilizes the mouth to feed and to explore his environment. This is also a period of rapid physical growth. Therefore much food must be ingested in this time, and the baby derives considerable erotic pleasure from the act of sucking and later from chewing his food. Depending on the amount of love and acceptance by family and parents at this age, the child associates his oral cavity with pleasure and security or anxiety and frustration.

The mouth not only is used for other erotic acts such as kissing, but it is active as the organ of speech with which a person may express either love or hate. Many aggressive impulses may be discharged through biting and chewing. Shakespeare's description of Richard III in *King Henry the Sixth* signifies that recognition of this fact is not a new finding:

Teeth hadst thou in thy head when thou wast born,
To signify thou camest to bite the world.

For a variety of reasons certain individuals remain somewhat locked at the oral stage in the subconscious mind. Hammerman (1954) discusses the consequences as follows:

This gives rise to patterns in the character structure of the individual as regards his behavior, his thinking, his emotional reactions and his unconscious fantasies, all of which are related to anxieties due to conflicts connected with unresolved oral problems. Some of the derivatives that may result from such unresolved oral conflicts are sexual perversions, problems of obesity, and various psychosomatic conditions, such as ulcers and asthma.

In other words, the patient may get "hung up" at one of these stages or return to it with all of its associations in times of anxiety.

Therefore, depending on the individual patient, the dentist may be viewed as a protector of the oral cavity or as a mutilator of this special area. The oral cavity has an erogenous potential; manipulating the oral tissues may result in erotic stimulation in some patients, whereas in others it may result in extreme horror and fears of sexual abuse. Consequently a rather bizarre range of reactions to the dentist and his efforts may be encountered. Although some patients may react with cooperation and appreciation accompanied by minimal anxiety, others may react with extreme anxiety, sweating, and even fainting associated with subconscious fantasies of abuse. Male patients may equate tooth loss with castration and faint to postpone or avoid the situation that provokes such thoughts. Females may equate dental procedures with sexual assault. Still others react to oral stimulation with erotic pleasure. *It should be made clear that these reactions are the extreme ends of a continuum of possible reactions; although rarely seen in a pure form in practice, they are nevertheless often noticed in small degrees in patients who mask their true feelings with well-constructed defense mechanisms.* Obviously such attitudes in a patient can be formidable barriers to proper motivation. They would also largely govern the dentist's personal conduct of the management of patients. Extreme hostility is generated by some of these patients in the dental situation. This should not be interpreted by the dentist as hostility necessarily toward him personally, but toward the situation in which the patient finds himself.

The practitioner who is aware of the emotional significance of the oral cavity should be able to interpret patient behavior more intelligently, save himself from some of the trauma of patient hostility, and therefore be better able to establish rapport and thus communicate with his patient. This would then be followed by reeducation, and hopefully a well-motivated, less hostile, more responsive patient would result.

Although the Freudian viewpoint helps in *understanding* the sometimes bizarre behavior associated with dental treatment, it offers the practicing dentist little advice on how to control patients' fears in the daily clinical situation (Ayer, 1972). Because Freudian psychoanalytic practice must deal with past instinctual behavior, much time is required for change to occur. The following two approaches can help the patient to overcome anxiety more rapidly.

Learning theory. Learning theory states that behavior is learned and as such can be unlearned or extinguished by aversive conditioning (Davidson, 1967). When applied to motivating patients to seek dental care it means that patients who are avoiding dental care because of fear can change their behavior if the punishment derived from dental neglect is greater than their fear of dental treatment. In time there will be a gradual suppression of their fear. Several pain-free "successful" appointments can initiate the change.

The learning theorist also knows that the patient's suppressed behavior or fear can reappear, and therefore positive rewards rather than punishments are recommended. When applied specifically to the motivation of patients it can be demonstrated to be a successful approach, especially when teaching control of periodontal disease by oral hygiene techniques. This will be discussed subsequently, but suffice it to say that it is as difficult to get a patient to seek dental care and follow an effective oral hygiene program as it is to get him to stop engaging in destructive habits such as thumbsucking or nailbiting. However, oral hygiene control measures are an activity that the patient must initiate rather than extinguish. Therefore the effects of seeking dental treatment and following effective control measures *must* bring noticeable advantage to the patient in terms that are *meaningful to the patient.* These could be freedom from pain, saving his teeth and his appearance, an odor-free mouth, lack of gingival bleeding, and so on.

Desensitization therapy. Another approach to reducing the patient's fear and hostility is desensitization therapy. Based on the premise that anxiety and relaxation cannot occur simultaneously, Wolpe (1964) states that "if a response inhibitory of anxiety can be made to occur in the presence of anxiety-evoking stimuli it will weaken the bond between these stimuli and the anxiety.'' Gale and Ayer (1969) discuss the technique as first teaching the patient to relax by the Jacobsen method (1938) and asking him, while relaxed, to visualize nonanxiety-evoking situations such as sitting in a favorite chair. The patient is then asked to list a hierarchy of anxiety-provoking dental stimuli ranked from mild to severe. He is asked to visualize the least provoking stimuli until he can do so without anxiety. He is then asked to visualize each successive point in the hierarchy while remaining relaxed. The basic desensitization premise illustrated here is that the stimulus situation previously linked with anxiety now becomes associated with relaxation.

Factors that influence patient motivation

Our youth-oriented society. In addition to the subconscious psychologic importance of the oral cavity there are many more obvious values placed upon the integrity of this area. Because our society is a youth-oriented one, those things that enable us to prolong our youth and retain our youthful appearance are much sought after and valued.

Teeth are the most important physical facial feature that, if lost almost single handedly give the impression of the onset of old age. Old age has been portrayed for centuries as a period of toothlessness with a collapse of vertical dimension in the face, subsequent characteristic changes in speech and facial form, and an increase in wrinkling.

Unlike some present-day European societies, where old age is viewed with respect, our society places little value on being old. Therefore from the aesthetic standpoint teeth are important, not purely for a superficial attractiveness, but also for a more deep-seated fear of aging.

Our desire to be physically attractive. Teeth are a major factor in preserving a pleasant facial expression that helps us retain our attractiveness to the opposite sex. Attractiveness in men and women is aided immeasurably by the presence of teeth—hopefully natural teeth.

Superstitions and folklore. Many times facts regarding teeth and the pathology associated with them are warped slightly or actually blatantly incorrect to the extent of preventing patients from receiving proper advice on retaining their teeth and preventing dental disease. Practitioners have repeatedly heard about the ''soft'' teeth or the familial susceptibility to decay or pyorrhea. Folklore also contributes its share of distortion to the truth. Some people in this country still believe that the way to arrest a toothache is to recite certain powerful incantations under a full moon. In certain sections of the southern United States the upper canine teeth are known as ''breeding teeth,'' and their loss is supposed to result in impotence for the unfortunate person.

For centuries teeth have enjoyed a reputation for possessing certain magical properties to cure ills and to afford protection from an adverse environment. Tonge (1965) indicates that this reputation is no doubt due to the fact that teeth are the most lasting parts of our bodies, as demonstrated by skeletal remains from all parts of the world. In present-day life some evidence of our respect for teeth still remains. We still use eruption of teeth as a measure of maturity in the child and reward him for the appearance and loss of certain teeth.

Self-discipline. Both caries and periodontal disease are by nature chronic and thereby slowly progressive. The practice of preventive measures to prevent future disease and discomfort requires considerable self-discipline by the patient.

Age. Another factor that may be a barrier to successful motivation is the fact that most periodontal patients are adults. Adults are more difficult to change from their habits of neglect because their previously held concepts must be overcome before learning can take place. On the other hand, an adult can learn from another's experience and can accept long-range goals better than a younger patient can.

According to Kydd (1959), adults, as opposed to children, have the following advantages in learning or appreciating new knowledge or concepts:

1. They can more readily accept or develop for themselves long-range goals.
2. They come to the learning situation a more complete being, able to relate learned material to past experiences.
3. They are often able to learn from another's experience.

Adults as learners have the following disadvantages in learning:

1. They have more set patterns, convictions, and habits that are often difficult to change or modify.
2. Their habits and convictions are obstacles to learning in that they are very difficult to unlearn.

• • •

Some patients, according to Moore (1963), are actually unsuited psychologically to undergo periodontal therapy. Therefore the dentist must remember that the prospective periodontal patient is usually an adult with his own past experiences, knowledge, and performance, which will definitely influence his acceptance or rejection of the dentist's recommendations.

NATURE OF DENTAL DISEASE AS IT AFFECTS MOTIVATION

We are discussing patient motivation with regard to periodontal health in particular and the patient's acceptance of our therapeutic endeavors and his responsibility. Emergency situations such as pulpal pain usually result in a rapidly developed need for relief of pain that activates the patient to action. Sudden loss of teeth, as in automobile accident, also serves as a great stimulus to the patient to seek rapid replacement of these missing parts.

Both relief of pulpal pain and replacement of missing teeth greatly improve the state of patient comfort and reduce anxiety. Such patients come to the office in pain and under stress, and they leave feeling relief after a relatively short time. Conversely, treatable periodontal pathology rarely causes pain, but periodontal therapy often does result in some pain and discomfort and is by nature of long duration.

Herein lies one of the major difficulties in realizing proper patient awareness of periodontal pathology and motivation for periodontal therapy. Periodontal disease usually does not cause pain in its early stages, when the treatment would be minimal and the prognosis would be best. When pain serves as a stimulus to action the periodontal condition may be in a terminal stage. Therefore there is only a slight chance of positive motivational value to be derived from pain in treatable periodontal disease. However, the discomfort encountered by previously pain-free patients after periodontal therapy may be made known to prospective patients and may serve as a countermotivational factor.

Another major difficulty encountered is that many dentists, even in this dentally enlightened country, are not particularly aware of early periodontal pathology. Therefore, as Marshall-Day et al. (1955) have brought out, much of the population of the United States is unaware of its widespread presence. According to Waerhaug (1966), people of all ages, all races, all countries, and all cultures suffer from periodontal disease.

Other dental practitioners, although very much aware of periodontal disease, have no strong convictions toward treatment because they believe in the doctrine of eventual and inevitable tooth loss. This doctrine, when applied to their practices, might be stated, "You are going to be toothless someday—why not now?"

An additional major factor is the lack of social pressure to maintain a clean healthy mouth. Most of us at some time have been refused admission to a restaurant or club for failing to wear a necktie or a jacket, but no one reportedly has been refused anything comparable because of an unhealthy or unclean mouth. As Friedman (1965) points out, dental troubles are socially acceptable and even expected.

If periodontal disease were caused by specific extrinsic factors such as poison, foreign bacteria, viruses, and so on rather than by one's own residual population of bacteria, more urgency would be generated in its control. This is not the case. Furthermore, it is difficult if not impossible to transmit periodontal disease to another person. In fact being afflicted with this condition is an unnewsworthy and uninteresting situation to be in and thus from a motivational standpoint is a situation almost devoid of factors that might arouse the patient to action.

The preventive philosophy of therapy and practice demands a well-informed, motivated patient, or it will fail in its objective of maintaining teeth for life. *Both the patient and periodontist must realize that periodontal disease* can be corrected, but the patient's plaque control must be effective. Control for the diabetic is self-administered dietary measures and medication. Control for the alcoholic is abstinence. Control for the dental patient is self-administered daily control procedures for the rest of his life. A

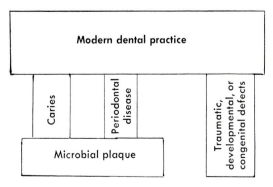

Fig. 19-1. Foundation of dental practice.

well-motivated patient is absolutely essential for success of such a philosophy. Modern dental practice, research, and teaching rest on the three supporting pillars of caries, periodontal disease, and traumatic, developmental, and congenital defects. Caries and periodontal disease are supported in turn by the foundation of microbial plaque (Fig. 19-1). Control of caries and periodontal disease depends on control of the plaque. At present an effective PDDC program relies heavily on daily thorough mechanical removal of plaque from the tooth surface and gingival sulcus by the patient.

INHERENT DIFFICULTIES IN PDDC PROGRAMS

Adequate oral hygiene is most important as a preventive and maintenance measure in the successful treatment of periodontal disease. Motivation of patients in this activity is very difficult. Some general factors that adversely affect successful performance of oral hygiene are the following: (1) lack of social pressure, (2) lack of pain in periodontal disease, (3) pleasures of eating and tasting food, (4) physical features of the oral cavity, (5) physical features of the bacterial plaque, (6) inefficient methods available, and (7) excessive time required. The first two factors have already been discussed and are of utmost importance in a negative way in encouraging poor oral hygiene.

General considerations

Pleasures of eating and tasting food. After eating an especially delicious meal the individual may enjoy certain rather pleasant tastes, which remain in the mouth long after the meal is over. The admirable and socially acceptable custom of lingering over coffee or other libations and nibbling sweets while indulging in pleasant conversation is a powerful countermotivational force against cleaning one's teeth. Besides, it is rather uncomplimentary to the host. Few persons prefer substituting the antiseptic taste of toothpaste for the psychologically gratifying taste of good food. Therefore the timeworn admonishment to brush one's teeth after each meal is very likely to meet with little success. Furthermore, this admonishment may only reinforce the well-accepted, but erroneous concept that the object of mouth and tooth cleansing is food removal. Patients and dentists laboring under this concept will have difficulty in appreciating the fact that it is the microbial plaque that must be removed at least once a day as a minimal acceptable level of oral cleanliness for disease control.

Physical features of oral cavity. If the patient, despite the strong countermotivational forces mentioned, does eagerly cleanse his teeth, the physical features of the oral cavity serve to make the process difficult.

If an artist-engineer were faced with the task of designing and building an object that was, among other things, difficult to cleanse, it is almost a certainty that he would not design anything so easily cleansed as an automobile windshield. He would, no doubt, produce something with many crevices, ledges, uneven surfaces, and complicated structure. If this were not enough to satisfy the requirement of being difficult to cleanse, he might fix the whole assembly permanently in a box with only one small opening and without sufficient illumination.

Clearly the oral cavity is such a dark box, with one small opening containing an apparatus that by its very nature is physically difficult to cleanse.

Physical features of bacterial plaque. Taking into account the physical features of the oral cavity and the difficulty that they introduce, one must now face the equally difficult physical features of the dental plaque. (1) It collects in the most inaccessible regions of the oral cavity; (2) it is invisible even in the best of light; (3) it is very tenaciously adherent to the tooth surface; (4) it forms continually; and (5) it utilizes sucrose from our diet.

In our Western culture, foods are heavily loaded with sucrose. Therefore partial control of the effect of plaque is by modification of diet.

Inefficient methods available. Most of the present methods utilized for oral hygiene are mechanical in nature. The toothbrush, floss, stimulators, abrasive toothpaste, and so on all act in a mechanical manner to remove plaque. Mechanical methods normally could be among the least desirable techniques for cleansing tenacious plaque from such a darkened, inaccessible labyrinth as the oral cavity. Yet mechanical techniques are presently used rather extensively because more practical methods such as chemical or electronic methods are not safe for intraoral use at the present time.

If periodontal disease were controlled by placing electrodes on the teeth with lead wires connected to a device with many dials, blinking red lights, and an oscilloscope or two, control programs would be downright interesting and might even result in a club or association's being formed akin to that of the CB radio following. However, because nothing really exciting or new has been added to the armamentarium and because existing instruments, brushes, floss, toothpaste, and so on have been around for a century or so, anything approaching enthusiasm must be generated from sources other than the instruments used. Paraphrasing the old idiom, one might say that familiarity with the instruments breeds contempt and avoidance.

Excessive time required. Due to the physical features of the oral cavity and dental plaque and the inefficient methods we are forced to use, the time required to properly cleanse the oral cavity is considerable.

Most patients would agree that cleansing an automobile windshield can be easily done in 1 minute. They would also agree that the windshield is well lighted, accessible, and therefore easily cleansed surface. The oral cavity is much more difficult to cleanse, and therefore patients agree that perhaps 5 to 8 minutes might be a reasonable time to spend in completing the task. However, most patients spend much less than 5 minutes on oral hygiene and one study cited, "The Ineffective Toothbrush," (Editorial, 1960) has shown that dental students spent an average of 45 seconds cleansing their mouths.

Although there is no real virtue in spending a fixed amount of time in oral hygiene, this example points clearly to the fact that adequate oral hygiene may take more time than patients have been conditioned to expect. Most people presently find it difficult to justify that much time because they have no pain, are not socially censured, and the aftertaste of a good meal is preferable to the medicinal taste of a toothpaste. It is for these reasons that the oral cavity is inherently difficult to cleanse physically and psychologically. Because it is difficult to cleanse, it stands as a definite obstacle in motivating people to perform adequate oral hygiene, which is a major requirement for successful periodontal therapy and dental disease control.

It should be noted that a commonly accepted occurrence of everyday life, for example, cleansing a windshield, when paralleled with a poorly understood or accepted concept like disease control, is an effective educational technique for making the new concept seem more reasonable and acceptable.

Patients resist change. New ideas, procedures, and routines can appear strange, threatening, and full of uncertainties even if they are improvements. People ask, "Will I be able to do it? Will I be able to adjust? If I fail, will I appear foolish, stupid or clumsy compared to other patients?" Another cause of resistance is the incon-

venience of change. Some patients become very resistant when told that they have to do something (Levoy, 1976).

Social values and pressures

Some of the more common ways in which behavior in general is modified by social pressures are laws, folkways, and mores practiced by society. If we fail to live up to the law, we are punished. If we fail to respect the folkways of our society, we are regarded as eccentric. As Cinotti and Grieder (1972) point out, violation of mores is a more serious offense because this is the area of moral and ethical behavior.

The acceptance or rejection of dental care is not socially important to the masses. Apathy toward the benefits of a healthy mouth likewise is not socially serious. Violation of laws, folkways, or mores of our society is not strongly related to dental health, so no primary motivation is likely to arise from this quarter. Some secondary motives, for example, appearance, do offer the possibility of motivating the public to seek dental health services.

Dental care has not yet taken on much social value, but there are a few factors that may assist in inducing an individual to follow better dental care. Society suggests that we should not offend others with body odor or halitosis or present a facial image with missing, broken, or stained teeth. No doubt this definitely helps the sale of mouthwashes and deodorants, but it may or may not force the patient to seek complete dental care (Everett, 1971).

Social pressures that might be important for use in motivation for dental health are *already known* by the advertising media and motivational researchers. However, dentistry is a profession that must use such information ethically. It is often necessary to make use of drives, needs, fears, and anxiety to force patients to act positively toward dental care. In our financially affluent society many people would rather spend their money on some prestige-producing product like a new car or a mink coat because prestige is "needed" by persons more than dental health is "needed."

Emergency care sells itself because the fears of pain and the need for self-preservation are active. *Preventive dentistry* is like any other intangible product such as vaccination for the prevention of communicable disease. The person must be persuaded to spend time and money to prevent possible disease in the future.

The principles of need creation should be utilized by dentists to gain a more rewarding practice financially as well as psychologically. In addition their patients would benefit more from less dental repair and more preventive practices.

It has been previously stated that periodontal disease does not result in much pain, and therefore little primary motivation is derived from it. Some motivational factors are not socially acceptable and are never openly admitted by patients because the patients feel embarrassed to admit their existence; e.g., patients might well desire to preserve their teeth because they want to be more attractive to members of the opposite sex, but the reason they admit is more likely to be that they hate going to the dentist, and therefore proper care will make this exposure minimal.

Status is one of the foremost social motives in our society. It operates with individuals as well as with groups. As Bauer (1960) puts it, ''The function of group influence is to reduce perceived risk by confirming the wisdom of choice.'' Some common status symbols in our society are riches earned or inherited, family tree, job, clothes, and social circle. Status-conscious persons seek such things to enable them to climb up the ladder to the next class. Therefore manufacturers spend millions of dollars on the promotion of certain brands of goods with snob appeal that are eagerly sought after by persons, few of whom have any real knowledge of the products that they are purchasing. The most expensive automobiles, according to *Consumer Reports* (1967), are usually bought for their prestige value, although they are supposedly promoted and purchased for their superior durability and craftsmanship.

In the field of dentistry, orthodontic bands and appliances have attained some of the aura of being a status symbol, and patients have been known to boast about the number of days or weeks that their periodontal dressing was in place. Thus presenting the prestige value of good dentistry and dental health is a sound procedure, if done in an ethical manner.

Status seeking is most prevalent in the middle class and in some people is an extreme form of neurotic behavior. Some people will spend to the edge of bankruptcy in pursuit of status. Thus Cinotti and Grieder (1972) imply that many such patients will readily agree to any fee to obtain the cosmetic benefits of treatment but are unable to meet the financial obligations.

The *desire for recognition* may motivate people into attention-getting behavior. Although similar to the status seekers, these people are interested only in attention, good or bad. One is reminded of the old show business saying that states, ''I don't care what you say about me, but spell my name correctly.'' The need for recognition may be an undesirable motive for seeking dental care because the motive is superficial relative to the real problem of dental health. In many patients, however, it serves as a secondary motive.

Other motivators mentioned by Blass (1958) include *dependency* upon the professional person for attention, *ego gratification* through an improved self-image, *fear of old age* and the role of loss of teeth in aging, *loss of beauty,* and *fear of dentures,* which is synonymous with old age and retirement, loss of function, and uselessness.

One of the most important factors is *fear of offending other people with bad breath.* The mouthwash and toothpaste interests probably have created and most certainly have capitalized upon this knowledge in our breath-conscious society. However, several important negative effects are derived from this. Many persons rely entirely upon these claims and leave their real dental problems untreated. In the case of periodontal disease, mouthwashes merely mask the odor of necrotic tissue and exudates. Other people, more suspicious by nature, are aroused by the implications of bad breath; but they are doubtful of the commercial claims and may seek professional advice. Once they have taken this step, further motivation is easier.

MOTIVATION: PURPOSE AND SOURCES

The need for a cooperative, knowledgeable, well-motivated patient in dentistry is threefold:

1. *The patient must accept the sole responsibility for a daily personal dental disease control program by oral hygiene, diet, and so on for the rest of his life.*

2. The patient should accept dental treatment and periodic recall examination as a adjunct to his PDDC program and accept it as a worthwhile investment of time and money in himself.

3. The patient should accept treatment and instruction.

Usually the topic of motivation is discussed in a manner that suggests that patients are motivated solely by dentists. Actually, the patient motivates himself. Although motivation comes from within each patient, the factors that lead to such motivation are influenced by the patient's past experiences, his family, his culture, his social standards and values, and most assuredly by the dental profession, that is, each dentist, his office, and his auxiliaries.

Furthermore, factors that affect a patient's beliefs about dental therapy may originate days, weeks, months, or years prior to the first actual visit or contact. The dentist and his patient might then be considered as two individuals, unknown to one another initially, both preparing themselves subconsciously for a future meeting in the dentist's office. Motives, desires, or needs originate with the patient and come from many sources. These needs are modified by the attitudes, knowledge, and philosophy of the particular dentist only after the patient first hears about him or contacts him. It is useful to remember that a patient will accept or refuse dental treatment for his own reasons, not necessarily those of the dentist.

Many persons are not motivated to accept periodontal care because they are not informed about the subject. An informed patient is more easily motivated than is an uninformed one. Therefore *some education of the patient* must occur in many instances prior to the arousal of specific needs in the patient. Conversely, before much learning can occur, the *individual must be somewhat* motivated to learn. Obviously, then, learning and motivation for learning must occur simultaneously.

For either learning or motivation for learning to occur in the patient, communication between the particular source of information and the patient must be established. *Therefore communication might necessarily precede motivation for learning and learning itself.* Communication must be established with the patient by a well-informed and *ethically motivated* source. Communication in this context connotes understanding of ideas, concepts, or information deficiencies that are discussed in a form that is meaningful, understandable, and pertinent to the patient.

From the preceding discussion *it now seems likely that learning, motivation for learning, and communication proceed together to arouse a need in the patient.* For purposes of further discussion each will be examined separately with the factors that affect it.

SOURCES OF INFORMATION ON PERIODONTAL THERAPY

It must not be assumed that the dentist is the sole source of information about dental disease and its treatment. It should be obvious that before a patient makes a dental visit oriented toward prevention, that is, a visit that is not provoked by pain, he must have already been informed to some degree about the dangers of neglecting his dental health. He might have been informed by any one of a great number of sources, some of which are listed as follows:

1. Family or friends
2. Mass media—television, radio, magazines
3. Past experiences—personal and family
4. Fear of future pain and discomfort
5. Other authorities—physicians, school teachers, nurses
6. Social and cultural background

At this point he may not be aware of the status of his periodontal health but be concerned only about the problems associated with dental caries.

The major source of information about periodontal disease should be the private practitioner of dentistry. Even though we often complain about the failure of many dentists to inform their patients about early periodontal disease and its treatment to save their teeth, the patient may still learn about periodontal disease and its end result at the time that he becomes toothless and a candidate for dentures. *By far the most frequent complaint made known to periodontists by patients about dentists is, "Why didn't he tell me I had this trouble?"*

We must assume that the patient has come to a dental office for some definite reason. The dental practitioner may then take steps to inform him through a suitable means of communication to arouse in him a need for the required periodontal therapy.

Another common method that a dentist may use to inform the population outside his office is to speak on behalf of dental health before groups of citizens at various places in the community. Although this is of some value, perhaps more attention should be focused upon informing and convincing the opinion makers in the community. Physicians and nurses are powerful opinion makers with regard to health practices in the community, and as such they should be ethically cultivated for the benefit that they can be in educating patients regarding dental health. Schoolteachers also should be informed and motivated positively toward dental health because, as Robinson et al., (1967) suggest, it is at the elementary school level that the most effective education is done and the most lasting attitudes are created. It must be restated that the profession must establish better communication and rapport with the masses.

In most decision-making situations a person is usually motivated for one of two reasons; namely, because his conscience dictates that the decision be based on a moral issue or because he feels pressure from an outside source, which has little to do with whether the situation is right or wrong. The decision of the dentist to inform a patient that he has periodontal disease should be initiated because it is right and is his duty as a professional.

Recently several successful lawsuits have resulted in widespread attention in the press. These suits were successful against several practitioners who were found negligent because they had not informed their patients that they had periodontal disease. *It is not required that the dentist treat a periodontal problem, but it is required that he inform his patients and refer them for treatment if they so desire.* A lawsuit is an undesirable way of informing the public about the widespread nature of periodontitis, but it is a very effective way of doing so.

ESTABLISHMENT OF COMMUNICATION: RAPPORT

The first task of the practitioner is to establish rapport with the patient, which then makes possible further development of communication, learning, and motivation. Obviously the fact that the patient is present in the office is evidence of some motivation on his part, but it may not be sufficient to make him aware of or accept periodontal therapy. The need may be very strong to accept tooth extraction because of pain or to have only operative dentistry performed to satisfy some aesthetic requirement. *The vast majority of patients do not wish to lose their teeth, merely the problems associated with them.* Their acceptance of extraction and dentures then may be due to the fact that no other solution to their problems has been presented to them. In other words, communication has been poor.

Despite their importance, history taking, clinical examination, and diagnosis must all wait because, according to Meares (1957), while they may all occur concurrently with rapport, *rapport must come first.*

Rapport is an emotional state in which logical, intellectual, or verbal factors may play only a small role. Expressions, gestures, and other nonverbal communication, however small, may assume symbolic value to the patient as the initial meeting with the doctor takes place. On the surface the patient may be reciting his symptoms and concerns, but underneath this veneer he is assessing the competence and trustworthiness of the doctor. Meanwhile the doctor should be es-

tablishing the emotional relationship with the patient that we know as rapport. Rapport is distinct from transference because the latter is a unilateral action on the part of the patient in which he reacts toward the doctor with feelings that he actually feels toward some other person, for example, his father. Some factors that favor formation of rapport are nature of the greeting, friendship, and attitude of the doctor.

The consultation may be routine for the dentist, but it is an event of major importance for the patient. Although a psychiatric interview may be carried on in either a warm, friendly or a cool, distant atmosphere, the latter is less applicable to the meeting of the dental patient and the dentist. Friendship often cannot be offered so well verbally as it can by actions; for example, the traditional seating of the doctor and patient on opposite sides of the desk may be avoided so that both will be equals in the discussion. Occasionally this seating of the doctor behind the desk is practiced if the authoritarian role of the doctor is required. Regardless of the technique utilized, its purpose is to establish an emotional bond between these two individuals. The bond should become stronger because doctor and patient now share the secret of how near the patient is to becoming toothless. MacKenzie (1965) adds that rapport between the dentist and the patient is an important variable in managing the reaction of the patient to discomfort or pain.

However, it is virtually impossible to establish rapport with an individual who lacks at least some motivation. This is common when the patient is brought to the office by relatives or friends rather than because he has a real desire of his own.

The doctor will attempt to appeal to a patient on either an intellectual or an emotional level. The choice of which approach to use will be discussed in relation to persuasion and suggestion. The patient may resist an offer of help from the dentist because he doubts the trustworthiness of anyone who apparently pushes his virtues and aptitudes too vigorously, or he may confuse this offer with a desire for personal gain on the part of the dentist.

Professional people should guard against talking down to a patient. Such a patient may exhibit hostility toward the doctor because he is irritated at having to come for help, and he may resent rapport because of its emotional quality. With such an aggressive patient the doctor may hastily respond to hostility with hostility and make rapport impossible or at least difficult.

Judgmental attitudes by the doctor are also to

be condemned because they prevent the patient from airing his feelings without criticism and defense of his neglect. The neglect may have been the result of lack of finances, misinformation, or extreme anxiety, all of which may be areas about which the patient is initially sensitive or indeed angry.

In considering further obstacles to rapport the dentist should note the difference between *sympathy* and *empathy*. Empathy, a great gift for a professional to possess, means that although we do not share the emotional feelings with the patient as in sympathy, we do appreciate how he is feeling. Empathy is a blend of interest and objectivity. Many times the more sensitive the individual happens to be, the more apt he is to possess a capacity for empathy. Lack of this qualification by the professional is an obstacle to formation of rapport with his patients or clients. In addition, sympathy precludes empathy because while interest is maintained, objectivity is replaced by subjectivity.

The incorrect use of *persuasion* and *suggestion* may also serve as a block to rapport. Persuasion implies an appeal to the person's reason via an intellectual approach, whereas suggestion utilizes an emotional approach and an uncritical acceptance of ideas. As Meares (1957) has suggested, the *two cannot be used concurrently,* or rapport may be subverted or lost. Choice of which approach to follow depends on a knowledge of the needs and values of the patient; for example, a scientist must be persuaded whereas a fashion model may be approached by suggestion.

Once rapport has been established, communication between the individuals is usually easily initiated, provided that language, terms, and methods used are compatible with the patient's level of education and his interest and capacity for understanding. Once this level has been established, the patient previously unaware of his periodontal condition may be rapidly educated and then be motivated himself to accept periodontal therapy. Failure to find the correct level on which to approach the patient with information nullifies the rapport almost instantly.

METHODS OF PATIENT EDUCATION

Trial-and-error learning. One method that we in dental practice cannot afford despite its possible value is trial-and-error learning. Cinotti and Grieder advocate other methods that may prove to be as effective yet more efficient. These are conditioning and insight learning.

Conditioning. The dental patient is conditioned by past experience to expect pain and discomfort before he visits the dental office. In our society the dentist is often portrayed in cartoons and lay articles as a threatening mutilator of the mouth who is to be feared. It has been stated by many that the most feared figure in our society is the psychiatrist and that the dentist is possibly a close second (Friedman, 1965).

In attempting to reeducate such patients many practitioners perform no treatment per se on the first visit but use it to establish rapport and communication and to commence the unlearning of old ideas and fears and the learning of old ideas and fears and the learning of new values. If several visits elapse without pain the former traumatic association is weakened, and the patient is conditioned to become less fearful in the dental situation. The dentist may then proceed with the full treatment that is needed. Such reeducated patients usually avoid or miss fewer appointments and have less anxiety generally. Conditioning may require several appointments, but over the period the patient's association with the dentist will be quite worthwhile.

Insight learning. If every patient came to the dentist with no previous dental experience or knowledge, patient education would be not only easy but almost effortless because no previous erroneous concepts would have to be unlearned. There would be no negative conditioning or avoidance reactions already established. Treatment could be started immediately, and insight learning could be instituted as treatment proceeded. Insight occurs when there is an instantaneous association between formerly unknown or poorly understood events and present happenings. In the process the individual avoids trial and error and the long-term building up of associations required in conditioning.

Both conditioning and insight learning are experienced when the initial appointments are devoted to reeducation in preventive measures.

SPECIFIC TECHNIQUES

Awareness. Awareness of the treatment plan must be created in the patient so that he participates in the proposed plan and knows its probable outcome. Furthermore, the patient must be aware of his responsibilities in the treatment plan, for example, disease control and payment of fees. He must also be convinced that his idea in coming to the dental office is a good decision and will be of benefit to him.

Repetition. From trial-and-error experience we are all aware that repetition is important if we wish to reinforce (Ferris and Winslow, 1970) and establish a certain response. This is certainly true in teaching a new method of disease control.

Praise and punishment. Of the two responses, praise and punishment, praise is more conducive to learning, but punishment can be used to initiate reaction; for example, suspension of treatment can be suggested as the result of the patient's failure to practice good oral hygiene to control his dental disease.

Guidance. Guidance may be vague and indirect, or it may be very direct. An example of the latter is a direct guiding of the patient's hand in executing a new flossing or toothbrushing technique. If the patient is required to follow a set of rules, the rules should be meaningful to him, and he should have a desire to follow them because he is convinced that he benefits directly. A patient is more apt to follow an effective program of personal dental disease control when he visualizes the reduction of bleeding and swelling that follow a week of personal effort.

• • •

It is wise to remember that the patient's education began long before he came to the office. He comes with preconceived ideas. The decor of the office, the atmosphere of the reception area; the background music, and the literature on the table all contribute. The assistant, the hygienist, and the secretary provide some initial contacts, which should be pleasant and efficient in gathering information about the patient. Many auxiliaries actually assist the patient in making a decision to accept the treatment plan. This is more apt to occur if the particular auxiliary is quite familiar with the details of the treatment plan and the results of it and is herself practicing disease control.

Armed with a history and a memo from the assistant, the dentist himself continues his educational efforts by consultation to establish rapport and communication. Education of the patient continues throughout the examination.

A useful list of objectives to be accomplished by the dentist in consultation would include the following:

1. Determine the patient's needs, motives, and desires.
2. Make the patient feel important and accepted.
3. Give the patient some recognition and attention as an active partner in the treatment plan.
4. Use visual aids (especially the patient's own mouth).
5. Be a good listener, especially in the earlier stages of consultation.

MOTIVATIONAL RESEARCH AND THE DENTAL PROFESSION: NEEDS AND GOALS

Motivational research is the study of the "why" of human behavior. Since all human behavior is initiated through needs, it can be said that human behavior is not spontaneous. Boyd and Westfall (1964) say that the terms "needs," "motives," "desires," "goals," "aspirations," "wants," "wishes," "hopes," "fears," and "frustration" are synonymous in relation to behavior and are the fabric of everyday life.

Knowledge of facts that exist in this area of study should be of interest to the dental profession because it deals with why people purchase or fail to purchase certain products and services from the psychosocial point of view. It is encouraging to see the subjects of psychology and sociology being introduced into the dental curriculum, although, as Grusky et al., (1967) note, some early experience has shown that these subjects are difficult to introduce and that student response may be somewhat negative. Although the pressure of a busy teaching schedule and the competition of other courses have been proposed as the reasons for the difficulty, it is quite likely that the preprofessional conditioning of the dental students to the present role of the dentist in our society is responsible for a negative response. The attitudes of dental students regarding the *basic role of the dentist* are largely drawn from the views and opinions held by their families, friends, and peers. The importance that the new student places on dental techniques far outdoes his interest in what dictates human behavior. Yet many of the most successful practices are established as much on human relations as on technical excellence. *We treat people not teeth.*

A motive or need refers to one of the more compelling determinants of a person's action designed to obtain certain goals. Needs are fixed but goals are always changing. We acquire new goals when we attain old ones or when we cannot attain old ones. Goals are flexible and are tailored to individual abilities. Unattainable goals will only discourage a patient and then become meaningless and unattractive and eventually be rejected

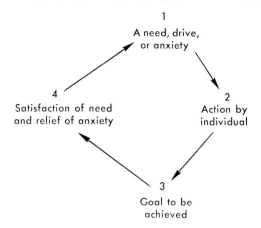

Fig. 19-2. Motivational cycle.

(Weiss, 1969). Motivation arises from tension systems that create a state of disequilibrium for that individual. This disequilibrium triggers a series of psychologic events directed toward selection of a goal that the individual anticipates will bring about release from the tensions. Patterns of action that he hopes will make the goal obtainable are also selected.

What Bayton (1958) calls *disequilibrium of an individual,* Meares terms *disquiet of mind,* which he defines as an urge to make a change to a more comfortable state.

Thus with the establishment of rapport and communication with the patient, followed by a learning experience by the patient, the result of the motivational cycle so far should be a state of anxiety, disequilibrium, or disquiet of mind in the patient sufficiently strong to compel him to act in a manner to relieve the anxiety. This relief of anxiety, or satisfaction of need, completes the motivational cycle (Fig. 19-2).

Therefore, incongruous as it may seem, the desirable end result of our relation with the patient to this point is anxiety or disquiet of mind in the patient relative to his dental health.

Whatever term is utilized to describe the state of mind that exists in a person who is making a definite selection of goals and methods of action to satisfy his needs does not matter nearly so much as does the understanding that such a force is necessary before a person will act in any manner.

Clawson (1958) states that consumers are influenced at some time, to some degree, and for some products or services by at least 600 different motives. Attempting to classify motives completely is beyond the scope of this discussion, but some simple division to clarify the source and relative importance of various drives or needs is in order.

Needs range from basic ones such as hunger and freedom from pain to ones that originate in highly complex social situations, for example, acceptance, recognition, leadership, and companionship. Silverman (1961) has described two main categories of needs: biologic and social. *Biologic needs* are basic ones that must usually be satisfied fully or serious consequences and even death result. However, *social needs* may be completely or partially realized without resulting death. Life continues even if the person is still anxious about unfulfilled social needs.

If we were dealing exclusively with basic drives, we would encounter little difficulty in getting a person to act. However, when the motivation evident in a person advised to practice better oral hygiene, the difference is outstanding because the patient does not really need good oral hygiene for its own sake to fulfill an urgent biologic requirement. Often, until the patient has suffered from a series of traumatic dental experiences, he is unwilling to adopt good dental care, professional or personal.

Many physiologic basic drives undergo modification and change from our social system and culture. We learn that there are socially acceptable ways of responding to various situations. Therefore often the modification in behavior of a patient will occur in response to some secondary drive. At the same time the modification in behavior also satisfies the basic drives rather by accident than by intent; for example, the patient may respond to a secondary drive for better and sweeter smelling breath by practicing better oral hygiene and simultaneously satisfy the more basic drive for self-preservation. Likewise good oral hygiene might be practiced to render the teeth less susceptible to caries and periodontal disease to avoid the more basic problem of pain.

Cinotti and Grieder (1972) classify drives or needs for dental services as follows:
1. Pain
2. Function—not able to chew properly
3. Aesthetics—appearance not compatible with position
4. Approval of self
5. Family pressure
6. Social pressure—has offensive breath
7. Status—neighbors and friends have had treatment
8. Fear—does not want bleeding gingiva and loose teeth

Blass (1958), who like Cinotti and Grieder is a dentist, classifies dental drives as follows:

1. To keep one's own teeth in comfort
2. To improve one's appearance
3. To keep one socially acceptable
4. To protect one's working ability
5. To improve one's health
6. To lengthen one's life-span

A simpler but more general classification of drives has been developed by Lawrence (1965) as follows:

1. Love of life and self-preservation
2. Need for romance
3. Need for self-esteem

Many common drives are noted in all these classifications in slightly different words.

Some of the more basic drives may be called "primary" motives, whereas others may be called "secondary." Meares would describe disquiet of mind, which is analogous to anxiety, as a primary motive. Reinforcing the primary motive might be a secondary motive; for example, a man might be anxious about maintaining his health (primary motive) so that he could earn more money or attain greater professional status (secondary motive).

Almost without exception the secondary motive is quite inferior to the *disquiet of mind*.

To trigger effectively a particular need into becoming a motivational force, it is necessary to have considerable knowledge of attitudes, sensations, assumptions, and images that prevail about a particular product or service. Although eating is biologically a necessity, the seller of a food product may decide not to use hunger as his basic appeal but, instead, to use social approval, economy, taste, or even pride. His choice will depend on what he knows of the attitudes, sensations, and images held by customers.

One way in which large producers of consumer goods ascertain these attitudes and images is by circulating questionnaires to the consumers, offering perhaps a chance at a prize as a reward for completing the questionnaire. One questionnaire (Consumer's Survey, 1966) recently received in the mail asked whether the consumer owned a color television set or a stereophonograph, the number of credit cards in family charge accounts, the number of magazines received, the number of airplane trips taken in the past year, if a domestic or international membership in a book and record club was held, if other purchases were made by mail, what sports were enjoyed, and the amount of education (including each family member).

Obviously such a questionnaire was pointed largely at modes of getting product information to the consumer because many questions were on the use of the various communication media—television, radio, magazines, the mail, and so on. Although the individual dentist could not afford such a venture, the local dental society and the American Dental Association should be more active in this field.

At the present time commercial products are often equated with youth, personal attractiveness, appeal to the opposite sex, action, athletic prowess, and, in the case of many common analgesics, relief from the tensions and anxieties of our frantic way of life. This frantic way of life is portrayed as something that should perhaps be followed if one is to succeed, by a member of the "in" crowd, and live the "good" life. Often it entails abuse of the body by eating, drinking, and smoking too much and by driving oneself to the extremes of human endurance both at work and at play. Such a portrayal then leads one to the obvious haven of rest through use of the right cigarette, beer, instant breakfast, hair spray, or analgesic.

For every 50 of these commercials perhaps one or two genuinely factual public service–type advertisements are seen. This is usually from an organization such as the American Heart Association or the American Cancer Society. The nature and quality of these latter presentations have been much less attractive from the point of view of artistic or emotional appeal or shock value than are the big budget commercials. It is encouraging to see the current utilization of truly effective factual need-creating presentations against smoking. The truth is that the advertisements on television and radio and in the magazines are opinion and attitude builders for our society and are backed by millions of dollars from the producers of consumer goods. We in dentistry must do more to teach prevention because it is all too obvious that we can never "drill and fill" our way around the problem.

The youth and adults whom we see and have difficulty in motivating today are yesterday's children, who have been bombarded for all their lives with such material and now have very set attitudes regarding many aspects of life, including dental care. Similarly, today's children are being assailed with an even greater flood of material, which they are building into the opinions and attitudes that they will hold when they become adults. It is clear that because most periodontal patients are adults, some of our difficulty in motivating them stems from the fact that we are starting too late in their lives. Robinson et al. (1967) have concluded that most of our educational efforts should be pointed toward today's child if tomorrow's adult is to be more easily motivated to accept the benefits of dental care.

Assuming that the dental profession through its organizations did direct more of its advertising to this age group, we would hope that the quality of its presentations, from the standpoint of appealing to youth, was improved and made more effective by the utilization of knowledge that was obtained at great expense by commercial interests; that is, the dental profession might use the same appeal to attractiveness, popularity, athletic prowess, success, and so on in the same short repetitive manner that is used in many television commercials.

SUGGESTIONS FOR MOTIVATING PATIENTS

Actions that dentists and the dental profession may take to improve the milieu in which the patient will motivate himself can be considered as either extramural or intramural procedures (Katz et al., 1972).

Extramural procedures

Because most periodontal patients are adults, and adults have beliefs that are often difficult to change, the profession should concentrate on informing patients when they are children. Extramurally this could be done by the dental profession through a more active participation in the health program at the elementary school level. It could be accomplished by supplying attractive audiovisual materials to the school, by participating in school functions, and by cultivating and educating the teachers, who are very powerful opinion makers in the child's life. Parents may be approached by other dentally educated opinion makers such as physicians and nurses. Therefore an active education program should also be aimed at these professionals.

The profession through its societies should increase its educational efforts through the mass media, using methods already proved to be effective by motivational research.

The dental schools should institute educational programs in the freshman year. These should be geared to reorienting the values and attitudes of incoming dental students as early as possible so that the new generation of dentists will possess no educational lack with regard to motivation of dental patients and the nature of dental disease and its control. All dental students and faculty should "possess" dental health and maintain it by personal control procedures.

All of these extramural activities must be presented in an ethical manner that is consistent with the established principles of communication, learning, and motivation.

If stories concerning dentistry are reported in the press and magazines (David, 1962; O'Brien, 1959; Snyder and Davids, 1958) and on television by third parties, dentists should assist the reporters in any way possible to make the reporting objective and factual. Often such presentations are less than correct or not objectively presented if left to the reporter. It is a good idea to see the final draft or script before it is presented to make certain that the facts are not obscured by the entertainment value of the piece.

Intramural procedures

Once the patient makes an appointment with the dentist, he has evidenced a certain amount of need, or the appointment would never have been made. After he arrives, stronger motivation is evidenced. Even though the patient has not come to the office for relief of pain, you may assume that he has come for the relief of some other anxiety (disquiet of mind).

After the suggestions made earlier in this chapter for establishment of rapport have been followed, communication and learning may then occur, and the patient may become motivated for complete dental care.

Kegeles (1963) has suggested a procedure for dealing with such a patient. He indicates that the following format is a useful framework in which to educate the patient relative to dental disease. For a patient to make a dental visit and to undergo treatment that is oriented toward prevention he must believe the following:

1. That he is susceptible to periodontal disease
2. That periodontal disease is personally serious
3. That there is something he can do to treat or correct the condition
4. To a lesser degree that the condition occurred due to natural causes

A patient must first believe that he is susceptible to periodontal disease before he can possibly consider the personal seriousness of it. Likewise he must accept his susceptibility and its seriousness before he can be required to consider whether any action that he may take will be beneficial in treating the problem.

If the patient accepts the fact that periodontal disease is serious for him, but does not accept the fact that he is susceptible to it, he will never take any beneficial action. Similarly, if he believes that he is susceptible, but that it is of no consequence, he will never agree to treatment. In like manner he may accept his susceptibility and its seriousness for him and yet not believe that periodontal therapy and oral hygiene will help him. He still will not take beneficial action.

Therefore Kegeles' outlines must be followed, in the order given, with each patient. Through factual information gleaned from suitable articles on the epidemiology of periodontal disease the dentist must develop a suitable presentation that will convince the patient that he has every right to expect that, as a member of the human race, he is susceptible to periodontal disease.

If the dentist is aware of some of the motives that compel men to action, he may similarly present the patient with factual information on the seriousness of tooth loss from the financial, hygienic, functional, esthetic, or psychologic aspects. The choice of approach depends on the patient's values in relation to his teeth.

Once the patient has truly accepted both his susceptibility and the serious nature of periodontal disease *he will probably ask the dentist* what he can do about treating the condition. *At this point a personal disease control program is outlined.* The individual dentist and his complete office staff should have their dental disease under control and should enthusiastically teach such a program to all patients (Katz et al., 1972).

Kegeles' last point states that the patient must believe that periodontal disease has occurred in his mouth due to natural causes. This means that the patient should accept his condition as a natural biologic sequence of events and not as a punishment evoked by God for some past sins. Occasionally, successful patient motivation is blocked by such a belief.

SUMMARY

Motivation of the patient comes from within himself in response to a need. He will act for his own reasons, not for the dentist's reasons, to seek dental care and to practice good oral hygiene. He acts to relieve an anxiety or disquiet of mind relative to his dental condition.

Factors that influence the patient's actions positively and negatively toward dental care include the pain involved, his state of knowledge, his previous dental experiences, his age, the social system and its influences, his subconscious fears, the dentist and his awareness of motivational psychology, and the emotional quality of dental

therapy. *Knowledgeable utilization of or compensation for these factors will make both patient and doctor more anxiety free in the stress-producing dental situation.*

The ideal approach is to initiate an educational program aimed at children that helps to establish proper habits of dental health at an early age. If these practices are well established in the child, there is a good chance that they will be continued in adult life. Allport (1937) attributes this to a process called "functional autonomy," which more simply stated means that habits formed early in life become so automatic that they may continue to be practiced long after the initial reason for their establishment is forgotten.

The education and enlistment of other professional authority figures, for example, teachers, physicians, and nurses, has not been exploited to the fullest. It is often more effective for respected opinion makers such as those just mentioned to boost dental health than it is for the dentist himself to do so.

The dental school curriculum should also be altered to include an early introduction of this knowledge to the freshman dental student so that the new generation of dentists does not unwittingly complicate its life's work through ignorance. All dental students and faculty members should themselves value dental health and be practicing dental disease control.

All patients cannot be motivated to the same degree. Each one will be motivated to a level sufficient to remove his disquiet of mind about his dental health. Therefore some patients are treated minimally, and others have full treatment. Failure to convince all patients to proceed with full dental treatment should not come as an unexpected shock to the informed practitioner.

Following a preventive philosophy of practice aids immeasurably in making dental health possible for more patients at the lowest cost. The dentist's practice will be more enjoyable, profitable, and psychologically rewarding. Furthermore, it will go immeasurably further in solving the dental needs of our country than the present reparative approach that is actually failing to meet the needs of the public. Such a dental disease control program is best introduced immediately after the examination and prior to any scaling or root planing. Once the patient sees the changes that occur after a week of proper self-administered care, he will be more apt to follow these procedures indefinitely. If the scaling is done prior to disease control, the patient is already conditioned to attribute any beneficial results to the dentist and his scaling. Therefore they will not continue the disease control program, but merely wait for the next recall appointment for another scaling. This one facet of treatment planning is most important for long-term patient motivation and performance of disease control procedures. All patients need to remotivate themselves every few months, at a recall visit to the office.

REFERENCES

Allport, G.: The functional autonomy of motives, Am. J. Psychol. **50:**141, 1937.

American Dental Association, Bureau of Economic Research and Statistics: A motivational study of dental care, J. Am. Dent. Assoc. **56:**434, 566, 745, 859 (editorial), 911, 1958, **57:**279, 1958.

Amsterdam, M.: Postgraduate notes, University of Pennsylvania, School of Dental Medicine, 1963-1964.

Awwa, I., and Stallard, R. E.: Periodontal prognosis — educational and psychological implications, J. Periodontol. **4:** 183, 1970.

Ayer, W., and Hirschman, R.: Psychology and dentistry, Springfield, Ill., 1972, Charles C Thomas, Publisher, p. xi.

Barclay, R.: A preventive philosophy of restorative dentistry, Dent. Clin. North Am. **15:**569, 1971.

Barclay, R.: Lecture to dental students, University of Pennsylvania, School of Dental Medicine, April 17, 1970.

Bauer, R. A.: Consumer behavior as risktaking. In Hancock, R. S., editor: Dynamic marketing for a changing world, Chicago, 1960, American Marketing Association.

Bayton, J. A.: Motivation, cognition, learning-basic factors in consumer behavior, J. Marketing **22:**282, 1958.

Blass, J. L.: Motivating patients for more effective dental service, Philadelphia, 1958, J. B. Lippincott Co.

Boyd, H. W., and Westfall, R.: Marketing research, rev. ed., Homewood, Ill., 1964, Richard D. Irwin, Inc.

Chaves, M., and Frichofer, H.: The future of the dentist, World Health, p. 39, November, 1966.

Cinotti, W. R., and Grieder, A.: Applied psychology in dentistry, ed. 2, St. Louis, 1972, The C. V. Mosby Co.

Clawson, J. C.: The coming break-through in motivation research, Cost and Profit Outlook II (5, 6), 1958.

Consumer Reports, Buick, Chrysler, Mercury, Oldsmobile, p. 273, May, 1967.

Consumer's survey: Circulated questionnaire, Westbury, N.Y., 1966, O. E. McIntyre, Inc.

David, L.: How to keep your teeth, American Legion Magazine **73:**24, 1962.

Davidson, P. O., Haryett, R. D., Sandilands, M., and Hansen, F. C.: Thumbsucking — habit or symptom? J. Dent. Child. **34:**252, 1967.

Derbyshire, J. C.: Patient motivation in periodontics, J. Periodontol. **41:**630, 1970.

Derbyshire, J. C.: How patients are motivated and taught to practice effective oral hygiene, Periodont. Abstr. **16:**99, 1968.

Derbyshire, J. C.: Methods of achieving effective hygiene of the mouth, Dent. Clin. North Am., p. 231, March, 1964.

Dunlap, I. E.: I hope you know what you're doing, Dent. Econ. p. 69, January, 1977.

Editorial: The dentist's personal health problems — and some remedies, Dent. Surv. p. 12, July, 1976.

Editorial: The ineffective toothbrush, Lancet **2:**42, 1960.

Everett, F.: Halitosis, Ore. Dent. J. **41:**13, 1971.

Ferris, R. T., and Winslow, E. K.: Reinforcing desired behavior with periodontal patients, Dent. Clin. North Am., p. 280, April, 1970.

Firestein, S. K.: Patient anxiety and dental practice, J. Am. Dent. Assoc. **93:**1180-1187, 1976.

Formicola, A. J., Witte, E. T., and Curran, P. M.: A study of personality traits and necrotizing ulcerative gingivitis, J. Periodontol. **41:**36, 1970.

Friedman, N.: Postgraduate notes on the psychologic significance of the oral cavity and teeth, University of Pennsylvania, School of Dental Medicine, March 5-6, 1965.

Gale, E. N., and Ayer, W. A.: Treatment of dental phobias, J. Am. Dent. Assoc. **73:**1304-1307, 1969.

Garn, R.: The magic of emotional appeal, Englewood Cliffs, N.J., 1959, Prentice-Hall, Inc.

Greene, J. C.: Review of the literature on oral health. In Ramfjord, S. P., Kerr, D. A., and Ash, M. M., editors: Proceedings of the World Workshop in Periodontics, Ann Arbor, 1966, University of Michigan Press.

Grusky, O., Sears, D. O., and Knutson, J. W.: Effect of a social science curriculum on attitudes of freshman dental students, J. Am. Dent. Assoc. **74:**769, 1967.

Hammerman, S. S.: Some psychiatric aspects of management of the dental patient, J. Conn. Dent. Assoc. **29:**14, 1954.

Howard, J. H., Cunningham, D. A., Rechnitzer, P. A., and Goode, R. C.: Stress in the job and career of a dentist, J. Am. Dent. Assoc. **93:**630-636, 1976.

Jacobsen, E.: Progressive relaxation, Chicago, 1938, University of Chicago Press.

Katcher, A.: Lecture to undergraduate dental students, University of Pennsylvania, School of Dental Medicine, 1964.

Katz, S. M., McDonald, J. L., and Stookey, G. K.: Preventive dentistry in action. Upper Montclair, N.J., 1972, DCP Publishing Company, pp. 121-276.

Kegeles, S. S.: Some motives for seeking preventive dental care, J. Am. Dent. Assoc. **67:**92, 1963.

Kydd, J. R.: How adults learn, New York, 1959, Association Press.

Lawrence, T. H.: How to get through to patients, Dent. Manage. **5:**46, 1965.

Levoy, R. P.: Are they challenging change in your office? Dent. Econ. pp. 67-69, July, 1976.

MacKenzie, R. S.: Psychodynamics of pain, J. Oral Med. **23:** 75-84, 1965.

Manhold, J. H., Jr.: Psychosomatic process in dental disease, Dent. Clin. North Am., pp. 609-621, November, 1962.

Manhold, J. H., Doyle, J. L. and Weisinger, E. H.: Effects of social stress on oral and other bodily tissues. II. Results offering substance to a hypothesis for the mechanism of formation of periodontal pathology, J. Periodontol. **42:**111, 1971.

Maslow, A. H.: Motivation and personality, New York, 1954, Harper & Row, Publishers.

Marshall-Day, C. D., Stephens, R. G., and Quigley, L.: Periodontal disease; prevalence and incidence, J. Periodontol. **26:**185, 1955.

Meares, A.: The medical interview, Springfield, Ill., 1957, Charles C Thomas, Publisher.

Moore, D. S.: Periodontal patient motivation in general practice, J. Can. Dent. Assoc. **29:**654, 1963.

O'Brien, R.: Protect your teeth from P.D. — and keep them, Reader's Digest **74:**88, 1959.

Quarantelli, E. L.: The dental student image of the dentist-patient relationship. Am. J. Public Health **51:**1312-1319, 1961.

Reed, O. K.: The why of preventodontics in general dentistry, J. Am. Soc. Prev. Dent. **1:**14, 1970.

Robinson, B. A., Mobley, E. L., and Pointer, M. B.: Is dental health education the answer? J. Am. Dent. Assoc. **74:**124, 1967.

Silverman, S. I.: Oral physiology, St. Louis, 1961, The C. V. Mosby Co.

Simpson, J. C.: Job hazard: dentists grow richer but feel the pressure: suicide rate is high, The Wall Street Journal, December 17, 1976, p. 1.

Snyder, D. E., and Davids, R. C.: Hang on to your teeth, Farm Journal **82:**32, 1958.

Stunkard, A.: Some psychological aspects of stress; implications for modern dentistry, J. Dent. Med. **11:**81, 1956.

Tonge, C. H.: Teeth hadst thou in thy head, inaugural lecture, University of Newcastle on Tyne, October 18, 1965.

Topics and Trends: Dental Surv., p. 12, July, 1976.

Waerhaug, J.: Review of the literature on epidemiology of periodontal disease. In Ramfjord, S. P., Kerr, D. A., and Ash, M. M., editors: Proceedings of the World Workshop in Periodontics, Ann Arbor, 1966, University of Michigan Press.

Walters, E.: How to live with failure and stress, Dent. Manage. pp. 20-24, October, 1976.

Weiss, R. L., Swearingen, R. V.: Chairside psychology in patient education. Washington, D.C., 1969, U.S. Dept. of Health, Education, and Welfare, p. 75.

W.H.O., Expert Committee on Dental Health: Periodontal disease, Technical Report Series no. 207, Geneva, 1961, World Health Organization.

Wolpe, J.: Behavior therapy in complex neurotic states, Br. J. Psychiatry **110:**28, 1964.

20 Temporary stabilization

VALUE OF TEMPORARY SPLINTING

A major objective in periodontal therapy is to minimize the amount of clinical crown exposed to the oral cavity and increase the amount of clinical root retained within its periodontium. The clinical crown can be defined as that part of the tooth that lies out of its support, and the clinical root can be defined as that part of the tooth that is within its support. In light of our present knowledge the periodontal clinician is more hesitant today to remove large areas of supporting structure than he was a few years ago. There is a greater emphasis on regenerative procedures whereby periodontal defects will repair themselves, thus negating the therapeutic removal of attachment apparatus. Other than the regeneration of lost parts of the periodontium, the only other means to effect changes in the clinical crown relative to the clinical root is to alter the tooth unit in some fashion. Generally this can be accomplished either by selective reshaping of teeth or by splinting weaker units to more stable ones.

Relative to selective reshaping of teeth, it is theoretically possible to remove a sufficient amount of clinical crown so as to significantly alter the clinical crown-to-root ratio in a favorable manner. This would in essence have a similar effect as regenerating a portion of the attachment apparatus. Although from a theoretic standpoint this may have merit, the clinician is often unable to achieve this for various reasons. For example, one may desire to reduce the clinical crown of an anterior tooth but may be limited by pulpal proximity, aesthetic demands, or the need for tooth length to meet the requisites of anterior incisal guidance. Reducing the heights of the posterior teeth may make the crown-to-root ratio more favorable but could potentially close the occlusal vertical dimension and place excessive forces on the anterior segment of teeth. It is a common finding that closing the vertical dimension of the posterior occlusion by 1 mm will manifest itself with a 3 mm closure in the anterior part of the mouth. One could see how this would complicate an already existing posterior occlusal collapse situation. This is especially true in those clinical cases where the occlusion is adjusted in the patient's maximum intercuspal position (that is, acquired occlusion).

It becomes rather obvious that it is extremely difficult to reduce the clinical crown of the natural dentition by selective reshaping on a consistent and routine basis to achieve the objective of minimizing the clinical crown and increasing the amount of clinical root. Some beneficial effect may ensue, but the clinician will always be limited by tooth position, cusp height, pulpal proximity, existing occlusal vertical dimension, anterior incisal guidance, and the aesthetic needs of the patient. As mentioned earlier, another approach to gaining more support would be to splint a number of teeth together whereby the principle of multiroot stabilization can be utilized.

This chapter will deal with the indications for temporary stabilization of teeth and various ways of achieving this end. It is important that one appreciate this phase of therapy and integrate it into the total scope of treatment of periodontal problems.

The temporary splinting of mobile teeth is often of value as a means of stabilization before, during, and after periodontal therapy. Immobilization of teeth during periodontal therapy adheres to the principle of fixation of movable parts to allow for tissue healing, thus permitting the therapist to evaluate better the progression and prognosis of treatment. Cohen and Chacker have noted, ''When large areas of attachment apparatus have been destroyed, the artificial support offered by temporary stabilization may allow a new, healthy tooth-bone relationship to be established.'' Therefore it would seem advisable that when the treatment plan is being formulated the need for stabilization be determined on the basis of the nature and extent of

535

Fig. 20-1. A, Occlusal periodontitis in 33-year-old white man. Mobility is significant on mandibular right second molar. Note thickened periodontal ligament space on mesial surface of mesial root in preoperative radiograph. **B,** Same area approximately 2 years postoperatively. Occlusion has been adjusted, treatment of inflammatory lesion completed, and mandibular fixed prosthesis inserted to stabilize segment. Note narrowing of periodontal ligament space on mesial surface of mesial root.

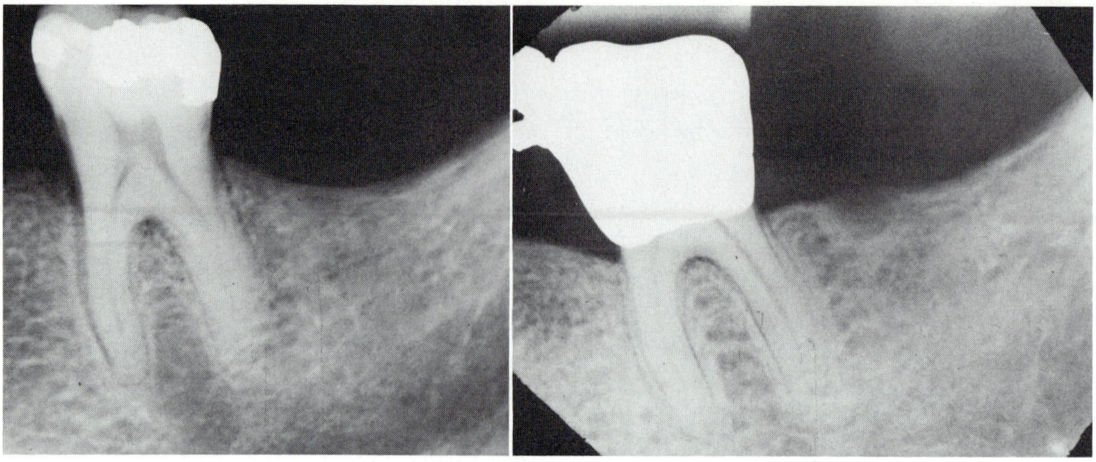

the destructive process present (Fig. 20-1). Kegel, Selipsky, and Phillips studied the effects of splinting on tooth mobility during initial therapy and concluded that the reduction of tooth mobility was the result of improved occlusal relationship and reduction of gingival inflammation. This points out that, in addition, it is important that occlusal relationships be initially corrected and again after definitive periodontal therapy.

The method utilized for stabilization may vary according to the overall projected treatment plan. However, certain essential factors should be considered: the mobility patterns of the teeth to be stabilized, the crown-to-root ratio of the involved teeth, the status of the remaining teeth in the arch, the nature and extent of the periodontal pockets, and the methods of therapy that will be employed. In some cases a permanent splint may be indicated to make the prognosis more favorable for retention of the involved teeth. When such a situation is present the most expedient solution may be to prepare the teeth and fabricate a provisional splint. In those cases where a restorative dentistry commitment has not been obtained from the patient, another form of temporary stabilization that does not require removal of the tooth structure should be employed.

A major consideration with any form of temporary stabilization is that it is only effective within the confines of the occlusion as it presents itself. In other words, it is extremely difficult or even impossible to effect a change in the occlusion via temporary stabilization. This presents a distinct

problem when one is confronted with a case where the existing occlusion is self-destructive. Probably this concern (other than durability) is the major difference between temporary stabilization and permanent splinting, whereby in the latter not only can individual tooth units be stabilized but also a change in the occlusion can often be effected.

It is generally believed today that forces in excess of physiologic limits produce specific changes in the attachment apparatus. As early as 1931, Gottlieb and Orban showed evidence of necrosis, hemorrhage, thrombosis, undermining resorption, thickening of the periodontal ligament space, loss of lamina dura, cemental tears, and root fracture all as a result of excessive forces. These findings have been confirmed in recent years by a number of investigators. In order for the lesion of occlusal traumatism to be better understood it has been subdivided into two main entities: primary and secondary occlusal traumatism. The primary type has been defined as a degenerative lesion of the attachment apparatus caused by excessive forces acting in the presence of adequate supporting tissues. Here the classic histologic signs of occlusal traumatism as first described may be noted. Barring any complicating factors such as periodontal pocket formation, the supporting tissues will be repaired when the force is removed or tempered. The secondary type, on the other hand, manifests itself usually after a long-standing periodontitis in which loss of supporting structure has become severe. Normal forces existent within the masticatory system such as those occurring during swallowing and mastication cannot be dissipated because of the excessive destruction of the attachment apparatus. It is in the situation of secondary occlusal traumatism that some form of splinting becomes a necessity.

It is important in the treatment of occlusal disorders that the clinician see resolution of the problem. Clinically, the classic sign of repair is of course a decrease in tooth mobility and, radiographically, the narrowing of the periodontal ligament space.

Amsterdam and Abrams have noted that teeth may demonstrate mobility in one or more directions: mesiodistally, buccolingually, circumferentially, and axially. "The prognosis of a tooth will be proportionate to the ability of the treatment to minimize or negate movement in all of these directions."

Temporary stabilization, acting in the form of a splint, will increase resistance to applied force, thus allowing the attachment apparatus to repair itself.

The functions of a temporary splint may be listed as follows:

1. To protect mobile teeth from further injury by stabilizing them in a favorable occlusal relationship
2. To distribute occlusal forces so that teeth that have lost periodontal support are not further traumatized
3. To retain teeth in the position to which they have been moved by orthodontic procedures
4. To prevent pathologic migration
5. To protect mobile teeth during periodontal procedures and to aid in healing
6. To aid in determining whether teeth with a borderline prognosis will respond to therapy

Cohen and Chacker have suggested that temporary immobilization be part of initial preparation of the dentition. Where indicated, certain salient points must be considered in utilizing a temporary splint procedure.

1. The occlusion of the dentition may be adjusted prior to the stabilization procedure. An exception could be in the situation where the remaining teeth are so mobile that they must first be stabilized in a favorable position and then occlusal adjustment be instituted. The basic objectives in the adjustment approach should allow for a stable maximum intercuspal position and freedom of mandibular movement to and from this position. Of course, the temporary restoration should be in harmony with the adjusted occlusion.

2. A sufficient number of sound teeth should be included so that the forces can be dissipated.

Often it is necessary to include both anterior and posterior segments for maximum stability. It is important to note that stabilization of a single posterior quadrant of teeth is most effective against mesiodistal movements. However, if the splint has a buccolingual movement, it is best stabilized by including the anterior teeth as well as the posterior teeth on the opposite side so as to achieve a crossarch splinting action.

3. The splints should be nonirritating to the gingival tissues, cheeks, lips, or tongue.

4. The splint should be as aesthetically pleasing as possible.

5. The splint should be constructed so as to allow for cleansing of the gingival tissues and teeth through routine oral physiotherapy techniques.

6. The splint should not impair or disturb the phonetic pattern of the patient.

7. If tooth structure is to be removed to facilitate construction of the splint, a restorative dentistry agreement must be obtained prior to any operative procedure. A possible exception would be the case of advanced periodontal disease with excessive tooth mobility in which the patient was unable to proceed with extensive restorative dentistry for financial reasons.

TYPES OF SPLINTS

Any categorization of restorations, of course, leaves much to be desired. However, we have taken the liberty of classifying them into basic types for purposes of discussion.

I. Temporary splints
  A. Extracoronal type
    1. Wire ligation
    2. Orthodontic bands
    3. Removable acrylic appliances
    4. Removable cast appliances
    5. Ultraviolet-light-polymerizing bonding materials
  B. Intracoronal type
    1. Wire and acrylic
    2. Wire and amalgam
    3. Wire, amalgam, and acrylic
    4. Cast chrome-cobalt alloy bars with amalgam, acrylic, or both
II. Provisional splints
  A. All acrylic
  B. Adapted metal band and acrylic

Temporary splints
EXTRACORONAL TYPES

Unfortunately almost all the extracoronal forms of stabilization have certain inherent disadvantages. They usually are a detriment to good oral physiotherapy because of their bulk, thus interrupting proper coronal forms. It is often difficult to perform various surgical procedures in these areas because of the nature of the appliance. The applicances frequently leave a great deal to be desired cosmetically.

Wire ligation. Wire ligation is probably the most commonly used type of stabilization (Fig. 20-2). It is easy to construct and rather sturdy. However, one of its basic limitations is that it can be utilized only where coronal form permits. Because of this shortcoming it has its greatest use in stabilizing the mandibular incisors. Hirschfeld suggests a loop tied at the cervical line on poorly contoured teeth to prevent slippage of the main wire. Often tooth-colored, self-curing acrylic is painted over the wire to obtain a more pleasing aesthetic result. Johnson and Groat have suggested a method that includes the use of 80-gauge brass mesh. After an interproximal tie is made, connecting the buccal and lingual segments of the mesh, the entire area is covered with acrylic. This method may offer the advantage of greater stability while producing a splint that is thin in a buccolingual direction and quite acceptable to the patient.

Orthodontic bands. Orthodontic bands tend to stabilize both anterior and posterior teeth and therefore have the advantage over wire ligation in that they are not as limiting. It is important to give proper attention to the contours of the bands and to check their relationship to the adjacent gingival tissue. Often the contacts between the teeth must be opened so that a band or bands can be inserted. Again, acrylic may be placed over the bands for cosmetic purposes. The bands may be welded directly or indirectly. When the multiple bands are welded together, it is necessary to have a common path of insertion so that the composite fit of the multiple bands is the same as the fit of each individual band (Figs. 20-3 to 20-5).

Removable acrylic appliances. The clinician must be aware of the fact that when he utilizes any form of acrylic appliance, the dimensional instability of the material may cause distortions to occur. It is imperative to check these appliances frequently and to make any necessary adjustments. It is also vital to check the path of insertion of the appliance, since the appliance must not be traumatic as it goes to its final seat.

External acrylic splint. Sorrin has described a removable acrylic splint that fits the contours of the teeth. This splint is cemented in place and, if properly constructed, does not irritate the lips,

---

Fig. 20-2. Stainless steel wire ligature for temporary splinting of teeth for stabilization is an extremely beneficial aid in periodontal therapeutics. It may be used especially in the anterior section, where aesthetics is a factor. Thin wire is not especially noticed (particularly when covered with quick-curing acrylic), yet stabilization is sufficient. Wire commonly utilized is two strands of 0.008 or 0.01 gauge. A heavier gauge wire may be used singly. One end of wire is placed interdentally, distal to last tooth to be splinted, and then again interdentally at other end of group of teeth. It is tied at open end by twisting with a hemostat. It should be adapted closely to teeth with any instrument. Arch wire should be positioned apical to contact areas but incisal to cingula. Interproximal wires are then inserted. This is done by placing a small section of wire through embrasure space, either above or below arch wire, returning it to labial side, thus engaging labial and lingual arch wires. When ends are twisted, interdental wire is tightened into place. After placement of all interproximal wires, each twisted end is carefully tightened as much as possible and cut as closely as possible without becoming disengaged. Cut ends are then bent into embrasure spaces so that splint will not be rough to lips or tongue. A modification of this technique is necessary when teeth are separated to extent shown in this illustration. Wire is twisted so that it engages tooth firmly until space is spanned. Arch wire is then continued labially and lingually to end of section to be splinted. This method holds separated teeth in place firmly, and splint does not become an orthodontic appliance. For the ligation to be effective it must be secure and tight. Since stainless steel wire tends to stretch, periodic attention is necessary, and, should any looseness be noticed, twisted ends of wires can be pulled out of embrasure spaces and tightened. An improvement over the wire splint is one that utilizes acrylic to cover wire. It is applied to splint with quick-curing material after area is completely dried. Some clinicians first apply a cement to the splint, over which they then place the acrylic. It is claimed that this results in better adherence. Acrylic is placed in a thin, striplike fashion both labially and lingually. Interdental ties should be covered completely, for splint must be smooth to the tongue and easily cleansed by a toothbrush.

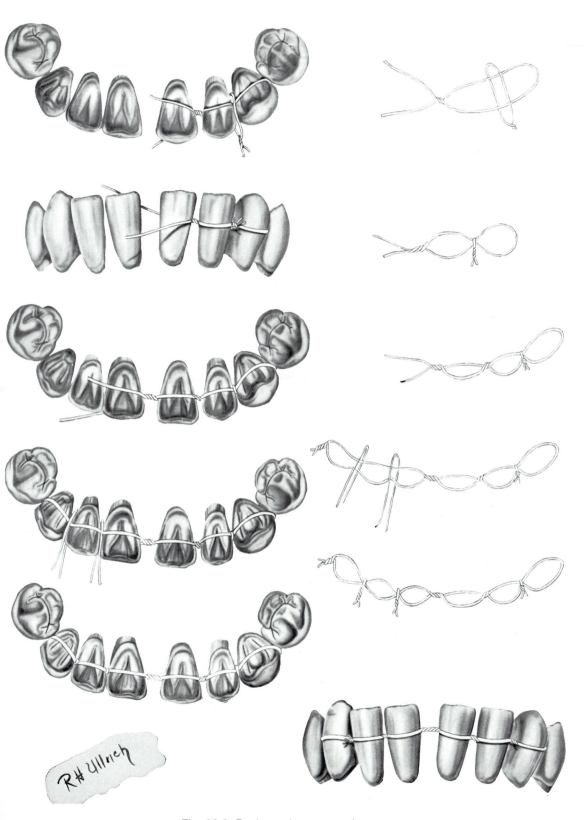

Fig. 20-2. For legend see opposite page.

cheek, tongue, or gingival tissues. Its main disadvantages lie in the inherent properties of acrylic.

Acrylic bite guards. Acrylic bite guards can be constructed in many ways, and they have a wide variety of uses. The most common type of appliance is one that covers the occlusal surfaces of the teeth (Fig. 20-6). For additional support the palate is often covered. Another appliance frequently used is the maxillary Hawley bite plane with a labial wire (Figs. 20-7 and 20-8). This appliance has an advantage in that the posterior teeth are freed of occlusal contact in all positions and excursions of the mandible. It can be used only when there is an anterior overbite so that the palatal bite plane can disarticulate the posterior teeth. When there is no overbite, a labial lip of acrylic over the maxillary anterior teeth will often suffice. An important consideration with all these appliances is that they must not obliterate the interocclusal distance (free-way space).

Removable cast appliances. The removable cast appliance is usually a rigid casting, either of gold or of chrome cobalt, made to fit around the teeth (Fig. 20-9). Friedman has suggested a useful variation utilizing a double continuous clasp casting. One end, usually the anterior section, is not joined but is left open so that the casting can be sprung over the undercuts and then ligated. The posterior end is continuous from the buccal to the lingual surface and is distal to the most posterior tooth. Another modification is an interlocking attachment on the distal end so that the appliance can be locked after being sprung over

the teeth. Obviously, with any form of removable splint, it is only effective if the patient wears the appliance.

Ultraviolet-light-polymerizing bonding materials. Recently developed restorative materials that are polymerized by ultraviolet light are proving very useful in providing stabilization of excessively mobile teeth. As Polson and Billen have stated, "Because the materials do not polymerize until they are exposed to ultraviolet light, they provide prolonged working times for placement, shaping, and contouring over extensive areas of enamel."

One of the more popular polymerizing kits is the Nuva System (Caulk, Division of Dentsply International Inc., Milford, Delaware). Basically the technique is a simple one and provides adequate stabilization if care is taken during the actual operative procedures. The technique for extracoronal stabilization is as follows:

1. If interproximal surfaces are involved, they should be "stripped" with sandpaper strips.
2. The surfaces to be treated are polished with a fluoride-free pumice.
3. The patient is asked to rinse. *Do not use any of the commercial mouthwashes—use only plain water!*
4. The teeth are isolated with cotton rolls or a rubber dam and thoroughly dried with an air syringe.
5. Tooth conditioner is then applied very carefully with a small paintbrush to the surfaces

---

Fig. 20-3. Welded stainless steel orthodontic bands offer a simple yet effective means of temporary splinting. Splint is made directly on teeth as illustrated. Two short pieces of orthodontic band material are welded together and placed interdentally between two premolars. Band material is then brought through contact areas, mesially for first premolar and distally for second. It is then adapted carefully to teeth and tightened by orthodontic pliers. Ends are squeezed together, and material is removed and welded at these joints. Bands are then returned to teeth and burnished. At the same time welded ends are folded over against labial portion of bands. After bands are removed, pointed areas are secured and welded. Molar band is made by welding another strip at interdental area, which is then adapted to tooth. Band is finished in same manner. After completion of welding of bands, splint is ground so that it can be well adapted to teeth. It is then cemented in place. Bands should fit accurately so that they will be secure without excess cement. Otherwise splint may loosen after breaking away of cement. Orthodontic band splint may be made on a cast in the following manner. An impression of teeth to be splinted is taken, and a stone model is poured. Contact areas of teeth on model are cut with a very thin disk. It is important that not too much be cut away, or bands will not fit into place. A band can be made for each tooth and then welded with others. Another method is to solder bands while they are on model.

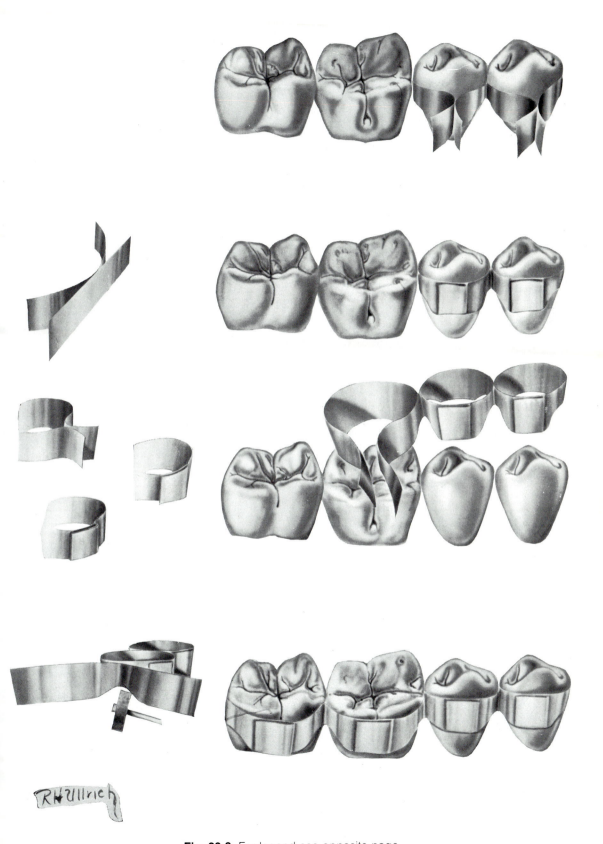

Fig. 20-3. For legend see opposite page.

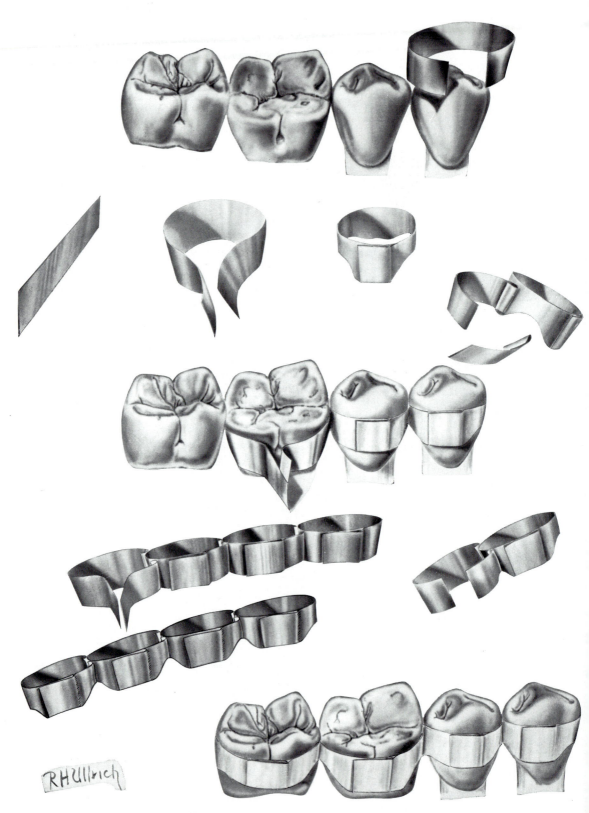

RHUllrich

Fig. 20-4. For legend see opposite page.

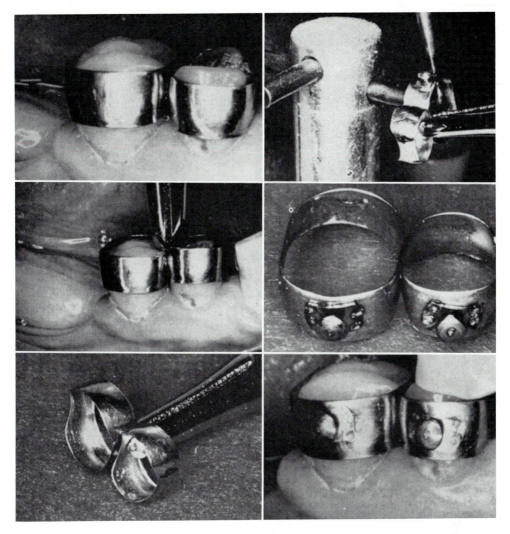

Fig. 20-5. An effective temporary splint may be constructed by uniting preformed ortho-dontic bands. This type of splint is applied more often on posterior teeth, but it can be uti-lized on anterior teeth as well. Individual bands are placed directly on teeth and are re-moved with aid of hemostat. Bands are then welded together. Orthodontic buttons may be added if minor tooth movement is anticipated. Another use of buttons is to ligate them to each other with wire for additional stability.

Fig. 20-4. Another method of fabricating an orthodontic band splint. It is especially useful in those instances in which contact areas are rather firm between some of the teeth to be splinted, thus not allowing for two thicknesses of band material interproximally; for ex-ample, in this case first molar is quite mobile, second molar is firmer than first but still a mo-bile tooth, and premolars are very firm. Effective splint must include four teeth. Premolars have no restorations, and contact is very firm. It will allow for placement of a single thick-ness of band material but not two thicknesses. In this instance such a splint is ideal. A band is made for the first premolar, and strips of band material are welded to band buccally and lingually to contact area. Two ends are then joined and welded. Thus band for second pre-molar has been made; only one thickness of material is present between premolars. Band splint is finished in same technique as that described previously. Note how bands are con-toured so that interdental cervical areas are not obliterated by bands.

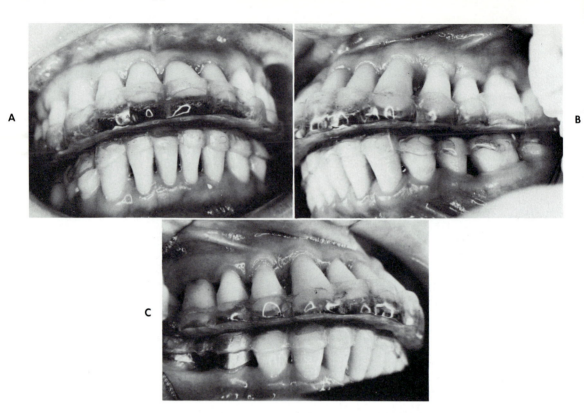

Fig. 20-6. Maxillary and mandibular night guards (description). **A,** Anterior view. **B,** Right side (mirrow view). **C,** Left side (mirrow view). Note simultaneous contact throughout posterior segments. Often free-way space will not allow for maxillary and mandibular night guards. Generally it is advisable to utilize a maxillary night guard in these cases. Occlusion should be adjusted beforehand to allow appliance to function in harmony free of any occlusal interferences.

that are going to be sealed. It is important that the conditioner not be applied with pressure.

6. After the conditioner has remained on for 1 minute, the teeth and surrounding tissues are rinsed with a water spray.

7. The teeth are again isolated and completely dried with an air syringe. Paper points, Stim-U-Dents, wooden wedges, or a rubber dam should be inserted interproximally.

8. A very thin coat of sealant is then applied to the etched surfaces with a small brush supplied in the kit. Dental floss can be used to clear the interproximal spaces of excess sealant.

9. Each sealed surface is exposed to the ultraviolet light for approximately 1 minute, holding the light as close to the surface as possible without touching the teeth. If the seal has not "set" by this time it should be exposed again to the light.

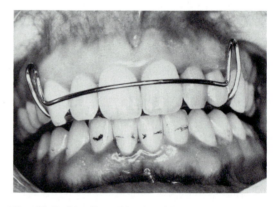

Fig. 20-7. Maxillary Hawley bite with labial bow. Note posterior teeth freed of occlusal contact. (Courtesy Dr. Garry Miller, Washington, D.C.)

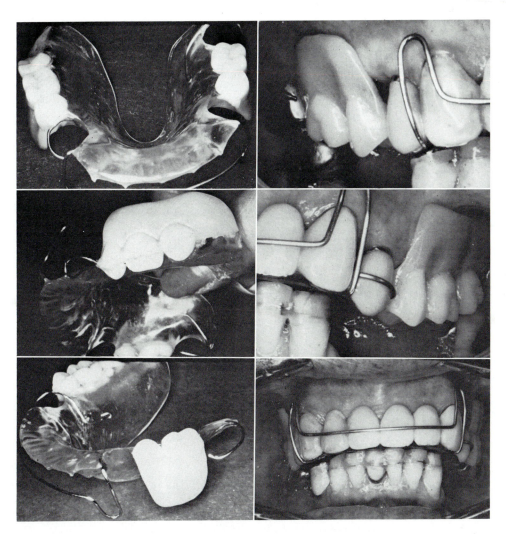

Fig. 20-8. Hawley bite plane is a removable acrylic appliance that may be used as retaining device for stabilization of periodontally involved teeth after active phase of orthodontic therapy; it may be used as a replacement of missing teeth to establish an occlusal pattern. The following conditions must be satisfied prior to clinical usage:

1. Palatal marginal periphery should be smooth so that an orthodontic force against tooth or teeth does not occur. Similarly on tissue and tooth side of appliance the area resting directly on palatal surfaces of teeth must be bubble free. Any excess may impinge traumatically on underlying tissue.
2. Design of appliance should be checked to verify that upon insertion and removal appliance is free of interference or imposed rotational torque due to undercuts.
3. Labial arch wire should be adapted closely to height of contour of six anterior teeth so that each tooth is in contact with it. When the appliance is seated, it should be free of mobility.
4. If a Hawley appliance with a flat palatal bite plane is being utilized, patient should exhibit maximum contact of six anterior teeth in centric relation and in all excursions, sufficient free-way space, and freedom of movement to and from centric relation without restraint.

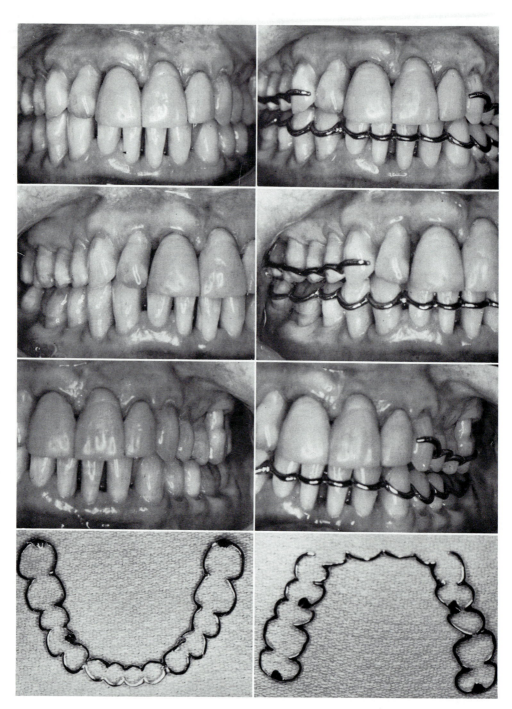

Fig. 20-9. Removable cast splint with occlusal rests. These splints may be constructed of either metal or clear acrylic. Appliance is rigid and does not irritate lips, cheek, or tongue. If aesthetics becomes a factor and metal is desirable because of its durability, one may eliminate maxillary anterior portion. This type of extracoronal splint has the advantage of being removable, allowing patient to cleanse thoroughly.

10. The filling material should only be placed in *1 mm increments,* shaped and contoured correctly, and then exposed to the light. Additional 1 mm increments are then applied and molded to the tooth surfaces. Each surface should be exposed to the light for approximately 1 minute.

11. The surfaces are then adjusted and recontoured with diamond stones, sandpaper disks, or rubber wheels and polished. Contouring is usually minimal if care is taken during the placement of the material.

12. The area is washed again, isolated, and air dried, and the sealant is again applied (as described in 8 and 9 above).

As stated previously it is extremely important to adhere to a strict regimen in order to ensure success. The following should be major considerations while performing this technique:

1. Plain water, not commercial mouthwashes, should be utilized.

2. The pumice used for polishing should be fluoride free. Fluoride apparently decreases the adhesive potential of the resin.

3. Teeth to be ligated must be thoroughly isolated and dried.

4. Do not apply the tooth conditioner with pressure—apply very carefully with a small paintbrush. After the conditioner has remained on for 1 minute, be sure to thoroughly wash the etched surfaces.

5. A new bottle of sealant should be used each day. This will assure the viscosity and flow essential for proper penetration. A very thin coat of sealant should be applied with a brush.

6. While the light is in use the patient should have the eyes closed and the operator should wear protective lenses. The sealant bottle should be covered and kept away from the operating area while the light is in use!

7. The filling material should be applied in 1 mm increments. Generally the light will not penetrate more than 1 or 1.5 mm of material (Fig. 20-10).

Combination splinting technique. Klassman and Zucker have described a combination wire-intracoronal splinting technique where 0.010 dead soft ligature is imbedded in prepared channels of the anterior teeth. The actual procedure for preparation of the channels and placement of the ligature wire is very similar to that described in the discussion on intracoronal types of stabilization. The use of the acid etch concept hopefully will circumvent the problems of the autocuring acrylics.

INTRACORONAL TYPES

Wire and acrylic. Obin and Arvins have described a technique of stabilization whereby wire (usually twisted in the form of a braid) is fixed with acrylic into channels prepared in mobile teeth. This approach can be utilized on the occlusal surfaces of posterior teeth and the lingual surfaces of anterior teeth. The technique offers advantages over the other forms of stabilization because there is greater control over coronal forms, occlusion, embrasure areas, and aesthetics. Unfortunately, because of the limited properties of self-curing acrylics, there is always the possibility of caries or breakage. This can be a very serious sequel of the technique if it is mismanaged or utilized as a permanent restoration. This technique had been varied by Kessler by placing threaded pins incorporated in the teeth along with wire and acrylic. This approach can be utilized more readily with anterior teeth. Of course, its major disadvantage is the possibility of recurrent caries. It therefore becomes imperative to have a restorative dentistry committment prior to the utilization of this form of stabilization. A possible exception to the rule would be in the advanced case of periodontitis compounded by secondary occlusal trauma, when a complicated and expensive restorative approach would not be feasible for the patient (for example, because of finances or health of patient). If the embedded wire-and-acrylic technique is utilized in such a situation, the possible consequences must be weighed carefully against the advantages.

Wire and amalgam. Because of the problems created by the use of acrylic, wire embedded in amalgam restorations seems to offer a more favorable prognosis. Lloyd and Baer have suggested the continuous amalgam splint as an easy, inexpensive, and effective method of joining together and immobilizing posterior teeth. A series of mesio-occlusodistal preparations are made in a quadrant of posterior teeth and then restored with amalgam that has wire embedded in it at the time of condensation. Prior to the procedure a buccal, lingual, and gingival matrix is fabricated in cold-cure acrylic to control proximal gingival contours. The authors note two possible disadvantages to this form of stabilization: (1) the confinement of the procedure to only posterior teeth and (2) the possibility of fracture (which will occur usually at the narrow part of the isthmus).

Text continued on p. 553.

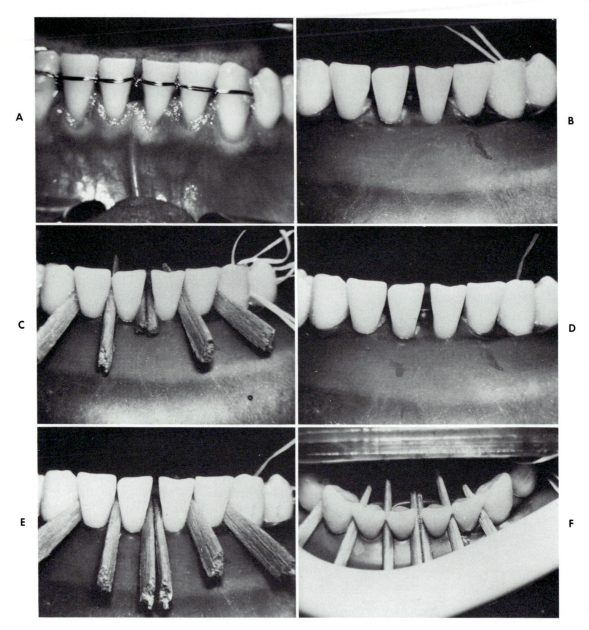

Fig. 20-10. A, Mandibular anterior area. Note extracoronal circumferential wiring that had been placed earlier in treatment. **B,** Teeth isolated with rubber dam. **C,** Wooden "wedges" placed interproximally to prevent bonding material from slipping gingivally. **D,** Areas to be bonded are conditioned (that is, "acid etched"). **E,** Wooden "wedges" again placed in preparation for sealant material. **F,** Incisal view of **E.**

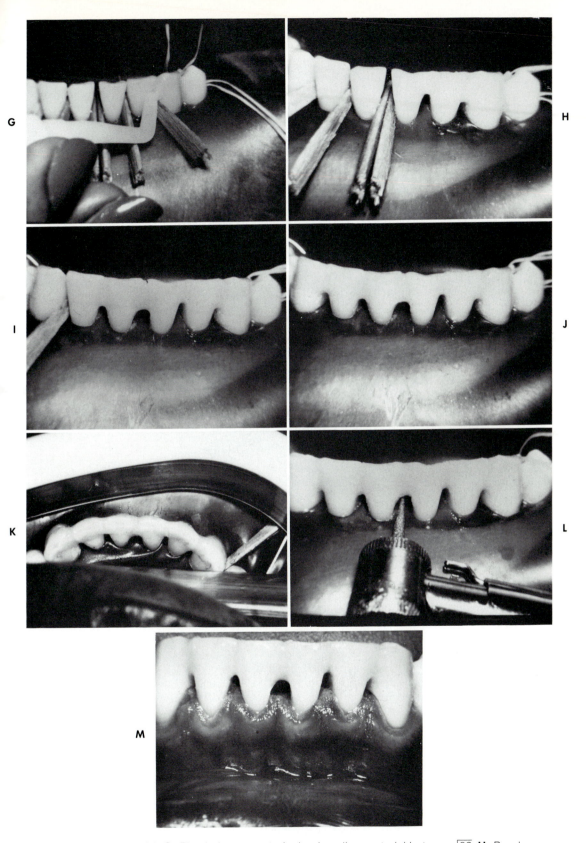

Fig. 20-10, cont'd. G, Plastic instrument placing bonding material between ⎯23. **H,** Bonding material contoured between ⎯123. **I,** Bonding material contoured between ⎯21|123. **J,** Bonding material contoured between ⎯321|123. **K,** Incisal view of **J. L,** Bonding material has been depolymerized with ultraviolet light source and contoured with a diamond stone interproximally. **M,** Completed bonding material after placement of sealant. (Courtesy Dr. Alan Rosenfeld, Chicago.)

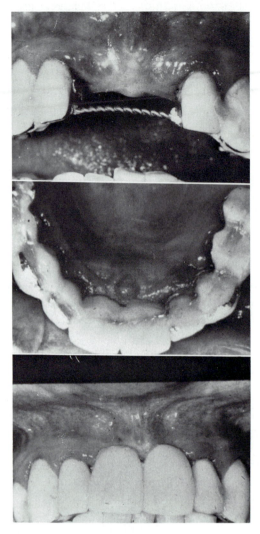

Fig. 20-11. A splint principle can be altered to restore missing teeth, thereby creating a more favorable aesthetic and occlusal form. Often it is necessary to stabilize mobile teeth in a mouth where anterior teeth are missing, thus causing an aesthetic problem. Channels can be prepared in remaining teeth on occlusal or lingual surface or both. A braided wire is then contoured and fitted into channel preparations so that it spans one quadrant to another. Wire is attached to remaining teeth by means of self-curing acrylic. Plastic denture teeth or processed teeth are utilized to restore missing segments. A channel is prepared in lingual aspect of anterior pontics or gingival aspect of posterior ones (or a channel is made directly into middle of tooth), and they are fitted over stabilizing wire and fixed in place with acrylic. To ensure optimal stability so as to allow for occlusal forces in maximum closure, it is wise to paint acrylic onto occlusal surfaces of posterior teeth and have the patient close into soft plastic. When plastic has set, it can be carved and shaped so as to allow as many of posterior teeth as possible to support forces of occlusion. If maxillary canines are present, one can add acrylic to their palatal surface and have the patient close. This will allow opposing teeth to strike canines along their long axis, thus permitting these key teeth to accept forces in a more favorable direction. Of course, it is necessary to check mandibular excursions so as to allow for freedom of movement to and from the position of maximum intercuspation.

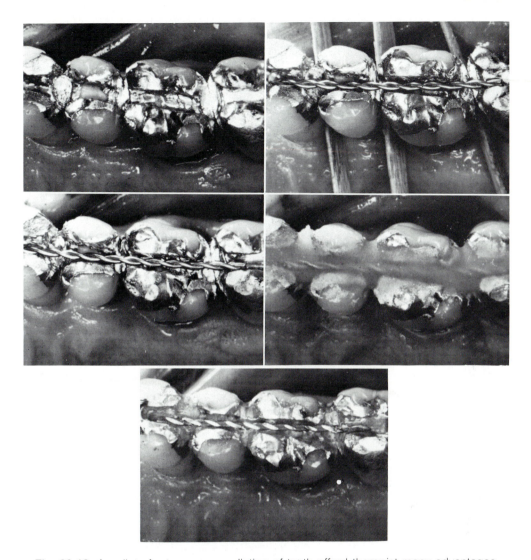

Fig. 20-12. A splints for temporary splinting of teeth afford therapist many advantages. These include maintenance of normal coronal contours of teeth, ability to establish an occlusal pattern, and production of an aesthetic result acceptable to the patient. A splint method may be employed in either anterior or posterior segment of arch. Material most commonly utilized is 0.020 or 0.010 dead soft wires twisted together to desired thickness. Teeth are isolated with either cotton rolls or rubber dam. A channel is cut horizontally, using a no. 35 or no. 37 inverted cone bur with class II preparation (placed interproximally, if added retention is desired). Channel extends mesiodistally through proximal margins of teeth to be included. After preparations are completed, endodontic paper points or Stim-U-Dents are inserted interproximally for protection of underlying gingival tissue. Sections of wire are measured and cut to fit mesiodistal extent of channels created. Self-curing acrylic is then placed in preparations and remoistened with the liquid monomer, using a sable hair brush. This will allow acrylic to flow into recesses of undercuts of channel. Small portions of polymer powder are painted successively into monomer wet channel slowly in a series of increments until channel is half filled. This portion of procedure is important to avoid trapping of air in preparation. A section of previously measured monomer wet wire is then seated to depth of preparation. Monomer and polymer are again added slowly until channel is overfilled. At this time patient is guided to terminal hinge position and closes to establish an occlusal pattern. After complete polymerization, A splint is polished with diamond stones, rubber wheels, and pumice. Care must be taken to provide a polished, finished surface with no trace of filling material extending beyond channel margins.

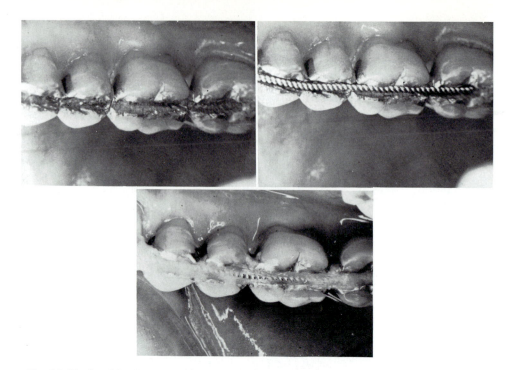

Fig. 20-13. Combination of wire and acrylic embedded in amalgam restorations. (Restorations by D. I. Trachtenberg, Philadelphia.)

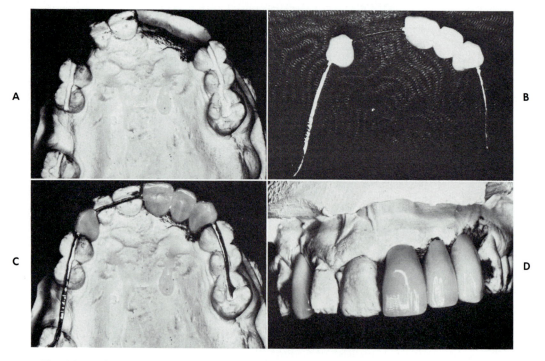

Fig. 20-14. Cast chrome-cobalt alloy and acrylic technique. **A,** Maxillary model prepared for chrome-cobalt bar; note grooves in teeth. **B,** Cast bar with acrylic teeth. **C,** Bar and teeth positioned on model. **D,** Anterior view of teeth on model.

A variation of this approach is to embed the wire in preexisting amalgam or gold restorations with acrylic (Fig. 20-11). The acrylic and wire embedded in amalgam or the amalgam-and-wire technique as described by Lloyd and Baer appears to have the advantage over the wire-and-acrylic method. Langeland and Langeland, utilizing tagged acrylic monomer in experimentally prepared cavities of monkey teeth, have shown the penetration of the monomer into the dentinal tubules next to the cavity. Another advantage of the wire and acrylic embedded in amalgam is that a greater degree of mechanical retention can be achieved for the plastic in the amalgam.

Wire, amalgam, and acrylic. Trachtenberg has combined the wire-and-amalgam and the wire-and-acrylic techniques (Figs. 20-12 and 20-13). This approach allows one to insert individual

compound amalgam restorations and finish their interproximal areas prior to insertion of the wire and acrylic. The author noted in an 18-month period of observation there had been no amalgam fractures or recurrent caries.

Cast chrome-cobalt alloy bars. Because of the disadvantages and weaknesses of threaded wire a number of clinicians have utilized cast chrome-cobalt bars for reinforcement. Baumhammers suggested condensing amalgam over a 14-gauge chrome-cobalt bar. He offered as an advantage increased strength of the splint but also noted that inherent to this technique were the usual problems of amalgam deterioration. Corn and Marks have expanded on this approach whereby a cast bar is fabricated on study casts prior to its insertion. A channel is made in the teeth to be stabilized and chromecobalt alloy bar cast. The bar is then

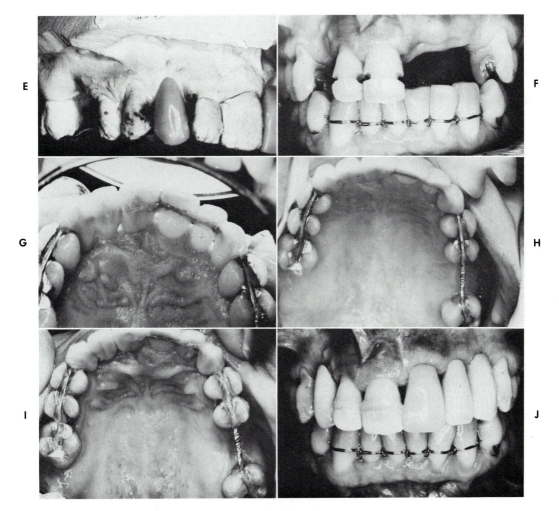

Fig. 20-14, cont'd. E, Right side view, canine on model. **F,** Teeth prepared. **G,** Bar and teeth positioned. **H** to **J,** Completed restoration, various views. (Courtesy Dr. H. Corn and Dr. M. Marks, Bristol, Pa.)

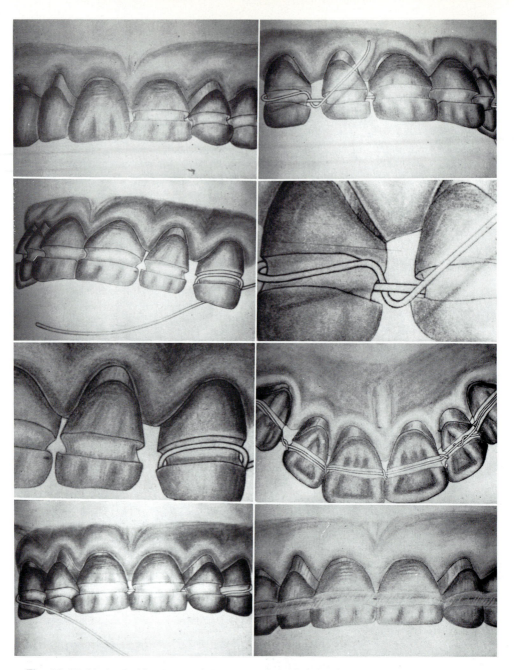

Fig. 20-15. Method of intracoronal temporary fixed ligation for anterior teeth utilizes horizontal circumferential wire with interproximal ties. This general principle has been in use for years as extracoronal method of stabilization. Basic principle of this splint is to induce rigidity for anterior segment of dental arch by permitting acrylic resin to harden into circumferential wire and undercuts of preparations. Rigidity produced seems to be much greater than rigidity of extracoronal circumferential wire splint. A groove is prepared on palatal, labial, and interproximal surfaces of teeth to be involved in splint. Precise location of grooves is dictated by (1) coronal limits of the pulp chamber position, (2) labiopalatal thicknesses of incisal thirds of teeth involved, and (3) relative degree of translucency of incisal thirds of teeth. After grooves are prepared, a continuous piece of 0.01 wire is wrapped around the most distal abutment and is then guided across palatal surface onto labial surface. Wire is passed interproximally gingival to palatal wire. It is taken back to labial surface coronal to palatal wire and is continued until distal tooth is reached. It is then joined with remaining free end. Wire is now completely covered with acrylic that is compatible in color with remaining tooth structure. Surface is highly polished (after paper points or Stim-U-Dents have been placed for protection of underlying gingiva). (Courtesy Dr. Jeffrey Ingber, Philadelphia.)

inserted with acrylic into grooves prepared in the natural dentition. This technique can be utilized both in the anterior and posterior parts of the mouth (Fig. 20-14).

The intracoronal type of temporary stabilization has served well for posterior teeth, but there are obvious disadvantages for the anterior segment. Because forces against the maxillary teeth are often generated in a labial direction, there is often noted a movement of the teeth away from the splinting mechanism. Realizing this problem, one could prepare a channel in these teeth on the labial, lingual, and proximal surfaces, utilize a circumferential wire ligation technique, and retain this with acrylic (Figs. 20-15 to 20-20). A major disadvantage to this means of stabilization is that the channels may prove to be undercut areas if the teeth are prepared for full crowns in the future. Again, the intraoral means of stabilization should be initiated only when the clinician appreciates the major disadvantages of these techniques. Ideally, it would be beneficial to have a future restorative dentistry commitment.

Provisional splints

The provisional splint is a restoration usually fabricated in acrylic as part of a restorative dentistry program. With this form of stabilization it is imperative that the patient go on to a permanent restorative program. Because of the nature of these splints, they offer the optimum in stabilization.

All acrylic. The all-acrylic type is probably the most common form of provisional splint. It is usu-

Text continued on p. 561.

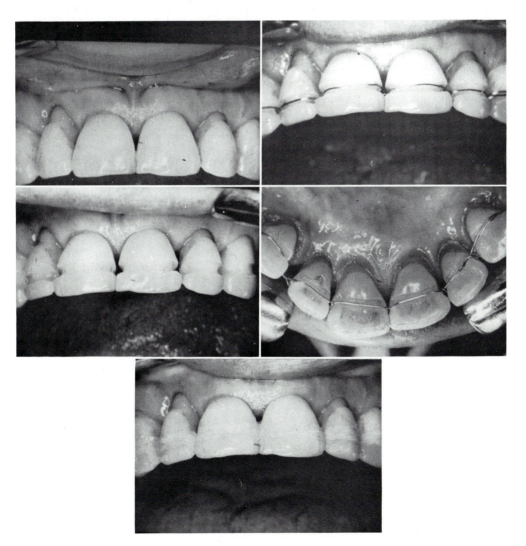

Fig. 20-16. Intracoronal temporary fixed ligation as illustrated in previous diagrams.

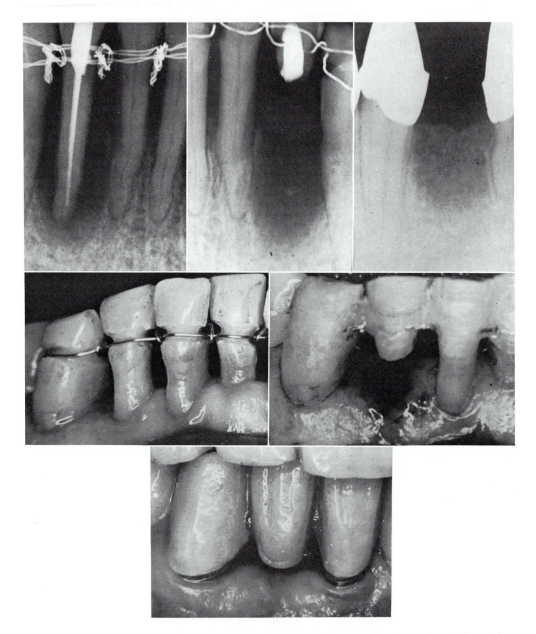

Fig. 20-17. Intracoronal splinting in area where strategic extraction is employed. In addition to previously mentioned advantages of this technique one can permit healing without patient's having to wear removable prostheses during surgical phase. (Restoration by D. I. Trachtenberg, Philadelphia.)

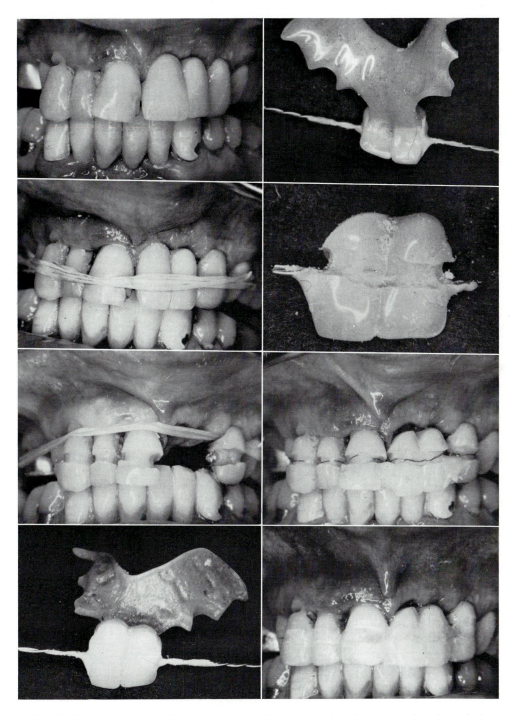

Fig. 20-18. Incorporation of a removable partial denture into intracoronal horizontal circumferential wire. Advantages include elimination of partial denture irritation to underlying tissue and negation of a phonetic problem, if one exists, due to acrylic covering the palate. If necessary, teeth can be moved into correct axial position and can be joined to the denture, thus providing stabilization of all periodontally involved teeth as well as retention of orthodontically repositioned teeth. (Courtesy Dr. Stanley Ross, West Palm Beach, Fla.)

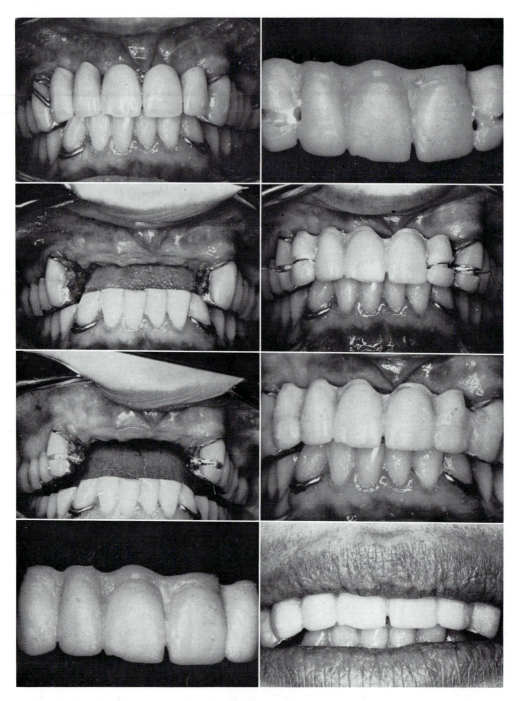

Fig. 20-19. Another variation of intracoronal temporary fixed ligation. Impression of existing partial denture is taken, enabling clinician to duplicate aesthetics when preparing acrylic shell for edentulous area. After completion of shell a groove is prepared on palatal, labial, and interproximal surfaces of abutment teeth and adjacent teeth of shell. A continuous piece of 0.01 wire is utilized as previously described. In addition to advantages of stabilization this variation negates irritation, which may arise from an ill-fitting partial denture. (Courtesy Dr. Stanley Ross, West Palm Beach, Fla.)

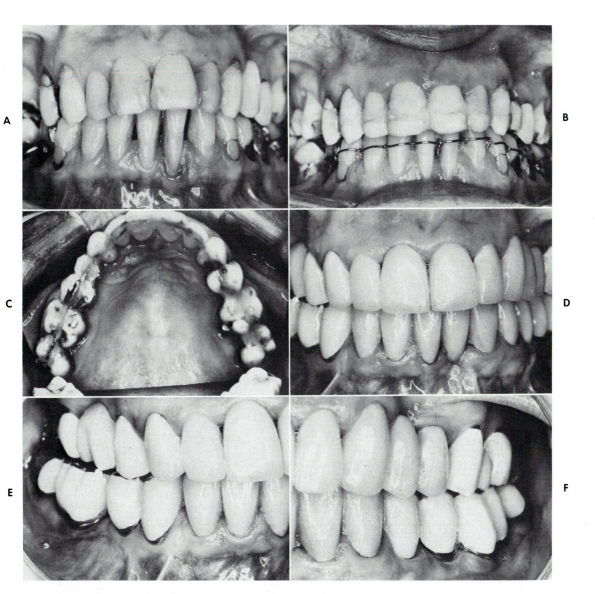

Fig. 20-20. A, Preoperative view; note flaring of maxillary anterior teeth. **B,** After initial periodontal therapy. Orthodontic movement of maxillary and mandibular teeth. Maxillary teeth temporarily stabilized with intracoronal wire-and-acrylic method; mandibular anterior teeth with external circumferential wire ligation technique. **C,** Palatal view of ligation technique. Note twisted wire and acrylic embedded in existing restorations in posterior teeth and intracoronal circumferential wiring with acrylic in anterior teeth. **D** to **F,** Various views of completed prosthesis. Maxillary and mandibular anterior teeth restored with porcelain fused to metal restorations and posterior teeth with acrylic veneer restorations over telescopic undercastings. Posterior segments "locked" to anterior portions with "dovetail" attachments. (Periodontal procedures completed by Dr. Garry Miller, Washington, D.C.)

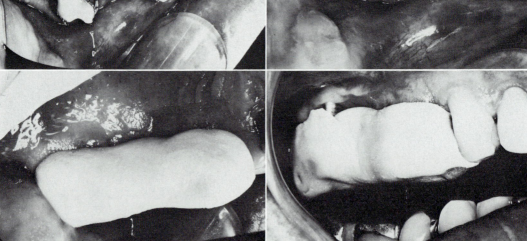

Fig. 20-21. Gold band–and–acrylic provisional restoration. **A,** Palatal view, maxillary right side prior to tooth preparation. (Periodontal procedure completed by Dr. Stanley Ross, West Palm Beach, Fla.) **B** to **D,** Various views of completed preparations. **E** and **F,** Gold bands fitted precisely to margination termination of preparation. Collar of gold left supragingivally. (Gold bands manufactured by J. M. Ney Co., Hartford, Conn.) **G** and **H,** Acrylic in a "doughy" state placed over preparations and gold bands.

ally fabricated from a premade shell, or it is done directly at the chairside. Its greatest limitation lies in its marginal adaptation.

Adapted metal bands and acrylic. Amsterdam and Fox have described the use of copper or gold bands fitted exactly to the subgingival termination of prepared teeth and then incorporated into self-curing acrylic. This technique fulfills all the objectives of a provisional restoration in that an exact marginal fit is achieved for maximum caries con-

trol and pulpal protection. Also, protective subgingival and supragingival coronal forms are more easily obtained, thus helping to achieve and maintain the health of the gingival tissue. Because of the added strength of the metal bands, frequent removal of the splints for various operative procedures (that is, impressions, coping transfers, assemblages) will not cause the splints to warp or the margins to become distorted (Figs. 20-21 and 20-22).

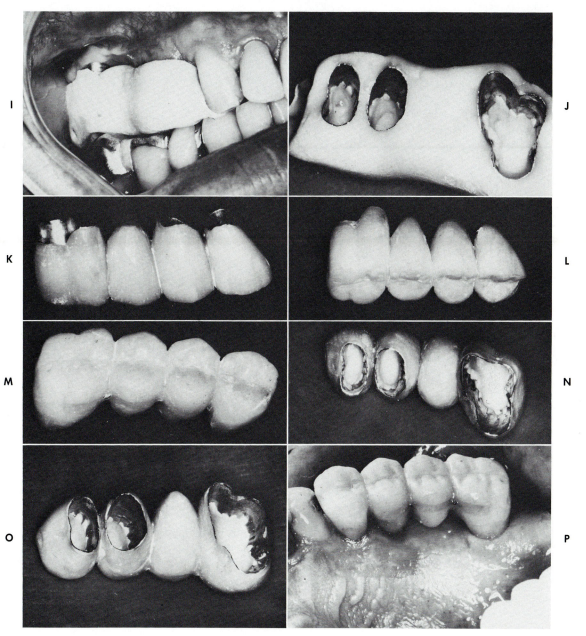

Fig. 20-21, cont'd. I, Patient biting in maximum intercuspal position. **J,** Acrylic mass with gold bands embedded after removal from teeth. **K** to **O,** Various views of completed provisional restoration prior to insertion into mouth. **P,** Palatal view of completed provisional restoration; note embedded wire in palatal surface for additional strength.

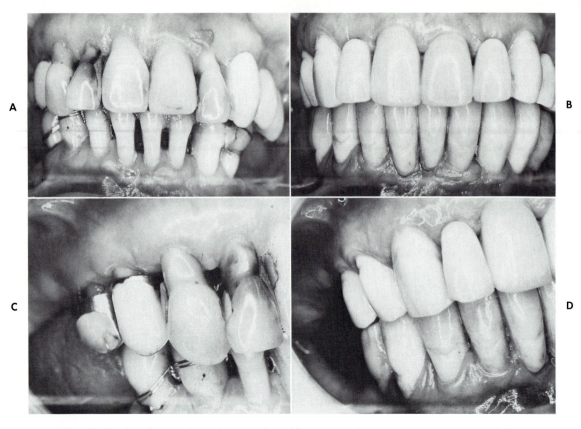

Fig. 20-22. Anterior provisional restoration with gold band–and–acrylic technique. **A,** Before, anterior view. **B,** Provisional, anterior. **C,** Before, right view. **D,** Provisional, right view.

REFERENCES

Amsterdam, M.: Periodontal prosthesis—twenty-five years in retrospect, Alpha Omegan, December, 1974.

Amsterdam, M., and Fox, L.: Provisional splinting—principles and techniques, Dent. Clin. North Am., p. 73, March, 1959.

Aspes, T., and McIlwain, J. E., Jr.: The multiple uses of acid-etch technics, Dent. Surv. **50:**25, 1974.

Baer, P. N., Malone, F. J., and Boyd, D. R.: A removable-fixed periodontal splint, Oral Surg. **9:**1057, 1956.

Barkam, L.: The case for metal ligatures in periodontia, J. Second District Dent. Soc. (N.Y.) **31:**341, 1945.

Bauhammers, A.: Fixed permanent amalgam splints using chrome-cobalt alloy reinforcement bars, J. Prosthet. Dent. **15:**351, 1961.

Bhaskar, S., and Orban, B.: Experimental occlusal trauma, J. Periodontol. **26:**270, 1955.

Buonocore, M. G., and Davila, J.: Restoration of fractured anterior teeth with ultraviolet-light-polymerized bonding materials: a new technique, J. Am. Dent. Assoc. **86:**1349, 1973.

Directions for Caulk Nuva-Seal Tooth Sealant: Milford, Del., June, 1976, The L. D. Caulk Company.

Cohen, D. W., and Chacker, F.: Criteria for the selection of one treatment plan over another, Dent. Clin. North Am., p. 3, March, 1964.

Corn, H., and Marks, M. H.: Strategic extractions in periodontal therapy, Dent. Clin. North Am. **13:**817, 1969.

Cross, W. G.: The importance of mobilization in periodontology, Parodontologie **8:**119, 1954.

Fenner, W., Gerber, A., and Muhlemann, H. R.: Tooth mobility changes during treatment with partial denture prosthesis, J. Prosthet. Dent. **6:**520, 1956.

Friedman, N.: Temporary splinting; an adjunct in periodontal therapy, J. Periodontol. **24:**229, 1953.

Glickman, I., Stein, R. S., and Smulow, J. B.: The effect of increased functional forces upon the periodontium of splinted and nonsplinted teeth, J. Periodontol. **32:**290, 1961.

Goldman, H. M., and Cohen, D. W.: Periodontal therapy, ed. 5, St. Louis, 1973, The C. V. Mosby Co.

Gottlieb, B.: Histologic considerations of the supporting tissues of the teeth, J. Am. Dent. Assoc. **30:**1872, 1943.

Graduate Periodontal Lectures, University of Pennsylvania, School of Dental Medicine, Graduate Division of Periodontology, 1963-1965.

Grupe, H. E., and Gromek, J. J.: Bruxism splint, J. Periodontol. **30:**156, 1959.

Hall, D. L., and Lindeberg, R. W.: Splinting of mandibular anterior teeth, Int. J. Forensic Dent. **22:**38, 1974.

Hirschfeld, L.: The use of wire and silk ligature, J. Am. Dent. Assoc. **4:**647, 1950.

Johnson, W. N., and Groat, J. E.: A new fixed temporary dental splint, Periodont. Abstr. **14:**2, 1966.

Kegel, W., Selipsky, H., and Phillips, C.: The effect of splinting on tooth mobility. I. During initial therapy, J. Clin. Periodontol. **6:**45, 1979.

Kessler, M.: A variation of the ''A'' splint, J. Periodontol. **41:**268, 1970.

Klassman, B., and Zucker, H. W.: Combination wire–composite resin intracoronal splinting rationale and technique, J. Periodontol. **47:**481, 1976.

Kronfeld, R.: Physiology of the human periodontal tissues under normal and abnormal occlusal conditions, Ill. Dent. J. **8:**13, 1939.

Kronfeld, R.: Structure, function and pathology of human periodontal membrane, N.Y. J. Dent. **6:**112, 1936.

Kronfeld, R.: Histologic study of the influence of function on the human periodontal membrane, J. Am. Dent. Assoc. **18:**1242, 1931.

Langeland, K., and Langeland, L.: Use of radioactive tracers to determine the protective effect of cavity liners, J. Dent. Res. **45:**1233, 1966.

Leff, A.: An improved temporary acrylic fixed bridge, J. Prosthet. Dent. **3:**245, 1953.

Lemmerman, J.: Rationale for stabilization, J. Periodontol. **47:**405, 1976.

Lloyd, R., and Baer, P.: Amalgam splint, Dent. Clin. North Am., p. 213, March, 1964.

Macapanpan, L. C., and Weinmann, J. P.: The influence of injury to the periodontal membrane on the spread of gingival inflammation, J. Dent. Res. **33:**263, 1954.

Muhlemann, H. R.: Ten years of tooth mobility measurements, J. Periodontol. **31:**110, 1960.

Munch-Hansen, E.: The pin splint, a removable splint fixation; a modification of von Weissengluh's Hulsenstiftschiene, J. Periodontol. **32:**322, 1961.

Obin, J., and Arvins, A.: The use of self-curing resin splints for the temporary stabilization of mobile teeth due to periodontal involvement, J. Am. Dent. Assoc. **42:**320, 1951.

Orban, B., and Weinmann, J.: Signs of traumatic occlusion in average human jaws, J. Dent. Res. **13:**216, 1933.

Overby, G. E.: Esthetic splinting of teeth by vertical pinning, J. Prosthet. Dent. **11:**112, 1961.

Overby, G. E.: Intracoronal splinting of mobile teeth by use of screws and sleeves, J. Periodontol. **33:**270, 1962.

Parfitt, G. J.: The dynamics of a tooth in function, J. Periodontol. **32:**102, 1961.

Polson, A. M., and Billen, J. R.: Temporary splinting of teeth using ultraviolet light–polymerized bonding materials, J. Am. Dent. Assoc. **89:**1137, 1974.

Riedel, R. A.: A review of the retention problem, Angle Orthod. **30:**179, 1960.

Sannell, C., and Feldman, A. J.: Horizontal pin splint for lower anterior teeth, J. Prosthet. Dent. **12:**138, 1962.

Shoushan, E. D.: A pin-ledge casting technique — its application in periodontal splinting, Dent. Clin. North Am., p. 189, March, 1960.

Simring, M.: Splinting theory and practice, J. Am. Dent. Assoc. **45:**402, 1952.

Simring, M., and Thaller, J. H.: Temporary splinting for mobile teeth, J. Am. Dent. Assoc. **53:**429, 1956.

Sorrin, S.: Use of fixed and removable splints in the practice of periodontia, Am. J. Orthod. **31:**354, 1945.

Stahl, S. S., Miller, S. C., and Goldsmith, E. D.: The effects of vertical occlusal trauma on the periodontium of protein deprived young adult rats, J. Periodontol. **28:**87, 1957.

Stern, I. B.: The status of temporary fixed-splinting procedures in the treatment of periodontally involved teeth, J. Periodontol. **31:**217, 1960.

Talkov, L.: The copper band splint, J. Prosthet. Dent. **6:**215, 1956.

Talkov, L.: Temporary acrylic fixed bridgework and splints, J. Prosthet. Dent. **2:**693, 1952.

Trachtenberg, D.: A combined amalgam-wire-acrylic splint, J. Periodontol. **39:**255, 1968.

Ward, H. L., and Weinberg, L. A.: An evaluation of periodontal splints, J. Am. Dent. Assoc. **63:**48, 1961.

Weinberg, L. A.: Force distribution in splinted anterior teeth, Oral Surg. **10:**484, 1268, 1957.

Wentz, F. M., Jarabak, J., and Orban, B.: Experimental occlusal trauma imitating cuspal interferences, J. Periodontol. **29:**117, 1958.

21 Tooth movement in periodontal therapy

A contributing factor to periodontal disease is tooth malposition. Two basic objectives in periodontal therapy are elimination or control of the etiologic factors and correction of the defects resulting from those etiologic factors. To ignore tooth malposition will compromise an optimal result or invite failure. Although responsibility toward aesthetics should not be minimized, the main goal of periodontal therapy is to restore function to the teeth and the periodontium. Some general considerations concerning tooth movement are discussed below.

Occlusal forces and landmarks. The teeth and the periodontium can best withstand the loading placed upon them if the forces are directed toward the vertical axis. However, for a compre-hensive evaluation one must not only recognize the axial inclinations of the teeth, but also evaluate tooth locations within the same arch (intra-arch) as well as relationships of the maxillary and mandibular components (interarch). In the retruded contact (RC) position, or centric relation, the bucco-occlusal line angle of the mandibular teeth should fall within the central fossa line of the maxillary teeth. In the maxillary arch the linguo-occlusal line angle should contact the central fossa line of the mandibular teeth (see Chapter 30). When these centric holding areas exhibit a marked discrepancy buccolingually, the malposed teeth should be repositioned when trauma from occlusion is diagnosed. In the presence or absence of periodontal disease, teeth can be moved successfully in adults as well as in children. A compromise in tooth malposition should not be accepted when an optimal result can be achieved by repositioning the indicated teeth.

"Minor" tooth movement and major orthodontics. It is generally accepted that the term "minor" tooth movement involves a single tooth or small segments of teeth. The mechanics of movement are usually accomplished by a removable acrylic-and-wire appliance or by several orthodontic bands, which generally result in a tipping action. In contrast, major orthodontics involves moving large segments of teeth or correcting entire arches, mainly with bracketed techniques. The brackets and arch wires allow for controlled bodily movement rather than tipping action. Another distinction is that of tooth movement in periodontal therapy for the adult as opposed to orthodontic tooth movement during growth and development for the adolescent.

Sequence of tooth movement procedures. A treatment program encompassing all facets of periodontal treatment and restorative dentistry should be planned in the following sequence:

I. Initial preparation of the dentition
   A. Emergency relief of pain

B. Removal of condemned teeth unless required to support an appliance
C. Therapy of the soft tissue lesion
   1. Instruction in plaque control and its reinforcement
   2. Removal of supragingival and subgingival deposits
   3. Control of the inflammatory lesion by curettage of the soft tissue pocket wall and removal of the granulomatous tissue and gingival fibers to the alveolar crest
   4. Correction of inadequate restorations to control the local etiologic factors (caries, food impaction areas, and so on)
   5. Exploratory surgery and root resection followed by endodontics when required
D. Therapy of the lesion of the attachment apparatus
   1. Correction of occlusal discrepancies
      a. Tooth movement establishing proper tooth position so that a stable occlusion can be developed through occlusal adjustment and restorative procedures
      b. Occlusal adjustment by selective grinding
   2. Provisional stabilization or immobilization
II. Reevaluation of the periodontium for further therapy. (It is necessary to determine the removal of strategic teeth that may delay therapeutic procedures or that may endanger the success of a restorative program. Reevaluations are conducted throughout treatment)
III. Pocket elimination
IV. Completion of therapy for the attachment apparatus lesion
   A. Final selective grinding
   B. Restorations by means of periodontal prosthesis
V. Night guards to control oral habits
VI. Continued periodontal maintenance and plaque control evaluations (Corn and Marks, 1969)

In summary, tooth movement procedures follow the control of the inflammatory lesions. Tooth movement would generally precede retention and stabilization procedures, occlusal adjustment, pocket elimination, and restorative dentistry.

Certain exceptions exist for this usual sequence of tooth movement. For example, hopeless teeth might be retained temporarily to act as anchorage for appliance retention. Another exception would occur when a marked discrepancy of 2 to 3 mm existed from the retruded contact position (centric relation, terminal hinge) to the intercuspal (IC) position (centric occlusion, acquired occlusion) with flared maxillary anterior teeth. Occlusal adjustment in the retruded contact position is first completed. This establishes maximum contacts of teeth posteriorly without a forward slip. Available intermaxillary space then exists between the mandibular and maxillary incisors to allow for retraction of the flared maxillary teeth. After tooth movement and retention in this instance, occlusal adjustment would be completed for all excursions. Proper case planning would determine the sequence of tooth movement.

Movement of the teeth with periodontal defects frequently modifies the gingival and osseous morphology. The subsequent surgical phases of therapy are then performed on the newly established tissue anatomy.

Indications and contraindications for tooth movement. The following is an outline of the indications for tooth movement, some of which overlap:

I. Periodontal
   A. Reduction of deep overbite or locked bite resulting in occlusal traumatism
   B. Correction of crowded teeth that do not allow for adequate plaque control
   C. Closure of open contacts prone to food impaction
   D. Correction of occlusal discrepancy in the presence of occlusal traumatism
   E. Improvement of landmark positioning (cusp tip to central fossa line) for occlusal equilibration
   F. Improvement or elimination of gingival and osseous defects
II. Aesthetic
   A. Closing diastemata
   B. Repositioning migrated or extruded incisors
   C. Correcting rotated teeth
   D. Realigning crowded incisors
   E. Correcting anterior crossbite or pseudoclass III malocclusion
III. Restorative
   A. Paralleling abutment teeth for a fixed bridge, partial denture, or A splints.
   B. Preparing the edentulous space for proper pontic size
   C. Preventing pulpal involvement in tooth preparation
   D. Allowing for adequate thickness of restorative materials on prepared teeth
   E. Reestablishing proper posterior occlusal plane
   F. Reestablishing incisal guidance
   G. Forcibly erupting teeth fractured at or below the gingival margin (Fig. 21-49).
IV. Other
   A. Moving adjacent teeth to make room for a locked-out tooth
   B. Retracting mandibular incisors to create intermaxillary space for retracting maxillary incisors
   C. Depressing teeth interfering with movement of an approximating tooth
   D. Intercepting early tooth drifting after extraction
   E. Realigning malposed teeth that have the potential for initiating habits (e.g., clenching, grinding, tongue thrusting) or affecting speech.

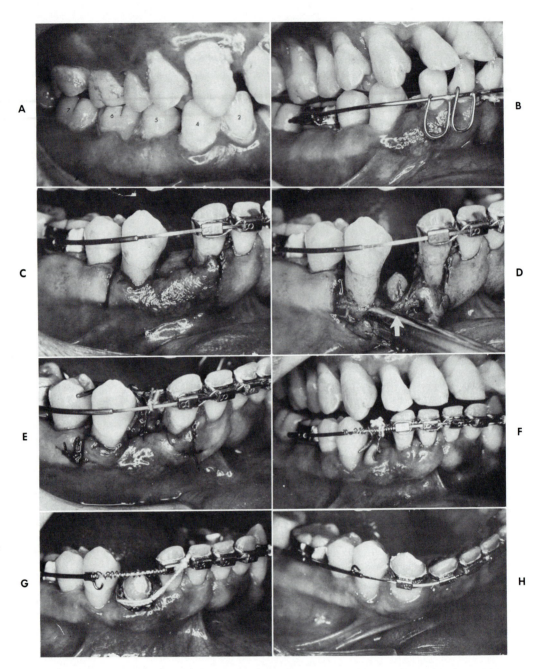

Fig. 21-1. A, Impacted mandibular right canine in 40 year-old-man. Note that lateral incisor, *2*, is in contact with first premolar, *4*. **B,** A 0.9 mm (0.036 inch) round gold labial arch wire with soldered crozat springs of 0.62 mm (0.025 inch) round gold wire moves incisors mesially. **C,** A 0.5 mm (0.020 inch) ribbon arch stabilizes incisors and maintains arch length. **D,** Impacted canine surgically exposed. Note intact distal alveolar crest remaining on incisor after tooth movement. This bony crest is also seen in Fig. 21-2. With proper tooth movement procedures, the bone moves with the tooth, and there should not be a loss of supporting bone. **E,** Hole drilled through lingual surface of canine to retain wire ligature that attaches light elastic ligature to arch. A metal pin with a loop from which elastics can be attached is now preferred and is placed into crown. **F,** Canine erupting after 3 months. **G,** Canine banded for rotating into position after 9 months. **H,** Canine in position after 14 months. (In conjunction with Alan Lauter and Charles Jonas, University of Pennsylvania.)

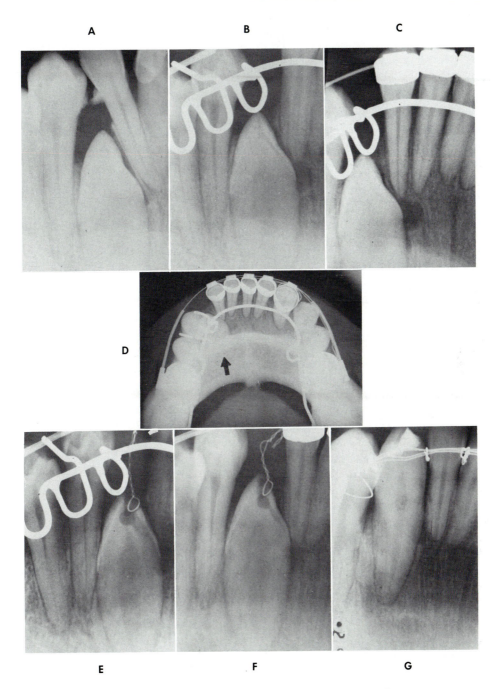

Fig. 21-2. Teeth of patient in Fig. 21-1. **A,** Impacted canine. Note lamina dura and height of intercrestal bone on distal surface of lateral incisor. **B** to **D,** Available space was created for canine. Loop lingual arch stabilized molar anchorage, and soldered crozat springs prevented premolars from drifting mesially. **E,** A hole was drilled into lingual surface of canine to secure steel ligature. **F,** Three months later. **G,** Canine in position after 24 months. Note incisor root resorption.

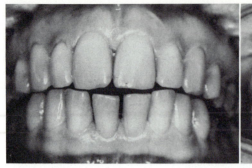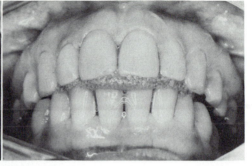

Fig. 21-3. Improper swallow with an anterior tongue thrust resulting in open bite and flared incisors. (In conjunction with Herman Corn, Levittown, Pa.)

Several considerations contraindicate tooth movement. These include the following:

1. No prior reduction of inflammation
2. Inability to stabilize and retain the new tooth position
3. No anticipated improvement of periodontal health after tooth movement
4. Lack of patient cooperation

Periodontal maintenance during tooth movement. Tooth movement appliances, whether fixed or removable, render oral hygiene procedures more difficult. Plaque retention is increased, necessitating a rigid plaque control program. Scaling and root planing supplemented with curettage may be required on a 1- to 3-month basis to minimize tissue inflammation. Hydrotherapy devices may be required to supplement the routine personal oral hygiene procedures.

ETIOLOGY, EXAMINATION, AND DIAGNOSIS OF TOOTH MALPOSITION

Etiology. The following is a classification of the etiology of malocclusions, modified after Moyers (1973):

I. Heredity, developmental
   A. Jaw size and shape—small, large, asymmetric, cleft, temporomandibular joint ankylosis
   B. Tooth size and shape—microdontia, macrodontia, peg-shaped teeth
   C. Tooth positions—impactions, eccentricities, crowding (Figs. 21-1, 21-2, and 21-7)
   D. Tooth number—supernumerary teeth, anodontia, oligodontia (Fig. 21-34)
   E. Abnormal exfoliation and eruption (Figs. 21-28 and 21-29)
   F. Tongue or muscle size and shape, frena (Fig. 21-34)
II. Habits
   A. Thumb and finger sucking
   B. Improper swallow with a tongue thrust (Fig. 21-3)
   C. Lip sucking and biting
   D. Nail biting
   E. Tooth to foreign object contact—pipe, pencil, bobby pin
   F. Clenching and grinding—depression
III. Diseases, local
   A. Periodontal, occlusal attrition
   B. Caries—early loss of primary teeth, loss of permanent teeth (Figs. 21-4 and 21-33)
   C. Nasopharyngeal
IV. Diseases, systemic
   A. Febrile—affecting incremental growth of bone
   B. Endocrine disorders—retarding or hastening growth, hormonal overgrowth of gingiva displacing teeth
   C. Dilantin sodium—gingival overgrowth displacing teeth (Fig. 21-5)

Classification of malocclusions. As emphasized previously, tooth malpositions must be evaluated relative to adjacent teeth in the same arch or intra-arch and to interarch relationship in the most retruded contact position (centric relation, terminal hinge). Malpositions should be corrected to this position rather than to the intercuspal contact or acquired occlusion. During the growth years tooth malposition as a result of jaw size discrepancy generally requires correction and retention with multibanded or multibracketed techniques under the guidance of an orthodontist. Frequently this allows for the control of jaw growth as well as control of tooth positioning. The malocclusions as described by Angle should be clearly understood (Fig. 21-6):

Class I (neutro-occlusion). The mesiobuccal cusp of the maxillary first permanent molar articulates with the buccal groove of the mandibular first permanent molar. This molar position, with tooth malpositions as crossbites or protrusions of the anterior teeth, is called a class I malocclusion. If the loss of teeth has resulted in drifting and distortion of the molar relationship, the

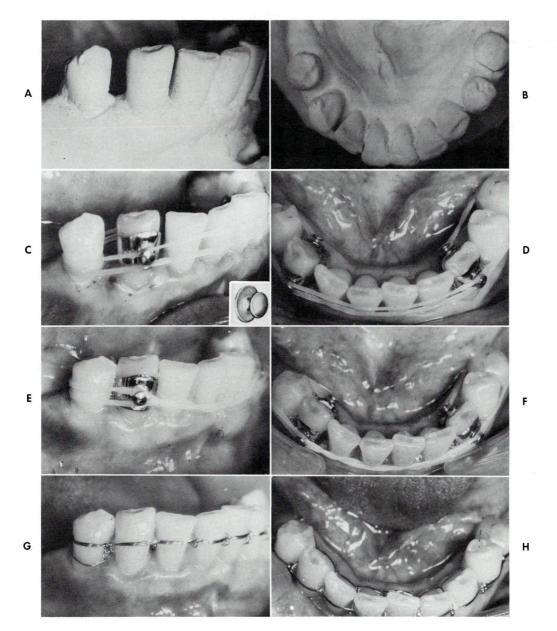

Fig. 21-4. A and **B,** Flaring of mandibular incisors and distal drifting of premolars due to loss of posterior teeth with resultant posterior bite collapse. **C** and **D,** Canines banded with buttons welded on labial and lingual surfaces. A 4 mm (³/₁₆ inch) regular elastic on right and 7 mm (⁵/₁₆ inch) regular elastic on left encircle premolars from labial and lingual buttons to move premolars mesially and to close open contacts. A 15 mm (⁵/₈ inch) light elastic from labial buttons on canines retracts incisors lingually. **E** and **F,** Premolars and incisors are in position. If incisor elastic tends to slip gingivally, it can be twisted to prevent its separation and to provide good position. **G** and **H,** Wire ligation for tooth retention. Note premolar cervical retaining wire. (**C** insert courtesy Rocky Mountain Dental Products Co., Denver.)

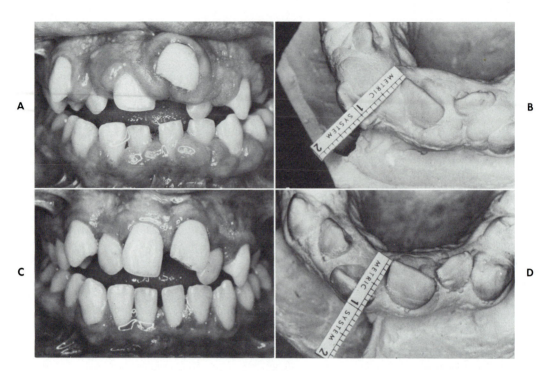

Fig. 21-5. A and **B,** Tooth displacement and open bite, resulting from Dilantin gingival hyperplasia concomitant with an incorrect swallowing pattern and anterior tongue thrust. **C** and **D,** Three months after gingivectomy. Central incisor discrepancy improved 4 mm without any active appliance therapy.

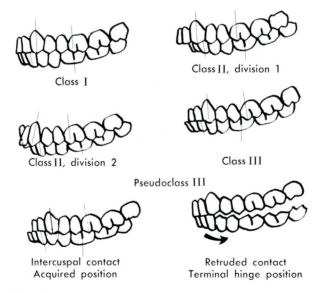

Class I

Class II, division 1

Class II, division 2

Class III

Pseudoclass III

Intercuspal contact
Acquired position

Retruded contact
Terminal hinge position

Fig. 21-6. Modified from Angle's classification of malocclusions. (Courtesy J. George Coslet, University of Pennsylvania.)

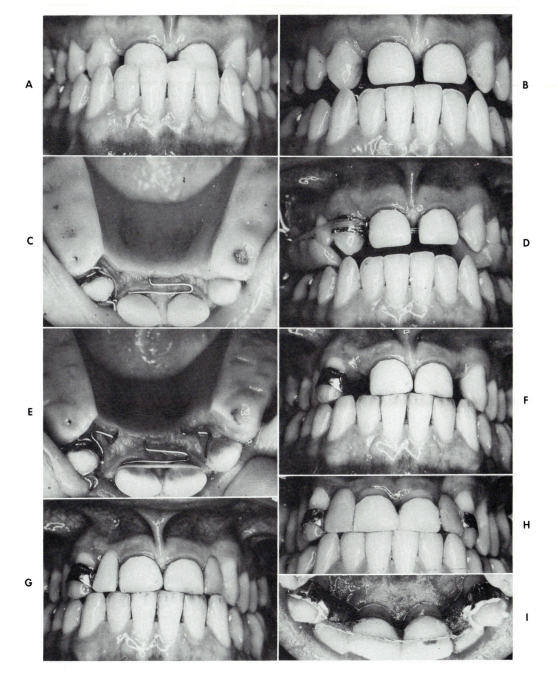

Fig. 21-7. A, Pseudoclass III with congenitally missing lateral incisors. **B,** In retruded contact position mandible is distally positioned, with incisors approximating edge-to-edge position. Interference in retruded contracting position is on right canines. **C,** Right maxillary canine is banded with hooks for rotation. A simple recurved spring lingual to central incisors is for labial movement. **D,** Posterior bite platform allows for sufficient anterior opening to correct canine and incisor crossbite. **E,** Recurved springs are added to provide canine labial movement. A 4 mm (³/₁₆ inch) light elastic moves central incisors mesially and reciprocally. **F,** Tooth movement completed, with incisors and canines in position after occlusal adjustment. Sufficient edentulous space has been created for lateral incisor pontic. **G,** A removable acrylic space maintainer with lateral pontics is worn during completion of periodontal therapy. **H** and **I,** Temporary bridge consisting of canine orthodontic bands, lingual soldered hooks, lateral incisor pontics, and a twisted wire and acrylic A splint is used for retention until a fixed bridge can be constructed. This eliminates the removable appliance, which tends to irritate tissues and to delay maturation of the gingiva. (In conjunction with Leonard Abrams and Alan Lautern, University of Pennsylvania.)

classification is based on the canine position, that is, the maxillary canine lying between the mandibular canine and the first premolar.

Class II (disto-occlusion). The mesiobuccal cusp of the maxillary first permanent molar articulates anteriorly to the buccal groove of the mandibular first permanent molar. The mandibular arch is in a position distal to the neutro-occlusion.

Division I—maxillary incisors are in labioversion.

Division II—maxillary central incisors are in normal anteroposterior position or in linguoversion, while the maxillary lateral incisors are tipped labially.

Subdivision—unilateral. One side may be in neutro-occlusion while the other is in disto-occlusion.

Class III (mesio-occlusion). The mesiobuccal cusp of the maxillary first permanent molar articulates posteriorly to the buccal groove of the mandibular first permanent molar. Often the posteriors are in cross-bite, and the maxillary incisors are in lingual crossibte. The mandibular arch is in a position mesial to the neutro-occlusion.

Pseudoclass III. In acquired or habitual occlusion the maxillary incisors are in lingual crossbite and apparently in a class III relationship. However, in the retruded contact position the mandible is distally positioned, and the incisors then approach an edge-to-edge relationship (Fig. 21-7).

Lischer (1912) describes the malpositions of individual teeth as follows: linguoversion, labioversion or buccoversion, mesioversion, distoversion, infraversion, supraversion, torsiversion (rotated on the long axis), axiversion (incorrect axial inclination), and transversion (incorrect sequence).

Overbite and overjet. The following is a list of terms and the situation to which each refers:

Deep overbite—excessive vertical overlap
Open bite—absence of occlusion locally

Adult	Adolescent
1. Adult is usually over 18 years of age.	1. Average age of treatment ranges from 10 to 15 years of age.
2. Skeletal growth and development of puberty and maturity is completed.	2. Skeletal growth and development is in progress (up to 20% in some adolescents during pubertal growth spurt).
3. Frequently there is periodontal disease with bone loss.	3. There is periodontal disease of soft tissue but rarely bone loss.
4. Often mobility patterns of the teeth with occlusal traumatism are diagnosed.	4. Rarely is occlusal traumatism seen. Mobilities may be noted immediately after orthodontics but is usually transient.
5. Primary needs are functional, and aesthetic needs are usually secondary.	5. Aesthetic needs are frequently the prime motivating factor, with functional needs secondary.
6. With tooth movement, elongation of the clinical crown is encouraged, permitting reduction of the clinical crown-to-clinical root ratio during occlusal adjustment and restorative dentistry.	6. Leveling and depressing of the teeth is preferred, and elongation of the teeth is generally contraindicated. Reduction of the clinical crown other than for minor adjustments is rarely planned.
7. Tooth movement is primarily accomplished with removable appliances, but occasionally with fixed.	7. Tooth movement is primarily accomplished with fixed appliances, but occasionally with removable.
8. In many instances teeth are missing, necessitating restorative dentistry after tooth movement.	8. Rarely are teeth missing, and restorative dentistry is generally not a consideration.
9. Because of occlusal traumatism and associated mobility patterns, anchorage may be a problem, and one may have to connect several posterior teeth in order to prevent movement of the anchor teeth.	9. Since tooth mobilities are generally not present, one can better evaluate the anchorage needs early in the tooth movement procedures.

Excessive overjet—excessive horizontal overlap
Crossbite—excessive overlap lingually, buccally, or
labially

Drifting. After the extraction of adjacent teeth in the same arch the potential for drifting of the permanent teeth often occurs in the following pattern:

Incisors—mesially	
Canine—mesially or distally	
First premolar—mesially or distally	← ←→ → ←
Second premolar—distally	1 2 3 4 5 6 7 8
Molars—mesially	

Occlusal plane. The anteroposterior occlusal plane can be gradual, excessive, flat, or reversed. The excessive curve may require leveling of the posterior teeth. The flat and reversed planes of occlusion may require posterior eruption to reestablish the normal or gradual curve of Spee. In patients who are excessive clenchers, the posterior teeth supporting the occlusion can be depressed. Associated with this, heavy pressure now produced by the mandibular incisors in contact with the lingual surface of the maxillary incisors can result in spacing and flaring. In this instance there would be loss of occlusal vertical dimension.

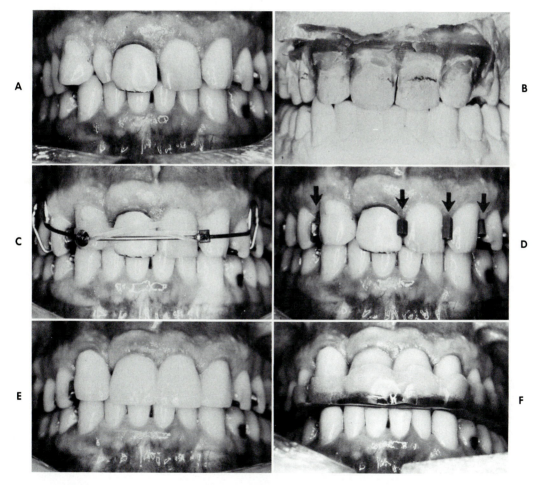

Fig. 21-8. A, In pretreatment picture one sees old acrylic veneer crown, several large defective silicates, and a peg lateral. If peg lateral were removed, would canine-to-canine distance be equally divided among remaining anterior teeth? **B,** Diagnostic setup was completed, removing anterior teeth with a saw blade, but separating teeth by breaking them at contact point to retain their proper mesiodistal width. **C,** Since setup was satisfactory, tooth movement was initiated with a Hawley appliance and use of several elastics from welded hooks on labial wire. **D,** Three days prior to tooth preparation, maxian separators were used to establish final equal spaces between each tooth *(arrows)*. **E,** Final anterior bridge. **F,** Maxillary guard to control nocturnal habits of clenching and grinding. (In conjunction with Herman Corn, Levittown, Pa., and Stanley Lipkowitz, Fairless Hills, Pa.)

ADULT VERSUS ADOLESCENT TOOTH MOVEMENT

Since orthodontic tooth movement in the past has been child oriented, it is important to differentiate the needs of the adult patient from those of the child. The boxed material is a partial list differentiating adult patients' needs from those of the adolescent (Marks and Corn, 1973).

BASIC PRINCIPLES FOR TOOTH MOVEMENT

Certain conditions must be realized before commencing successful tooth movement procedures.

1. The patient must understand the indications for the tooth movement, be desirous of such therapy, and agree to cooperate throughout its duration. Failure results when these are not made clear initially.

2. Intra-arch and interarch space must be available or obtainable. Intra-arch space can be created by stripping, by moving adjacent teeth, by extraction, or by arch expansion.

In cases of posterior bite collapse where a minimal anterior slip is present from retruded contact to intercuspal contact position and the maxillary incisors have flared, a maxillary Hawley appliance with an anterior bite platform is used (Fig.

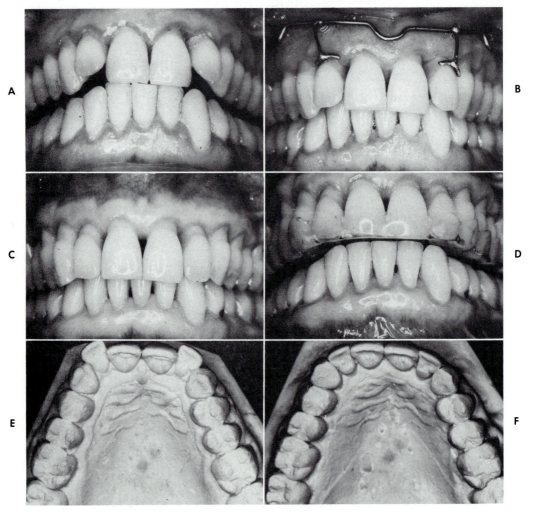

Fig. 21-9. A, Class II, division II, malocclusion but well articulated posteriorly. **B,** A high, labial appliance with J springs exerts lingual pressure on the lateral incisors. Better action is obtained if the spring contacts further down on labial surfaces. Available space is obtained by stripping maxillary incisors and canines. Stripping of mandibular incisors would be contraindicated because these teeth are square shaped with long contact points. **C,** Tooth movement completed in 4 months with continual stripping. **D,** A maxillary bite guard is constructed to control clenching and grinding habits and to retain new tooth position. A Hawley retainer was worn for 6 months after tooth movement and before bite guard was made. **E** and **F,** Occlusal view of models before and after tooth movement. Note narrowed incisors and canines.

21-40). The resulting posterior eruption creates *interarch* space anteriorly for the retraction.

In other circumstances the maxillary anterior teeth are flared and the mandibular anterior teeth contact heavily in the intercuspal position (centric occlusion). However, a forward slip of 1 mm or more exists from retruded contact to intercuspal contact position. Occlusal adjustment establishing maximum posterior contacts in the retruded contact position creates interarch space anteriorly for retraction of the flared maxillary anterior teeth.

If available intra-arch space is questionable, a diagnostic setup by cutting and repositioning the teeth on the study model is an aid (Fig. 21-8).

Measurements of the thickness of the enamel on the x-ray films is imperative. At the contact point the average enamel width is 0.5 mm, which will limit the amount of stripping. Tapering teeth with occlusally or incisally placed contact points are suitable for enamel stripping (Figs. 21-9 and 21-10), whereas square-shaped teeth with long, broad contact points are generally contraindicated for this procedure. This is frequently seen with mandibular incisors (Fig. 21-9). When crowding exists, the removal of a mandibular incisor will rarely achieve a stable tooth arrangement and relapse is common.

3. Adequate anchorage must be planned to pre-

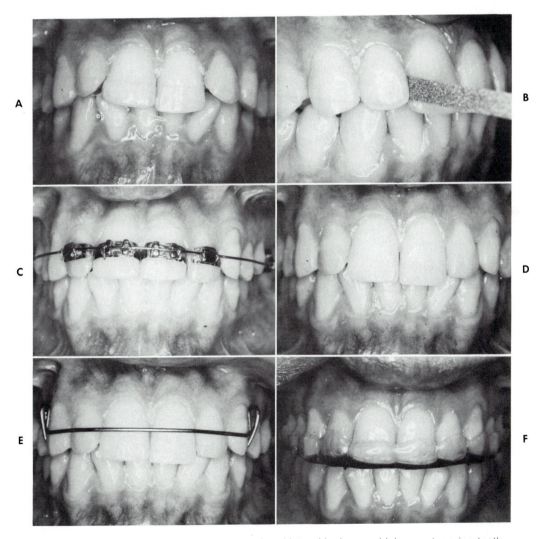

Fig. 21-10. A, Wide enamel cap on central and lateral incisors, which were tapering teeth. **B,** Enamel being reduced with a metal strip. **C,** Fixed edgewise arch with bands on central and lateral incisors and first molars to intrude as well as to retract incisors. **D,** Tooth movement completed. Note level gingival margins compared to **A.** Controlled intrusion is more difficult with a removable appliance. **E,** Hawley retainer, with labial wire contacting su face of each anterior tooth, was worn for 1 year. **F,** Bite guard. (In conjunction with Jerome Sklaroff, University of Pennsylvania.)

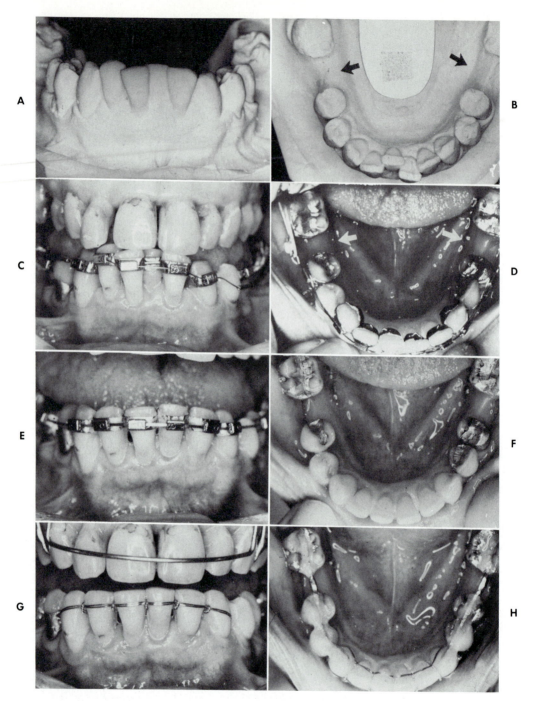

Fig. 21-11. A, Mandibular incisors crowded and extruded. Full splinting was indicated, with retention of maximum number of teeth. Fixed appliance therapy was indicated for leveling incisors and rounding out arch. **B,** Occlusal view. Note size of edentulous space. **C,** Six anteriors, second premolars, and molars were banded for Johnson twin arch. Single wire was used initially. **D,** Occlusal view after 8 months. Arch is rounded, and premolars are retracted distally for anterior spacing. Note decreased edentulous space. **E,** Rectangular arch is placed for retention and stabilization after tooth positioning. **F,** All orthodontic bands removed. Note spaces remaining interproximally from double thickness of band material, which was 0.07 mm (0.003 inch) thick. **G,** Anterior spacing was closed with wire ligation tightened periodically. **H,** Posterior segments were stabilized with A splint cast bar from canines to second molars. (In conjunction with Herman Corn, Levittown, Pa.)

vent its slippage. This will be discussed in the section on Essentials of Anchorage.

4. Infection and inflammation must be controlled prior to tooth movement as noted under Sequence of Tooth Movement Procedures.

5. The occlusion must not interfere with the freedom of tooth movement. When required, a maxillary Hawley appliance with an incisal bite plane or in selected cases a posterior acrylic platform may be used. These will disarticulate the potential interfering tooth inclines (Fig. 21-19).

6. If tipping of the teeth with removable appliances would create unfavorable axial inclinations, then bodily movement with fixed appliances should be considered (Fig. 21-34).

7. No tooth movement should be started unless the retention and stabilization phases have been fully planned.

ESSENTIALS OF ANCHORAGE

Newton's third law states that for every action there is an equal and opposite reaction. This principle is basic to the discussion of anchorage. For successful tooth movement the anchor units must resist movement. Pressure placed on one tooth will produce movement on other teeth unless the threshold force is below that needed to initiate displacement of the anchorage.

Sources. Sources of anchorage include the roots and their cementum, the attachment apparatus of the periodontal ligament, the supporting bone, the palatal and lingual mucosa, the occlusion of the teeth, and the skull.

Locations. There are three basic locations for anchorage. Anchorage that is located within the same arch as the teeth being moved is designated as *intramaxillary* (Figs. 21-1, 21-4, 21-7, 21-8 to 21-10, 21-15, 21-17, and 21-18). When teeth or appliances in one arch are used to move teeth in another arch, the location is referred to as *intermaxillary* (Figs. 21-19, 21-28, 21-35, and 21-38). Extraoral anchorage, consisting of head or cervical straps or caps, is generally not practical for adult patients.

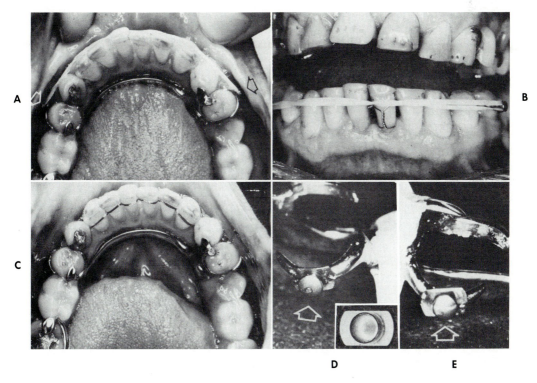

Fig. 21-12. A, Existing mandibular partial denture is used to retract flared incisors. Buttons were welded to buccal arm of clasps. **B,** An 18 mm (¾ inch) light elastic was stretched across incisors. Note wire ligature tie to prevent elastic from slipping gingivally. **C,** Retracted incisors were retained with wire ligation, and buttons were removed. **D** and **E,** Closeup view of welded buttons. (In conjunction with Herman Corn, Levittown, Pa.; **D** insert courtesy Rocky Mountain Dental Products Co., Denver.)

Categories. Anchorage has been categorized, based on single or multiple teeth and resistance to tipping or bodily movement, as follows:

1. Simple—the anchor teeth have the potential for tipping, but have a greater resistance to movement than do the malposed teeth.
2. Stationary—the anchor unit has the potential to move bodily rather than to tip, allowing for greater resistance to slipping.
3. Single—one tooth is involved.
4. Compound anchorage—two or more teeth are involved.
5. Reciprocal—the potential to resist movement between the two units is equal. This is planned only when both units are to be moved together or apart equal distances (Fig. 21-34).

Selection. The following considerations in the selection of suitable anchorage will avoid pitfalls during tooth movement therapy:

1. The greater the number of teeth used, the more resistant to movement the anchor unit will be (Figs. 21-11 to 21-14).

2. Stability will be dependent on the shape of the roots, their unit area of attachment, the amount of bone remaining, whether the roots are single or multiple, and the convergency or divergency of the roots.
3. The use of acrylic-and-wire removable appliances will splint the multiple anchor units together and add the bony resistance of the maxilla or mandible.
4. The anchor units should be widely separated and bilaterally situated if possible.
5. Resistance to slipping will be dependent on the quantity, direction, and duration of force that the anchor units must withstand.

Slipping of anchorage. At each appointment one must check the original diagnostic study models to determine the progress of the tooth movement and the possible slipping of the anchorage. If the anchorage units are displacing, immediate changes must be undertaken. Some modifications include the following:

1. Decreasing or eliminating the forces (Often the anchor teeth will return to their original

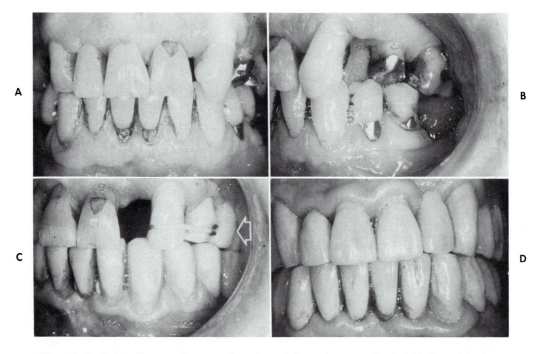

Fig. 21-13. A, Maxillary canine was tipped mesially and encroached within lateral incisor space. **B,** Note severe tipping of canine and nonparallelism of future abutments. **C,** Premolar and molar were splinted, with a gold band and an acrylic provisional splint now acting as anchor unit. Hooks were embedded with quick-cure acrylic in buccal surface, a 4 mm (³/₁₆ inch) elastic was used to retract the canine, and a mesial groove was placed to prevent elastic from slipping. **D,** After tooth movement and completion of periodontal therapy a full maxillary splint was completed. (Courtesy Leonard Abrams, University of Pennsylvania.)

positions; if they do not, the anchor teeth in turn must be moved)
2. Adding teeth to the existing anchor units by ligation or banding, using opposing arch for anchorage (Figs. 21-28 and 21-35)
3. Modifying the appliance design by adding clasps and rests
4. Constructing a new and more stable appliance
5. Relining an old appliance with cold-cure acrylic directly in the mouth can increase its stability

6. Overlaying quick-curing acrylic on the occlusal surfaces
7. Using an Adam's clasp rather than the conventional ring clasp will markedly increase the stability where molar teeth lack good undercut areas (Figs. 21-15 and 21-19)

APPLIANCES

The two classes of tooth movement appliances are the removable and the fixed. The removable appliance can be taken out by the patient for plaque removal and placement of elastics. However, the

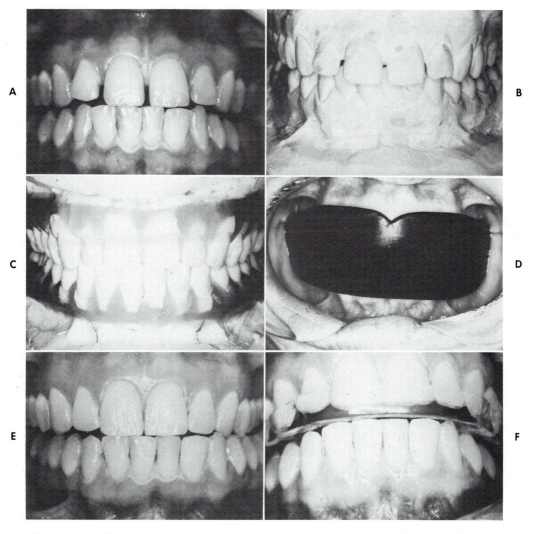

Fig. 21-14. A, Patient required a fixed multibanded technique for optimal tooth positioning, but this was unacceptable. **B,** Study models were mounted on an articulator. **C,** Teeth were cut from stone models and repositioned in wax. From this setup a tooth positioner was fabricated. **D,** Positioner was adjusted in mouth. It was worn only at night for 8 hours and ½ hour three times daily for exercising. After 8 months of tooth movement it was worn as a retainer. **E,** Tooth movement and occlusal adjustment completed. **F,** Maxillary night guard was finally made for retention. (Courtesy George Coslet, Jerome Sklaroff, and Garry Miller, University of Pennsylvania.)

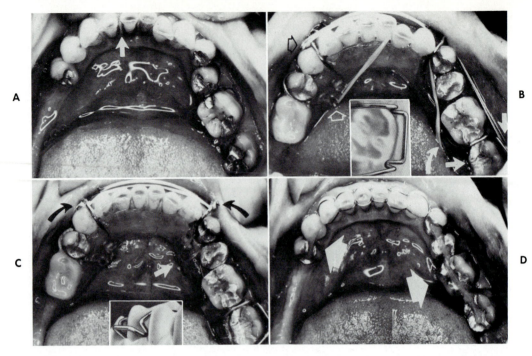

Fig. 21-15. A, Incisors overlapped, with open contact *(arrow)*. Mandibular left premolar is in buccoversion. A full mandibular splint was indicated because of advanced secondary trauma. **B,** Mandibular Hawley appliance was constructed with an Adam's clasp (insert) on second molar for increased stability. Hooks and cleats *(arrows)* were placed for retaining elastics. A 7 mm (5/16 inch) elastic aligned incisors and moved first premolar lingually. **C,** An 18 mm (3/4 inch) light elastic from soldered hooks lingually retracted incisors. **D,** Retention was achieved by **A** splinting posterior teeth *(arrows)* and wire ligating anteriors. (Restorative dentistry in conjunction with Joseph Wolfson, Trenton, N.J.; **B** and **C** inserts courtesy Rocky Mountain Dental Products Co., Denver.)

fixed appliance is not removable by the patient, since the bands are cemented or brackets are bonded directly to the teeth and connected with an arch wire.

Removable appliances

Removable appliances consist of an acrylic base, clasps on the anchor teeth, and generally a labial bow, depending on the movement desired. Most are modifications of the original Hawley (1919) retainer. The acrylic is preferably of the clear type in order for the operator to see the tails of the clasps and springs when removing acrylic and checking for their possible interference. Clear acrylic also allows one to see the tissue blanch if a pressure area exists beneath the acrylic appliance.

For the patient's comfort the acrylic must be kept thin and highly polished, with no blunt ends. The usual clasp designs include the Adam's clasp (Fig. 21-19), the circumferential or ring clasp (Fig. 21-32), the T or J clasp (Figs. 21-24 and 21-54), and the interproximal ball clasp (Fig. 21-45). The clasp wire is generally round stainless steel, 0.8 or 0.9 mm (0.032 or 0.036 inch) in diameter for rigidity. Rests of 0.62 or 0.75 mm (0.025 or 0.030 inch) are used on occlusal surfaces to prevent further tooth extrusion during therapy (Fig. 21-19). Rests are also designed for mandibular removable appliances to keep them tooth borne rather than tissue supported when possible. In selected cases hopeless teeth are retained during the tooth movement phase for appliance retention and then extracted after completion of tooth movement.

The precise placement of the acrylic and wires should be indicated on an accurate stone model. The mesiodistal measurement of the canine loop formed from the Hawley labial bow is drawn half the width of the canine. This allows for either shortening or lengthening of the arch width from canine to canine. The apical curve should not extend beyond the free gingival area, since a long loop apicocoronally does not add any versatility

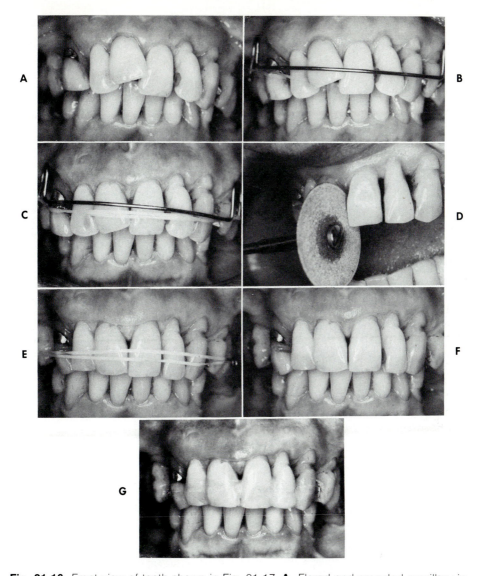

Fig. 21-16. Front view of teeth shown in Fig. 21-17. **A,** Flared and crowded maxillary incisors. **B,** Continuous Hawley appliance with loops at premolar areas. Note 7 mm ($5/16$ inch) heavy elastic moving right lateral incisor and canine distally. **C,** Now central incisors are being retracted palatally. **D,** Stripping creates additional space to facilitate movement. These teeth had thick enamel caps. **E,** From hooks embedded in **A** splints an 18 mm ($3/4$ inch) light elastic retracts incisors palatally. **F,** Tooth movement completed. Final movement can be accomplished with original appliance if it is stable. **G,** Intracoronal **A** splint stabilization. (From Marks, M. H., and Corn, H.: Dent. Clin. North Am. **13:**229, 1969.)

to its adjustment and can interfere with the mucobaccal fold. This is a common error in appliance design for the beginner. The labial arch wire should lie in the middle third of the anterior teeth, contacting the maximum number of labial surfaces when no labial movement is planned. Placement at the gingival third has the potential for elongation, whereas placement at the incisal third has the potential for tipping and intrusion. Clasp design must not interfere with occlusion. When a

wire crosses occlusal surfaces, the opposing model will indicate the optimal opening between contacting teeth.

The labial bow serves several purposes other than for tooth movement:

1. A guide to determine amount of movement from one appointment to the next. One can see space that develops and then determine the amount of movement (Figs. 21-16 and 21-17).

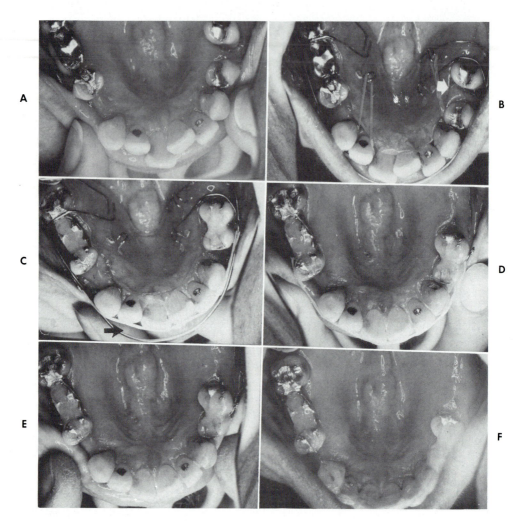

Fig. 21-17. Palatal mirrow view. **A,** Flared and crowded maxillary incisors. Note open contact between maxillary left premolars. **B,** Continuous Hawley appliance with palatal cleats and elastics to move right lateral incisor, canine, and left first premolar distally. Note open contact between left premolars *(arrow).* **C,** Posterior segments are splinted and an 18 mm (¾ inch) light elastic produces palatal movement of incisors and condenses arch. Some enamel stripping has been done to facilitate movement. Note space existing between incisors and labial arch wire indicating degree of palatal retraction *(arrow).* **D,** Hooks were placed into posterior **A** splints to complete incisor retraction. As an alternative this can be completed with original appliance if it is stable. **E,** Tooth movement is completed (compare with **A**). **F,** Stabilization by means of intracoronal **A** splinting. Wire ligation or provisional splints are alternatives. (From Marks, M. H., and Corn, H.: Dent. Clin. North Am. **13:**229, 1969.)

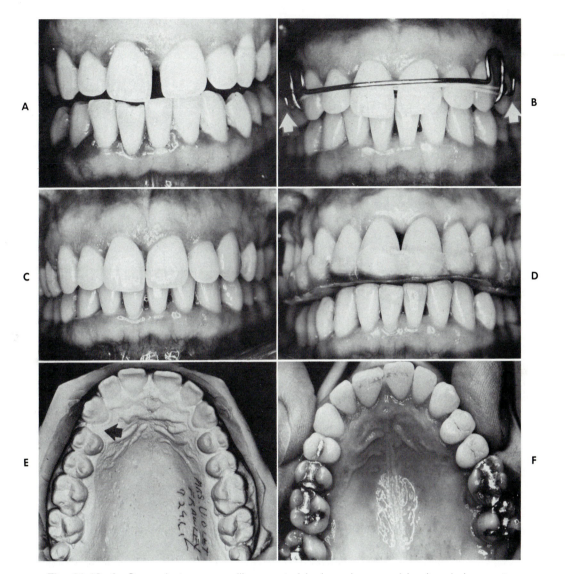

Fig. 21-18. A, Space between maxillary central incisors increased in size during past several years. Infrabony defect is present on mesial of right central incisor. **B,** After scaling, root planing, curettage, and instruction of plaque control, a maxillary Hawley appliance was made. Note distal hooks soldered to canine loops *(arrows)* from which elastics are placed to retract anterior teeth. In this case labial wire is used as a guide to determine amount of movement between visits and finally as a retainer after movement is completed. Only elastics move teeth. **C,** Tooth movement is completed after 3 months. Appliance was modified as a retainer and worn for 6 months during which occlusal adjustment was completed. **D,** Maxillary night guard was then made. **E** and **F,** Occlusal views, before and after movement. All anterior spaces closed including space between right canine and first premolar. Only proper wire placement will allow for space closure. (In conjunction with Herman Corn, Levittown, Pa.)

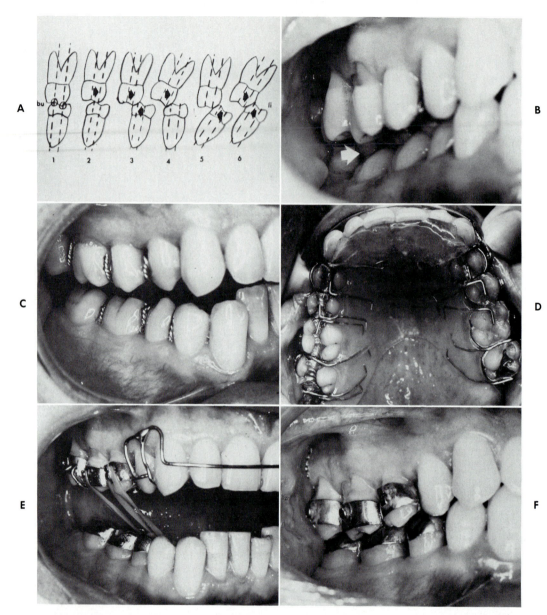

Fig. 21-19. A *1,* Proper occlusal landmark positioning of bucco-occlusal and linguo-occlusal line angles in their respective central fossa line areas. **A** *2,* Small discrepancy of landmark positions and, as a matter of convenience, maxillary tooth is moved. This frequently is observed when examining mandible in intercuspal position and then in retruded contact position. **A** *3,* Full crossbite, and axial positions indicate movement of upper and lower teeth simultaneously. **A** *4,* Maxillary tooth movement. **A** *5,* Mandibular tooth movement because of axial positions. **A** *6,* Movement of teeth in both arches, since both have poor axial positions. **B,** Crossbite is present similar to **A** *5.* **C,** Brass ligature separatures used 3 days prior to banding to gain sufficient space to place multiple bands. **D,** Maxillary Hawley with anterior bite platform is placed to disarticulate posterior teeth during movement. Multiple rests will prevent maxillary teeth from extruding and keep them in their positions while mandibular teeth move. **E,** Crossbite elastics used in conjunction with bite plane. **F,** Crossbite corrected, occlusion adjusted to gain maximum contacts of posterior teeth in retruded contact position, and bite plane discontinued. Interdigitation will prevent crossbite correction from relapsing. (**A** modified from Geiger, A., and Hirschfeld, L.: Minor tooth movement in general practice, ed. 3, St. Louis, 1974, The C. V. Mosby Co., p. 46.)

2. After teeth are moved with an elastic, which gives a light continuous force, the Hawley wire can be shortened by adjusting the canine loops to allow the wire to contact the labial surfaces and act as a retainer (Figs. 21-18 and 21-35).

3. In a Hawley appliance with an incisal bite plane, the Hawley bow acts as a clasp, helping to retain the appliance (Fig. 21-19).

The indications for the Hawley retainer with an anterior bite platform are as follows:

1. Disarticulating the posterior teeth, allowing for noninterference of posterior tooth movement such as crossbite correction (Fig. 21-19) or uprighting (Fig. 21-44)

2. Disarticulating the posterior occlusion in patients with temporomandibular joint syndrome (myofacial pain), allowing the muscles to function without restraint from tooth-to-tooth contacts (Fig. 21-20)

3. Decreasing the anterior deep overbite, allowing for posterior eruption (Figs. 21-40 and 21-42)

4. Determining the comfortable occlusal vertical dimension in a patient with posterior bite collapse (Figs. 21-35 and 21-40)

5. Disarticulating the posterior teeth where the mandibular first premolars would contact the Hawley wire as it passed between the maxillary canine and the first premolar

The design of the labial bow and clasps of the Hawley bite plane should allow for the eventual removal of the acrylic platform, with the continual wearing of the appliance without occlusal interferences. It is often best to taper the wearing of an appliance prior to its complete removal. This may be done over several days or weeks by wearing nightly, every other night, and so on.

Fixed appliances

Fixed appliances are selected when optimal control and bodily movement are imperative for movement in a mesiodistal direction. The bands are made of stainless steel with welded or soldered attachments. The usual band material thickness is 0.07 mm (0.003 inch) for anterior teeth, 0.1 mm (0.004 inch) for premolars, and 0.12 mm (0.005 inch) for molars. If the contact points are tight,

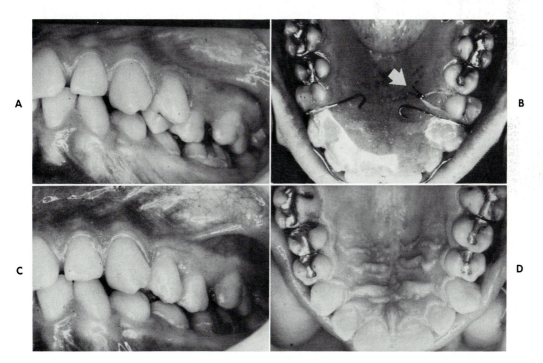

Fig. 21-20. A, A 17-year-old-girl exhibited right temporomandibular joint syndrome in conjunction with a left maxillary first premolar in buccal crossbite. **B,** Hawley bite plane was inserted to disarticulate posterior occlusion, resulting in elimination of pain and allowing for crossbite correction. Note palatal cleat *(arrow)* retaining a 4 mm (³/₁₆ inch) heavy elastic and moving premolar palatally. **C,** Crossbite is corrected, and joint pain has ceased. **D,** Corrected premolar (palatal mirror view). (In conjunction with Jacob Salzman, University of Pennsylvania.)

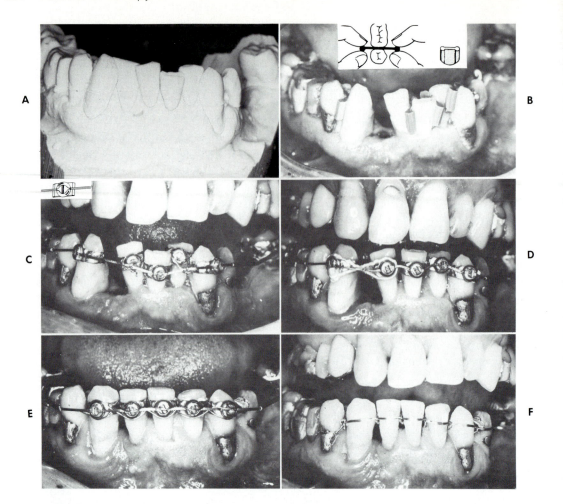

Fig. 21-21. A, Crowded mandibular incisors. Complete periodontal prosthesis was indicated because of secondary trauma. Mandibular right lateral incisor was hopeless, and its removal was planned to gain available space to realign remaining incisors. **B,** Hopeless incisor was removed, and rubber maxian separators were placed 3 days prior to making bands. **C,** Johnson twin arch appliance was selected to effect bodily movement. **D,** After 3 months incisors are leveling and rounding out. **E,** Tooth movement is completed after 6 months, and a rectangular arch is used for stabilization and retention with a figure 8 wire ligature tie. **F,** Bands are removed, and anteriors are wire ligated for completion of periodontal therapy. (In conjunction with Herman Corn, Levittown, Pa., and Herman L. Press, Fairless Hills, Pa.; **B** and **C** inserts courtesy Rocky Mountain Dental Products Co., Denver.)

separation must be planned several days prior to band construction and cementation. Separation can be accomplished with brass ligature (Fig. 21-19), rubber separators (Fig. 21-21), or various metal clips. The sizes of the arch wires vary with the techniques and stages of movement.

Advantages and disadvantages of each appliance

I. Removable appliances
  A. Advantages
    1. Ease of construction and repair
    2. Removable for plaque control
    3. Removable by patient if discomfort is excessive
    4. Minimally unaesthetic
    5. Greater ease of buccolingual movement
    6. Tipping and elongating the clinical crown that can be shortened to improve the crown-root ratio
  B. Disadvantages
    1. Necessity of relying on patient to wear as prescribed
    2. Bulky; can interfere with speech and function
    3. Rarely achieve bodily tooth movement
II. Fixed appliances
  A. Advantages
    1. Ease of construction and repair

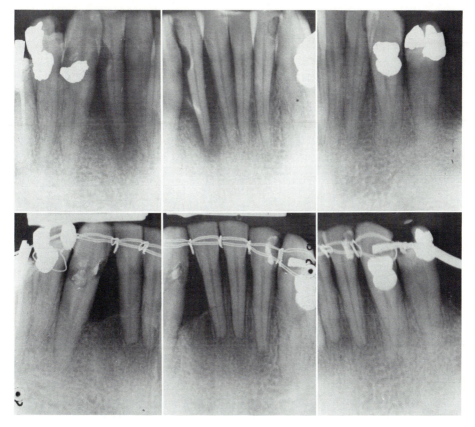

Fig. 21-22. Before and after tooth movement of patient in Fig. 21-21.

2. Controlled bodily movement
3. Slight bulk, with little interference of function
4. Necessity for patient cooperation minimized

B. Disadvantages
  1. Favor plaque retention; personal oral hygiene difficult
  2. Unaesthetic with anterior brackets
  3. Patient discomfort relieved primarily by dentist
  4. Difficult to effect slight movement in buccolingual direction.

In certain instances the placement of orthodontic bands with attachments and pressure exerting mechanisms such as elastic ligatures will eliminate the need of a removable appliance and the patient's active part in the tooth movement. With some adult patients the best designed removable appliance is rejected completely or is worn only intermittently. This would indicate the use of fixed appliances under maximum control of the operator (Fig. 21-22).

ACTIVATING MECHANISMS AND ATTACHMENTS

The activating mechanisms or attachments can be embedded in the acrylic by means of a retentive tail, or they can be soldered or welded to the fixed appliance (Hirschfeld and Geiger, 1966). Available methods for anchoring activating mechanisms are as follows:

1. Removable acrylic-and-wire appliances, which are usually modifications of the Hawley retainer (Figs. 21-7, 21-8, 21-9, 21-15, 21-16, 21-18, 21-20, 21-24, 21-25, 21-27, 21-32, 21-40, and 21-47)
2. Wire ligation (Fig. 21-33)
3. Orthodontic bands with steel ligature, elastic ligature, or elastic (Figs. 21-4, 21-19, and 21-28)
4. Orthodontic bands with arch wires (Figs. 21-1, 21-10, 21-11, 21-21, 21-34, 21-35, 21-38, 21-41, and 21-43)
5. Existing removable partial denture (Figs. 21-12 and 21-25)
6. Existing fixed bridge (Fig. 21-13)
7. Hooks and ties to acrylic provisional splints (Fig. 21-13)
8. Hooks and ties to acrylic-and-wire A splints
9. Rubber tooth positioner (Fig. 21-14)
10. Other appliances, for example, Schwarz

plate, Nord expansion plate, Crozat removable appliance, split plate, and many other variations

Springs. Metals, within their elastic limit, tend to resist distortion and return to their passive state. Spring shapes may be straight (Fig. 21-24), recurved (Figs. 21-7 and 21-23), helically looped (Fig. 21-45), recurved with a helical loop (Fig. 21-41), J or T shaped (Figs. 21-9 and 21-24), or open (Fig. 21-25); or there may be variations of these, depending on the therapist's imagina-tion. They are constructed of 0.55 or 0.62 mm (0.022 or 0.025 inch) diameter stainless steel round wire or 0.55 mm (0.022 inch) diameter gold spring wire. The thinner and longer the action arm of the spring, the lighter and more prolonged the net pressure. Generally springs should be dis-placed 1 to 3 mm when the appliance is inserted.

There are several wire-bending and utility pliers (Fig. 21-59), including the no. 139 angle wire-bending plier, the no. 201 clasp-adjusting plier, the no. 110 How plier, and the no. 74 Young

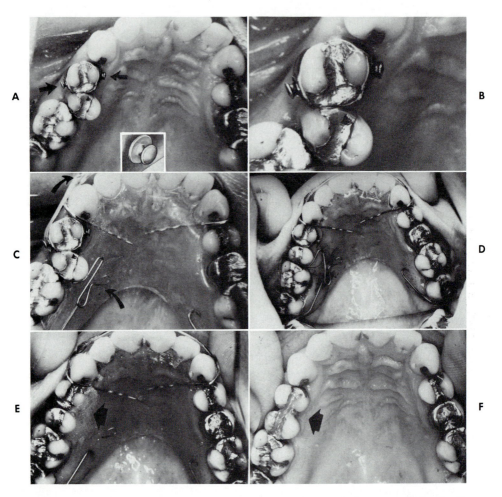

Fig. 21-23. A, Second premolar in linguoversion and first premolar rotated distally. Cor-rection of rotation required banding first premolars with welded buttons on midbuccal and lingual surfaces. **B,** Closeup view of tooth malposition. **C,** Maxillary Hawley appliance was inserted, and hook was soldered on labial wire to hold buccal elastic for rotation. A 0.55 mm (0.022 inch) recurved gold spring wire was embedded in acrylic for buccal pressure on second premolar. **D,** First premolar is rotated in position, and second premolar is in good buccal alignment. **E,** Recurved spring was removed, and quick-cure acrylic was added for retention. **F,** A wire-and-acrylic **A** splint is placed into class II amalgams for sta-bility. (In conjunction with Herman Corn, Levittown, Pa.; **A** insert courtesy Rocky Mountain Dental Products Co., Denver.)

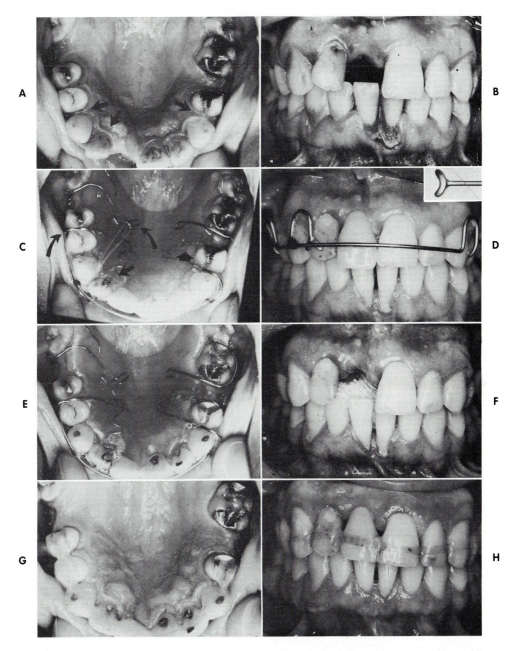

Fig. 21-24. A, Open contacts between first premolars and canines. Note rotated lateral incisor (palatal mirrow view). **B,** Front view. Note rotated lateral incisor. **C,** Maxillary Hawley appliance replaces missing central incisor. Palatal cleat and soldered buccal hook retain a 7 mm ($^5/_{16}$ inch) light elastic to move canine distally for space closure. Mesial ring clasp is around each molar. Helical spring is used for mesial movement of first premolar. Straight spring with a looped end for pressure on mesiolingual corner of lateral incisor is used for rotation. **D,** T spring is soldered to labial wire for pressure on distolabial corner of lateral incisor to effect rotation. **E** and **F,** Tooth movement completed. **G** and **H,** A splint was placed from premolar to premolar, replacing missing central incisor. (In conjunction with Herman Corn, Levittown, Pa., and Joseph Wolfson, Trenton, N.J.; **D** insert courtesy Rocky Mountain Dental Products Co., Denver.)

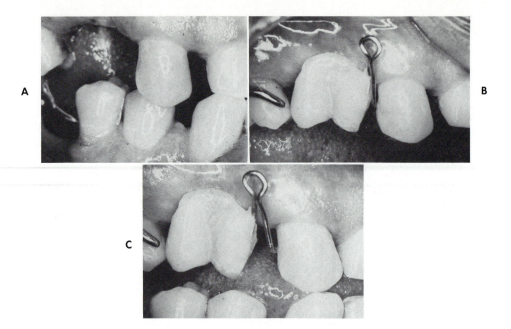

Fig. 21-25. A, Maxillary canine was indicated for mesial movement to reduce interproximal infrabony defect and to enlarge edentulous space for two premolar pontics. **B,** Opening loop cured into old partial denture for canine movement. **C,** Canine in position. A new partial denture was eventually made. (Courtesy Garry Miller, University of Pennsylvania.)

loop-bending plier. The experienced operator bends most wires with his fingers, using the pliers for holding the wire. Nicks or sharp bends, which weaken the wire, are to be avoided.

Elastic ligature thread. Elastic ligature thread is used for separation, retractions, extrusions, rotations, and small space closures. There are two types. One consists of tightly wound, moisture resistant nylon and rubber. It resists breakdown and continues to function without replacement for 2 to 4 weeks. The other is a silk elastic ligature that contracts by shrinkage after being moistened.

The elasticized thread is made in light, medium, and heavy strengths for use on anteriors, premolars, and molars, respectively. Its action is similar to that of rubber dam elastics, since the force is constant. However, it does not require the dexterity of the patient, since it is tied in place and not used with removable appliances (Fig. 21-33).

Rubber dam elastics. Rubber dam elastics are fabricated from tubes of latex and are cut of uniform wall thickness to provide a predictable pressure from one batch to another (Fig. 21-26). Sizes vary from 3 mm (⅛ inch) to 18 mm (¾ inch) (Fig. 21-27), and wall sizes are light, medium, and heavy. A pressure of 90 to 180 g (3 to 6 oz) can be measured by the Dontrix stress and tension gauge (Fig. 21-37). Their action depends on the elastic return to the undeformed state.

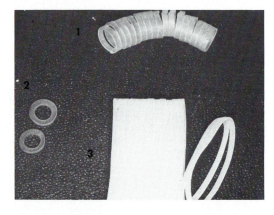

Fig. 21-26. *1,* Rubber dam elastic, 4 mm (³/₁₆ inch) heavy; *2,* rubber bands, no. 2 regular; *3,* rubber dam elastic, 18 mm (³/₄ inch) light.

Rubber bands. Rubber bands are made from heavier rubber than are the rubber dam elastics, and they are used more commonly for intermaxillary pressures during correction of class II and III malocclusions and crossbites. For crossbites they are often used in a triangular fashion when reciprocal movement is not desired and the anchor unit must be increased (Figs. 21-28 and 21-29). They are removed during meals and plaque control and are changed four times daily—after each meal and at bedtime (Fig. 21-19).

Cleats and loops. Cleats and loops are small hooks that are embedded in the acrylic of remov-

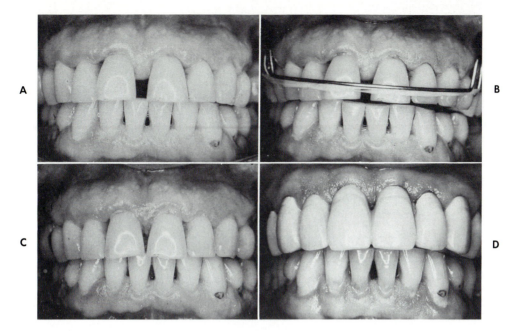

Fig. 21-27. A, Flared maxillary incisors, producing large diastema between central incisors with sufficient interarch and intra-arch space. **B,** Maxillary Hawley appliance with distal hooks soldered on labial bow for retaining an 18 mm (¾ inch) light elastic. **C,** Tooth movement completed. Retention was accomplished by A splinting. **D,** Periodontal prosthesis was planned after periodontal therapy. (In conjunction with Herman Corn, Levittown, Pa., and Stanley Lipkowitz, Fairless Hills, Pa.)

able appliances (Figs. 21-20, 21-24, and 21-30), or they are embedded in provisional splints soldered to metal bands and wires (Fig. 21-31). Their function is to anchor one end of the elastic while the other end encircles the tooth or the attachment on a banded tooth. With the Hawley-type appliance optimal placement and stretching of the elastic are obtained when the cleats are embedded halfway between the tooth and the midline of the palate. Elastic placement can be facilitated by placing dental floss through the center of the elastic, thereby adding a handle for stretching the elastic around the tooth. The smaller 4 mm (³/₁₆ inch) elastics are difficult initially to grasp with the fingers.

Expansion screws. The expansion screws are available in various types and dimensions (Schwartz and Giatzinger, 1966). They are useful for single or sectional correction of posterior crossbites. They are also used for distally driving maxillary molars small distances when a premolar is locked palatally. They are small and flat in overall dimension. Each turn of the guide pin 360 degrees results in 0.8 to 0.9 mm opening or expansion (Fig. 21-32). Three or four turns are planned every 1 to 2 weeks.

The palatal or lingual cleats are made of small stainless steel round wire of 0.5 or 0.55 mm

(0.020 or 0.022 inch) diameter. The cleats are difficult to bend if they are made of larger diameter wire. They can be manufactured and stored in advance to be quickly cured in the acrylic appliance as needed. If the tongue becomes irritated by the cleat a small piece of carding wax can be placed over the exposed end to produce a smooth surface.

Many variations of hooks and loops are manufactured for soldering and welding to bands and arches.

Stainless steel ligature. Dead soft 0.25 mm (0.010 inch) diameter ligature wire is used to ligate anchor teeth. Slight anterior open contacts can be closed by anterior wire ligation. In turn, the ligated anterior segment can be used as an anchor unit to move distally drifted premolars with elastic ligature (Fig. 21-33). The premolars can then be retained by wire ligation to the anterior teeth. Often a polished groove placed on the distal surface will prevent wire displacement on bell-shaped teeth as premolars (Fig. 21-4, *G*). The anterior teeth, with their lingual concavities, lend themselves readily to retention of wire ligation, whereas the posterior teeth, with their convexities, interfere with the stability of extracoronal wiring.

With fixed arches teeth can be rotated or moved to the main arch by wire ligating. The arch is

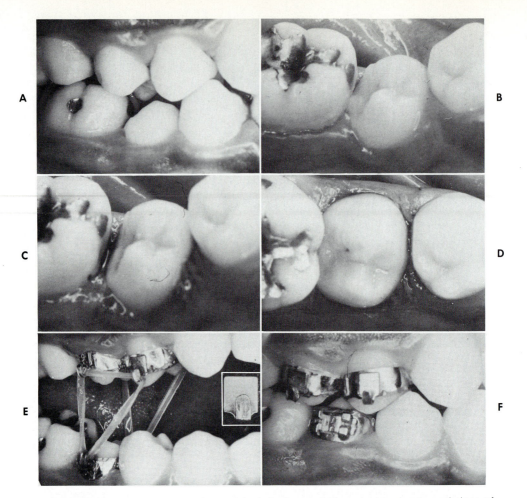

Fig. 21-28. A, Mandibular second premolar is locked out of occlusion due to early loss of second deciduous molar, resulting in mesial drift of first permanent molar prior to eruption of premolar. B, Locked out premolar (lingual mirror view). C, Stripping was performed on mesial surface of first molar and on distal surface of premolar (lingual mirror view). D, Stripping was also performed on mesial surface of second premolar and distal surface of first premolar (lingual mirror view). E, Stainless steel bands with hooks (insert) were welded on buccal and lingual surfaces. Triangular elastics increase maxillary anchorage. Note that elastics are exerting force both buccally and lingually. F, Edgewise bracket was welded on mandibular band for a wider horizontal elastic purchase. (In conjunction with Garry Miller, University of Pennsylvania; E insert courtesy Rocky Mountain Dental Products Co., Denver.)

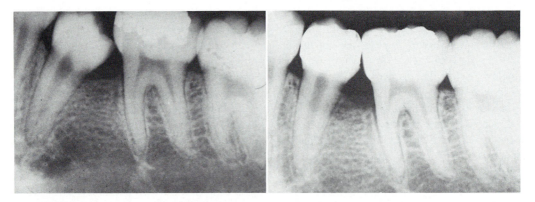

Fig. 21-29. Before and after tooth movement in Fig. 21-28. Note leveling of cementoenamel junctions. Thick enamel cap permitted adequate stripping to gain available space for tooth movement.

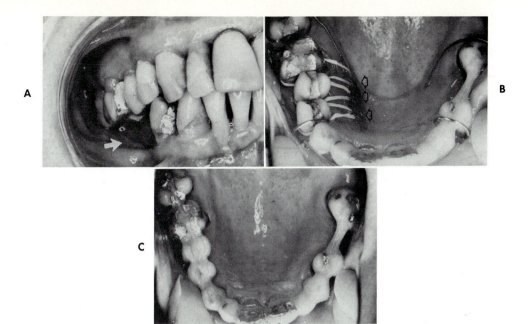

Fig. 21-30. Lingual cusps of maxillary second premolar and molars are buccal to crest of mandibular edentulous ridge. **A,** Premolars and molars were indicated for palatal movement for proper landmark positioning with future prosthetic appliance. **B,** Maxillary Hawley appliance with palatal cleats held 4 mm (³/₁₆ inch) heavy elastics for palatal movement. Two premolars and first molar were repositioned and then **A** splinted before second molar was moved palatally, using last cleat. **C,** Retention was obtained after tooth movement with a full maxillary **A** splint. Periodontal prosthesis was planned after periodontal therapy was completed. (In conjunction with Herman Corn, Levittown, Pa., and Stanley Lipkowitz, Fairless Hills, Pa.)

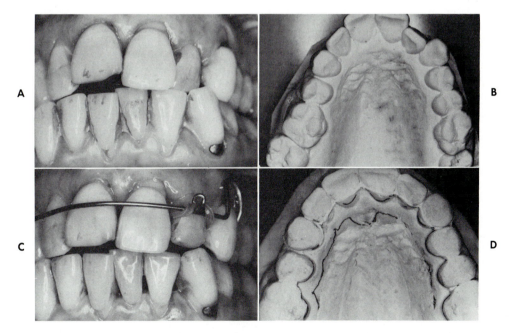

Fig. 21-31. A, Result of 2 years of major orthodontic therapy 6 years prior to initiating periodontal therapy. Patient rejected retreatment by orthodontist for present relapse. Occlusal adjustment was impossible with left maxillary lateral incisor in lingual crossbite. **B,** Occlusal view of original study model, showing lingual crossbite. **C,** Maxillary Hawley appliance with soldered hook was used to move lateral incisor labially with a 4 mm (³/₁₆ inch) light elastic prior to initiating occlusal adjustment. **D,** Occlusal view of night guard model, showing lateral incisor in position. (In conjunction with Herman Corn, Levittown, Pa., and Joseph Wolfson, Trenton, N.J.)

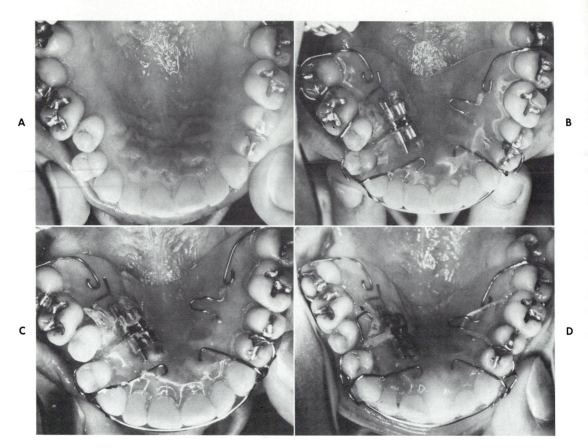

Fig. 21-32. A, Maxillary right second premolar is locked palatally with insufficient space for repositioning. **B,** Maxillary right third molar has been extracted. Opening screw placed in anteroposterior position will move second premolar and molars distally a small distance. Screw is opened 3- or 4-quarter turns weekly. Remaining body of appliance is anchored by teeth and palatal tissues. **C,** After sufficient space is created, a recurved spring beneath appliance is activated to move second premolar buccally. **J** spring has moved first premolar palatally several millimeters. **D,** Final tooth position. Note appliance was connected by quick-cure acrylic after distal movement was sufficient. Appliance now serves as a retainer until occlusal adjustment is completed. (In conjunction with Herman Corn, Levittown, Pa.)

slightly distorted, and its return to the passive state produces the desired movement.

Coil springs. Open or closed coil springs are used on fixed arches to move teeth bodily (Figs. 21-34 and 21-47). Open coil springs are frequently used to drive teeth distally, with the anchor unit being all of the banded or bracketed teeth attached to the arch wire anteriorly. Often the anchorage must be backed up by the use of intermaxillary elastic, bringing in the opposite arch for increased stability. Careful measurement of the elastic force and the open coil spring must produce a net distal molar movement and must avoid anterior slippage of the anchor segments (Fig. 21-35).

Acrylic platforms. The anterior incisal platform incorporated into the Hawley appliance disarticulates the posterior segments and encourages erup-

tion of the posterior teeth. The anteroposterior width of the platform should be kept about 1 mm lingual to the contact of the mandibular incisors in centric relation. Its thickness should allow up to 1 mm posterior opening, and all the mandibular incisors should uniformly contact the plane when possible in all excursions (Figs. 21-40 and 21-42).

The posterior bite platform is used to depress posterior teeth or to produce sufficient opening anteriorly for correction of anterior crossbites (Fig. 21-7).

FORCE APPLICATION DURING TOOTH MOVEMENT

Histologic changes. With gentle forces the periodontal ligament is compressed on the pressure side but remains vital. The bone reveals frontal

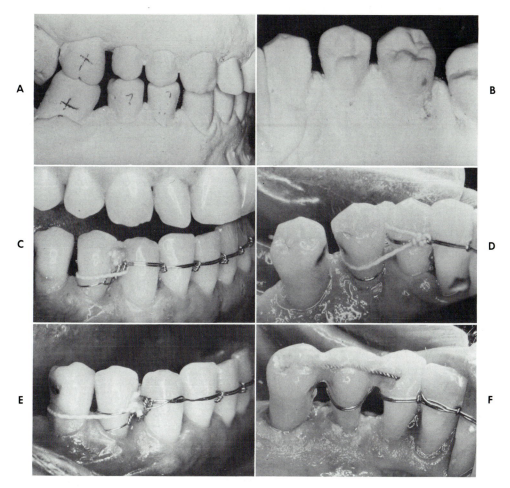

Fig. 21-33. A, Distal drifting of mandibular premolars due to loss of mandibular first molar. **B,** Lingual view on study model. **C,** Wire ligation of mandibular anterior teeth to act as anchor unit. Light elastic ligature tied around first premolar for mesial movement. **D,** Tied elastic ligature (lingual mirror view). **E,** Elastic ligature ties around second premolar for mesial movement. **F,** Premolars and canine were A splinted for stability. (In conjunction with Herman Corn, Levittown, Pa.)

and rear resorption by osteoclasts in Howship's lacunae. On the tension side there is a stretching of the fibers, initiating new bone formation.

If the forces are excessive, the periodontal ligament on the pressure side is crushed, resulting in hemorrhage and thrombosis with necrosis of the tissue. These changes are similar to those of occlusal trauma. No frontal resorption occurs, since the cells of the periodontal ligament are destroyed, and rear resorption from within the marrow spaces must occur. These changes take much longer, and therefore the movement is much slower. The tension side exhibits a tearing of the fibers and hemorrhage (Fig. 21-36).

With this brief histologic description in mind one can understand that relatively light forces in adults are required for optimal tooth movement. There is a tendency for the inexperienced prac-

titioner automatically to increase the force application if tooth movement is not occurring. However, the force may have been excessive initially, and the pressure should be *decreased* rather than increased to avoid crushing the periodontal ligament on the pressure side.

Rate of movement. The rate of movement is related to the reactivity of the bone and varies with individual teeth. Movement of 1 mm per month is considered satisfactory (Reitan, 1953), although teeth in secondary trauma may move a greater distance due to the excessive bone loss and the lack of resistance to movement. The amount of movement should be noted at each visit by checking the original study models.

Magnitude of forces. When possible, the force placed on a tooth should be measured. It must be reemphasized that light, not heavy, forces are the most effective and least traumatic to the supporting apparatus (Fig. 21-37).

Light force—60 to 120 g (2 to 4 oz) (Fig. 21-37)
Medium force—120 to 180 g (4 to 6 oz)
Heavy force—over 180 g (over 6 oz)

In theory the force is on a unit area of the periodontal ligament and bone and is not the absolute force applied in ounces or grams. A multirooted tooth will require more force than will a single-rooted tooth or one with marked bone loss. In contrast to tipping, more force is needed to move a

tooth bodily, since a larger area of the periodontium receives the pressure. With these principles in mind one can then intelligently select the correct magnitude of force for the specific requirement.

Force application. Moyers (1973) has described force application as continuous and intermittent. Continuous force is maintained at a near constant level with elastics and springs. Some auxiliary springs may diminish in their force as the tooth moves. Reitan (1947) has described the decelerating continuous force. In this instance a

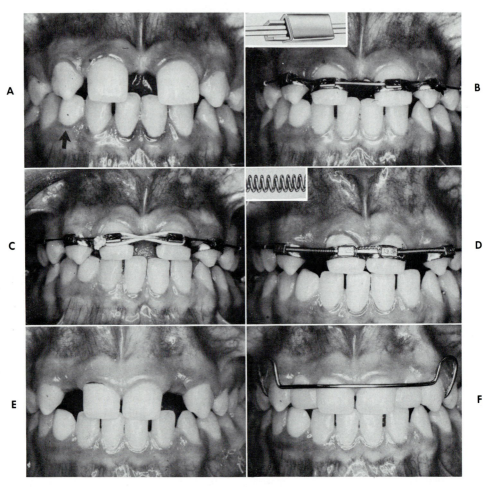

Fig. 21-34. **A,** Congenitally missing maxillary lateral incisors. Note retained mandibular deciduous canine. Aesthetics was prime consideration for tooth movement in this instance. Since bodily movement was required to bring central incisors together, fixed appliance therapy was indicated. **B,** Johnson twin arch appliance was used with Johnson brackets and caps (insert). **C,** Central incisors were moved reciprocally with light elastic ligature. **D,** Canines were moved distally with open coil springs to close open contacts between canines and first premolars. **E,** Tooth movement completed. Note remaining space between incisors from double thickness 0.07 mm (0.003 inch) band material. **F,** Hawley retainer with lateral pontics to be worn until an anterior bridge is made. (In conjunction with Soona Jahina, University of Pennsylvania; **B** and **D** inserts courtesy Rocky Mountain Dental Products Co., Denver.)

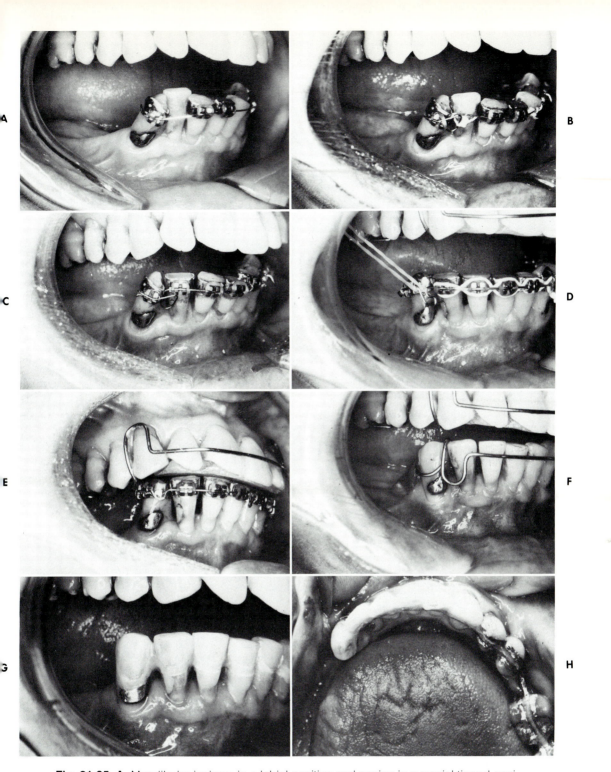

Fig. 21-35. A, Mandibular incisors in a labial position and canine in a mesial tipped position. Initial fixed appliance therapy with 0.014 round stainless steel arch. **B,** Large loop mesial to canine to begin distal movement when activated. **C,** Distal movement has begun for canine, and anterior spacing has permitted banding of remaining anteriors. Because of lack of anchorage in right mandibular quadrant, anteriors have flared slightly with only intra-arch anchorage. **D,** Class III mechanics (elastic running from lower anterior to upper posterior) 7 mm (⁵⁄₁₆ inch) heavy elastic attached to an **L** hook in the 0.016 round stainless steel arch wire retracts entire lower arch lingually and distally. This movement took about 4 months. Figure 8 elastic ligature thread begins to close interproximal spaces during class III retraction. **E,** Lower anterior retraction almost completed. Upper Hawley bite plane used to establish vertical dimension. **F,** Lower Hawley retainer after debanding to retain new tooth position and close residual band spaces. Fixed bridge in lower arch planned initially as final restoration. **G** and **H,** Lower arch stabilized with a cast vitallium bar and acrylic to prevent any relapse.

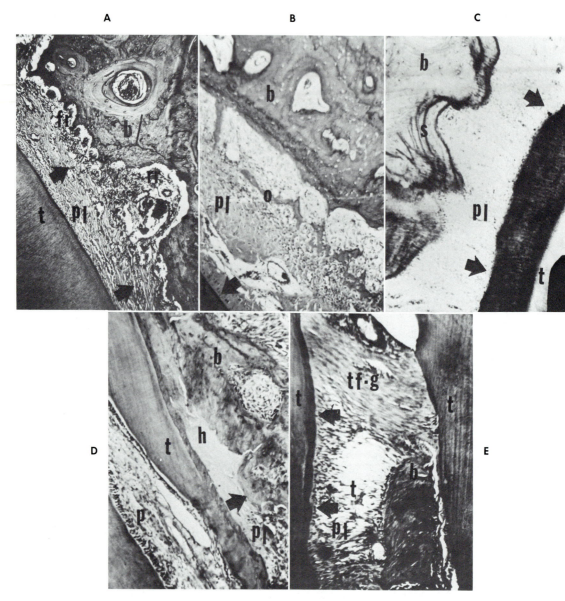

Fig. 21-36. A, Normal pressure side, tooth, *t,* moving toward alveolar bone, *b (arrows).* Frontal resorption, *fr,* occurring within periodontal ligament space, *pl.* Osteoclasts resorbing bone in Howship's lacunae. Rear resorption, *rr,* also occurring with marrow space not broken through to periodontal ligament. Periodontal ligament fibers running parallel to tooth rather than perpendicular. **B,** Normal tension side, tooth moving away from alveolar bone. Periodontal ligament space is widened and new bone, or osteoid, *o,* is forming within periodontal ligament on tension side. **C,** Normal, tension side stained to show striations, *s,* within bone representing increments of bone formation within periodontal ligament on tension side. Arrows show direction tooth is moving. **D,** Excessive force on pressure side resulting in hyalinization of the periodontal ligament. *P* represents pulp and arrow is direction tooth is moving. **E,** Excessive force on tension side resulting in tearing, *t,* of fibers within periodontal ligament. Transseptal fibers of gingival group, *tf-g,* are still intact. (Courtesy D. Walter Cohen, University of Pennsylvania.)

strong force is applied continuously, but its size diminishes rapidly. This occurs when a tooth bracket is ligated to an arch wire. The tooth is moved to the arch wire and is then splinted by it when the force has been dissipated. This mode of force application allows for the reorganization of the tissues between appliance adjustment.

Intermittent force is seen with the inclined plane or incisal bite platform. It may be heavy or light, but its duration is short only when the tooth is brought into contact with the acrylic.

Root resorption. A slight degree of root resorption is not significant if the amount of root surface lost for attachment of the periodontal liga-

ment is small compared to the remaining total square area.

Two types of root resorption can be noted. The first type, microresorption, is confined to the cementum and generally heals by the deposition of new cementum. It is not detectable radiographically. The second type, progressive resorption, involves increasing apical root end resorption and is the result of heavy apical pressure. This root resorption can be seen on x-ray film. A third type, idiopathic root resorption, is not related to tooth movement. Should it be present, it will often progress further with active tooth movement.

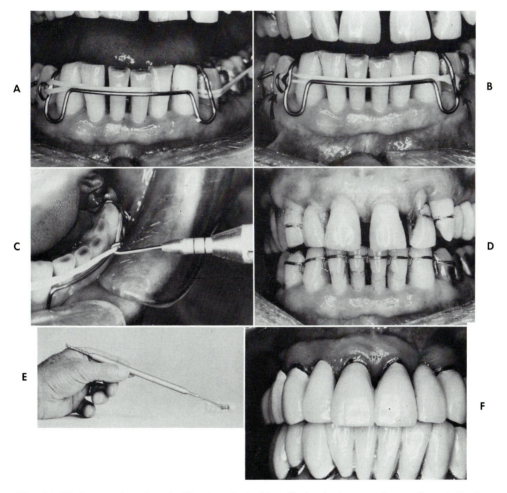

Fig. 21-37. Teeth of patient in Fig. 21-15. **A,** Mandibular incisors to be realigned. **B,** A 9 mm (³/₈ inch) light elastic is held by a welded button and a soldered hook to retract incisors. **C,** Dontrix stress gauge is used to measure force applied in ounces. Each vertical mark represents 28 g (1 oz). Elastic utilized produces 70 to 84 g (2½ to 3 oz) of pressure. This is measured just as elastic is disengaged from tooth. **D,** Mandibular incisors are wire ligated after tooth movement. **E,** Opposite end of Dontrix (held in hand) is used to measure pressure of the springs. **F,** Periodontal prosthesis. (In conjunction with Herman Corn, Levittown, Pa., and Joseph Wolfson, Trenton, N.J.; **E** courtesy Rocky Mountain Dental Products Co., Denver.)

PATIENT MANAGEMENT DURING TOOTH MOVEMENT

Patient orientation. The patient should first understand the indications for repositioning the teeth. The aesthetic considerations and means of retention should be thoroughly discussed to avoid any misunderstanding during this phase of periodontal therapy. The patient must be discouraged from frequently removing the appliance, thereby producing an interrupted or jiggling movement of the teeth. The total treatment plan should be clarified with the patient at the outset, and the restorative commitment for periodontal prosthesis or its contingency should be realized.

Clinical problems and follow-up. The appliance should be passive at the insertion visit, with few exceptions. This allows the patient to become accustomed to the initial discomforts of pressure, aesthetics, and speech. All occlusal interferences and acrylic impingement on the gingiva are removed. The appliance must be worn day and night, but this may be flexible during the first week. It is removed for thorough cleansing after each meal and upon arising. The appliance may be removed during meals. This management nets a total force application of 22 hours daily. The patient soon learns the path of insertion. The appliance is removed by the clasps rather than by the arch wire or springs.

After the patient has adapted to the appliance, the visits are scheduled at 2- to 3-week intervals, depending on the individual requirements. The patient must be seen between scheduled appointments if pain is present from excessive pressure, occlusal prematurities, excessive tooth mobility, or temporomandibular joint syndrome. Any situation that compels the patient to interrupt wearing the appliance should be quickly corrected to avoid patient discouragement. This is one major area where patient management varies markedly between the child and the adult. The ease with which the adult can become discouraged with tooth movement and appliance therapy has resulted in many orthodontists limiting their acceptance of adults.

Pain may not occur until several hours after activation. If the forces are gentle, the discomfort should subside after 1 to 2 days, and thereafter the patient should be relatively comfortable. Pressure on the gingiva or mucosa causes ulceration. Decreasing the force application and relieving the adjacent acrylic will offer relief. The appliance may have to be discontinued for several days if the pain has been severe. Topical anesthetic oint-

ments are useful for tissue ulcerations until healing has occurred after adjustment. The lidocaine (Xylocaine) and Orabase combination has excellent pain-relieving and adhesive qualities.

Tissue changes. The gingiva often becomes inflamed during appliance therapy as a result of plaque retention. When necessary, plaque control procedures may be supplemented with hydrotherapy devices that use a jet or water under pressure to flush out food accumulations. If the acrylic does not intimately contact the tissues and if a space results, debris will collect, and the appliances may be unstable and irritate the tissues. When this situation exists the appliance should be relined with quick-curing acrylic directly in the mouth.

Ligation with stainless steel wire or elastic leads to plaque retention. Ligations can loosen or slip into the gingiva and must be tightened or replaced without delay. Decalcification or caries can result from ligatures or cemented bands.

Hyperplastic tissue prior to or as a result of tooth movement is commonly resolved with curettage and careful oral hygiene. If it persists and inhibits tooth movement, its removal is required.

Gingival recession can result on the labial, buccal, or lingual surfaces from excessive movement which destroys the radicular bone.

X-ray studies are invaluable during and after tooth movement to determine the following:
1. Axial position of roots
2. Possible leveling or eliminating of vertical osseous defects
3. Loss of alveolar interproximal bone
4. Root resorption
5. Thickened periodontal ligament space
6. Loss of lamina dura
7. Cemental tears (unusual)
8. Internal resorption (unusual)

DIRECTIONS OF TOOTH MOVEMENT

Teeth can be moved in all planes of space—mesial, distal, facial (buccal and labial), lingual, palatal, and rotational. Depression and eruption may also occur, and the tooth can move bodily or be tipped, or both.

Movement in a mesial and distal direction can be accomplished with springs, rubber dam elastics, rubber bands, elastic ligature, and stainless steel wire. These activating mechanisms can be used with either fixed or removable appliances. The activating mechanisms should generally be kept coronal to the cingulum to prevent them from sliding gingivally. Well-controlled springs can be placed near the gingival margin and with light force can effect a near bodily movement with minimal tipping. Elastics can be retained with stainless steel ligature or a spur attached to a band if it tends to slide gingivally due to the convergence or divergence of the tooth axis.

Movement in a facial, lingual, or palatal direction is accomplished in a similar fashion as in a mesial or distal direction. In addition, intermaxillary elastics and the Hawley labial wire, are used.

Tongue depressors, inclined planes, and rubber tooth positioners (Fig. 21-14) are effective in children but are rarely tolerated in adults.

Rotational movements can occur around an axis in the center of the tooth or an axis located at one corner. In most instances rotations require bracketing with attachments to effect force in an arc. Pressure in opposite corners with a removable appliance can produce rotation, but good control is minimized (Fig. 21-24).

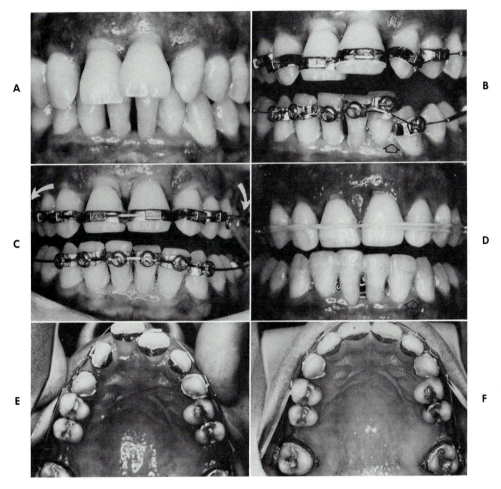

Fig. 21-38. A, Maxillary and mandibular incisors required leveling and rounding out. It was felt that this could best be accomplished with fixed appliance therapy, affording maximum control and anchorage. Johnson fixed appliance was used, and a single wire was placed at initial visit. Note discrepancy of mandibular left lateral incisor and canine. **C,** In 4 months arches were leveled, twin arch in maxilla and ribbon arch in mandible. Class II elastics, upper anterior to lower posterior, were used to retract maxillary incisors *(arrow).* **D,** Movement in mandibular arch completed. Retention was achieved with **A** splinting due to advanced secondary trauma. Note relationship of mandibular lateral incisor and canine in comparison to **B.** Maxillary bands were removed, and residual spaces from band material were closed. Maxillary posterior teeth were **A** splinted, and a brass ligature hook was bent over and under an interproximal space to retain an 18 mm (¾ inch) light elastic for anterior retraction. **E** and **F,** Comparison of initial and 4-month tooth relationships. Maxillary arch was eventually **A** splinted also. (In conjunction with Herman Corn, Levittown, Pa.)

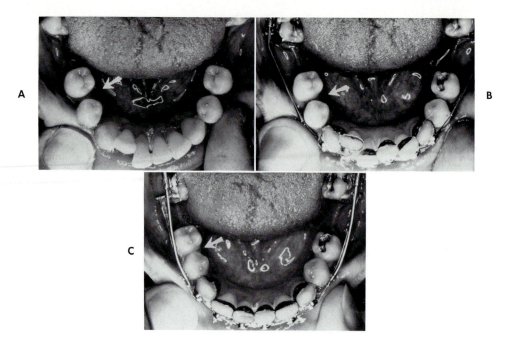

Fig. 21-39. Teeth of patient in Fig. 21-38. Note **A,** before **B,** during, and **C,** after tooth positions. As incisors leveled and rounded out, premolar open contacts closed *(arrows).* Four months' duration.

Depression of teeth is difficult becasue the entire periodontium resists the force. It takes longer than movement in other directions, and the requirements for anchorage are increased. With the acrylic-and-wire bite plane the intermaxillary masticatory pressure potentially depresses the occluding incisors. With multibracketed techniques the intramaxillary arch wire levels the teeth and the cementoenamel junctions if bracket placement is equidistant from the incisal edges (Figs. 21-38 and 21-39). The equal and opposite force has the potential for extruding the anchor molars. Therefore it is essential that careful planning of the anchorage teeth be thorough whether with an acrylic base and clasps or with banded posteriors.

Eruption can be accomplished by elastic ligatures, elastics, bite planes, and fixed arches. One must first determine the cause of the infraversion and then the available space for erupting. Some teeth are locked out of occlusion by the approximating ones, whereas others may be impacted with teeth having drifted into the available spaces. The force must be carefully controlled so as not to extrude the anchor segments or cause pulpal damage from too rapid eruption. The acrylic bite plane allows for eruption of those teeth not in occlusion. The duration of time may vary from 6 to 12 months and frequently longer.

POSTERIOR BITE COLLAPSE AND LOSS OF OCCLUSAL VERTICAL DIMENSION

When posterior teeth have been removed, particularly the first molars, and not replaced, there is a tendency for those teeth adjacent to the edentulous space to tip into it. The shifting of those portions of the teeth that support the posterior occlusion results in loss of occlusal vertical dimension. The mandibular anterior teeth that initially were in light or no contact with the palatal surfaces of the maxillary anterior teeth now contact heavily, resulting in flaring of the maxillary anterior teeth. The open contacts frequently initiate an adult or secondary tongue-thrusting habit, and the mandibular anterior teeth can also flare. The usual sequence of tooth movement is as follows (Figs. 21-40 and 21-42):

1. Retraction of the mandibular incisors, and closing of the open contacts if present.

2. Mandibular incisors are ligated with wire if retraction was necessary or occlusal traumatism was present.

3. A maxillary Hawley appliance with an anterior bite platform is inserted to keep posterior teeth out of occlusion potentiating posterior eruption. Some clinicians feel anterior depression may also occur. The acrylic platform should be flat and allow complete freedom of movement in all

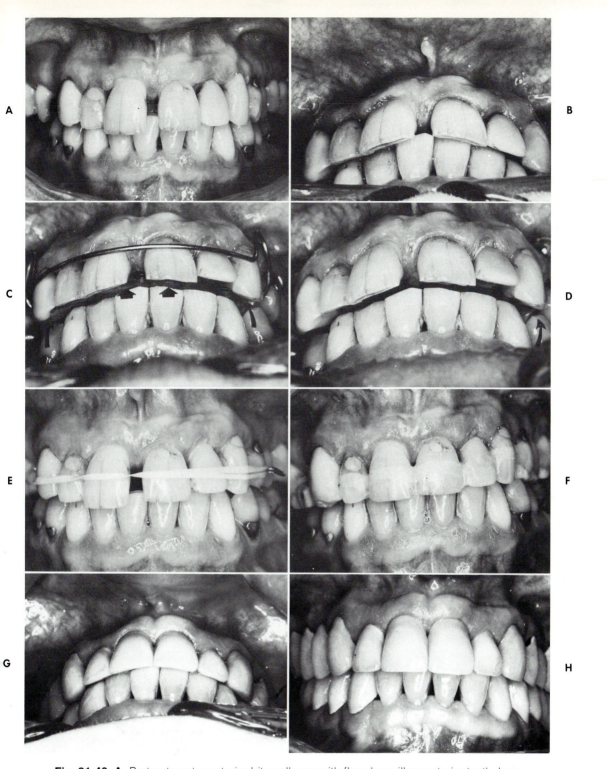

Fig. 21-40. A, Pretreatment, posterior bite collapse with flared maxillary anterior teeth, loss of vertical dimension. **B,** View from below, intercuspal contact or acquired or habitual occlusion. **C,** Maxillary Hawley appliance with anterior bite platform *(arrows)*. Posterior occlusion disarticulated 0.5 to 1 mm. **D,** Eruption of posterior teeth results in a space between mandibular and maxillary teeth and a change in vertical dimension. Note left premolar in occlusion *(arrow)*. **E,** Posterior segments have been A splinted at new vertical dimension and embedded hooks retain elastics for anterior retraction. This eliminates Hawley appliance. Alternatives would be the continued use of the Hawley after eliminating the bite platform or placement of posterior provisional splints with buccal hooks for retaining elastics. **F,** After anterior retraction, retention completed by intracoronal A splinting. Alternative would be use of anterior provisional splint. Intracoronal stabilization permits optimal bilateral stabilization when secondary occlusal traumatism is present on anterior and posterior teeth. **G** and **H,** Restorative dentistry completed. Anterior views showing overjet and overlap and showing interdental embrasures and restored tooth form, respectively. (In conjunction with Herman Corn, Levittown, Pa. and Leonard Juros, Willingboro, N.J.)

excursions. Its thickness should keep the posterior teeth out of contact for approximately 1 mm. The time necessary for sufficient eruption ranges 6 to 12 months or longer.

4. The posterior occlusion is now stabilized at the new occlusal vertical dimension and occlusal adjustment begun to gain maximum contacts of the posterior teeth. Anterior excursive movements are not adjusted until after the maxillary anterior tooth movement has been completed. The clinician will now note sufficient space between the mandibular and maxillary anterior teeth into which the maxillary anterior teeth can be retracted.

5. The anterior platform can be relieved or eliminated as the case dictates and the maxillary anterior teeth retracted palatally with elastics.

6. The maxillary anterior teeth can be stabilized with wire ligation, **A** splinting, or provisional splinting as indicated.

7. Now, occlusal adjustment can be completed for the anterior excursions (Marks and Corn, 1977).

In those cases where uprighting of tipped molars is necessary, this is accomplished after the mandibular anterior teeth are retracted and stabilization and a Hawley appliance with a bite plane is in place.

CROWDED MANDIBULAR ANTERIOR TEETH

Crowded mandibular anteriors often result in poor gingival form because of broad and irregular contact points and eviction of the gingival papillae. Osseous defects are most difficult to correct due to the proximity of the roots. If splinting is indicated, tooth preparation is virtually impossible, and replacement with adequate bulk of restorative material usually impinges on the tissues. Invariably the slipped contact points and the anterior component of force results in extrusion of the incisors. Plaque control is difficult for even the most conscientious patient.

Orthodontists find that relapse is common after the correction of crowded incisors and that in some situations permanent retention with canine bands and a soldered lingual arch is required. The latent downward and forward growth of the mandible, which has been observed in many patients during the second decade, rather than the presence of the third molars placing anterior pressure on the arches, has been indicated as an etiologic factor. However, differences of opinion concerning this growth and development remain.

If fibrotic gingival tissue or minimal osseous defects are present, surgery will usually suffice, and the irregular tooth position can be maintained. When tooth movement is required, the arch length from canine to canine must be measured. If the incisors have a tapering form, stripping can be considered. However, these teeth are generally square shaped, with long contact points from the incisal edge to the gingival margin contraindicating stripping. If a class II malocclusion is also present with a deep overbite and full orthodontic treatment is contemplated, the crowding is corrected by gaining available space through premolar extraction, driving the posterior segments distally, or by expanding the arch. If full orthodontic therapy is not practical, then extraction of one incisor may be considered (Fig. 21-41). After the canine arch length has been recorded, a diagnostic setup is achieved by cutting the teeth from the diagnostic model and waxing the desired positions. A very fine saw blade is used after each tooth has been numbered. Excess remaining space will result in an unstable relationship so that in some instances splinting must be planned if one tooth is to be removed.

DEEP OVERBITE

Clinical findings with the deep overbite include (1) trauma to the maxillary palatal gingiva, (2) wear facets on the labial surface of the mandibular incisors and on the lingual surface of the maxillary incisors, (3) trauma to the labial gingiva of the mandibular teeth, with lingually inclined maxillary incisors, and (4) locked bite anteriorly, producing excessive anterior force upon the maxillary incisors and potentiating migration and mobility patterns (Fig. 21-42).

The correction of the deep overbite with a removable posterior overlayed appliance is contraindicated. The outcome is further depression of the posterior teeth, with further deepening of the already existing overbite.

As previously discussed, the deep overbite due to extruded mandibular incisors can be corrected by depression with fixed appliance techniques. Retention may be achieved with wire ligation, occlusal adjustment, and a night guard. Splinting may be a contingency if these are not satisfactory for retention.

MESIALLY INCLINED SECOND AND THIRD MOLARS

Etiology. The common cause of the mesially tipped second or third permanent molar is the

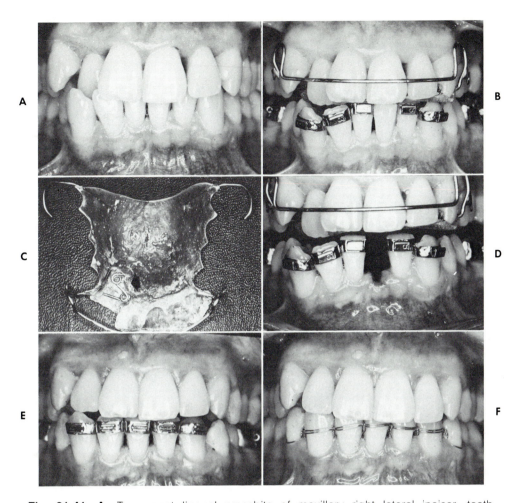

Fig. 21-41. A, To correct lingual crossbite of maxillary right lateral incisor, tooth movement in mandibular arch was necessary to obtain proper overbite and overjet relationships. **B,** Maxillary Hawley bite plane was inserted with a double helical recurved spring to move the incisor labially. The platform disarticulated the potential interfering tooth inclines. Bands were placed on mandibular incisors. Mandibular left central incisor was selected for extraction in order to gain available space for realignment. **C,** Tissue side of Hawley appliance. Note spring *(arrow)* and molar ring clasps. **D,** Mandibular incisor was extracted, and fixed appliance was immediately inserted. **E,** With light elastic ligature, incisors were realigned over 6 months. Forces were kept very light (54 g [2 oz] or less), and bodily movement was achieved with fixed arch and brackets. **F,** Bands were removed, and final spaces were closed and retained with wire ligation. (In conjunction with Herman Corn, Levittown, Pa.)

loss and nonreplacement of the first permanent molar.

The following clinical findings are commonly seen:

1. Mesial infrabony defect with plaque retention
2. Forces of occlusion not directed toward the long axis of the molars
3. The distal marginal ridge above the plane of occlusion, interfering in the retruded contacting and protrusive positions

4. Extrusion of the opposing first or second molar
5. Narrowing or obliteration of space previously occupied by the first molar

Indications for uprighting. The indications for uprighting the mesially tipped second or third molar or both include the following:

1. Decreasing the infrabony defect (This occurs by [a] an alteration of the relationship of the tooth to crest, [b] partial fill of the infrabony pocket in conjunction with curettage

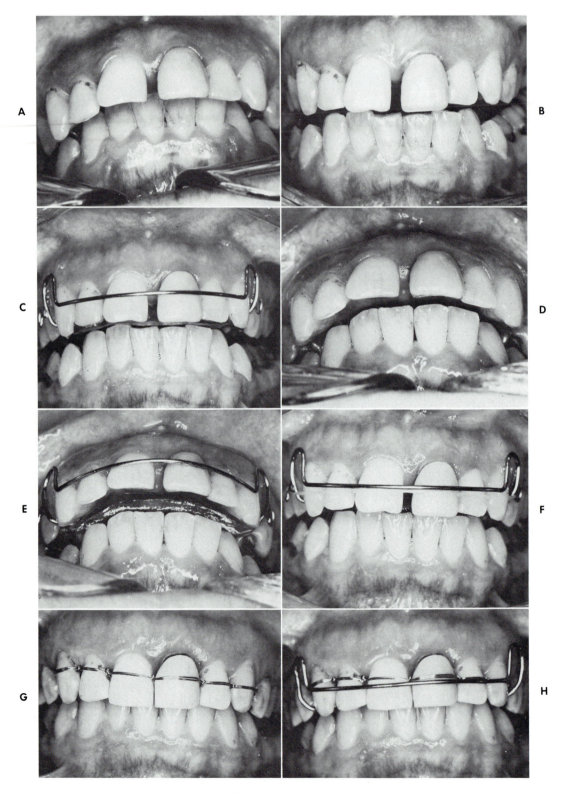

Fig. 21-42. For legend see opposite page.

and plaque control, or [c] a combination of both.)

2. Redirecting occlusal forces toward the long axis of the molars
3. Establishing proper pontic space for future restorative dentistry
4. Paralleling abutment teeth for restorative dentistry
5. Permitting better access for plaque control on the mesial surface

X-ray evaluation of inclined molars. Figs. 21-43 and 21-44 emphasize the importance of evaluating the tooth position radiographically as well as clinically. The x-ray examination will show the relative degree of tipping detween the molars and the teeth anteriorly and finally demonstrate when the tooth roots are nearly parallel. Frequently it is impossible to determine if a molar is tipped by simply observing the crown clinically. Any prior restoration will have the mesial marginal ridge built into occlusion, and this will obscure the true axial position of the molar. During the mechanics of uprighting, follow-up x-rays will indicate when uprighting is completed and the improvement of the mesial infrabony defect. Six

months is the average duration of time for uprighting molars.

Planning stabilization after uprighting. The method of choice is the **A** splint (Fig. 21-45) for the following reasons:

1. It is extremely effective and functional and can be accomplished with the minimum of chair time by the dentist, and consequently with a minimum of cost to the patient.
2. There is no time delay to allow for relapse if a provisional splint has to be made in a laboratory and another appointment is needed for its preparation and placement.
3. It eliminates the need for tooth preparation prior to periodontal surgery if a provisional splint is planned. After periodontal surgery the crown margins of the provisional splint will be supragingival and the teeth must be repreparaed. The provisional splint then must be remade.
4. If finances limit the patient's plan for a fixed bridge, then the **A** splint can be placed into class II amalgams, minimizing the problem of caries during maintenance. In this treatment program the amalgams are placed *be-*

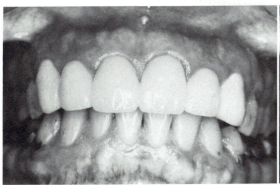
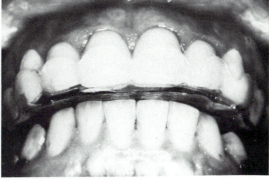

I   J

Fig. 21-42. A, Pretreatment, class II, division I, malocclusion. Posterior occlusion, although not in class I relationship, is well articulated buccolingually with forces of occlusion directed toward long axes of teeth. Maxillary left central incisor acrylic veneer crown is to be replaced. Patient is dissatisfied with anterior aesthetics. **B,** Note dual plane of occlusion usually seen with deep overbite case. Only maxillary anterior teeth planned to be retracted. **C,** Maxillary Hawley appliance with anterior bite platform to allow for posterior eruption and possible mandibular anterior depression. **D,** Twelve months necessary to develop sufficient spacing between mandibular and maxillary anterior teeth. **E,** Patient continues to wear the appliance but acrylic is removed from palatal surfaces of maxillary anterior teeth to allow elastic to retract them. Note line from white arch marking pencil to guide amount of acrylic to be relieved. **F,** A 7 mm (5/16 inch) regular elastic used for retraction. **G,** Retention by wire ligation after space closure. **H,** Hawley modified to aid in retention and will be used during the restorative procedures. A maxillary bite guard is planned to aid in retention after Hawley is discontinued. **I,** Anterior fixed bridge, **J,** Maxillary guard to control clenching and tongue habit. (In conjunction with Herman Corn, Levittown, Pa., and Stanley Lipkowitz, Fairless Hills, Pa.)

fore bracketing and uprighting to avoid any relapse from the time of the completion of uprighting to placement of the **A** splint. When a cast Vitallium bar is used, processed teeth can be added if required.

However, in selected cases the provisional splint allows the operator to establish the occlusal plane

and vertical dimension that may be impractical with the **A** splint (Fig. 21-44).

Mechanics of uprighting mesially inclined molars

1. Bands are made for the canine, second premolar (first premolar added for additional anchorage where necessary), and tipped molar.

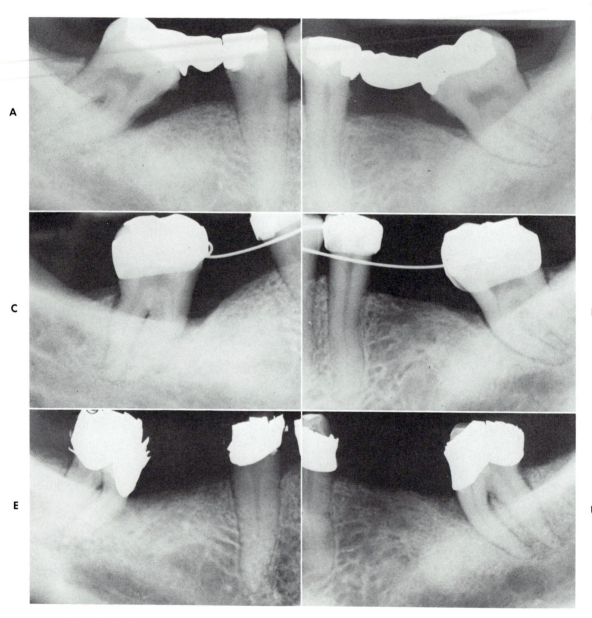

Fig. 21-43. X-ray films of case in Fig. 21-44. **A** and **B** show marked mesial tipping of mandibular second molars with mesial infrabony defects. Inlay bridges had initially been made. On right, gingival margin of Mo inlay for second molar has a defective gingival seat. **C** and **D** show partial uprighting of second molars after 3 months with Broussard uprighting spring in place. **E** and **F** show second molars stabilized with gold band provisional splint. Note radiographic improvement of mesial alveolar crests of both molars. During periodontal surgery only small shallow craters remained. (In conjunction with Herman Corn, Levittown, Pa., and Leonard Abrams, Philadelphia.)

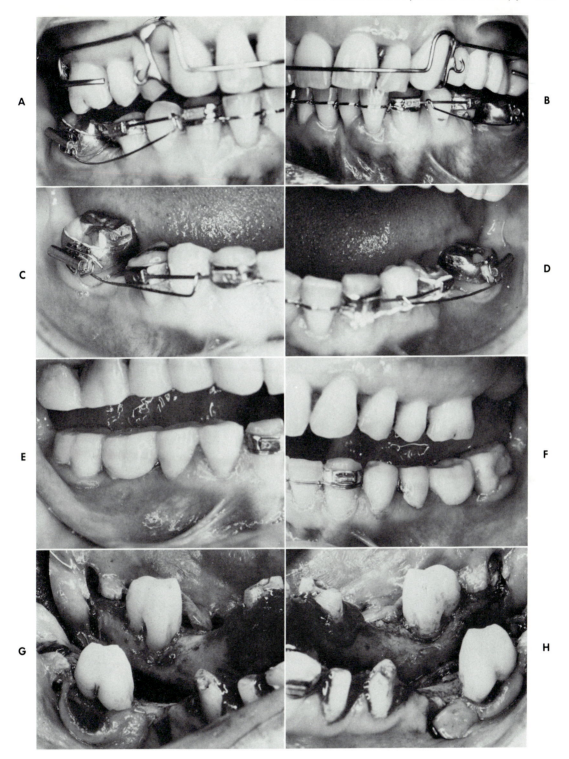

Fig. 21-44. Clinical case in Fig. 21-43. **A** and **B,** After defective bridges were sectioned and pontics removed, tipped second molars were banded with preformed stainless steel molar bands, and Broussard buccal tubes with a vertical slot were welded. A Hawley bite plane was placed in maxillary arch to disarticulate posterior teeth during uprighting. Sectional arch was placed between banded canine and second premolar to support Broussard uprighting spring. **C** and **D,** Second molars are upright after 4 months. **E** and **F,** Provisional splints were used to retain and stabilize second molars. A splints can be used for stabilization. **G** and **H,** Note shallow mesial defects that remained after uprighting. Initially 6 to 7 mm was probed prior to treatment.

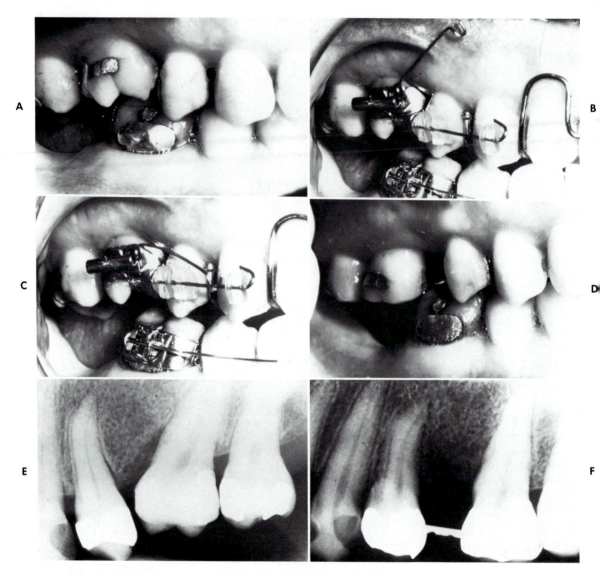

Fig. 21-45. A, Mirrow view of upper left second and third molars mesially tipped into missing first molar and second premolar space. **B,** Second molar was banded with welded Broussard buccal tube containing a vertical slot. Plastic edgewise brackets were bonded to upper left canine and first premolar. A sectional arch of 0.016 round wire was secured with clear A1 Alastik (Unitek). A Broussard uprighting spring of 0.40 mm (0.016 inch) round wire was bent similar to that in Fig. 21-46 but in opposite direction to fit into upper arch. Note activation of end of spring into vestibule. A Hawley appliance with an anterior bite platform disarticulated teeth during tooth movement to minimize occlusal traumatism. An interproximal ball clasp secured removable Hawley appliance on left side. A ring or Adam's clasp could not be used on molars since they were being moved. **C,** Uprighting spring was then activated by securing loop onto sectional arch. Interproximal ball clasp rests lingual to sectional arch wire and loop. **D,** After approximately 6 months second and third molars were uprighted, shortened, and **A** splinted for retention and stabilization. **E,** Original x-ray film of mesially tipped upper left second and third molars. **F,** X-ray film of molars uprighted and **A** splinted.

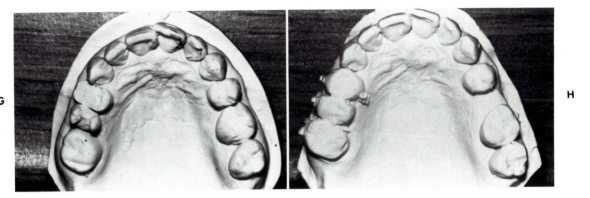

Fig. 21-45, cont'd. G, Original study model, occlusal view. **H,** Study model after uprighting completed. Note pontic space developed after uprighting molars. (In conjunction with S. Heller, University of Pennsylvania; **A** and **B** courtesy Rocky Mountain Dental Products Co., Denver.)

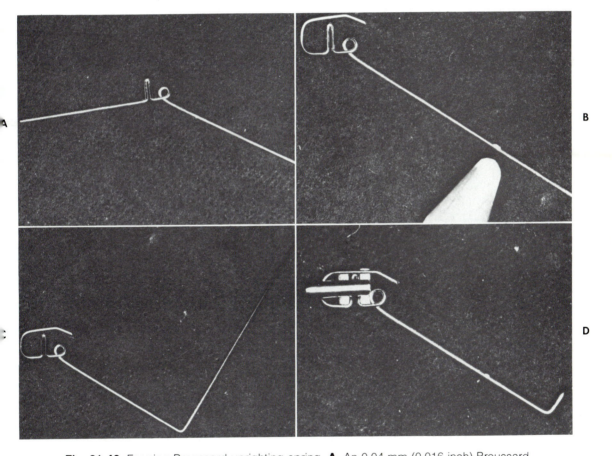

Fig. 21-46. Forming Broussard uprighting spring. **A,** An 0.04 mm (0.016 inch) Broussard uprighting spring made by Rocky Mountain Dental Products Co., Denver. **B,** Distal portion of spring is bent in a C to lock around and within tube. Helix points occlusal. Arch marking pencil marks furthest distance mesially that loop can be made and remain free sliding on sectional arch. **C,** To make loop, wire is bent occlusally 90 degrees and then bent over a pliers lingually to form loop. Excess wire is removed and end polished. **D,** Broussard uprighting spring locked around Broussard buccal tube.

2. Weld an edgewise bracket to canine and premolar band that will accept a sectional arch. Brackets bonded to the canine and premolars are frequently used in place of cemented stainless steel bands with wedged brackets.

3. Place 0.40 mm (0.016 inch) round stainless steel sectional arch secured to the bracket by 0.25 mm (0.010 inch) stainless steel ligature wire (Fig. 21-45) or an A1 Alastik.

4. Weld a Broussard buccal tube with vertical slot (RM-A165) to the molar band keeping the buccal tube parallel to the occlusal surface of the molar.

5. Form the locking portion of Broussard uprighting spring (Fig. 21-46) to fit within and around the molar tube.

6. Measure anteroposterior length of spring to loop over the sectional arch as far forward as possible (this gains maximum potential of the spring) and bend an open loop lingually (Fig. 21-46)

7. The spring is locked into and around the slot of the molar buccal tube; the action arm anterior to the helix should rest in the base of the vestibule; the Broussard spring is activated by placing it occlusally over the sectional arch between the canine and premolar just distal to the canine bracket, allowing for distal movement of the loop during uprighting.

The same technique is used when upper mesially inclined molars require uprighting (Fig. 21-45, *A*). The premolars and canine are used as the anchor teeth with welded or bonded edgewise brackets that accept a round sectional arch wire. The uprighting spring is bent in the same fashion but in reverse of the lower spring, as seen in Fig. 21-46. The major change occurs in the retention

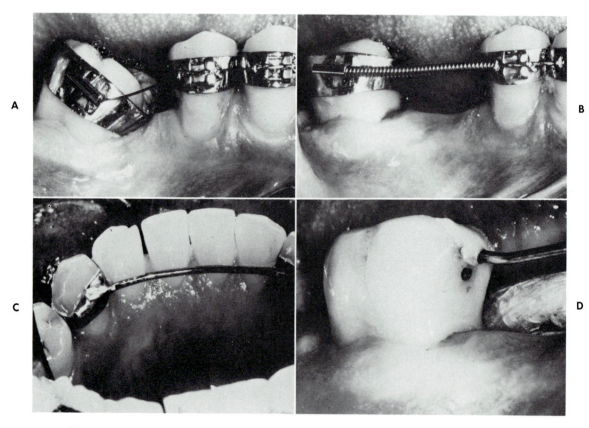

Fig. 21-47. A, Another method of uprighting tipped second molar includes use of arch wire rather than uprighting spring and, when indicated, incorporating open coil spring in **B. C,** Since anchor units have a force placed upon them in an anterior direction rather than in an apical direction, potential for mesial slippage of canine is present. This problem can be managed by banding opposite canine and increasing anchorage with a soldered lingual arch between canines. **D,** Molar uprighted and stabilized with an **A** splint. (Courtesy I. Stephen Brown, University of Pennsylvania.)

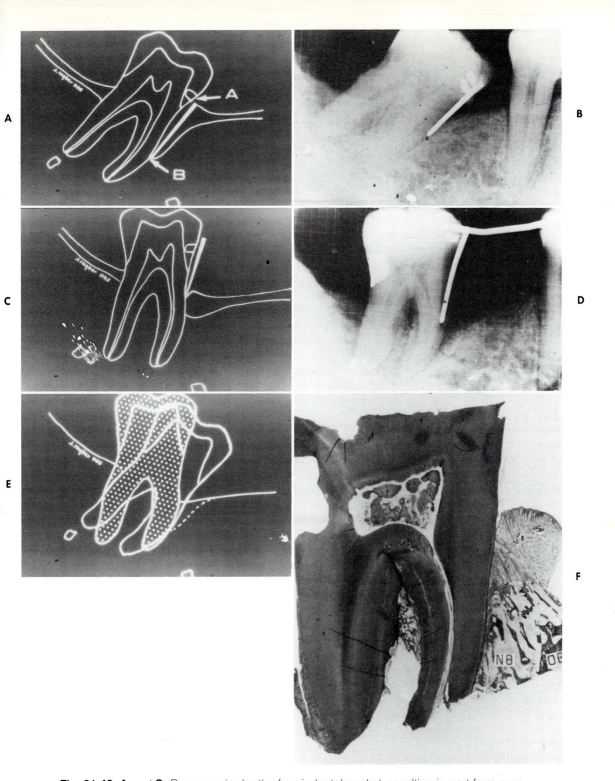

Fig. 21-48. A and **C,** Decrease in depth of periodontal pocket, resulting in part from eversion of pocket wall as mesially inclined molar is uprighted. **B** and **D,** X-ray film of a human clinical case before and after uprighting molar and **A** splint stabilization. **E,** Mesially tipped molar superimposed upon uprighted molar. **F,** Human histologic slide of case shown in **B** and **D.** Osteoid or new bone, *NB,* has formed on mesial or tension side. Old bone, *OB,* remains intact. Although new bone has formed as is classically seen on tension side, there is apparently no coronal increase or reattachment of additional new bone. Reduction of soft tissue pocket depth is result of eversion of pocket epithelium that morphologically becomes ridge epithelium. (**A, C,** and **E** from Brown, I. S.: J. Periodontol. **44:**742, 1973; **B, D,** and **F** from Brown, I. S.: J. Periodontol. In press.)

of the maxillary Hawley bite plane. For the conventional Hawley removable bite plane, a ring clasp or Adam's clasp is designed around the remaining molars. However, since the maxillary molars are to be moved, they cannot be clasped. The appliance is secured with interproximal ball clasps that seat lingually to the arch wire and loop of the uprighting spring (Fig. 21-45, *A* to *C*). Retention and stabilization is achieved by

splinting or provisional splinting where the restoration of clinical crown form is required early in therapy.

A second method of uprighting molars uses an open coil spring on a sectional arch that extends through the molar buccal attachment (Fig. 21-47). Since the open coil spring has a mesial component of force against the anchor teeth as well as a distal force against the mesially inclined molar,

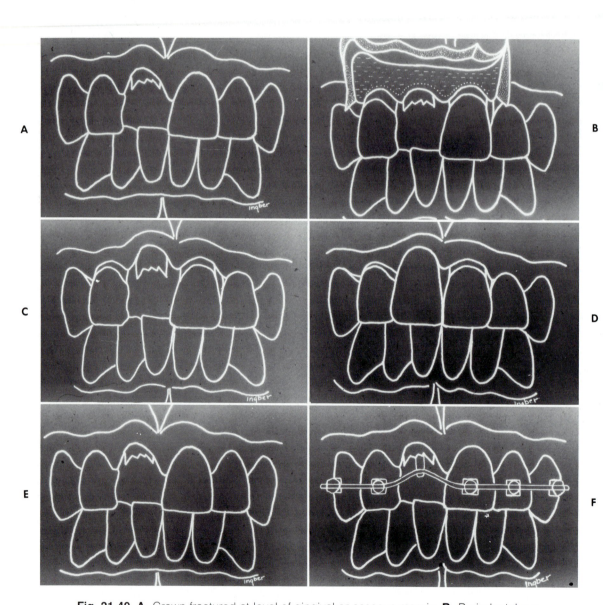

Fig. 21-49. A, Crown fractured at level of gingival or osseous margin. **B,** Periodontal surgery to expose sound tooth structure for adequate restoration. **C,** Osseous surgery results in sacrifice of bone on adjacent teeth, and aesthetic deformities may result. **D,** Final restoration after surgery may produce long clinical crowns and open embrasures. **E,** Fractured crown to be managed with forced eruption instead of usual periodontal surgery. **F,** Sectional orthodontic appliance is activated by engaging a temporary post that has been cemented in prepared root canal.

the potential for the canine to slip forward is present. This problem is compensated for by using additional anchorage of a canine-to-canine fixed lingual arch (Brown, 1973).

A third method of uprighting mesially inclined molars uses an "L" or "T" loop (Vanarsdall, 1977). This technique tends to keep the tipped molars within the same plane as the premolars and canine and often produces mesial root movement.

However, the use of the Broussard uprighting spring with its disto-occlusal component of movement, a form of forced eruption, is preferred when a mesial infrabony defect exists and maximum improvement with tooth movement prior to periodontal surgery is desired.

Anchorage consideration. Since the maximum number of periodontal ligament fibers resist tooth movement in an apical direction, the depressing

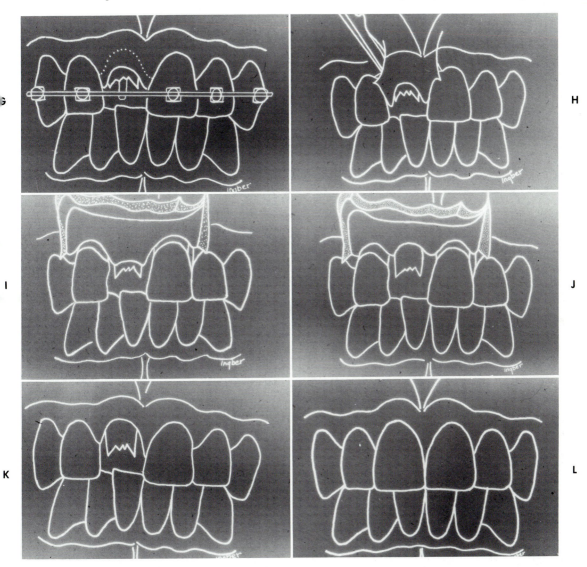

Fig. 21-49, cont'd. G, Gingival margin and root segment have been erupted to a position further coronal relative to adjacent teeth. Dotted line represents position of preoperative gingival margin. **H,** Periodontal surgery is employed after a period of stabilization to reposition gingival complex to approximate preoperative gingival margin. **I,** Flap design involving adjacent teeth if osseous defects on other teeth are to be managed concurrently. Osseous margin has followed coronal movement of teeth. Note angular crests. **J,** Angular crests are corrected, which exposed sound tooth structure without sacrificing bone on adjacent teeth. **K,** Flap sutured to approximate gingival margins on adjacent teeth. **L,** Final restoration placed, producing acceptable aesthetics. (From Ingber, J. S.: J. Periodontol. **47:**203, 1976.)

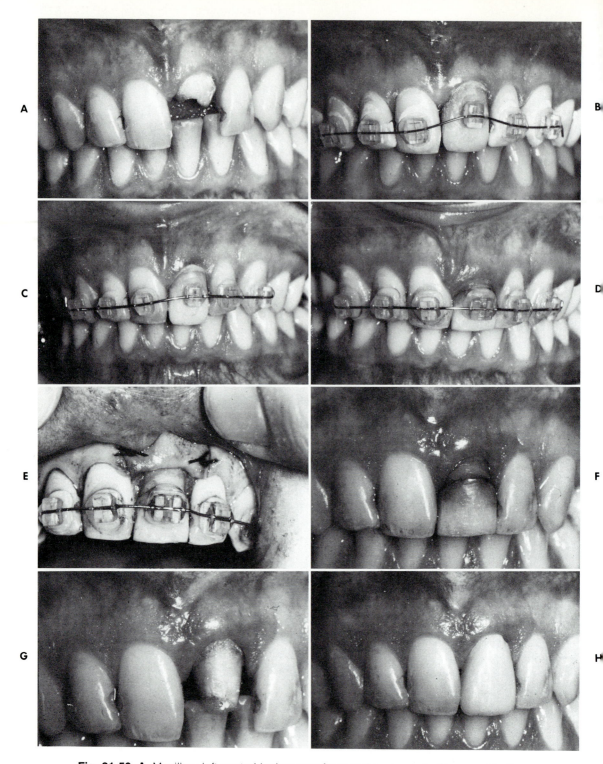

Fig. 21-50. A, Maxillary left central incisor was fractured as a result of trauma. Tooth was prepared for a full crown restoration; however, tooth was fractured below gingival margin. **B,** A metal band temporary restoration was cemented. A sectional appliance was bonded directly to teeth and activated. Note relative positions of mucogingival junction and gingival margin. **C,** Some eruption has occurred since 0.014 arch wire wants to return to its undistorted state. **D,** Approximately 4 mm of eruption was obtained in 6 weeks, at which time tooth was stabilized in appliance. It appears that position of mucogingival junction has remained relatively stable, while gingival margin has moved coronally. **E** and **F,** Full-thickness flap was elevated to reposition gingival margin apically to approximate adjacent teeth. **G,** Tooth is reprepared for final restoration. There is now adequate crown length as a result of forced eruption. **H,** Final restoration was inserted and adjusted to minimize occlusal stress. (From Ingber, J. S.: J. Periodontol. **47:**203, 1976.)

effect placed on the premolars and canine is above the threshold force for intrusion of these teeth. However, the molar is being tipped distally and fewer periodontal ligament fibers resist this tipping movement. Even if the anchorage units did intrude, this would not appreciably effect the future utilization of these teeth as abutments. Anterior rather than intruding forces should be avoided because of the potential of mesial slippage of the canine (Fig. 21-47).

When opposing molars are present, a Hawley appliance with an anterior bite plane is used to disarticulate the opposing teeth during movement. The duration of time averages 6 months. The patient is seen at 3-week intervals during adjustments at which time the occlusion is checked and interferences relieved as the molar is uprighting.

Effect of orthodontic therapy on periodontal defects of mesially inclined molars. In December 1973 Brown presented in the *Journal of Periodontology* the rationale for the improvement of periodontal defects when a mesially inclined molar is uprighted. He states:

Clinical evidence presented in this series suggests that those principal fibers of the gingiva which are attached to the tooth are probably displaced in the direction of the tooth movement and are then reorganized after a prolonged period of retention . . . leads the investigator to postulate that the marked reduction in the soft tissue pocket depth in this group occurred as a result of distal displacement of the attached fiber bundles apical to the epithelial attachment, causing a substantial portion of the pocket wall to become essentially *everted*. This would explain the leveling of the soft tissue defect and the apical positioning of the new gingival margin [Fig. 21-48].

If a portion of the mesial infrabony defect present on the tipped molar has three osseous walls, some reattachment may occur following an effective plaque-control program, root scaling, root planing, and soft tissue curettage. This curettage would remove the ulcerated crevicular lining of the pocket, the underlying connective tissue, and the entire gingival fiber apparatus down to the alveolar bone. This enucleation of the entire soft tissue content of the pocket is similar to that described by Prichard (1965).

FORCED ERUPTION

As a result of subgingival and subcrestal fractures, caries, or restorative pins an isolated nonrestorable tooth can occur. The usual periodontal surgical management exposes sound tooth structure (Ingber, 1974) (Fig. 21-49). In the anterior

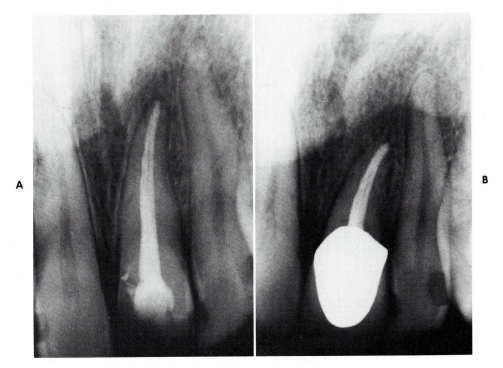

Fig. 21-51. Preoperative, **A,** and postoperative, **B,** radiographs of case in Fig. 21-45, **C.** (From Ingber, J. S.: J. Periodontol. **47**:203, 1976.)

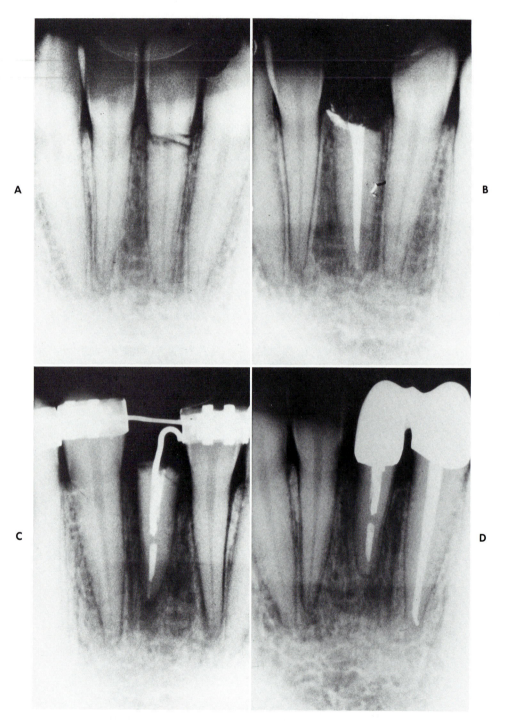

Fig. 21-52. A, Radiograph of subcrestal fractured lower incisor. **B,** Endodontics completed. **C,** Forced eruption with fixed sectional arch. **D,** Incisor crowned with canine that subsequently became endodontically involved.

part of the mouth, aesthetics may be compromised. Gingival and osseous surgery usually involves adjacent teeth to achieve a blend of gingival and osseous contours.

Forced eruption moves the isolated tooth, gingiva, and supporting structures coronally farther than the adjacent teeth. Periodontal surgery to expose sound tooth structure will then not compromise the adjacent teeth (Ingber, 1976) (Figs. 21-49 to 21-53).

PSEUDOCLASS III

The anterior crossbite must be examined with the mandible guided into retruded contact position (Fig. 21-6). If the mandibular incisors approach an edge-to-edge position, the malocclusion is a pseudoclass III. A posterior bite opening appliance is indicated to disarticulate the anterior crossbite and allow for anterior tooth positioning without incisal interference. Existing circumstances will dictate whether the maxillary anteriors are to be moved labially or the mandibular incisors are to be retracted lingually or both (Fig. 21-7). After tooth movement occlusal adjustment of the incisal inclines should stabilize the resulting overbite (Marks and Corn, in press).

CLASS II AND III MALOCCLUSIONS

Correction of class II and III malocclusions requires the services of an orthodontist. The treatment requires multibanded techniques, and full segments must be repositioned. Usually 2 years or longer is required. Often a discrepancy in jaw size exists in addition to the disparity in tooth position. In some instances splinting can compensate for the tooth position, but this complicates the restorative dentistry and may result in unnecessary compromises.

RETRACTION OF MAXILLARY ANTERIOR TEETH WITH NO POSTERIOR ANCHORAGE

The problem. One occasionally encounters a patient who has lost all of his maxillary molars

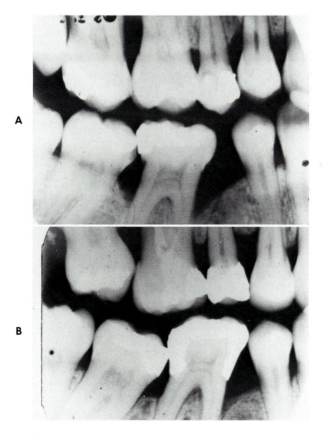

Fig. 21-53. A, Initial radiograph prior to complete fixed orthodontics. Note infrabony pockets on distal aspect of upper first premolar and mesial and distal infrabony defects on lower first molar. **B,** Two years after orthodontics. Note leveling of infrabony defects. No periodontal surgery had yet been completed. (In conjunction with Richard Kahn, Willingboro, N.J.)

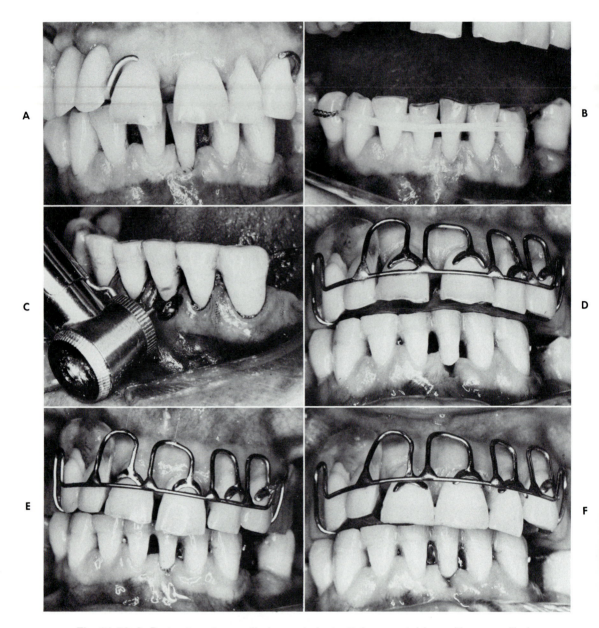

Fig. 21-54. A, Pretreatment, mandibular posterior teeth in acceptable position, mandibular anteriors flared labially and spaced, all maxillary teeth missing except central incisors, and left lateral incisor and canine. Maxillary anterior teeth are to be retained for final restoration. **B,** Mandibular posterior teeth have been stabilized by **A** splinting and embedded hooks anchor elastic that retracts incisors. **C,** Mandibular incisors are now included in **A** splinting, resulting in bilateral stabilization. Mandibular left central incisor was hopeless and root is removed leaving clinical crown remaining attached within intracoronal **A** splint. **D,** Maxillary Hawley with anterior bite platform, soldered **J** clasps to be used as springs for individual movement. **E,** Only maxillary left central incisor has been moved palatally with remaining teeth and palate anchoring appliance. **F,** Next right central incisor followed by lateral incisor have been retracted palatally. Canine was determined to be in acceptable position.

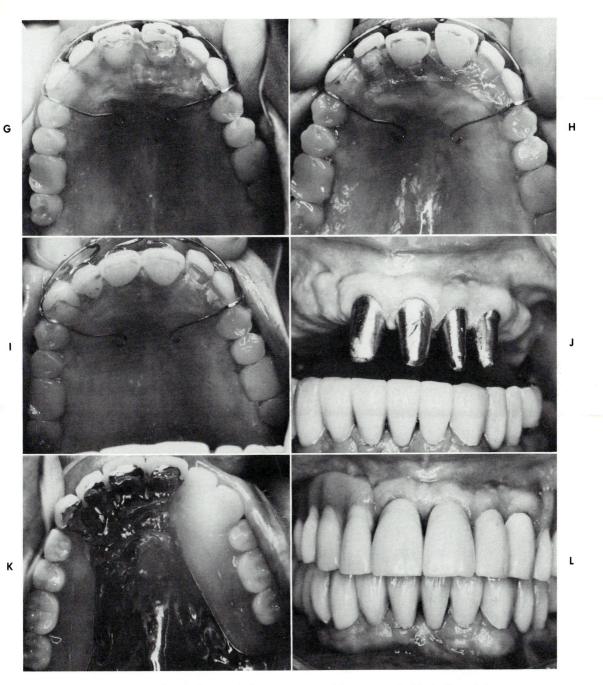

Fig. 21-54, cont'd. G to **I,** Occlusal views of sequential movement. **J** to **L,** Complete mandibular fixed splint with a maxillary sleeve coping partial denture. Should any of the remaining maxillary abutments be lost, they can easily be added to partial denture without constructing a new restoration. (In conjunction with Herman Corn, Levittown, Pa., and Stanley Lipkowitz, Fairless Hills, Pa.)

and premolars. Because of the loss of occlusal vertical dimension and posterior bite collapse, the pressure from the mandibular anterior teeth results in flaring of the maxillary anterior teeth. In many instances the mandibular anterior teeth have also migrated labially. The retraction of anterior teeth when no posterior teeth remain presents a serious problem of anchorage. Adequate anchorage is obtained by constructing a removable appliance that encompasses the maximum edentulous area. Frequently the acrylic covering the lingual surfaces and the incisal edges and extending onto the labial surfaces of the anterior teeth is necessary. This removable appliance also establishes the occlusal vertical demension by using acrylic teeth as pontics or acrylic bite blocks (Fig. 21-54).

Since the position of the mandibular teeth dic-

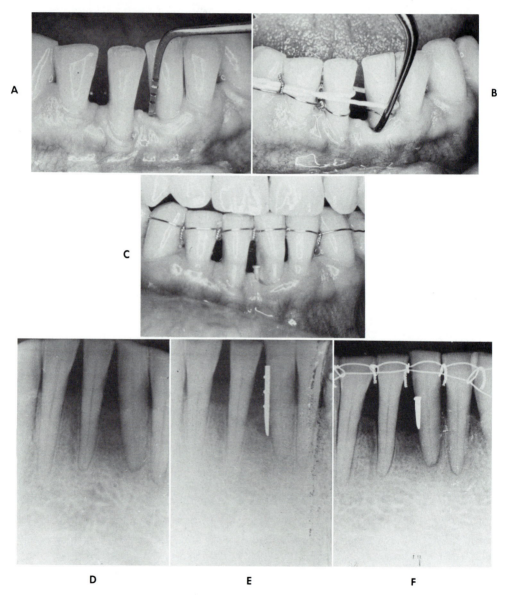

Fig. 21-55. **A,** Open contacts between central incisors, with an infrabony defect. **B,** Tooth movement was performed with elastic ligature. Individual wires helped to prevent elastic ligature from slipping apically. Frequent curettage was performed. **C,** After tooth movement, retention was achieved with wire ligation, and original defect was markedly reduced. **D,** Roentgenogram taken April 1963. **E,** June 1966, when treatment was begun. **F,** January 1967, after tooth movement and wire ligation stabilization were completed. (Courtesy Dennis Winson, University of Pennsylvania.)

tates the position of the maxillary anterior teeth, the following is the sequence of tooth movement (Marks and Corn, in press):

1. Stabilization of mandibular posterior teeth (assuming tooth position is acceptable)
2. Retraction of the mandibular anterior teeth
3. Stabilization and retention of the mandibular anterior teeth
4. Retraction of the maxillary anterior teeth
5. Retention and stabilization of the maxillary anterior teeth

Several principles must be highlighted:

1. The impression taken for the removable appliance must encompass the maximum tissue-bearing area.
2. Only one tooth is moved at a time initially with the remaining teeth and mucosa supporting the appliance.
3. The lightest force is used to move teeth in order to minimize appliance displacement, approximately 56 g (2 oz).

Construction of the maxillary removable appliance. In order that the impression encompass the maximum tissue-bearing area, the impression tray should be muscle molded. This can be accomplished with soft wax, compound, or mortite. The final borders of the appliance should be clearly drawn on the study model to include the junction of the hard and soft palate. A wax bite is taken to relate the maxillary and mandibular models on the articulator. A shade is selected for the molar and premolar pontics. If an occlusal vertical dimension can be established that creates space between the maxillary and mandibular anterior teeth, then an occlusal platform can be bypassed. However, in most cases a bite platform is a necessity, since protrusive excursion will result in a labial vector of force.

Force placement. A lingual or palatal force can be achieved by the use of palatal cleats with elastics around the teeth or the use of labial springs. Springs are preferred, since they can be activated and one does not have to rely on the patient to change the elastics four times daily. However, springs are less aesthetic.

One tooth is moved at a time. The most distal remaining teeth are usually selected first, alternating to the midline. After a tooth is retracted, the appliance is adjusted to passively hold this tooth in its new position and act as an anchor unit.

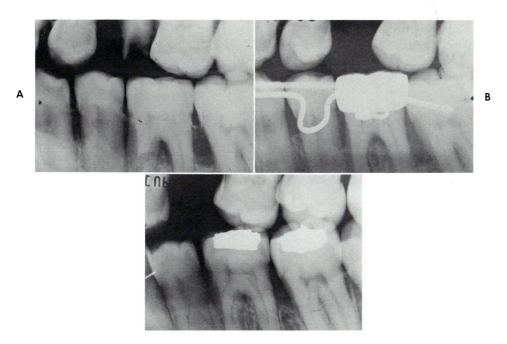

Fig. 21-56. Teeth of patient in Fig. 21-1. **A,** Original x-ray film of mandibular left first molar prior to therapy. **B,** One year after tooth movement was begun. Frequent curettage was performed. Note increased density of bone in bifurcation. **C,** Two years after tooth movement was begun. Bands were removed, and an occlusal filling was placed. Note density of bone in bifurcation and leveling of crest between first and second molars. There may have been some slipping of molar anchorage over the 2 years. Tooth is slightly extruded. No surgery for osseous defects was performed.

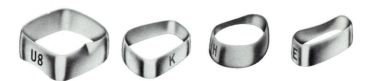

Fig. 21-57. Preformed bands for molars, premolars, canines, and incisors of many sizes. A large selection is necessary because of tooth size variation. These are seamless. (Courtesy Rocky Mountain Dental Products Co., Denver.)

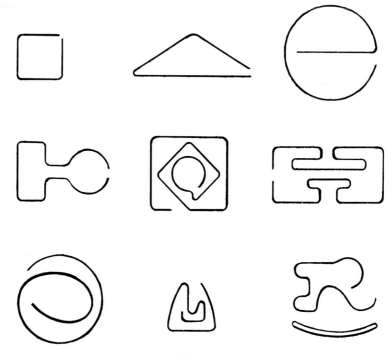

Fig. 21-58. Wire-bending exercises. (Courtesy University of Pennsylvania School of Dental Medicine, Department of Orthodontics.)

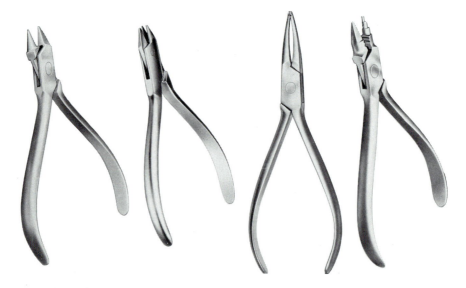

Fig. 21-59. No. 139 angle wire-bending pliers. No. 201 clasp-adjusting pliers. No. 110 How pliers. No. 74 Young loop-bending pliers. (Courtesy Rocky Mountain Dental Products Co., Denver.)

If the appliance begins to displace with the force application and sore spots develop, several suggestions can be considered:

1. Decrease the magnitude but continue the force.
2. Eliminate force until sore spots are comfortable, then initiate lighter force.

Fig. 21-54 is an example of maxillary anterior retraction with only four teeth remaining.

MOVING TEETH INTO OSSEOUS DEFECTS

When teeth are moved into osseous defects after complete débridement of the pocket, there is the potential for eliminating or reducing the depth of the original defect. Root planing and soft tissue curettage are performed at each visit when the patient is seen for an adjustment. If the osseous defect is not eliminated, it becomes narrow, which renders it more favorable for reattachment procedures (Figs. 21-55 and 21-56).

RETENTION

The clinician should not begin tooth movement therapy unless he can stabilize and retain the new tooth position. The final tooth position is dependent on the balance of forces acting on the teeth for stability. Drifting and replapse occur when the forces are unbalanced. Occlusal equilibration must be considered part of every retentive program of tooth movement regardless of its simplicity or complexity. Ideally retention should be required only for the time necessary to allow the tissues to return to a physiologic state and the transformation of the bone and periodontal ligament fibers to maturity. If the factors causing the original malocclusion are not eliminated, permanent retention is required. If a balance of forces is achieved, 3 to 6 months of retention is required with the original tooth movement appliance in a passive state or a Hawley retainer. Tapering of the appliance rather than complete withdrawal is preferred.

Means of retention include the following:

1. Occlusal adjustment
2. Wire ligation — anterior teeth
3. Maxillary and mandibular Hawley retainers
4. Maxillary and mandibular bite guards
5. Interlocking restorations — amalgams, inlays, crowns, pin splints, welded orthodontic bands (Fig. 21-57), A splints
6. Removable partial dentures
7. Wire and acrylic Sorrin splint, continuous cast splint

WIRE-BENDING EXERCISES

Fig. 21-58 is a group of wire-bending exercises to acquaint the therapist with the use of standard wire-bending pliers and 0.8 mm (0.032 inch) round stainless wire generally used for Hawley removable acrylic appliances. Start at the upper left, using an arch-marking pencil to guide the bends. All the figures should be kept flat on a plane surface.

Fig. 21-59 shows common pliers used in adult orthodontics for wire bending and adjustments.

SUGGESTED INSTRUMENTS AND SUPPLIES

Instruments
Wire-bending pliers, no. 139
Double-beak band-forming pliers, anterior no. 155
Double-beak band-forming pliers, posterior no. 157
How pliers, straight no. 110
A crown-and-bridge scissors, curved
Band-removing pliers, no. 347
Band pusher, no. 300
Wire cutter, heavy duty
Dontrix
Arch-marking pencil
Hemostat

Supplies
Premolar blanks, 3.175 × 0.102 mm (0.125 × 0.004 inch)
Molar blanks, 4.572 × 0.127 mm (0.180 × 0.005 inch)
Cuspid blanks, 3.801 × 0.076 mm (0.150 × 0.003 inch)
Broussard buccal tube with vertical slots, no. A165
Broussard uprighting spring, 0.406 mm (0.016 inch)
Edgewise bracket, no. A50
0.813 mm (0.032 inch) round stainless steel wire, no. E18
0.406 mm (0.016 inch) round stainless steel wire, no. E9
J clasp 0.6 mm, no. G40
Wire solder, 25 gauge, 2 dwt., no. H22
Flux for soldering, no. J41
0.254 mm (0.010 inch) stainless steel wire ligature

REFERENCES

Adams, C. P.: The design of removable appliances for mesio-distal movement of teeth, Dent. Pract. **5:**191, 1955.

Adams, C. P.: The design and construction of removable orthodontic appliances, ed. 2, Bristol, 1957, John Wright & Sons, Ltd.

Alexander, P. C.: Orthodontic procedures in periodontal therapy, J. Periodontol. **28:**46, 1957.

Altemus, L. A.: Mechanotherapy for minor orthodontic problems, Dent. Clin. North. Am., p. 303, July, 1968.

Anderson, G. M.: Practical orthodontics, ed. 9, St. Louis, 1960, The C. V. Mosby Co.

Anderson, J., Hoffman, L., and Hoffman, J.: Tongue thrust and deglutition: some anatomical, physiological and neurological considerations, J. Speech Hear. Disord. **30:**105, 1965.

Andreasen, G. F.: A review of the approaches to treatment of impacted maxillary cuspids, Oral Surg. **31:**429, 1971.

Angle, E. H.: Classification of malocclusion, Dent. Cosmos **41:**248, 1899.

Atherton, J. D.: The gingival response to orthodontic tooth movements, Am. J. Orthod. **58:**179, 1970.

Atherton, J. D., and Kerr, N. W.: Effect of orthodontic tooth movement upon the gingivae, Br. Dent. J. **124:**55, 1968.

Batenhorst, K. F., Bowers, G. M., and Williams, J. E.: Tissue changes resulting from facial tipping and extrusion of incisors in monkeys. J. Periodontol. **45:**660, 1974.

Beagrie, G. S., Thompson, G. W., and Basu, M. K.: Tooth position and anterior bone loss in skulls, Br. Dent. J. **129:** 471, 1970.

Begg, P. R.: Begg orthodontic theory and technique, Philadelphia, 1965, W. B. Saunders Co.

Begg, P. R.: Light wire arch technique, Am. J. Orthod. **47:** 30, 1956.

Bell, W. R.: Study of applied force as related to the use of elastics and coil springs, Angle Orthod. **21:**151, 1951.

Berlinger, A.: Ligatures, splints, bite planes and pyramids, Philadelphia, 1964, J. B. Lippincott Co.

Bernstein, M.: Orthodontics in periodontal and prosthetics therapy, J. Periodontol. **40:**577, 1969.

Bien, S. M.: Orthodontic procedures in the treatment of periodontal disease, Int. Dent. J. **3:**78, 1952.

Brown, I. S.: Effect of orthodontic therapy on periodontal defects, J. Periodontol. **44:**742, 1973.

Breitner, L.: Bone changes resulting from experimental orthodontic treatment, Am. J. Orthod. and Oral Surg. **26:** 521, 1940.

Corn, H., and Marks, M. H.: Strategic extraction in periodontal therapy, Dent. Clin. North Am. **13:**817, 1969.

Cross, W. G., and Yuktanandana, I.: The role of orthodontics in periodontal treatment, Dent. Pract. **7:**388, 1957.

DeAngelis: Observations on the response of alveolar bone to orthodontic force, Am. J. Orthod. **58:**284, 1970.

Dickson, G. C.: Orthodontics in general dental practice, ed. 2, London, 1964, Pitman Medical Publishing Company, Ltd.

Dummett, C. O.: Orthodontics and periodontal disease, J. Periodontol. **22:**34, 1951.

Edwards, J. G.: A surgical procedure to eliminate rotational relapse. Am. J. Orthod. **57:**35, 1970.

Edwards, J. G.: A study of the periodontium during orthodontic rotation of teeth, Am. J. Orthod. **54:**441, 1968.

Fischer, B.: Clinical orthodontics, Philadelphia, 1955, W. B. Saunders Co.

Fogel, M. S.: Adult orthodontics as related to periodontal disease and occlusal reconstruction procedures (abstract), N.Y. J. Dent. **27:**159, 1957.

Geiger, A. M.: Orthodontics; an aid in restorative dentistry for the adult patient, N.Y. State Dent. J. **25:**111, 1959.

Geiger, A., and Hirschfeld, L.: Minor tooth movement in general practice, ed. 3, St. Louis, 1974, The C. V. Mosby Co.

Geoffrion, P.: Clinical application of the twin-wire mechanism, Paris, 1962, Julien Prelat.

Gianelly, A. A.: Force induced changes in the vascularity of the periodontal ligament, Am. J. Orthod. **55:**5, 1969.

Gianelly, A. A., Ruben, M. P., Frankl, S. N., and Turner, H.: Alveolar bone resorption and periodontal vascularity, Periodontics **6:**220, 1968.

Gianelly, A. A., and Goldman, H. M.: Biologic basis of orthodontics, Philadelphia, 1971, Lea & Febiger.

Goldstein, M. C.: Orthodontics in crown and bridge and periodontal therapy, Dent. Clin. North Am., p. 449, July, 1964.

Goldstein, M. C.: Adult orthodontics and the general practitioner, J. Can. Dent. Assoc. **24:**26, 1958.

Goldstein, M. C.: Oral rehabilitation for the adult through orthodontics, Fortn. Rev. Chic. Dent. Soc. **33:**11, 1957.

Goldstein, M. C.: Adult orthodontics, Am. J. Orthod. **39:** 400, 1953.

Gottlieb, B.: Orthodontic treatment of wandering teeth in cases of diffuse atrophy, Dent. Outlook **28:**551, 1941.

Graber, T. M.: Orthodontics: principles and practice, Philadelphia, 1966, W. B. Saunders Co.

Gresham, H.: A manuel of orthodontics, Christchurch, New Zealand, 1957, N. M. Peryer, Ltd.

Hawley, C. A.: A removable retainer, Int. J. Orthod. **5:**291, 1919.

Hemley, S.: The clinical significance of tissue changes incidental to tooth movement, Am. J. Orthod. **41:**5, 1955.

Hemley, S.: The incidence of root resorption of vital permanent teeth, J. Dent. Res. **20:**133, 1941.

Hemley, S.: Bite plates, their application and action, Am. J. Orthod. **24:**721, 1938.

Henry, O. J.: The Crozat removable appliance and some of its advantages, Int. J. Orthod. **12:**261, 1926.

Hirschfeld, I.: Food impaction, J. Am. Dent. Assoc. **17:**1504, 1930.

Hirschfeld, L.: The use of wire and silk ligatures, J. Am. Dent. Assoc. **41:**647, 1950.

Hirschfeld, L., and Jay, J.: Minor tooth movement by means of rubber dam elastics, J. Am. Dent. Assoc. **50:**281, 1955.

Hotz, R.: Orthodontics in everyday practice, Berne, 1963, Hans Huber.

Hutcherson, J. B.: Repositioning and permanent retention of adult teeth, Ann. Dent. **16:**12, 1957.

Ingber, J. S.: Forced eruption. II. A method of treating nonrestorable teeth — periodontal and restorative considerations, J. Periodontol. **47:**203, 1976.

Ingber, J. S.: Forced eruption. I. A method of treating isolated one and two wall infrabony osseous defects — rationale and case report, J. Periodontol. **45:**199, 1974.

Jarabak, J. R.: Technique and treatment with the light wire appliance, St. Louis, 1963, The C. V. Mosby Co.

Johnson, J. E.: The construction and manipulation of the twin wire mechanism, Am. J. Orthod. **27:**202, 1941.

Kesling, H. D.: Philosophy of the tooth positioning appliance, Am. J. Orthod. **31:**297, 1945.

Lischer, B. E.: Principles and methods of orthodontics, Philadelphia, 1912, Lea & Febiger.

Lundstrom, A.: Introduction to orthodontics, New York, 1960, McGraw-Hill Book Company.

Lusterman, E. A.: The interrelationship of periodontics and orthodontics, J. Am. Dent. Assoc. **59:**28, 1959.

Macapanpan, L. C., Weinmann, J. P., and Brodie, A. G.: Early tissue changes following tooth movement in rats, Angle Orthod. **24:**79, 1954.

Marks, M. H.: Tooth movement in periodontal therapy. In Periodontal therapy by Goldman, H. M., and Cohen, D. W., editors: ed. 5, St. Louis, 1973, The C. V. Mosby Co.

Marks, M. H., and Corn, H.: The integration of adult tooth movement into a comprehensive periodontal treatment program. In H. L. Ward, editor: A periodontal point of view, Springfield, Ill., 1973, Charles C Thomas, Publisher.

Marks, M. H., and Corn, H.: Adult tooth movement: alteration of the occlusal vertical dimension preparatory to tooth movement, Alpha Omegan, Dec. 1977, pp. 54-61.

Marks, M. H., and Corn, H.: Adult tooth movement, uprighting mesially tipped mandibular second and third molars. In press.

Marks, M. H., and Corn, H.: Adult tooth movement, management of the pseudo-class III malocclusion. In press.

Marks, M. H., and Corn, H.: Adult tooth movement, retraction of the maxillary anterior teeth with no posterior anchorage. In press.

Marks, M. H., and Corn, H.: The role of tooth movement in periodontal therapy, Dent. Clin. North Am. **13:**229, 1969.

Massler, M.: Changes in the lamina dura during tooth movement, Am. J. Orthod. **40:**364, 1954.

McCoy, J. D., and Shepard, E. E.: Applied orthodontics, ed. 7, Philadelphia, 1956, Lea & Febiger.

Mershon, J. V.: Possibilities and limitations in the treatment of closed bites, Am. J. Orthod. **23:**581, 1937.

Moyers, R. E.: Spacing between the maxillary central incisors, Alpha Omegan **46:**80, 1952.

Moyers, R. E.: The periodontal membrane in orthodontics, J. Am. Dent. Assoc. **40:**22, 1950.

Moyers, R. E., and Bauer, J. L.: The periodontal response to various tooth movements, Am. J. Orthod. **36:**572, 1950.

Neustadt, E.: The correction of tooth malposition as a factor in the treatment of periodontal disease, N.Y. J. Dent. **1:**14, 1931.

Oliver, O. A., Irish, R. E., and Wood, C. R.: Labiolingual technique, London, 1940, Henry Kimpton.

Oppenheim, A.: Artificial elongation of teeth, Am. J. Orthod. and Oral Surg. **26:**931, 1940.

Pearson, I. E.: Gingival height of lower central incisors orthodontically treated and untreated, Angle Orthod. **38:**337. 1968.

Posselt, U.: Studies in the mobility of the human mandible, Acta Odontol. Scand. **10**(suppl.):10, 1952.

Posselt, U., and Nohrstrom, P.: Orthodontic treatment of functional disturbances in the adult dentition, Odontol. Tskr. **68:**450, 1960.

Prichard, J. F.: Advanced periodontal disease — surgical and prosthetic management, Philadelphia, 1965, W. B. Saunders Co.

Reitan, K.: Tissue rearrangement during retention of orthodontically rotated teeth. Angle Orthod. **29:**105, 1959.

Reitan, K.: Tissue reaction as related to the age factor, Dent. Pract. Dent. Rec. **74:**271, 1954.

Reitan, K.: Clinical and histologic observations on tooth movement during and after orthodontic treatment, Am. J. Orthod. **53:**721, 1967.

Reitan, K.: Tissue changes following experimental tooth movement as related to the time factor, Dent. Pract. Dent. Rec. **73:**559, 1953.

Reitan, K.: The initial tissue reaction incident to orthodontic tooth movement as related to the influence of function. An experimental histological study on animal and human material, Acta Odontol. Scand. **9**(suppl.):6, 1951.

Reitan, K.: Continuous bodily tooth movement and its histological significance, Acta Odontol. Scand. **6:**115, 1947.

Renfroe, E.: Technique training in orthodontics, Ann Arbor, 1960, Edwards Bros.

Riedel, R. A., and Kraus, B. S.: Vistas in orthodontics, Philadelphia, 1962, Lea & Febiger.

Salzmann, J. A.: Orthodontics, vol. I, Principles and prevention; vol. II, Practice and techniques, Philadelphia, 1966, J. B. Lippincott Co.

Schwartz, A. M., and Gratzinger, M.: Removable orthodontic appliances, Philadelphia, 1966, W. B. Saunders Co.

Scopp, I. W., and Bien, S. M.: Principles of correction of simple malocclusion in the treatment of periodontal disease, J. Periodontol. **23:**135, 1952.

Shapiro, M.: Orthodontic procedures in the care of the periodontal patient, J. Periodontol. **27:**7, 1956.

Shepard, E. E.: Technique and treatment with the twin-wire appliance, St. Louis, 1961, The C. V. Mosby Co.

Sillman, J. H.: Serial study of good occlusion from birth to 12 years of age, Am. J. Orthod. **37:**481, 1951.

Sorrin, S.: Interesting case of orthodontic-periodontic treatment, J. Dent. Med. **10:**182, 1955.

Sternlicht, H. C.: Tooth movement in periodontal disease, Tex. Dent. J. **77:**4, 1959.

Strang, R. H. W., and Thompson, W. M., Jr.: Textbook of orthodontia, Philadelphia, 1958, Lea & Febiger.

Straub, W.: Malfunction of the tongue, Am. J. Orthod. **48:**426, 1962.

Straub, W. J., and Peterson, L. N.: Combined periodontic and adult orthodontic therapy, Acad. Rev. **6:**90, 1958.

Subtelny, J. D., and Subtelny, J. D.: Malocclusion, speech and deglutition, Am. J. Orthod. **8:**790, 1962.

Sved, A.: Growth of the jaws and the etiology of malocclusion, Int. J. Orthod. **22:**218, 581, 1936.

Tarpley, B. W.: Technique and treatment with the labio-lingual appliance, St. Louis, 1961, The C. V. Mosby Co.

Tulley, W. J., and Campbell, A. C.: A manual of practical orthodontics, ed. 2, London, 1965, John Wright & Sons, Ltd.

Vanarsdall, R. L.: Uprighting the inclined mandibular molar in preparation for restorative treatment, Continuing Dental Education Series, vol. 1, no. 2, Philadelphia, October 1977, University of Pennsylvania Press.

Weinmann, J. P.: Bone changes related to eruption of teeth, Angle Orthod. **11:**83, 1941.

White, T. C., Gardiner, J. H., and Leighton, B. C.: Orthodontics for dental students, ed. 2, St. Louis, 1967, Warren H. Green, Inc.

Wilson, W. L.: A critical analysis of orthodontic concepts and objectives, Am. J. Orthod. **43:**891, 1957.

22 Drugs in periodontal therapy

It is impossible to conduct a practice of periodontics at the highest professional level without a considerable knowledge of clinical pharmacology. Although drugs are seldom curative in treatment of periodontal disease, they represent important adjunctive measures.

The periodontist, or for that matter any dentist, has two major areas of concern in drug use. *First,* he must be sufficiently knowledgeable about the drugs he uses or prescribes to ensure their safest and most effective use. *Second,* he must realize that many of his patients are taking drugs on medical prescription or by self-medication. He should know what agents each patient is using and how they are modifying the patient's responses and possibly imposing changes in the handling and treatment of the case. Although the latter concern is of great importance, it is beyond the scope and intent of this chapter to consider *all* drug groups. The discussion in this chapter will be limited to drugs actually used or prescribed by the periodontist. More complete reference texts should be consulted for the coverage of additional drug groups and a greater in-depth consideration of all drugs (DiPalma, 1971; Goth, 1978; Holroyd, 1978).

The drugs most frequently employed by the periodontist are those that are effective in the management of infection, pain, and anxiety. These agents (antibiotics, analgesics, and sedatives) will be discussed from the standpoint of their indications, special problems, and specific clinical pharmacology. Other pharmaceutical preparations that will also be discussed include muscle relaxants, postoperative dressings, mouthwashes, and desensitizing agents.

ANTIBIOTICS

Antibiotics are not innocuous drugs. Their use should be justified on the basis of a clearly established need, and they should not be substituted for adequate local treatment. Indications for the use of antibiotics in periodontics can be categorized as *prophylactic* and *therapeutic* and will be discussed on that basis.

Prophylactic indications

The only unquestionable prophylactic indication for antibacterial agents in the practice of periodontics is in the prevention of subacute bacterial endocarditis (SABE) (AHA, 1977). However, the use of antibiotics to prevent postoperative infections, enhance surgical results, and reduce postoperative discomfort has been recommended and will be discussed.

Prophylaxis against SABE. It is well known that antibiotic prophylaxis is needed to prevent SABE in patients with rheumatic or congenital heart disease who are to experience procedures likely to precipitate a bacteremia. The current recommendations of the American Heart Association (1977) are presented in the boxed material.

The AHA (1977) states that this regimen should be instituted for *any procedure that causes bleeding.* Obviously, then, prophylaxis is indicated in cases of surgery and of scaling and curettage and even in most cases of polishing by rubber cup and heavy probing of pockets. How about the 1-week postoperative change of surgical dressings? In most cases, I do not believe antibiotic prophylaxis is necessary for dressing changes when the procedure was not extensive, healing has been normal, and gentle removal and replacement of a dressing can be attained. However, if in doubt, cover.

Prevention of postoperative infection. Since the beginning of antibiotic therapy, clinicians have attempted, with a basis of considerable logic, to prevent postoperative infections by administer-

PHARMACOLOGIC PROPHYLAXIS AGAINST BACTERIAL ENDOCARDITIS*

Regimen A or B should be used in cases of rheumatic or acquired valvular heart disease, most congenital heart disease, idiopathic hypertrophic subaortic stenosis, and mitral valve prolapse syndrome with mitral insufficiency. Only Regimen B should be used in cases of patients with prosthetic heart valves.

REGIMEN A

Parenteral/Oral

Adults: 1,000,000 units crystalline penicillin G *mixed with* 600,000 units procaine penicillin G given IM, 30-60 minutes prior to dental procedure. This to be followed by 500 mg penicillin V q6h for 8 doses.

Children†: 30,000 units/kg aqueous cystalline penicillin G mixed with 600,000 unts procaine pencillin G given IM, 30-60 minutes prior to dental procedure. This to be followed by 500 mg penicillin V (250 mg for children under 60 lbs) q6h for 8 doses.

Or

Oral

Adults and children over 60 lbs: 2 Gm penicillin V, 30-60 minutes prior to procedure followed by 500 mg q6h for 8 doses.

Children under 60 lbs†: 1 Gm penicillin V, 30-60 minutes prior to procedure, followed by 250 mg q6h for 8 doses.

For patients allergic to penicillin

Use Vancomycin (see Regimen B).

Or

Adults: 1 Gm erythromycin 90-120 minutes prior to procedure followed by 500 mg q6h for 8 doses.

Children†: 20 mg/kg erythromycin 90-120 minutes prior to procedure followed by 10 mg/kg every 6 hours for 8 doses.

REGIMEN B

Adults: Same as parenteral/oral schedule Regimen A *plus* 1 Gm streptomycin IM when parenteral penicillin given.

Children†: Same as parenteral/oral schedule Regimen A *plus* 20 mg/kg streptomycin IM when parenteral penicillin given.

For patients allergic to penicillin

Adults: 1 Gm vancomycin IV over 30-60 minutes starting 30-60 minutes prior to procedure. This to be followed by 500 mg erythromycin q6h for 8 doses.

Children†: 20 mg/kg vancomycin IV over 30-60 minutes (total dose should not exceed 44 mg/kg/24 hrs) 30-60 minutes prior to procedure. This to be followed by 10 mg/kg erythromycin q6h for 8 doses.

*Lecture Guide prepared by Holroyd from a statement by the Committee on Prevention of Rheumatic Fever and Bacterial Endocarditis of the American Heart Association, Circulation **56:**139A, July, 1977. For more complete coverage of this subject one should read the entire AHA statement.

†Doses for children should not exceed recommendations for adults for a single dose or for a 24-hour period.

ing antibiotics prophylactically. Over the years many types of surgery have been routinely "covered" by antibiotics with the hope of reducing the incidence of postoperative infections. There have been a number of attempts to evaluate the effectiveness of this approach. Karl and co-workers (1966) conducted a well-controlled, double-blind study. They observed 150 cases of a similar type of surgery in which half the patients in the study received an antibiotic and half received a placebo. A wound infection rate of 18.5% was observed in patients receiving antibiotics prophylactically and of 12.9% in the control, or placebo, group. Johnstone (1963) studied the prophylactic use of antibiotics in over 1,000 cases of general surgery and reported that "prophylactic antibiotics not only failed to prevent, but also were in fact associated with an increase in the infections of all types." These results are typical of numerous medical studies.*

Paterson and co-workers (1970) evaluated antibiotic prophylaxis in 488 cases of oral and maxillofacial surgery. They found that patients treated prophylactically with antibiotics had an overall postoperative infection rate of 15.38%, whereas those receiving no antibiotics had an infection rate of 9.9%. Although the basis for selecting patients to receive or not to receive antibiotics was unclear, this study certainly tends to be consistent with reports in the medical literature. Curran and co-workers (1974) observed 133 cases of bone-impacted lower third molar extractions in 68 patients. Half the cases received antibiotics prophylactically. In the group given antibiotics, 15.1% of the patients and 7.8% of the sockets became infected. In the group *not* receiving antibiotics, 14.3% of the patients and 8.7% of the sockets became infected. There was no statistical difference between the groups. The authors concluded that "the use of prophylactic antibiotics in third molar surgery is unnecessary unless specific systemic factors are present."

I have previously summarized the subject of prophylactic antibiotics in the control of postoperative infections in regard to periodontal surgery as follows:

Most patients who undergo periodontal surgery are not going to develop a postoperative infection. Infections that do evolve might have been prevented by prophylactic antibiotics if the invading organism was susceptible to the particular drug selected. It is apparent from medical studies that some individuals who would not have developed a postoperative infection may do so if prophylactic antibiotics are used. The mechanism of this may be related to alterations in the normal flora which were induced by the antibiotic. Thus, in the final analysis, one must balance the infections he prevents with antibiotics against the infections he causes with antibiotics. If the medical literature on this subject accurately reflects the situation in periodontal surgery, the gains and losses in using antibiotics to prevent postsurgical infection are

approximately equal. One's capacity to gain more than he loses from using antibiotics to prevent postsurgical infections is likely to be proportional to his ability to predict the likelihood of a postoperative infection in a particular case. [Holroyd, 1971]

Enhancement of surgical results. Many practitioners prescribe antibiotics routinely in osseous graft cases and when they attempt to establish a new attachment at a more coronal level. Although some logic underlies such use, no significant research evidence is available to indicate that antibiotics are necessary or even helpful in obtaining the desired result (Holroyd, 1971). Stahl (1962) reported that rats receiving antibiotics showed more crestal bone repair than did control rats in the early stages of healing; he stated, however, that "the beneficial potential of these drugs did not, under our experimental conditions, influence ultimate repair levels." In another study Stahl (1963a) concluded that antibiotics enhance connective tissue reattachment in rats, but he later reported that the benefits noted had been the result of an effect of the antibiotic on pulpal repair rather than on the reattachment potential of the soft tissue (1936b). Stahl (1964) has also observed that protein-deprived rats treated with antibiotics following gingival wounds exhibited more crestal osteogenesis than did a control group. However, the superimposition of a nutritional deficiency makes it difficult to apply these results to the clinical use of antibiotics. Schafer and co-workers (1964) have also reported a favorable effect of antibiotics on healing following osseous contouring in dogs.

Although the foregoing authors have made significant contributions to the understanding of the effect of antibiotics on wound healing, their findings cannot be considered adequate justification for the use of antibiotics to enhance the results of periodontal surgery. In this area the use of antibiotics continues to be highly speculative.

Reduction of postoperative discomfort. Ariaudo (1969) has reported the results of a double-blind study which indicated that lincomycin (Lincocin), 500 mg every 6 hours for 2 days prior to and 4 days after surgery, reduced the incidence of malaise, edema, necrosis, and pain following periodontal surgery. However, DeMarco and Kluth (1972) in a similar double-blind study using clindamycin (Cleocin), 150 mg 1 hour prior to surgery and every 6 hours thereafter for 5 days, found no advantage to this use of antibiotics. Consequently, we must conclude that there is no

---

*Cole and Bernard, 1961; Editorial, 1966; Hogman and Sahlin, 1957; King, 1961; Lachdjiam and Compere, 1957; Laylor, 1960; Marshall, 1959; McKittrick and Wheelock, 1954; Petersdorf and Merchant, 1959; Petersdorf et al., 1957; Pulaski, 1961; Weinstein, 1955.

adequate evidence at this time to justify the use of antibiotics to reduce postoperative discomfort.

Therapeutic indications

Therapeutic indications presuppose an existing infection. The clinician must accept the fact that not all infections require antibiotic therapy. The decision to use antibiotics therapeutically must be based on a consideration of both the nature of the infection and the general health of the patient. I have previously provided the following guidelines:

1. It is obvious that severe, acute, rapidly spreading infections should be treated with antibiotics. The less severe, localized infections where drainage can be established or where other local treatment is highly effective will, in most cases, especially in the healthy patient, be resolved without the use of antibiotics.

2. Evidences of systemic involvement, such as an elevated temperature, general malaise, and lymphadenopathy, frequently indicate a need for antibiotics.

3. Infections in patients with certain systemic conditions that predispose to the spread of infection generally require antibiotic therapy. Examples of such systemic conditions are (a) uncontrolled diabetes, (b) leukemia, (c) agranulocytosis, (d) aplastic anemia, (e) Addison's disease, (f) depressed natural defense mechanisms as a result of therapy with adrenal steroids and immunosuppressive and cytotoxic drugs, (g) history of rheumatic or congenital heart disease, and (h) debilitation by age or disease.

4. Infections involving the region of the upper lip and nose can be serious because of venous drainage into the cavernous sinus. Antibiotics may be advantageous for combating infections in this region that would otherwise not require antibiotic therapy.

5. The basis of a decision to use or not to use antibiotics [in treating an active infection] is essentially a balancing of those factors that tend to require their use against those factors that tend to obviate the need for them. [Holroyd, 1971]

Antibiotics of choice

In certain oral infections, such as acute necrotizing ulcerative gingivitis (ANUG), the etiologic agent is relatively predictable on the basis of the diagnosis. Penicillin, erythromycin, and the tetracyclines are all effective against ANUG. In this case the antibiotic of choice (Holroyd, 1978, 1971) is selected on the basis of the diagnosis. In preventing subacute bacterial endocarditis we are primarily concerned with *Streptococcus viri-*

dans. Penicillin is the antibiotic of choice, since it is highly effective against that organism. In this case the drug is selected on the basis of what is known about the infection. Unfortunately, periodontists must treat many infections in which the etiologic agents cannot be accurately predicted on the basis of the symptomatology. Ideally in these cases material from the infection would be cultured and sensitivity tests carried out to determine which antibiotic is effective against the specific etiologic agent. However, for practical reasons, periodontal infections are usually treated without the benefit of sensitivity tests. Most bacteria that are causative agents in periodontal abscesses and postoperative infections are grampositive organisms and within the antibacterial spectra of the penicillins, the cephalosporins, erythromycin, and to some extent the tetracyclines. Sensitivity tests will show that any of these antibiotics will be effective on the culture plate against most bacteria sampled from periodontal infections. Consequently, when an antibiotic is indicated, the periodontist is justified in starting treatment with one of these drugs before obtaining the results of the sensitivity tests. The primary advantage of sensitivity tests is that they will let the clinician know within 12 to 24 hours if he is dealing with a pathogen that is insensitive to the most commonly effective drugs.

When an antibiotic is selected without the benefit of sensitivity tests the choice is essentially between a penicillin, a cephalosporin, erythromycin, and possibly a tetracycline. The selection of a specific antibacterial agent should be based on a knowledge of the pharmacology of the individual drugs. The following brief resume summarizes the most important clinical pharmacology of the antibiotics of primary concern to the periodontist. More complete sources should be consulted for an expansion of this discussion.

The penicillins. The selection of penicillin (Holroyd, 1978, 1973, 1971, 1970) as the drug of choice in oral infections should be based on a consideration of the points discussed in the following paragraphs. This discussion pertains more completely to the most frequently prescribed penicillins—penicillin G and phenoxymethylpenicillin (penicillin V)—than to the newer, semisynthetic penicillins. Special considerations and exceptions relative to the newer drugs will be discussed separately.

Although the penicillins have a relatively narrow antibacterial spectrum, they will "hit" most oral infections. Their great bactericidal potency is of especial value in life-threatening infections. (A bactericidal antibiotic, as opposed to a bacteriostatic agent, is capable of killing pathogenic organisms without the assistance of the body's defense mechanisms. This factor may be all important if the patient's reserves of strength are depleted.) The penicillins are also extremely important in severe infection because they are almost entirely nontoxic, and therefore extremely high blood levels can be used with minimal hazard. (This is not completely true of the semisynthetic penicillins, which will be considered more specifically later.) No other antibiotics have such a low toxicity. Thus the penicillins must be considered the preferred drugs for the treatment of most severe oral infections (AHA, 1977).

Unfortunately, bacteria readily develop resistance to the penicillins. In addition the penicillins are perhaps the most allergenic drugs currently being administered. The more the penicillins are used indiscriminately, the larger will be the number of pathogens that develop resistance to the drugs and the number of persons who are allergic to them. The poor judgment shown in using these life-saving antibiotics when they are not specifically indicated should be obvious (AHA, 1977).

I have concluded that penicillin should be used "(1) in severe infections, (2) when body defenses are impaired, (3) where drug toxicity is particularly significant, as in infants, small children, the elderly, the debilitated, pregnant women, and those with liver and kidney impairment. Special consideration of an alternative to penicillin should be exercised for patients who exhibit a tendency to become sensitized readily, such as those with asthma and multiple allergies. The above presupposes, of course, that the infective agent is within the antibacterial spectrum of penicillin." [Holroyd, 1973]

The semisynthetic penicillins, methicillin, oxacillin, nafcillin, cloxacillin, and dicloxacillin, are penicillinase resistant. Consequently, they are specifically useful against penicillinase-producing staphylococci that would not be responsive to the other penicillins. They are more toxic than the other penicillins and will generally be less effective than penicillin G against nonpenicillinase-producing bacteria. These drugs should be reserved for use against penicillinase-producing bacteria and therefore should not be used unless the clinician has a definite indication, as by antibiotic sensitivity tests, that a specific need exists for a penicillinase-resistant drug.

Carbenicillin is a semisynthetic penicillin that is not penicillinase resistant. Its special clinical use, for which it should be reserved, is in the treatment of infections by *Pseudomonas aeruginosa* and sensitive strains of *Proteus*.

Ampicillin, another semisynthetic penicillin, is not penicillinase resistant, but has a slightly broader spectrum that includes a few gram-negative bacteria, notably *Hemophilus influenzae*. The involvement of gram-negative bacteria in dental infections appears to be increasing, and sensitivity tests may indicate a need for ampicillin in some cases. Ampicillin should not be considered as either a routine substitute for penicillin G or V or a broad-spectrum drug. Its use in dentistry should be based on specific evidence that it will be effective when penicillin G or V is ineffective.

The cephalosporins. The cephalosporins are potent bactericidal agents against many gram-positive and gram-negative pathogens, including penicillinase-producing staphylococci. Their basic chemical structure is similar to that of penicillin, and they probably have a similar mechanism of action. The cephalosporins are usually well tolerated. Most adverse reactions to oral forms are gastrointestinal in nature; hematologic, renal, and hepatic tolerances are quite favorable. Although many patients allergic to penicillin are also allergic to the cephalosporins, these drugs should be considered excellent substitutes when penicillin cannot be used and a bactericidal potency is particularly desirable.

Erythromycin. Erythromycin has a slightly broader antibacterial spectrum than penicillin. Recent studies have shown it to be effective against a higher percentage of oral infections than penicillin. Some of this increased effectiveness is due to its activity against some staphylococci that are resistant to penicillin.

Erythromycin is essentially a bacteriostatic drug, but it may be bactericidal at some concentrations against certain bacteria. Bacterial resistance to erythromycin develops, but not as frequently nor as quickly as with penicillin. Allergy has not presented a problem. Adverse reactions to erythromycin are usually mild. Side effects are most frequently gastrointestinal in nature and include abdominal cramps, nausea, vomiting, and diarrhea. Allergic reactions are not frequently seen, and adverse effects on the hematologic and renal tissues have not been observed. Hepatic impairment has occasionally been associated with the use of erythromycin estolate (Ilosone). Symptoms indicative of intrahepatic cholestasis have been observed after a few days of treatment but usually have developed only after 1 or 2 weeks of use. Erythromycin should be considered as the antibiotic of choice for oral infections when a potent bactericidal effect is not necessary, especially in the relatively healthy patient.

The tetracyclines. Although the tetracyclines are broad-spectrum antibiotics, they will "hit" a significantly smaller percentage of oral infections than the penicillins, cephalosporins, and erythromycin. The tetracyclines are strictly bacteriostatic drugs. Bacterial resistance develops relatively slowly but is being seen clinically with greater frequency. Allergy has not presented a significant problem.

Serious adverse effects to the tetracyclines are seldom observed. Gastrointestinal upset, stomatitis, glossitis, xerostomia, and candidiasis are generally related to local irritation and to alteration in the oral, gastric, and enteric flora. These reactions usually disappear quickly when the drug is withdrawn. The incidence of gastrointestinal disturbances can be reduced by taking the drug with a small amount of food in the stomach. However, a full meal, especially one that includes calcium products, would significantly reduce their absorption. Photosensitivity reactions are infrequent but may occur. The tetracyclines have a definite potential for liver damage, especially at high doses and in pregnant women. Their potential for kidney damage contraindicates their use in patients with renal impairment. The tetracyclines become incorporated in calcifying tissues and may produce a permanent discoloration of teeth and enamel hypoplasia if administered during the last trimester of pregnancy or early childhood. Consequently, the tetracyclines should not be used during pregnancy or early childhood unless other drugs with less adverse effects are not likely to be effective.

Lincomycin and clindamycin. Although lincomycin and clindamycin should be effective against most oral infections, the high incidence of severe diarrhea and serious pseudomembranous colitis associated with these drugs should restrict their use in oral infections to cases in which sensitivity tests have indicated that other, less toxic, drugs would not be effective.

ANALGESICS

The first considerations in pain control are to prevent discomfort by proper local procedures and to eliminate the *cause* of pain already present. Analgesic drugs (Holroyd, 1978, 1973) are only secondary to these efforts.

The selection of an analgesic for any particular case is essentially a matter of matching the potency of an analgesic against the severity of the pain present or anticipated. This rather simplistic concept becomes complicated when you consider the importance of the emotions on pain and pain control. Although it is beyond the intent of this chapter to discuss the "psychology of pain control," certain points should be mentioned with a view toward initiating further thought and consideration by the reader.

One must never lose sight of the fact that the psychologic makeup of a patient is an extremely important factor in the selection of the proper analgesic. Healthy patients have approximately the same capacity to perceive pain, but their reaction to what they perceive may vary widely. Discomfort that requires no analgesic in one patient may require aspirin or acetaminophen in another and even codeine, meperidine, or morphine in others. Thus knowing one's patients is of considerable value. Predisposition toward a greater reaction to pain has been said to be associated with emotional instability, fatigue, youth, the female sex, fear, and apprehension (Monheim, 1969). Fear and apprehension are of particular significance and are the basis of the potentiation of analgesics by sedatives.

The clinician should understand the psychologic aspects of pain control and take advantage of them whenever possible. Many individuals will obtain greater benefit from an analgesic if they expect it to be effective or if they have found it to be effective in the past. The clinician should assert his confidence that a particular agent will give prompt relief. The confidence the patient has in his dentist will then be conveyed to the analgesic. Similarly, it may not be wise to belittle an over-the-counter analgesic in which the patient has established confidence.

A range of analgesic potencies will be required in alleviating discomfort from periodontal infections and temporomandibular joint dysfunction as well as varying degrees of postoperative discomfort, but proper local treatment will usually allow complete pain control with mild analgesics such as aspirin or acetaminophen. Only in extensive cases, where local treatment is restricted or when the patient is hypersensitive to discomfort, are more potent analgesics required. Routine postoperative discomfort often requires no analgesic, and when one is required, aspirin or acetaminophen is frequently adequate. Only in extensive osseous cases, where there has been heavy trauma, where wound closure has been inadequate, or again where the patient is hypersensitive to discomfort, will more potent agents be required.

Aspirin. Most pain of periodontal origin can be effectively controlled by aspirin alone (650 mg [10 grains] every 4 hours). Analgesic, antipyretic, and anti-inflammatory effects are provided. Many practitioners are too quick to go to more potent drugs with greater toxicity and more troublesome side effects and could make a greater use of aspirin alone. However, the clinician should be aware of the adverse effects of this drug. Aspirin causes gastric irritation, especially if taken on an empty stomach, and should be avoided in people with ulcers or other gastrointestinal difficulties. Many individuals are allergic to aspirin and obviously should not be given this drug or any combination product containing it. Aspirin is known to prolong prothrombin time and inhibit platelet function. However, this is not likely to be clinically significant in the practice of periodontics except in patients with peptic ulcer, hemorrhagic disease, or those on anticoagulant therapy. The practitioner should also be aware of the clinically important aspirin drug interactions that have been demonstrated, notably those with the coumarin anticoagulants and the sulfonylurea hypoglycemics. The clinician should also recognize the danger of aspirin overdose in infants and children.

Acetaminophen. When aspirin should be avoided, acetaminophen (Tylenol, Tempra, Nebs) is an excellent substitute. In the same dosage as aspirin (650 mg [10 grains] every 4 hours) this drug equals aspirin in analgesic and antipyretic potency. At this time acetaminophen is not believed to have anti-inflammatory effects. It is not known whether the absence of this effect is important in situations with a significant inflammatory component, as in most dental cases requiring an analgesic. Although acetaminophen appears to have the same drug interactions as noted earlier for aspirin, it does not have the adverse gastrointestinal effects or the antiprothrombin and antiplatelet effects of aspirin. Acetaminophen should also be safe in cases of aspirin allergy.

Combination products. When aspirin and acetaminophen are thought to be inadequate, certain combination products should be considered. Many practitioners employ the propoxyphene (Darvon) or ethoheptazine (Zactane) preparations. Neither of these drugs provides an antipyretic effect when used alone, and their analgesic potencies are quite vague. Propoxyphene hydrochloride is probably superior to a placebo in doses of 65 mg or more,

but is of questionable efficacy in doses under 65 mg (Beaver, 1965). Undoubtedly, propoxyphene adds something to the aspirin with which it is ordinarily used, especially when a suggestible patient allows the attainment of a significant placebo effect. The psychologic value of prescribing propoxyphene may considerably enhance the drug's effectiveness. The new preparations, propoxyphene napsylate tablets and suspension, offer no potency advantage over the older propoxyphene HCl in capsule form. The potency of ethoheptazine is more vague than that of propoxyphene, but ethoheptazine probably shares propoxyphene's "placebo advantage" when used with aspirin. Although propoxyphene and ethoheptazine may cause some gastrointestinal distress, they are quite safe in therapeutic doses. One should note, however, that propoxyphene is highly subject to abuse, and numerous overdose deaths have occurred.

The most definitive method of increasing the analgesic potency of aspirin or acetaminophen is to prescribe these drugs with the narcotic codeine, either separately or in one of the numerous combination products available. The usual preparations include 325 mg aspirin or acetaminophen with 30 mg codeine per tablet and an adult dosage of 1 to 2 tablets every 4 to 8 hours. When prescribing codeine the practitioner should be aware of the numerous side effects that are associated with its use at even the 30 to 60 mg dose level, namely, sedation, emesis, nausea, and constipation.

Other combination products increase analgesic potency by taking advantage of the fact that a calm, sedated patient is less reactive to pain. Various products, such as Fiorinal, add a barbiturate to an analgesic combination. Prescribing one of these combinations or a sedative or minor tranquilizer with a separate analgesic agent may be especially helpful in the highly anxious patient or in one who is likely to have difficulty in adjusting to the wearing of a periodontal surgical dressing.

Whenever the practitioner contemplates the use of a multiple entity preparation, he should be aware of the therapeutic effects and adverse potentials of each ingredient. These effects and potentialities must be considered additive and in some cases may be potentiating.

Analgesics for severe pain. In cases of severe pain it will be necessary to go to the drugs listed in Table 16. These agents are potent, provide sedation, and can be used parenterally to obtain a rapid onset. The adverse effects of these drugs are highly significant and should be familiar to

Table 16. Potent analgesics*

Drug	Preparations	Route	Usual adult dose (mg)
Pentazocine lactate (Talwin)	30 mg/ml	Intramuscular, subcutaneous, intravenous	30
Pentazocine HCl	50 mg tablets	Oral	50 to 100
Meperidine HCl	25, 50, 75, and 100 mg/ml	Intramuscular, subcutaneous	50 to 100
	50 and 100 mg tablets	Oral	50 to 100
	50 mg/5 ml elixir	Oral	50 to 100
Morphine sulfate	8, 10, 15, and 30 mg/ml	Subcutaneous	10 to 15

*From Holroyd, S. V.: Control of pain and infection, Dent. Clin. North Am. **17**:417-427, 1973.

the clinician before he prescribes any of them.

The more common adverse effects of these drugs include nausea, vomiting, constipation, dizziness, and headache. All are subject to abuse, and high doses may significantly depress respiration and increase intracranial pressure. Pentazocine has also been associated with rather unusual effects, including hallucinations, delusions, and visual disturbances. With these as with other drugs the clinician should consult more complete reference texts to ensure that he is totally familiar with their adverse effects.

SEDATIVES

I have previously presented the following introduction to the use of sedatives in dental practice in *Clinical Pharmacology in Dental Practice.*

Patients approach dentistry with varying degrees of anxiety. Some are completely relaxed even when anticipating rather extensive procedures. On the other hand, some are highly apprehensive about even the simplest procedure. Most lie somewhere between these extremes. We owe to our patients the most pleasant experience possible within the limits of safety. Inducing relaxation in a patient allows the accomplishment of more fruitful work with less trauma to both patient and dentist.

Working with a relaxed patient is not only a matter of pleasantness and convenience; with some patients it may be a matter of life and death. McCarthy (1971) has recently pointed out that sudden unexpected death is not uncommon, occurs even in people who appear to be in good health, and can be brought on by emotional stress. He points out that this is strong justification for adequate pain-anxiety control for dental patients. In view of the fact that the well-known sedative-hypnotic drugs are not very dangerous, their use may be beneficial to both patient and dentist in many cases.

Prior to a consideration of the sedative-hypnotic drugs, certain generalizations should be made. Although any precise degree of sedation can be obtained by intravenous titration, this requires special training and experience on the part of the practitioner. Since few dentists are so experienced, oral sedation is currently the principal method of reducing anxiety in dental patients. This presents a most fundamental problem: sedation by orally administered drugs will not provide consistent or highly predictable results. Many factors influence the blood level obtained from orally administered drugs. Additionally, variations are seen in patient responses to similar blood levels. Because of the variations and lack of predictability from oral sedation, many practitioners continually switch from drug to drug hoping to find the ultimate agent or dose that will provide ideal sedation. Neither the ultimate drug nor the dosage is there, so I suggest that they discontinue their search. The greatest consistency will be found in staying with one or two drugs, knowing these well, and knowing how they affect different types of patients. In the long run, this will yield greater benefits than "jumping" from drug to drug.

It is not the intent of this chapter to review all available sedative drugs. Only those that appear to have special application in the practice of periodontics will be discussed.

Barbiturates. The barbiturates are effective, safe, available in numerous forms that are convenient to administer, and can provide either short or prolonged durations of action. They have been used in great quantities over many years; consequently, problems associated with their use are well known. The most appropriate barbiturates for preoperative sedation in the practice of periodontics are the short-acting barbiturates, secobarbital (Seconal) and pentobarbital (Nembutal). Preparations for oral, rectal, intramuscular, and intravenous administration are available. An adult oral dose of 100 to 200 mg taken 30 to 60 minutes before the appointment should provide sedation in most patients for 2 to 3 hours.

Sedative and hypnotic doses of the barbiturates are quite safe. However, central nervous system depression may be exaggerated in elderly and debilitated patients and in those with impaired liver or kidney function. The practitioner should also remember that the sedative effects of the barbiturates are additive to sedation produced by alcohol and other central nervous system depressants. This fact and its significance should be made quite clear to the patient.

Although some individuals are allergic to these drugs, serious reactions are rare. Acute poisoning with barbiturates accounts for several hundred deaths annually in the United States. Some of these overdose cases are intentional (suicide) and some are accidental. Consequently, no more of a drug than necessary should be prescribed at any one time. The clinician should also remember that the chronic use of barbiturates can lead to habituation and addiction.

Nonbarbiturate sedatives. The nonbarbiturate sedatives, such as chloral hydrate, paraldehyde, ethinamate (Valmid), methaqualone (Quaalude) and many others, provide no special advantage in the practice of periodontics and will not be discussed.

Minor tranquilizers. The minor tranquilizers produce sedation and some degree of muscle relaxation without as much sleepiness as is observed with the barbiturates. They also have a greater safety relative to overdose than do the barbiturates. In many instances they will provide adequate oral sedation for anxious periodontal patients. It is more effective to start patients on these agents the night before the dental appointment to ensure a good night's rest and to obtain an early blood level.

Meprobamate (Miltown, Equanil) in the adult dosage (400 mg every 6 hours) will provide mild sedation and muscle relaxation in most individuals. Although meprobamate is an extremely safe drug, its long-term use can lead to addiction, and recently a possible teratogenic effect has been suggested. Hypotensive episodes have also been seen in the elderly.

Either chlordiazepoxide (Librium) or diazepam (Valium) will provide mild sedation and muscle relaxation in most individuals when taken in the recommended adult dosage (5 or 10 mg three or four times daily for chlordiazepoxide; 2 to 10 mg two to four times daily for diazepam). Both are extremely safe drugs. However, their long-term use can lead to addiction, and recently possible teratogenic effects have been suggested for both drugs. The principal differences between these drugs are that diazepam appears to have a greater margin of safety relative to overdose and a slightly shorter duration of action and is a more potent muscle relaxant.

MUSCLE RELAXANTS

Centrally acting skeletal muscle relaxants are used in the practice of periodontics to relieve muscle spasm of local origin. A large number of drugs are available. As noted earlier the minor tranquilizers meprobamate, chlordiazepoxide, and diazepam can be used as muscle relaxants. Other effective agents include carisoprodol (Rela, Soma), chlorzoxazone (Paraflex), mephenesin, orphenadrine citrate (Norflex), and methocarbamol (Robaxin). Since pain frequently accompanies muscle spasm, a number of muscle relaxants are available in combination with analgesics. These include a combination of orphenadrine citrate, aspirin, phenacetin, and caffeine (Norgesic) and of chlorzoxazone and acetaminophen (Parafon Forte).

In view of the fact that in the practice of periodontics there is no compelling reason to select one of these agents over the other, dosage and adverse effects will not be discussed. The clinician who selects a specific muscle relaxant should apprise himself of the dosage rates and the adverse potentialities of the drug selected.

POSTOPERATIVE DRESSINGS

Periodontal postoperative dressings are placed over surgical sites to protect the wound area, increase patient comfort, maintain a relatively clean area to abet healing, and provide some degree of bacteriostasis and hemostasis. A periodontal dressing should be (1) soft and plastic after mixing (to allow for easy placement), (2) bland, smooth, and nonirritating (so as not to irritate the tongue or oral mucosa), (3) nonabsorptive (to prevent absorption of liquid and any other materials), and (4) resistant to pressure without fracturing and becoming loose.

Most periodontal dressings consist of a powder and liquid that are mixed into a puttylike consistency. The powder usually consists primarily of zinc oxide with a powdered rosin, tannic acid, and kaolin. Shredded asbestos was once a common ingredient but should no longer be used because of recent evidence of its respiratory dangers to both patient and doctor. The liquid is essentially eugenol with or without other substances such as peanut, cottonseed, or olive oil. These zinc oxide–eugenol packs are ready for use immediately after mixing but may also be wrapped in foil and frozen for days or weeks of storage. Most dressings become firm 30 to 45 minutes after being placed in the mouth.

Some people believe eugenol to be sufficiently irritating to the tissues to recommend the use of noneugenol dressings, especially on exposed bone. Although eugenol-containing packs do not appear to present a significant problem, two noneugenol dressings that are available include the following ingredients:

I. Noneugenol, fat-bacitracin dressing (Baer et al., 1960)
  A. Powder
    1. Zinc oxide
    2. Rosin
    3. Zinc bacitracin
  B. Ointment
    1. Zinc oxide
    2. Hydrogenated fat
II. Coe-Pak (Eisenbrand, 1962)
  A. Tube 1 paste
    1. Metallic oxides
    2. Lorothidol
  B. Tube 2 paste
    1. Nonionizing carboxylic acids
    2. Chlorothymol

The use of bacitracin in periodontal dressings appears to allow a cleaner postoperative field (Baer et al., 1958). The clinical significance of this, if any, is not clear. Tetracyclines have also been evaluated as constituents of periodontal dressings (Fraleigh, 1956). The tetracyclines offered no advantage but were associated with the appearance of ulcerations and tissue discomfort in a number of the subjects. With the exception of bacitracin the use of antibiotics in periodontal dressings is not recommended.

MOUTHWASHES

The mouthwash is a valuable agent for flushing the mouth and teeth mechanically and for helping to dislodge debris or to irrigate inaccessible areas. Normal saline solution is as effective in this regard as any other mouthwash. Some mouthwashes with flavoring agents may be desirable in patients who consider flavor important. Other mouthwashes, such as Cepacol, provide both flavor and a topical local anesthetic effect, which may be desirable when an obtundent action would be particularly helpful.

Over the past few years a great deal of effort has been directed toward the use of oral rinses to prevent or destroy bacterial plauqe. There is no question that the toothbrush, dental floss, and much motivation are not the ultimate plaque control measures. Undoubtedly the pharmacologic approach to plaque control offers the most complete answer. Parsons has reviewed the use of antibiotics, enzymes, chlorhexidine, dextran, quaternary ammonium compounds, phosphoamidase, organic and inorganic fluorides, and commercial mouthwashes. He concludes: "At present there is no chemotherapeutic agent that can be safely administered for long-term control of bacterial plaque. Antibiotic compounds can be considered only for short-term plaque control due to their systemic side effects and limited spectrum of activity. All other compounds are limited in their usefulness due to (1) local or systemic side effects that are unpleasant or toxic, (2) lack of clinically significant effectiveness, and (3) inadequate experimental evidence." [Parsons, 1947]

DESENSITIZING AGENTS

Hypersensitivity of exposed root surfaces is a common dental complaint. This pain is usually precipitated by mechanical touching of the area, by heat or cold, or by sweet or sour foods. Root hypersensitivity may result from occlusal trauma or may be caused by the irritation of organic matter in exposed dentinal tubules. When occlusal trauma is the cause, occlusal adjustment is the treatment. The treatment of sensitivities due to the irritation of exposed dentinal tubules must begin with the removal of plaque and other irritants in the area. If the establishment of excellent plaque control does not alleviate the discomfort, other efforts should be made. A wide variety of agents have been applied to sensitive roots. I have previously discussed some of the numerous agents that have been employed in cases of root hypersensitivity in *Clinical Pharmacology in Dental Practice.*

Glycerin. One of the most simple treatments for root hypersensitivity has been to burnish glycerin into the cleaned and dried sensitive area with a ball burnisher or orangewood stick. The results are not highly predictable, and the mechanism of action is unknown. It is likely that any favorable effects result from the burnishing action rather than from any direct effect of the glycerin.

Sodium fluoride. Various mixtures of sodium fluoride have been applied to hypersensitive root areas. Although results have been neither consistent nor highly impressive, success has been obtained in some cases. There is no evidence that the more exotic mixtures of sodium fluoride are any more effective than straight 2% topical solution applied by cotton swab or placed in pumice for rubber cup application to clean, dry root surfaces.

Stannous fluoride. A number of stannous fluoride mixtures have also been applied to hypersensitive root areas. There is no evidence that the more exotic mixtures of stannous fluoride are any more effective than straight 10% topical solution applied by cotton swab or placed in pumice for rubber cup application to clean, dry root surfaces. The application of a 9% stannous fluoride paste should be equally effective or ineffective.

Adrenal steroids. Bowers and Elliott (1964) evaluated the effectiveness of a prednisolone preparation against root hypersensitivity. They found that one or two applications of the following solution "appeared effective in the treatment of sensitivity due to incisal (occlusal) fractures, extensive occlusal adjustment or odontoplasty, periodontal surgery and post scaling and root planing procedures."

Components	Percentages by weight
p-Chlorophenol	25
Metacresyl acetate (Cresatin)	25
Gum camphor	49
Prednisolone	1

The solution was applied with a cotton pellet to clean, dry sensitive areas. This prednisolone solution deteriorates rapidly and is not likely to be effective after 90 days. Sensitivity resulting from gingival recession was reduced but not so dramatically as in other cases. Although no side effects of the prednisolone solution were observed in this study, an effort should be made to limit systemic absorption by restricting the solution to tooth surface as much as possible.

Prichard (1965) and others have used an ophthalmic solution of prednisolone (Metimyd) successfully. This 0.5% prednisolone solution is applied to clean, dry tooth surfaces. Each milliliter of this ophthalmic solution contains 5 mg of prednisolone acetate, 100 mg of sodium sulfacetamide, and preservatives. It is available in 5 ml bottles. The antibacterial action of sulfacetamide would have no purpose if this solution were used for desensitization. Although no studies are available, it might be equally effective and more rational to eliminate the unnecessary but active ingredient sulfacetamide by using an ophthalmic solution that contains 0.5% of prednisolone as the only active ingredient. Such a solution is available (Optival) in 5 ml bottles.

One should become familiar with the pharmacology and precautions related to adrenal steroids prior to their use. In view of the broad pharmacologic effects of systemically absorbed adrenal steroids, these drugs should not be used for root hypersensitivity unless contact with soft tissues can be minimized. This is not likely to be possible in cases of generalized hypersensitivity.

Home brushing of hypersensitive areas with concentrated saline solutions and 0.5% stannous fluoride have been recommended. The results are not well documented.

Desensitizing toothpastes deserve some discussion. Many practitioners believe that optimal effects occur when office treatment is followed by the use of a desensitizing toothpaste. The degree of usefulness of these pastes is rather vague.

Until further double-blind comparisons of desensitizing dentifrices are available, it is not possible to assess the practical superiority, if any, of special desensitizing dentifrices over regular dentifrices. Unquestionably, improved tooth cleaning is effective against root hypersensitivity regardless of the type of dentifrice used.

REFERENCES

AHA: Prevention of bacterial endocarditis, Circulation **56:** 139A, 1977.

Ariaudo, A. A.: The efficacy of antibiotics in periodontal surgery: a controlled study with lincomycin and placebo in 68 patients, J. Periodontol. **40:**150, 1969.

Baer, P. N., Goldman, H. M., and Scigliano, J.: Studies on a bacitracin periodontal dressing, Oral Surg. **11:**712, 1958.

Baer, P. N., Sumner, C. F., and Scigliano, J.: Studies on a hydrogenated fat–zinc bacitracin periodontal dressing, Oral Surg. **13:**494, 1960.

Beaver, W. T.: Mild analgesics, Am. J. Med. Sci. **250:**577, 1965.

Bowers, G. M., and Elliott, J. R.: Topical use of prednisolone in periodontics, J. Periodontol. **35:**486, 1964.

Cole, W. R., and Bernard, H. R.: A reappraisal of the effects of antimicrobial therapy during the course of appendicitis in children, Am. Surg. **27:**29, 1961.

Curran, J. B., Kennett, S., and Young, A. R.: An assessment of the use of prophylactic antibiotics in third molar surgery, Int. J. Oral Surg. **3:**1, 1974.

DeMarco, J. J., and Kluth, E. V.: The use of Cleocin in post-surgical periodontal patients, J. Periodontol. **43:**381, 1972.

DiPalma, J. R., editor: Drill's pharmacology in medicine, ed. 4, New York, 1971, McGraw-Hill Book Co.

Editorial, N. Engl. J. Med. **275:**335, 1966.

Eisenbrand, G. F.: A method for making an efficient and adherent periodontal pack, Dent. Digest **68:**210, 1962.

Fraleigh, C. M.: An evaluation of topical terramycin in post-gingivectomy pack, J. Periodontol. **27:**201, 1956.

Goth, A.: Medical pharmacology, ed. 9, St. Louis, 1978, The C. V. Mosby Co.

Hogman, C. F., and Sahlin, O.: Infections complicating gastric surgery, Acta Chir. Scand. **112:**271, 1957.

Holroyd, S. V.: Clinical pharmacology in dental practice, ed. 2, St. Louis, 1978, The C. V. Mosby Co.

Holroyd, S. V.: Control of pain and infection, Dent. Clin. North Am. **17:**417, 1973.

Holroyd, S. V.: Antibiotics in the practice of periodontics, J. Periodontol. **42:**586, 1971.

Holroyd, S. V.: Clinical pharmacology of antibiotics of dental importance, Dent. Clin. North Am. **14:**711, 1970.

Johnstone, F. R. C.: An assessment of prophylactic antibiotics in general surgery, Surg. Gynecol. Obstet. **116:**1, 1963.

Karl, R. C., Mertz, J. J., Veith, F. J., and Dineen, P.: Prophylactic antimicrobial drugs in surgery, N. Engl. J. Med. **275:**305, 1966.

King, G. C.: The case against antibiotic prophylaxis in major head and neck surgery, Laryngoscope **71:**647, 1961.

Lachdjiam, M. O., and Compere, E. C.: Postoperative wound infections in orthopedic surgery, Int. Surg. **28:**797, 1957.

Laylor, G. W.: Preventive use of antibiotics in surgery, Br. Med. Bull. **16:**51, 1960.

Marshall, A.: Prophylactic antimicrobial therapy in retropubic prostatectomy, Br. J. Urol. **31:**431, 1959.

McCarthy, F.: Sudden unexpected death in the dental office, J. Am. Dent. Assoc. **83:**1091, 1971.

McKittrick, L. S., and Wheelock, F. C.: The routine use of antibiotics in elective abdominal surgery, Surg. Gynecol. Obstet. **99:**376, 1954.

Monheim, L. M.: Local anesthesia and pain control in dental practice, ed. 4, St. Louis, 1969, The C. V. Mosby Co.

Parsons, J. C.: Chemotherapy of dental plaque—a review, J. Periodontol. **45:**177, 1974.

Paterson, J. A., Cardo, V. A., Jr., and Stratigos, G. T.: An examination of antibiotic prophylaxis in oral and maxillofacial surgery, J. Oral Surg. **28:**753, 1970.

Petersdorf, R. G., Curtin, J. A., Hoeprick, P. D., Peeler, R. N., and Bennett, I. L.: Study of antibiotic prophylaxis in unconscious patients, N. Engl. J. Med. **257:**1001, 1957.

Petersdorf, R. G., and Merchant, R. K.: A study of antibiotic prophylaxis in patients with acute heart failure, N. Engl. J. Med. **265:**565, 1959.

Prichard, J. F.: Advanced periodontal disease, Philadelphia, 1965, W. B. Saunders Co.

Pulaski, E. J.: Antibiotics in surgical cases, Arch. Surg. **82:**545, 1961.

Schafer, T. J., Collings, C. K., Bishop, J. G., and Dorman, H. L.: The effect of antibiotics on healing following osseous contouring in dogs, Periodontics **2:**243, 1964.

Stahl, S. S.: The healing of a gingival wound in protein-deprived, antibiotic-supplemented adult rats, Oral Surg. **17:**443, 1964.

Stahl, S. S.: The influence of antibiotics on the healing of gingival wounds in rats. II. Reattachment potential of soft and calcified tissues, J. Periodontol. **34:**166, 1963a.

Stahl, S. S.: The influence of antibiotics on the healing of gingival wounds in rats. III. The influence of pulpal necrosis on gingival reattachment potential, J. Periodontol. **34:**371, 1963b.

Stahl, S. S.: The influence of antibiotics on the healing of gingival wounds in rats. I. Alveolar bone and soft tissue, J. Periodontol. **33:**261, 1962.

Weinstein, L.: Chemoprophylaxis of infection, Ann. Intern. Med. **43:**287, 1955.

23 Healing of periodontal surgical wounds

CLINICAL REQUIREMENTS FOR EFFECTIVE HEALING

There are several clinical prerequisites for the promotion of effective healing after periodontal surgery. These include the following:

1. The application of initial therapy prior to surgical intervention.
2. The selection of a surgical approach specific for the cure of the particular inflammatory lesion.
3. The type of tissue environment that exists after surgery has been performed, that is, the tissue topography in relation not only to the surrounding soft tissues but also relative to the teeth and underlying bone.
4. The degree of fibrosis of gingiva prior to and after surgery.
5. The method by which the surgical wound is protected in the postoperative period.
6. The maintenance of the dentition and the periodontium by the patient and the dentist, daily and in periodic office visits.

Importance of initial therapy; physiologic tissue form

Rapid and effective healing after periodontal surgery is largely dependent on the attention given to the correction of the local environment and to the removal of locally active irritants. Thus all the applicable facets of initial therapy should be performed preoperatively, augmented if required during the surgical procedure, and continued by the dentist and maintained by the patient after therapy.

Initial therapy accomplishes several objectives. It removes primary irritants such as bacterial plaque, calculus, and food debris, which usually results in a decrease in the severity of inflammation and induces containment of the inflammatory process. Containment implies the limitation of inflammation to the marginal tissues by connective tissue deposition, within the gingival corium and peripheral to the destructive zone of the inflammatory process. Comparable repair may take place not only within the periosteal aspect of gingiva and alveolar mucosa, but also relative to supporting and alveolar bone. Containment also connotes an amelioration of the intensity of the inflammatory process, limiting collagenolysis, reducing vascularity and edema, and changing the character of the inflammatory cell infiltrate to a "chronic" and presumably immunologically protective one. In the latter context, recent studies have indicated that a lymphokine, derived from circulating human lymphocytes (T cells) of patients with periodontal disease, when coincubated in vitro with rat calvarium in a viable tissue culture system, may induce tissue resorptive or formative responses or both. The data suggests that the presence of chronic inflammation of low intensity is allied to the tissue repair coincident with periodontal disease and, by extrapolation, to the healing after periodontal surgery. The resultant tissue, its health clinically improved, is more amenable to surgery. The "pretreated" tissue incises well because it is relatively dense and firm; there are few tissue tabs and irregularities because the tissue is not friable. This in turn decreases the necessity for correction of the wound site at the time of dressing change or thereafter. Healing is thus facilitated because the reparative process is not interfered with postoperatively. It should also be noted that topographic irregularities of a surgically created connective tissue surface in the form of tabs, tears, crevices, and so on act to retard epithelialization, as migrating epithelial cells do not have sufficient amoeboid vigor to ascend high, irregular hills. Epithelial cells will tend to accrue at the base of the "hill" in disturbed clusters, while the exposed connective tissue remains inflamed, with a tendency for the formation of punctate areas of unepithelialized, red, bleeding, granulation tissue. Where narrow, irregular tissue rents exist there are comparable consequences of defective healing, since epithelial cells ordinarily fail to enter tissue recesses, possibly related to the anaerobic or hypoxic environment of the defects.

Tissue conditioning by initial preparation tends also to reduce bleeding during the surgical procedure, since vascularity has been decreased, easing the performance of the operation and allowing the procedure to be more deliberately and skillfully performed. A decrease in surgical time may also be possible, limiting surgical and psychic trauma to the patient. These are important factors for the minimization of postoperative discomfort. The procedures tend also to be less arduous for the surgeon.

Initial therapy also serves to provide a clean atmosphere for the healing process. When, for example, opened or defective proximal tooth contacts have been repaired or damaged restorations have been replaced, there should be few or no areas for the lodgment of irritants against the tissues. The root surfaces and the cementoenamel junctions must be smooth and devoid of irregularities that may engender plaque accumulation or aid in its attachment; bacterial plaque is the most significant etiologic agent in the propagation of the inflammatory disease state. The postsurgical application of fastidious oral hygiene by the patient and the dentist appears to be directly allied to the effectiveness of healing.

There is new evidence that the root surface, altered adversely by the action of inflammatory exudates, provides an area of marked irregularity and porosity that favors the accumulation of inflammatory exudates. When such segments of cementum or dentin are removed, pulverized, suspended in an aqueous vehicle, and subsequently brought into association with fibroblasts in an in vitro assay system, cytotoxic effects are noted. The severity of cytotoxicity generally parallels the severity of periodontal inflammation at the in vivo site. Investigations of the nature of the accrued exudate indicate the presence of such substances as endotoxins, prostaglandins E_1 and E_2, and hydrolytic enzymes (e.g., acid phosphatase). These substances are generally allied with the resorption of both hard and soft tissues. Additionally, endotoxin has been demonstrated to have direct cytotoxic effects and to engender damaging immunologic reactions. While little or no direct evidence exists relative to the deleterious effects of exudate components on the healing after periodontal surgery, it is reasonable to assume that such effects can and do occur.

There is also a developing body of evidence that the chemically resorbed and molecularly altered root surface is a poor substrate for the formation and mineralization of the new cementum needed to provide soft tissue attachment during postsurgical healing. Actually, a root effectively debrided so that its face is mineralized and microirregular appears to be a most favorable substrate for the apposition of cementoid, mineralizing to cementum. This will be detailed later in the chapter.

The period of initial preparation provides for a period of patient education into the need for continuous oral hygiene and furnishes time for the patient to secure facility in physiotherapeutic procedures. Thus the patient can make a more effective contribution to the healing process and to the prevention of recurrent disease.

The concept of *physiologic tissue form* as an essential aspect of periodontal surgery was introduced by Goldman, who recognized the importance of the local tissue environment in the preservation of periodontal health. Goldman felt that the morphology of the gingiva postoperatively was of utmost concern for expeditious healing and for the prevention of future inflammation in the area. Therefore the healed gingival surface required certain attributes that permitted ready *self-*

cleansing (i.e., food and debris clearance from the marginal area) and that allowed the patient to perform effective oral hygiene measures (Fig. 23-1):

1. The gingival margin should be thin and beveled, adapted tightly to the tooth, while extending mesiodistally in a smooth parabolic curve. The sulcular wall should be short and intrinsically well collagenated to promote its tight adherence to the tooth. In a general context the sulcular wall, that is, the "free gingiva," should have the cross-sectional form of an equilateral triangle. Wherever possible the gingival margin should be protected by cervical tooth convexities or the axial form of the tooth root, if the new tissue margin rests on the radicular surface.

2. The interdental gingiva should be formed by a pyramidally shaped confluence of the gingival margins of adjacent teeth. The tip of the peak should preferably be located coronally to the adjacent gingival margins, thereby obviating the possibility of reverse marginal architectural form. The interdental soft tissue pyramid should additionally be designed to have a slope of approximately 45 degrees (with the tissue tip pointed interdentally) and an interdental vertical groove

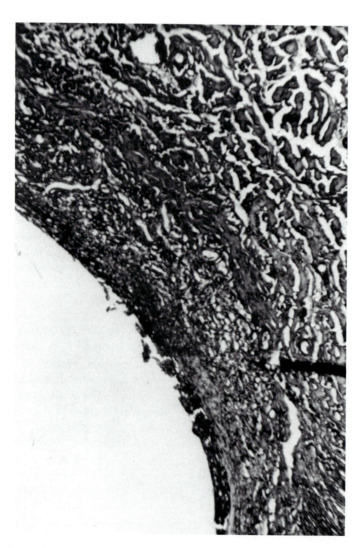

Fig. 23-1. Photomicrograph illustrating disruption of the junctional epithelium with subjacent inflammation. Cross-sections of circular fibers can be seen in upper portion of photomicrograph.

that forms a sluiceway in an occlusoapical direction. In certain instances the interdental col form no longer remains, with only *one* tissue peak or a convex tissue surface present after healing, *permitting this area to be covered with a keratinizing oral epithelium* (Fig. 23-2). These qualities permit sanitation of the interdental areas and provide a measure of physical protection against the recurrence of gingival inflammation.

3. Physiologic form also necessitates that there be an adequate zone of attached gingiva and that its surface be shaped to allow the unimpeded passage of foreign substances from the marginal and interdental areas toward the vestibular and lingual fornices. Attached gingiva is strongly linked by a collagenous attachment to tooth and bone and its

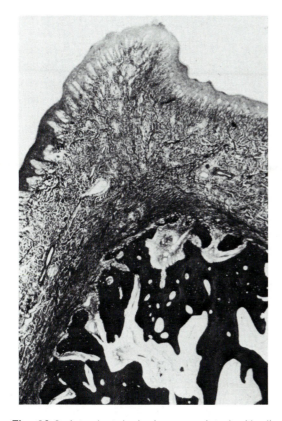

Fig. 23-2. Interdental gingiva associated with diastema between teeth. Covering epithelium displays a keratinizing effect. Its connective tissue corium is dense, with well-organized pattern of collagen distribution. Density and rigidity of tissue corium, combined with its secure bond to underlying bone and cementum, are prime determinants of epithelial keratinization. Comparable morphology and tissue characteristics may be seen after elimination of interdental col form by surgical procedures.

epithelium should be a keratinizing one; these characteristics contribute to the resistance of the periodontium to disease-producing agencies and to the spread of the inflammatory process. After healing, a shallow intact gingival sulcus should be present, but difficult to enter except with a fine tapered probe. The epithelial adherence and adaptation of the sulcular wall is a function of the fiber attachment to the tooth, the density and organization of the circular group of gingival fibers (Fig. 23-3), the degree of maturation of gingival connective tissue, the tonus of the gingival wall provided by tissue fluid and intravascular blood pressures, and an indefinitely defined epithelial "cementation" to the tooth surface. In the context of this thesis, tissue maturation implies the *ratio* of collagen to tissue matrix; the greater the collagen-matrix disparity, the denser the tissue complex. Vascularity and cellularity tend to be coincidently reduced. The term "maturation" also connotes the degree of sulfation of such matrix components as chondroitin as well as the extent of collagen insolubility and resistance to physiologic resorption as part of tissue turnover. The process of maturation appears to be related directly to the age of the individual. Therefore, in a general context, the objectives of the surgery are (1) pocket elimination and (2) the development of physiologic tissue form for disease prevention. *These also constitute requirements for proper healing.* Rationally applied and properly executed, the plastic surgical measures bring about cosmetic improvement for pleasing aesthetics by eliminating tissues that are disfigured by fibrous enlargement and irregular recession and resorption.

Successful application of periodontal surgery demands that the incisional and tissue-shaping portions of the procedure be carried out in tissue that is *free* of overt inflammatory manifestations —hyperemia, exudation, edema, and so on— and is thus in the relatively quiescent, fibrogenic phase of the inflammatory process. To achieve such qualities all procedures composing initial therapy should be performed prior to surgical treatment. Such procedures as scaling (calculus and plaque removal) and tooth surface preparation and smoothing, by planing and polishing, should be carried out as fully as possible before subjecting an area to gingival surgery. It has been established that edematous and often hemorrhagic tissue is difficult to handle surgically; such tissue is friable, tearing or shredding during incision, and often bleeds profusely, tending to obscure the surgical site. The results of incisional, excisional,

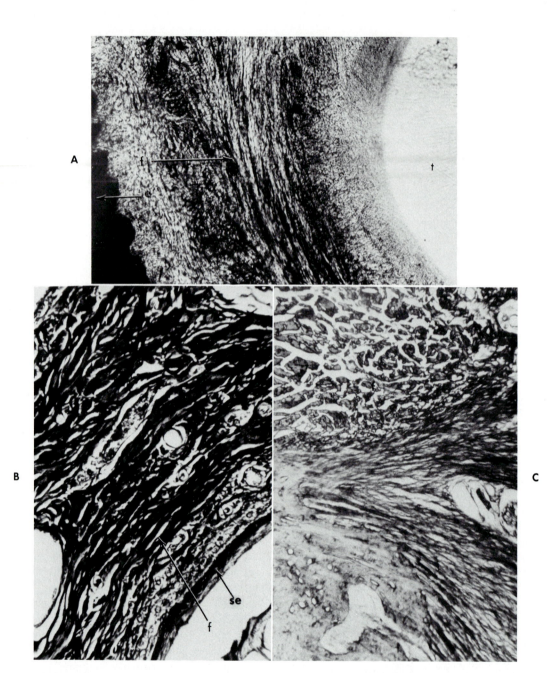

Fig. 23-3. Cross section, **A** and **B,** and buccolingual section, **C,** of circular fiber system, important for support of gingival wall. May be conserved, in partial measure, in surgical methods such as in flap surgery. *t,* Tooth; *f,* circular fibers; *e,* gingival epithelium; *se,* sulcular epithelium. **A,** Light striae represent circular fibers, whereas interspersed dark zones are areas of loose connective tissue between circular fiber bundles. **B,** Circular fibers, *f,* appear dense and distinct; they are poorly soluble, resistant to resorption physiologically, and under the influence of gingival inflammation and functional stress. **C,** Cross section of circular fiber complex, *f,* at upper portion of photomicrograph. Although definitive studies have not been accomplished to ascertain extent of retention of this fiber system postsurgically, methods employed in periodontal flap surgery—internal bevel and repositioning of the bulk of the gingival corium—are designed to maximally conserve fiber system.

and plastic procedures, performed in edematous tissue, are difficult to predict and maintain. Facile surgical performance and stable tissue form postoperatively are predicated upon execution of the surgery in densely fibrous tissue. Initial therapy, besides converting the inflammatory process to a clinically less severe one—reducing edema, erythema, and so on and augmenting fibrogenesis in the tissue—may be sufficient therapy in some cases to bring about resolution of the inflammatory process and acquisition of acceptable tissue form, thus minimizing the need for surgical intervention. The inflammatory lesion must be negated, since it may tend to be self-perpetuating and furnish cause for continued disease.

Tissue environment for tissue resection and shaping

Once the gingiva has been incised the resultant wound surface should be smooth. To achieve this end, the cut, made within gingiva, should be precise and deliberately executed (Fig. 23-19, *B*). Hesitation in drawing the knife through the tissues prompts tissue irregularity. This does not imply that the surface undulations produced in such procedures as gingivectomy and gingivoplasty or indirectly by internally beveling, splitting, or shaping a flap are interferences to healing. The surface irregularities that impede or retard healing are those that are more infinitely localized and harsh. They may be sharply inclined hillocks, narrow depressions, tissue tears, or tags.

In the healing after all periodontal surgical procedures there is a fundamental need for early epithelialization. Epithelium is protective to the subjacent tissues, shielding it against mechanical, chemical, bacterial, and enzymatic irritation and therefore permitting concomitant connective tissue repair to occur. The keratinizing epithelium of gingiva may be particularly efficacious in this regard.

The source of the epithelium required to cover a gingival incisional or excisional area is the epithelium peripheral and adjacent to the wound site (McHugh and Persson; Ramfjord and Costich, 1963; Engler et al.). Early in healing—often 24 to 36 hours after surgery—cells of the surrounding epithelium begin to migrate over the wound. This has been likened to an ameboid type of cell movement, with the transient formation of pseudopods to self-propel the cells (Winter). Whether this is a truly active type of propulsion remains to be elicited, for mitotic activity within the adjacent epithelium, temporally lagging shortly behind the initial cell movement, may tend to express cells laterally toward and centripetally over the wound site. Yet active cell migration is a distinct possibility since epithelial cells contain intracytoplasmic filaments of contractile proteins that are confluent with each other and with the epithelial cell membranes. The cells' muscular system consists of actin and myosin. The contraction and relaxation of the chemical filaments in an oriented repetitive fashion, along with glycolytic processes requiring ATPase to provide for energy requirements, contribute to cell movement. Regardless, the movement of epithelial cells occurs at a relatively predictable rate, 0.5 to 1 mm of lateral progress per day; it does so *under* the surface blood or fibrinomembranous coagulum and just subjacent to the "polyband" that adjoins the clot. Epithelial cells tend to move in a moist interstitial fluid environment reinforced by fibrin, reticulum, or collagen strands. This progress also is aided materially when there are few or no physical impedances to the movement. Cell migration is hindered when a deep crevice, a sharp hill, or an irregular fault is encountered; thus individual areas of denuded gingival corium, periosteum, and granulation tissue may persist and complicate the reparative process. These would be manifested clinically as small or minute reddish zones that bleed with little provocation, as localized areas of tenderness, or as zones demonstrating inflammatory hyperplasia. In areas of bone exposure produced by laceration of gingiva or periosteum, not only may healing of soft tissue be impaired, but bone may also resorb or sequester, possibly leading to loss of essential periodontal support of a tooth. Thus delayed healing and continued inflammation are promoted. Lesions comparable to pyogenic granulomas may develop if particulate material, calculus, or bacterial plaque are impacted onto the tissue. This likelihood is increased when healing is retarded.

Attention should therefore be given clinically to the following measures that minimize defects: (1) sharp, deliberate incision in fibrotic tissue, (2) excision of marginal and surface tissue projections, (3) planned instrumentation (e.g., contouring with rotary diamonds to obviate crevicing; skiving with knives to create a smooth blending of the incisional site with peripheral tissue) to ensure a "free-flowing" surface, (4) thinning and contouring tissue flaps when required and permissible, (5) alteration by osteoplasty of bone form to reduce undue deformity, and (6) postsurgical protection of the wound with a nonirritating, adherent surgical dressing, stressing avoidance of brittle cements, whose particles may lacerate the wound and the abrasion that could be incident to a loose dressing. The cement may also act as a brace or stent to maintain desired tissue placement and adaptation, particularly in association with surgical methods designed to reposition gingiva and alveolar and vestibular mucosae. At times, without such reinforcement, flap evulsion from the apical aspect of the surgical site may occur.

Role of collagenation. Physiologic architectural form is generally considered a prime objective of periodontal therapeutics. This necessitates, as part of the surgical operation, the establishment of certain morphologic attributes that are important for self-cleansing and more effective oral hygiene (and thus the prevention of recurrent disease), as well as for improved aesthetics and more harmonious dentogingival relationships. Briefly restated, they include thin, parabolically curved gingival margins, pyramidal and beveled interdental soft tissue form, shallow sulci and tight marginal adaptation, blending of marginal and attached gingiva, retention or creation of an adequate zone of attached gingiva, and so on. The topographic attributes appear to be best created and maintained in tissue that is dense and thus well collagenated, firm, and relatively free of edema and hemorrhage. Otherwise stated, there is a requirement that plastic procedures be performed in tissue that is fibrotic if one is to expect that the established contours will be reasonably well preserved posttherapeutically. The degree of predictability of results appears to be at least in part proportionate to the degree of fibrosis and in inverse relationship to the extent of tissue hypertrophy and edema. Initial preparation is integral to the creation of the fibrogenic state.

Protection of surgical wound. Healing appears to be improved, within limits, by the postoperative protection of the wound. Various types of surgical cements have been employed. Most are formulated for close adaptation to the wound, adherence to tooth surfaces and contiguous dressing, and with adequate flowability to lock into interdental areas, improving retention. Some cements containing eugenol, chlorothymol, eucalyptol, and so on are compounded to provide a topical anodyne effect and may be mildly antiseptic. Bacterial and fungal overgrowth may take place at the tissue-dressing interface. In this regard it has been shown that tetracycline-containing surgical dressings promote superficial *Candida albicans* infection. A primary effect of such

infection is epithelial necrosis and desquamation, including retardation of postsurgical reepithelialization of the wound. Tannic acid powder may be incorporated for surface hemostasis. There is a nearly universal trend toward the use of bland, semirigid dressings devoid of essential oils and with slight resiliency. Eugenol is considered by some not only as a substance capable of producing soft tissue necrosis but also able, when in proximity to bone, to induce its resorption. The surface resiliency of the dressing reduces, to an extent, direct mechanical irritation to the wound. All surgical dressings are designed to quickly acquire firmness and rigidity.

It is especially important that the wound be sheltered during early recollagenation and the period of epithelialization, essentially offering protection against topical irritants such as rough or granular substances, acidic or highly seasoned foods, and toothbrush abrasion. The dressing can also act as a restraining wall, limiting the likelihood for overgranulation of the wound by containing the reparative process. Therefore if exposure is restricted, there is usually a minimum of topical irritation with a limitation of bleeding and postoperative pain, and improved healing. Effective healing, however, can occur without a dressing in position (Orban and Archer; Persson); barring abrasion or laceration there does not appear to be temporal retardation of the process. The surgical cement may be of considerable importance in the so-called closed (flap) procedures in maintaining the repositioned tissues in close approximation to receptor sites. Poor or indifferent flap adaptation may allow for exudate or blood clot to accrue in excessive thickness, delaying flap or graft attachment and producing a greater likelihood of ectopic tissue localization and poor tissue form. Exudate must drain or be phagocytized and digested by tissue macrophages in order to yield renewed approximation; there may be temporal retardation consistent with its thickness. The areas occupied by clot and produced by malposed tissue may heal or fill with connective tissue, increasing gingival or mucosal thickness and altering postoperative form.

Debridement effects. Curettage of the soft tissue lesion in gingivitis and marginal periodontitis removes the ulcerated and hyperplastic pocket epithelium and the subjacent diseased gingival corium down to bed of firm, uninvolved connective tissue; in the case of osseous lesions all the inflammatory tissue included in the bony defect is removed to the periodontal ligament and the osseous surfaces (and marrow cavities). After this phase of debridement the periodontal ligament is found to be exposed at the bone crest and at all interfaces of the periodontal ligament with the intraosseous lesion. For example, in the case of the three-walled osseous infrabony pocket, located on the proximal aspect of a tooth, periodontal ligament faces the debrided lesion from the buccal, lingual, and apical bony walls. Should a two-walled infrabony pocket be present on the proximal portion of a root, the exposure of the periodontal ligament would be J shaped.

During this debridement, which must be thoroughly accomplished, the root surface is also prepared for the deposition and attachment of new cementum, a process that is imperative for the reattachment of tissue flaps and for the acquisition of new attachment. There is a growing body of biologic evidence that indicates that the physical nature of the root surface, particularly the hydrated, mineralized state, is a primary factor that is topically inductive for cementogenesis in healing.

This mechanical debridement also removes enzymes that originate from the resident bacterial flora as well as those hydrolytic enzymes derived from degenerating tissue cells. Certain streptococci and staphylococci produce hyaluronidase that attacks the tissue ground substance, binding for cells and fibers, changing a viscous, relatively impermeable tissue matrix to a pervious, watery one. Streptococci, *Clostridium histolyticum,* and *Bacteroides melaninogenicus* produce a collagenase that acts upon the collagen fiber systems, degrading the collagen as infinitely as to its peptide constituents. *Bacteroides melaninogenicus, Veillonella, Neisseria, Vibrio,* and spirochetes of the gram-negative pocket flora, upon lysis, release endotoxins capable of inducing tissue necrosis, attacking epithelium and connective tissue, and seriously impairing vascularization to the area. Studies at Boston University have established a direct and linear correlation between the amount of endotoxin in the gingival exudate and in bacterial plaque and debris and the severity of the inflammatory state.

Lysosomes of cells are known to be a fundamental source of intrinsic degrading enzymes. For example, degenerating leukocytes are a source of proteolytic enzymes, and their removal would decrease the availability of collagenases and proteolytic substances.

Thus debridement serves as an agency for the removal of a multiplicity of etiologic factors, which may have engendered the lesion or which may conceivably impair the healing process.

TISSUE BIOLOGY RELATED TO WOUND HEALING

To appreciate fully the complex yet orderly reparative processes occurring in the periodontium after instrumentation and surgery, it is essential to review and understand the structure, synthesis, biochemistry, and physiology of its components. Connective tissues are the bases of gingiva, alveolar mucosa, periodontal ligament, bone marrow, blood and lymphatic vessels, nerves, and bone. Vital interactions take place between epithelia and adjacent connective tissues, blood and lymphatic structures and the surrounding tissue milieu, and bone and its ensheathing periosteum and endosteum. These involve, for example, the transport of a vascular transudate—containing amino acids, simple carbohydrates such as glucose, cationic elements such as calcium (Ca^{++}), sodium (Na^+), and potassium (K^+), hormones, vitamins such as ascorbic acid, and water—necessary for the metabolism and hydration of both cellular and extracellular aspects of the tissues associated with the vasculature (Fig. 23-4). The transudate derived from the subepithelial capillaries and venules of attached gingiva and alveolar mucosa supplies the lamina propria, traverses the epithelial basement membrane, enters the epithelial intercellular substance, and thence passes into

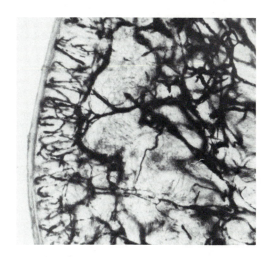

Fig. 23-4. Dye-stained transudate derived from subepithelial capillaries of attached gingiva, producing tissue darkening in this section. Network of blood vessels associated with gingiva's periosteum can be seen at far right, whereas peripheral vascular plexus subjacent to gingival epithelium can be discerned at left of section.

epithelial cells either by diffusion or via pinocytotic vesicles for their utilization. A portion of the transudate may also diffuse through the matrix of the connective tissue and be comparably employed by connective tissue cells such as the fibroblasts, while still maintaining gelation of the matrix. Compromise, then, of vascularization to the outer aspects of the tissue's corium may affect directly the status of both connective tissue and epithelium. There is therefore strong emphasis in periodontal surgery today on procedures that stringently conserve afferent blood supply (and by implication, venous and lymphatic drainage) to the different parts of the periodontium. Noteworthy are those procedures aimed at periosteal conservation; it must be recognized that this tissue furnishes the prime vascularization to itself, alveolar mucosa, gingiva, adjacent bone, and, when bony septa are thin and compact, periodontal ligament. We will point out later the essentiality of periosteum in reparative processes associated with irritation, inflammation, and surgery.

Connective tissues are composed of both fibrillar and amorphous elements synthesized by enclaved cells. They are also both physically and enzymatically resorbed by cells and cellular products found within the milieu. The principal fibrillar structure is collagen, a fibrous protein, formed by the dominant cell of connective tissue, the fibroblast. This same cell type also synthesizes lesser amounts of delicate reticulum (argyrophilic) strands comparable in composition and structure to collagen, possibly elastic fibers, and the bulk of the extracellular or interfibrillar matrix. The various fibers and cells are actually situated in and surrounded by the three-dimensional matrical gel, a binding and, although amorphous, an organizing substance. In the latter context it should be recognized that the viscosity of this gel is variable, increasing in a dense, well-collagenated connective tissue and, conversely, decreasing in a loose, less fibrous area. The corium of attached gingiva is usually representative of an area of high matrical viscosity, whereas the connective tissue phase of alveolar mucosa is associated with a greater degree of fluidity and lesser gelation. The subepithelial zones of attached and marginal gingiva, bone marrow, inner aspects of periosteum, and the perivascular zones of periodontal ligament also fall into the latter category. Interestingly, these are also the *zones of greatest number and synthetic capacity of cells.*

The fibroblast is of mesenchymal origin and is derived from the stem cell of connective tissue, the *undifferentiated mesenchymal cell*. The latter, a reserve cell, is particularly abundant in loose connective tissues, thus in perivascular sites, lamina propria, periosteum, and so on. When examined by light microscopy it appears as a plump, nearly rounded but fusiform cell with a large, distinctly outlined but lightly staining nucleus. Cytoplasmic granularity, crudely indicative of the presence of ribosomes and thus synthetic activity, is weak or sparse. When viewed via electron microscopy its endoplasmic reticulum is poorly granular and incompletely developed, mitochondria are few with broad undulations of their cristae, and the Golgi system is indistinctly outlined and saccular.

Remarkable changes take place after injury or in association with irritation. The undifferentiated mesenchymal cell undergoes mitosis, forming a greater primordial cell population. A number of these cells will develop into fibroblasts that when active, undergo decided change. Nuclear chromaticity is greater, while its size, related to overall cell area, is less; affinity for basic stains such as hematoxylin increases. Cytoplasmic area is greater and is marked by exceptional granularity. The bulk of the granules are evidenced by increased tinctorial intensity; the polyribonucleotides, affiliated with an ultrastructural rough endoplasmic reticulum, are vividly elicited by the stain pyronin, whereas mitochondrial constituents may be reflected by supravital staining methods such as Janus green. Ultrastructural examination reveals a highly developed system for protein transport and synthesis, the endoplasmic reticulum; this canalicular maize is adjoined by numerous clusters of ribosomes (polyribosomes), sites of amino acid aggregation into peptides and polypeptide linkages. Mitochondria are abundant, apparently increasing by independent mitochondrial replication within the cell's cytoplasm, and demonstrate more numerous and steeper invaginating cristae. Mitochondrial activity is associated with energy-producing processes, particularly aerobic glycolysis (citric acid cycle of carbohydrate metabolism) and oxidative phosphorylation, the formation of high energy yielding adenosine triphosphate from adenosine monophosphate and diphosphates. Creatinine phosphate esters are hydrolyzed to make phosphate ions available. The Golgi complex, a system of cytoplasmic vesicles, becomes more highly developed; if one recognizes that these saccules constitute a packaging and transport system for substances synthesized at the ribosomal sites, one can understand their development.

The Golgi complex also functions in the addition of carbohydrate to peptides, the peptides having been synthesized earlier at polyribosomal sites. For example, the collagen molecule is composed of small amounts of sugars such as glucose, galactose, and fucose in combination with amino acids; the number of amino acid residues predominates over the carbohydrate residues in a ratio of 500:1. Yet despite the minimal amount of simple sugars present, their presence appears to be fundamental to collagen integrity. Thus when tropocollagen is released from the cell it is a glycoprotein rather than a pure protein. In some instances the Golgi vesicles with accrued glycopeptides and a lipid additive are released from cells such as osteoblasts and odontoblasts as matrix vesicles, which in turn become substrates for mineral accrual within osteoid and dentinoid matrices. Mineral accumulates within the matrix vesicles in the form of calcium phosphate in amorphous and apatite forms. When the vesicles are filled with mineral their limiting membranes rupture, and the vesicular-mineral aggregates become nucleating sites within the tissue matrix. Epitactic expansion of mineralization proceeds very rapidly once these nidi form at "calcification fronts." Thus the Golgi system is *uniquely* important as a site of carbohydrate addition to protein and as a basis for mineralization of tissue matrices.

Using histochemical means such as autoradiography, one may visualize the dynamic nature of cellular processes, particularly the fibroblast. Ubiquitous and unique to collagen and reticulum is the hydroxylated amino acid hydroxyproline. Proline is the precursor amino acid. Employing radioactively tagged proline, such as proline ^{3}H (tritiated proline) or proline ^{14}C, introduced intravenously or intraperitoneally in appropriate volume and concentration into laboratory animals, an investigator may document the process of collagen (protein) formation by the fibroblast. Recognizing that the amino acid quickly circulates throughout the body and is found in vascular transudates, uptake in active cells may begin within minutes of its introduction into the circulation. The speed of dissemination throughout the animal is evidenced by the fact that the radioactive material may be found in sulcular fluid as early as 30 seconds after injection intravenously.

The process of autoradiography demonstrates diffusion and pinocytotic uptake through the cell membrane and accumulation within 30 minutes in the ribosmal areas of protein synthesis. Over the subsequent 3 to 24 hours the radioactive, incorporated amino acid may be discerned successively in the endoplasmic reticulum, the Golgi complex (where carbohydrate is added; double isotopic labeling, for example, with proline ^{3}H and glucose ^{3}H, will demonstrate this phenomenon), in association with the inner aspect of the cell membrane, and thence in close affiliation with the *outside* of the cell membrane, indicating transmembrane passage of a collagen precursor containing proline (Fig. 23-5). The extracellular transport may possibly be accomplished by passage of "secretory vesicles" through the cell's plasma membrane via a process simulating reverse pinocytosis. The labeled proline is then noted incorporated into the collagen and reticulum fibers of the connective tissue. Proline in nonhydroxylated form may be found in noncollagenous tissues or areas such as enamel matrix during tooth formation, in epithelial cells for endogenous protein synthesis and during formation of the epithelial phase of basement membrane, and within dentinal tubules as part of dentinal fluid. Proline is utilized also by cells (possibly smooth muscle) of the tunica media of arterioles and arteries in the formation of their elastic laminae.

Comparable proline utilization is seen by cells concerned with the formation of fibrillar constituents of calcifiable connective tissues, that is, osteoblasts (bone), odontoblasts (dentin), and cementoblasts (cementum). Proline is present in hydroxylated form in these tissues. In a similar way *the amino acids glycine and betaine (lysine) are utilized, including their hydroxylation, in collagen formation.*

The collagen fiber, present in connective tissues, is composed of laterally aggregated fibrils. The fibrils appear to be bound together in bundle (fascicle) form and surrounded by sulfated protein-polysaccharides, essentially chondroitin sulfate. These are acid mucopolysaccharides, demonstrable by alcian blue dye and by Hale's colloidal iron technique. Glycoproteins are also present at the cementing sites, particularly in association with reticulum and young, more weakly aggregated collagen; these may be elicited by the periodic acid–Schiff technique. Using the Mallory trichrome method for connective tissues, newly formed, immature (young) collagen reacts with the aniline blue dye, whereas older (greater maturity, greater cross-linking between peptide chains) collagen appears to have a strong affinity for orange G. In this and the Masson's method, reticulum is poorly demonstrable with acid stains

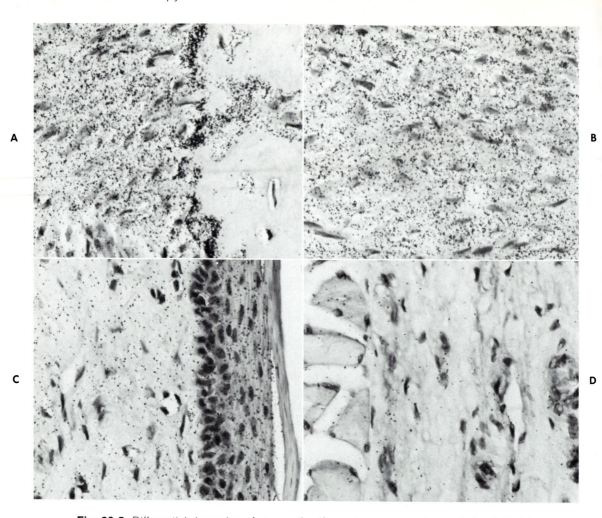

Fig. 23-5. Differential dynamics of connective tissue turnover can be partially elicited by autoradiographic means after administration of an amino acid in isotopic form (proline ³H), which is a precursor of collagenous elements. In this experiment, periodontal tissues were examined 24 to 48 hours after intraperitoneal injection of proline ³H to adult mice. Most pronounced utilization of amino acid can be seen in **A** in periodontal ligament (left side of section), in vascular channel site (right center), and along periodontal ligament aspect of alveolar bone. In **B** there is a more or less uniform distribution of substance in periodontal ligament, but particularly in its alveolar aspect and in association with collagen fibers and perivascular reticulum. **C,** Little proline is utilized in the gingival corium, whereas in **D,** representing connective tissue of alveolar mucosa, there is also a paucity of collagen synthesis. (From De Moraes, F., and Carniero, J.: Personal communication.)

and is best elicited by techniques such as silver nitrate impregnation. Reticulum is especially prevalent in young connective tissues, in early aspects of connective tissue repair, and in lamina propria and perivascular zones. The fibers are fine, delicate, "cotton candy" in nature and indifferently dispersed in the tissue. Conversely, collagen tends to be well arranged with palisading of fibers and a bundle type of orientation.

Recent biologic and clinical data indicate that allogeneic connective tissues such as gingiva, dura mater, and sclera may be used in lieu of gingival autografts in periodontal reconstructive surgery; these investigations are preliminary. The antigenicity of collagen, especially the more stable and physiologically insoluble types, may be minimized by special processing of the connective tissue graft material prior to application to the host. In a *general context* the soft tissue graft, after procurement from the donor individual, is program-frozen, subsequently freeze-dried (ly-ophilized), and stored under sterile conditions until the time of application to a receptor area. The experimental results using this procedure have been equivocal. In animal investigations we have treated homografts via a method complex that includes freezing with liquid nitrogen, gamma irradiation (2.5 to 3 megarads from a cobalt 60 source), and sterile storage under anaerobic conditions until use. Such irradiation fully sterilizes the tissue, obviating bacterial, fungal, and viral agents and their infectivity. In addition the tissue's collagen is made more insoluble and stable via the addition of H^+ cross-links between its polypeptide chains, and its antigenicity is essentially eliminated. Since all cellular components are rendered nonviable by denaturation, the graft actually functions at the host site in an allostatic-prosthetic fashion. It is attached to receptor periosteum by reparative activities of periosteal origination and covered by epithelium originating from the mucosa or gingiva adjacent to the graft. Studies are needed to document the neovascularization and the renewal of the cellular population of the connective tissue phase of the graft. Gamma-irradiated aortic valves (cadaver derived) have been utilized extensively and successfully in the replacement of incompetent aortic valves in humans; immunologically mediated tissue rejection has not been a problem despite the fact that patients do not receive immunosuppressive therapy, thus testifying to the lack of antigenicity of the donor tissue. Interestingly the valvular transplants after 5 to 7 years display mineralization, at times rendering the valve leaflets functionally incompetent and necessitating their replacement. Investigations are needed in this regard to ascertain the fate of scleral grafts after transplantation to periodontal infrabony defects. Biologic data suggest that the collagen of bone is significantly more insoluble than that of connective tissues; collagen stability may thus be a requisite for its mineralization.

In connective tissues such as alveolar mucosa, but not in attached gingiva, some *elastin* may be seen in the form of elastic fibers. These are highly refractile cylinders when viewed via polarized light, thinner than collagen fibers, and homogenous and nonfibrillar when seen through the light microscope. At times they may appear short and thick (6 μm); in association with arteries they may appear as long wavy fibers. Particularly useful for the elicitation of elastin are the stains aldehyde fuchsin, orcein, or resorcin-fuchsin, which do not ordinarily stain collagen. There is some evidence, however, that resorbing or altered collagen (deaminated, acetylated) may also be stained by these methods; in areas where elastin is not customarily seen (as in the corium of attached gingiva), these staining techniques may be useful for demonstrating collagen alterations associated with such conditions as inflammation, orthodontic tooth movement, and wound healing.

Under the electron microscope there is *no* axial periodicity evidenced for elastin (collagen has definitive periodicity of 64 nm; tropocollagen, about 280 nm) nor is any type of structure clear; it is therefore amorphous. Unique to the composition of elastin are the amino acids desmosine and isodesmosine; these have been related to the unusual rubberlike elasticity of the substance. Actually the fibers will stretch to 150% of their original length, tending to rebound when tensional force is released. This quality is obviously especially significant and vital in the elastic membranes of the aorta and arterial system. *Whether the minimal quantity of elastin found in such areas as alveolar mucosa and periodontal ligament imparts elasticity and pliability to these tissues is a matter of conjecture;* the structural arrangement of alveolar mucosa (a loose, hydrated connective tissue, its fibers relatively few and poorly oriented and with an abundant ground substance) would be more likely to impart such "elastic" qualities to the tissue. When compared to insoluble collagen, which is readily converted to soluble gelatin by heating in boiling water, elastin is nearly inert. It is resistant to acids and alkalis, but it can be solubilized by heating with boiling water in the presence of acids. Elastin is attacked by enzyme preparations containing elastase, such as those derived from flavobacterium and mammalian pancreas. It is not affected by trypsin, chymotrypsin, or pepsin. In connective tissues the substance is apparently secreted by fibroblasts, whereas in blood vessels, medial smooth muscle cells have been implicated in its synthesis.

Ground substance of connective tissue. The embedding substance for cells and fibers of connective tissue exists in the form of an amorphous, homogenous gel that secures hydration from vascular transudates. It is of course a universal component of connective tissues. It does, however, vary in the extent of gelation and thus of viscosity — young, new, or structurally loose connective tissues are rich in matrix and display a greater degree of fluidity than older or more collagenous connective tissues. The ground substance of tumors, such as myxomas, is especially great in quantity, imparting a soft, often mushy consistency to these masses. Abundant ground substance is seen in the marginal gingiva of children, especially when passive eruption is incomplete; this may help to account not only for the soft texture and compressibility of these tissues, but also for their more facile retractability from the tooth and for the overt ballooning associated with inflammatory edema. The ground substance of newly forming connective tissues after periodontal surgery is also notable for its abundance and diminished viscosity.

Conversely, dense connective tissue hyperplasias such as hereditary diffuse gingivofibromatosis, the "aging" dental pulp, the hyperfunctional periodontal ligament, and gingiva in an advanced stage of healing show lesser quantities of matrix with a greater degree of apparent viscosity. Sulfation is also increased; chondroitin sulfate is the principal protein-polysaccharide present.

Histochemically, the ground substance, when newly secreted or found in loose connective tissues, stains metachromatically with toluidine blue, whereas denser, older, or more mature connective tissue matrices either stain very weakly or not at all. Young matrices show little if any affinity for alcian blue or colloidal iron, whereas more mature, dense tissues show alcianophilia and attraction to colloidal iron because of their greater content of acid and sulfated protein-polysaccharides, particularly in association with the fibers of the tissue. Thus older matrices tend to reflect greater viscosity, are diminished quantitatively, and show increased sulfation and poor affinity for toluidine blue. In the latter context it should be noted that the nonsulfated protein-polysaccharides, hyaluronic acid and chondroitin, are extremely prevalent in loose connective tissues, and the water-binding capacity, especially of hyaluronate, may help to augment the tissues' hydration.

Interestingly, there is an inverse relationship between tissue density and the extent of vascular patency and transudation. Patent blue violet in aqueous solution, a highly diffusible dye, when injected intra-arterially (at existing intravascular

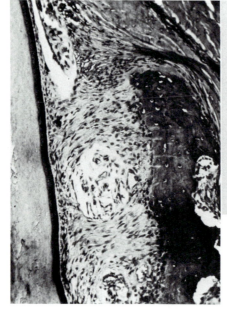

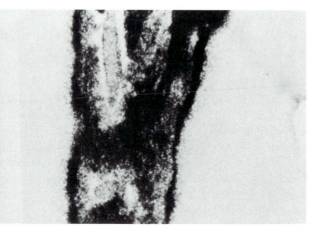

Fig. 23-6. Periodontal ligament is a dynamic tissue. **A,** Marked cellularity of attachment apparatus and crestal phase of periodontal ligament in a human specimen (4-year-old child). **B,** Uptake and utilization of proline ^{14}C in collagen and bone synthesis in crestal phase of periodontal ligament in a nonhuman primate (2-year-old monkey). Amino acid was administered 48 hours prior to sacrifice; thus, there is minimal intracellular proline ^{14}C localization, with greatest portion of amino acid incorporated into newly synthesized connective tissue. After surgical injury, periodontal ligament reacts in a prolific manner, producing all connective tissue components necessary for significant repair, such as marginal reattachment of a flap to tooth and bone.

pressure) in experimental animals produces deep and extensive vital staining of loose or new connective tissues or both (Fig. 23-6) and a relative paucity of staining in denser matrices or tissues. Such measures have been used to document the diffusion of tissue fluids from receptor or host sites to free autogenous soft tissue grafts, a process vital to the sustenance and success of the grafting procedure. Interestingly, transudation and exudation *into* the graft are especially marked in the first 4 to 7 days after the procedure. The graft actually becomes clinically and histologically edematous (increased dye staining). With the establishment of vascular and lymphatic anastomoses between recipient site and graft, edema and staining decrease. The measure, using intravenously injected fluorescent dyes or patent blue violet, is also used clinically in humans to determine the ''vitality'' of tissues such as large skin grafts, either pedicle or free.

Connective tissue matrices may be enzymatically degraded. In normal tissues, fibrocytes (functionally termed ''fibroclasts'') produce enzymes that are responsible for the physiologic degradation of collagen and ground substance attending connective tissue turnover. The enzymes, such as collagenase and hyaluronidase, appear to act at or near normal tissue pH and are ordinarily formed and released by fibroclasts in very small quantities. It is not known whether certain fibroblasts are specifically programmed to perform resorptively or if all tissue fibroblasts are pluripotentially capable of alternating between formative, resorptive, and static activities. Fibrocytes have also been seen to have collagen particles, with characteristic cross striations (64 nm) within their cytoplasm, suggesting a possible phagocytic function. Bacterial hyaluronidase (i.e., β-hemolytic streptococcus in origin) will hydrolyze hyaluronic acid. Hyaluronidase may also be derived, in the inflammatory process or during early connective tissue repair, from the acid hydrolase collection of mast cells and invading neutrophils and monocytes (tissue macrophages). When the lysosomal enzymes of such cells are released into the extracellular zones, they may include chondroitin sulfatases, nonspecific proteases, cathepsins (proteolytic), and so on capable of degrading both matrical and fiber binding substances. Bacterial and neutrophilic (also monocyte and mast cell) derived enzymes can attack the fibrillar elements of the tissue. Collagenases capable of such activity are released from gram-negative microorganisms (i.e., *Bacteroides melaninogenicus*), anaerobic

streptococci, and so on. Proteolytic enzymes of cellular derivation (collagenases, aminopeptidases, cathepsins, proteases) may also affect the cross and terminal linkages between polypeptide chains to produce segmentation visually and biochemically of collagen and reticulum.

The synthesis of elements of ground substance by fibroblasts may be followed autoradiographically in a manner comparable to that described for the synthesis of collagen precursors. Glucose (H_3 or C_{14}) is a progenitor ingredient of both hyaluronate and chondroitin, whereas the formation of sulfated polysaccharides (chondroitin SO_4) may be followed by employing intravenously or intraperitoneally administered isotopic $NaSO_4$.

Connective tissue cells. Mention should here be made of the pluripotentiality of differentiation of the undifferentiated mesenchymal cell. Mesenchymal cell offspring include the osteoblast (odontoblast, cementoblast), fibroblast, the mononuclear macrophage, the mast cell, and, by mitosis and fusion, the osteoclast. There is a substantial body of evidence indicating that tissue macrophages and osteoclasts are primarily derived from monocytes, which emigrate extravascularly into lesional sites. Many humoral substances, for example, endotoxin, prostaglandins E_1 and E_2, and osteoclast-activating factor, appear to convert (''turn on'') the cells to resorptive activities. Additional comments are necessary regarding the activity of the fibroblast in the repair process. Osteoblasts, essentially fibroblasts located in association with a bone surface, appear as rounded or cuboidal cells aligned in a monolayer on the face of previously existing bone. Like the fibroblasts, they display a granular, pyroninophilic cytoplasm indicative of polyribonucleotide presence and protein synthesis. Mitochondria and the Golgi system are usually abundant; the endoplasmic reticulum is complex and studded with granularity. Histochemically, enzymes of the tricarboxylic acid cycle—malic, isocitric, and to a lesser extent succinic dehydrogenase activity—can be elicited. β-Hydroxybutyric dehydrogenase activity, as in the fibroblast, denotes the utilization of this ketonic acid, presumably returning it to the acetyl-CoA and Krebs cycle metabolism. Interestingly, deficiency of ascorbic acid, essential for collagen synthesis, leads to defects in the enzyme systems of the cells; *all collagen-producing cells are involved in the impairment.* Bone (osteoid) formation is accompanied by high alkaline phosphatase synthesis and employment by osteoblasts; conversely, alkaline phosphatase is weakly or negatively demonstrable when bone formation is retarded.

The fundamental sources of osteoblasts within periodontal tissues are the inner layer (cambium) of periosteum, endosteum lining the vascular channels and peripheralized in the marrow spaces, the thin connective tissue lining of haversian canals, the periodontal ligament, and the perivascular progenitor cells of marrow. Endosteum and periosteum actually serve as a "dynamic functional membrane" enclosing and in juxtarelationship to bone. Osteoblasts are not only responsible for the synthesis of the bone matrix, which is then converted to bone by mineralization, but also participate in providing the nutritional supply to cells enclaved *within* bone, for example, osteocytes. Cellular extensions of osteoblasts penetrate osteoid, communicate with osteocytic canaliculi, and thus provide cytoplasmic portals for the "feeding" of osteocytes. This is comparable to the extension of odontoblastic processes into dentinal tubuli. *Interestingly, the body of gingiva — the corium external to periosteum — is relatively deficient in its indigenous cell population (mesenchymal and fibroblastic) and thus may be but a minor participant in the repair not only of underlying tissues such as bone and ligament but also of itself. It serves best as a nearly inert scaffold material for epithelial migration and cover, and for attachment to tooth and bone via dynamic periosteum, periodontal ligament, and endosteum (when available at orifices or within vascular channels).*

The secretory products of osteoblasts are categorized as osteoid. The substance stains eosinophilic, separated from subjacent bone by resting lines attracting basic stains (as hematoxylin). Osteoid, like reticulum, is also susceptible to silver impregnation; fine, heterogenously dispersed argyrophilic fibrils can be seen within the material. Fibrils may also be periodic acid–Schiff positive, indicating the presence of protein-polysaccharide–containing complexes. Its matrix is that of connective tissue with comparable composition and tinctorial qualities. It appears that both the matrical substance and the fibrils (collagen and reticulin) of osteoid are capable of mineralization, the mineral being derived from available tissue fluids that are supersaturated, and thus metastable, relative to mineral — $CaPO_4$ essentially, and in its hydroxyapatite form. Collagen can demonstrate intrafibrillar mineral deposits; axial periodicity of 64 nm appears to be a requisite for deposition of mineral. Protein-polysac-

charides of the osteoid matrix have been said to attract and physically bind cations (Ca^{++}) by the process of chelation leading to nucleation (a "seed" of protein-polysaccharide-mineral) and subsequent crystal lattice formation. Direct cellular participation in the mineralization does *not* appear to be necessary except to produce a connective tissue amenable to mineralization from the extracellular milieu. However, updated studies show that osteoblasts, via the elaboration of secretory vesicles that as matrix vesicles subsequently mineralize within osteoid, actually furnish the nucleating sites upon which crystal lattices of mineral develop and expand. The osteoblast-derived matrix vesicles provide the seeds for epitactic mineral deposition. Introduction of mineral, experimentally or clinically, into operative sites to provide sources of calcium salts for mineralization reactions appears to be unnecessary for the process. *What is more important is to have adequate vascularization to the site and thus an availability of mineral-containing vascular transudates.* Thus, for example, removal of the dense transseptal fiber system overlying bone in infrabony defects is required to facilitate the process of new bone formation and new attachment (Fig. 23-7). Removal of the connective tissue barrier allows for concomitant connective tissue and vascular ingrowth as well as opening avenues for the diffusion of fluids into the defect. Substances such as Dilantin, calcium hydroxide, and plaster of paris particles, if they are productive of bone formation, do so by being phagocytized by formative cells and subsequently inducing protein and polysaccharide synthesis at ribosomal sites. *Alien substances may also provoke chronic in-*

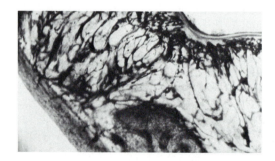

Fig. 23-7. Microcirculation of periodontium. Linear network represents blood vessels of gingiva that are most abundant and complex subjacent to its epithelia. Although not discernible in this specimen, periosteal vascularization is extensive and furnishes primary vascular source for gingiva and alveolar mucosa.

flammation of low intensity, which in turn is responsible for reactive tissue formation, for example, connective tissue and bone. Glycopeptides of lymphocytic origin may serve to activate formative cells such as osteoblasts and fibroblasts. The material, then extruded (i.e., connective tissue or osteoid) from the cell, undergoes mineralization from serumal or humoral fluid. It is also conceivable, although speculative, that highly alkaline substances such as CaOH and plaster of paris alter or degrade elements of the tissue into which they are placed, with subsequent uptake (phagocytosis) of the modified tissue substance into fibroblasts and induction of their synthetic capacities. The phenomenon of "induction" requires further and thorough investigation. At Boston University preliminary studies attest to the potential of low-voltage, direct continuous electric currents in the induction of connective tissue and bone formation. Decalcified allogenic bone transplants, autografts of hematopoietic marrow, allogenic grafts of frozen and irradiated red marrow, and so on are being investigated for their osteogenic potential. In this context, allogeneic grafts of attached gingiva, quick frozen and subjected to 2.5 to 3 megarads of gamma radiation, have been shown to survive in alien animal hosts and to act as collagenous scaffolding for periosteal fibergenesis and for epithelial migration and cover. The cells of the graft do not appear to survive functionally.

The tissue *mononuclear macrophage,* a scavenger and debriding cell, is particularly important in tissue repair. Derived by mitosis or differentiation from the blood monocyte, it, *like the fibroblast,* migrates on connective tissue and fibrinoid strands toward and into the wound. It is responsible in part for the phagocytosis and digestion of cellular debris, bacteria, particulate exogenous matter, collagen remnants, and so on. These cells also align themselves peripheral to and within the blood clot, aiding substantially in its removal. Enzymes derived primarily from neutrophils participate actively in clot dissolution and its preparation for phagocytosis by the mononuclear cell. The histiocyte (mononuclear macrophage) often resembles the fibroblast, is notable for its concentration of hydrolytic enzymes (such as acid phosphatases, collagenases, proteases, lipases, cathepsins) and may demonstrate intracytoplasmic inclusions of phagocytized debris. Experimentally, the introduction of carbon particles (30 nm) into the tissues leads to rapid mobilization of phagocytic cells of this category; the foreign substance can be seen within the cells for protracted time periods as the ingested substance resists enzymatic disposal.

Mast cells appear to be indigenous in small numbers to gingival connective tissues, particularly in perivascular sites and in the subsulcular lamina propria. They increase in chronic inflammatory states and may be especially prevalent during the first 7 to 10 days of healing after surgery. The cell, probably of mesenchymal origin, yet structurally and functionally comparable to the blood basophil, appears as a markedly granular, ovoid to round cell with a large, deeply staining (basophilic) nucleus. In fact, cytoplasmic granularity, particularly after toluidine blue or thionine staining, is often so extensive as to completely fill the cytoplasm and obscure the nucleus. The cells synthesize histamine by the decarboxylation of the amino acid histidine and may be a connective tissue source of heparin and the sulfated protein-polysaccharide heparitin sulfate. The mast cell may also be replete with lysosomal enzymes of proteolytic, glycolytic, and lipid-destroying potentials. Thermal, traumatic, chemical (i.e., detergents), and other irritants may elicit degranulation of the mast cell with release of histamine and the hydrolytic enzymes into the tissue. The immediate hypersensitivity response (humoral) is also in part dependent on the presence, activity, and degranulation of the cells. It is well established that antigen-humoral antibody (reagin, immunoglobulin E) reactions in association with the cell membrane lead to release of the cell constituents into the extracellular area. Histamine is a powerful vasodilating peptide, producing increased venular and capillary patency via relaxation of the arteriolar medial smooth muscle in the precapillary zones and vascular permeability. It is thus productive of hyperemia and edema. Antihistamines given prior to and after periodontal surgery may *possibly* assist in the reduction of the effects of histamine released during and after surgery. Other vasoactive kinins associated with tissue injury and healing are of plasma (alpha globulin) and pancreatic origins and are released at the site of injury by the action of trypsin or trypsinlike substances on the polypeptide substrates. Bradykinin is a most important, prevalent nonapeptide with sustained activity and may be related to the early postsurgical inflammatory process. Aprotinin (Trasylol), a protease inhibitor, has recently been found to antagonize bradykinin activity.

The *osteoclast* (cementoclast, odontoclast) is

the primary cell affiliated with the resorption of bone. There is also some evidence available that *osteocytes* participate in the enzymatic degradation of the perilacuner bone; these fundamentally proteolytic enzymes are formed in the cell and contained within intracytoplasmic packets termed "lysosomes." Notable also are the hydrolytic enzymes such as acid phosphatase, β-glucuronidase, and aminopeptidase. The perilacuner resorption can be demonstrated by faintly irregular enlargement of the lacunae and by diminished staining reactions for sulfated acid protein-polysaccharides (alcian blue), glycoproteins (periodic acid–Schiff), collagen (aniline blue), and reticulin (silver nitrate). *Thus a cell that was once formative (osteoblast) can be converted to one with destructive potential (degranulating osteocyte).* Osteocytes also function beneficially in intralacunar formation of osteoid and in the physiologic perilacunar resorption of bone matrix; they are thus vital to bone turnover dynamics.

The osteoclast is a multinucleated giant cell derived from mitosis and fusion of locally available undifferentiated mesenchymal cells. These processes are readily demonstrable experimentally by utilizing autoradiography of histologic specimens after administration of a DNA precursor to the experimental subject. Most often used is the pyrimidine analogue, thymidine ^3H, which is employed by progenitor cells for nucleic acid synthesis during DNA replication just prior to cellular mitosis. The aggregation of cells into osteoclasts occurs adjacent to bone surfaces, the derived giant cells in intimate approximation to bone. In most histologic specimens the cells are located in resorptive bays (Howship's lacunae) in bone. Histochemically, osteoclasts are remarkable for their high concentration of acid phosphatases, nonspecific esterases, nonspecific proteases, aminopeptidases, β-glucuronidases, cathepsins, lipases, and glycolytic substances; these enzymes are concerned, when released from the osteoclast extracellularly, with the lysis of bone. In order for organic bone matrices to be affected by enzymes of osteoclastic origin, they must be demineralized first. The osteoclast appears also to develop rather intense anaerobic metabolism of carbohydrate to form lactic acid, citrate, and the H^+ ion. These organic acids contribute to bone resorption by furnishing an extracellular acidic environment favoring bone demineralization. They apparently bind bone mineral via a chelating process and thus withdraw calcium salts from their affiliations with bone collagen and matrix.

There is little information to denote active phagocytosis on the part of the cell. The parathyroid hormone, parathormone, a factor regulating in part the withdrawal of mineral from bone and its renal excretion, thus establishing physiologic concentrations of calcium and phosphate within serum, appears to do so by labilizing the lysosomes of the osteoclast. There is consequent extracytic transfer of acid hydrolases. Other substances of endogenous origin, for example, osteoclast-activating factor (OAF) and prostaglandins E_1 and E_2, are also important mediators of bone resorption, especially in relationship with inflammatory states. In this context prostaglandin content of periodontal exudates parallels the clinical and radiologic extent of bone resorption in marginal periodontitis.

The osteoclast is easily recognized in histologic specimens because of its large size, irregular morphology, numerous deeply stained nuclei, granular cytoplasm, and its localization next to bone. In the normal attachment apparatus, subjected to homeostatic bone appositional-resorptive processes, osteoclasts are rarely observed despite the fairly rapid turnover cycle of the tissue. However, when inflammation or injury supervene, the formation and activity of osteoclasts are engendered. *Interestingly, the "prolific" tissues of the periodontium—those capable of the greatest formative potential—are the tissues that give rise to osteoclasts; these are periosteum, endosteum, and periodontal ligament* (Fig. 23-8). The early reparative process (about the first 2 or 4 days) after periodontal surgery often shows little osteoclastic activity, particularly if the periosteum has been involved in the surgical procedure. The subsequent 7 to 10 days may be marked by bone resorption as the mitotic and generative capabilities of the tissue return. *Procedures retaining periosteum in situ or with minimal surgical traumatization and manipulation or both tend to conserve bone by preserving the periosteum's fibrogenic and osteogenic abilities; much of the vascularization to adjacent bone is also retained. This thesis will be expanded in the section dealing with repair after "periosteal conservation" surgery.*

The special role of the *plasma cell* in healing may be difficult to promulgate. It does engage in the early and intermediate phases of tissue repair and is affiliated with the inflammatory response. The cells, of B-lymphocyte origin, appear first in perivascular sites as ovoid bodies with fairly distinct cell membranes (especially

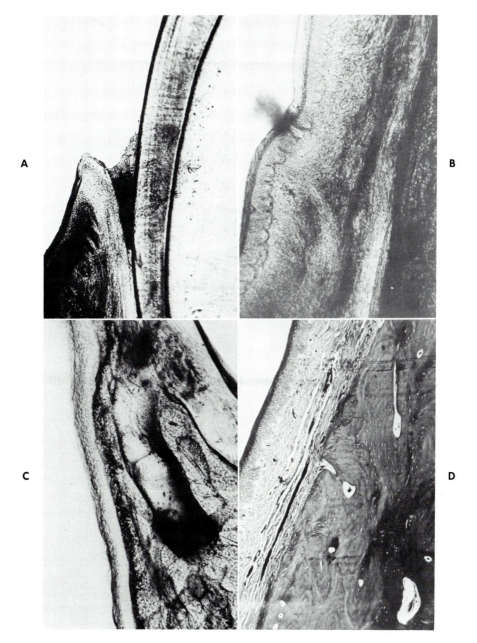

Fig. 23-8. After perfusion of cervical lymphatics to demonstrate lymphatic pathways in periodontal tissues, perfusate (flowing in a reverse pathway through gingiva) eventuates in gingival sulcus, **A,** while distending unattached gingival cuff from tooth. Thin, incompletely formed and weakly collagenated tissue tends clinically to be more easily retracted. This may be undesirable, since it may favor submarginal accrual of bacterial plaque with consequent initiation of inflammation. **B** and **C,** Periosteal lymphatics and lymph pathways, important in removal of fluid excesses and particulate debris from gingiva, mucosa, and bone. **D,** Example of periosteal blood vessels, in this instance closely following bone surface. When periosteal conservation techniques of surgery are employed in therapy, principal periosteal blood and lymph vessels are preserved. They also serve as springboards for vascular and lymphatic regeneration and extension.

with iron-hematoxylin staining procedures). The nucleus is positioned with eccentric polarity and surrounded by a weakly staining halo of cytoplasm; it may appear large and centrally granular or vesicular. Characteristic, however, are nodular clusters of deeply staining chromatin (DNA) aligned along the inner aspects of the nuclear circumference. The cytoplasm of this differentiated cell (it does not have mitotic ability) shows distinct and prominent granularity, characteristic of cells that are synthetically active. Mitochondria are plentiful and their cristae are complex and granular (via ultramicroscopy). Pyroninophilia is marked, indicating polyribosomal accumulation; ultrastructural evaluations elicit extensive development of granular endoplasmic reticulum, Golgi complex, and lysosomes. Protein synthesis by the cell is often striking; it is concerned with the formation of gamma globulins —particularly immunoglobulins G and M—that are reactive with either exogenous (bacterial) or endogenous (tissue) antigens. Antibody formation can be graphically demonstrated using fluorescent antiglobulins that are permitted to react with tissue specimens; granular cytoplasmic fluorescence within plasma cells is characteristic.

Plasma cells appear to be nearly ubiquitous in small numbers to the subsulcular connective tissue of clinically and otherwise histologically normal gingiva, are numerous in cellular infiltrates in chronic inflammation in association with lymphocytes and mononuclear macrophages, and are abundant in the granulation tissues of healing wounds. Antigens may be phagocytized by such cells as monocytes and mononuclear macrophages and "processed" intracellularly; antigenic information (probably ribonucleic acid complexes) is then transferred to approximating lymphocytes, which are converted in peripheral tissues to antibody-producing plasma cells. Lymphocyte transformation either to large, "activated" lymphoblasts (cellular immunity) or to plasma cells appears to take place primarily within lymphoid tissues (lymph nodes). One may extrapolate from this information that the role of the plasma cell in healing is concerned with the ultimate negation of microorganisms and their products. Also, tissue proteins and polysaccharides rendered "foreign" by surgical injury and inflammation may elicit plasma cell immunoglobulin production. These globulins may in turn affiliate with antigens, increasing their susceptibility to phagocytosis and removal from the injured site. Much study is required of immunologic processes during the

healing of oral wounds; our scientific information is more descriptive than analytic. It is well known, for example, that systemic administration of such drugs as prednisolone and azathioprine (Imuran) interferes with cellular immunologic processes; such substances could be utilized to elicit directly and indirectly the roles played by plasma cells, lymphocytes, and so on in healing.

While it is not within the purview of this paper to discuss either general or periodontal immunobiology, it may be apropos to discuss the lymphocyte's role in cellular and humoral immunologic processes and the known and hypothetical roles of lymphocyte-derived factors in inflammatory and reparative processes. While the B-lymphocyte is primarily concerned with the facilitation of humoral (antibody-mediated) immunity and tends to be "fixed" within lymphoid and connective tissues, especially after activation by macrophage-processed antigen, the T-lymphocyte (thymic derived) is concerned with immunologic memory, the elaboration of a variety of effector substances collectively designated as lymphokines, and the recruitment of cells required for antigen disposal. The majority (75% or more) of circulating lymphocytes are of the T type. The T-lymphocyte has recently been implicated in a rather unique function—that of antigen recognition with subsequent activation of B-lymphocytes. B-lymphocytes, under thymic control, may then synthesize immunoglobulins specific for the negation of the specific antigen recognized by the T cell or may undergo structural and functional metamorphosis to become plasma cells. The plasma cells may then synthesize and release antibodies (IgG, IgM, IgA, IgE) for specific resistance to alien or altered self-components. The T cell may also provide an enzyme that can cause plasma cells to switch from IgM to IgG production. This latter phenomenon may possibly be seen in acute necrotizing ulcerative gingivitis, where in the initial days of the infection serumal IgM levels are elevated and IgG levels are depressed. On the fifth to seventh day IgG blood levels increase significantly while IgM blood levels become markedly reduced. A T-lymphocyte factor may split the pentamer molecule, IgM (900,000 mol. wt.), to its monomeric form, IgG (160,000 mol. wt).

The T-lymphocyte is ubiquitous to chronic inflammatory infiltrates. As the acute phase of postsurgical inflammation subsides, about 2 to 4 days after injury, and is supplanted by chronic inflammation, large numbers of lymphocytes, plasma cells, and macrophages are dispersed throughout the topical and outer aspects of the wound. The T-lymphocytes *may* aid in the healing process by their production and secretion of a macrophage-activating factor (promotion of their enzymatic and phagocytic débridement of the wound), a migration-inhibiting factor (maintaining macrophages at the center of action of the wound), osteoclast- and fibroclast-activating factors, and, importantly, osteoblast- and connective tissue–activating pep-

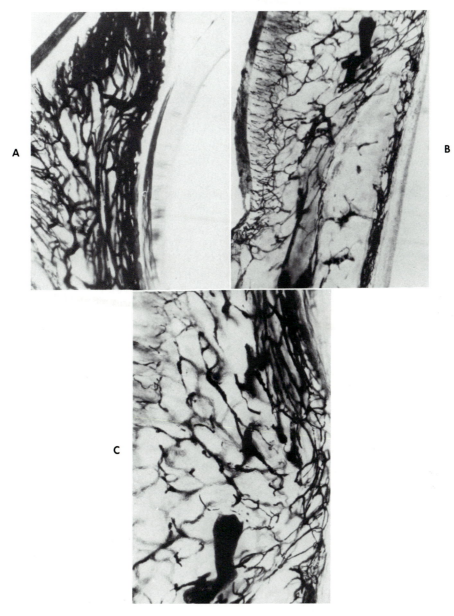

Fig. 23-9. Studies of microcirculation to gingiva and alveolar mucosa demonstrate a horizontal plexus of blood vessels subjacent to sulcular and junctional epithelia (extending vertically in center of **A**), and a combined horizontal and vertical arcade of vessels under the gingival epithelium (left of **A**). **B,** Prominent periosteal vasculature with extensions into a weakly vascularized buccal septum. Periodontal ligament's vessels are elaborate in number and distribution and can be seen as reticulated band between bone and tooth. **C,** Indicative of diminished vascular supply to central portion of gingival corium (central portion of **C**). Note vascular plexus at right, just external to cementum within gingiva. Vessels communicate with those of periodontal ligament. (From Janson, W., Ruben, M. P., Kramer, G. M., and Bloom, A. A.: J. Periodontol. **40:**707, 1969.)

tides. The latter substances, glycopeptides of multiple but low molecular weights, after release from T-lymphocytes diffuse with exudates through the tissues and are presumed to be phagocytized by or bound to surface receptors of fibroblasts, osteoblasts, cementoblasts, and so on. Reparative processes are thus initiated and maintained. The persistence of low-intensity chronic inflammation with T-lymphocyte presence and participation may be a prime requisite for healing and a concomitant to the resorption of hard and soft tissues that invariably attends surgical procedures.

Tissue vascularization. All the body tissues are reliant upon the nutritive and hydrating elements ferried to them via their vasculature. For example, water is vital to cellular chemistry and metabolism, since all matter is either suspended or dissolved in a fluid milieu. Water is also required for the dynamic maintenance of the intracellular gelation state, imparting bulk, form, and appropriate spatial relationships between cell constituents *and* between the cell and its environment. Water is integral to the viscosity of the gel state of ground substance, to the "cementation" of collagenous molecules and fibrils, and to the transport of substances to, through, and away from the tissue site. There is, then, a state of dynamic equilibrium between intravascular and extravascular zones, and between extracellular and intracellular sites, maintained via fluid transport.

The units of the vasculature participating directly in such activity include blood capillaries, venules, and lymphatic channels (Fig. 23-9). The capillary bed of a particular connective tissue, in a general context, is morphologically extensive. Close examination discloses a reticulated network of vessels reaching *every aspect of the tissue* (Fig. 23-9). Actually, tissue cells are rarely if ever more than 50 μm away from a capillary; diffusion of transudates to cells with subsequent cellular uptake via pinocytosis is ordinarily very rapid. It has been estimated, however, that only a small fraction of these channels are open or patent at any given time. The structural organization of the connective tissue, its degree of function, the presence of disease, and the quality and amount of irritants derived from disease processes are representative factors that regulate the type and quantity of patent vessels, intravascular rheology, and movement of matter through vascular walls. Dense connective tissues, such as the *intermediate* zone of the gingival corium, display a relative paucity (Fig. 23-9, *C*) of vessels; yet in the *same* tissue complex (attached gingiva) in the loose con-

nective tissue subjacent to the epithelium there is, physiologically, an unusually great display of operating vessels. The same is true of the lamina propria adjacent to sulcular epithelium and epithelial attachment and the connective tissue of the inner aspect of periosteum. These areas of pronounced vascularization are also the zones of the greater cellular metabolic and formative activity. Thus a balance exists between the structural quality, metabolic activity, and the extent of a tissue's microcirculation.

Capillaries are constructed of a simple, thin, and nearly flat monolayer of endothelial cells encased in a basement membrane and surrounded and contained by perivascular connective tissue. The density and thus the rigidity of the connective tissue containing collagen *inversely* regulates, in significant measure, vessel size, luminal patency, and degree of transudation. Patency and transendothelial fluid movement are also controlled *directly* by the intravascular hydrostatic pressure in relationship to its pressure gradient with that of the intercellular zone. Normally, capillary pressure approximates 28 mm Hg, whereas that of tissue fluid varies between 6 and 8 mm Hg; thus a difference of 20 to 22 mm Hg exists.

Endothelial cells are maintained in approximation not only by a balance between intraluminal pressure and the restricting action of peripheral basement membrane and connective tissue, but also by *dynamic* occlusion of their approximating cell walls—zonula occludens. Neither desmosomes nor intercellular bridges are found. It is felt that despite apparent contact, a minute linear space of about 8 nm intervenes, through which the serumal phase of blood moves. The width and number of patent "slits" varies physiologically (as in increased function) and pathologically (as in inflammation). Processes comparable to those theorized for the "dynamic adherence" of epithelial attachment to tooth may possibly be operative in interendothelial sites (Chapter 1). These include the intercellular presence of glycoproteins (histochemically demonstrable by the periodic acid–Schiff reaction) and ionic bonding of negatively charged plasma membranes by Ca^{++} and so on. The surface charge of cells appears to be produced by neuraminic acid, a sialoprotein; neuraminidase treatment of cells eliminates the negative surface potential. It has also been shown that endothelial cells of venules may phagocytize minute particulate substances, transport them in intracytoplasmic vesicles to the outer aspect of the cell, and then, via "reverse phagocytosis" or "reverse pinocytosis," excrete the material to the basement membrane area. This process may be demonstrated experimentally using carbon or ferritin tracers in vivo; it may assist in the transport of cells (e.g., small lymphocytes) from the intraluminal to extraluminal zones in inflammatory and immunologic states.

The basement membrane of capillaries is usually thin and difficult to demonstrate with commonly employed stains. However, it is periodic acid–Schiff positive, indicating carbohydrate, reacts with silver nitrate for reticulin, shows limited sudanophilia for lipid, and engages lightly with colloidal iron for acid mucopolysaccharides. Ultrastructurally it is comparable in form to the epithelial basement membrane and separated by a thin electron-lucent space from endothelium. Fenestrae, or "pores," may possibly be present, allowing for transudation and export of fine particulate matter from the vessel; however, they have not been convincingly elicited. One can only extrapolate from the rheology of fluid passage that such "pores" are existent. Active movement of large bodies, such as neutrophils, occurs; this may, however, be facilitated (1) by the activity of chemical mediators of the inflammatory process (such as histamine, bradykinin, and prostaglandins and (2) by the lytic action of neutrophilic acid hydrolases on interendothelial substance and basement membrane.

Contained within the basement membrane one may occasionally see outstretched thin cells resembling fibroblasts; these are pericytes, or Rouget cells. Pericytes have been implicated as providing a contractile function because of their location and arrangement external to the endothelium. They may also constitute a stem cell population for the replacement of lost or damaged endothelial cells; pericytic proliferation may also play a part in the formation of new blood vessels that dominate the healing surgical wound.

Endothelium shows sparse intracellular enzyme activity, particularly of acid hydrolases. Most endothelial cells exhibit striking, histochemically elicited, adenosine triphosphatase (ATPase), possibly synonymous with high mitochondrial metabolism of carbohydrate (such as glucose). This histochemical method is valuable for the demonstration of the cells and is useful in the documentation of microvascularization.

Vascular transudates are composed of the serumal aspect of blood, meaning that macromolecular material such as fibrinogen is excluded. Generally, substances with a molecular weight of

under 50,000 to 60,000 are allowed to pass. This relationship is by no means rigid; trace amounts of such molecules as albumin, hemoglobin, and low-molecular-weight α-globulins are customarily found in transudates. Ubiquitous to transudative fluids are water, amino acids, simple sugars such as glucose, and serumal cations and anions, the most important of which are Na^+, K^+, Ca^{++}, Mg^{++}, Cl^-, PO_5, and CO_3. Selective permeability exists.

The removal of fluid from the tissue is accomplished by joint action of the venular phase of the microcirculatory bed and the lymphatics (Fig. 23-10, *A*). Their structure is grossly comparable to that of the blood capillaries. However, lymphatics are notable for the paucity of basement membrane (it may be nonexistent), weak occlusion between endothelial cells (30 to 50 nm for lymph vessels), absence of pericytes, and sparse

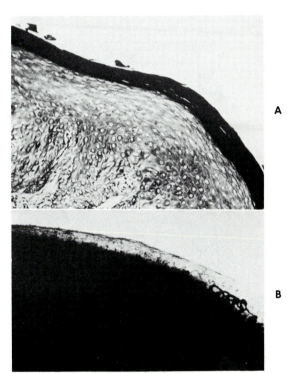

Fig. 23-10. Gingival keratinization is a desirable physiologic and postsurgical attribute; it affords a barrier to ingress of exogenous irritants (generally only lipid soluble and ionizable substances will enter epithelium) and appears to inhibit outward movement of tissue fluid into oral cavity, tending to maintain tissue hydration. **A,** Gingival keratinization is distinct and is relatable to nature of connective tissue corium. **B,** Keratinizing epithelial effect is a satisfactory hindrance to transepithelial passage of a vascular transudate.

or loose encompassing connective tissue. Tissue solutes tend to reenter the circulatory system through the venular and lymphatic circulation, whereas macromolecular materials, such as cell debris, high-molecular-weight immunoglobulins (e.g., immunoglobulin M—mol. wt. 900,000), and lipid, are preferentially removed via the lymphatics. Their potentially great ''pore'' size usually permits facile transport of fluid and molecular substances into their lumina. Tissue hydrostatic pressure, usually somewhat greater than that within venules and lymphatics, is of cooperative assistance. Substances are returned to the venous system in the head and neck from draining lymphatics by the thoracic and right lymphatic ducts. Macromolecular tissue debris, present either as a consequence of physiologic resorptive processes or as an accompaniment of pathologic conditions, may also be disposed of by phagocytosis. In connective tissues both banded and nonbanded segments of collagen fibrils have been seen intracellularly within cells resembling fibroblasts, while comparable phagocytosis and intracellular digestion are effected by macrophages in inflammation, wound healing, and traumatic lesions.

The lymphatic terminal arcades in periodontal tissues have recently been displayed via perfusion methods (Fig. 23-9). They undoubtedly play an essential role in normalcy. Lymphatics become more overt and patent during inflammation, with conditions producing lymphatic obstruction (i.e., staphylococcal infections), and in the primary, early, and intermediate phases of wound healing (up to 12 to 14 days). Sulcular fluid is comparable in composition to that of lymph; the gingival sulcus and epithelium may constitute a ''lymphatic area'' (Fig. 23-9, A). The lymphatics of the periodontium are distributed with the blood vasculature and are especially evident in gingival lamina propria, alveolar mucosa, periosteum, marrow, and alveolar phase of periodontal ligament (Fig. 23-9, A to C).

The formation of new capillaries (and lymphatics) during inflammatory processes (as in pyogenic and reparative granulomas) and in wound healing is especially prolific. In healing, new vessels arise, beginning 3 to 4 days after injury and continuing for an additional 10 to 15 days, by proliferation of the endothelia (possibly pericytes also) of existing vessels. Buds of endothelial cells can first be seen, arising from the sides and ends of severed or damaged vessels. Then cell masses —shoots, cords, clusters—extend outward from the original vessel forming irregular networks of nonlumenized vessels. These vessels anastomose with other newly forming capillaries and extend to join other available capillaries. Once the junction occurs, blood and blood plasma begin to course irregularly between the endothelial cells. The new blood and lymph vessels are extremely permeable to both particulate and fluid material. Tissue edema and extravasation of formed blood elements are common. Lumina form as the solid cell masses begin to carry serum, plasma, or blood. At first the new capillary may have several cell layers. However, the capillary endothelial wall becomes progressively thinner, finally acquiring a monolayer structure. The surrounding connective tissue, at first loosely and poorly organized because of an abundance of ground substance and weak collagenation, gradually acquires increasing gelation and oriented fiber arrangement. Perivascular reticulum and collagen are not only arranged longitudinally but also circularly, a factor indirectly regulating the extent of vascular patency.

Nerves and their regeneration. The pattern of distribution of neural supply to periodontal tissues grossly parallels that of its vasculature and lymphatics. Thus larger nerve assemblies are seen in association with periosteal, intraseptal, and pulpally directed vessels. Lateral arborations of smaller caliber, generally myelinated, extend respectively into the gingival corium and bone, marrow and periodontal ligament, and ligament and dental pulp. Plexi and terminations of fine, dominantly nonmyelinated filaments are located within the gingival lamina propria, endosteum, inner phase of periosteum, and in the indifferent connective tissue of the ligament.

Each filament is composed of an extension of a nerve cell body, located in either the central nervous system or ganglia; actually its core—the axon—is a product continuously synthesized within the cell body. In the formation of neural filaments the secretory product (protein primarily) flows peripherally within a tube composed of the outer membrane of neuroectodermal cells—the Schwann cell, absent within the central nervous system (substituted by processes of connective tissue cells) but universal to all peripheral nerves either as myelin or neurilemmal sheaths. These sheaths are ultrastructurally lamellar and are comprised of lipoprotein. Nerve fibers, except at or very near effector or receptor sites, tend to be arranged in fascicles bound internally and circumscribed by connective tissue.

When nerves are severed in periodontal surgery, the axons and myelin or neurilemmal sheaths *distal* to the incision are actually divorced from the cell body and undergo rapid disintegration, a droplet type of degeneration. Macrophages of connective tissue phagocytize and digest the remnants of necrotic axons and sheaths. As connective tissue and vascular repair begin, the cells of the Schwann sheath of the proximal (central nervous system connected) stump proliferate, growing irregularly distally into the granulation tissue of the healing wound. They form planes of orientation for the *flow* of axon protein into clefts or slits between them and then encompass the regenerating axons as neurilemmal or myelin tubes, replicating the original formation of the nerves. The *rate* of axonic extension to form new distal nerve stumps approximates 1 mm per day. Droz documented the synthesis and peripheral flow of axon protein via autoradiographic techniques (Leblond and Warren). Comparable investigations are in progress at Boston University. Histochemically, nerve distribution and regeneration may be demonstrated by $AgNO_3$ (after pretreatment of sections with collagenase) and with Luxol fast blue and Sudan black for lipid-containing modalities. Sympathetic innervation to the vasculature of the periodontium normally and during tissue repair has not been investigated. Methods do exist for the demonstration specifically of catecholamines either utilized or synthesized at medial myoneural junctions of arteries and arterioles.

Epithelium. The progenitor basis for epithelial replication lies in its basal cell population. Mitosis and tissue turnover occur physiologically at a fairly uniform rate, within a *given* area of the oral cavity, but some variation exists between *different* zones (Chapter 1). For example, the replication cycle of junctional epithelium is approximately 5 days, while that of the surface of attached gingiva is 10 or more days. The cycle is also influenced by such factors as species, body temperature, time of day, age, hormones and vitamin availability, degree of function, and hydration. Striking effects are produced during inflammation and as a consequence of wounding.

As new epithelial cells are produced by mitosis within the basal layer, excess cells — those beyond the territorial capacity of the basal zone — tend to be expressed outward into the epithelium. This appears to be a passive phenomenon, nonpreferential for either progenitors or siblings. Prior desmosomal adherences are provisionally dissolved but are reacquired and lost dynamically

as cells move into and through prickle cell layers and thence into granular cell lamellae. In parakeratotic and keratotic layers, attachment plaques are lost, facilitating eventual cell desquamation into the oral cavity. In nonkeratinizing epithelia, flattened cells are shed from the free surface of the tissue. Against hard dental surfaces — enamel and cementum — epithelium does not display its keratinizing potential and will simulate the cell character and shedding pattern seen in the *nonkeratinizing variety*. The epithelial conversion induced at its interface with a hard surface is of *primary* importance not only in the development of the dentogingival relationship but also in the planning and the execution of periodontal therapy.

One must *first* recognize that the keratinizing quality of certain epithelia is genetically determined, manifested first in the fetus and later revealed and extended in the postnatal and later periods of life. Thus, for example, the epithelium of attached gingiva in situ or transferred en bloc to other areas (e.g., to labial mucosa) will continue to display the keratinizing effect. Conversely, nonkeratinizing epithelium such as that of buccal or alveolar mucosa when in situ or transplanted to the zone of attached gingiva will continue to manifest the nonkeratinizing quality. There are indications, within the structure of epithelial *basal* cells, of this potential for keratinization, for example, the numerous and well-oriented intracytoplasmic tonofilaments that later form the mat upon which polyribosomes are deposited when the granular cell phase is reached. Yet when the epithelium of attached gingiva at the gingival margin "turns" into the sulcus, its surface qualities change; its basal cell potential for intracellular keratinization does not become manifest. A comparable gingivodental interface is formed at the *contact* areas between adjacent teeth — thus the lack of keratinization of col epithelium. If we exclude primary gingival development from consideration by removing original sulcular and col epithelium and a *portion* of the epithelium of attached gingiva by gingivectomy, and then observe the postexcisional healing, we would see the reacquisition of the keratinizing cover of attached gingiva and the failure of keratinization in contact with the tooth. This replication of original development would take place despite the fact that the *source* of these epithelia is the same — the keratinizing epithelium at the *edge* of the incision. These observations point then to biologic considerations that are fundamental and of extreme importance in periodontal surgery and in the prevention of renewed disease:

1. The propensity of epithelial tissue to display either parakeratinization or orthokeratinization is largely determined by the nature of the connective tissue substrate upon which it is situated. Dense connective tissues, with a high fiber-matrix ratio, maximal matrix viscosity, diminished vascularization, and decreased tissue fluid content favor the development of keratinization of the overlying epithelium (e.g., attached gingiva). Conversely, loose connective tissues with low collagen-matrix proportions, enhanced vascularization, and tissue hydration are associated with nonkeratinizing epithelia (e.g., alveolar mucosa) (Fig. 23-11).

2. Epithelial keratinization will be manifested relative to dense connective tissues regardless of the epithelial source. Thus epithelium of alveolar mucosal derivation (nonkeratinizing) will exhibit a keratinizing effect when combined with gingival

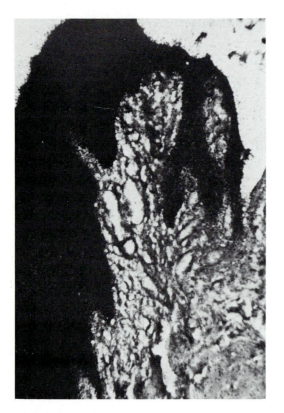

Fig. 23-11. Autoradiograph of marginal gingiva after proline ^{14}C administration parenterally. Tissue fluids are labeled with isotope; thus transudates entering epithelium are discernible after diffusing across basement membranes. At top left corner and top right area fluid is leaving tissue, indicating loss from nonkeratinizing and erosive epithelial surfaces.

connective tissue both in vitro and in vivo. Gingival epithelium when brought into alliance with mucosal connective tissue will convert to the nonkeratinizing type.

3. Epithelium in abutment with enamel, dentin, cementum, and artificial substances such as porcelain, plastics, and gold loses its capacity for keratinization. The inability of the junctional, col, and sulcular epithelia to keratinize has been allied to a "disturbed" connective tissue marked by deficient collagenation, haphazard connective tissue fiber orientation, and evidence of fibroblastic degeneration. These findings may be causally related to a minimal inflammatory state present in the connective tissue, a near universal situation at these sites, or to the presence of sparse numbers of immunocompetent cells and macrophages. Immunocompetent cells and macrophages are known at other body locations to produce and release factors that may cause the following tissue alterations: (1) macrophages $\rightarrow$ collagenase, hyaluronidase and (2) lymphocytes (T type) $\rightarrow$ prostaglandins, bradykinin. Epithelial cells abutting dental surfaces usually have smooth topography, while the free surfaces of keratinizing epithelium display plicated (wrinkled) cell membranes. Are there variations of cell hydration and cytoplasmic viscosity that determine the surface nature of epithelial cells?

4. When tooth-abutting epithelium is exposed to the oral environment, for example, col epithelium when teeth are separated orthodontically, it will gradually transform, in the absence of inflammation, into the keratinizing variety as the col morphology is gradually changed to one of convexity. If interdental gingiva is surgically shaped so that it is convex and shy of contact with the proximal tooth contact, the healed area will demonstrate an epithelial cover of the keratinizing type.

5. A number of studies have indicated that both sulcular and col epithelia serve as tissue portals for the entrance of irritative and potentially antigenic moieties into the gingival connective tissue—these include bacterial hyaluronidase, proteins such as albumin and endotoxin and tracer particulate matter such as peroxidase and ferritin—and thus may incite inflammatory and immunobiologic reactions. This faculty may be associated with the nonkeratinizing nature of the epithelia and the lack of physical and chemical protection that could be afforded by a stratum corneum. In the latter context the *outer* keratinizing effect places definite limitations on the nature and the

amount of material that may traverse the stratum corneum and enter the other phases of the epithelium or subsequently diffuse into the subjacent epithelium and connective tissue. Generally, only lipid-soluble and dissolved and nonionized substances will cross the barrier zone of a keratinizing epithelium from the external environment into the tissues. Surgical procedures should therefore be designed to minimize the square area of epithelial contact with the tooth; this may be an important physical factor in the prevention of renewed inflammatory disease.

Shallow sulci and rigidity of the sulcular wall, as a reflection of gingival connective tissue density, inhibit the intrasulcular accumulation of bacterial plaque and debris and thus reduce the possibility of gingival disease. Prevention of epithelial contact with zones of dental approximation allows the fullest expression of epithelial keratinization, a quality deigned to be protective against irritation and injury.

Connective tissue in the healing process. The first few days (up to 4) of connective tissue healing are dominated by the inflammatory reaction to the surgical procedure. Severance of epithelium and a fraction of the underlying corium of connective tissue is accompanied by bleeding derived from cut and injured blood vessels; arterioles, capillaries, and venules make up the microvasculature of periodontal tissues. Vascular injury connotes bulk movement of and perviousness to the macromolecular portions of blood and increased fluid transport through existing vessel walls. These include such plasma fractions as albumin, fibrinogen, α-globulins and β-globulins, immunoglobulins, as well as the formed elements, for example, erythrocytes, monocytes, leukocytes, and platelets. An aggregate of these—in hydrated and gel form—is the *blood clot,* formed extravascularly on the wound surface, adjacent to the injured wall, or severed ends of blood vessels, and in faults, notably clefts, within the tissue corium. The fibrin clot also intervenes between tissue flap and bone or periosteum, acting to promote a tenuous tissue adherence at the site. The clot furnishes a viscous provisional seal controlling hemorrhage and limiting exudation; its interface with underlying or contiguous tissue also serves as a pathway for the escape of the exudate.

The clot, fibrin based, also acts to orient a mat of leukocytes (the polyband). These cells, both viable and nonviable in character, are found immediately adjacent to the clot; many are also dispersed throughout the clot matrix and are usually difficult to identify because of their tendency to undergo autolysis or to be destroyed by the surrounding exudate. The collection of leukocytes peripheral to the clot may contribute to its dissolution and to clearance of an avenue for epithelial cell migration to occur over the connective tissue corium under the clot or for new connective tissue to form at the interface zone. The neutrophil, other granulocytes, and monocytes are well endowed with the acid hydrolases of lysosomal derivation; these enzymes have at minimum a duopotential: (1) for endocytic digestion of foreign material (i.e., bacteria) and antigens and (2) for extracellular tissue hydrolysis. These digestive substances are potentially proteolytic, demineralizing, lipid destroying, and glycolytic relative to clot and tissue components. In the postsurgical inflammatory state the blood clot is enzymatically dissolved and phagocytized and digested by mononuclear macrophages; the residuum is shed from the wound surface as clot fibrinolysis occurs as a portion of the wound exudate. A portion of the exudate is also removed from the wound area via patent lymphatics, although early in the postsurgical period (0 to 4 days) partial lymphatic blockade is commonly present. In the regenerative phase of healing, lymphatics become important avenues for disposal of both liquid and particulate portions of the exudate.

The connective tissue of the wound reflects early engorgement with tissue fluid and hemorrhagic exudate, resulting in displacement and disorientation of its fibrillar, vascular, and cellular constituents. This is a physical or mechanical process augmented by alterations induced by fluid intrusion between the fibers and by the action of hyaluronidase, chondroitin sulfatase, and so on on the protein-polysaccharide binding and supporting substrates of the tissue. Collagen fibers are split longitudinally into fibrils by comparable processes; chondroitin sulfate forms the cementing medium between them and is depolymerized by cell-derived hydrolytic enzymes. Thus in histologic analyses, affinity for alcian blue or colloidal iron would be diminished or absent in the region of the fibers, since these dyes are specific for acid protein-polysaccharides. Haphazardly distributed collagen and reticulin fibrils are seen dispersed on a pale granular background.

Collagen fibrils are further damaged by segmentation derived from the activity of collagenases, nonspecific proteases, aminopeptidases, etc., severing end- and cross-linkages between collagen and tropocollagen molecules. Collagen may actually be reduced to its polypeptide, peptide, and amino acid constituents. These alterations, including the loss of axial periodicity, may to a large extent be demonstrated via electron microscopy. Light microscopically analyzed sections reveal fibril fragmentation into short segments and amorphous and granular forms that may be adjoined by neutrophils (later by monocytes and histiocytes). As collagen is altered — by deamination, acetylation, and so on — it loses its usual affinity for aniline blue, orange G, acid fuchsin, and so on and may often be stained by dyes considered to be specific for elastin; thus aldehyde fuchsin and orcein may delineate regressive changes in collagen.

Biochemical assays of new connective tissue wounds produced by incision demonstrate reductions in the total amounts of both insoluble and soluble collagen. Concomitantly, tissue hydroxyproline content is diminished. When collagen synthesis becomes progressively more extensive and dynamic, there is substantial improvement in the tissue content of soluble collagen; hydroxyproline concentrations concurrently increase. In radioisotopic studies of connective tissue healing, proline ^{14}C accumulation within collagen appears to be greatest 7 to 21 days after wounding. There appears to be a substantial temporal delay in the formation of significant quantities of insoluble collagen at a connective tissue wound site as evidenced by the degree of cross-linkage between collagen's polypeptide chains and the quantitative increase in the connective tissue's tensile strength. After 3 months wound tensile strength is inferior to that of comparable uninjured tissue. Persistence of a low-intensity, chronic inflammatory state may be integral to the continuation of collagen and matrical synthesis by fibroblasts (osteoblasts, cementoblasts.).

The inflammatory process in relationship to mineralized surfaces — cementum, bone, dentin — may also elicit the collagen resorption patterns just described; a demineralizing action is also evidenced prior to matrix and collagen hydrolysis. The acidity of the resorptive milieu may contribute to the destructive process; lactic acid and citric acid synthesis and release by inflammatory cells and osteoclasts may lead to demineralization via the process of chelation.

The acute inflammatory reaction is also characterized by cellular destruction. Tissue fibroblasts, endothelium (including pericytes), mesenchymal cells, and so on are usually damaged or eliminated at the site of injury. Cell membranes become indistinct and are lost; cytoplasmic organelles decrease and lose their fine structure to variable extents, indicating reduced or absent metabolic and formative activities. Mitochondria, for example, appear swollen, lose their cristae (and associated granules), cease replicating, and thus decrease in number; the mitochondrial metabolic mill may function poorly or not at all.

Nuclear structure and activity are also adversely affected. Mitosis may cease. Nucleoli (RNA) are deficient or defective. Chromatin (DNA) may clump, become granular, and be indifferently distributed. The nuclear membrane, usually of a characteristic trilamellar nature, becomes homogeneous; segmentation may also occur here. As nucleic acids are progressively depolymerized and destroyed, nuclear staining by the Fuelgen (DNA) and pyronin (RNA) reactions is comparably modified. Nuclei become morphologically irregular, shunken, and split — thus pyknotic and amorphous via light microscopy.

When cells are destroyed their constituents — nuclear, cytoplasmic, and membrane — are scattered into the exudate of the site. Cellular lysosomal enzymes, thus released, contribute to the *lytic potential of the exudate* and in this way may further the destructive phase of inflammation.

Cellular debris, like its fibrillar counterpart, is also phagocytized and digested by scavenger cells: the monocyte-macrophage cell series. It is conceivable that this debris, once phagocytized and "processed," may serve as antigens to stimulate *later* antibody synthesis by local plasma cells *or* as antigens to excite cell-mediated (lymphocytic) immunologic reactions. Both types of reactive cells, plasma cells and lymphocytes, become progressively more prominent in the inflammatory and healing processes on the third and fourth day after wounding and thereafter. The chronic infiltrate wanes in intensity as collagenation increases. The antigenic information is "passed" from phagocytic cell to plasmoblast or lymphocyte. These are probably RNA polymers that after transfer act as inducers or templates for RNA synthesis by the recipient cells. In the case of plasma cells the RNA synthetic products are largely immunoglobulins, whereas in the case of transformed lymphocytes the secretory products are termed "lymphokines." After extracytic transfer into the tissues these substances may incite osteoclasts, fibroclasts, monocytes, macrophages, and so on to resorptive activity and activate cells such as macrophages to phagocytize and digest antigenic substances.

It has been hypothesized that altered epithelial and connective tissue components may be phagocytized by mononuclear macrophages, processed, and then transferred to tissue mesenchymal cells, leading to their mitosis and differentiation, with subsequent synthesis of connective tissue elements (collagen, reticulin, matrix constituents, and so on). Such transfer is also accomplished with comparable subsequent synthetic activity to already existing fibroblasts and osteoblasts. Endothelial proliferation may also be similarly produced. Thus the "processed tissue" acts as an inductor for cellular proliferation and the formation of new tissues in the healing wound. Inflammation, then, can function as a sword and also as an olive branch, setting the stage for repair. Inductor materials presently under investigation include calcified and surface demineralized particles of compact bone, dentin, and cementum; hematopoietic (red) marrow homogenates of transitional epithelium; T-lymphocyte-derived fibroblast- and osteoclast-activating factors (glycopeptides); polyribonucleotides; and such exogenous substances as phenytoin sodium (Dilantin sodium) and carrageenan (Irish moss).

Prostaglandins, generically a group of fatty acids found in nearly all body tissues, are considered to be locally acting "wound hormones" largely but not exclusively formed by cells at the site of injury. For example, prostaglandins E_1 and E_2 are synthesized by fibroblasts and mononuclear cells at areas of chronic inflammation. Prostaglandins E_1 and E_2 may encourage collagen biosynthesis and the hydroxylation of amino acids indigenous to collagen (proline $\rightarrow$ hydroxyproline; glycine $\rightarrow$ hydroxyglycine).

These lipid compounds may participate in wound healing by activating and halting cyclic adenosine monophosphate (AMP) synthesis. Cyclic AMP can induce cell mitosis, for example, of undifferentiated mesenchymal cells, epithelium, and so on, necessary for tissue repair.

A number of tissue cells—epithelium, lymphocytes, fibroblasts, and so on—form and liberate growth-inhibitory substances that function best in the presence of corticosteroids and epinephrine. Chalones act by inhibiting DNA synthesis and mitosis. Lymphocyte-derived chalones may retard the immune response; T-lymphocytes stimulated in vitro by a mitogen (phythemagglutinin) undergo rather predictable blastogenesis and transformation into "activated" lymphocytes. In the presence of chalones these human lymphocyte changes are inhibited.

Wound repair appears to be based upon *competition* between cellular and chemical agents stimulatory to repair and upon substances and cells that retard proliferative and synthetic processes or produce tissue resorptive change.

Epithelialization. When the face of the surgical wound is exposed to the oral cavity or the tooth or both, epithelialization must occur because it is essential for connective tissue protection and for efficiency of healing. This process may commence very soon after the surgery is performed. The blood clot is usually well established 6 to 12 hours postoperatively. The outer, or superficial, portion contiguous to the surgical dressing or the oral cavity rapidly acquires an amorphous character. Fluid occupies and seeps from the clot-wound interface. This fluid carries with it a large number of neutrophils, some of which accumulate at the undersurface of the clot; these cells also seem capable of independent active movement and migrate to the area on collagen and fibrin strands. The source of regenerative epithelium is that which is located peripheral to the wound. Epithelial cells begin their migration over the wound bed, generally 24 to 36 hours after injury, and travel best in the moist environment *subjacent* to the blood clot and the adjacent band of neutrophils (the polyband) (Fig. 23-12). They actually move over the connective tissue corium, *beneath* the polyband, employing surface fibrin, reticulum residual collagen, and the essential *hydrated* tissue matrix as strata upon which to travel. This mode of travel has been likened to an ameboid type of movement, with transient formation of pseudopods to "self-propel" the cells. Whether this is a truly active type of propulsion remains to be clarified, for mitotic activity within the adjacent epithelium, temporally lagging briefly behind the initial cell movement, may tend to "express" cells laterally toward and over the wound site. Regardless, the cell migratory rate is quite predictable, 0.5 to 1 mm of lateral progress per day. The cell migratory pattern has been compared to a "caterpillar track"—a rolling-over phenomenon. Cells of the prickle (spinous) layers of laterally contiguous epithelium furnish a progenitor source—losing contact adhesion by desmosomal dissolution—migrating over underlying basal cells and implanting onto the "bared" connective tissue. As the first cells accomplish this they are followed by comparable epithelial cells, which in turn roll over them and fix (adhere) to the connective tissue corium. The initial monolayer of implanted prickle cells becomes the

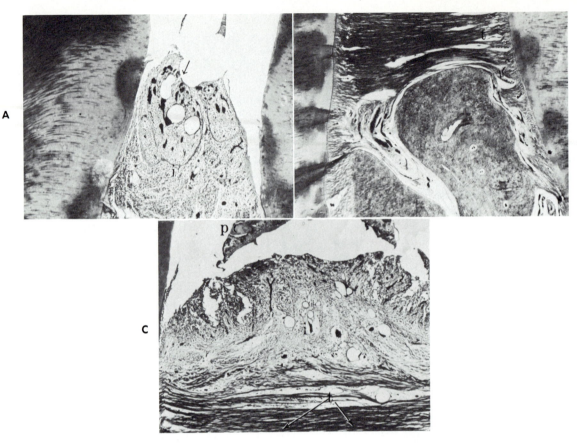

Fig. 23-12. Interdental gingiva involved by inflammatory process. Evident in **A** are collagen resorption, detachment of fibers from cementum and migration of junctional epithelium onto cementum, and increased patency and dilation of vasculature. **B,** Note preservation of transseptal fiber complex subjacent to zone of tissue resorption. We project that this area, as well as crestal aspects of periodontal ligaments, will react productively in the face of characteristically smoldering inflammatory process tending to contain inflammatory exudate and inhibiting its spread into bone marrow and periodontal ligament. Transseptal fiber zone may behave as a periosteum in healing after surgery. **C,** Plaque, *p,* in association with resorbed phase of interdental gingiva. Effective healing requires removal of zone of tissue resorption and epithelial necrosis as well as meticulous plaque, debris, and calculus control. *i,* Inflamed gingival margin; *t,* transseptal fibers.

basal cell layer of the epithelium of the wound and gradually acquires the morphology and mitotic potential of basal epithelium. As the repair of connective tissue commences (3 to 4 days postoperatively), fibroblasts of the subepithelial granulation tissue can be expected to synthesize reticulin and protein-polysaccharides of the connective tissue phase of the basement membrane and provide its early annexation to the connective tissue corium; fine, delicate, irregularly oriented reticulum fibrils can be seen extending from the corium into the basement membrane area (Fig. 23-13). There is evidence that epithelial cells may also participate in basement membrane area synthesis, secreting a granular amorphous glycoprotein that

forms the epithelial phase (segment) of the basement membrane. This process has been demonstrated by autoradiography utilizing amino acid (proline ^{3}H) and carbohydrate (glucose ^{14}C) precursors (Fig. 23-14).

When the initial coverage by epithelium has been provided, migration ceases (contact inhibition) as a primary epithelializing event and is supplanted by the mitotic process as a means for increasing epithelial thickness and rete peg formation (in masticatory mucosa). The implanted prickle cells have "redifferentiated" to basal cells and the process of epithelial replication commenced with an inward → outward cell migratory pattern. Keratinization, as an intracellular process

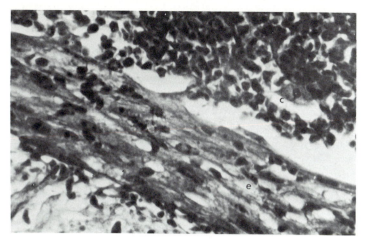

Fig. 23-13. Epithelial migration, *e*, under blood clot and neutrophilic polyband, *c*, an important event in healing of all surgical procedures involving soft tissues. There is some evidence that epithelial cells form and release collagenase (Fullmer) and other proteolytic enzymes and that epithelial cells during wound healing (Ross) act in a phagocytic capacity, digesting erythrocytes, fibrin, and other substances in their path.

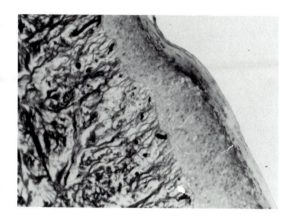

Fig. 23-14. Ordinarily, reticulum (argentophilic) fibers extend from gingival lamina propria into basement membrane zone adjacent to epithelium, serving to "anchor" epithelial to connective tissues. In this postsurgical specimen (periosteal retention type of mucogingival surgery), these reticulum fibers are renewed, presumably ensuring a tenacious bond of epithelium to connective tissue substrate. (Mallory trichrome stain; × 100.) (From Novaes, A. B., Kon, S., Ruben, M. P., and Goldman, H. M.: J. Periodontol. **41:**685, 1970.)

of keratohyalin synthesis, is often evidenced as early as 14 to 17 days postoperatively, whereas the surface keratinizing effect may not be manifest until 28 to 42 days postsurgically.

The keratinizing events appear to be a genetically determined epithelial quality, modified by the local or somatic environments. Basal cells reflect ultrastructurally their propensity to produce or differentiate into keratin-producing cells; basal cells of nonkeratinizing epithelia show a deficiency of poorly aligned tonofilaments. The tonofilaments appear to provide, especially in the granular cell population, the matrix on which keratohyalin granules are deposited, once synthesized at ribosomal sites. An additional concept indicates that the process of keratohyalin granule formation represents degeneration of cytoplasmic structures, such as effete mitochondria and Golgi vesicles. In keratinizing epithelia, granular cells display a paucity of functional mitochondria, mitochondrial degeneration, as evidenced by loss of cristae and "granular" aggregations on their surfaces, mitochondrial accumulation of mineral (e.g., amorphous $CaPO_4$) as well as the histochemically demonstrable presence of acid hydrolases (e.g., acid phosphatase, nonspecific esterase, β-glucuronidase). Hydrolytic enzymes are present both intracellularly and extracellularly and may be prime contributing factors to cellular degeneration and formation of the overlying stratum corneum. Cells of this lamella are nonfunctional; their cytoplasmic organelles, if present, are found in an altered and resorbed condition. The corneal layer is notable for lipid and mineral accumulation, generally allied with degenerative and dystrophic cellular modifications. Recent evidence points to the fact that epithelial keratinization is markedly dependent on the nature of the connective tissue substrate. Dense tissue, especially that rigidly bound to underlying bone (as in gingiva), is physically inductive of keratinization of overlying epithelium. Conversely, loose connective tissue substrata (as in buccal and alveolar mucosa) appear to be inhibitory to the keratinizing effect.

The presence of keratinizing epithelium in the zone of attached gingiva and the conversion of a nonkeratinizing epithelium postsurgically may not be related to direct physical stimulation of epithelial tissue, but may be influenced by its environment. Thus epithelium situated in approximation to a dental surface does not display a keratinizing effect. When a diastema is present between adjacent teeth the interdental gingiva is structurally identical to gingiva at the buccal and lingual aspects of the teeth, being composed internally of dense connective tissue and topically of keratinizing epithelium.

The precise processes responsible for epithelial change in relationship to physical environment, that is, its interfaces, and for the determination of epithelial specificity by the quality of its connective tissue substrate are not clear. It may well be that the nature of epithelium as regards keratinization is ultimately related to its interactions with the connective tissue, and that exposure of the outer face of epithelium to the oral cavity leads to basic modifications in the connective tissue, which in turn determines the epithelial status.

It is tempting to postulate that epithelial enzyme synthesis and activity are related to the variable structure and density of the connective tissue. For example, keratinizing epithelium of gingiva reflects histochemically the synthesis of significant amounts of acid hydrolases while nonkeratinizing epithelia do not. Actually, nonkeratinizing epithelia display predominantly oxidative rather than hydrolytic enzyme synthesis and activity. Since the two types of epithelia, in pure form, rest on distinctly different types of connective tissue, the extent of tissue vascularization and the concomitant availability of nutrients and hydrating fluids derived by transudation from vessels and diffusing into epithelium may be related to epithelial synthetic activity and quality. Thus keratinization and hydrolytic enzyme activity of gingival epithelium may not only be interrelated but may also be influenced by the diminished vascularization of the tissue's corium. Conversely, oxidative enzyme content and the lack of keratinization of mucosal epithelium may be reflections of the more elaborate vascularization of mucosal connective tissue, with consequent increase in epithelial nutrition and hydration. Keratinization may be a physiologic degenerative

process induced by "negative" signals from the connective tissue. The hypothesis could also be extended to include deficiencies of—

1. Neural-derived epithelial growth factors
2. Chalones, that is, epithelial antimitotic regulatory peptides
3. Trophic factors of fibroblastic origin
4. Humoral fluids necessary to serve as transport vehicles for oxygen, nutrients, hormones, and trophic substances from the connective tissue into the epithelium

DIFFERENTIAL PARTICIPATION OF PERIODONTAL TISSUES IN HEALING AFTER SURGERY

The tissues of the periodontium may be divided into two broad categories on the basis of their contribution to the healing response: (1) dynamic and (2) the comparatively hypodynamic on both appositional and resorptive levels. Although a paucity of studies exist related to the physiologic stability or turnover cycles of periodontal tissues, there is some evidence that the structures composing the attachment apparatus—periodontal ligament and the endosteum of alveolar vascular channels and of marrow of supporting bone—exhibit rapid replacement cycles and thus corresponding cell vitality on both mitotic and synthetic bases. Tissue turnover also implies resorption of its constituents at a rate roughly coincident with that of apposition. In the absence of influential disease processes, the continuation of function with transmission of occlusal forces to these structures is sufficient to maintain equilibrium between formative and destructive processes. Cementum is excluded from this consideration as its sustenance is dependent on contiguous periodontal ligament and gingival corium. There is no evidence available for its "replacement cycle." The possibility of mineral and water uptake and removal exists.

Under the influence of surgical injury both periodontal ligament and endosteum can usually be relied on as predictable and enthusiastic suppliers of regenerative tissue, not only for self-replacement, but also for formation of tissues to attach gingiva to tooth and bone. In the first 2 to 3 days of the healing process, however, these tissues, along with the inflammatory exudate, are responsible for some resorption of collagen, marrow, bone, and so on. With the waning of the acute inflammatory state and the initiation of the chronic inflammatory process and repair, these areas literally jump into action as progenitors of reparative

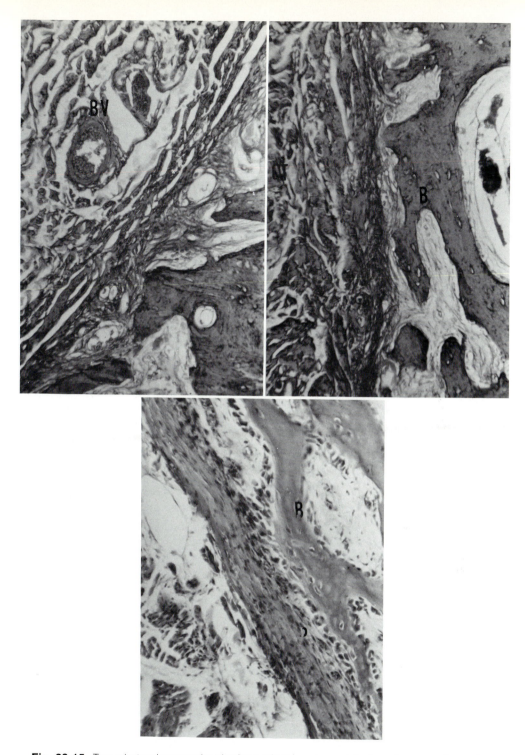

Fig. 23-15. Top photomicrographs depict periosteum-bone interface in zone of attached gingiva. Outer phase of periosteum is fibrous and forms a continuum with group C (3) fibers of the gingiva, which insert into cervical cementum. The inner aspect of periosteum consists of a delicate maze of collagen and reticulum fibers that are either inserted directly into bone surface or are in continuity with endosteal lining of vascular channels and superficially located marrow cavities. Bone surface in relationship to gingiva is remarkable for a large number of indentations, irregularities, and perforations that provide additional physical anchorages of gingiva to bone. Lower photomicrograph displays periosteal dynamicity relative to bone formation in developing alveolar process of 6- to 7-month-old fetus. Comparable activity *may* be evident in reparative processes accompanying periodontal surgery.

tissue—productive for collagen and its ground substance substrate, blood vessels, lymphatics, nerves, bone, and so on.

Many periodontal surgical procedures are founded upon this unusual regenerative capacity. For example, in new attachment procedures designed for repair of infrabony defects, deliberate effort is exerted in their débridement to expose *periodontal ligament and marrow* with minimal surgical trauma. Full mucoperiosteal flap positioning to or just coronal to the osseous crest (and exposed periodontal ligament) takes advantage of the potential of the periodontal ligament for flap reattachment; this placement also recognizes the limited expanse of the coronally directed tissue generation from this source (about 1 to 2 mm). When vascular channels or marrow spaces are sufficiently available at the bone crest, marginally and interdentally, their endostea exhibit a striking ability for production of granulation tissue. For example, regeneration interdentally of a soft tissue cover for bone after full mucoperiosteal flap procedures is markedly dependent on new tissue arising from crestal bone and periodontal ligament. Comparable repair occurs at the outer surfaces of facial and lingual cortices of the alveolar process. However, highly cortical bone may have a deficiency of such tissue reservoirs; flap reattachment to areas with a limited number of vascular channels may be retarded. In these instances, flap reattachment requires the centripetal ingrowth of reparative tissue from periosteum at the edge of flap retraction or must await delayed and limited production of regenerative tissue from the periosteum of the flap.

Available studies indicate that when a full-thickness mucoperiosteal flap is dissected from a cortically constituted bone surface, its periosteum becomes productive on about the tenth postsurgical day. This finding implies that the inner cambium of periosteum is damaged or destroyed by the surgery and that a new cambium lamella, or its equivalent composed of granulation tissue, originates from the loose connective tissue located perivascularly in the interstitial portion of the outer fibrous layer of periosteum (Figs. 23-15 to 23-17). Thus there may be ingrowth from these progenitor sources. During the period of formation of this renewed cambium zone, flap attachment to the bony surface is at best tenuous. Where periodontal flaps are applied to "gingival bone," bone subjacent to the gingival corium, flap reattachment occurs quickly with outgrowth of granulation tissue from exposed marrow cavities, vas-

Fig. 23-16. Scanning electronmicrographs of buccal surface of bone in area of gingiva. Soft tissue removed from autopsy specimens of mandible by autoclaving technique, and subsequent application of proteolytic enzymes to effect complete digestion of residual connective tissue. Osseous surface (top photograph) is markedly irregular with random placement of pits, grooves, ridges, and hills—reminiscent of Martian surface. Majority of pits represent openings of vascular channels, communicating in vivo between periosteal phase of gingiva and marrow cavities. There are innumerable smaller, punctate depressions that are sites where Sharpey's fibers were incorporated into bone. Center photograph is an enlargement of "gingival bone." Openings seen in center and at left again depict orifices of vascular canals. They are lined, when soft tissue is present, by endosteum that is affixed externally to periosteum and internally to endosteum of marrow cavities. During healing processes, after bone exposure in periodontal surgery, endosteum may furnish reparative (granulation) tissue needed to cover denuded bone. After full-thickness mucoperiosteal flap surgery, residual periosteum and endosteum are reservoirs for granulation tissue needed to reattach gingival portion of flap to bone; such proliferative activity begins about 3 to 4 days postsurgically. Bone and soft tissue resorption coincide to varying degrees, as both endosteum and periosteum have pluripotentiality during normalcy, disease, and healing processes. Bottom photograph dramatically exhibits a single vascular channel. It is peripheralized by an extremely irregular bone surface; microridges may be indicative of linear areas of calcified collagen fibers where Sharpey's fibers extend from bone surface into periosteum. Accessory vascular channels, portals for entrance of blood vessels into haversian canals, mark inner surface of "large" canal seen at center. Pocked, perforated, rough quality of "gingival bone" thus represents (1) a secure, internal anchorage for gingiva and (2) an exceptionally prolific source of reparative tissue during healing by virtue of extensive amounts of exposed endosteum. (In conjunction with Dr. C. Pameijer.)

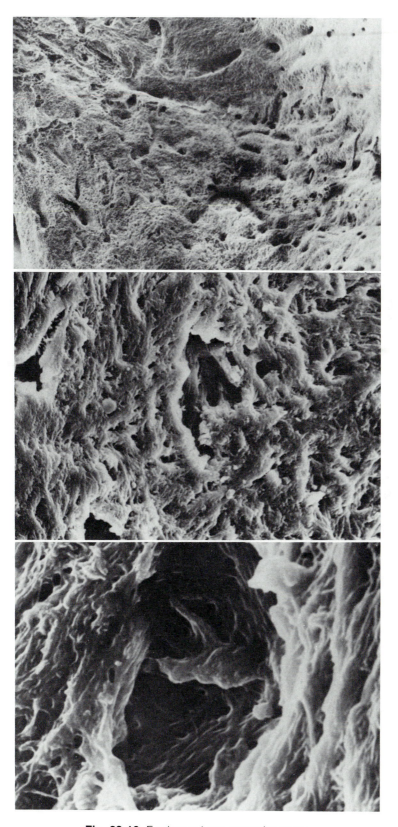

Fig. 23-16. For legend see opposite page.

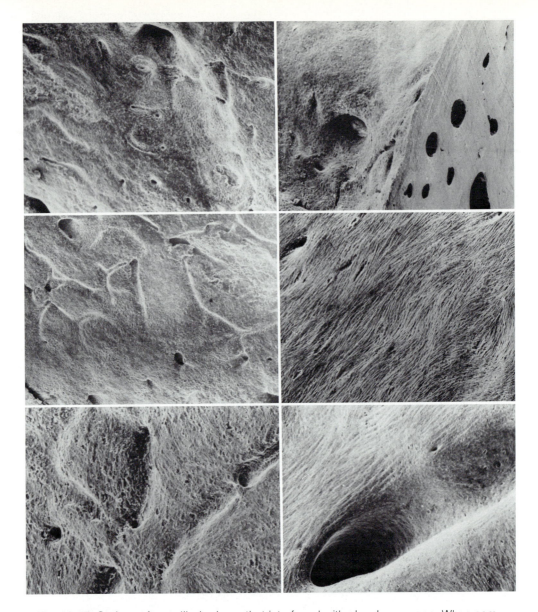

Fig. 23-17. Surface of mandibular bone that interfaced with alveolar mucosa. When compared to "gingival bone," "mucosal" bone is relatively smooth, has a more undulating topography, and presents a markedly diminished number of vascular channels. Large, darkened depressions seen in left top and center photomicrographs are orifices of vascular channels that in intact specimen communicated between periosteum and bone marrow. They are lined by endosteum. Bottom left photograph reveals punctate depressions that correspond to sites where collagen fiber bundles of periosteum (Sharpey's fibers) attach to bone. Specimen sectioned tangentially (top right) demonstrates osseous surface at left and largely compact and dense quality of cortical plate of "mucosal" bone at right. Surface of bone in zone of alveolar mucosa tends to be deficient in number of vascular channels and, concomitantly, availability of endosteum. Thus when periosteum is separated from this type of bone in periodontal surgery, it appears that flap reattachment postsurgically is largely reliant on periosteal rather than endosteal sources of reparative tissue. Melcher has indicated delayed contribution of periosteum to repair when it is divorced even temporarily from bone at time of surgery; this lag phase of periosteum may be associated with periosteal injury at time of surgery. It may be more advisable, so as to ensure earlier, more predictable, periosteal participation in healing, to leave it in situ when flaps are retracted. This necessitates a "split flap" approach in zone of alveolar mucosa. Center right photograph (approximately × 2400) denotes ridged surface of bone in zone of alveolar mucosa, while lower right electronmicrograph displays not only smooth morphology of "mucosal" bone, but also stoma of a vascular channel. Linear depression at right accommodates blood vessel that extended parallel to bone surface in vivo.

cular channels, and crestal periodontal ligament. This flap attachment is *not* initially reliant on periosteal activity. Actually, both full- and partial-thickness gingival flaps are affixed to this type of bone with equal rapidity. The fixation is relatively tenacious.

When partial-thickness mucosal flaps are made, leaving periosteum in situ over smooth, dense bone surfaces, periosteal reparative activity is ordinarily initiated by the fourth postsurgical day and continues dynamically over the ensuing 3 to 4 weeks, providing ready attachment of overlying tissues to the periosteal receptor area. Ruben, in a detailed retrospective analysis of periosteal participation in the healing of partial-thickness gingivomucosal flaps, free gingival autografts, and equivalent donor site areas of laterally repositioned split-pedicle flaps, has observed the following in 60- to 85-day postsurgical specimens:

1. Increased periosteal tissue density, for example, fibrosis, at the soft tissue-bone interface.
2. Significant increases in the number of Sharpey's fibers (as compared to untreated control areas) extending from periosteum into surface bone.
3. Diffuse topical bone formation, the equivalent of an external callus, over the original bone surface.

These findings may further substantiate that an intact periosteum is essential for earlier and more secure repair.

During the development of the alveolar processes and the largely coincident eruption of teeth, the periosteum (including transseptal and group 3 fiber complex areas) constitutes a major osteogenic source for building crestal bone and the outer cortical plates of the jaws. It also contributes to self-production and maintenance. The cells of its inner cambium not only provide the collagenous and matrical elements convertible by mineralization to bone but also secrete the reticular and collagenous attachments (Sharpey's fiber) anchoring periosteum to bone. This osteogenic and fibrogenic capacity wanes when developmental processes become quiescent; therefore periosteal activity is physiologically minimal in late adolescence and adulthood.

In the "fully" developed state of the alveolar processes, periosteum subserves several important functions:

1. It forms a variably rigid attachment for gingiva to bone because of its density, numerous fibrous insertions into bone, and its confluence with endosteum of vascular channels.

2. It provides attachment linkage of alveolar mucosa essentially to *cortical* bone of alveolar processes and jaws. These do not appear to be as tenacious as in the relationship of attached gingiva to subjacent bone. The Sharpey fiber insertions here appear to be more frail, to be fewer with greater spacing over the cortical surface, and to have a shallower penetration into the bony cortex.

3. It carries the principal vascular supply and lymphatic drainage for alveolar mucosa and gingiva. Additionally, it contributes to the vascularization of adjacent bone, joining with branches of intraseptal vessels to provide liberal blood supply to cancellous bone. Many of the blood vessels coursing from periosteum to cortical bone are of a minute caliber. They arise from an extensive and delicate vascular plexus located in the inner phase of periosteum and enter bone's haversian canals directly, joining with an elaborate microvascular arcade within *cortical* bone. Fluids also diffuse from periosteum's extravascular connective tissue, as a transudate, into bone principally into and through a canalicular maze. In this way bone matrix is hydrated, mineral is added to and withdrawn homeostatically within bone, and osteocytes receive nutrients and release wastes. *When osseous septa are thin and largely or completely composed of compact bone, the periosteal blood supply may constitute the principal one to the septum.* Any condition or surgical procedure substantively interfering with periosteal integrity may place the osseous septum in ischemic jeopardy.

4. It contains prominent neural fibers, generally myelinated, that liberally arborate into gingiva, mucosa, periosteum, and bone marrow.

5. It responds, generally in an appositional manner by fibrogenesis or osteogenesis, to exigencies derived from overlying gingiva and mucosa. Thus the inflammatory response in marginal gingiva is usually contained and restricted from progress through attached gingiva to alveolar bone by the capacity of periosteum (and periodontal ligament) to "repair" in the face of irritation.

Despite its routine performance of these essential functions, periosteum is a *sleeping giant* only mildly stirred on a generative level by functional stimuli and gingival inflammatory processes. *When surgical injury assails periosteum, it quickly springs to action, joins, and often exceeds periodontal ligament and endosteum in cellular dynamicity, both appositionally and resorptively oriented.*

In repair of periodontal wounds the periosteum has a marked capacity for the following:

1. Fibrogenesis, osteogenesis, and secretion of

protein-polysaccharide complexes of the matrices of connective tissue, bone, and blood vessels.

2. Endothelial proliferation and the formation of new vascular and lymphatic vessels. Both initiate at 3 to 4 days postsurgically and continue strongly and coincidentally with the genesis of collagen and ground substance of connective tissue. This hyperplasia plateaus at 14 to 17 days postoperatively, wanes somewhat, and then replateaus at 30 to 35 days at the 17-day level.

3. When maintained intact on bone (as in partial-thickness flap techniques), the periosteum is responsible for bone resorption crestally and on outer aspects of alveolar plates for periods ranging up to 14 to 17 days. Resorption is superseded by osteogenesis derived from the *same* periosteum. With periosteal conservation in situ the pendulum can usually be counted on to swing in favor of an overall appositional response with minimal sacrifice of bone crest or periphery.

4. After both partial-thickness and mucoperiosteal flap surgery, periosteum at the *border* of flap retraction often responds by providing literally a "river of regenerative tissue" moving centripetally into the wound. This tissue is responsible for gingival and mucosal reattachment to periosteum, bone, and possibly to tooth with the assistance of tissue derived from periodontal ligament.

5. Its vasculature responds rheologically and by dilatation and permeability to provide hydration and nutritive materials to adjacent tissues and to itself in the healing process. This is especially apparent in the sustenance of free gingival autografts and partial-thickness pedicle grafts that are completely or strongly dependent on periosteum of the recipient site, especially during the first week after grafting. *Periosteal blood vessels also serve as progenitors for new blood vessels required to link to those of the graft* (Fig. 23-10, *B*). We also project that comparable lymphatic anastomoses occur, assisting substantially in removing exudate and cellular and other debris from the graft.

6. It is a springboard for nerve regeneration into overlying gingiva, mucosa, or graft and into subjacent bone. These processes have not been documented in periodontal tissues. Extrapolation from the medical and basic sciences would support a hypothesis that wound healing, as an overall efficient and completed process, would be impaired without adequate neural supply to the part and without adequate neural regeneration at the site. Growth factors may be released from nerve endings that are trophic (stimulatory) to reparative processes. These are generally glycopeptides and peptides of low but mixed molecular weights. For example, an epidermal growth factor (EGF) has been demonstrated and is felt to be of neural origin. Comparable substances that activate fibroblasts may also be of neurogenic derivation; connective tissue repair may be in part related to an intact nerve supply.

This thesis points to the essentiality of periosteum in normalcy, inflammatory disease, and reparative processes.

The *corium* of attached gingiva, that is, the connective tissue area situated between periosteum and the thin lamina propria subjacent to epithelium, is considered to be a highly stable connective tissue. It is usually composed of mature, largely insoluble collagen arranged in dense and well-oriented layers. The matrical component of the tissue is highly viscous while minimal in amount and relatively rich in sulfated protein-polysaccharide complexes. Its vascularization is low, with but a few vessels of small luminal caliber and limited transudative quality. Histologic examination also denotes a paucity of formative cells (fibroblasts) and a limited progenitor cell population. Thus we are describing a tissue with low collagen and matrical turnover, a tissue of restricted solubility and maximal stability, and a tissue probably dependent, in a nearly parasitic manner, on contiguous and more vital periosteum and lamina propria.

These qualities render the body of the corium of attached gingiva to be a rigid, strong, stable complex, one best suited to be a scaffolding material. It can be shaped, detached and replaced, transposed, and so on with reasonable assurance that its structural qualities will be retained postsurgically. On these bases it is an ideal foundation for gingivectomy and gingivoplasty, since there is a strong likelihood that it will not become hyperplastic after partial resection and that the morphology (physiologic form) placed in the tissue will be retained in the stable tissue postoperatively. Such connective tissue also provides a stable graft material either as part of a flap or in free transposition; a vascular, hydrated, strongly regenerative foundation in the form of periosteum or periodontal ligament is vital for graft survival and attachment. Gingival connective tissues, to be utilized as autografts, may be frozen and stored. Unless program-frozen is employed in conjunction with graft glycerolization to inhibit intracellular ice crystal formation (causing cells to burst and die), its cells do not remain viable. The tissue, however, may be used for grafting. Its survival and attachment to the receptor site is dependent entirely on the host periosteum; reepithelialization takes place from epithelial progenitor sources located peripheral to the graft. It thus serves in an autoprosthetic capacity. Frozen and irradiated gingiva may be allotransplanted and incorporated at a receptor area, serving as a sterile, minimally immunogenic, molecularly stabilized (H^+ cross-links between polypeptide chains of collagen molecules are increased by irradiation), cell-free "prosthetic" connective tissue. Comparable results have been claimed for preserved sclera and dura mater (the inner lamella that sheaths the brain is used). Both are dense, hypovascular, hypocellular connective tissues. Scleral tissue *may* undergo mineralization in intraosseous sites. Fundamentally gingiva is a passive tissue; it requires aggressive associations.

The outer phase of the gingival corium — that adjacent to epithelium — is a thin band of loose connective tissue with liberal vascularization and cellularity. This lamina propria of attached and marginal gingiva turns inward at the gingival crest and continues subjacent to sulcular and col epithelia. Its prime physiologic purposes appear to be those of providing (1) hydration and nutrition to epithelium via its extensive blood vessel network, (2) anchoring of epithelium through fibrils extending from connective tissue into basement membrane zone, and (3) furnishing a stem mesenchymal cell population for differentiation into fibroblasts, to mast cells with normalcy and with inflammation, and to mononuclear macrophages that act as phagocytic and digestive impediments to the ingress of irritants into the tissues. Macrophages, however, are considered to be principally derived from blood monocytes, which enter extravascular aspects of connective tissues in great numbers in chronic inflammatory states. They have also been discerned in attachment apparatus loci with occlusal traumatism and in tissues involved in wound healing. The origination of macrophages relative to the traumatic lesion has not been elicited.

In the healing after periodontal surgery (particularly that associated with gingivectomy, gingivoplasty, curettage, and periosteal retention type of mucogingival surgery) the lamina propria displays a striking ability for formation of reparative granulation tissue. It is joined by regenerative tissue derived on a limited scale from underlying gingival corium, especially from the loose connective tissue surrounding blood vessels. There is much evidence for a major contribution of new tissue from the lamina propria bordering the wound, with centripetal inward "movement" over the wound bed. Actually the combination of renewed lamina propria and epithelial cover constitutes the bulk of new tissue generated in the healing of these gingival resective procedures; the underlying corium is the scaffold.

CURETTAGE

There has been a relative paucity of documented histologic studies pertaining to the healing of the gingival wound after the curettage procedure (Fig. 23-18). An understanding of the basic elements of healing is complicated when both scaling and curettage are performed at the same time. Although it appears clear that some inadvertent tissue débridement does occur during subgingival scaling and when rotary diamond stones are used during the preparation of a tooth for crown-and-bridge prosthesis, it is also apparent that complete healing usually does not occur from these procedures alone because of the unpredictability of the efficacy of the débridement (Goldman, unpublished data). From a clinical and histologic point of view, therefore, the term "curettage" must refer *only* to the deliberate and systematic treatment directed at the surgical débridement of the soft tissue side of the pocket wall. The procedure removes the chronically inflamed, ulcerated lining in an effort to eliminate inflammation and obtain shrinkage of the tissue by establishing drainage of exudate and by promoting fibrosis. Available evidence tends to suggest that when indicated, gingival curettage may be performed as a separate and definitive procedure to distinguish it from the inadvertent and usually incomplete tissue débridement attending scaling and root planing procedures. The definitive approach accomplishes the desired clinical goals and may be expected to result in more efficient and complete healing.

Historically, there have been numerous approaches, both chemical and mechanical, for the performance of definitive gingival curettage; these have included electrocautery, chemical dissolution, and mechanical débridement. The sharp curet or blade, however, has remained the method of choice. Recent evidence suggests that gingival curettage can be more adequately performed by the use of surgical blades rather than with sharp curets. Accordingly, a technique described as an excisional new attachment procedure (ENAP) has been advocated as a method of choice for curettage operations. This method ensures direct visualization of the surgical site and consequently more effective management of the soft tissues and the root surfaces. Clinically, improved and reliably predictable healing patterns and enduring results have been noted with this approach. A parallel healing study on rhesus monkeys revealed the formation of a long epithelial attachment, little or no new connective tissue reattachment, and a corium relatively free of inflammation. At a recent symposium Stahl (1977) delineated the variability of the soft tissue–tooth interface, claiming the (1) lack of predictability of repair by cementogenesis, especially at distances greater than 1 mm from attachment apparatus (that is, periodontal ligament, an important reparative source), (2) a more marked propensity for healing by the interposition of reparative tissue between the collagen of soft tissue and collagen purposely or inadvertently left in situ on the root surface, (3) the common finding at supracrestal areas of connective tissue adaptation (adhesion) to the root surface; and (4) the derivation of an epithelial (junctional-sulcular)-tooth interface at more marginal areas. Such a postsurgical result appears to be clinically satisfactory and temporally durable,

providing that the soft tissue wall is densely collagenated and thus rigid and essentially self-supporting. On the basis of this and previous long-term longitudinal studies it has been suggested that a curettage approach is as efficacious as pocket elimination for the treatment of periodontal disease provided that good plaque control is permanently and professionally maintained. There is apparently very little difference between the ENAP procedure and the Widman flap; both are essentially surgical curettage techniques. Although reduction or elimination of gingival inflammation occurs by this method, the possibility of pocket elimination by way of reattachment appears somewhat negligible. Within recent years the use of ultrasonics has become available as an additional method of performing gingival curettage and is now often employed.

Reattachment after gingival curettage, with a more coronal connective tissue attachment of gingiva to cementum than that which was present preoperatively and with a concomitantly located sulcular base and epithelial attachment, is not reliably obtained. If one recognizes that the gingival corium is a relatively stable collagen complex with its cell population mitotically and syn-

Fig. 23-18. Sequence of events in healing of gingiva after curettage. **A,** Control specimen. Junctional and sulcular epithelia, *se,* are on enamel surface. In instances of gingival inflammation, epithelium displays both hyperplasia and ulceration while adjacent connective tissue would evidence such facets of inflammation as collagen resorption, vasodilation, and vascular permeability or an aggregation of exudate and inflammatory cell infiltrate. Line, *i,* extending from outer aspect of gingival epithelium, *e,* to cemental surface is representative of line of tissue incision with curet and could represent lateral boundary of zone of tissue destruction characteristic of gingivitis. **B,** Area of gingival curettage just after surgical procedure (0 hour) in which tissue was debrided and plaque and calculus were removed. Wound surface is haphazardly covered by a thin blood clot, *c.* Note at *o* the area of tissue laceration produced by instrumentation. Such areas may tend to exhibit poor connective tissue healing, as gingival reparative response usually tends to be minimal and unpredictable; area may epithelialize with deepening of sulcular base or may remain unepithelialized and repaired by indifferently oriented and sparse connective tissue. **C,** Two-day postsurgical specimen. Interface zone between wound and tooth is covered at *c* by a thin blood clot. **D,** Two days after surgery; initial phase of epithelialization of wound, primary epithelial source being that of the outer, marginal aspect of tissue. Clot has partially lifted from its contact with wound, and epithelium is migrating and intruding under coagulum. **E,** Six days after surgery; sulcular and junctional epithelia have been renewed; gingival epithelium does not keratinize when in contact with a natural or artificial (acrylic, ceramics) hard surface. **F,** Higher magnification of blocked area in **E.** Note that epithelium, *se,* is thin (four to five cell layers). Blood vessel in center of photomicrograph displays marked perviousness, and extravasated red blood cells can be seen in the tissues. Newly formed capillaries tend to be very fragile, and minute tissue hemorrhage may be manifested as a result of tissue manipulation. All specimens, with the exception of **D,** have been stained with hematoxylin-eosin, whereas Mallory trichrome method was applied to **D.**

thetically quiescent—aroused minimally to activity even with injury—one can understand the paucity or failure of cementoid and collage synthesis necessary to provide the added attachment. Actually the limits of lateral and apical débride-

ment of the connective tissue fall within this area of gingival stability and relative inactivity.

Should the curettage involve the periosteal aspect of the gingiva or expose the periodontal ligament, more dynamic and extensive connective

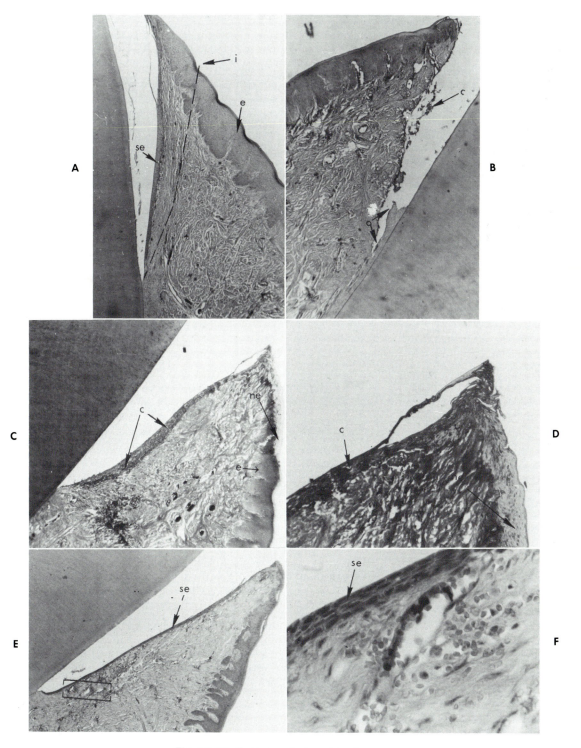

Fig. 23-18. For legend see opposite page.

tissue production could be expected along with gingival reattachment, but rarely more than 1.5 to 2 mm from the ligament. But then we are no longer adhering to the definition of gingival curettage and would be involved with *flap* considerations.

Effective curettage and subsequent healing are based on the removal of the ulcerated pocket wall and subjacent connective tissue. With this procedure there is a surgical débridement of the ulcerated and hyperplastic epithelium as well as the contiguous zone of damaged connective tissue downward and outward to the firm and inner aspect of the gingival corium.

In general, healing under circumstances of surgical curettage occurs as in virtually any other surgical wound repair, involving epithelialization of the sulcular wall and collagenation and resolution of inflammation in the gingival connective tissue.

The use of a sharp curet or blade transforms a previously chronically inflamed gingival lesion to a surgical wound that heals in the following ways: (1) gingival wall shrinkage, which is markedly enhanced by the increased drainage of tissue fluid exudate, (2) epithelialization of the wound bed of exposed connective tissue from the adjacent oral epithelium, and reestablishment of the epithelial attachment, (3) formation of a new lamina propria subjacent to the new sulcular lining and epithelial attachment, and (4) a return to the original quality and distribution of the microvascularization of the tissue.

The removal of pocket epithelium is one of the salient features of healing because connective tissue must be exposed to disclose the sources of connective tissue repair and to provide a morphologic foundation for reepithelialization. The pocket epithelium also is capable of releasing cellular hydrolytic enzymes potentially damaging to itself and to adjacent connective tissues. A number of studies have reported wide variations in the predictability of success with respect to complete removal of the epithelial lining of the pocket wall during the curettage procedure. The lack of unanimity in opinion may largely be related to the surgical methodology—the excisional techniques apparently being the more efficacious. Some epithelial cells may be left unintentionally where there has been or is marked inflammation with subsequent formation of rete pegs penetrating deeply into the connective tissue. Although the complete removal of these few cells would be ideal, their presence does not appear to be detrimental to the ultimate result. In addition the epithelial attachment, which is almost always removed without any special attempt to do so, may become readily reestablished as the remainder of the sulcular lining heals. Attempts at total removal of the pocket and junctional epithelia by gingival curettage may produce a separation of healthy connective tissue from the root surface. It is uncertain whether this damage would allow for epithelial proliferation into the region or whether connective tissue reattachment (a more desirable phenomenon) or adherence would be the permanent result during healing. These possibilities suggest the need for careful instrumentation during the procedure. Total removal of the epithelium and the epithelial attachment appears to be possible but apparently difficult and unpredictable.

The complete elimination of pocket epithelium, including the coronal margin, results in a wound that is initially covered by a blood coagulum, which is then replaced by healing epithelium. The clot is instrumental both in correcting the irregularities of connective tissue caused by curettage and in mediating a provisional adherence of gingiva to tooth.

The clot that fills the gingival sulcus after the curettage operation is the temporal precursor of the regenerative healing process. Granulation tissue, which consists of newly formed blood vessels, connective tissue fibroblasts, and some inflammatory cells, forms subjacent to the clot and may replace it in part as it resorbs and sequesters. Removal of the blood clot postsurgically occurs by both enzymatic and phagocytic activity. In the early phases of the clot's presence neutrophilic enzymes begin a dissolution process that is completed when the accumulating macrophages phagocytize the clot's residual elements. Circulating monocytes arrive at healing sites via transendothelial pathways. They appear to become metabolically, phagocytically, enzymatically, and digestively active at tissue (extravascular) locations. Epithelial cells arising from epithelium at the gingival margin initially migrate over and through the fluid exudate subjacent to the clot and external to the debrided corium. The granulation tissue forms between the epithelium and the primary wound bed.

Gradual maturation of the granulation tissue is evidenced by a marked reduction in small blood vessels, a decrease in number and maturation of fibroblasts, and the development of distinct collagen fibers and reticulum.

The removal of pocket epithelium and underlying inflamed connective tissue appears to enhance the potential for soft tissue attachment or adherence to the root surface. More rapid repair may also be expected following incisional or mechanical débridement of the tissues, the resultant smooth connective tissue surface favoring rapid and effective epithelialization. The excision of pocket epithelium and the resorptive inflammatory locus in connective tissue and the débridement of the root surface altered by and containing inflammatory exudates eliminate in large measure substances (e.g., hydrolytic enzymes and endotoxin) detrimental to repair.

The size of the wound surface appears to play a significant role in healing. A relatively small, smooth wound surface tends to encourage epithelialization when compared to a large, irregular one; in a large, irregular wound the process tends to be slower and more incomplete. Large wounds that may exist in deeper pockets (over 4 to 5 mm) tend not to epithelialize. From a practical point of view, therefore, the use of very sharp instruments in relatively shallow pocket regions would appear to be most desirable for this procedure. Large wounds that result from deeper pocket areas would be expected to heal much more slowly since irregular, broad surface regions involve a greater complexity of tissue response, and the surgeon must deal with greater surface area in removing inflamed surface tissue element. In this manner also, relatively shallow, edematous tissue responds more readily to inflammatory control than those areas characterized by fibrous tissue coincident with long-standing inflammation; gingival wall and general tissue shrinkage are enhanced by increased exudative drainage.

After an initial lag of 12 to 24 hours, migration of epithelium begins from the existing epithelium of attached gingiva. The rate of cell migration approximates 0.5 to 1 mm per day over the wound surface. New epithelium begins to cover the exposed gingival corium within 2 to 3 days after curettage and is complete in 7 to 10 days. Epithelial cells move in a fluid stratum subjacent to the blood clot and its contiguous band of leukocytes (polyband). The prickle cells of the keratinized epithelium at the periphery of the wound initiate a migration of cells that give rise to the new nonkeratinized epithelium of the dentogingival junction. Recent investigations have shown that these new epithelial layers are identical to the cells found in normal dentogingival areas. Thus the belief that epithelial specificity is largely determined by the connective tissue substrate rather than by innate properties of the cell itself is strengthened.

A marked acute inflammatory reaction of the gingival corium develops within hours close to the wound surface and continues during the first days after surgery. The cells of the acute inflammatory response, namely, the neutrophilic leukocytes and macrophages, are responsible for removal of cellular debris and for tailoring of the connective tissue surface to permit smooth passage of the migrating epithelial cells. There is a coincidence of diminishing inflammation and epithelialization; by the third to fourth day after surgery and certainly by the time the epithelium has been renewed the inflammatory response has subsided and the reparative phase of inflammation has supplanted the initial destructive one. At about 4 days, as inflammation becomes more chronic and epithelialization progresses, collagenation (including matrix formation) begins in the subepithelial area to eventually form a new and thin lamina propria. Connective tissue that is damaged during surgery heals, and its fibers, although somewhat immature in arrangement, width, staining characteristics, and so on, appear well organized in about 2 weeks. The formation and reorganization of the connective tissue fibers is the product of vascular proliferative and fibroblastic elements of the reparative phase of the inflammatory response. It has recently been shown that the fibroblast is also capable of resorption and ingestion of collagen, thus more fully explaining its role in the remodeling of connective tissue damaged during surgery.

Some degree of chronic inflammation can be observed in the healed tissue, at times for several weeks after the procedure. It is associated with bacterial plaque. The presence of local irritants could cause a modification of tissue response with consequent impairment in the healing process.

The vascular reaction in the gingiva is initially one of marked vasodilation and increased permeability. Both these aspects show considerable diminution within 3 to 4 days. As healing progresses, there is a further reduction in the number of vessels until the tissue eventually assumes an appearance of normalcy, with the subsulcular area showing prominent reticular vascularity. New subsulcular and marginal vessels are formed that simulate the appearance of those found in normal gingiva.

Healing of gingival curettage performed with

the ultrasonic instrument produces a wound surface resembling that of heat coagulation and mechanical débridement. Goldman has considered healing after ultrasonic curettage more satisfactory in many respects than that after hand instrumentation. After 14 to 16 days of healing (up to 6 weeks) he found not only a more substantive decrease in the inflammatory cell infiltration, but also in many instances a virtual absence of even a "chronic" cellular infiltrate. He also commented as to the more efficient and complete epithelialization seen after ultrasonic instrumentation.

Immediately after use of the ultrasonic device one finds a smooth, debrided pocket wall with many areas of coagulation. Fused collagen fibers stain basophilic. Superficial cellular morphology is altered. Flattened and hyperchromatic perivascular cells are evident in residual areas of inflammation over a short distance from the wound surface following the course of the blood vessels. Collagen fiber bundles in the subsurface lamina propria show some degree of separation. Regenerated epithelium, after a 2-week period, tends to be shorter and thinner and demonstrates fewer rete peg ridges when the tissue has been debrided with the ultrasonic instrument. Both hand and ultrasonic curettage effectively remove epithelium and connective tissue; ultrasonic curettage possibly removes more of the affected gingival corium. After a 2-week period there seems to be little clinical difference between hand and ultrasonic curettage, although optimum healing appears to be reached more quickly after ultrasonic instrumentation.

From both clinical and histologic points of view, curettage ideally produces a sulcular wound that is both smooth and continuous throughout and free of laceration and ulceration. Although disturbances in healing may be suspect of systemic influences, a more likely and frequent cause may be related to residual calculus retention or recent plaque accumulation.

After the procedure the clinical alterations immediately apparent are the presence of a marginal blood clot, oozing of blood and exudate, and color changes in the marginal gingiva to hues of bluish red or purplish red. Extended digital pressure may be important in the formation of a very thin blood clot in the sulcular area; a thin coagulum is resorbed rapidly and improves the potential for more rapid healing and reepithelialization. The day after the procedure the marginal gingiva and a portion of the attached gingiva are edematous and swollen, with persistence of discoloration. On the following day the coloration of the tissue is not as distinct, but now a lighter bluish red. Edema is still present as is some evidence of the clot at the dentogingival interface. At 4 to 6 days the gingival appearance is strikingly improved with reduced edema, greater rigidity and adaptation of the gingival wall, and concurrent shrinkage. By 7 to 10 days the gingival margin has acquired a pale orange-pink coloration and gradually loses its smooth topography, indicating the presence of greater surface keratinization and improved collagen formation and organization in the underlying corium. A firm pink gingival margin that resists bleeding on palpation is evident at 10 to 14 days.

Clinical findings may suggest almost total healing in about 10 days. Epithelialization may be complete by this time. The connective tissue phase of repair, however, is a considerably slower process, as indicated by the presence, after 21 days, of immature and poorly arranged collagen fibers below the new epithelium. The tissue may not exhibit diffuse firmness until this time. The presence of plaque or calculus on the root surface or absorbed endotoxin some distance from the cemental surface may delay healing or promote new inflammation. Also inadequate surgical technique with blunt instruments may result in ragged and uneven connective tissue wounds. The irregular wound surface must first be smoothed by the inflammatory repair system before epithelium can migrate over the connective tissue. This results in delayed healing and patient discomfort in the postoperative period. In addition the continued presence of plaque, adsorbed endotoxin, or calculus on the roots will also delay healing and promote further inflammation at and at some distance from the root surface. Thus thorough preparation of the root surface is a sine qua non to successful curettage.

GINGIVECTOMY-GINGIVOPLASTY

The primary response after gingival resection, either by gingivectomy or gingivoplasty (Fig. 23-19), consists of an acute inflammatory reaction marked by such events as neutrophilic infiltration, vasodilation and vascular injury, collagen resorption and matrix liquefaction in the gingival connective tissue, and edema and exudation. This is followed by a gradual waning of the inflammatory state, the commencement of epithelialization, connective tissue repair including vascular proliferation and redistribution, and resorption and remodeling of the subjacent bony septa (although this latter aspect is not a universal component of the tissue reaction to the surgery). In essence the reparative phenomenon is grossly composed of the formation of a lamina propria of connective tissue and a new epithelial sheath over the area of excision. Additionally, the marginal triangle of gingiva is renewed; this consists of the restoration of the epithelial adherence to the tooth, a minimal expanse of intact sulcular epithelium, and an outer (facial, lingual, palatal) oral epithelial cover. These epithelia enclose a pyramidal zone of connective tissue. Although initially the oral aspect of the epithelium does not reflect its keratinizing potential, it usually does so by the twenty-eighth postoperative day. The epithelium in approximation and adherence to the tooth does not display parakeratinization or orthokeratinization, despite its origination from the same epithelial progenitor as the oral epithelium.

Studies relating to the repair of the gingivectomy-gingivoplasty wound have become considerably more detailed in recent years, since improved techniques for observing cellular activity (e.g., radioisotopes) and particularly microvascularization have become available. These investigations have provided an opportunity to monitor healing over a period of several months when necessary. The more significant observations have been concerned with the elucidation of the patterns of repair, the progenitor sources of reparative tissue, the response of tissues not directly involved in the surgery, and the influences of extraneous or exogenous processes on healing.

The surgical procedures of gingivectomy and gingivoplasty produce open surface wounds that are similar not only in the physical qualities of the wound itself but also in the reparative processes. Although the rationale and indications for these two procedures may differ, from the standpoint of healing they may be considered to be virtually one entity.

The refinement of technique is important in this surgical procedure not only from a technical aspect but from a healing standpoint as well. A basic gingivectomy is performed with a beveled incision that attempts to end at the bottom of the measurable pocket (the base of the epithelial attachment). Although clinical examination indicates that the entire pocket wall, including the epithelial attachment, may have been removed, histologic evaluation may demonstrate that the exact end of the incision cannot always be predicted. The epithelial attachment is usually completely removed with the incisional end in the connective tissue just apical to the epithelial attachment. Recent evidence confirms that pocket depths measured clinically are recordings of the distances between the gingival margin and a point just inside the most coronal part of the connective tissue attachment, just subjacent to the apical limit of the junctional epithelium. Therefore although various clinicians differ concerning the depth of the incision, most would agree that whenever possible a gingivectomy should not extend beyond the bottom of the clinically detachable crevice. Individualized exceptions may exist, particularly when it is necessary to gain access to localized areas of inflammatory bone involvement.

The end of the incision may also produce inadvertent notching in the root surface that may affect the position of the new epithelial attachment. Apical migration of the epithelium occurs when notches are made close to the bottom of the pocket. When these irregularities are located apical to the prior epithelial attachment, connective tissue tends to fill into these spaces and thus inhibit epithelial migration. There is therefore a tendency for a tooth to lose some gingival attachment each time a gingivectomy is performed. The gingivectomy is not singular in this regard, however, and, at least initially, all periodontal surgical procedures are responsible for some loss of gingival attachment.

The root planing part of the gingivectomy must also be performed with care, since severence of connective tissue attachment may occur during this aspect of the procedure. Cemental scaling and curettage is usually followed by a downgrowth of new epithelial attachment instead of connective tissue attachment. This may produce a permanent loss of gingival attachment.

As mentioned, a cleanly incised gingivectomy wound produces an initial inflammatory reaction followed by relatively quick epithelialization that takes place over a smooth bed of connective tissue. The connective tissue becomes increasingly more collagenous and less vascular. With progressive healing the gingival epithelium manifests its keratinizing potential, whereas that epithelium in approximation to the tooth either in the sulcular or col areas does not reflect a keratinizing effect.

The initial response to injury produced by a gingivectomy is that of hemorrhage followed by the formation of a serofibrinous exudate and blood clot covering the wounded area. Cut vessels can be observed in direct contact with the blood clot and the surface of the wound immediately after the surgical procedure. The blood clot that forms over the wound fills the irregularities of the surgical site, and its outer surface roughly acquires the form of the excised tissue. Some leaking vessels may be seen in contact with the clot. Perfusion studies have shown that the clot generally retains and contains the perfused material but may also show a considerable amount of permeability. This allows materials like carbon black (and thus exudate) to pass through it, accumulate on the surface at the clot-tissue interface, and seep from the peripheral margins of the wound.

The clot, however, does tend to contain fluid within the gingival corium, a condition considered instrumental for early epithelialization. Epithelium migrating over the wound surface subjacent to the clot does so more expeditiously when this interface area is well hydrated. Diminished hydration is consistent with retarded epithelialization.

Epithelialization of the wound comes from two major areas: (1) epithelium at the wound margins and (2) possibly remnants of the epithelial attachment. If the incision is such that the entire epithelial attachment is removed during the surgical procedures, epithelium (of attached gingiva) at the margins of the wound provide the prime source of new epithelium to cover the wound surface. If on the other hand some epithelial attachment has remained, the possibility of epithelial migration from both sides exists, thus providing dual epithelial sources. Where this latter condition is present it is presumed that epithelialization of the wound is considerably faster. Postincisional presence of epithelial attachment, that is, pocket epithelium, implies that the entire breadth of the pocket wall has not been removed and that a segment of the detachable pocket wall remains.

Healing after gingivectomy involves also the formation of a linear zone of granulation tissue over the cut surface of the gingival corium. This area of granulation tissue is overlaid by new epithelium derived from that peripheral and contiguous to the wound surface. In essence this layer of granulation tissue is converted to a new lamina propria that lies in contiguity with the outer aspect of the "old" gingival corium remaining after gingivectomy excision. Histologically the connective tissue bed appears to be composed of a stable, relatively insoluble collagen; this state may substantiate the often observed success of gingivectomy-gingivoplasty not only in the resection of diseased tissue, but also in the attainment of stable physiologic tissue form after surgery. The existence of a smooth wound bed with the absence of irregularities, tissue tags, and tears tends to promote rapid epithelialization and the development of the new lamina propria.

The sequence of the regeneration of epithelium when observed in primates and dogs shows an initial response of necrosis at the wound margin concomitant with an acute inflammatory reaction as the surface of the wound is covered by a blood

Fig. 23-19. Healing after gingivectomy. **A,** Control specimen, dog. Apical base of junctional epithelium (epithelial attachment) is, in this instance, located at cementoenamel junction. Line, *i,* illustrates line of incision extending from gingival surface to base of epithelial attachment. **B,** Immediately after incision, wound surface is covered by a thin blood clot that extends into rents and defects in tissue corium. **C,** Two-day postoperative specimen. Blood clot, *c,* overlays wound surface. At lower left note beginning of epithelial migration under clot; progenitor epithelial source is that of adjacent tissue not directly involved in surgery. **D,** In this magnification of a portion of **C,** notice blood clot and patent vessels leading toward wound surface. This is from an animal perfused, just prior to sacrifice, with carbon suspension; carbon particles are extravascular and within clot, evidencing vascular permeability and fragility. **E,** Epithelium, *e,* wedging between wound surface and blood clot, *c.* Clot is gradually resorbed and sequestered. **F,** Seventh postsurgical day. Sulcular epithelium, *se,* has been partially renewed whereas face of wound (at left) is covered by a thin epithelium, *e,* that has migrated in a centripetal pattern over wound from its periphery. Vascularity is marked, and chronic inflammatory cell infiltrate persists perivascularly and adjacent to epithelia. **G,** Sixteen days after surgery. Wound site essentially repaired by development of new lamina propria and epithelium over zone of excision. It is unusual for epithelial keratinizing effect to be manifest so early in healing process. Studies in humans indicate that keratinization—either parakeratinization or orthokeratinization—may be more predictably seen approximately 30 to 45 days after surgical procedure. (From Novaes, A. B., Kon, S., Ruben, M. P., and Goldman, H. M.: J. Periodontol. **40:**359, 1969.)

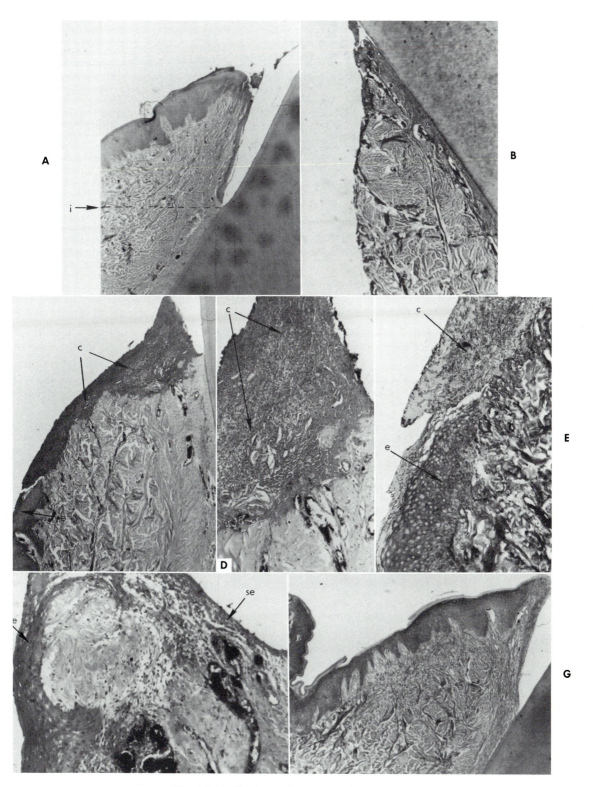

Fig. 23-19. For legend see opposite page.

clot. Epithelial tissue adjacent to the wound margin shows distinct changes within a few hours marked by the presence of scattered chromatin masses from ruptured cells and pale-staining prickle cell layers with indistinct intercellular bridges. Basal cell layers appear relatively unchanged. Normal morphology of epithelial cells is seen at at the wound margin in about 9 to 18 hours, at which time they begin to cover the wound surface by migration from the prickle cell layers. Distinct movement of epithelial cells begins to cover over the wound between 12 and 24 hours after surgical excision. The migration of epithelial cells from the wound margin is an early phenomenon that occurs well in advance of increased synthesis of DNA by epithelial cells in this area. Increased DNA synthesis is observable in approximately 2 mm of epithelium at the wound margin by 24 hours. Cells for initial migration from the wound margin are provided, therefore, by the increased mitosis in this epithelium. After about 2 to 3 days, however, both the basal cells and the wound margin produce cells necessary for migration. This occurs as a stratification at the original wound margin.

Epithelialization of exposed gingivectomy wounds occurs in centripetal fashion from the epithelial periphery of the wound. Cells of the prickle cell layer lose their attachment to adjacent cells and roll over one another in ''caterpillar'' fashion, gradually implanting themselves over the entire wound surface. Once implanted the prickle cell acquires mitotic potential and assumes the role of a typical basal cell. The stage is now set for differentiation of epithelial cell layers normally found in gingival tissue. Electron microscopic observations confirm the formation of a basement lamina between the epithelium and the connective tissue. Immunofluorescent and autoradiographic studies support the contention that the basal lamina is primarily an epithelial product.

The nature of the underlying connective tissue will determine the final differentiation of the overlying epithelium. When the connective tissue is densely collagenous, the covering epithelium will be of the keratinized type, that is, masticatory mucosa. Ultrastructurally, cytofilaments are seen to become bundled in the upper cell layers, membrane coating and keratohyalin granules appear, intercellular spaces are reduced in the superficial layers, and a stratum corneum is formed. When the underlying connective tissue is less dense, such as that found subjacent to crevicular epithelium, spaces between the epithelial cells remain wide, upper cell layers develop membrane-bound granules in their cytoplasm, and prominent Golgi apparatus is formed, but no stratum corneum develops.

As the basal cell layers become more active, DNA activity at the wound edge tends to decrease. The completion of epithelial healing occurs with mitotic activity at some distance from the wound border. This observation plus the finding that DNA synthesis decreases steadily and markedly after the first day lends doubt as to whether the wound margin plays any role in the completion of epithelial healing. It appears more likely that the stimulus for final epithelial regeneration comes either from within the epithelium or from the exposed or incompletely covered connective tissue.

Concomitant with epithelial healing the connective tissue also undergoes significant and observable changes. Immediately after the surgical procedure the excised corium wound is covered by a thick blood clot. The thickness and surface morphology of this structure resembles that of the excised tissue. The clot that covers the dense, well-collagenated, irregular surface caused by the incision plays a significant role in provisionally correcting these irregularities and producing a smooth outer surface.

Within a few hours of the surgical procedure an acute inflammatory reaction occurs, as evidenced by a marked migration of polymorphonuclear cells into the clot and to the surface region of the wound. On the surface area a thin layer of connective tissue gradually becomes filled with polymorphonuclear leukocytes. The external layer, therefore, within 12 to 25 hours shows a blood clot, a subjacent polyband, and superficially disorganized and edematous connective tissue, with collagen fragmentation. The stratum of clot and polyband appears to serve a protective function over the wound area until regenerating epithelium covers the surface. As epithelialization of the wound progresses, the clot loses its attachment to the connective tissue and is eventually shed in part into the oral cavity. This process is facilitated by appropriate phagocytic and enzymatic action at the clot-tissue interface on the part of the neutrophilic leukocytes of the polyband and the macrophages. Polymorphonuclear leukocytes virtually tend to disappear after the protection of the wound surface by epithelium. Lymphocytes may prevail, however, for several weeks after healing. It is currently believed that the lymphocyte, an important part of the immunologic system, is able to control effector cells such as the macrophage and fibroblast by means of the lymphokines that it produces. These effector cells are integral to the healing process and would necessitate the continued presence of their controllers until healing is complete. A similar enduring presence of lymphocytes has been noted in healing of periapical infections after endodontic therapy even after clinical and radiologic evidence have long confirmed successful therapy. Migrating epithelium wedges its way between the surface coagulum and underlying viable connective tissue. There is recent evidence to indicate that epithelium is capable of phagocytosis, facilitating wound débridement.

In healing, proliferation of connective tissue begins later than that of epithelium. Although premitotic activity (tritiated thymidine in a monkey) in epithelium reaches a peak in 24 to 36 hours, connective tissue peaks of premitotic activity are not achieved for at least 3 to 4 days. Connective tissue proliferation is initiated away from the margin of the wound. As soon as epithelium covers the wound, however, cells under the basement membrane assume further production of connective tissue. This activity proceeds to produce a vascular granulation tissue within 3 to 7 days.

Collagen formation and improved tissue organization develop gradually over a 3- to 4-week period, as inflammation with attending vascularity decreases, even though clinically the gingival surface may appear "completely" healed in 2 to 3 weeks after surgery. Collagen production in granulation tissue occurs after the proliferation of fibroblasts that arise locally in perivascular, periosteal, and lamina propria regions.

The general pattern of healing after gingival resection therefore involves the formation of a new lamina propria over the cut surface of the gingival corium. The extremely vascular layer of granulation tissue provides the progenitor for a new lamina propria over which epithelial renewal occurs. As healing progresses the granulation tissue is transformed into a new gingival lamina propria. This is evidenced by a progressive decrease in vascularity, an organized pattern of connective tissue elements, and a conversion of epithelium that becomes markedly similar in structural configuration and keratinization to resemble normal gingiva. The healing process, generally rapid and uncomplicated, maintains the desirable tissue contour produced in the gingivoplastic phase of the operation.

New sulcus formation after gingivectomy occurs as the result of epithelial progression into the shallow crevice present between the tooth and developing marginal soft tissue. It appears that there is a physiologic constancy of width of gingival attachment to the root above the crest of bone (about 1 to 1.55 mm) and that there is a renewal of the expanse of this attachment after surgery.

At about 21 days the surface epithelium may appear normal. The vascularity of the area decreases and connective tissue reflects an improvement of collagen in quantity and organized distribution. A few inflammatory cells may be seen to persist, particularly in the subsulcular area. These are dominantly lymphocytes and plasma cells. Since other qualities consistent with inflammation are no longer evident, we must assume that these cells are providing immunologic protection at the site.

The removal of the sulcular and junctional epithelium during gingivectomy necessitates the formation of a new dentogingival relationship. This occurs when the centripetally migrating epithelium reaches the root surface, and its further movement is inhibited. Cell differentiation can now occur, and all the elements of a healthy dentogingival junction will form. Any factor, including excessively traumatic surgical technique, that impedes healthy connective tissue attachment to the cementum may promote continual apical migration of epithelium with eventual inadvertent pocket formation.

Firm epithelial adherence to the root surface is delayed until inflammation is no longer apparent and until collagen synthesis (and connective tissue rigidity) is advanced. Experimental observations (monkeys) have shown further that mitotic activity in the attachment epithelium does not return to preoperative levels until some 4 to 5 weeks after surgery. Once this "epithelial seal" is established, inflammation, which has persisted with waning intensity to this time in the connective tissue, tends to disappear. Since after completion of wound epithelialization there appears to be a temporal lag before the epithelium seals against the tooth surface, the use of a periodontal probe into the sulcular area for several weeks after the surgical procedure would appear to be contraindicated.

On an ultrastructural level, healing of the dentogingival junction involves the formation of hemidesmosomes against the root surface and on the connective tissue side of the epithelial cells prior to the appearance of the basal lamina. The hemidesmosomes will adapt or attach to the root surface whether it is composed of cementum, dentin, enamel or any combination of these substances.

Inflammation in connective tissue after gingival resection may be associated with a transient effect on alveolar crest in the form of resorptive activity at about 7 to 12 days after the surgery. Distinct osteoclastic activity, at the periosteal phase of the gingiva, is apparent at this time, although the process does not appear to produce a permanent defect. At about 14 to 18 days postsurgically a reversal pattern is usually observed with the formation of a well-defined osteoblastic layer.

Since the sulcular area may require a longer period of time for complete epithelialization, it is apparent that a delay in healing may be produced by the presence of inflammation. A program of meticulous oral hygiene would therefore appear to be not only justified but crucial. The presence of plaque and food debris adjacent to the newly forming sulcus may cause retarded healing, with the persistence of gingival inflammation.

Recent well-controlled clinical studies indicate that gingivectomy is not the treatment of choice in instances in which underlying osseous defects must be managed. When compared to Widman and apically repositioned flap procedures used to treat similar defects, the gingivectomy approach resulted in a net loss of attachment. This confirms earlier observations that the gingivectomy modality should only be considered in situations where pockets are suprabony or when the gingival tissue is hyperplastic.

MUCOGINGIVAL SURGERY

Studies relating to the healing of mucogingival surgical techniques have become extremely numerous over the past several years, with a wide variety of clinical approaches having been introduced to cope with periodontal disease involving the gingiva and the contiguous alveolar mucosa. The recognition of the histologic nature of these tissues has prompted the use of techniques that are designed to retain tissue or create a functionally adequate zone of gingiva where it is missing or where a surgical procedure such as gingivectomy would remove most or all of the attached tissue. Gingiva appears to be well adapted to withstand the functional stresses of friction and pressure to which it is normally exposed, whereas alveolar mucosa may be poorly adapted to such function. Emphasis, therefore, has been placed on approaches that are designed to manipulate these delicate tissues in order to conserve them along with their underlying structures.

Correlation of healing mucogingival wounds in experimental animals and in human beings has presented a remarkable consistency of observations relating to these procedures. The findings clearly indicate that the most favorable postoperative results from the point of preservation of periodontium, repair, and attainment of objectives are best accomplished with various flap procedures. Wounds that involve the exposure of underlying alveolar process and root structure tend to give far better repair if they can be covered completely by fully mature tissue or at least remain with some degree of periosteal retention.

Numerous studies have further recognized the resorptive implications of osseous exposure. It has become increasingly obvious that there is virtually no surgical modality used in periodontal therapy that does not affect the underlying osseous structures. The extent of the involvement may be of little clinical consequence or may have significant qualitative and quantitative effects. To a large degree this is dependent on both the original nature of the osseous scaffolding and the surgical procedure used. As a result, osseous surgery and the covering of bone have undergone considerable modifications in approach. By preserving much of the vascular nutrition to the cortical layer of bone, resorptive activity can be kept to a minimum. The flap therefore allows alveolar bone to receive its own biologic dressing and allows for maximized preservation and conservation of periodontium. With this in mind, flap elevation should be executed with due regard for the maintenance of flap integrity and viability. Flap necrosis may well result in destructive changes in the underlying bone that by far overshadow the problem flap elevation was originally intended to correct.

In broad terminology the two major types of flaps used in most mucogingival procedures are based on the elevation of the entire complex of tissue, including periosteum (full thickness), or the raising of only a portion of this tissue (partial thickness). Partial-thickness flaps allow periosteum and some connective tissue fibers to remain attached to root or bone or both.

Experimental studies have shown that repair of epithelium and connective tissue is much the same irrespective of whether the full- or partial-thickness approach to flap surgery is used. There is, however, a marked difference in the reaction of alveolar bone. Although bone resorption is seen in both instances, that seen with full-thickness flaps may be more severe and penetrating, often leading to permanent deformation. The greater physical, biologic, and infective insult that occurs when full-thickness flaps are used is thought to be responsible for this phenomenon. This pernicious process may have no clinical significance in areas where bony septa are thick, but may lead to total disappearance of alveolar plates in regions in which it is thin. As it is not possible to predetermine the amount of bone that will be lost with either procedure, it may be advisable to use the partial-thickness approach when the roots are prominent in the arch and when the associated alveolar plates are expected to be thin and vulnerable.

Full-thickness flaps

Full-thickness mucoperiosteal flaps (Figs. 23-20 to 23-25) have been used for several decades as approaches for débridement and pocket elimination in the management of moderately deep periodontal pockets where the soft tissue walls are of a fibrotic character. The importance of this

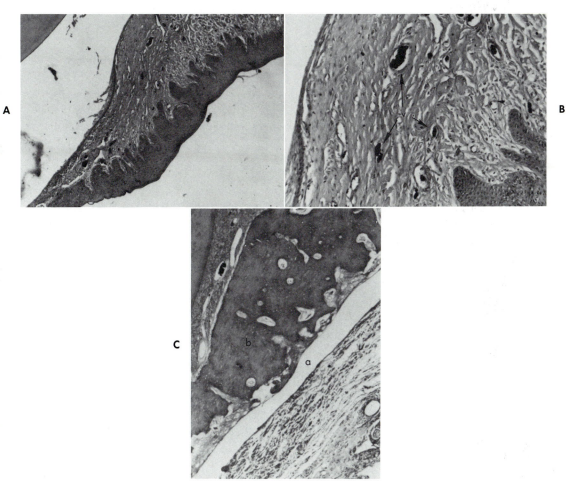

Fig. 23-20. Sequence of healing process shown in Figs. 23-20 to 23-25. Full-thickness mucoperiosteal flap, dog. **A,** Gingival portion of tissue flap within minutes after it has been returned and sutured to approximate tooth and bone. Sulcular and junctional epithelia were inadvertently permitted to remain. **B,** Higher magnification of gingival corium depicted in **A.** Vascular patency, *v,* may be augmented as earliest phase of postsurgical inflammatory response. Little observable change in gingival connective tissue, since it is remarkably stable. **C,** Lack of attachment of flap to bone; linear area, *a,* is usually occupied by blood clot. Whereas clinically a full-thickness flap was executed, histology demonstrated residual connective tissue on bone surface, extending into its vascular channels and marrow. This tissue may react productively and assist in reattachment of flap to bone septum.

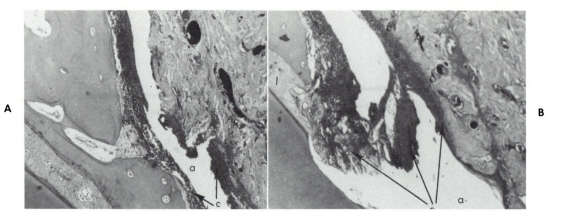

A

B

Fig. 23-21. Full-thickness mucoperiosteal flap healing process, dog; second postsurgical day. **A,** Absence of a bond, *a,* between flap and bone. Dark fragmented band, *c,* is blood clot. **B,** Blood coagulum, *c,* over crest of periodontal ligament, *l,* Blood clot is resorbed enzymatically via such agencies as neutrophilic acid hydrolases, phagocytized by mononuclear macrophages, and is sequestered (in part) in exudate from wound.

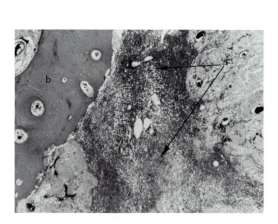

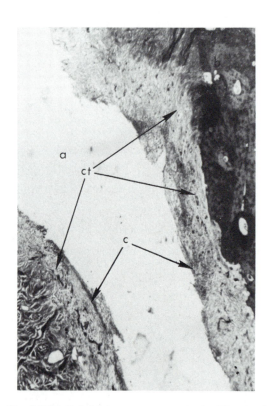

Fig. 23-22. Full-thickness mucoperiosteal flap healing process, dog; fourth postoperative day. Blood clot, *c,* still persisting between face of bone, *b,* septum, and soft tissue. Vacuoles are seen within clot, and its elements tend to be dispersed, indicating more advanced resorption of blood clot. Irregularities on surface of bone (lower part) are resorptive bays induced by action of osteoclasts, since some periosteum was residual on bone at time of surgery. It is progenitor tissue in this area for osteoclasts. Topical etching of bone adjacent to clot may be enzymatically produced by hydrolytic constituents of exudate.

Fig. 23-23. Full-thickness mucoperiosteal flap healing process, dog; 6 days after surgery. Tissue flap has separated from bone due to inadequacy of production of reparative tissue needed for flap reattachment. This is a problem of particular concern when flap is retracted from highly cortical bone surface with few available endosteal sources of granulation tissue; flap reattachment is here largely dependent on centripetal ingrowth of reparative tissue from periosteum at edge of flap retraction and later from periosteum of flap. *c,* Remnants of blood clot; *ct,* sparse, new connective tissue; *a,* space between flap and bone.

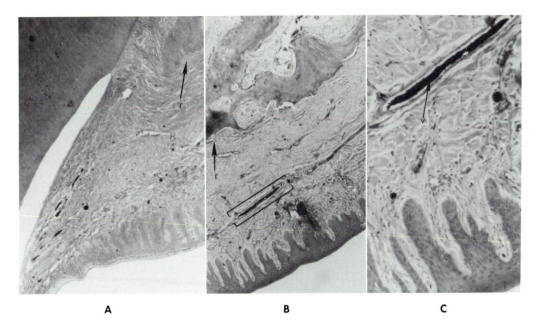

Fig. 23-24. Full-thickness mucoperiosteal flap healing process, dog; 12 days after surgery. Flap has been reattached to bone and tooth. **A,** Tissue corium is moderately hypervascular but retains original density. Epithelium is intact, including parakeratotic outer zone. Arrow points to area of resorption, *r,* of bone crest. **B,** Irregular resorption of facial aspect of septum yet soft tissue is attached to bone; resorption and repair can coexist, especially when osteoclastic activity and inflammation are in waning stage. **C,** Periosteal vasculature is well maintained and functional. Arrow points to perfused blood vessel.

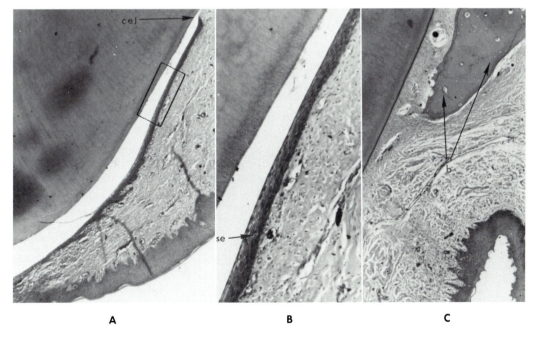

Fig. 23-25. Full-thickness mucoperiosteal flap healing process, dog; 85-day postoperative section. Flap had been positioned at time of surgery in relationship to enamel surface. This is not desirable, since it may result in a long tissue approximation to tooth, that is, unattached gingival cuff capable of being retracted from tooth. **A** and **B,** At variable magnifications, thin nature of the crevicular epithelium, *se,* and minimal subepithelial aggregate of inflammatory cells. Marginal aspect of tissue wall is very thin and should be clinically flaccid. **C,** Intact, renewed fixation of soft tissue complex to bone and tooth. Surface topography, *b,* of bone septum is smooth. Reattachment of flap is not only mediated by periosteal activity, but also via productivity of exposed periodontal ligament.

procedure has been emphasized over the past several years, and access to bone for the correction of osseous lesions and malformations has also been stressed. As a result a considerable number of wound-healing studies have been performed to evaluate not only the initial tissue damage and reaction, but also the sources and mode of attachment of regenerative soft tissue and bone. By use of a full-thickness mucoperiosteal approach, both attached gingiva and alveolar mucosa are separated from the underlying root and alveolar process by blunt dissection, thus exposing osseous tissue for indicated treatment. In the dissective process the periosteum may be inadvertently divided, particularly in the area of attached gingiva; the cellular layer (cambium) remains essentially on the bony surface, and the fibrous layer is retained as part of the reflected soft tissue. In some instances the cambium is eliminated by the mere interposition of a periosteal elevator at the soft tissue-bone interface. Healing occurs by both primary and secondary intention, since the flap is readapted to cover the margin of radicular bone in a more apical position than its original level.

Healing of full-thickness flaps occurs in a relatively rapid sequential manner. As the flap is replaced with but minimal vascular damage in its desired position, there is the formation of a blood clot over exposed bone and the inner connective tissue surface. This clot, with fibrin strands in a parallel arrangement relative to the wound, is interposed between the flap and the underlying osseous surface. A great deal of significance has been placed on the thickness of the blood clot; a thick coagulum has been associated with incomplete or imperfect adaptation of the soft tissue to the underlying bone. Since the clot must be resorbed and replaced by connective tissue during the healing process, it is evident that a thinner clot is considerably more desirable than one that is thick and thus retardant to rapid attachment of soft tissue to bone. The weakest part of the adherence between flap and bone occurs in the area of the fibrin clot. This adherence, mediated by the blood clot between soft and hard tissue, is not substantial enough to hold them together. The clot contributes very little, in fact, to maintaining the flap in position; during the first 7 to 10 days of the healing process close flap approximation to bone tends to accelerate healing because (1) a lesser amount of interposed reparative tissue is necessary for attachment and (2) there is a lesser amount of clot to be resorbed.

Although initial flap adhesion is mediated by fibrin and other viscous elements of the blood coagulum, epithelium in the area of the epithelial attachment appears to provide the initial marginal readaptation of the mucogingival complex. The strength of epithelium to root surface may indeed be greater than that which exists between epithelial cells. It can be demonstrated that epithelial cells will separate from one another much more easily than from cementum.

Within a few days the fibrin (blood) clot undergoes resorption and is replaced concomitantly with new connective tissue. Its fibers appear in the form of reticulum and collagen that become increasingly well organized as connective tissue is formed to provide an increasingly firm attachment of soft tissue to tooth and bone. Recent data also suggests the possibility of tenacious connective tissue *adaptation* to tooth surfaces.

Although a significant bone resorptive phase is a primary event, bone formation subsequently coincides with resorption and finally the process appears to become purely appositional. The initial loss of crestal bone *may* therefore be temporary and may be expected to regenerate entirely or remodel and stabilize at a minimally lower level. Cementum also may show initial resorption, particularly in areas where the root has been curetted. New cementum formation, however, tends to be much slower and less extensive than that of bone. Continued cementogenesis coronal to the osseous crest mediates the new connective tissue attachment as well as repair of the treated root surface in the adjacent vicinity to the periodontal ligament and bone crest.

It has been noted that the cemental contribution to repair is a sluggish and often unpredictable process and that it may be advisable to retain existing viable connective tissue on root surfaces during flap surgery rather than to plane those surfaces clean. This approach has been advocated in the belief that the retention of Sharpey's fibers will allow more rapid connective tissue reattachment, by permitting new connective tissue of the repair process to unite with the retained collagenous fibers, rather than awaiting new cementogenesis before this can occur. "Scar" formation of this type may have the added advantage of limiting epithelial migration during the repair of flap wounds. The use of this technique implies that definitive root planing be confined to those areas coronal to the retained connective tissue attachment.

The histologic sequence of healing of full-thickness mucoperiosteal flaps shows that the initial fibrin clot that separated the soft tissue and alveolar process and tooth remains essentially for about 3 to 4 days, after which it begins to become gradually resorbed. It is usually completely replaced at 6 to 7 days by the concomitant development of young connective tissue (reparative tissue) derived from marrow spaces and vascular channels of bone, the crestal aspect of periodontal ligament, and the periosteal connective tissue of the mucosa at the apical and lateral aspects of the flap. At this time the edge of the flap is sharply demarcated, with a distinct band of granulation tissue present between the flap and bone and flap and tooth. This budding tissue is characterized by the presence of marked endothelial proliferation and many young fibroblasts that are beginning to produce new collagen in the form of fine fibrils, forming a delicate lacelike or indifferent pattern. Although connective tissue synthesis has distinctly commenced at 6 to 7 days, the joining of the corium of the flap to bone and tooth is still a very tenuous one.

New connective tissue is essentially formed from the existing connective tissue cells of the bone and soft tissue. More specifically it appears to arise from at least four major areas: (1) growth from the periodontal ligament, (2) extension from endosteum of vascular channels and marrow, (3) proliferation from the periosteum of the flap at the periphery of its detachment from bone, with centripetal ingrowth of connective tissue, and (4) ingrowth from the fibrous aspect of periosteum. Although the periodontal ligament is not markedly visibly altered in the very initial stages of healing, one can expect to find early marginal disorganization of this structure as well as an increase in its vascularity; inflammation may be evident at its crestal phase. It exhibits (4 to 7 days) new connective tissue cells, many fine collagen fibrils, and a distinct vasoproductive reaction. Intense fibroblastic activity may be significantly observable by 6 to 7 days. The periodontal ligament is undoubtedly the prime source of the early connective tissue reattachment to tooth and marginal bone. At this time also there is evidence of new collagen fibers emanating from periosteum at the periphery of the flap to form a phase of the granulation tissue interposed between flap and subjacent hard and soft tissues. Hence there is a need for close adaptation between these areas.

The wound area initially exhibits marked inflammation, as evidenced by the heavy infiltration of polymorphonuclear leukocytes. These cells diminish in intensity and number after about a week and are replaced by lymphocytes, plasma cells, and macrophages that are indicative of a change to a diminished state of inflammation. There is a temporal coincidence between chronic inflammation and repair.

Revascularization of the wound area generally tends to follow the pattern of new connective tissue formation. Beginning revascularization is observable at about 2 to 3 days by marked vasodilation in the flap. Although dilation of the flap vessels constitutes the initial response, this vascular change tends to decrease during the first week and thereafter. At this time a significant number of budding and sprouting capillaries can be identified within the granulation tissue at the interface between flap and bone. The vasoproliferative reaction gradually diminishes between the first and second week; thereafter an improved organization is apparent. The new fibroblastic population is derived from undifferentiated reserve connective tissue cells, whereas capillary formation is dependent on endothelial and pericytic proliferation and migration.

The periosteum will more readily contribute to wound repair if its two layers have not been seriously damaged during surgery. In this regard it has been noted that the periosteum, and in particular the inner, relatively quiescent cambium, may be stimulated to fibrogenic, osteogenic, vascular proliferative, and neural trophic activity by surgical trauma. This is demonstrated by the veritable stream of repair tissue that arises in the periosteum at the lateral borders of flap wounds and "flows" centripetally under the replaced flap. As a result of these phenomena it has been advocated that osteoperiosteal flaps be utilized in periodontal surgery to incorporate into the flap the full reparative potential of the periosteum. In preliminary clinical trials in which the periosteum of donor site tissue was surgically stimulated with sharp needles 8 to 10 days prior to laterally positioning osteoperiosteal full-thickness flaps, very encouraging results were obtained when the coverage of denuded roots was attempted (Goldman and Smukler). (Melcher in earlier investigations ascertained the surgical vulnerability of periosteum and its delayed contribution to the healing process after elevation from bone and subsequent replacement and advocated the osteoperiosteal flap as a method of surgical conservation of periosteum's reparative qualities.)

The surface epithelium of the flap reflects an essentially normal appearance after the first few days of healing, although the basal cell layer at the cut margin exhibits a marked increase in mitotic activity. These cells begin a migratory process over the connective tissue surface under the blood coagulum and at 1 week have usually approximated the root surface initiating the epithelial attachment and the sulcular lining.

The reaction of bone to a full-thickness mucoperiosteal flap procedure is one of initial topical resorption followed by eventual repair at the affected areas. Resorption is apparent at about 3 to 4 days on the periodontal ligament and crestal surfaces of the alveolar septa, as evidenced by the presence of large multinucleated cells adjacent to these resorptive bays in bone. Empty lacunae at the bone surface are indicative of osteocytic dissolution at this site. The intensity of osseous resorption tends to increase markedly over the entire first week, peaking at about 8 to 10 days after the procedure. Osteoclastic resorption of the outer aspect of a septum is delayed until granulation tissue is interposed between flap and bone, since this is a fundamental source of precursors to the osteoclast. Other progenitors include the endosteum of bone and reparative tissue derived from the periodontal ligament.

The amount, pattern, and severity of bone destruction may be directly related to both the anatomy and histology of the osseous tissue present. Resorption tends to be most widespread and intense in areas where septa are thin and are composed of two plates of compact bone fused together, for example, the labial septa of the mandibular incisors and overprominent radicular surfaces. A lesser overall destructive pattern is evident where cancellous or supporting bone is present between the outer cortical plate and alveolar bone proper. This latter situation is far more desirable and more subject to efficient repair, since marrow spaces and other vascular sites are readily available for contributions to the eventual healing process. Areas composed primarily of compact bone over a radicular surface may be subjected to more permanent loss, depending on the thickness of this tissue over the root area; a thin septum tends to be more substantially influenced by resorptive processes. In any event the *initial* resorptive pattern, whether with compact or cancellous bone, appears to be limited to the crestal and periodontal surfaces.

Healing at about 10 to 12 days shows a changing pattern with respect to bone. Resorption of the periodontal crestal areas is still active but to a lesser degree, giving way to signs of repair, manifested by the apposition of osteoid tissue on these surfaces. Concomitant with bone formation in these previously noted areas, the periosteal aspect, which has been relatively dormant to this time, now exhibits active resorption; it reaches its most extensive activity at about 10 to 14 days, after which the intensity of the reaction tends to decrease. Resorption and bone formation also exist simultaneously at the 14- to 21-day period. There is therefore a contrast of areas of active bone build-up on the periodontal surface and predominant resorption on the periosteal surface. Apposition is evidenced in histologic sections by reversal lines and osteoid tissue, with numerous osteoblasts adjacent to the surface, whereas resorption is revealed by cupped-out or eroded areas of osteoclastic activity.

During the second postoperative week the soft tissue portion of the wound exhibits significant signs of healing and maturation, with the observation of loosely arranged collagen fiber bundles replacing much of the fine fibrils previously present. Numerous fibers, although loosely structured and somewhat disorganized, appear to line up in a somewhat parallel arrangement relative to the periosteal surface of bone.

Collagen fibers in relation to bone appear, at about 2 weeks, to assume a pattern consistent with that seen normally. In the crestal area, as bone shows significant signs of repair, collagen bundles acquire an oblique distribution different from the more parallel formation previously present. Periodontal ligament fibers are still not well oriented at about 14 days, and the new collagen fibers of this area are becoming incorporated into developing cementum, although the relationship at this stage is an extremely tenuous one. Reformation of cementum is a comparatively minimal process. Initial active resorption of cementum and exposed dentin gives way to repair of these tissues and eventually results in new attachment by an apparent active cellular process. It is possible, as with bone, to go through phases of initial resorption, then concomitant resorption and formation, and later a predominantly formative stage. As periodontal ligament and supracrestal fibers form, they are incorporated intimately into this calcifying tissue. Root resorption tends to be more pronounced in areas where cementum has been completely planed from the area. Cementogenesis may be marked in areas of root irregularity produced by instrumentation.

The healing pattern at about 3 weeks is one in which repair dominates the general biologic picture. A thickening and regenerating connective tissue covers the crest of bone, although the periosteal surface may still show signs of both osteoblastic and minimal osteoclastic activity. Osteoblasts are aligned on the periodontal ligament side of the septum and on bone surfaces surrounding the marrow spaces. New bone formation is evidenced by the presence of osteoid and by reversal lines demarcating it from previously formed bone. Orientation of supracrestal and periodontal ligament fibers is not more distinct.

Healing after a 4- to 5-week period consists essentially of maturation and repair of all the tissues involved. Uneventful healing progresses with variably complete re-formation of bone that had been lost from the crest and buccal aspect of the osseous septum. By 2 to 3 months one would expect to see the flap firmly reattached to the tooth via dense, organized, connective tissue and cementum. Tissues affected by the surgery have fundamentally regenerated. Epithelium of attached gingiva shows distinct rete peg formation, whereas that of the sulcus is thin and free of rete projections. Bone apposition *may* have been intense enough to reestablish the original height of the bone septa. The extent of loss of osseous crest is relatable to the original quality and thickness of bone. When this is thin—composed essentially of two cortices—such septa may show significant loss of width and height and may not completely regenerate. A thicker septum therefore gives a more favorable response; some septal thickness may be lost but the height of bone may be retained. Cortical bone forming a thin septum may, on the other hand, show significant resorption, and healing to the presurgical level may not take place.

When full-thickness flaps are raised beyond the mucogingival line and subsequently replaced, the clinical observations during the first week exhibit a tissue that is bluish red in appearance. Because of the edema of the initial inflammatory response, the tissue gives a shiny appearance with loss of stippling. Exudation and oozing are present. The tooth may exhibit some degree of mobility and be tender to palpation or percussion. The flap has a very tenuous early attachment that improves in tenacity with time. Although a well-adapted flap may be found on the buccal or lingual surface, the interradicular septal region is covered by edematous tissue. Where interdental gingival coaptation has not been secured, the area of osseous exposure heals by secondary intention with granulation tissue derived from underlying bone and periodontal ligament. This tissue binds flaps to bone and tooth and secures the attachment of buccal to lingual soft tissue.

The success of flap operations may depend on multiple clinical considerations such as anatomy, correct flap positioning, adaptation and maintenance, and prevention of bacterial plaque accumulation. Where there is a strong and high muscle insertion, it is possible that a space may be created between the flap and the tooth or the flap and the bone by the bulk and pull of the musculature. The correct repositioning of the flap together with the necessary means to maintain it in place during the first few weeks is critical for proper healing. Loose sutures or muscular activity may create spaces filled with a large clot that could be temporally detrimental to reattachment. Digital pressure applied to the flap for several minutes immediately after surgery is one means of obtaining good adaptation postoperatively of soft to hard tissue and avoiding space ("pseudocyst") between the wound surfaces. Protection of the area via a rigid dressing, which may also act as a stent, and proper oral hygiene create an environment that encourages epithelialization of the crestal soft tissue, promotes formation of a new epithelial attachment and sulcular epithelium, and keeps inflammation to a minimum. Proper flap adaptation allowing for shallow sulcular depth along with thin contour of gingival tissue may be helpful to maintain good gingival health during the postoperative period.

Partial-thickness flaps

The literature in recent years contains a large number of clinical and histologic studies concerned with the use of partial-thickness mucogingival surgery (Figs. 23-26 to 23-30). The basic rationale for this therapeutic procedure is to attempt to create an increased width of attached gingiva or gain access to underlying bone for osseous surgical techniques. Although there are numerous variations in approach, the fundamental surgical procedure consists in splitting gingival tissue by sharp dissection, thus separating a soft tissue flap from underlying periosteum and connective tissue covering bone. Surgery of a partial-thickness gingival flap involves the reflection of gingiva from periosteum by a delicate dissective process, allowing no area of bone to be exposed. The flap portion, consisting of gingival epithelium, a significant portion of lamina propria, and corium, may be designed so that the connective tissue attachment to the alveolar process and the tooth need not be disrupted. After the indicated therapy

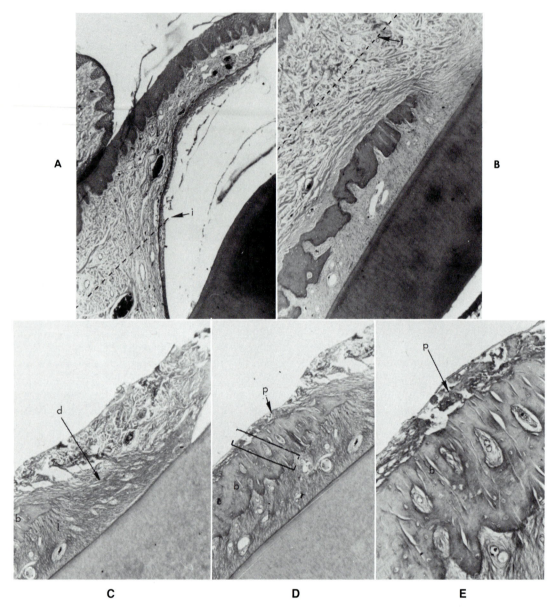

Fig. 23-26. Representative events in healing of periosteal retention type of mucogingival surgery is shown in Figs. 23-26 to 23-30; dog. Comparable repair can also be seen at donor sites for free gingival grafts and laterally repositioned partial-thickness flap. **A,** Control specimen. Gingival cuff approximates enamel. Line of projected incision, *i,* while resecting outer aspect of gingiva, leaves periosteum in attachment to bone, and in some specialized instances, to tooth. **B,** Control tissue, comparable to presurgical site. Dotted line, *i,* at left, continues incision through gingiva and will eventuate in alveolar mucosa. **C** to **E,** Area immediately after surgical intervention. Note that a thin periosteal sheath, *p,* covers bone, *b.* **C,** Thin segment of gingival corium remains attached to cementum and may later serve as a substrate for development of additional gingiva. It would not be clinically favorable to allow marginal gingiva to remain in situ over enamel as **C;** incision should terminate at cementoenamel junction. (From Novaes, A. B., Kon, S., Ruben, M. P., and Goldman, H. M.: J. Periodontol. **41:**685, 1970.)

the flap is replaced at the desired level, which may or may not cover the connective tissue remaining on the alveolar process.

The historical development of partial-thickness periodontal surgery occurred when it became clear that there was a need for special techniques in the treatment of problems that affect the postoperative architecture of the mucogingival area (Goldman). Prior to this time bone denudation procedures often resulted in a substantial loss of supporting structures, particularly bone. Subsequent wound-healing studies showed these approaches to be destructive, particularly to radicular bone, causing significant and often serious anatomic deformities. Other investigations eventually indicated that a biologic covering over bone may be desirable. Current evidence infers that much less bone, if any at all, is lost by the replacement

of either a full- or partial-thickness flap over bone. Experimental healing studies indicate that osteoclastic activity under partial-thickness flaps begins at about 4 days and continues for approximately 2 weeks after surgery. When full-thickness flaps are utilized, osteoclastic resorption begins at about the seventh to fourteenth day postsurgically and may continue thereafter. In general it is believed but poorly substantiated that osseous resorption under full-thickness flaps is of a greater intensity and more enduring nature than that found with the partial-thickness approach. This may be of great clinical significance where radicular bony septa are thin, but of less import when they are broad. Leaving connective tissue attachment to tooth and radicular bone has proved to be a far more conservative approach while still obtaining the desired objective, such as the

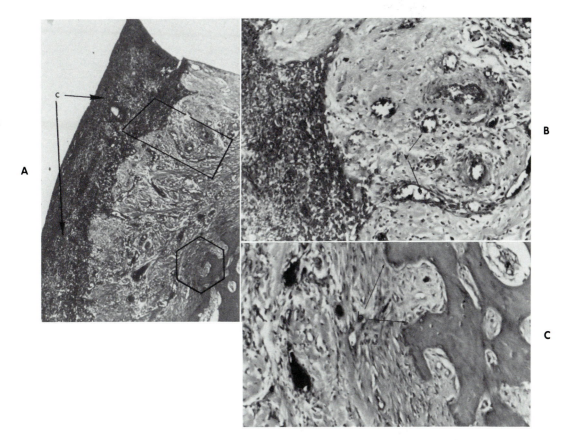

Fig. 23-27. Reparative sequence of periosteal retention procedure, dog; fourth postoperative day. **A,** Wound surface is covered by blood clot, c, which extends in podlike form into connective tissue clefts. **B,** High-power magnification of rectangular zone seen in **A.** Notice numerous patent blood vessels and perivascularly located inflammatory cell infiltrate. **C,** Magnification of hexagonally outlined bone septum in **A.** Periosteal blood vessels are intact and functional. Periosteum extends into irregular bays on bone surface; it is very cellular with evidence of osteoblastic activity, b. (From Novaes, A. B., Kon, S., Ruben, M. P., and Goldman, H. M.: J. Periodontol. **41:**685, 1970.)

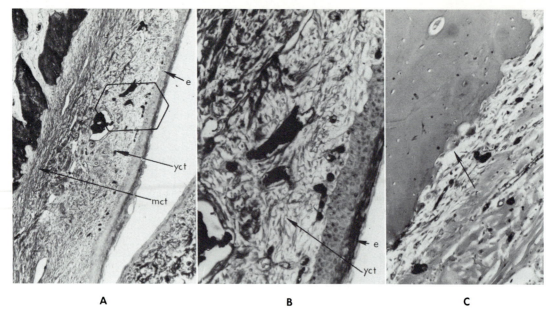

A   B   C

Fig. 23-28. Reparative sequence of periosteal retention procedure, dog; seventh post-surgical day. **A,** At a survey magnification, zone of connective tissue, *yct,* with overlying epithelium, *e,* has developed external to periosteal aspect, *mct,* of alveolar mucosa and gingiva. This young, highly vascular loose connective tissue has its origination from periosteum present subjacently and at periphery of wound. **B,** In greater detail connective tissue, *yct,* which has formed external to periosteum. It is highly cellular and vascular, with indifferently oriented reticular and collagenous fibrils dispersed in a very edematous matrix. Characteristically, epithelium, *e,* is thin and tenuously bound to connective tissue. Keratinizing effect will be manifest as connective tissue substrate becomes more rigid and viscous. **C,** Surface of bone manifests effects of osteoclastic action with resorptive notches at times containing multinucleated cells. (From Novaes, A. B., Kon, S., Ruben, M. P., and Goldman, H. M.: J. Periodontol. **41:**685, 1970.)

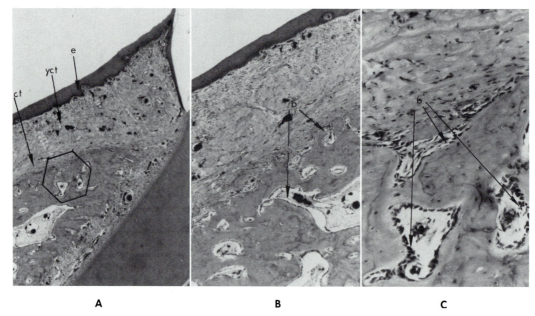

A   B   C

Fig. 23-29. Reparative sequence of periosteal retention procedure, dog; twelfth day; gingival area. **A,** Gingival corium has increased in thickness as a result primarily of formation of new connective tissue, *yct.* This reparative tissue is very vascular (note multitude of perfused, patent vessels). There is also considerable cellular activity in periosteal phase of gingiva, *ct.* Epithelium, *e,* is thin, nonkeratinized, and devoid of rete pegs. **B** and **C,** Hexagonal area of **A.** There is much osteoblastic, *b,* and fibroblastic activity in both periosteum and endosteum of marrow sites. (From Novaes, A. B., Kon, S., Ruben, M. P., and Goldman, H. M.: J. Periodontol. **41:**685, 1970.)

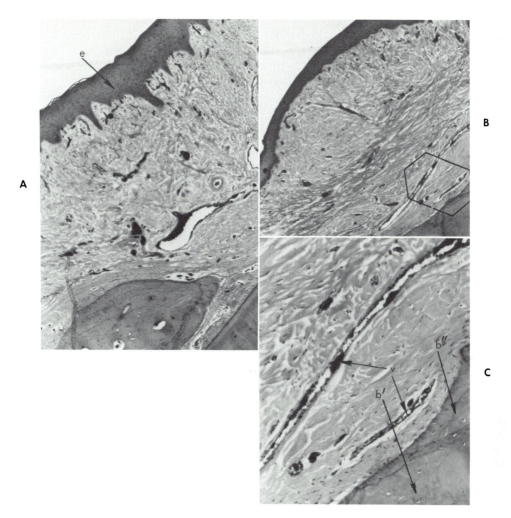

Fig. 23-30. Reparative sequence of periosteal retention procedure, dog; quality of repair of a zone of periosteal exposure 85 days after surgery. **A,** Epithelium, *e,* although thin and with irregular rete extensions into connective tissue, is complete and manifests outer zone of parakeratosis. Lamina propria, just adjacent to epithelium, is composed of loose connective tissue without undue vascularity. **B** and **C,** Note well-structured gingival corium that has formed external to periosteal (group C) fibers that were left in situ at the time of surgery; intact functional vasculature, *b',* within the entire soft tissue complex; and regular, presumably remodeled, topography of external face of bone, *b".* (From Novaes, A. B., Kon, S., Ruben, M. P., and Goldman, H. M.: J. Periodontol. **41:**685, 1970.)

development of an adequate band of attached gingiva.

Given a sufficient depth of vestibular fornix this procedure may be definitely advantageous in areas where teeth are in prominent positions in the arch. Malposed teeth may result in presurgical problems such as an absence of radicular bone, a thin radicular plate of bone, a dehiscence, or a fenestration of the radicular surface. Preservation of tissue over these areas may alleviate or prevent potentially permanent deformities.

With the development of numerous types of partial-thickness periodontal procedures, an in-

creasing amount of attention has been redirected to the exact nature of periosteum in an attempt to more clearly understand the basis upon which numerous clinical procedures are used.

From a histologic viewpoint, periosteum consists of two main portions: an outer layer, which is rich in vessels and nerves and shows a dense arrangement of collagenous fibers, and an inner layer (cambium) in which the fibers are loosely arranged, the cells are numerous, and the blood vessels are relatively numerous and minute (Weinmann and Sicher). Healing of partial-thickness wounds depends largely on the nature and thickness of periosteum and its retained connective tissue covering, the nature and thickness of radicular bone, and position of the flap in relation to its presurgical location.

Although the various clinical techniques concerning retention of periosteum may differ widely, the initial cellular reaction to this type of wound is similar. This occurs whether it is in relation to the surface of exposed connective tissue or interposed between wound surfaces of the flap. In these areas there is initially an accumulation of a blood clot composed of fibrin, polymorphonuclear leukocytes, erythrocytes, and cellular debris. The *initial* reaction in periosteum, its connective tissue covering, and alveolar crest may be minimal, with little disorientation of collagen bundles of the intact lamina propria, no unusual osteoclastic activity, and a normal cellular pattern of periosteum. The soft tissue flap, on the other hand, may show a marked inflammatory response within a short period of time with noticeably dilated vessels containing erythrocytes and marginating polymorphonuclear leukocytes. The sequential histologic findings will differ somewhat from this point in time, depending on the nature of the procedure.

All things being equal, replacement of the flap to approximately its original position so that no wound surface is exposed produces a distinctly less pronounced reaction than if connective tissue is left exposed. When the wound edges, both composed of connective tissue, are placed in close approximation to one another, healing is by "primary intention," and the pro tempore flap "attachment" occurs by the mediation of a clot comprised of a reticulum of fibrin containing many polymorphonuclear leukocytes and erythrocytes. A marked proliferation of endothelial cells and young fibroblasts migrating into the clot soon is apparent at the margins of the wound area. Since close coaptation of the epithelial edges is virtually impossible, the split in this area is readily apparent even while connective tissue edges are active with respect to one another. The epithelial break, however, becomes less evident early, since basal epithelial cells begin to become active and migrate across exposed connective tissue after an initial 24-hour lag period. This may be described as a slipping or sliding of cells over one another as a bridge is created across the defect over the clot. This epithelial regeneration may effectively seal the wound within a few days, although the dimension from the basal cell layer to the surface epithelium is thin for several days after the initial

closure. Continuous proliferation quantitively restores the thickness of the tissue in the area to normal. Eventual observation of this area shows that basal and prickle cell layers regenerate completely, although the upper strata of epithelium may reveal some lack of cellular maturation resulting in a surface defect. Gingival epithelial proliferation in experimental animals such as dogs indicates complete restoration in 14 days to the preoperative level. The presence of surface keratinization is indicative of eventual maturation of the tissues. While epithelium is regenerating, the underlying connective tissue is highly cellular and differentiation of many cells occurs. Connective tissue proliferation is evident as the incision area becomes filled with numerous young fibroblasts and new, somewhat disoriented, collagen bundles. In the region of the wound area there is more advanced repair in the superficial layers than the advanced reconstruction seen in the deeper layers at the same time. Collagen fiber bundle formation lags behind somewhat in the deeper areas when compared to the superficial gingival zone. Capillary orientation tends to parallel the vestibular surface of bone in a manner similar to that of collagen fibers. This parallel bundle arrangement with respect to alveolar bone remains this way until full maturation of collagen bundles several weeks later. When this occurs there is fiber reorientation as the bundles become perpendicular to the vestibular plate. Associated with connective tissue proliferation, the periosteum shows marked proliferation, the periosteum shows marked activity with cellular differentiation and numerous newly formed blood vessels. This increased periosteal activity results in the histogenesis of osteoclasts and later osteoblasts.

The response of bone to this surgical procedure is one of initial resorption followed by eventual apposition. Osteoclastic resorption is markedly evident primarily on the periosteal surface between 4 and 8 days, after which it diminishes. Activity finally ceases at about 28 days when the most intense phase of osteoblastic metabolism is evident in the vestibular plate and crestal areas. Actually osteoblastic activity becomes quite apparent within a few days after the surgery. At this time marked proliferation of endosteal tissues produces a type of osteophytic bone. The most intense osteoblastic activity is not apparent for some time, until, as mentioned, osteoclastic activity decreases. By several weeks all tissues appear to regenerate themselves and show a functional repair with or without an anatomic deformity. Much may depend in this respect upon the technique used, the delivery of handling the tissues, and whether or not inadvertent bone exposure may have occurred.

If the surgical procedure is such that only a portion of the wound area is recovered — as may occur if more attached gingiva is desired — and a portion of the area of periosteal retention is left exposed, this area of exposed connective tissue is covered by a clot and shows a markedly increased inflammatory reaction within a 2- to 4-day period. By this time there is significant vascular dilation and a marked number of acute inflammatory cells extending into periosteum and bone proper. The exposed connective tissue wound is covered by cellular debris, bacteria, and fibrin strands. The originally thick collagen bundles of lamina propria and corium show a state of progressive disorientation and degeneration, although osteoclastic activity is not significant as yet. The thickness of the retained tissue over periosteum appears to determine the early reaction to the fibers immediately adjacent to this bone covering. After an initial degenerative and lag period at the margins of epithelium there appears to be distinct mitotic activity in the basal layer at 2 to 3 days, since the cells show migration over the connective tissue surface and invasion into the clot as they travel to cover the surface. Epithelialization of this exposed area requires 7 to 10 days, depending on the total connective tissue surface involved. Epithelium appears to cover this exposed wound surface at the rate of about 0.5 to 1 mm per 24-hour period after an intial lag of about 24 hours prior to the beginning of epithelial cell movement. Progressive mitotic activity in the basal cells produces an early thin layer over the wound that thickens as a prickle cell layer and surface parakeratotic cell layer are produced. By approximately 21 days the epithelium appears essentially normal in appearance. Rete peg formation may be variable.

After the initial reaction of connective tissue to surgical injury there is evidence of repair and new connective tissue formation replacing the clot as early as 3 to 4 days as epithelialization progresses. The proliferation and maturation of new tissue originally appears to arise from the periodontal ligament, marrow spaces, and periosteal surface of bone. Cellular elements occupy areas in dense collagenous connective tissue fibers in spaces provided by the disorientation of these bundles. Fiber bundles adjacent to the periosteum, while not disoriented, may show evidence of inter- stitial edema. In these edematous spaces one may find many large mononuclear perivascular cells that have been referred to as reserve cells, progenitor cells, or pluripotential cells. It has been suggested that undifferentiated perivascular cells are the source of specialized tissue cells that may be mobilized early (first few hours) after surgical intervention and that may be involved in specialized functions such as fibrogenesis, osteoclasia, osteogenesis, or tissue débridement. Within a few days proliferation of these cells is evident among collagenous fibers near the wound edge, in the periosteal connective tissue area, and in marrow spaces. Fibroblastic proliferation produces many new immature collagen fiber bundles that are oriented in a parallel arrangement relative to the surface of the tooth. This is readily apparent between 1 and 2 weeks. This orientation changes at about 3 to 4 weeks as new fiber arrangements are organized in a pattern perpendicular to the tooth surface and similar to the mature bundles present prior to the injury.

The reaction of osseous tissue to an area of connective tissue exposure compared to one where the flap is replaced is one of degree of destruction and rapidity of repair to restoration of anatomic form. The sequence of healing as well as its pattern is essentially the same, although flap retention and replacement appear to provide a more advanced stage of tissue repair and maturation. Osteoclastic activity appears within 4 to 8 days, when connective tissue is exposed, and may persist for some time longer. The resorptive pattern occurs primarily at the crestal and periosteal surfaces. Concomitant resorption and repair are evident at an early time. Within a few days after the injury, repair in marrow spaces is apparent even though this activity is some distance from the wound. Osteoblastic activity is marked along the periosteal surface 2 to 3 weeks after the injury. Both marrow spaces and the periosteal surface show significant amounts of osteoid formation and osteoblasts lining these and marrow surfaces. Repair predominates at 3 to 4 weeks and little osteoclasia is evident after this period. This repair process essentially results in complete restoration of the alveolar process.

Final healing shows that this type of tissue restoration may be expected to produce a functional repair with a slight anatomic deformity of the dentogingival junction slightly apical to its preoperative position.

One of the most important advantages of the partial-thickness approach is that a relatively intact, surgically stimulated periosteum is left in intimate contact with the underlying alveolar bone at the surgical site. This improves the potential for relatively rapid repair and the replacement of bone, lost in the osteoclastic phase of wound healing, by the surgically activated and overlying periosteum. In contrast the full-thickness flap results in disruption of the potentially reparative cambium of the periosteum. This periosteal repair and replacement can only occur when (1) the centripetally ingrowing periosteal repair tissue, from the periphery of the wound, reaches the involved area and (2) a new cambium of periosteum is formed from residual microislets of loose connective tissue localized within the outer fibrous phase of periosteum. This is corroborated by the delayed repair phenomenon noted during full-thickness flap surgery.

Alveolar process repair can be expected to produce healing that shows a functional restoration and approximates the presurgical anatomic form. However, crestal and periosteal surface resorption may decrease the height and thickness of this bony form.

From the clinical point of view several meaningful factors appear to emerge. The amount of connective tissue retained over the periosteum appears to play a significant role in the resorptive and reparative process. The replacement of a partial-thickness flap to cover the wound surface produces a distinctly less pronounced cellular reaction than if the connective tissue remains exposed. In the partial-thickness approach the presence of periosteum permits accurate suturing of the flap to the wound surface and ensures optimal covering of the exposed tissues. Areas that have a thick alveolar process and in which thick connective tissue is retained produce active resorption on both the periosteum and periodontal ligament. These patterns of resorption may produce a slight loss in vertical height but a significant thinning of the alveolar process. The surgical technique, particularly with respect to tissue manipulation and contact of bone, may also play a role in the healing process. Contact with underlying bone by the surgical knife produces a reaction similar, although isolated, to that which one finds in a denudation procedure. The fibrin clot, present in the wound made by the knife, is in contact with the surface of the alveolar process. Osseous tissue in this area has a necrotic appearance because of the lack of cells in lacunae, but osteoclastic activity does not predominate and may in fact not be present even though active resorption

is occurring elsewhere. This bone is eventually removed by undermining resorption from adjacent periosteum. This reaction is somewhat intensive during the first week but decreases thereafter. Knife penetration, very near to or in contact with bone, results in necrosis of the superficial layer of vestibular alveolar bone and its periosteum. Should this occur on marginal radicular bone, a permanent resorptive pattern may ensue. If this develops in the interproximal area the result may not be significant due to the anatomy and nature of the cancellous bone present.

Pedicle flaps

The correction of isolated gingival and periodontal resorptive defects by the translocation of gingiva via pedicle-type gingivomucosal flaps is a well-accepted therapeutic procedure in mucogingival surgery (Figs. 23-31 to 23-34). Commonly referred to as "attached pedicle grafts," "pedicle flaps," or laterally repositioned flaps, the transferred tissue's apical base remains in continuity with and attached to alveolar mucosa. Since periosteum carries the principal vascular supply to gingiva and alveolar mucosa, it should be noted that a variability of impairment of the flap's vascular supply will exist in accordance with the type of flap that is utilized. Should the flap be mucoperiosteal, (full thickness), flap blood supply will be essentially preserved. However, if the flap is of partial thickness, leaving periosteum in situ at the donor area, the only remaining direct vascularization to the graft will be those vessels coursing apico-occlusally within that portion of alveolar mucosa that is *external* to periosteum; this flap type is strongly reliant not only on its diminished internal circulation but also upon that of the receptor area. In this context the flap could be designated as an attached pedicle *graft* because of its strong reliance upon host site periosteum and periodontal ligament for (1) early nutrition and hydration via diffusion of exudates, (2) neovascularization, and (3) attachment to the root surface and surrounding periosteum. In a general context the full-thickness flap is more desirable from the standpoint of facile and rapid repair. This concept will be detailed later in this discussion.

Historically the "sliding flap" operation was based on the elevation of full-thickness (mucoperiosteal) pedicle flaps for eventual lateral positioning to receptor sites. The total exposure of bone, dehiscences, and fenestrations at the donor sites during these procedures often resulted in

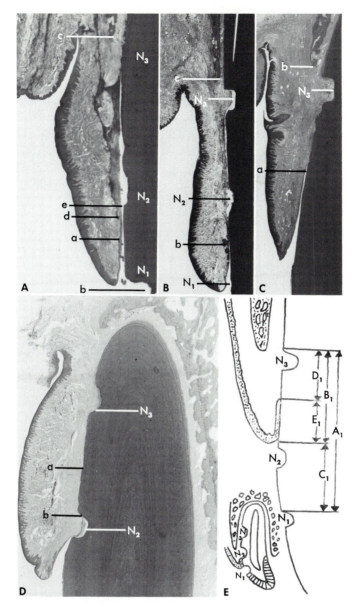

Fig. 23-31. Repair of a dentogingival defect with a pedicle flap. N_1, Level of marginal gingiva before creation of experimental defect. Crown notch. N_2, Crestal level of alveolar bone before creation of experimental defect. N_3, Level to which alveolar bone was reduced. Apical root notch. **A,** Two-day postoperative specimen; maxillary canine area, dog. Pedicle flap and fibrin clot, *a*, is adapted to tooth and periosteum of vestibular bone. *b*, Level of marginal gingiva prior to creation of periodontal defect; *c*, lowered bone crest level; *d*, spicule of bone from donor site is present in pedicle flap, curetted root surface is evident; *e*, artifact space. Hematoxylin-eosin stain. **B,** Six-day postoperative specimen; maxillary canine area; dog. Pedicle flap extends to coronal notch, N_1. *b*, Bone spicules; *c*, alveolar crest. Hematoxylin-eosin stain. **C,** Twenty-eight-day postoperative specimen; maxillary canine area; dog. *a*, Attached epithelial cuff; *b*, alveolar bone crest is only slightly apical to notch. Connective tissue and epithelial attached cuff covering tooth are of equal length. Hematoxylin-eosin stain. **D,** Ninety-day postoperative specimen; maxillary canine area; dog. *a*, Very long connective tissue attachment of pedicle flap to tooth; *b*, long epithelial attachment cuff that is longer than that of unoperated control specimens. Hematoxylin-eosin stain. **E,** Pedicle flap repair. A_1, Length of experimentally created defect; B_1, length of attachment of pedicle flap to tooth; C_1, amount of atrophy of mechanical displacement; D_1, amount of new connective tissue attachment to tooth; E_1, amount of new epithelial attachment to tooth. (**A** to **D** ×12.) (From Wilderman, M. N., and Wentz, F. M.: J. Periodontol. **36:**218, 1965.)

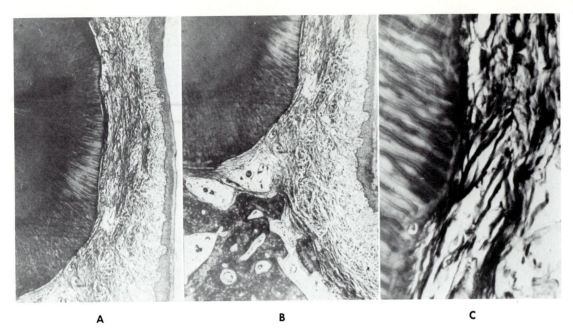

A   B   C

Fig. 23-32. Healing associated with transfer of laterally repositioned full-thickness muco-periosteal flap to cover exposed root surface is shown in Figs. 23-32 to 23-35; dog; 28 days after surgery. Cross-sectional views of tooth and periodontal tissues. **A,** Flap in association with debrided root surface. Notice cemental and dentinal irregularities. Dark striae within gingiva and paralleling root are periosteal fibers. Epithelium is atrophic but viable. **B,** Periodontal ligament and alveolar bone lateral to exposed tooth surface. Tissue flap is secured to bone as a consequence of both periosteal and endosteal production of bone and collagen. Loose connective tissue occupies buccal phase of periodontal ligament, which may also constitute a reparative source. **C,** Higher magnification of den-togingival interface; gingival fibers aligned parallel to and tenuously attached, via ce-mentoid, to dentin.

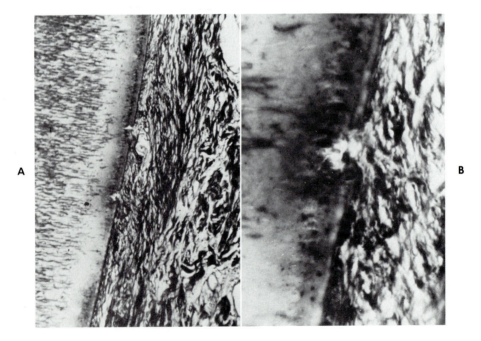

A   B

Fig. 23-33. Healing of laterally repositioned full-thickness mucoperiosteal flap; dog; 42 days. **A** and **B,** Deposition of new collagen and cementoid required to anchor gingival complex to root. Periodontal ligament located peripheral and adjacent to osseous de-hiscence and periosteum of flap provide cellular sources of regenerative tissues. If pedicle graft was of partial-(split-) thickness variety, repair would be dependent on periodontal ligament and periosteum of receptor site. **B,** Dark zone on root is cementoid.

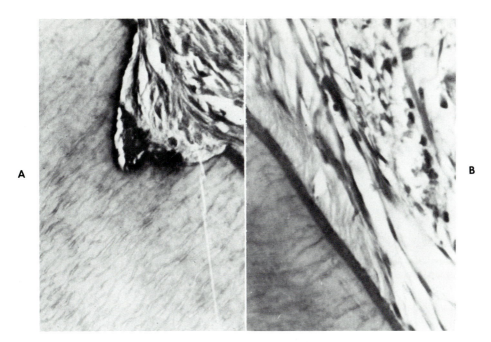

Fig. 23-34. Healing of laterally repositioned full-thickness mucoperiosteal flap, dog. Root surface irregularities, with exposure of mineralized dentin, cementum, or both, appear to be physically inductive of cementum (osteoid) formation and may be the first and the histologically more secure sites of soft tissue attachment to root. Careful root surface preparation at time of surgery, with removal of altered cementum, bacterial plaque, calculus, and debris, may serve to provide this type of receptor area, thus improving predictability of successful outcome of surgery. **A,** Connective tissue and new cementum in notch. **B,** Collagen fibers of pedicle graft appear to be annexed to root by both osteoid and collagen (reticulum).

inordinate osseous resorption and new cleft formation after healing. To obviate these pernicious effects the use of partial-thickness flaps was advocated. This approach, while preventing possible harmful effects at the donor site, has been seen to adversely affect the predictability of the procedure in those instances in which coverage of denuded roots is attempted. Recently developed techniques include both partial- and full-thickness flaps lateral to and united with one another within a single flap. Correct lateral positioning of this type of flap will ensure simultaneous coverage of the vulnerable donor site with the partial-thickness section and of the root surface with the full-thickness element. In this way surgical advances, based on sound biologic rationale, have helped overcome two seemingly irreconcilable problems.

Intact vascular, neural, and lymphatic systems are prerequisites for the healing of periodontal wounds, as are the enthusiastic suppliers of reparative tissue such as the periodontal ligament, periosteum, endosteum, and lamina propria surrounding the lesions (receptor site tissue). The lateral or centripetal ingrowth of these tissues over radicu-

lar or exposed bone surfaces is generally only 1 to 2 mm. This seriously affects the survivability of partial-thickness gingivomucosal flaps or autogenous gingival grafts, which are so greatly dependent on receptor site reparative responses. Mucoperiosteal flaps, on the other hand, have *almost intact, included, vascular* and neural supplies and relatively quiescent periosteum that may be surgically nudged into activity, thereby providing a veritable river of fibrogenic, osteogenic (cementogenic), vascular proliferative tissue and neural trophic, reparative tissue. Recent clinical and statistical evidence of the successful use of mucoperiosteal laterally positioned pedicle grafts for the treatment of denuded root surfaces confirms the foregoing observations. Further, newer investigations in which periosteum has been stimulated into activity some time prior to ''sliding flap'' surgery have produced even more encouraging clinically and histologically verified results.

The success of the procedure is dependent on the maintenance of an *adequate vascular supply* to the transposed tissue from its base, a potentially highly reactive periosteum, eager and responsive recipient site tissues, and the rapid development of connective tissue attachment between the flap and the hard and soft tissues of the receptor site. An early and firm connective tissue attachment is critical to prevent epithelial migration along the inner surface of the flap. In order to utilize fully the reparative potential of the donor and receptor site tissues, careful performance of the surgery is mandatory. Prior to the transposition of the pedicle flap complex the receptor site is prepared so as to remove the pocket wall laterally and apically. Based on the assumption that adequate root preparation is integral to the deposition of new cementum in reattachment procedures, the root surfaces should be extensively scaled and planed. Receptor site sources of reparative tissue such as the periodontal ligament and periosteum also should be adequately exposed. Close adaptation and fixation of the pedicle flap should ensure rapid healing with connective tissue continuity between the flap and root or osseous surface and effective exclusion of epithelial migration other than that which occurs with normal sulcular formation.

Although there are variations in clinical approach, the essential reactions in the healing of pedicle flaps are similar, and a sequential pattern can be observed using a partial-thickness dissection. Observations in experimental animals show an initial clot interposed between the flap and the tooth with fibrin strands arranged in a somewhat parallel alignment with respect to the surface of the tooth. A layer of exudate containing red blood cells is observable between the fibrin clot and tooth. Inflammation at this stage is minimal.

Observation of histologic sections obtained at 2- and 4-day intervals shows a more distinctive clot arrangement consisting of a definite fibrin arrangement parallel to tooth and bone, increased numbers of polymorphonuclear leukocytes in the clot and connective tissue, and signs of epithelial migration a short distance along the gingival margin surface. Where the epithelium is in contact with the tooth, a fibrin clot may be absent.

If flap preparation is by blunt dissection, bone fragments may be retained within the soft tissue. Well embedded in collagen fiber bundles, the bone spicules are separated from the tooth either by the fibrin clot or by a combination of the clot and some connective tissue. These bone spicules are not evident after 21 days. Root planing during the surgical procedure may also result in the finding of cementum particles within the clot at this early period.

The initial stages of flap adaptation just described change to a process of proliferation, particularly of connective tissue, 4 to 6 days postoperatively. Originating from loose connective tissue around the flap vasculature and consisting essentially of numerous capillaries, fibroblasts, lymphocytes, and polymorphonuclear leukocytes, this young tissue appears to arise in the deeper areas of the wound around the alveolar crest and move coronally toward the gingival margin as the clot is being sequestered and resorbed.

Young proliferating connective tissue, present from the alveolar crest region to the gingival margin of the soft tissue, by 6 days shows a distinct line of demarcation with respect to it and mature collagen fiber bundles within the flap. Fibroblastic proliferation, in parallel arrangement and in close adaptation to the root surface at 6 days, extends along the entire inner flap surface to the gingival margin by the tenth day. Remnants of the clot and evidence of acute inflammation are virtually nonexistent at this time. Active collagen formation is present throughout this area.

Although the epithelium at the flap margin initially increases in thickness, there is little observable migration along the root surface during the first week after the procedure. Apical proliferation, however, appears to be greatest during the 10- to 14-day postoperative period. Further apical movement is not observable after about 21 to 28 days — a phenomenon that some investigators have attributed to cementoid deposition and connective tissue attachment. This combined epithelial and connective tissue activity eventually results in the formation of a new gingival margin, sulcus, and epithelial attachment. Since the initial active migration of epithelium along the root surface is not a desirable phenomenon, the removal of sulcular epithelium and epithelial attachment as part of the surgical procedure appears to be advantageous to the final result.

The reaction of bone to a pedicle flap procedure is one primarily of osteoclastic resorption. This is first seen along crestal and periosteal surfaces at about 4 days, increasing somewhat in intensity and reaching an apparent peak by 6 days. Although a 4-day histologic specimen shows the greatest resorptive activity along the periosteal surface with the presence of many osteoclasts and Howship's lacunae, observation at 6 days finds alternating areas of resorption and apposition along this border. The process diminishes considerably and by 14 days there is virtual cessation of resorptive activity. Bone activity along the periodontal ligament surface throughout appears to depend in large part on the depth of penetration of the inflammatory process. The end result of the resorptive process appears to be a slight decrease in crestal height and a thinning of the alveolar septum.

The healing process at 21 days and beyond is essentially one of attachment and tissue maturation. It is approximately at this 3-week period that the first overt sign of cementum formation is evident by the presence of cementoid, most frequently on exposed dentin, notches, and defects created by the surgery along the root surface. Where cementum has not been completely removed by root planing, cementoid deposition can be seen but not to the extent of that observed where dentin is exposed. There is some evidence at 21 days and beyond that the presence of cementoid at the area of the epithelial attachment may have limited the proliferation of epithelium along the root surface. By 28 days, cementum in the form of cementoid is evident along the entire root surface, and one may observe an occasional few collagen bundle fibers embedded into the cementoid tissue. Distinct collagen fibers are now present with fibroblasts in the flap itself in the reparative area, showing a parallel arrangement to the root surface. Bone formation shows its most active phase during the 21- to 28-day period, with periosteal and periodontal osteoblastic activity repairing the resorbed alveolar crest. Crestal bone loss, as observed in experimental animals, rarely appears to exceed 1 mm of vertical height, but varies inversely with septal thickness.

Observation of the surgical area after 90 days shows the presence of collagen fiber bundles in the new connective tissue at right angles between the root and original flap, although some of these bundles are still parallel to the root surface. Cementoid is still forming actively on the surface of previously calcified and calcifying cementum. Apposition of bone at the alveolar crest is minimal at this time with little or no active resorptive process present.

At about 6 months collagen fiber bundles, now oriented at right angles to the root surface and passing between cementoblasts, are observed embedded in cementoid. This pattern of alternating bundles of connective tissue fibers between cementoblasts along the root surface is similar to that seen prior to the surgical procedure.

From a clinical point of view the success of a pedicle flap procedure would appear to depend on several significant factors. (1) The flap must be readily adapted and stationary with little or no tensional pull exerted upon the tissue. (2) There should be close proximity of the tissue to the root surface itself with as little clot present between the flap and soft and hard tissues as possible. This may more readily ensue by using digital pressure with a wet gauze on the transferred tissue as well as a proper postoperative covering that may act as a stent. Healing will be enhanced, since a thin clot may be more readily replaced, and possibly allow for more rapid healing and a more predictable result. (3) The removal of sulcular epithelium and the epithelial attachment appears to encourage the potential for success, since epithelialization of the inner aspect of the flap can only come from the margin, thus allowing a longer period for connective tissue and root surface to form a more intimate union. (4) The inclusion of bacteria, endotoxin, and other inflammatory products in cementum associated with periodontal disease, plus the fact that new cementum formation occurs more readily on hard, calcified structures, necessitate fastiduous root planing and scaling if successful pedicle grafting is to be performed. (5) The use of the modified full-thickness –partial-thickness approach to pedicle grafting obviates the pernicious effects of complete bone exposure at the donor site and enhances the attachment of grafts to denuded roots and bone in the receptor site.

BIOLOGY OF BONE: CORRELATIONS WITH WOUND HEALING

It is not possible in this chapter to summate adequately the comprehensive wealth of data concerning this vitally important tissue. Bone may be considered the structural bulwark of the periodontium, forming an investing, supportive, and retentive housing for the teeth as well as a segment of the tissue complex, the attachment apparatus, which receives, absorbs, and transmits forces that are primarily of occlusal derivation. In the latter context bone assists materially in sustaining dentition during function. Dental, glossal, labial, and buccal forces, transmitted through dentition and periodontal ligament to alveolar and supporting bone under conditions of structural and functional normalcy, are imperative to the preservation of a "steady state." This homeostatic condition is one in which equilibrium is maintained between bone resorption and osteogenesis, with conservation of morphology, topography, and internal trabeculation, enclaving a formative (and resorptive) and space-filling marrow complex, while providing dense yet structurally resilient cortices for the attachment of gingiva, alveolar mucosa, and periodontal ligament. The cortices frame and strengthen the alveolar processes and serve as anchorages for facial and accessory masticatory musculature via intervening periosteum. Muscle function is instrumental in the preservation of cortical bone.

Under dysfunctional circumstances, for example, occlusal traumatism and hypofunction, imbalances between appositional and resorptive processes tend to produce not only morphologic defects but also structural and formative inferiority of the linkages between bone and dentition. The metabolism of bone is also integrated intimately with that of the entire body. Thus when endocrine, metabolic, hematologic, immunologic, neoplastic, nutritional, and other deviations from the norm occur, mandibular, maxillary, and facial bones often participate in and reflect the systemic disease's skeletal manifestations. It is not unusual, for example, for the alveolar processes to show resorptive and osteomalacic lesions of hyperparathyroidism, the osteoporosis and marrow defects of chronic hemolytic anemias and hematologic malignancies, the exaggeration of periodontal disease allied with the immunologic and cellular metabolic aberrations of juvenile diabetes mellitus, or the impairment of osteoid (and collagen) synthesis concomitant with nutritional (protein, vitamin C, and so on) deficiencies.

Bone is a dynamic tissue with great demands for function, hydration, nutrition, and systemic and local health in order to survive. It is a living complex that is unusually susceptible to injury. Its life is irrevocably bound to the integrity of enclosed marrow and endosteum and investing periosteum and periodontal ligament. These soft tissues carry the vascular supply and venular and lymphatic drainage of bone, provide the principal neural filaments that are sensory and trophic for bone, supply bone's formative and resorptive cells, and are sources of matrices mineralizable to bone.

All bone surfaces are covered by living connective tissue "membranes" that are attached to bone by reticulum and collagen fibers. Actually a large majority of the fibers not only serve in anchoring capacities, but are also part of the structural bone matrix. The bone matrix, as initially formed and elaborated by osteoblasts, is composed of the protein-polysaccharide ground substance that enclaves bone's fibrillar elements. It appears that the entire matrix is calcifiable with rapid postsecretory mineral deposition occurring not only throughout the ground substance but also within and surrounding the collagen and reticular fibers.

It is generally agreed that the thin matrix fibers are fully mineralized with aggregation of calcium phosphate, in amorphous and hydroxyapatite forms, in the interstices of the helices of the collagen molecules, and in intermolecular locations. Ultramicroscopic evaluations reveal crystalline mineral aggregates not only at these locations but also at interfibril and perifiber areas. Thick bundles of collagen fibers, extending from periosteum, endosteum, and periodontal ligament into bone, may be incompletely mineralized particularly in their core, or central, portions. Analogous mineralization characteristics are seen where gingival and periodontal ligament fibers enter and are confluent with acellular (fibrillar) cementum; at these locations complete or nearly complete fiber calcification exists. Where periodontal ligament's cemental fibers are embedded in cellular cementum the biphasic pattern of mineralization can be discerned.

Bone's "living membrane" fully veneers vascular channels, marrow cavities, and the outer and periodontal surfaces of bone. It is ordinarily discerned as a delicate, cellular, connective tissue lamella at endosteal locations extending into and peripheralizing fatty and vascular marrow. Thinner and more delicate ramifications of endosteum are seen at the surfaces of haversian canals, again in tenuous linkage to adjacent bone and surrounding the capillary-venular microcirculatory vessels, which provide the most intimate of bone's nutritive and hydrating supply. Osteocytes in lacunar locations are rarely more than a few micrometers either from a blood vessel or from canaliculi, which serve as the finite channels of transudate movement from blood vessel to osteocyte. Thus osteocyte viability and function are maintained, and the mineralized state of bone is preserved; calcium and phosphate appear to be constantly removed and replaced in bone by a delicate homeostatic process designed to preserve the product of calcium and phosphate in blood and tissue fluids. Periosteum is the counterpart of endosteum located on the external aspects of bone. The inner, cambium portion of periosteum is in reality the structural and formative analogue of endosteum and is often found to be continuous with endosteum via vascular channels extending from the periosteal surfaces of bone to marrow areas. Like endosteum it should be considered a functioning, viable membrane essential to the structural integrity and the "living" quality of bone.

Additional comments should be made regarding bone cells since an understanding of cell types, their biologic qualities, and their dysfunctional and pathologic behavior is fundamental to an appreciation of healing processes after periodontal surgery. Aberrations of repair, including their clinical and biologic genesis, are usually based on deviations of cell behavior. Effective clinical prevention and correction of healing complications require extensive knowledge of cell and tissue biology.

The undifferentiated mesenchymal cell of periosteum, endosteum, and periodontal ligament is considered to be the primordium for all of bone's formative and resorptive cells. It therefore has functional and structural pluripotentiality. It may differentiate along several pathways to osteoblast, osteocyte, fibroblast, fibrocyte, "fibroclast," macrophage, osteoclast, and so on. Prior to differentiation the mesenchymal cell has mitotic capacities. Since all postmitotic cells do not differentiate to become synthetic or resorptive, a reserve cell population is in continuing residence in bone's living membrane. The undifferentiated mesenchymal cell is difficult to discern with routine light microscopy utilizing commonly employed staining methods. It simply presents as a fibroblastlike cell with a large, pale, vesicular nucleus and a cytoplasm deficient in structure and granularity. Ultramicroscopic assay is particularly remarkable for deficiencies not only of endoplasmic reticulum, but also of polyribosomes, Golgi complex, and mitochondria. The deficiencies are not absolute, since they are functioning cells primarily in an endocytic manner. Mitosis and differentiation may be initiated and stimulated by a wide variety of events and substances. Variations in tissue electrical potential induced by function or functional change have been demonstrated to dictate cell type and activities at specific tissue sites. For example, where bone and collagen tend to be or are deformed, even momentarily, negative electrical tissue potentials are established at sites of bone concavity. Negativity lends to positive osteoblastic and fibroblastic activity, with bone or connective tissue formation. Positive electrical effects are produced in tissues in juxtaposition to zones of bone convexity; bone and connective tissue resorptive change mark the production of positive piezoelectrical charges.

In instances of periodontal inflammation, especially the chronic, low-intensity variety typifying most areas of periodontal disease, peptides of mononuclear cell origination (possibly T-lymphocytes), when transferred to the mesenchymal cell, may not only induce mitosis but may also be the determinants of the paths of differentiation and activity of the offspring cells. Thus reactive fibroplasia and osteogenesis commonly seen in periodontal inflammatory lesions have their origination at least partially in the particular type(s) and amount(s) of lymphokines released from the mononuclear cells of inflammation. Conversely, bone and connective tissue resorptive factors (peptides) are formed and liberated from comparably appearing mononuclear cells in more or less direct correlation with the severity of inflammatory states. Other substances (e.g., parathormone, prostaglandins E_1 and E_2, bacterial endotoxin) are causally and quantitatively related to bone and soft tissue resorption.

Since periodontal wound healing is so closely allied to inflammatory processes, it may be reasonably assumed that comparable humoral and local cellular factors play important roles in the processes of repair on both appositional and resorptive levels. The dependence of repair upon chronic inflammation appears to be an important biologic tenet.

Osteoblasts are usually aligned adjacent to bone surfaces. Interposed between the monolayer of osteoblasts and previously formed bone, tissue examination commonly reveals a thin lamella of newly synthesized bone matrix; it is of osteoblastic origination as is its primary synthetic product, osteoid. Osteoid as initially secreted is nonmineralized and composed of collagen, reticulum, and essentially nonsulfated protein-polysaccharide ground substance. It is liberally hydrated and being extremely pervious to tissue fluids allows for their free transfer from endosteal vessels into bone's interior; the pathways are through the uncalcified, or incompletely mineralized, matrix and along the canaliculi communicating from bone's surface via intermediary canaliculi to intralacunar areas. Mineralization of osteoid occurs rapidly, the source of mineral being tissue fluids that are supersaturated and thus metastable relative to bone mineral (primarily but not exclusively $CaPO_4$ in amorphous acid hydroxyapatite form). It has been estimated that 90% to 95% of bone maturation by calcification occurs within 3 weeks after extracytic release of osteoid from osteoblasts. Recent data also implicates the osteoblast (odontoblast, cementoblast, ameloblast) in mineralization processes. Several events occur within these cells preparatory to the extracellular release of glycoproteins that, within bone matrix, appear to initiate its mineralization:

1. Polypeptides are formed at polyribosomal

areas adjacent to endoplasmic reticulum from amino acid precursors. The process is dictated by messenger RNA of nuclear origin.

2. The peptides are then transferred to Golgi vesicles, at supranuclear locations, where carbohydrates are annexed. The glycoproteins are packaged in lipoprotein sheaths and begin a rapid intracytoplasmic journey to the cell's plasma membrane. The lipoglycopeptide package is designed as a *secretory vesicle*. Interestingly, mineralization of the vesicles is initiated intracellularly with amorphous $CaPO_4$, tending to reduce the lipid concentration of the vesicles.

3. The secretory vesicles, via exocytosis, are released into the previously synthesized but unmineralized portion of osteoid as *matrix vesicles*.

4. Matrix vesicles spread through osteoid, accruing additional mineral as amorphous $CaPO_4$ and as $CaPO_4 \cdot H_2O$.

There are phenomenal numbers of matrix vesicles within osteoid. As they migrate toward previously mineralized bone through osteoid pathways, the matrix vesicles accumulate additional mineral to such an extent that when reaching a calcification front at the osteoid-bone interface they are so laden with mineral that they literally burst, exposing "mineral seeds" to humoral fluids within the tissue's matrix. The ultramicroscopic glycopeptide-mineral complexes are the nucleating sites for subsequent epitactic deposition and growth of mineral within the ground substance and within the reticulum and collagen fibrils and fibers of the tissue.

Osteoblasts, as well as other formative cells such as odontoblasts and cementoblasts, are notable for the aerobic employment of carbohydrate via the citric acid cycle especially within their mitochondria, the conjugation of carbohydrate (e.g., fucose, galactose, glucose) with protein in their Golgi complexes, highly developed and complex endoplasmic reticulum studded liberally with polyribosomes, the synthesis of enzymes, such as alkaline phosphatase, which appear to be vital not only to energy production but also to the synthesis of cyclic adenosine monophosphate (cyclic AMP) (an important intermediary in CHO metabolism), and, fundamentally, the construction from multiple raw materials of both the fibrillar and matrical substrates of bone (also dentin, cementum, enamel). They are differentiated cells that are functionally specialized. What is most striking is that they exert their maximal, most predictable formative capabilities when they are associated with previously mineralized bone, which serves as the locale of a "mineralization front" when it interfaces with osteoid (cementoid, dentinoid).

This points to a fundamental biologic concept applicable directly to the rendition of periodontal therapy. If the therapist wishes to induce bone formation to obviate an intraosseous lesion, he must remove all soft tissue (e.g., inflammatory tissue) that peripheralizes the defect and blankets the osseous and dental surfaces of the lesion. While the sources of reparative tissue are exposed marrow cavities and periodontal ligament—a proliferative phenomenon leading to centripetal ingrowth of granulation tissue into the bony void—the reparative tissue will only mineralize into bone where it is affiliated with already mineralized bone. The formation of cementoid, mineralizing to cementum, also demands root surface preparation to the extent that mineralized dentin or cementum is exposed at the time of surgery. Recent data also suggests that the exposed mineralized tooth surface undergoes superficial demineralization 1 to 2 days postsurgically. However, this ultrathin lamella of demineralized dentin or cementum (and by extrapolation, bone) is subsequently remineralized from the available tissue fluids. Once remineralized, cementogenesis (osteogenesis) takes place. Artificial demineralization clinically via acid treatment of the debrided root surface may accomplish the same purpose. In vivo, such demineralization may be the consequence of topical acid activity, as postsurgical inflammatory exudates contain lactic and citric acids. Citric acid appears to be an avid demineralizing agent.

Osteocytes are derived from osteoblasts and are located with lacunae of bone. When osteoblasts elaborate bone matrix they not only release this material from their proximal (toward bone) surfaces but also pericytically. They thus become entrapped within osteoid. Canalicular processes extend from the cells into the surrounding milieu; intraosseous canaliculi of osteocytes intercommunicate, and osteoblastic processes extend into the surface portion of osteoid to connect with their intraosseous counterparts. Intercellular communication has been demonstrated via the employment experimentally of radioactive amino acids and iodinated ^{131}I serum albumin and via immunoassay methods. Osteocytes are functional cells but are not capable of mitosis. Receiving fluids and nutrients from without the lacunae, they perform essentially aerobically when located close to marrow, endosteum, and periosteum. Deeper within lamellar and trabecular bone and within cementum (as cementocytes) their function diminishes; the less the availability of nutrition and hydration and the more hypoxic the lacunar environment, the more anaerobic will be the function of the osteocytes and the more likely will be their synthesis of hydrolytic enzymes (e.g., acid phosphatase, chondroitin sulfatases and so on). The more secluded the cells' location within hand tissues, the more evident will be perilacunar bone (and cemental) resorption (osteocytic osteolysis) and disintegration of osteocytes (and cementocytes) within their lacunae. Osteocytes have a limited potential for osteogenesis.

Osteoclasts are resorptive entities originating within bone's living membranes from precursor mesenchymal cells or by extravascular fusion of blood-derived monocytes. They are large, multinucleated cells derived from the fusion of connective tissue's reserve cells. Ordinarily they are seen in proximity to bone (cementum), situated in concave depressions in the bone's surface. Thus a portion of the cell abuts bone, while the remaining portion interfaces with soft tissue. A number of clinical and biologic events and substances induce osteoclast formation and activity. The most fascinating is a lymphokine, *osteoclast-activating factor*, released from T-lymphocytes in chronic inflammatory states. OAF has been eluted from human circulating lymphocytes in amounts more or less directly related to the severity of tissue (periodontal) inflammation. When brought into association with living bone (including periosteum) in in vitro assay systems, OAF of human lymphocyte origin will cause osteoclastic development, activity, and thus bone and tissue resorption. Parathormone, prostaglandins, and endotoxin act comparably. Osteoclasts perform via enzymatic activity; they also produce and liberate extracellularly large quantities of demineralizing acids. Demineralization appears to precede enzymatic hydrolysis of bone (cementum, dentin) matrices. The hydrolytic enzyme complements of osteoclasts are outstanding in variety and quantity and include acid phosphatase, hyaluronidase, β-glucuronidase, collagenase, cathepsins, sulfatases, lipases, and carbohydrate hydrolyzing agents. Their acids have been noted as H^+ ion, citric, isocitric, lactic, and so on. Additionally, a phagocytic function has been ex-

pressed; it is probably minimal and secondary to the cells' major methods of operation. In periodontal surgery the greater the therapeutic exposure and involvement of bone or its "membranes," the greater the likelihood of hard tissue resorption. Interestingly, osteoclastic activity is associated with the onset of chronic inflammation seen initially 3 to 4 days postsurgically. As chronic inflammation wanes, osteoclast activity diminishes. The persistence of low-intensity, chronic inflammation may, however, be a prime requisite for repair by tissue apposition.

Recently the macrophage has been incriminated in tissue resorption. It is a dynamic cell that typifies chronic inflammation, being present in large numbers in chronic inflammatory infiltrates. The macrophage of connective tissue (and bone) is largely but probably not exclusively of hematologic origin. The precursor is the monocyte. Macrophages appear to be activated and maintained at inflammatory and injured sites by "peptide factors" of lymphocyte origination. There is a growing mass of evidence that the macrophage not only acts phagocytically as a negator of tissue debris, bacteria, antigen-antibody aggregates, and so on, but also as an effector of tissue resorption. Bone may well be included in its list of prey. The macrophage's enzyme complements rival those of the osteoclast and the neutrophil in type and quantity. Much emphasis is presently being placed on the collagenolytic potential of this sometimes predator cell. As such it may participate in both hard and soft tissue resorption. Much study is required of the degree and variability of macrophage activity in periodontal inflammation, occlusal traumatism, tissue transplantation, and wound healing.

Bone resorption

The process of bone resorption, either as a physiologic or pathologic phenomenon and as a concomitant to periodontal wound healing, is unusually complex and impossible to ally with a single, simple inducing factor. It has been previously stated that mononuclear cells (e.g., T-lymphocytes) present within chronic inflammatory infiltrates synthesize and release extracellularly low-molecular-weight glycopeptides and peptides (17,000 mol. wt.), which provoke the formation of osteoclasts from precursor mesenchymal cells or monocytes or both via cellular fusion and presumably mediate, by chemical provocation, their subsequent resorptive activity. The demineralizing effects of osteoclast-derived acids and the enzymatic and hydrolyzing bone matrix resorptive changes of osteoclast-originating acid hydrolases have been correlated directly with the severity of periodontal inflammation and the amounts of osteoclast-activating factor capable of being eluted from circulating lymphocytes. It is entirely possible that less overt but quantitatively equivalent osteocytic osteolysis may be produced by the same T-lymphocyte factor, functionally OOF, or osteocytic osteolysis factor.

In a rather obscure but important publication, Raisz has indicated that the "same" osteoclast-activating factor may in a slightly different osseous microenvironment be responsible for the induction of osteogenesis or that the eluted OAF may contain a peptide fraction that initiates osteoblastic (fibroblastic, odontoblastic, cementoblastic) activity. Thus in the periodontium bone apposition and resorption may take place in nearby microareas of the attachment apparatus.

Additional substances of significance in the mediation of soft tissue and bone resorption are fatty acids, generically termed "prostaglandins," which provoke osteoclasts, osteocytes, fibroblasts, and so on to engage in resorptive processes. Prostaglandins E_1, and E_2, in in vitro bioassays, appear to activate both osteoclastic resorption and osteocytic osteolysis. Tissues cultured from dental cysts and tissue exudates from established periodontal inflammatory lesions resorb bone in vitro by releasing indomethacin-sensitive prostaglandin E_2. Indomethacin is an inhibitor of prostaglandin synthesis; acetylsalicylic acid may act comparably.

Inflammatory lesions may additionally contain leukocytes (e.g., neutrophils) that release lysosomal hydrolases, which in turn damage bone matrix and dental tissues (e.g., cementum, dentin). Certainly the so-called angry macrophages, ubiquitous to resolving acute as well as chronic inflammatory processes, may be active in connective tissue and bone resorption when they release comparable hydrolases into the extracytic milieu.

The complexity of tissue resorption is further emphasized by recent data that notes the interaction of prostaglandins with complement (C') and with collagenase. When the terminal components of complement (e.g., C6) are activated by antigen-antibody complexes or via the alternative pathway (e.g., direct endotoxin-induced C3 production), synthesis of prostaglandin E_1 is induced, and bone resorption takes place in in vitro bone culture systems.

Macrophages stimulated by endotoxins of dental plaque or by products of activated lymphocytes form and liberate collagenases that are in part responsible for the primary degradation of collagen observed in periodontal lesions (and, by extrapolation, healing wounds). Endotoxin is an alternative complement (C') pathway activator. Macrophages (and neutrophils) also secrete elastase, a broad spectrum protease that can hydrolyze native collagen as efficiently as collagenase. The glycoproteoglycans of connective tissue and bone matrices are enzymatically resorbed by macrophages.

The "two-fisted" resorptive activity of the macrophage tends to be counterbalanced in chronic periodontal inflammatory states and progressively superseded in healing wounds by fibrosis and osteogenesis. Activated macrophages or T-lymphocytes or both form and secrete one or more substances that stimulate mitosis of mesenchymal cells, bring about fibroblastic and osteoblastic differentiation from precursor mesenchymal cells, and increase collagen and matrical synthesis by fibroblasts (osteoblasts, odontoblasts, and so on).

Detailed characterization of the cellular and chemical factors involved and intimate correlations between in vitro and in vivo resorptive and appositional tissue changes are obviously essential in future evaluations of the nature, behavior, and chronology of periodontal disease and the healing processes attending periodontal therapeutics.

Bone marrow

Special attention should be given to the correlated structure, function, and dynamics of hematopoietic marrow inasmuch as autogenous heterotopic transplantation of this tissue has on a diminishing basis become an exotic yet standard and predictable method for inducing new attachment in periodontics. In orthopedics and oral surgery, because of the often massive nature of osseous defects, red marrow (hematopoietic) grafting has a broader range of necessary applicability. As in all rational periodontal therapy the benefits to be derived from the utilization of the surgical procedure must exceed the potential untoward consequences, both physical and psychic, that may ensue at or after surgery. Since hematopoietic autografting requires both hematologic and intraoral surgery, that is, twin surgical interventions, it should be obvious that the periodontal lesions that are to be corrected must be of sufficient magnitude in size and number and intractable by any other more facile and less complex therapeutic approaches to warrant the procedures. The state of the entire dentition and the need for its preservation are also important considerations.

The hematologic system, while diffuse and multiple in localization and extraordinarily large and complex, is in reality one of the most vital organs of the body. If one could withdraw all red marrow from all bones of the adult, measure its volume, and then add the area of accessory portions of the hematologic system, for example, spleen, reticuloendothelial system, thymus, and lymph nodes, the combined cubic tissue volume would easily double that of the liver. The reticuloendothelial system, thymus gland, and lymph nodes are included in the tissue complex because all lymphocyte progenitors of T and B cells have their ultimate origin in the stem cell of marrow. The tissue and intralymphatic macrophages are largely if not exclusively derived from blood monocytes, which in turn originate from primordial marrow precursors.

In fetal life nearly all marrow of all bones is of the hematopoietic type. In prenatal and early postnatal periods, for example, the marrow of the jaws, facial bones, calvarium, long bones (e.g., tibia, femur, and so on) is overwhelmingly of this nature. With advancing age, except in such bones as those of the skull, sternum, ribs, ileum, vertebrae, and so on, there is a gradual replacement of red marrow by the fatty, yellow type. Thus in the adult mandible all or nearly all marrow cavities are occupied by endosteum, loose connective tissue, many blood vessels, nerves, lymphatics, and fat cells. Islands of red marrow may persist, generally unpredictably, in mandibular retromolar bone, the condylar head, and in the maxilla at intratuberosity sites. The transition from red to yellow marrow begins at about 4 years of age, even at such areas as the diaphysis of long bones, until approximately 18 years of age the primary sites of hematogenesis are located in flat bones, the mandible and maxilla being excluded. From the standpoint of availability, in quantities adequate for transplantation and with the least surgical trauma, the ileum is the preferred source.

All marrow cavities are internally veneered by endosteum, previously described as a cellular, loose, vascular connective tissue in attachment via fibrillar collagenous insertions to the contiguous bone. Emphasis was also placed on the biologic multipotentiality of the tissue—particularly its capacities for connective tissue and bone synthesis and resorption (see discussion on Bi-ology of Bone: Correlations with Wound Healing). The vascular networks of hematopoietic marrow are unique in that the afferent arteriolar and capillary circulations continue into complicated venous sinusoids, which in turn empty into collecting venules and small veins. The formation of blood cells occurs external to the sinusoids in colonies, and with normalcy and at the appropriate stages of maturation the formed elements of the blood enter the sinusoids via interendothelial areas. The sinusoidal collecting system has been compared to a sieve or strainer. The sinusoids are lined internally not only by endothelial cells but also by phagocytic members of the reticuloendothelial system. The sinusoids do not have basement lamina. The nerve supply to marrow is extensive and ample with fine neurofilaments located in both endosteum and in the body of the marrow.

The marrow cell population may be subdivided into many categories, including the following:

1. Multipotential stem cells dedicated to hematopoiesis
2. Monopotential daughter cells committed to separate futures as erythrocytes, granulocytes, thrombocytes, monocytes, lymphocytes, and so on
3. Pluripotential stem cells that give rise to cells that are formative and resorptive for connective tissue and bone, such as—
   a. Osteoblasts
   b. Fibroblasts
   c. "Fibroclasts" (Ten Cate et al., 1976; Ten Cate and Freeman, 1974)
   d. Osteoclasts
   e. Macrophages
4. Cells committed to angiogenesis and neurogenesis, especially after injury

There may be self-perpetuating groups of osteogenic precursor cells. They number about 10^{-5} of nucleated cells of the marrow.

The intraosseous microenvironment is especially important for cell renewal and differentiation. There is suggestive evidence that the cells responsible for bone marrow renewal and regeneration appear to be cells that morphologically and kinetically resemble small mononuclear cells (the lymphocyte). The precise patterns of marrow cell differentiation are probably dictated by humoral substances that act in a stimulatory manner. It is most interesting and undoubtedly of much importance in red marrow autografting that the effects of the humoral stimuli are modified in variable "inductive microenvironments." The studies of Trentin show that colonies of red marrow cells implanted on the splenic surface are essentially erythroid, while comparable colonies of cells placed in central splenic *or* bone marrow microenvironments are largely myeloid and thrombocytoid. The periodontal microenvironment *may* be such as to encourage osteoblast and fibroblast activities and to discourage hemopoiesis when red marrow is implanted into intraosseous defects.

The monopotential stem cells — erythroblasts, myeloblasts, monoblasts, megakaryocytes, and possibly lymphoblasts — are capable of mitosis with continuing renewal and differentiation of a portion of either or both maternal and offspring cells. The most widely studied activators of mitosis and differentiation are humoral and polypeptide carbohydrate in composition. For example, erythropoietin (formed in kidney) is specifically related to red cell formation. There are also leukopoietins and thrombopoietins, which are necessary for granulocyte and thrombocyte formation. It has been shown recently that differentiation of thymocytes, within the thymus gland, from marrow precursors, and thymocyte multiplication are controlled by a stimulatory humoral substance (thymopoietin), which is elaborated by epithelial cells within the gland. This is a most important and suggestive example of epidermal-mesenchymal interactions.

When red marrow is subjected to specific amounts of irradiation, as via thymidine ^{3}H or gamma irradiation using cobalt 60, nearly all marrow cells that are synthesizing DNA are destroyed by the irradiation. However, doses that negate the unipotential stem cells and their lineage do *not* destroy the pluripotential stem cell population. Although they are resting and apparently unaffected by the irradiation, they are considered to be the *reserve* cell marrow population. They may be activated by injury to the marrow, with marrow depletion, and after heterotopic transplantation from medullary donor to intralesional recipient sites.

In the microenvironment of the debrided intraosseous periodontal lesion, both fresh and thawed hematopoietic marrow are capable of inducing an unusual degree of tissue repair. The transplanted tissue, however, not only consists of red marrow, but also of endosteum and osseous trabeculae. The latter tissues, via their included or contiguous cells, may be partially responsible for attachment apparatus repair. Bone fragments also act as multiple nidi or foci for osteogenesis.

Fresh autografts of hematopoietic marrow, containing multipotential mesenchymal stem cells, may also give rise to resorptive cells such as osteoclasts, fibroclasts, and macrophages. The results of this phenomenon have been manifested at the graft-root interface as root resorption. Ankylosis precedes and accompanies root resorption. Such data emphasize both the pluripotentiality of bone marrow and the vagaries of biologic processes that beneficially or adversely influence the success of clinical therapy (see discussion on Osseous and Marrow Autografts and Schallhorn, 1972, 1968, 1967; Schallhorn and Hiatt, 1972; Schallhorn et al., 1970).

Reaction of bone to therapeutic procedures

The use of surgical procedures for the correction of various types of bone deformities resulting from inflammatory periodontal disease is a widely accepted therapeutic approach in periodontal therapy. The periodontal literature is replete with experimental animal and human studies concerned with the removal or modification of bone lesions and the means by which the surgical intervention heals. Correlation of these investigations has presented an overwhelming amount of evidence that the most desirable postoperative response and therapeutic results can be obtained when the surgical sites are recovered by soft tissue after their manipulation. Mucoperiosteal flaps are generally used in association with osseous surgery, not only to gain access to and improve visibility of bone, but also to protect underlying structures during healing in order to minimize the resorptive process and inhibit postoperative sequelae of pain, hemorrhage, infection, and so on. Since numerous studies have recognized the resorptive implications of osseous exposure, the use of procedures that leave bone exposed after surgical intervention is no longer considered a desirable approach. It should be emphasized at this time that even temporary (limited to the operative tenure of the surgical intervention) bone exposure is commonly accompanied by postsurgical resorption. These resorptive sequelae are generally of minimal significance when the exposed interdental, interradicular, buccal, or lingual bone septa are composed of trabecular bone and sheathed with denser cortices. These septa are broad or thick, and while some topical and internal resorption may occur, it does not ordinarily lead to significant loss of septal height. Thus the periodontal ligament attachment to the tooth would be preserved. The

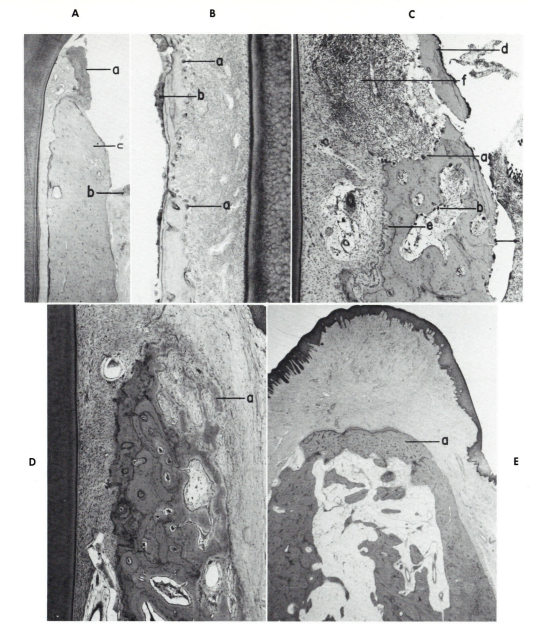

Fig. 23-35. Histogenesis of repair after mucogingival surgery. **A,** Two-day postoperative specimen, mandibular radicular area; dog. *c,* Exposed compact vestibular plate of bone showing few marrow spaces; *a,* blood clot is present at severed dentogingival junction; *b,* blood clot at wound edge with inflammation beneath it. Hematoxylin-eosin stain. **B,** Six-day postoperative specimen, after denudation, maxillary radicular area; dog. *a,* Osteoclastic activity is occurring all along periodontal surface of alveolar bone. Inflammation is evident in periodontal ligament. *b,* Bacterial plaque is present on exposed bone surface. Hematoxylin-eosin stain. **C,** Ten-day postoperative specimen, after denudation; dog. *a,* Undermining resorption occurs at crest; *b,* resorption in marrow space; *c,* wound edge indicating frontal resorption; *f,* former periodontal space, inflammation in young proliferating connective tissue; *d,* sequestrum is almost exfoliated and covered on surface by bacteria; *e,* apposition of bone is evident below exposed area of periodontal space. Hematoxylin-eosin stain. **D,** Twenty-eight-day postoperative specimen, mandibular radicular area; dog, after denudation. *a,* Osteophytic bone trabeculae formation at lowered labial alveolar crest in radicular area. Hematoxylin-eosin stain. **E,** Ninety-three-day postoperative specimen, after denudation; mandibular interdental area; dog. *a,* Complete regeneration of interdental septum. Marrow tissue is of a normal fatty type. Epithelium is thick and contains only a few ridges. Hematoxylin-eosin stain. (**A** and **E** ×12; **B** to **D** ×50.) (From Wilderman, M. N., and Wentz, F. M.: J. Periodontol. **31**:283, 1960.)

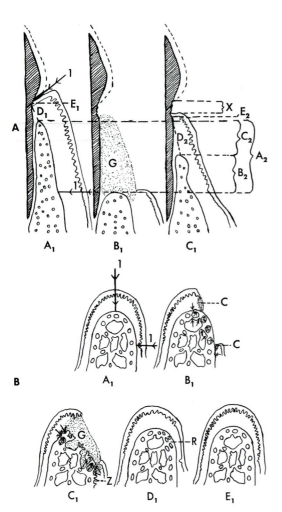

Fig. 23-36. Histogenesis of repair after mucogingival surgery. **A,** Operative site at radicular area. A_1, Normal; B_1, 6 to 10 days; C_1, 95 to 185 days. *i*, Incision, epithelium and connective tissue removed, baring bone; A_2, 5 mm bone exposure and resorption; B_2, 2.5 mm new bone formation; C_2, 2.5 mm loss of bone; D_1, original connective tissue attachment; D_2, new connective tissue attachment; E_1, original epithelial attachment on cementoenamel junction; E_2, epithelial attachment apical to cementoenamel junction; *X*, epithelium at lower level; *G*, young connective tissue. **B,** Operative site at interdental area. A_1, Normal; *L*, direction of incisions. B_1, Two to four days, direction of resorption; *c*, blood clot and exposed bone between blood clots. C_1, Six to ten days, direction of resorption; *G*, young connective tissue; *Z*, trabeculae at the formation of coarse fibrillar bone. D_1, Twenty-eight days; *R*, trabeculae, bone formation at wound; E_1, 95 to 185 days; return to normal. (From Wildermann, M. N., and Wentz, F. M.: J. Periodontol. **31:**283, 1960.)

bone septa may be permanently or temporarily thinned. In those cases where bone is thin and largely if not exclusively composed of dense cortical-type bone, even a minimal degree of postsurgical resorption may eventuate in a through-and-through pattern with loss of septal height and periodontal attachment for the tooth. Such defects are more likely to occur in areas where roots are prominent with corresponding thin buccal radicular bone. (Ruben has measured bone dimensions at such sites and found that under conditions of tissue normalcy, bone may be as thin as 0.16 mm.)

Preservation of periosteum in situ over bone does not in itself guarantee its structural and dimensional integrity. All periodontal surgery is accompanied by postsurgical inflammation, initially of a variably acute type, and later, beginning on the third or fourth postoperative day, by chronic inflammation. At first resorption may be mediated by acidic and hydrolytic exudates (e.g., of neutrophilic origination), while the resorption of bone effected during chronic inflammation may be related to macrophage activity and the release of tissue resorptive factors (e.g., osteoclast-activating factor) produced by and liberated from activated lymphocytes. These substances apparently diffuse after release into and through periosteum to bone surfaces where they activate resorptive cells (i.e., macrophages, osteocytes, osteoclasts, fibrocytes). Periosteal conservation in situ *may* reduce resorptive processes but may not obviate them. Much depends on (1) bone thickness, (2) the degree and temporal period of inflammation, and (3) "periosteal" thickness and fiber density, providing dimensional and structural limitations to exudate diffusion toward bone. There are *no* pat or carte blanche answers to this important and intriguing problem. It may be found, however, that inadvertent exposure of some areas may occur, resulting in an interesting sequence of events.

The reactive pattern of bone to exposure or denudation depends in large part on the anatomy of the tissues involved. Surgical bone exposure may occur primarily in three regions: (1) the radicular area, (2) interproximally between adjoining teeth, and (3) the interradicular zones. Marginal radicular bone often consists of narrow fused plates of compact bone with few if any marrow cavities. This is particularly true in mandibular incisor and cuspid areas at their labial aspects and in the buccal septa of mesiobuccal roots of maxillary molars. More apically, spongy bone becomes progressively more evident as the cortical plates tend to diverge. In the interdental and interradicular areas, on the other hand, the outer layer of compact radicular plate has a definite pattern of underlying spongy bone with numerous marrow spaces present. Thin septa, however, in any of these regions are composed primarily of compact bone with a direct relationship between the extent of trabeculation and the width of the septum. The architecture of interdental and interradicular bone where roots are flattened proximally or are located in close approximation to each other reflects a paucity of supporting trabeculae and minimal enclaved marrow; these septa are highly cortical and unduly vulnerable to resorption attending marginal periodontitis, occlusal traumatism, the periodontitis-occlusal traumatism complex, and periodontal and oral surgery with a consequent loss of attachment apparatus at the site.

Histologic observation of bone exposed after surgery shows the immediate formation of a clot over the affected area, particularly over the cut surfaces of adjacent soft tissue. The blood coagulum present in relationship to soft tissues in a conglomerate of the formed elements of the blood and cellular and tissue debris dispersed is a fibrin matrix; it is of a gellike consistency. The clot supervening on bone is a complex of exudate and cellular and tissue debris, loosely complexed with fibrin. It should really be considered a semiclotted exudate. Both types are bordered by a definite band of viable and nonviable granulocytes (the polyband). Exposure of a cortical plate, including the removal of periosteum, results in the eventual necrosis and resorption of a portion of this osseous surface. The early aspects of topical bone resorption may well be mediated by hydrolytic enzymes derived from this band of neutrophils, as these cells are richly endowed with hydrolases capable of resorbing the collagenous, protein-polysaccharide matrix of bone. Since the tissue milieu is acidic — lactic and citric acids are ubiquitous to the granulocytes with both intracellular and extracellular dispersal — demineralization of bone occurs. This process antecedes matrix resorption. While grossly superficial in clinical and microscopic evaluations, histochemical and ultrastructural analyses indicate the topical and intracanalicular localization and diffusion of resorptive enzymes (e.g., acid phosphatase) as well as surface irregularities of bone. The superficial phase of bone reveals demineralization (loss of crystal structure of collagen and matrix) with splaying of collagen fibers into

their fibrillar constituents and loss of axial periodicity of collagen molecules. In areas where vascular channels communicate between the bone surface and marrow cavities and haversian canals, comparable resorptive changes may be noted relative to their walls. In effect these orifices and canals are broadened. Osteocytes, present in the more superficial lacunae of bone, reflect necrotic change. Perilacunar matrix may also be affected; this is termed "osteocytic osteolysis" and appears to be mediated by hydrolytic enzymes formed and released from these cells. The degraded bone and cellular and fibrillar remnants are later removed by macrophage action when a cover of granulation (reparative) tissue forms over the previously denuded bone surface. The granulation tissue is of periosteal and endosteal origin with centripetal lateral ingrowth from peripherally located periosteum (and periodontal ligament, where exposed) and outgrowth from exposed marrow cavities and vascular channels. Even with the presence of this ostensibly "protective" soft, reparative tissue, bone resorption may be expected to continue but with diminishing intensity and effect. The persistence of chronic-type inflammation, particularly with lymphocytes and macrophages dominating the cellular infiltrate, can be expected to lead to three patterns of bone involvement generally occurring in tandem:

1. Resorption
2. Resorption and formation
3. Formative (appositional)

While the first two steps of this sequence tend to occupy a 2- to 3-week period beginning at the third to fifth postsurgical day, little is known as to the reasons for the waning of resorption and the substitution concurrently and thereafter of repair. Preliminary data suggest that at first "angry macrophages" have a tissue resorptive potential; this is replaced by macrophage activity aimed at phagocytosis and débridement of the wound. It has been hypothesized and partially substantiated that T-lymphocytes present in the granulation tissue produce and release "cell-activating factors" that may activate and halt the various functional capabilities not only of macrophages but also of osteoclasts, osteoblasts, fibroclasts, fibroblasts, endothelium, and so on. The primary or fundamental regulatory process is unknown. As inflammation decreases, but continues with low-grade, protracted chronicity, repair by apposition continues.

If osseous surgery has been performed, the reaction may be expected to be more intense, since numerous subjacent marrow spaces may have been exposed. Marked inflammation may be seen early in the soft tissue wound and crestal phase of the periodontal ligament. Viable bone may exist under the superficial necrotic plate. During the 2- to 10-day period after surgery one may note an increased intensity of undermining resorption, which has its origin in vascular canals and particularly from marrow spaces beneath the exposed bone. The bone resorption is mediated primarily by osteoclasts, which are ordinarily located in resorptive bays in the bone's surfaces. Additional bone loss may be produced via actions of osteocytes and macrophages. All forms of bone resorption are effected by hydrolytic enzymes liberated from cells, regardless of the cell type involved, acting in an acidic environment favorable to bone demineralization.

During this period active resorption may also be seen over the radicular area at the periodontal surface of the alveolar bone, eventuating in a widening of the periodontal ligament space. This first results in a widening of the ligament at the expense of bone. The pattern of resorption in this area continues until there may be through-and-through loss of the exposed bone septum with concomitant lowering of the osseous crest. As this occurs periodontal ligament is deprived of its bony attachment. It reflects fiber resorption, matrix dissolution, vasodilation and vasodestruction, edema, and the presence of a tissue inflammatory infiltrate. Although neutrophils may be present, particularly perivascularly, the predominant cell population is composed of macrophages, lymphocytes, plasma cells, and fibroclasts. In the interproximal and interradicular areas resorptive activity eventually also effects the loss of crestal and vestibular compact bone surfaces, causing the exposure of marrow spaces and giving a configuration of a flat slope.

Repair of bone becomes most active during the twenty-first to twenty-eighth day period after the surgical procedure. Relatively complete restoration of crestal height is evident in the interdental and furcation areas where numerous marrow spaces remained open after completion of the active resorptive process. Over the face of roots, unlike in the broad bone areas often present interproximally and interradicularly, the resorption may have been confined to a thin compact septum, which is incapable of internal rebuilding. Reconstruction occurs so that only a minor portion of the bone may be rebuilt, giving a resultant lower bone level.

The histologic sequence of osseous exposure shows that bone gives initial evidence of degeneration along the crest and at outer phases of the buccal or lingual septa; numerous empty lacunae are seen within 2 days after the procedure. Both osteocytes and osteoblasts undergo enzymatic degradation and disintegration. Although little or no osteoclastic activity is evident at this time, increasing numbers of these cells begin to appear until they are markedly apparent at 6 to 8 days; osteoclast-mediated resorption continues for 10 to 14 days, after which this activity begins to subside. Bone apposition becomes apparent about 2 weeks postsurgically when osteogenic cells, usually originating in marrow areas and derived from mesenchymal precursors, begin deposition of collagenous precursors (osteoid). This process continues strongly for 2 to 3 weeks. Consisting of large amounts of osteoid, with enclosed osteocytes and topically located osteoblasts, the new bone gives an appearance of coarse fibrillar trabeculae termed "woven bone." This pattern is observable in radicular, interproximal, and interradicular areas and occurs at about the same time that bone along the periodontal ligament face of the septum is re-forming. By 4 weeks the periodontal ligament width is commonly restored to a width and structural character consistent with its preoperative state. By 3 months postoperatively a compact bony plate may be partially restored, although it does not appear as fully mature bone due to an irregular fiber arrangement and indifferent lamellation. At this time the constituents of the periodontal ligament appear normal and in good relationship to a layer of cementoid along the root surface. Interproximal and furcation areas may have regenerated almost completely, while the radicular surface may have lost much of the original height of bone exposed.

The initial connective tissue reaction at the wound margins is one of marked inflammation evidenced by large numbers of polymorphonuclear leukocytes and extensive vasodilation, edema, and so on. By the fourth to fifth day after surgery, beginning proliferation of granulation tissue, which will eventually comprise a new gingival covering for bone, is evident primarily from the exposed periodontal ligament and the lateral wound edges. Periodontal ligament cellularity, with concomitant productivity, may be so pronounced that the crest of the septum is covered within a few days (that is, by 10 to 12 days) by reparative tissue. Granulation tissue expands by proliferation from exposed marrow spaces of the interdental and furcation areas as well as the periodontal ligament of the radicular area. This budding tissue joins that derived from the lateral wound edges and ultimately blends, at about 14 days, with the alveolar mucosa or gingiva at the apical base and the lateral edges to the wound. During the early stages of healing, this tissue appears hyperplastic and irregular. It is friable and bleeds quite readily. It is incompletely epithelialized.

Epithelium, originating from the wound margins, migrates over the developing connective tissue. There is often a 7-day delay in the process because of the lack or incompleteness of the bed of connective tissue. It completely covers the area in about 2 to 3 weeks, depending on the size of the wound; it is present as an atrophic, nonkeratinized epithelium at this stage with a well-developed basal cell layer adjacent to a thin basement lamina (periodic acid–Schiff positive). A definitive prickle cell layer may not be observable for 25 to 28 days. The epithelium may not regain its preoperative appearance for as long as 6 months. A system of gingival collagen may be present by 2 to 3 weeks, although its fibers tend to have a parallel arrangement with respect to the root and bone. The tissue corium, at first edematous and laden with poorly organized reticulin and collagen, may acquire an organized arrangement at a 6-month postoperative time. There is substantive evidence that it will maintain a resemblance to a dense scar tissue without regaining the anatomy found physiologically in gingiva.

The ultimate result of bone exposure is such that the *radicular* area shows soft tissue repair at the dentogingival junction with a residual anatomic bone deformity. As much as 50% of the original radicular attachment apparatus may be lost. Ordinarily the site of maximal loss of periodontal attachment will be located in relationship to the most buccally prominent segment of the root of the tooth. Gingival tissue above the bone crest may exceed its original length and thus compensate somewhat for the reduced bone level. Because of the nature of bone present, other areas such as furcation and interproximal locations may show virtually complete repair of bone and soft tissue. Again, the original anatomy of the site is a prime determining factor in the response to the surgery. Where bone is thin, the site is composed of compact bone. In labial, buccal, lingual, and palatal sites, such bone septa interface on one side with periodontal ligament and on the opposite surface with periosteum.

Interdentally and interradicularly, in areas of root proximity, the thin bone septum is bilaterally faced with periodontal ligament and buccally and lingually veneered by periosteum. The primary vascular supply to such thin, compact bone is derived from its periosteum (periodontal ligament may also be considered as a periosteum in the context of vascular supply and as a reparative source) (Fig. 23-37). While such osseous septa may have internally derived vascular sources (i.e., from marrow cavities to haversian canals), these are generally minimal and may not be sufficient to maintain nutrition and hydration to bone's enclaved cells. The consequence is bone necrosis, its extent depending on the degree of deprivation of vascularization, the extent of surgical trauma, the duration of acute postsurgical inflammation, the lack of marrow availability within the septum, the presence and extent of concurrent occlusal traumatic effects in adjacent periodontal ligament(s), the extent of denudation, and the pace of development of granulation tissue over the previously exposed periosteal bone surfaces. Regretfully, bone resorption does not cease even when bone is revascularized and covered by reparative granulation tissue; in a most general context, however, the presence of a soft tissue cover, for example, periosteum, endosteum, and granulation tissue, as well as the onset and continuation of a state of chronic rather than acute inflammation, is an ameliorating factor in bone necrosis and resorption.

The presence of endosteum, lining marrow cavities and vascular channels, is essential for the internal reconstruction of bone. The remodeling and structural redevelopment of the outer surfaces of bone are reliant upon periosteum that surrounds the area of bone exposure. There is lateral and centripetal ingrowth of granulation (reparative) tissue over the bone surface from this source. It is joined by granulation tissue derived from *available* periodontal ligament and marrow areas, completing a multidirectional pattern of "periosteal" neodevelopment. There is no evidence that areas of completely resorbed *thin* bone are ever rebuilt; the loss should be considered permanent. Thicker osseous septa have a greater potential for repair because of internally located marrow and endosteum; these are dynamic sources of the new tissue required for reconstruction of previously lost attachment apparatus and alveolar processes. Of prime additional consideration is the amount of postsurgical bone resorption in relationship to the *dimensions* of the bone septum.

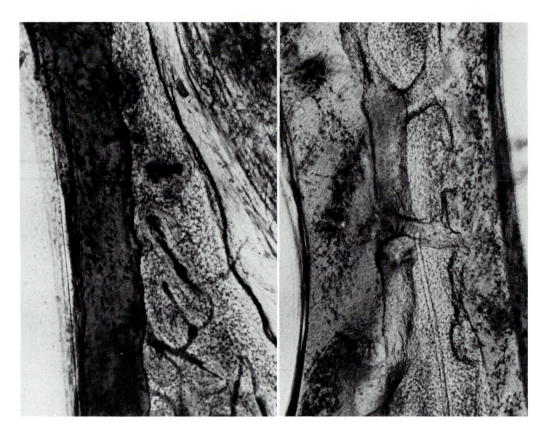

Fig. 23-37. At left, nature of radicular bone, in this instance at buccal aspect of a mandibular first premolar. At its superior aspect, plate of bone is *very* thin, about 0.4 mm, while apical phase of bone septum is considerably thicker and reveals a multiplicity of marrow cavities and vascular channels. Under influence of inflammatory exudates, spreading periosteally but in interface with bone, thin phase will tend to resorb through and through and lend to horizontal and essentially irreversible bone loss. When resorption involves thicker portion of radicular septum, pattern of resorption may change to an angular type with formation of intrabony (infrabony) pockets. In occlusal traumatism, comparable patterns of bone resorption may occur but pocket formation is not produced in occlusal traumatism. Should inflammation coexist or supervene with occlusal traumatism in same locale, resorption lesion could be derived from *dual* etiologies. At right, interdental septum in a transversely sectioned specimen; at far left and far right are roots of adjacent teeth. Central linear band is osseous septum with periodontal ligaments bilaterally situated. Septum varies in width from 0.5 to 0.7 mm and is largely constituted of cortical bone. Proximal surfaces of roots are flattened and approximately 1.5 mm apart. Such bony areas also tend to resorb completely, with little potential for effective repair after therapy aimed at negating either periodontal pocket or occlusal traumatic lesion should either or both be present at site. (From Ruben, M. P., Prieto-Hernandez, J. R., Gott, F. K., Kramer, G. M., and Bloom, A. A.: J. Periodontol. **42:**774, 1971.)

For example, 1 mm of bone resorption buccolingually where the osseous septum is 1 mm thick will eliminate the attachment apparatus at that site. However, the same amount of buccolingual resorption when the septum is 2.5 mm thick will result primarily in a reduction of septal thickness but without a loss of periodontal attachment for the tooth.

Although the differences between human and experimental observations are not always comparable because of size of the area of bone exposure, amount of inflammation presurgically, and the presence or absence of a periodontal dressing, it is quite obvious that bone exposure, particularly along root surfaces, often produces highly undesirable sequelae with the potential for blatant loss of periodontal attachment. These considerations lend credence to the use of techniques now avail-

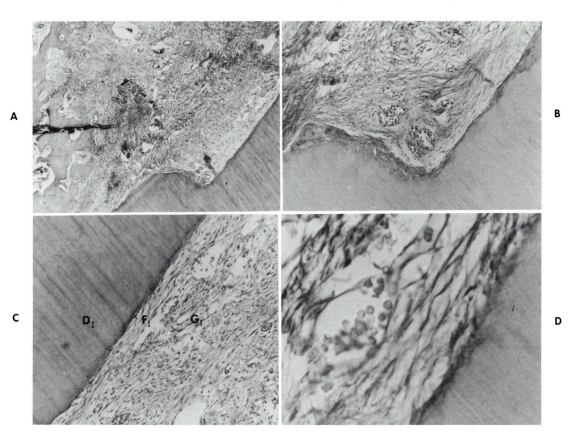

Fig. 23-38. Representative events in healing occurring after infrabony pocket therapy in dog are shown in Figs. 23-38 to 23-45. (Development of new attachment.) Twenty-one days after surgery. **A,** Osseous defect contains very vascular connective tissue complex derived via endosteal hyperplasia from adjacent marrow areas and through productive activity of contiguous periodontal ligament, exposed deliberately in débridement of pocket. **B,** Notice reticulum and collagen fibers of granulation tissue both oriented parallel to root and attached by osteoid to dentin. It is most interesting that greatest amount of osteoid deposition is on areas of root irregularity. **C,** Axial surface of root shows irregular lattice of collagen fibers, *F,* compromising fibrillar phase of granulation tissue, G_1, in association with surface of dentin, D_1, whereas **D** (photograph reversed) depicts early attachment of collagen fibrils to root; attachment is obviously frail.

able to minimize or obviate postoperative inflammatory and resorptive phenomena. These are procedures that conserve periosteal and gingival tissues and recognize the extreme lability of bone—a lability in direct proportion to its exposure and manipulation in relationship to its original (presurgical) structure and form.

Healing after surgical treatment of infrabony pocket

From the standpoint of reconstructive healing, new attachment or reattachment connotes the development of all or a portion of the attachment apparatus previously lost as a result of periodontal inflammation or a combination of the inflammatory process with an occlusal traumatic lesion.

Thus it represents positive repair of an infrabony pocket after it has been suitably converted by débridement to an osseous defect—a surgical wound (Figs. 23-38 to 23-45).

In general the surgical débridement of the lesion entails complete removal of the contained inflammatory tissue. Chronically inflamed tissue is curetted laterally or circumferentially to its osseous walls, to the cemental surface of the tooth, and apically to the bony floor of the defect to periodontal ligament. The periodontal ligament is additionally exposed proximate to the tooth, at its *full* available interface with alveolar bone. Thus, for example, a three-walled infrabony defect on the proximal aspect of a posterior tooth (which has proximal, buccal, and lingual walls, with the

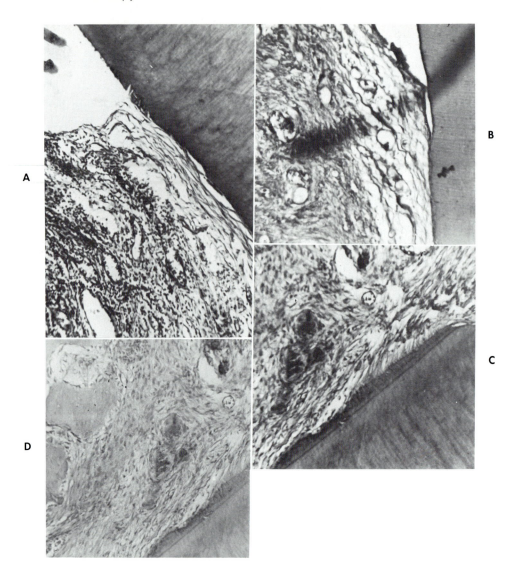

Fig. 23-39. Healing after curettage of infrabony pocket, dog. Full-thickness flap approach. Twenty-first day. **A,** At site between flap and tooth, interposed collagen is sparse, essentially unattached, and oriented parallel to root. At left, dense inflammatory cell infiltrate around focal zone of necrosis (suture site?). **B,** Paucity of fibrillar elements intervening between flap (at left) and tooth. It is our opinion that flap reattachment is largely dependent on proliferation of reparative tissue from marrow and periodontal ligament areas and that there is an inverse relationship between the quantity and quality of reparative tissue and *distance* of flap from these progenitor areas. In **C,** just apical to **B,** inflammation persists, whereas in **D,** somewhat apical and lateral to **C,** connective tissue is abundant and bone production (at periphery of defect, but at *left* in this section) is active. Note osteoblasts along edges of bone trabeculae.

cementum as a fourth surface) has periodontal ligament facing the defect from the lingual, apical, and buccal aspects and can in a geneal way be morphologically classed as a U- or V-shaped exposure. Recognition of this pattern of exposure of the periodontal ligament is fundamental to an understanding of the proper rationale of treatment and healing of infrabony defects. The periodontal

ligament physiologically is a dynamic tissue with fairly rapid turnover (replacement cycle) and with a delicate balance between the appositional and resorptive process. Under the influence of injury it can acquire even greater generative potential and contribute markedly to repair of the surgical site. There is some observational data indicating that the periodontal ligament, after surgical ex-

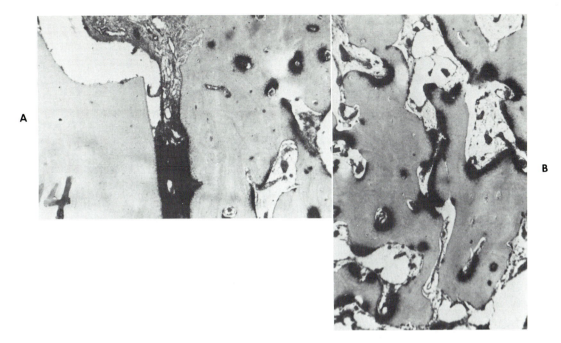

Fig. 23-40. Healing of infrabony pocket, dog. Periodontal ligament and marrow areas exposed in periodontal surgery exhibit marked propensity for formation of reparative tissue (granulation tissue of healing wound) required for new attachment, reattachment of flaps to tooth and bone, and so on. These autoradiographs graphically illustrate this dynamic property of periodontal ligament, **A,** and endosteum, **B.** Experimental animal was injected parenterally with proline ^{14}C 48 hours prior to death. **A,** Notice at top left-center isotopic labeling of granulation tissue within infrabony defect. Two weeks after surgery.

posure, provides the segment of reparative tissue that forms on the prepared root surface and serves as the progenitor of the new periodontal ligament. This outgrowth of granulation tissue from intact periodontal ligament, contiguous to the defect, probably does not exceed 2 mm from any single linear area of exposure. However, where ligament is present buccally and lingually in interface with the debrided defect, one can reasonably expect about 4 mm of outgrowth in a buccolingual direction. This lamella of new tissue is joined by reparative tissue originating from the *apical* periodontal ligament. There is experimental evidence noting that the exclusion of periodontal ligament participation in repair obviates the formation of a new periodontal ligament and sets the stage for the ankylosis of newly formed bone to the root surface. While not a universal finding, ankylosis tends to be associated with root resorption, which if progressive may eventuate with loss of a portion of the tooth and in extreme instances pulpal involvement. Pulpal involvement has been observed when fresh red marrow and bone autografts are employed in new attachment procedures.

The granulation tissue of periodontal ligament derivation not only provides replacement periodontal ligament, but is also the source of cells concerned with the deposition and mineralization of cementoid on the root, a process integral to new *attachment* and the reattachment of gingival flaps to the root. The proliferation of reparative tissue from crestal, exposed periodontal ligament acts to unite the soft tissue flap to the root and to underlying attachment apparatus, since it interposes between the flap and the tooth. On one side the new connective tissue is linked to gingival connective tissue, while in proximity to the root its inner aspect is joined to the debrided cemental or dentinal surface via new cementum. Very recent data confirm that osteoid, cementoid, and dentinoid will undergo mineralization only when deposited on a *mineralized* substrate of bone, cementum, or dentin. Interestingly, osteoblasts, cementoblasts, and odontoblasts form and secrete glycopeptide- and lipid-containing products, which are packaged as "secretory" and (later) matrix vesicles. Updated studies by Ruben suggest that the therapeutically debrided and planed root surface initially undergoes superficial demineralization and resorption of the cemental matrix that enclaves embedded collagen and reticulum fibers. This process is both acid and enzyme activated (for example, citric acid and elastase) and is manifest within 48 hours after surgery. Interestingly, collagen and reticulum, intrinsic to cementum (and dentin), is largely spared. Studies by Franck and Cimasoni denote the "remineralization" of this lamella with subsequent deposi-

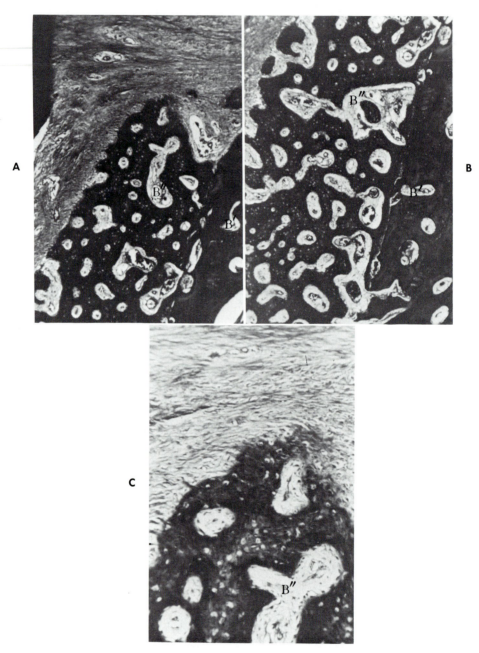

Fig. 23-41. Healing of infrabony pocket, dog. New attachment, 42 days after surgery. **A,** Trabecular bone, *B'*, has nearly filled infrabony defect. **B,** In higher magnification, one may readily see original osseous wall, *B'*, which has served as a scaffolding for deposition and attachment of new bone, *B"*, and marrow. Periodontal membrane may be seen at left in **A** and **B;** its fibers are in hypofunctional arrangement, yet tissue is very cellular, indirectly indicating continuing synthetic activity of cells. **C,** Crest of developing osseous phase of new attachment. It is very cellular with abundant lacunae and included osteocytes.

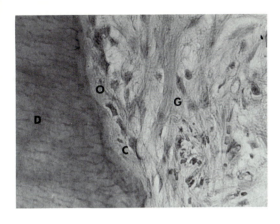

Fig. 23-42. Healing of infrabony pocket, dog. Forty-two days. Newly formed periodontal membrane, *G*, attached to dentin, *D*, by cementoid, *O*. Notice cementoblasts, *C*, situated in proximity to osteoid.

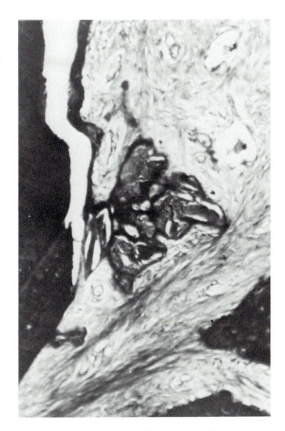

Fig. 23-43. Healing of infrabony pocket, dog. Inclusion of cementum and dentin chips within healing osseous lesion. Osteoid has formed *minimally* on their surfaces. Thin lamella of cementum has formed on axial aspect of root, but has separated from dentin as artifact of histologic preparation. Forty-two-day postoperative specimen.

tion of a new cementum external to the remineralized tooth structure (dentin).

The matrix vesicles diffuse through either tooth or bone matrix, gathering mineral while in transit. As the mineralizing vesicles reach and accumulate at the matrix-tooth or matrix-bone interface, at an area termed the "calcification front," the mineralized matrix vesicles become so laden with mineral that they appear to "explode." Thus hordes of nucleating sites for subsequent epitactic mineral crystal deposition are provided, the mineral (as $CaPO_4$ in both amorphous and apatite forms) precipitating from available tissue fluids and exudate. Once the initial lamella of new matrix undergoes this transformation into a mineralized state, the process of matrix formation and mineralization is repeated. The collagen and reticulum of osteoid and cementoid undergo comparable mineralization as matrix vesicles localized along and within their fibrils. Therefore the careful and fastidious débridement of the lesion creates an optimal environment for regeneration.

In histologic analysis of infrabony inflammatory lesions there is the nearly universal observation of a blanket of connective tissue—a modified transseptal fiber system—over bone. While it may reflect in part the persistence and directional reorientation of the original transseptal fiber complex, it is primarily a zone of reactive fibroplasia. Periodontal inflammation is usually a low-grade, chronic process inductive not only of resorptive tissue changes but also of connective tissue (and bone) apposition. While in the long run resorption tends to be greater with progressive loss and detachment of periodontal tissues from the teeth, shorter term evaluations indicate that tissue formation may nearly equal tissue resorption. This near-equalization may account for the ordinarily slow progression of inflammatory periodontal disease.

It should be reemphasized that cells (e.g., lymphocytes) associated with chronic inflammation may release peptides (RNA complexes), which in turn activate osteoblastic and fibroblastic activities. There are also angiogenetic, neurotrophic, and epithelial growth factors operative in inflammatory states; they are considered to be of mononuclear cell derivation. Conversely, in the biphasic inflammatory condition, mononuclear cells (e.g., T-lymphocytes) are considered to be sources of resorption-inducing agents.

The transseptal fiber system is often well laminated, variably dense, and continuous with the endosteum of the adjacent marrow spaces and,

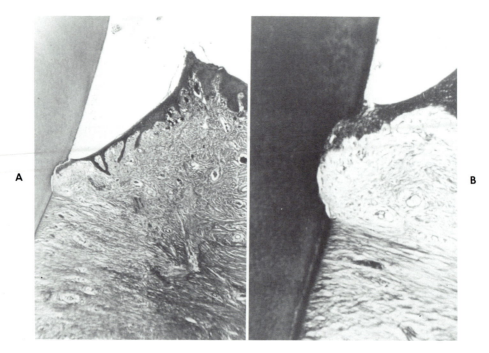

Fig. 23-44. Healing of infrabony pocket, dog; 42 days. Reattachment of mucoperiosteal flap to root. **A** and **B**, New sulcular and junctional epithelia have formed inner aspect of gingival cuff. Epithelium is just apical to cementoenamel junction, having migrated into defect in root. There is mild, marginal inflammatory reaction in gingiva. Note collagenous bridge (at lower left of **A**) extending from collagen of flap (dark fiber complex at lower right) to root cementum. Delicacy of this bridging fiber complex can be discerned in **B.**

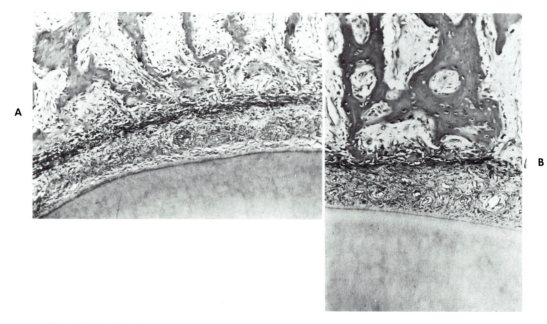

Fig. 23-45. Healing of infrabony pocket, dog. Cross section of tooth and developing attachment apparatus 60 days after treatment. Trabecular bone, enclaving very cellular marrow, can be seen at top of **A.** Particularly striking in both photomicrographs is linear formation of alveolar bone, lateral to periodontal ligament. Fibroblasts and osteoblasts synthesize collagen and matrical substance in this platelike pattern; it subsequently mineralizes. Interposition of periodontal ligament between bone and tooth is inhibitory to ankylosis.

at the coronal periphery of the defect, with the periosteal aspect of the gingiva. It is also affixed to the cementum and may blend lightly with the periodontal ligament. Removal of this "sheath" appears to be integral to "new attachment" Divestment of this complex allows for the participation of both *periodontal ligament* and the *endosteum* of marrow spaces and vascular channels in repair. With this band of tissue excised, vascular transudates (exudates in the early healing process) and regenerative tissue may enter the defect from these prime progenitor areas. Additional contributions in healing, which are thought to be slight, may also be derived from the overlying gingival flaps and the periosteum at the edge of flap retraction. The differential participation of the various tissues of the periodontium in the healing process is not entirely clear. There is no doubt, however, as to the potential wealth of healing derived from endosteum and periodontal ligament.

Detailed root surface preparation also appears to be a vital phase of the surgery. However, it should be emphasized that new attachment of connective tissue to the prepared dental surface requires the deposition of a mineralizing osteoid enclaving collagen and reticulum fibers. Cementum that is altered by the inflammatory process by proteolysis and demineralization, adherent masses of bacterial plaque and calculus, and accumulations of exudate are considered to be inhibitory to the formation of osteoid (cementoid) and cementum. Both dentin and cementum divested of the undesirable substances may serve as scaffolding for newly formed cementum. Interestingly a roughened yet debrided surface appears to favor earlier and more extensive apposition of a mineralizing connective tissue (cementoid) (see boxed material on p. 728).

The early events in the healing of osseous defects are merely modifications of those that are coincident with any other periodontal surgical wound. These include hemorrhage and the subsequent formation of a fibrin clot within the lesion and within the superficial portions of the periodontal ligament and marrow. The blood coagulum is believed to constitute a provisional seal of the surgical site (see discussion on tissue biology related to wound healing), to provide intrinsic and surface pathways for wound exudation, and to serve as a topical viscous gel for orientation of a leukocytic polyband. The accumulated neutrophils appear to be important in the phagocytic and enzymatic dissolution of the clot.

Within 30 to 60 minutes an inflammatory state begins to dominate the early postoperative period. It is marked by an inflammatory cell infiltration, predominantly neutrophilic, adjacent to the clot and in the nearby periodontal ligament and marrow areas. The infiltrate changes in character and intensity over the next several days, with a progressive dominance of lymphocytes, plasma cells, monocytes, and mononuclear macrophages over neutrophils. There are concomitant reductions in the number of cells and modifications of their localization in the tissues. Usually by the third to fourth day postoperatively these modifications are evident. By the fourteenth to seventeenth day the infiltration is minimal and consists essentially of lymphocytes, plasma cells, and macrophages.

There are also vascular alterations with substantive increases in the number of patent blood vessels, as well as in their permeability, in the periodontal ligament, endosteum, marrow, and periosteum. Thus exudation is promoted. Vessels at the wound surface are actually severed in the surgical procedure, resulting in both vasoconstrictive and leakage phenomena. These changes are gradually supplanted by vasoproductive reactions, since the acute inflammatory lesion is converted to the chronic inflammatory condition associated with active repair. Angiogenesis is believed to be stimulated by low-molecular-weight proteins (glycopeptides) formed by activated lymphocytes, with subsequent uptake by endothelial cells.

Initially, the inflammatory *exudate* with its strong neutrophilic component and acidic pH is locally destructive for collagen, cells, and connective tissue matrix, bone, and so on. Its quantity is great and its viscosity exceeds that of physiologic transudates and tissue fluids. Diminishing exudation relies on diminishing inflammation and on repair and becomes progressively less in the first 3 to 4 days after surgery. Exudate fills the marrow areas, vascular channels, the interface between wound bed and clot, and the crestal phase of periodontal ligament and is responsible for early displacement and breakdown of matrical, cellular, and fibrous elements at these sites. The blood clot may also be permeated by exudate, a process that may favor dissolution of the "fibrinous gel."

Connective tissue resorption at the marrow, endosteal, ligament, and other areas results in collagen fiber fragmentation, liquefaction (variable) of ground substance, cellular destructive changes, segmentation of vascular sheaths, and so on. The degeneration is favored by the release, from inflammatory (neutrophils) and other cells, of acid hydrolases and by the acidity of the local tissue

---

BIOTHERAPEUTIC PHILOSOPHY IN ROOT SURFACE PREPARATION

A knowledge of the nature of the cemental alterations produced by periodontal inflammation is of paramount importance in the provision of a biologic basis for root surface preparation in periodontal therapy. It now appears that suprabony pocket elimination with subsequent re-attachment of gingival flaps to the tooth surface at or near the crest of bone in juxtaposition to the marginal aspects of the periodontal ligament is predicated on the formation of cementum onto a fastidiously prepared root surface. In a like context, new attachment procedures aimed at the negation of infrabony pockets demand the deposition of new cementum on previously debrided cementum or dentin to attach the newly formed periodontal ligament complex to the tooth.

The basic elements of this revised biotherapeutic philosophy include the following:

1. *All* soft (bacterial plaque, debris, exudate) and hard (calculus) deposits should be removed from the root. There seems to be no doubt that their presence is a barrier to the formation and mineralization of new cementum.

2. The root surface should be debrided so as to effect removal of all cementum (and dentin, if modified) altered by the inflammatory process. The "damaged" root surface may act as a nidus for exudate accumulation. It is conceivable that many of the components of exudate, including bacterial toxins and neutrophil- and macrophage-derived hydrolytic enzymes as well as the acid character of the material, can be cytotoxic to cells formative of cementum and thus inhibit or destroy their synthetic activities.

3. The postdebridement root surface should be mineralized and topically "etched" or irregular. A mineralized surface of either tooth or bone appears to be physically inductive of cemento-genesis and osteogenesis, respectively, including the mineralization of the deposits. Once the first lamellae of cementoid and osteoid are formed the surface of previously debrided mineralized substrate appears to serve as the locale of a *calcification front* of the cemental (and osteoid) matrix. Topical irregularities of the prepared root surface may serve to provide a more secure physical anchorage for the new tissue.

4. The debrided dentin or cemental surface can be treated with inorganic or organic acids such as 0.6N hydrochloric acid, citric acid, or phosphoric acid. This treatment may possibly enhance subsequent cementogenesis, including its bond to the tooth. In a similar vein, topical demineralization of particles of autogenous and allogeneic compact bone may render these elements more inductive or receptive of new bone formation on their surfaces. Interestingly the artificially demineralized peripheral zone of bone tends to remineralize from tissue fluids, which provide $CaPO_4$ in amorphous and apatite forms needed for the process. Only then is new osteoid deposited and subsequently mineralized.

5. In the repair of the surgical site, granulation tissue derived primarily from contiguous exposed areas of periodontal ligament expands by proliferation onto the treated root. It may well serve as the progenitor of the "new" periodontal ligament, covering the previously exposed root; thus its cells act in a cementogenic capacity. This sheath of new connective tissue is inhibitory to ankylosis and thus retardant to root resorption.

6. It is axiomatic in periodontal therapy that the supragingival root surface, which will continue to be exposed to the oral environment, should be thoroughly debrided and polished. Such a surface can be markedly inhibitory to plaque and debris attachment. Cementum or dentin thus prepared and exposed to saliva and gingival fluids *may* become hypermineralized (and hard) and structurally resistant to attack by bacterial and inflammatory products.

---

environment. Collagen resorption and matrical regressive changes may also be mediated by macrophages. Macrophage action is both phagocytic and enzymatic.

Bone resorption appears to be part and parcel of the early postsurgical state. Osteolysis, produced by release of acid hydrolases from osteocytes with accompanying perilacunar resorption,

may occur very soon after injury (within minutes to hours). However, bone resorption affiliated with osteoclasts does not occur significantly until the waning of the acute inflammatory state; it is really an accompaniment to primary repair and thus may be delayed until the fourth and subsequent days. Areas notable for resorption include periodontal ligament regions (generally outer and superficial), trabeculae of marrow spaces, and walls of vascular channels. Osteoclastic activity persists with decreasing intensity and generally ceases to be of consequence by the end of the second week of healing. The role of the macrophage in both hard and soft tissue resorption should be stressed again. Macrophages tend to be ubiquitous to chronic inflammatory infiltrates. Even though these cells may not be in juxtaposition to resorbing bone, their liberated enzymes may diffuse through connective tissues to reach bone surfaces.

In retrospect the healing process during the first several days after surgery consists of initial hemorrhage, fibrin clot, the acute inflammatory event in all of its ramifications, and a generally deleterious effect at the immediate surgical site on both the hard and soft tissue elements. If treatment is based on a scientific rationale and is carried out skillfully and carefully, if exogenous irritants are barred from the wound, and if there are no participating adverse systemic influences, the regenerative phase will now predominate.

From the fourth postoperative day there is an extensive elaboration of the regenerative tissue with a change of the quality of the granulation tissue contained within the surgical defect. Activity now centers on the gradual conversion of a vascular connective tissue (granulation tissue) to bone in trabecular form and to marrow. The adjacent bone marrow, initially composed of inflammatory connective tissue with numerous dilated vessels and manifesting extensive edema, now undergoes conversion, and osteoblasts are seen in increasing numbers on the trabecular surfaces. At a later time there is a slow transformation of marrow to a fatty type, although one still finds the presence of endosteum and areas of fibrous tissue. The change in marrow is to a mixed fibrolipid type. As this develops there is a decrease in vascularity and edema.

Bone regeneration essentially occurs from the base and sides of the defect and extends toward the tooth as irregular projections that are readily anastomosed to each other by connecting trabeculae; thus a lattice of bone develops. Adjacent to the tooth is a variably wide band of connective tissue that has fibrils attached to the tooth via cementoid (mineralizing to cementum). The fibers "entering" the tooth are haphazardly oriented and aligned crudely parallel to the root; they are delicate and "lacelike" or cotton-candy-like in arrangement. This loose connective tissue is also continuous with the adjacent periodontal ligament

and the endosteum of the new trabeculae and thus with marrow. As regenerating bone "approaches" the tooth, a "plate" of alveolar bone is ultimately formed parallel to the root surface (in all dimensions) (radiologically a lamina dura); it is a cribriform plate with vascular channels and an endosteal lining continuous with marrow and with the new periodontal ligament. There is concomitantly a slow conversion of connective tissue of the progenitor periodontal ligament from a loose, edematous, vascular complex to a more organized membranous tissue resembling a hypofunctional periodontal ligament. It is estimated that over a period of many months there may be the establishment of a ligamentous structure resembling that seen associated with a tooth in a functional state.

During this regeneration of the attachment apparatus, reparative phenomena are occurring in overlying gingiva. The process is comparable to that noted in the healing of an apically repositioned mucoperiosteal flap. The prime reattachment of the flap to tooth is reliant primarily on reparative tissue derived from the crestal aspect of the periodontal ligament adjacent to the osseous defect and from the connective tissue complex (granulation tissue) of the healing bone defect. This tissue is actually interposed between flap and tooth, uniting the essentially stable original collagen fiber complexes of the gingiva to the tooth. Thus it is responsible for the attachment, via connective tissue and cementum, of the gingiva to the tooth. Attachment can be expected over a distance of 1 to 1.5 mm — at times 2 mm — above (coronal to) the ligament and defect. There may also be contributions of reparative and attaching tissue from endosteum of marrow spaces and vascular channels exposed at the crests and outer margins (buccal and lingual) of bone septa, and from the periosteum of the gingival flaps. The former is probably more predictable and reliable.

The epithelial cover of this regenerating tissue (at flap-tooth interface) originates from the epithelium of the flap and migrates under the resorbing blood coagulum. As it approaches the tooth a provisional sulcus and epithelial adherence to the tooth are formed (see discussion of epithelium). This may well be termed a "sliding" adherence, for as the osseous defect fills with granulation tissue and then attachment apparatus and supporting bone, this epithelium *may* move coronally under the influence of the increased bulk of the regenerative tissue. This is, in reality, a phenomenon that is the *reverse* of that seen occurring

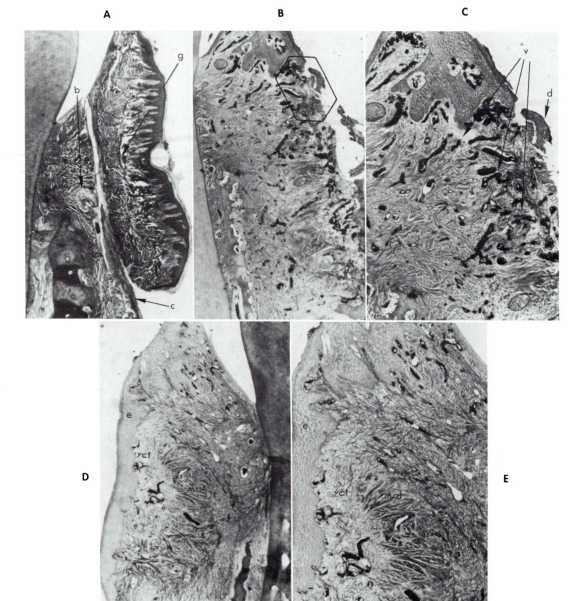

Fig. 23-46. Development of blood supply to split-thickness free gingival autografts. Perfused section, dog. **A,** Zero-hour specimen. Grafted tissue is in close opposition to underlying tissues. There is no graft attachment except possibly that afforded by intervening blood clot. *b,* Connective tissue bed, in this instance both periosteal and gingival. *g,* Graft; *c,* blood clot. **B,** Seven-day specimen, showing rich vascularization of graft, marginal gingiva, and cervical phase of periodontal ligament. Note topical resorption of buccal septum. Vascularization of recipient tissue and of corium of graft is extensive. **C,** Seven-day specimen, higher magnification of **B**. Note epithelial atrophy and necrosis with epithelial desquamation at outer central portion of graft, *d. v,* Vessels filled with carbon black. **D,** Thirteen-day specimen. Peripheral vascular plexus has been restored. Note blending of young, *yct.* and mature, *mct,* connective tissues. Gingival epithelium, *e,* is intact and has been renewed. **E,** Thirteen-day specimen, higher magnification of **D**. Note sharp distinction between mature, recipient site and young, new connective tissue, as well as comparatively marked vascularity with bridging capillaries. Epithelium is at left and is thin and nonkeratinizing. (From Janson, W., Ruben, M. P., Kramer, G. M., and Bloom, A. A.: J. Periodontol. **40:**707, 1969.)

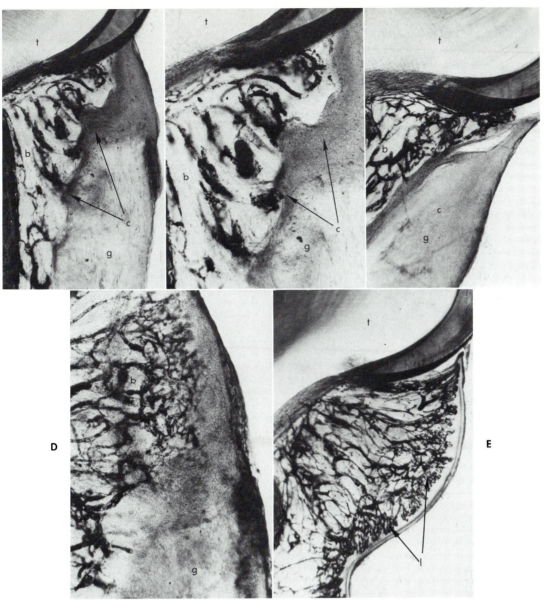

Fig. 23-47. Development of blood supply to split-thickness free gingival autograft. Perfused, dog. **A,** One-day postoperative specimen, cleared section. Graft, *g,* in close adherence to host site. Carbon black (indicative of blood vessel perviousness when extravascular) has not entered graft but is present at interface of graft with connective tissue. *b,* Well-vascularized host side; *g,* graft in opposition to it. No ink-filled vessels are seen in transplant; thus graft is avascular at this stage of healing. *c,* Clot; *t,* tooth. **B,** One-day, higher magnification of **A;** cleared section. Perfused specimen. Clot, *c,* exists between graft and connective tissue bed. Note dilation of vessels of periosteum and gingival corium (top center). **C,** Two-day specimen, cleared section. Animal perfused with carbon suspension. Graft is in close apposition to host site and lacks vascularity. Note prominent vasculature of gingival corium. Only adherence provided for graft is possibly by blood clot. There is initial vasoproliferative reaction at outer aspect of receptor site; transudate (exudate) diffuses into graft from receptor area's blood vessels. *b,* Vascularity of remaining periosteal aspect; *g,* graft; *c,* blood clot; *t,* tooth. **D,** Four-day specimen, cleared section. Perfused, showing increased patency of its vessels at bed-graft interface. Since exudates are also labeled with diffusible dye (patent blue violet), it is evident that the graft appears "darkened" due to uptake of perfusate from receptor area. Notice striking vascular proliferation at top center. *b,* Connective tissue bed; *g,* graft. **E,** Ten-day specimen, cleared section, perfused. Evidence of vascular "take" of graft to receptor site. *l,* Subepithelial capillary loops are arranged in a disorganized pattern. (From Janson, W., Ruben, M. P., Kramer, G. M., and Bloom, A. A.: J. Periodontol. **40:**707, 1969.)

in the gingival and periodontal inflammatory state where severance of the gingival fiber attachment to cementum, connective tissue matrix hydrolysis, and cemental resorption by proteolysis and demineralization lead to epithelial migration in an apical direction on the root surface.

FREE SOFT TISSUE AUTOGRAFTS
Gingival autografts

The transplantation of sections of attached gingiva from one site in the oral cavity to another in the same individual for the correction of several clinically significant defects is now a widely used and accepted procedure in periodontal therapy (Figs. 23-46 and 23-47). Free gingival autografts have been successfully utilized clinically to increase the width of attached gingiva, extend the depth of the vestibular fornix, dissipate muscle pull, and cover small areas of denuded root that have resulted from gingival recession. Although there are a number of variations in approach, the procedure of gingival grafting essentially consists of the removal of an appropriate amount of tissue from a donor site and its application to a prepared recipient bed. Unlike flap surgery where a blood supply is retained, the vascular connections of a free graft are completely severed. Success of the procedure depends in large part on the establishment of an adequate circulation to the grafted tissue. The prime technical problem involved in the "take" or survival of a graft concerns the assurance that the transplanted tissue will be adequately nourished in its new position. Permeable, thin graft tissue allows for the nourishment and hydration by way of diffusion mechanisms via tissue fluid until the graft is vascularized. Vascularization appears to occur either by capillaries' ingrowth into the graft from the recipient site or by blood vessels in the transplant becoming connected to capillaries in the bed for the graft. It is more likely that a dual process of revascularization occurs.

Until recently there has been a paucity of material in the periodontal literature relating to the healing of free autogenous gingival grafts. It was reasonably assumed that healing of such wounds did not differ markedly from that of other mucosal or skin areas. Although there may be many technical variations in clinical approaches, the essential aspects of the healing process of a free gingival autograft are related to early graft nutrition, hydration, and renewal of its vascularization. Graft acceptance to the host area is based essentially on establishment of early "circulation" be-

tween the two tissues for the retention of graft vitality. In addition revascularization provides a permanent circulation. The recipient area is also responsible for the development of a firm connective tissue attachment between host and graft, resulting in a functionally vital attached gingiva at the new site.

Autogenous gingival grafts of a split-thickness variety that include only the outer phase of the gingival corium appear to be more desirable than full-thickness grafts that contain a greater bulk of connective tissue. A thin tissue ensures that tissue fluids will have the opportunity to diffuse easily and early from the recipient bed into the graft. A well- but not densely collagenated tissue allows not only for hydration and nutrition but also for the proliferation of blood vessels into the graft in areas of loose connective tissue between collagen bundle fibers and around blood vessels. There is a tendency, with continuing repair, for the thin connective tissue graft to increase in thickness and density. This structural change appears to be related to periosteal osteogenesis (a thin, linear callus forms external to the original osseous face) and fibrogenesis and to connective tissue formation within the corium of the graft. Biologically these processes are best seen 60 to 85 days after surgery. Thinner grafts therefore appear to have a better prognosis, since they can be more easily maintained by diffusion and vascularize more readily. In addition, thick donor tissue that may come, for example, from the palatal region may include a submucosa rich in loose connective tissue, fat, or glands that could act as a physical barrier to diffusion and vascularization and to the ingrowth of connective tissue from receptor periosteum. When this occurs the removal of this submucosa is most desirable, if not critical, to the success of the procedure.

The host site also presents several cogent considerations for graft success. The literature on reconstructive surgery strongly indicates that the receptor area should consist of periosteum or thin connective tissue in order to provide an adequate source of reparative connective tissue and blood vessels. A recipient bed with the potential capacity for the rapid formation of granulation tissue will provide vascular outgrowth for eventual graft vascularization. Tissue placed on an area unable to form blood vessels and connective tissue will not survive in its new location and will be lost.

The application of a free soft tissue autograft in a host area results in gingiva that clinically reflects a blanched whitish appearance shortly after its placement and immobilization. Histologic examination of the area at this time in experimental animals shows a distinct blood clot formed between the transplanted tissue and the periosteal and connective tissue bed. There is no true graft attachment at this time except possibly that which may be afforded by the intervening blood clot and the sutures placed at strategic locations. The interface zone between the graft and recipient site consists of periosteal and gingival mats of connective tissues in approximation to one another. During the first 48 hours the wound area exhibits a marked inflammatory response that is evidenced in the recipient site by the presence of dilated capillaries congested with blood elements, disorganization of connective tissue, and substantial inflammatory cell infiltration. Red blood cells and cellular and tissue debris are also present. The connective tissue wound margins of both graft and host site are not only in approximation to one another but may appear somewhat fused by a matrix of a fibrin network. Although marked inflammatory activity is evident early at the recipient site, the graft shows no such reaction. Its vasculature is neither established nor patent. The degree of inflammation at the recipient site appears to be limited in area by the density of periosteal connective tissue, although perivascular edema and separation of fibrous elements occur.

The most critical period in graft healing appears to be during the first 48 hours. There is no evidence of actual vascularization of the transferred tissue prior to this period. Patency of the graft vessels does not appear to exist before the third postoperative day, at which time perfusion studies show some indication of "filled" vessels; nutrient supply during the first 48 hours (or longer) therefore must come from other means. The graft is maintained during this period by fluid diffusion from the vessels of the periosteal bed. The evidence for this concept lies in the observations of a lack of patency of graft vessels and the presence of a blood clot between surfaces of the graft that may be pervious in nature. Survival of the graft, including its cells during this period, requires hydration and nourishment that must occur by avascular nutrition. Fluid penetration from the underlying tissue to the transplanted tissue has been demonstrated in a number of microcirculatory studies. The mechanism appears to be comparable to that which exists in skin grafting and which has been referred to as "plasmatic circulation." Observations of sequential healing indicate that, indeed, after having diffused into the graft, the

fluid accumulates until it is removed by new vessels (veins and lymphatics) growing into it from the host site. Beginning at the first day after transplantation, the grafted tissue appears edematous up to about the sixth day. Remission of edema appears to coincide with the establishment of venous and lymphatic anastomoses and the initial connective tissue annexation of graft to receptor site.

The thickness of the clot between the graft and its bed may significantly affect the success of free autogenous grafts. Since revascularization and renewed attachment is dependent on close approximation of the connective tissue wound surfaces, the presence of bleeding and subsequent hematoma formation may separate the transferred tissue from its bed and result in graft necrosis. Adequate hemostasis of the host area becomes necessary before and after the graft is placed in position to prevent estrangement between the two tissues. The presence of a thick clot inhibits nutritional diffusion and retards rapid capillary penetration into the graft, ultimately resulting in its failure to survive. Since the graft is maintained during the first few days postoperatively *only* by fluid diffusion from the host bed, a thinner clot is helpful, if not critical, in maintaining the nutrition and hydration of the transplanted tissue. From a clinical point of view therefore, digital pressure exerted against the graft for several minutes after its immobilization usually results in thin clot formation. Total displacement of blood between the two tissues is difficult, if not impossible, particularly since irregularities exist along the two connective tissue wound surfaces. These areas may act as reservoirs for blood pooling, ultimately creating localized microhematoma formation. A thin fibrin clot also may aid in anchoring somewhat the "free" tissue and allow diffusion of metabolites and waste products through it while encouraging revascularization by rapidly proliferating capillaries.

By the third postoperative day a minimal degree of vascularity may be evident in the transplanted tissue. This becomes exhibited clinically by the gradual change in color from one that has been blanched — associated with initial absence of blood from its vessels — to a gradual return of circulation and pinkish coloration. Histologically, the endothelium is active at the surviving cut ends and periphery of blood vessels in the host bed, giving rise to cells that form into new capillaries. (The process of endothelial proliferation is presented in the discussion on Biology of Bone:

Correlations with Wound Healing.) Revascularization of the grafted tissue appears to be reestablished by means of an anastomosis between those vessels inherent to the graft and vessels proliferating into the graft from the receptor site. There exists some controversy, however, as to whether this new vasculature joins with the previously existing one in the graft. At this period in healing there is marked patency and dilation of the periosteal blood vessels and particularly in that portion of the graft adjacent to the periodontal ligament. The periodontal ligament indeed appears to be one of the main sources for revascularization when it is part of the wound bed. Blood flow through the vessels of the graft at this time appears somewhat sluggish.

The degenerative processes evident during the first 2 days, showing essentially epithelial desquamation and connective tissue disorganization and collagenolysis within the corium, undergo a slow reversal process with the beginning of fibroplasia. By the fourth day postoperatively there are voluminous communications present at the graft-bed interface as a network of fine capillaries extend toward and into the graft. The blood clot at this site is gradually resorbed; concomitantly it is replaced by loose connective tissue. No patent vessels are evident, however, at the outer, central portion of the graft; there is continued evidence in this area of ischemic necrosis and some epithelial desquamation. Except for this outer central poorly vascularized area, a new thin layer of epithelium has proliferated over the external surface, originating from the adjacent gingiva and alveolar mucosa and covering the connective tissue that still shows signs of disorganization; *where the graft is thin and intimately applied to receptor zone, the original graft epithelium may persist.*

At 6 to 7 days there is a striking and significant increase in the numbers of vessels between the graft and the recipient bed that generally tend to run in a horizontal direction, that is, perpendicular to graft from the receptor site. Some early signs are evident that vessels begin to assume a reticular arrangement in the loose connective tissue of the junctional zone. There is also a decided increase in the numbers of vessels at the graft's outer periphery. The graft itself reflects remarkable vascularization. The only area still not showing vascularization is that of the central, outer zone of the transplant, since vessels have not fully entered and developed in this region.

Distinct early connective tissue formation at the junctional site is evident. The graft epithelium, while still showing isolated signs of desquamation, is generally intact, although it is thin and devoid of rete pegs. Both basal cell and prickle cell layers are showing signs of regeneration and there is evidence of increased mitosis, although some intercellular and intracellular edema is evident.

Infiltration of inflammatory cells among the organized collagen bundles of both the graft and recipient tissue is present, particularly in an area near the dentogingival junction. Cellular infiltrate will persist with waning intensity and eventual spotty distribution during the first 17 to 21 days of healing.

Continuing modification of epithelium and connective tissue is evident at 10 days after the surgical procedure. There is a significant increase in the number of fibroblasts and a concomitant decrease in the inflammatory response in the connective tissue areas of the graft and wound bed (now joined), as shown by the presence primarily of lymphocytes and plasma cells, with few polymorphonuclear leukocytes in and about the capillary network. Collagen fiber bundles in the graft are becoming more definitively oriented to the radicular aspect of alveolar bone and root surface of the tooth. There is significantly high cellular activity in areas of the periosteum, periodontal ligament, and subepithelial zone and comparatively lower activity in the connective tissue proper. A renewed peripheral vascular plexus has been established within the graft; one may observe rete formation of blood vessels, particularly below the epithelium of the original graft.

Histologically, increasing maturation of the area continues for several weeks. By 14 days the epithelium shows some degree of thickness and a suggestion of the cellular and intercellular character that it had exhibited prior to the surgery. Moreover, an indication of the incipiency of keratinization is apparent with keratohyalin distribution in the granular cell layers. By 28 days the epithelium has a relatively normal appearance with a surface keratinizing effect, increased thickness, and rete peg formation. Although the gingival connective tissue appears young and shows wavy immature collagen bundles and much reticulin, the area of the dentogingival junction gives a more normal appearance. Concomitant with an increase in connective tissue and its improved organization is a decrease in vascularity. Characterization of the dentogingival junction to that approximating normalcy does not occur for about 4 to 6 weeks.

The reaction of alveolar bone to a free gingival

graft procedure appears to be comparatively minimal and may be related to some degree to the amount of connective tissue constituting the receptor site. An initial resorptive reaction by osteoclastic activity on the outer and crestal aspects of the alveolar process reaches a peak at about 8 days. Compared to periosteal retention and mucoperiosteal flap investigations, however, the amount of osseous resorption is significantly less in intensity and distribution. By 14 days postoperatively the osseous reaction is of a predominantly osteoblastic nature. The periodontal ligament area, however, shows some resorptive activity at 8 to 10 days; it is not prolonged and begins a reversal pattern at 14 days. It is essentially normal in character at 21 to 28 days with the presence of osteoid tissue at the crestal and radicular aspects of the alveolar process. Bone on the opposite side of the tooth shows no evidence of significant osteoclastic or osteoblastic influence throughout the healing phases. Final healing indicates that repair of the graft at the dentogingival junction proceeds without eventual deformity.

The clinical implications of available healing studies relating to autogenous gingival grafts establish the concept that there is definite biologic acceptance, attachment, and incorporation of the tissue by adjacent tissues with no evidence of graft rejection. It would appear that success of the procedure depends primarily on the qualities of donor and receptor tissues. Transplanted gingival tissue should be thin and as closely approximated to the underlying connective tissue bed as possible to facilitate fluid diffusion, rapid clot resorption, and early bridging from the receptor periosteum to the graft by a vascular and connective tissue complex. The presence of any significant space between the connective tissue surfaces may result in hemorrhage or exudation that could limit the initial hydration and nutrition of the graft that are essential during the first 2 to 3 days after surgery. Should this occur, a delay in revascularization is possible, with consequent partial or total necrosis of the transplanted tissue. Graft epithelium may degenerate and be desquamated during the first 2 to 3 days; if this occurs, a new epithelium will regenerate over the graft within several days. Epithelial desquamation does not necessarily indicate failure of the procedure. Finally, a graft should not be placed upon an avascular surface, since fluid diffusion during the first 48 hours (or longer) serves to keep the tissue ''vital.'' Placing a graft, for example, over a large avascular root area increases the potential for partial or total

necrosis and thus failure of attachment. This factor becomes a significant consideration when planning for the repair of denuded root regions, as it has been demonstrated that only in those cases where the lesions are 2 mm or less in depth and width can predictable root coverage be expected. A cortical area of denuded bone is also an unfavorable receptor area not only because it cannot provide a fluid source but also because it *cannot predictably* elaborate the reparative tissue required for graft attachment. It has been reported that free autogenous gingival autografts placed over alveolar bone do survive and eventually exhibit less mobility than those placed over loosely attached periosteum. The report does not, however, indicate precisely what the nature of the bony surface was or whether any decortication was undertaken prior to graft placement. It would seem important to know whether a blood supply emanating from the endosteum could be developed rapidly enough to help sustain the graft's vitality in the initial stages of healing.

Connective tissue autograft

There is accumulating evidence based on human and animal studies that autogenous gingival dense connective tissue may be used successfully in gingival reconstructive procedures in lieu of the classically described gingival (epithelium-connective tissue) autograft. The dense collagenous tissue may be obtained from the inner aspects of palatal flaps, edentulous ridge flaps, or retromolar and tuberosity areas and transplanted to properly prepared mucogingival receptor sites. Tissue obtained in this manner permits total closure of the donor site wound after the tissue has been removed and obviates many of the postsurgical complications that may be associated with the open wounds left at the donor site when classically described techniques are used.

For the most part the healing processes are similar to those seen in gingival autograft procedures. Epithelialization commences at the surrounding mucosal and gingival margins of the receptor site at about the second or third postoperative day and progresses centripetally until initial epithelialization is complete on the seventh to tenth day. Keratinization, which is accompanied by typical changes in surface character and color of the graft, commences about 4 weeks postoperatively. It is believed that the keratinization process is not only phenotypically determined but also related to the nature of the connective tissue substrate. Thus the keratinization process seen with this procedure may be associated with the increased collagen density of the connective tissue substrate, reduction of the matrical element, decreased vascularity and fluid content, and the progressive abatement of the surgical inflammatory reaction.

It has been substantially postulated that the nature of nonkeratinizing epithelium, that is, the junctional epithelium, is related to a "disturbed" connective tissue substrate that is seen with inflammation. In addition alterations in physical environment may also have an effect. Epithelium in contact with teeth does not normally display a keratinizing effect, and yet should a tooth be moved orthodontically and the unkeratinized junctional epithelium exposed to the oral environment, it will soon become keratinized. The precise mechanisms of this phenomenon are not clear, but it may well be that connective tissue status influences the character of the epithelium.

It may be further postulated that epithelial enzyme synthesis and activity are also related to the variable collagenous nature of adjacent connective tissue. Histochemically, keratinizing epithelia are known to elaborate acid hydrolases (for example, nonspecific esterases, acid phosphatases), while nonkeratinizing epithelia do not. In fact nonkeratinizing epithelia exhibit mainly oxidative enzyme activity. This occurrence is even more interesting since nonkeratinizing epithelia have loose connective tissue substrates, while keratinizing epithelia rest on dense connective tissue. Should the character of the connective tissue substrate affect the availability of nutrient and hydrating fluids to the epithelium, it may be inferred that keratinization and hydrolytic enzyme activity of gingival epithelium are related to the diminished vascularization of the tissue's corium. On the other hand, lack of keratinization and predominantly oxidative enzyme activity may be associated with more elaborate vascularization of the connective tissue substrate and increased hydration and nutrition to the epithelium. Therefore keratinization may be looked upon as a degenerative process induced by properties of the connective tissue substrate.

PERIOSTEAL FENESTRATION

The periosteal fenestration technique is generally employed today as an adjunct to the free gingival autograft procedure. In this context the incision and separation of periosteum at or near the apical margin of the graft may induce fixation of the border of the grafted tissue to underlying periosteum and bone. This is especially required where the vestibular fornix is shallow and the alveolar mucosa unduly movable in relationship to subjacent cortical bone and periosteum and where the presence of intramucosal musculature requires not only control of its activity but also its obviation, as it is a barrier to "gingival" development at the site.

Analyses of the histostructure of alveolar mucosa, including its interface with adjacent periosteum and bone, reveal that the mucosal complex is composed of randomly oriented collagen and reticular fibers, rarely in bundle array, dispersed with blood vessels, tissue fluids, and protein-polysaccharide ground substance. It is surmounted by nonkeratinizing epithelium (a quality largely determined by the physical consistency of the connective tissue) and is tenuously linked to contiguous periosteum. A salient feature of alveolar mucosa is the inclusion either of the *body* of facial or accessory masticatory musculature or of the confluence of their fascial insertions with periosteum. When one applies these findings to clinical practice it should be apparent that to convert mucosa to a "gingival equivalent" tissue it would be necessary to dissect and displace mucosa from its periosteal attachment as a prelude to gingival autografting procedures, thus eliminating the soft, pliable, muscle-encumbered barrier to gingival development. Such a dissection, which exposes periosteum, also permits the necessary participation of periosteum in the postsurgical healing process.

The linkage between periosteum and bone in the area of alveolar mucosa often appears to be structurally inferior. Evaluations of the external aspects of buccal, labial, and lingual osseous septa, in juxtarelationship to mucosa's periosteum, indicate that these aspects of the alveolar processes are constituted of cortical bone, often inordinately thick and dense in the adult, with a sparse number of communications via vascular channels between periosteal and endosteal phases of the septum. The fiber-mediated attachment of periosteum to such bone is notable for the paucity of fibers, including their narrow diameters, shallowness, and relative diffuseness of insertion. The inferior nature of the periosteum-bone attachment becomes more marked as the distance from the mucogingival junction becomes greater. Thus on a clinical level the mobility of periosteum related to bone becomes more apparent as the vestibular fornix is approached.

Although extensive and detailed analyses of the

postoperative effects of periosteal fenestration are few, it may be reasonably inferred from the studies of Carranza and Melcher that subperiosteal deposition of reparative tissue will occur lateral to the slitlike periosteal window, eventuating as fibrosis (increased connective tissue density) of the periosteal component with concomitant conversion of the innermost portion of periosteum, that contiguous to the face of the septa, to osteoid mineralizing to bone. Ruben has noted comparable transformation in the nature of periosteum and its linkage to bone in surgical procedures where periosteum is left in situ (i.e., free gingival graft, periosteal retention procedure, split-mucosal flap, and so on). It may be reasonably concluded that in the region of alveolar mucosa, periosteal preservation in situ is fundamental not only to the maintenance of the primary, variably tenuous periosteum-bone bond, but also to its postsurgical enhancement. The superimposition of periosteal fenestration may not only improve the tenacity of periosteal-bone attachment but also may lead, in the healing of the surgical rent, to the formation of granulation tissue, which will serve not only to repair the fenestration, but also to strongly bind overlying tissue (i.e., gingival autograft, split-mucosal flap) to both periosteum and bone. It is on these biologically based premises that we proposed the clinical employment of the combined surgical procedure—split-mucosal flap with periosteal fenestration—to provide security of posttherapeutic attachment of mucosa by "scar tissue" to subjacent periosteum and bone. Ancillary benefits that may be derived include negation of muscle influence, deepening of the vestibular fold, and augmented fibrosis and attachment of periosteum to cortical bone. Periosteal fibrosis may also teleologically serve as a structural barrier to the spread of inflammatory exudates within periosteum and at the periosteum-bone interface should inflammation again ensue, thus tending to "contain" the inflammatory process.

OSSEOUS AND MARROW AUTOGRAFTS

The use of free or contiguous osseous autografts for the correction and reestablishment of a portion of the attachment apparatus previously lost through periodontal disease has recently received much attention. In the past, numerous substances such as plaster of paris, ivory, calcium phosphate, and inorganic heterogenous bone have been used, all with equally poor results. Inorganic bone did not appear to induce osteogenesis unless in intimate contact with the host bone and did not appear to be predictably nonantigenic, whereas other materials caused a foreign body reaction to occur, resulting in exfoliation of the implant with attendant severe inflammation. Implanted calcium salts were rapidly removed via the lymphatics and circulatory channels. These substances neither formed an osteogenic base nor provided a source of calcium salts for young proliferative connective tissue required for the formation and calcification of newly forming bone. Research in the field indicates that the production of new bone is the result of active periosteal, endosteal, and marrow cells rather than fibroblasts that have other specific functions.

The types of procedures used clinically are distinguished according to their vascularization. In the first instance the osseous tissue being transplanted has been completely severed from its blood supply (free osseous tissue autograft), whereas in the other type of procedure the vascular supply is retained with the tissue (contiguous osseous tissue autograft).

The process of repair of a contiguous osseous autograft is one of conjecture. The possibilities include (1) ankylosis, (2) reattachment, and (3) transplant resorption utilized for the formation of new bone.

There also exists a relative paucity of histologic studies in the periodontal literature regarding the healing of autogenous bone grafts. It has seemed reasonable to assume that healing in the oral cavity would not differ markedly from that observed in other areas where transplantation of osseous material has been widely used. Clinical grafting techniques for reestablishing the coronal aspect of the attachment apparatus have been directed toward the use of compact bone, cancellous bone, and hematopoietic bone marrow. A considerable amount of discussion has evolved concerning the fate of each of these implant materials.

When a graft of compact bone is placed in a freshly prepared recipient site, most of the osteocytes present die, with the possible exception of the surface osteocytes. Once the blood supply has been severed, osteocytes must obtain all their nourishment via tissue fluids through canaliculi. Therefore only those osteocytes that are close to functioning capillaries or tissue fluid will survive. Osteocytes present near the surface under these conditions have the best opportunity for continued existence in newly transplanted bone. In addition, the osteogenic cells in a surface position have a better opportunity for survival, since they are contiguous to and immersed in tissue fluids. Theoretically it is possible that the dead osteocytes release during cytolysis an inductive organic substance capable of promoting osteogenesis in the underlying connective tissue. Although the surface cells may survive and possibly contribute to osteogenesis, most of the active bone formation comes from the area and milieu into which the graft has been placed. This process appears to occur by the proliferation of cells from the osteogenic layer (cambium) of periosteum, endosteum, and marrow of the host bone that are brought outwardly in granulation tissue toward the graft forming new trabeculae that eventually unite with the graft. After the union of graft and host the general processes of resorption and replacement occur concurrently. Resorption takes place both along the outer surfaces of the transplant between areas where the trabeculae of new bone have become joined and on the inner surfaces of haversian canals. Little resorption occurs along the walls of the graft's haversian canals until these areas have functional blood vessels secured by ingrowth of granulation tissue; this process may not ensue for several weeks. A functional vasculature is necessary for resorption, deposition, and maintenance of bone. Graft "turnover" may take a considerable amount of time to occur; nonviable bone must be resorbed from a free surface, whereas new osseous tissue must also be deposited on a free surface.

Although the chance of osteocyte survival is no greater in a cancellous bone transplant than in a compact graft, the possibilities of endurance and growth of the covering and lining cells of cancellous fragments is considerably greater than that of compact bone. Osteocytes, however, do not survive in this situation even if the cancellous trabeculae are transplanted into an area close to functioning capillaries, since the circulatory mechanism within the bone is insignificant and inadequate. Covering and lining cells survive and grow, since the cancellous trabeculae are covered with osteogenic cells; there exists therefore a high proportion of surface cells (osteoblasts) to bone cells (osteocytes).

In compact bone the opposite situation occurs, since a poor surface cell population is present. This situation is especially true relative to bone chips. Stimulation of host osteogenic cells, osteoblasts, and undifferentiated mesenchymal cells to initiate growth into the graft and lay down bone on their many surfaces may be induced by existing cancellous bone and tooth fragments. Both dentin and cementum have been implicated as furnishing loci of bone formation. Cancellous fragments may also create new centers for osteogenesis if these are transplanted into an area with an adequate vascular bed that provides surface cells with sufficient tissue fluid.

Histologic studies relating to the healing of periodontal lesions with the use of autogenous marrow are scarce. Although this approach has recently received widespread clinical attention and use, the mechanism by which osteogenesis is stimulated remains unclear.

In theory, autogenous hematopoietic bone marrow would appear to be an ideal implant substance. It provides both a nonantigenic bony scaffolding, since it contains fragments of trabecular bone and large numbers of viable cellular elements that could augment the potential for "take" or reorganization of the area into which it is placed. It has been speculated that bone may be expected to generate from several possible sources, including (1) bone spicules within the graft, (2) endosteum not separated from the marrow, (3) marrow cells themselves, and (4) the receptor site tissue. Although it has been a consistent finding that hematopoietic marrow stimulates bone formation when transplanted, the exact mechanism by which this occurs is as yet unclear. At the present level of knowledge, there is little justification for the view that bone spicules alone may be primarily implicated as a source for bone formation in hematopoietic marrow grafting. Bony spicules that are produced by fragmentation of trabeculae provide limited opportunity for cellular survival and may not supply an osteogenic source for new bone formation; their osteocytes are noncontributory. The endosteum of the donor site may be introduced with the marrow graft and act as a possible source of osteogenic cells. The undifferentiated mesenchymal cells of the donor tissue (the stem cell of the marrow) may differentiate into osteoblasts at the recipient area to form new osseous tissue. The undifferentiated mesenchymal cells differentiate into osteoblasts, when transplanted, because of an uncertain stimulatory material. This stimulus may be the inductive effect of damaged recipient bone tissues upon the cells; it may be the removal of an inhibitory system present within the progenitor marrow that prevents these cells from differentiating into osteoblasts; or it may be an inductive mechanism present in the recipient site that leads to osteoblastic proliferation. The fourth concept indicates that the donor marrow cells may undergo disruption and liberate an inductor substance that acts as a stimulus for the undifferentiated mesenchymal cells of the receptor site to differentiate into osteoblasts. RNA polymers have been considered as inductor agents.

Marrow obtained from the maxillary tuberosity region and lateral or posterior superior iliac crest are often comparable and appear to lend themselves well to autogenous implantation into periodontal defects. The tuberosity area offers greater operative convenience and patient acceptance, and the clinical results, in contained or semicontained lesions, may be prognostically equal. The incidence of hematopoietic marrow in tuberosity bone in the adult is minimal at best.

The scarcity of histologic material available on marrow grafts suggests the regeneration of a new periodontal ligament, to a previously exposed root surface, as well as of alveolar bone. Hypercementosis may occur at the graft site when the root has

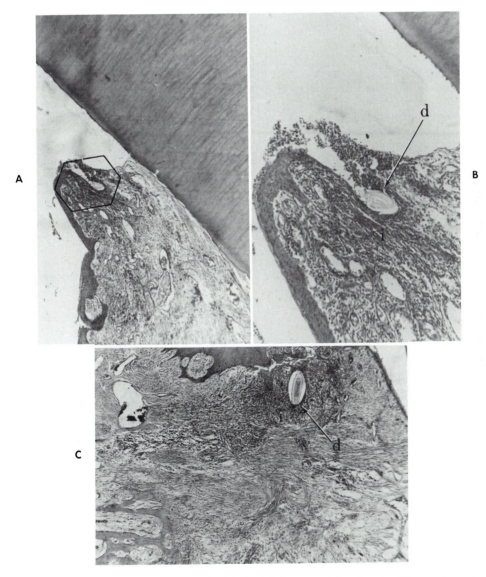

Fig. 23-48. Foreign substances imbedded, *d,* into wound, leading to inflammatory reaction, *i,* and retarded epithelialization. Epithelium will not migrate into deep tissue faults, over areas of debris impaction, *d,* or over sharp irregular projections of tissue. Note intense accrual of inflammatory cells (and by inference, exudate) around impacted debris, *d,* in **B** and **C.** Such reactions may also be associated with unresorbed suture material, particularly gut type, that may persist up to 60 days in tissue.

been extensively planed prior to the implant. The possibility of active root resorption in the region of the implants has been another finding. The stimulatory activity of the transplant material may possibly be overreactive to the point of being undesirable; as in other dynamic reparative tissues (periosteum, marrow, periodontal ligament), primordial cells may eventuate with either formative or resorptive capacities. With the availability of long-term studies, it may be possible to have a clear understanding of the dynamics of marrow graft wound healing as well as the ultimate fate of the grafted material itself.

COMPLICATIONS OF HEALING PROCESS AFTER PERIODONTAL SURGERY

In the majority of instances healing after periodontal surgery progresses uneventfully and efficiently with acquisition of treatment objectives. At times postsurgical problems arise that retard healing, promote continuance of inflammation, induce necrotic or hyperplastic responses, generate malformations and tumorlike lesions, or are associated with postoperative bleeding or exudation, and so on. In a general context, a few of the prominent ways of obviating undesirable sequelae to therapy include applicable and careful as well as skillful surgical technique leading to smooth wound surfaces free of dedritus, intimate coaptation and adaptation of gingival and mucosal flaps to receptor areas, postoperative protection and reinforcement of the tissues, prevention and control of infection, minimization of bone exposure and manipulation consistent with treatment rationale, and preservation of periosteal integrity. The following discussion of the more prevalent and unwanted ill effects and their causation may be of assistance in clinical practice (Figs. 23-48 to 23-51).

Retarded epithelialization. Retarded epithelialization after curettage, gingivectomy-gingivoplasty, mucoperiosteal flaps, and so on may be productive of chronic ulceration or erosion. This circumstance may be due to (1) rough and irregular wound surfaces and tissue tags, producing a situation wherein epithelial cells are retarded in their migration by morphologic tissue faults; (2) foreign substances embedded in the wound (such as caiculus, tooth fragments, bacterial plaque, food, bristles of tooth brush, hair, and periodontal dressing); (3) donor epithelium required for re-epithelialization is distant to the wound site with temporal delay in epithelial coverage; and (4)

hyperplastic connective tissue substratum due to the production of irregular granulation tissue or infection, etc. The consequent *clinical effects* include bleeding and exudation, necrotic surface with fibrinomembranous cover, irregular hyperplastic hyperemic and edamatous tissue, and discomfort.

Failure of epithelial keratinization. Epithelium fails to exhibit keratinization when the connective tissue edge of the incision is in alveolar mucosa or a comparable zone. It is located in a soft, pliable, movable tissue with or without included musculature. There appears to be a direct relationship between connective tissue density, rigidity, tightness of bond to underlying bone, etc. and clinical quality of epithelial surface. With densely collagenated, well-organized tissue, diminished vascularization and consequent decreased hydra-

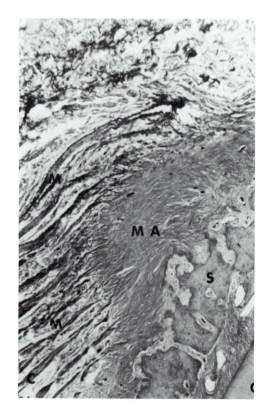

Fig. 23-49. High muscle insertion with dense fibrous attachment to bone. *M,* Muscle; *MA,* thick periosteum, furnishing fibrous attachment of muscle to bone septum; *S,* bone; *C,* tooth. Failure to excise or detach and properly apically reposition muscle may be responsible for postoperative flap evulsion by virtue of muscle activity. Bulkiness of tissue complex may inhibit proper apical displacement and attachment.

tion favor the acquisition of a *clinically* "keratinizing" surface.

Donor epithelium may *not* be available for early coverage of the surgical site. Since epithelial cells migrate over smooth wound surfaces at the rate of 0.5 to 1 mm per day, broad exposure of connective tissue may lead to a protracted period of reepithelialization. During this time inflammation will persist within unepithelialized gingival or partially epithelialized mucosal connective tissue with both hyperplastic and resorptive sequelae. For example, the tissue surface may become irregularly lobulated because of exuberant formation of granulation tissue. This tissue is easily damaged (e.g., by topical abrasive action of food), producing even greater tissue irregularity, pain, and bleeding. Such macerated tissue morphology will in turn prevent epithelial coverage. With the persistence of inflammation (usually chronic), bone resorption, effected primarily by periosteal cells, will continue to a variable degree. Loss of an osseous portion of the attachment apparatus may ensue. Thin bone septa are especially vulnerable to irreversible loss.

In this regard, for example, the mesiodistal extent of the wound in relationship to its superoinferior expanse should be considered together in the prognosis of the rapidity of wound epithelialization. A narrow area of surgical exposure of connective tissue will tend to be rapidly reveneered with epithelium. For example, a gingivoplasty site 5 mm wide occlusoapically, even though extending over a broad area mesiodistally, will be covered primarily by epithelium of apical (gingiva or alveolar mucosa) derivation, with primary completion of epithelialization at the sixth to tenth postsurgical day. On the other hand, a wound with a broad apico-occlusal dimension (e.g., 10 mm) with a mesiodistal extent over the area of the same number of teeth will not ordinarily be epithelialized until the eleventh to twentieth postsurgical day, despite the fact that there is centripetal migration of epithelial cells from donor sites occlusal, apical, mesial, and distal to the wound. The epithelial source may have been excised in performance of surgery and is perhaps too distant from the wound surface.

Epithelium will not display its keratinizing potential when in the association or contact with a dental surface or restoration. For example, if re-

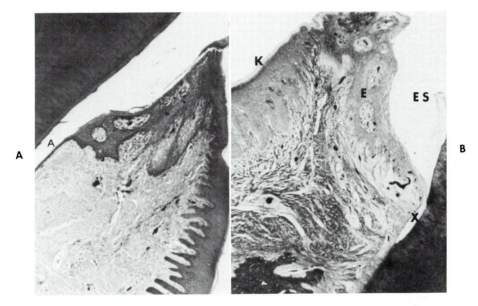

Fig. 23-50. Failure of tissue flap to reattach to tooth. **A,** Note space between soft tissue and tooth, *A.* **B,** No reattachment, *X,* in a full-thickness flap. Thirty-one days after procedure. Sulcular epithelium, *E;* keratinized epithelium, *K.* Flap has been placed coronally on enamel at *X* in **B** and partially on enamel in **A.** There is a growing body of evidence that reattachment of gingival corium to root surface and bone is reliant at cervical area of root upon reparative potential (with outgrowing granulation tissue) of periodontal ligament and available endosteum and periosteum. This "outgrowth" from attachment apparatus sources rarely exceeds 1.5 to 2 mm, thus minimizing or obviating gingival reattachment beyond this distance.

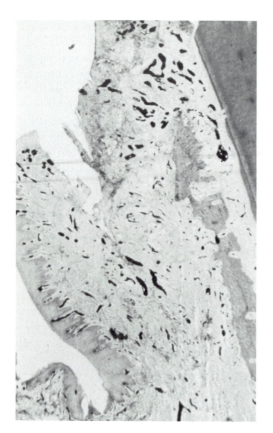

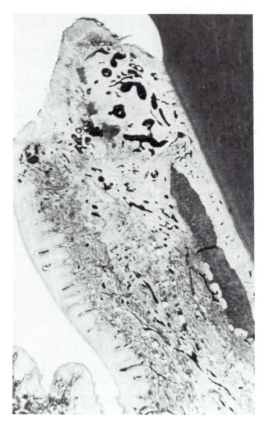

Fig. 23-51. Poor adaptation of split-thickness flap to receptor site leading to cleavage at interface zone. Notice resorption of thin buccal septum of bone despite fact that it was not exposed by surgery. At upper portion of specimen there is vascular mass of unepithelialized granulation tissue; since flap was displaced, primary epithelial source was unavailable. Such problems may be affiliated with suture breakage, movement of periodontal dressing, inclusion of muscle mass within flap without adequate provision for securing in new site, and so on.

Fig. 23-52. Flap detachment from receptor zone. Area occupied by hyperplastic and edematous tissue resembling pyogenic granuloma. May lead to poor tissue form when healing is more advanced.

generated interdental tissues after surgery approximate the contact areas of teeth, the keratinizing effect will not be manifest where the epithelium is in apposition to the tooth, and the morphology and epithelial characteristics of the col will be recreated.

Other factors detrimental to keratinization may include the presence of bacterial plaque or debris with continuing inflammation, the conditions previously indicated as responsible for retarded epithelization, and systemic influences such as hyperestrogenism, hypoestrogenism, pregnancy, vitamin B complex deficiency, and pernicious anemia. It may be difficult to precisely incriminate somatic factors unless other more frank or pathognomonic clinical or laboratory manifestations are

evident. The *clinical effects* include a smooth and shiny gingival surface that is hyperemic, turgid, and so on rather than pink, stippled, "dry," and coarse. The usual sharp demarcation between attached gingiva and alveolar mucosa may be dulled or obviated because of the change in tissue texture and topical qualities.

Flap displacement and evulsion. Flap displacement and evulsion (Figs. 23-52 and 23-53) may occur as a result of retardation or failure of the tissue flap to reattach to bone or tooth and marginal aspect of the periodontal ligament, for example, the mucoperiosteal flap may be situated over highly cortical bone; the coronal portion of the flap may be placed on enamel or on cementum at an inordinate distance from the periodontal ligament and the marrow areas of crestal bone. It should be stressed that coronally or laterally directed proliferation of regenerative tissue from the periodontal ligament or crestal bone is generally limited to 1 to 1.5 mm and that flap or graft attachment to tooth (dentin or cementum) beyond

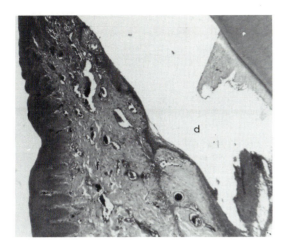

Fig. 23-53. Full-thickness flap, *f,* displaced, *d,* due to suture breakage early in healing process. Flaps should not be approximated to enamel at time of surgery. At best, epithelialized or incompletely epithelialized crevice will result, often in tenuous adherence to enamel, lending to tissue retractability and intracrevicular accumulation of bacterial plaque and debris.

this limit is both unpredictable in occurrence and tenuous in quality.

Additional factors that may be responsible for ectopic flap position include the inadequate adaptation of the tissue complex to underlying receptor area occurring as a result of an inadequate number of sutures or their improper placement, suture breakage, or pack displacement or loss. Hematoma or undue accrual of exudate may exist between flap and tooth/bone or periosteum, in the case of a partial-thickness flap, and raise the tissue flap from its approximation to the recipient zone.

The clinical reflection of such an occurrence may include the development of poor or undesirable tissue form, the presence of hyperplastic unepithelialized granulation tissue at marginal and interdental areas, shallowing of vestibular extension and inadequacy of zone of attached gingiva, retarded healing and continuance of inflammation and periodontal pockets, and bone and periosteal exposure with resorption and necrosis.

Bone exposure. The untoward postsurgical sequelae of bone exposure may be caused by deficiencies of vascularization. Ordinarily periosteal preservation in situ or flap replacement onto bone, after exposure, provide microvascular sources of hydrating and nutritive fluids that are sufficient to minimize (but not obviate) resorption, necrosis, and sequestration. Resorptive and necrotizing

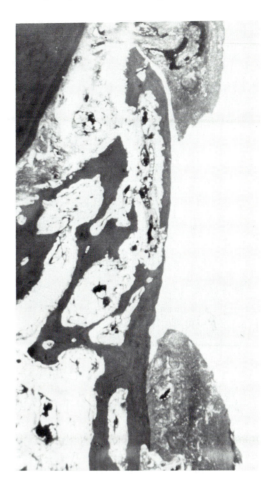

Fig. 23-54. Extensive endosteal bone resorption coincident with flap necrosis and bone exposure. Thin cortex may sequester, resulting in substantial thinning of septum and loss of bone height. Note striking resorptive changes, not only within osseous septum, but also in zone of periodontal ligament (top left). Inflammatory exudate has "destroyed" this portion of periodontal ligament, including its reparative potential.

bone changes are especially notable where bony septa are very thin; labile bone sites are commonly encountered, for example, where manidibular and maxillary cuspid roots are prominent because of tooth placement or root curvature (Fig. 23-54). Such bone has a diminished vascular supply internally because of its cortical nature (with few marrow spaces) and may be left when shorn of periosteum with only a blood supply from adjacent periodontal ligament. This reduced vascularization may be inadequate for the sustenance of viable bone cells or hydration of bone's crystal structure. Resorption of the cortical plate may occur from the periodontal ligament or, where cortex overlies marrow areas, from endosteal tissue. At times,

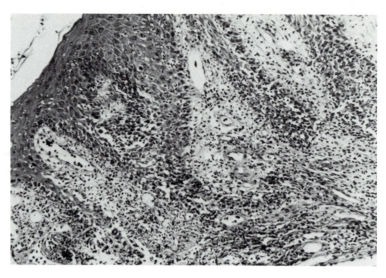

Fig. 23-55. Pyogenic granuloma. Epithelium is hyperplastic with considerable intercellular edema, lysis of its basal (and other) cells, and intraepithelial penetration of leukocytes. Intense inflammatory infiltrate consists largely of neutrophils. Collagen resorption and edema are marked. Such reactions are usually allied to calculus, plaque, or debris impaction, intrusion of particles of periodontal dressing, and bacterial or fungal infection.

sequestration of thin septa or cortices may occur with loss of valuable support for the tooth.

Periodontal abscesses, pyogenic granulomas, and giant cell reparative granulomas. *Postoperative infection* is an uncommon complication of periodontal surgery. It appears that infection is more likely to occur in association with bone exposure, flap displacement, where periodontal lesions are the result of pulp degeneration, in association with sutures and particles of impacted dedritus, in areas of tissue laceration and impaired vascularization, and where calculus and bacterial plaque have been accidentally impacted into the tissues (Figs. 23-55 and 23-56). There is incomplete but convincing evidence also that certain systemic disease states enhance the potential for postoperative infection; these include diabetes mellitus, atherosclerosis, and malignancy. Also, therapeutic use of antineoplastic and immunosuppressive drugs and corticosteroids may increase the potential for infection and impairment of wound healing. There is a growing fund of evidence that diabetes mellitus, especially in its juvenile-onset form, leads to defects in both cellular and humoral (antibody) immunity, encouraging infective processes and aberrant and retarded healing. The rapidity of progress of periodontal inflammation and thus the severity of the lesion may also be enhanced. The phagocytic functions of granulocytes and macrophages may also be compromised in diabetes mellitus, lower-

ing the tissue defenses against microbiologic agents. The "lazy phagocytic syndrome" has recently been allied to the inadequacy of entrance of nutrients into the cells. Insulin is necessary for this process; thus insulin deficiencies can lead to cellular malnutrition. Corticosteroids (e.g., prednisone) depress cellular (T cell) immunity and T cell assistance of humoral immunity (helper function). The primary effects of other chemotherapeutic substances (e.g., azathioprine) are upon B cell and plasma cell synthesis of antibody.

Pyogenic granulomas appear as florid, hyperplastic masses with a soft, often mushy, consistency. Their surfaces are ulcerative or erosive with formation of a fibrinomembranous cover. Bleeding and exudation are common, whereas discomfort is variable. Most of these lesions appear to be related to enclaved debris. Removal of the irritant and excision of the mass usually suffice for correction of the problem.

Periodontal abscesses comprise areas of tissue necrosis within gingiva, mucosa, or marrow and present as soft tissue enlargements due essentially to exudate accumulation. The mass may be diffuse or focal with a surrounding zone manifesting intense inflammatory characteristics; pain is variable, since neural filaments may be destroyed by enzymatic processes. The exudate may be responsible for considerable hard and soft tissue lysis; if bone and marrow are involved, resorption and sequestration may be found. The bacterial com-

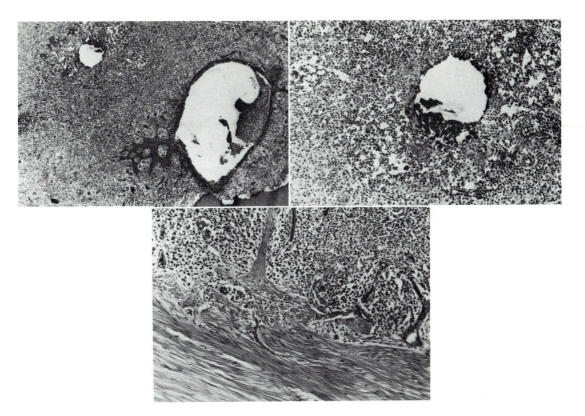

Fig. 23-56. Periodontal (gingival) abscess after surgery. Suture site (tissue void in photo) in gingival flap. Necrosis just adjacent to suture with surrounding severe inflammatory reaction.

ponents of the lesion are of a mixed nature; streptococci, staphylococci, filamentous strains, and gram-negative genera (such as *Veillonella* and *Bacteroides*) may individually, but usually conjointly, participate. Bacterial products—exotoxins and endotoxins—as well as the acid hydrolases of the neutrophilic tissue infiltrate may be responsible for the destructive character of the condition. In physically debilitated patients, fungi and unusual bacterial strains may be causative factors. More often than not, local factors consisting of many varieties of debris should be considered as the prime etiology.

Giant cell reparative granulomas constitute modified or aberrant healing responses with overproduction not only of connective tissue but also of blood vessels and overlying epithelium. The rapid expansion of the hyperplasia may also be inductive of overlying epithelial atrophy or subject the lesion to irritative or traumatic insult; ulceration and surface erosion with concomitant inflammation may supervene. Reparative granulomas are considered to be of periosteal origin and due primarily to encased foreign substances. The histopathology is noteworthy in that there are numerous multinucleated giant cells aligned in the periosteal phase of the lesion, at times associated with bone resorptive processes. These hyperplasias are of variable morphology and size, but most often tend to be sessile and lobulated, thus resembling a red raspberry, when affiliated with surgical wounds. Pain is not a consistent effect, and most lesions are noted by the surgeon during postoperative visits. Excisional biopsy to subjacent bone is required.

Increased tooth mobility. Tooth mobility often ensues after periodontal surgery. Excisional procedures, particularly with flap retraction and accompanying removal of interdental soft tissues, actually divest a tooth of gingival and periosteal support on a temporary basis. Although initial reattachment may be evident in the first 10 to 14 days after surgery, more advanced collagenation and renewal of the gingival attachment to tooth and bone may require 30 to 45 days or more. Mobility may persist, usually on a diminishing level, during this period.

More flagrant tooth movement, often with displacement, may occur if a rapid pattern of bone resorption, including loss of periodontal attachment, occurs. These unanticipated resorptive errors may take place as sequelae to bone denudation, the loss of thin but supportive septa by resorption, osteoplastic procedures of a traumatic or contaminated nature, postoperative infection including periodontal abscess and localized osteomyelitis, secondary occlusal traumatism, communication with periapical lesions of pulpal derivation, and periosteal necrosis accompanying local ischemia.

At times postoperative inflammation integral to the early phase of healing may be augmented or protracted. This may delay the onset of repair or it may extend the process into tissues directly fundamental to tooth attachment. For example, inflammatory reactions within the periodontal ligament leading to collagen and bone resorption, edema, fiber disorientation, and so on may be responsible for transitory tooth mobility. This inflammatory change may be extensive in association with treatment of infrabony pockets where manipulative procedures actually encroach on or are immediately adjacent to periodontal ligament and contiguous bone. In infrabony pocket therapy there is actual divestment of a transseptal fiber complex to expose bone, marrow, and periodontal ligament; deliberate attempts are made to expose these areas and thus encourage them to act as progenitor reservoirs for regenerative tissue. The inflammatory response may be profound, and the clinical consequences may be temporarily marked.

ACKNOWLEDGEMENT

Assisted by the investigative efforts of Dr. Waldyr Janson, Professor and Chairman, Department of Periodontology, Faculdade de Odontologia, Universidade de Sao Paulo at Bauru, Brazil; and Dr. Arthur B. Novaes, Faculdade de Odontologia, School of Dentistry, Ribeirao Preto, Brazil.

REFERENCES
General principles

Abell, R.: Permeability of blood capillary sprouts and newly formed blood capillaries, Am. J. Physiol. **147**:237, 1946.

Abercrombie, M.: Behavior of cells toward one another. In Montagna, W., and Billingham, R. E., editors: Advances in the biology of skin: wound heailng, New York, 1964, The Macmillan Co.

Alba, Z. C., and Ferrigno, P. D.: Postoperative healing in rat periodontium, Abstract no. 193, I.A.D.R. Program and abstract of papers, 1963.

Ambrose, E. J.: The surface properties of mammalian cells in culture. In The Proliferation and spread of neoplastic cells, Baltimore, 1968, The Williams & Wilkins Company, p. 23.

Ambrose, J. A., and Detmore, R. J.: Correlation of histologic and clinical findings in periodontal treatment, J. Periodontol. **31**:238, 1928.

Anderson, H. C.: Calcium accumulating vesicles in intercellular matrix of bone. In Hard tissue growth, repair, and remineralization, Ciba Symposium 11, Amsterdam, 1973, Associated Scientific Publishers.

Anderson, H., Heyden, G., and Fejerskov, O.: Histochemistry of the epithelium in excisional palatal wounds of guinea pigs, Scand. J. Dent. Res. **82**:588, 1974.

Angelakos, E. T., and King, M.: Histochemical demonstration of catecholamine uptake by adrenergic nerve fibers, J. Histochem. Cytochem. **13**:282, 1965.

Batchelor, J. R., Casey, T. A., Werb, A., et al.: HLA matching and corneal grafting, Lancet **1**:7959, 1976.

Beckwith, T. D., and Williams, A.: Regeneration of periodontal membrane in the cat, Proc. Soc. Exp. Biol. Med. **25**: 713, 1928.

Belanger, L. F.: Resorption of cementum by cementocyte activity ("cementolysis"), Calcif. Tissue Res **2**:229, 1968.

Bentley, J.: En vivo incorporation of labeled amino acids during early stages of collagen synthesis, Biochem. Biophys. Res. Commun. **10**:517, 1959.

Bernier, J. L., and Kaplan, H.: The repair of gingival tissue after surgical intervention, J. Am. Dent. Assoc. **35**:697, 1947.

Billingham, R.: The immunobiology of tissue transplantation, Int. Dent. J. **21**:478, 1971.

Birn, H.: The vascular supply of the periodontal membrane, J. Periodontol. **1**:51, 1966.

Block, P., Seiter, I., and Oehlert, W.: Autoradiographic studies of the initial cellular response to injury, Exp. Cell Res. **30**:311, 1963.

Box, H. K.: Studies in periodontal pathology, Toronto, 1924, Canadian Dental Research Foundation.

Brophy, D., and Lobitz, W.: Injury and reinjury to the human epidermis. II. Epidermal basal cell response, J. Invest. Dermatol. **32**:495, 1959.

Bullough, W. S., and Laurence, E. B.: The energy relations of epidermal mitotic activity adjacent to small wounds, Br. J. Exp. Pathol. **38**:278, 1957.

Bullough, W. S., and Laurence, E. B.: A technique for the study of small epidermal wounds, Br. J. Exp. Pathol. **38**: 273, 1957.

Butcher, E. O., and Klingsberg, J.: Age, gonadectomy and wound healing in the palatal mucosa of the rat, Oral Surg. **16**:484, 1963.

Cabrini, R. L., and Carranza, F. A., Jr.: Alkaline and acid phosphatase in gingival and tongue wounds of normal and vitamin C deficient animals, J. Periodontol. **34**:74, 1963.

Calman, J., and Davies, A.: The effect of methotrexate (Amethopterin) on wound healing. An experimental study, Br. J. Cancer **19**:505, 1965.

Carneiro, J., and de Moraes, F. F.: Radioautographic visualization of collagen metabolism in periodontal tissues of the mouse, Arch. Oral Biol. **10**:833, 1965.

Carneiro, J., and Leblond, G. P.: Role of osteoblasts and odontoblasts in secreting the collagen of bone and dentin, as shown by radioautography in mice given tritium-labelled glycine, Exp. Cell Res. **18**:291, 1959.

Carranza, F. A.: A technic for reattachment, J. Periodontol. **25**:272, 1954.

Carranza, F. A., Carranza, F. A., Jr., and Carraro, J. J.: Periodontal parodontal disease; local therapy, Int. Dent. J. **7**:209, 1957.

Carranza, F. A., Jr., and Cabrini, R. L.: Histoenzymatic behavior of healing wounds, J. Invest. Derm. **40**:27, 1963.

Carranza, F. A., Jr., and Cabrini, R. L.: The healing of oral wounds; a histoenzymatic analysis, Periodontics **1**:70, 1963.

Clemmesen, T.: The early circulation in split skin grafts, Acta Chir. Scand. **124**:11, 1962.

Converse, J. M., Ballantyne, D. L., Rogers, B. O., and Raisbeck, A. P.: Plasmatic circulation in skin grafts, Transplantation **4**:154, 1957.

Converse, J. M., and Rapaport, F. T.: The vascularization of skin autografts and homografts, Ann. Surg. **143**:306, 1956.

Crandon, J. H., Lennihan, R., et al.: Ascorbic acid economy in surgical patients, Ann. N. Y. Acad. Sci. **92**:246, 1961.

Cutright, D. E.: The proliferation of blood vessels in gingival wounds, J. Periodontol. **40**:137, 1969.

DeVito, R. V.: Healing of wounds, Surg. Clin. North Am. **45**:441, 1965.

Droz, B.: Fate of newly synthesized proteins in neurons. In Lebond, C. P., and Warren, K., editors: Radioautography in investigating protein synthesis, New York, 1965, Academic Press, Inc.

Droz, B., and Leblond, C. P.: Axonal migration of proteins in the central nervous system and peripheral nerves as shown by radioautography, J. Comp. Neurol. **121**:325, 1963.

Dunphy, J. E.: Repair of tissues after injury, Ann. N.Y. Acad. Sci. **73**:426, 1958.

Dunphy, J. E., and Udupa, K. N.: Chemical and histochemical sequences in normal healing of wounds, N. Engl. J. Med. **253**:847, 1955.

Eastoe, J. E.: Composition of collagen and allied proteins. In Ramachandran, G. N., editor: Treatise on collagen, vol. 1, New York, 1967, Academic Press, Inc.

Edel, A.: Clinical evaluation of free connective tissue grafts to increase width of keratinised gingiva, J. Clin. Periodontol. **1**:185, 1974.

Editorial: Dacron used as synthetic fascia in reconstruction of coracoacromial ligaments. In What's happening in medicine, Postgrad. Med. **55**:40, 1974.

Ellegaard, B., Karring, T., and Löe, H.: The fate of vital and devitalized bone grafts in healing of interradicular lesions, J. Periodont. Res. **10**:88, 1975.

Engler, W., Ramfjord, S. O., and Hiniker, J.: Healing following simple gingivectomy. A tritiated thymidine radioautographic study. I. Epithelialization, J. Periodontol. **37**:36, 1966.

Epstein, W., and Sullivan, D.: Epidermal mitotic activity in wounded human skin. In Montagna, W., and Billingham, R. E., editors: Advances in biology of skin, vol. 5, New York, 1964, The Macmillan Co.

Fawcett, D. W.: The fine structure of capillaries, arterioles and small arteries. In Reynolds, S. R. M., and Zweifach, B., editors: The microcirculation, Urbana, 1959, University of Illinois Press.

Fisch, U.: Lymphography of the cervical lymphatic system, Philadelphia, 1968, W. B. Saunders Co.

Freedman, E.: A preliminary report on pigskin grafts in oral surgery, Int. J. Oral Surg. **3**:269, 1974.

Freidenstein, A., and Kurolesova, A.: Osteogenic precursor cells of bone marrow in radiation chimeras, Transplantation **12**:99, 1971.

Freidenstein, A., and Lalykina, K.: Lymphoid cell populations are competent systems for induced osteogenesis, Calcif. Tissue Res. **4**:105, 1970.

Fullmer, H.: Collagenase and periodontal diseases, J. Dent. Res. **50**(suppl.):290, 1971.

Fullmer, H. M.: The histochemistry of the connective tissues, Int. Rev. Connect. Tissue Res. **3**:1, 1965.

Fullmer, H. M., and Gibson, W.: Collagenolytic activity in gingiva of man, Nature **209**:728, 1966.

Galbreath, J. C., and Hinds, E. C.: Steroids and antibiotics in wound healing, Abstract no. 195, I.A.D.R. Program and abstract of papers, 1963.

Garrett, J. S.: Cementum in periodontal disease, Periodont. Abstr. **23**:6, 1975.

Gelfant, S.: Initiation of mitosis in relation to the cell division cycle, Exp. Cell Res. **26**:395, 1962.

Gelfant, S.: The energy requirements for mitosis, Ann. N.Y. Acad. Sci. **90**:536, 1960.

Genco, R.: Immunoglobulins and periodontal disease, J. Periodontol. **41**:196, 1970.

Glickman, I., Turesky, S. S., and Manhold, J. H.: The oxygen consumption of healing gingiva, J. Dent. Res. **29**:429, 1950.

Glucksmann, A.: Cell turnover in the dermis. In Montagna, W., and Billingham, R. E., editors: Advances in biology of skin, vol. 5, New York, 1964, The Macmillan Co.

Glucksmann, A., Howard, A., and Pelc, S. R.: The uptake of radioactive sulphate by cells, fibres and ground substance of mature and developing connective tissue in the adult mouse, J. Anat. **90**:478, 1956.

Goldberg, M., and Callender, R.: Hydrocortisone and healing and repair, J. Dent. Res. **40**:675, 1961.

Gottlieb, B.: The new concept of periodontoclasia, J. Periodontol. **17**:7, 1946.

Gould, B. S.: Collagen biosynthesis. In Gould, B. S., editor: Treatise on collagen, vol. 2, part A, New York, 1968, Academic Press, Inc.

Gould, B. S.: Ascorbic acid and collagen fiber formation, Vitam. Horm. **8**:89,. 1960.

Grant, L.: The sticking and emigration of white blood cells in inflammation. In Zweifach, B. W., Grant, L., and McCluskey, R. T., editors: The inflammatory process, New York, 1965, Academic Press, Inc.

Greenlee, T. K., Jr., Ross, R., and Hartman, J. L.: The fine structure of elastic fibers, J. Cell Biol. **30**:59, 1966.

Grillo, H. C.: Derivation of fibroblasts in the healing wound, Arch. Surg. **88**:218, 1964.

Grillo, H. C.: Aspects of the origin, synthesis, and evolution of fibrous tissue in repair. In Montagna, W., and Billingham, R. E., editors: Advances in biology of skin, vol. 5, New York, 1964, The Macmillan Co.

Grillo, H. C., Watts, M. B., et al.: Studies in wound healing. I. Contraction and wound contents, Ann. Surg. **148**:145, 1958.

Gross, J.: Studies on the formation of collagen. IV. Effect of vitamin C deficiency on the neutral salt-extractible collagen of skin, J. Exp. Med. **109**:557, 1959.

Henning, F. R.: Epithelial mitotic activity after gingivectomy, J. Periodont. Res. **4**:319, 1969.

Hershon, L. E.: Elaboration of hyalouronidase and chondroitin sulfatase by microorganisms inhabiting the gingival sulcus: evaluation of a screening method for periodontal disease, J. Periodontol. **42**:34, 1971.

Hiatt, W. H., and Schallhorn, R. G.: Human allografts of iliac cancellous bone and marrow in periodontal osseous defects. I. Rationale and methodology, J. Periodontol. **42**:642, 1971.

Hiatt, W. H., Solomons, C. C., and Butler, E. D.: The induction of new bone and cementum formation. II. Utilizing a collagen extract of ox bone, J. Periodontol. **41**:274, 1970.

Holthuis, A.: Free autogenous gingival grafting in periodontal therapy, Periodont. Abstr. **22**:103, 1974.

Horton, J., Raisz, L., et al.: Bone resorbing activity in super-natant fluid from cultured peripheral blood lymphocytes, Science **177**:793, 1972.

Howes, E.: The rate and nature of epithelization in wounds with loss of substance, Surg. Gynec. Obstet. **76**:738, 1943.

Hunt, T. K., Twomey, S., et al.: Respiratory gas tensions and pH in healing wounds, Am. J. Surg. **114**:302, 1967.

Hurley, L. A., Stinchfield, F. E., et al.: Role of soft tissues in osteogenesis, J. Bone Joint Surg. **41A**:1243, 1956.

Hurst, R.: Regeneration of periodontal and transeptal fibers after autografts in rhesus monkeys: a qualitative approach, J. Dent. Res. **51**(suppl. 5):1183, 1972.

Hyden, H.: The neuron. In Brachet, J., and Mirsky, A. E., editors: The cell, vol. 4, New York, 1961, Academic Press, Inc.

Ivanyi, L., and Lehner, T.: Stimulation of lymphocyte trans-formation by bacterial antigens in patients with periodontal disease, Arch. Oral Biol. **15**:1089, 1970.

Jackson, L., Wallace, S., Farb, S. N., and Parke, W. W.: Cervical lymphography, Laryngoscope **73**:926, 1963.

Janson, W., Ruben, M. P., Kramer, G. M., and Bloom, A. A.: Development of blood supply to split thickness, free gingival autograft, J. Periodontol. **40**:707, 1969.

Joseph, J., and Townsend, J.: The healing of defects in im-mobile skin in rabbits, Br. J. Surg. **48**:557, 1961.

Karring, T., Ostergaard, E., and Löe, H.: Conservation of tissue specificity after heterotopic transplantation of gingiva and alveolar mucosa, J. Periodont. Res. **6**:282, 1971.

Kellen, E. E., and Gorlin, R. J.: Effect of diphenylhydantoin sodium and analogue on wound healing, J. Dent. Res. **39**:665, 1960.

Kinmonth, J. B.: Lymphangiography in man, Clin. Sci. **11**:13, 1952.

Kohl, J. T., and Zander, H. A.: Morphology of interdental gingival tissues, Oral Surg. **14**:287, 1961.

Langeland, K., Rodriques, H., and Dowden, W.: Periodontal disease, bacteria, and pulpal histopathology, Oral Surg. **37**:257, 1974.

Larato, D. C.: Alveolar plate fenestrations and dehiscences of the human skull, Oral Surg. **29**:816, 1970.

Leblond, C. P.: Renewal systems. In Price, D., editor: Dy-namics of proliferating tissues, Chicago, 1958, The Uni-versity of Chicago Press.

Leblond, C. P., and Greulich, R.: Renewal of epidermal cell population. In Montagna, W., and Billingham, R. E., edi-tors: Advances in biology of skin, vol. 5, New York, 1964, The Macmillan Co.

Leblond, C. P., and Warren, K. B.: Use of radioautography in investigating protein synthesis, New York, 1965, Aca-demic Press, Inc.

Libassi, P. T.: Two for the cellular seesaw, The Sciences, vol. 15, December, 1974.

Lundquist, G. R.: The zero crevice in the management of periodontal involvement, J. Am. Dent. Assoc. **27**:837, 1940.

Mancini, R. E., Villar, O., Stein, E., and Fiorini, H.: A histochemical and radioautographic study of the participation of fibroblasts in the production of mucopolysaccharides in connective tissue, J. Histochem. Cytochem. **9**:278, 1961.

Matsumoto, T., and Soloway, H.: Tissue adhesion and wound healing. Observation of wound healing by microscopy and microangiography, Arch. Surg. **98**:226, 1969.

McHugh, W. D., and Persson, P. A.: Fluorescence mi-croscopy of healing gingival epithelium, Acta Odont. Scand. **16**:205, 1958.

Malm, J., et al.: Results of aortic valve replacement utilizing irradiated valve homografts. In Blanchard, S., et al.: Aortic valve disease, changing concepts in assessment and man-agement, Ann. N.Y. Acad. Sci., vol. 147.

Marangoni, R. D., Glaser, A. A., et al.: Effect of storage and handling techniques on skin tissue properties, Ann. N.Y. Acad. Sci. **136**:439, 1966.

Melcher, A. H.: Repair of wounds of the periodontium: in-fluence of periodontal ligament on osteogenesis, Arch. Oral Biol. **15**:1183, 1970.

Mergenhagen, S. E., Tempel, T. R., and Snyderman, R.: Immunologic reactions and periodontal inflammation, J. Dent. Res. **49**:256, 1970.

Miles, A. A., and Miles, E. M.: The state of lymphatic capil-laries in acute inflammatory lesions, J. Pathol. Bacteriol. **76**:21, 1958.

Montagna, W., and Billingham, R. E., editors: Advances in biology of skin, vol. 5, New York, 1964, The Macmillan Co.

Morris, M. L.: The implantation of human dentin and cemen-tum with autogenous bone and red marrow into the sub-cutaneous tissues of the rat, J. Periodontol. **40**:259, 1969.

Myers, M. B., Cherry, G., and Heimberger, S.: Augmentation of wound tensile strength by early removal of sutures, Am. J. Surg. **117**:338, 1969.

Nachmansohn, D.: Proteins in excitable membranes, Science **168**:1059, 1970.

Nathaniel, E. J. H., and Pease, D. C.: Collagen and basement membrane formation by Schwann cells during nerve re-generation, J. Ultrastruct. Res. **9**:550, 1963.

Neiders, M. E., and Weiss, L.: The electrical charge at sur-faces of isolated, human, epithelial gingival cells, J. Peri-odontol. **42**:761, 1971.

Neumann, W. F., and Neumann, M. W.: Chemical dy-namics of bone mineral, Chicago, 1958, University of Chicago Press.

Novaes, A. B., Ruben, M. P., et al.: The development of the periodontal cleft, J. Periodontol. **46**:701, 1975.

Ochstein, A. J., Hansen, N. M., and Swenson, H. M.: A comparative study of cyanoacrylate and other periodontal dressings on gingival surgical wound healing, J. Periodontol. **40**:515, 1969.

Oliver, R., and Löe, H.: Microscopic evaluation of the healing and revascularization of free gingival grafts, J. Periodont. Res. **3**:84, 1968.

Orban, B., and Archer, E. A.: Dynamics of wound healing following elimination of gingival pockets, Am. J. Orthod. **31**:40, 1945.

Ordman, L. J., and Gillman, T.: Studies in healing of cu-taneous wounds, Arch. Surg. **93**:911, 1966.

Orekhovitch, V. N., Shpitkiter, V. O., Kazakova, O. V., and Mazourov, V. L.: The incorporation of C^{14} labeled glycine into the α and β components of procollagen, Arch. Bio-chem. Biophys. **85**:554, 1959.

Patterson, W. B.: Wound healing and tissue repair, Chicago, 1956, University of Chicago Press.

Pease, D. C.: The basement membrane: substratum of histo-logical order and complexity, Proc. Fourth Int. Conf. Elec-tron Microscopy **2**:139, 1958.

Persson, P.: The healing process in the marginal periodontium after gingivectomy with special regard to the regeneration of epithelium, Odont. Dent. Pract. **11**:427, 1961.

Prudden, J. F.: Wound healing produced by cartilage prepara-tions, Arch. Surg. **89**:1046, 1964.

Ramfjord, S. P., and Costich, E. R.: Healing after simple gingivectomy, J. Periodontol. **34**:401, 1963.

Ring, J. R.: Alkaline phosphatase activity of healing gingival wounds in the rat, J. Dent. Res. **31**:329, 1952.

Rizzo, A. A.: Absorption of bacterial endotoxin into rabbit gingival pocket tissue, Periodontics **6**:65, 1968.

Robertson, P. P., and Simpson, J.: Collagenase: current concepts and relevance to periodontal disease, J. Periodontol. **47**:29, 1976.

Robertson, W. V.: The biochemical role of ascorbic acid in connective tissue, Ann. N.Y. Acad. Sci. **92**:159, 1961.

Robertson, W. V.: Ascorbic acid and the formation of collagen, J. Biol. Chem. **201**:689, 1953.

Robinson, P.: Possible roles of diseased cementum in periodontitis, J. Prev. Dent. **2**:3, 1975.

Ross, R.: Wound healing: recent progress—future direction, J. Dent. Res. **50**(suppl. 2):313, 1971.

Ross, R.: The fibroblast and wound repair, Biol. Rev. **43**:51, 1968.

Ross, R.: Studies of collagen formation in healing wounds. In Montagna, W., and Billingham, R., editors: Advances in biology of skin, New York, 1964, The Macmillan Co.

Ross, R., and Benditt, E. P.: Wound healing and collagen formation. V. Quantitative electron microscope radioautographic observations of proline-H^3 utilization by fibroblasts, J. Cell Biol. **27**:83, 1965.

Ross R., and Benditt, E. P.: An autoradiographic study with the electron microscope of healing wounds, I.A.D.R. **41**:71, 1963.

Ross, R., and Benditt, E. P.: Wound healing and collagen formation. II. Fine structure in experimental scurvy, J. Cell. Biol. **12**:533, 1962.

Ross, R., and Benditt, E. P.: Wound healing and collagen formation. III. A quantitative radioautographic study of the utilization of proline-H^3 in wounds from normal and scorbutic guinea pigs, J. Cell. Biol. **15**:99, 1962.

Ross, R., and Benditt, E. P.: Wound healing and collagen formation. I. Sequential changes in components of guinea pig skin wounds observed in the electron microscope, J. Biophys. Biochem. Cytol. **11**:677, 1961.

Rothman, S., editor: The human integument, Washington, D.C., 1959, American Association for Administration of Science.

Rovin, S., Costich, E., Fleming, J., and Gordon, H.: Healing of tongue wounds in germ free and conventional mice, Arch. Path. **79**:641, 1965.

Sato, M.: Histopathological study of healing process after surgical treatment for alveolar pyorrhea, Bull. Tokyo Dent. Col. **2**:45, 1958.

Schallhorn, R.: Postoperative problems associated with iliac transplants, J. Periodontol. **43**:3, 1972.

Schallhorn, R., and Hiatt, W. H.: Human allografts of iliac cancellous bone and marrow in periodontal osseous defects. II. Clinical observations, J. Periodontol. **43**:67, 1972.

Schallhorn, R., Hiatt, W., and Boyce, W.: Iliac transplants in periodontal therapy, J. Periodontol. **41**:566, 1970.

Schilling, J.: Wound healing, Physiol. Rev. **28**:374, 1968.

Schoefl, G. I.: Studies on inflammation. III. Growing capillaries: their structure and permeability, Virchow. Arch. Path. Anat. **337**:97, 1963.

Schoefl, G. I., and Majno, G.: Regeneration of blood vessels in wound healing. In Montagna, W., and Billingham, R. E., editors: Advances in biology of skin, vol. 5, New York, 1964, The Macmillan Co.

Schroeder, H. E., and Listgarten, M. A.: The fine structure of the developing epithelial attachment of human teeth, Basel, 1971, S. Karger.

Schultz-Haudt, S. D., and Aas, E.: Dynamics of periodontal tissues. II. The connective tissues, Odontol. Tidskr. **70**:397, 1962.

Schultz-Haudt, S. D., and From, S.: Dynamics of periodontal tissues. I. The epithelium, Odontol. Tidskr. **69**:431, 1961.

Selvig, K. A.: Attachment of plaque and calculus to tooth surfaces, J. Periodont. Res. **5**:8, 1970.

Shapiro, M.: Acceleration of gingival wound healing in non-epileptic patients receiving diphenylhydantoin sodium, Dent. Abst. **5**:219, 1960.

Smith, D.: The chemical structure of the periodontium, J. Dent. Res. **41**:250, 1961.

Smith, L. R.: The role of epithelium in the healing of experimental wounds, J. Dent. Res. **37**:187, 1958.

Spector, W. G.: The mechanism of inflammation. In Rook, A., editor: Progress in the biological sciences in relation to dermatology, New York, 1960, Cambridge University Press.

Stahl, S. S.: Healing of gingival tissues following various therapeutic regimens—a review of histologic studies, J. Oral Ther. **2**:145, 1965.

Stahl, S. S.: Long-term healing sequences following gingival injuries in rats, Periodontics **2**:97, 1964.

Stahl, S. S.: Healing of gingival wounds in female rats fed a low-protein diet, J. Dent. Res. **42**:1511, 1963.

Stahl, S. S.: Morphology and healing pattern of human interdental gingivae, J. Am. Dent. Assoc. **67**:48, 1963.

Stahl, S. S.: Pulpal response to gingival injury in adult rats, Oral Surg. **16**:1116, 1963.

Stahl, S. S.: Soft tissue healing following experimental gingival wounding in female rats of various ages, Periodontics **1**:142, 1963.

Stahl, S. S.: The healing of an experimentally induced wound in female rats, J. Dent. Med. **17**:68, 1962.

Stahl, S. S.: The effect of a protein-free diet on the healing of gingival wounds in rats, Arch. Oral Biol. **7**:551, 1962.

Stahl, S. S.: The effects of repeated injuries on gingival healing in rats, Oral Surg. **15**:1172, 1962.

Stahl, S. S.: Gingival healing after occlusal injury, Dent. Prog. **2**:202, 1962.

Stahl, S. S.: The healing of gingival wounds in male rats of various ages, J. Dent. Med. **16**:100, 1961.

Stahl, S. S.: Healing gingival injury in normal and systemically stressed young adult male rats, J. Periodontol. **32**:63, 1961.

Stahl, S. S.: Response of the periodontium, pulp and salivary glands to gingival and tooth injury in young adult male rats. I. Periodontal tissues, Oral Surg. **13**:613, 1960.

Stahl, S. S.: Effect of oral somatotropic hormone injections upon gingival wounds in rats (abstract), J. Dent. Res. **38**:725, 1959.

Stahl, S. S.: Effect of somatotropic hormone on gingival wounds in normal and protein deprived rats, J. Periodontol. **30**:158, 1959.

Stahl, S. S., Sandler, H. C., and Cahn, L. R.: The effects of protein deprivation upon the oral tissues of the rat and particularly upon periodontal structures under irritation, Oral Surg. **8**:760, 1955.

Stahl, S. S., Soberman, A., and DeCesare, A.: Gingival healing. V. The effects of antibiotics administered during the early stages of repair, J. Periodontol. **40**:521, 1969.

Stahl, S. S., Weiner, J. M., Benjamin, S., and Yamada, L.: Soft tissue healing following curettage and root planing, J. Periodontol. **42:**678, 1971.

Stambaugh, R., and Gordon, H.: Connective tissue influence on mucosal keratinization (abstract), J. Dent. Res. **52:**355, 1973.

Stern, I. B.: Electron microscopic observation of oral epithelium. I. Basal cells and the basement membrane, Periodontics **3:**244, 1955.

Sullivan, J. D., and Epstein, W. L.: Mitotic activity of wounded human epidermis, J. Invest. Dermat. **41:**39, 1963.

Ten Cate, A. R., Deporter, D. A., and Freeman, E.: Role of fibroblasts in remodelling of periodontal ligament during physiologic tooth movement, Am. J. Orthod. **69:**155, 1976.

Ten Cate, A. R., and Freeman, E.: Collagen remodelling by fibroblasts in wound repair, Anat. Rec. **179:**543, 1974.

Thilander, H.: Effect of leucocytic enzyme activity on structure of gingival pocket epithelium, Acta Odont. Scand. **21:**447, 1963.

Toto, P. D., and Abati, A.: The histogenesis of granulation tissue, Oral Surg. **16:**218, 1963.

Turesky, S. S., and Glickman, I.: A histochemical evaluation of gingival healing in experimental animals on adequate and vitamin C deficient diets, J. Dent. Res. **33:**273, 1954.

Turner, H., Ruben, M. P., Frankl, S. N., Sheff, M., and Silberstein, S.: Visualization of the microcirculation of the periodontium, J. Periodontol. **40:**22, 1969.

Viziam, C. B., Matolsty, A. G., and Mescon, H.: Epithelialization of small wounds, J. Invest. Dermat. **43:**499, 1964.

Weatherell, J. A.: Sulfated mucopolysaccharides and calcification. In Blackwood, H. J. J., editor: Bone and tooth symposium, New York, 1964. The Macmillan Co.

Weinmann, J. P., and Sicher, H.: Bone and bones, ed. 2, St. Louis, 1955, The C. V. Mosby Co.

Weiss, P. A.: The biological foundations of wound repair, Harvey Lectures **55:**13, 1959.

Weiss, P.: Guiding principles in cell locomotion and cell aggregation, Exp. Cell Res. **8**(suppl.):260, 1961.

Weiss, R., Stahl, S. S., and Tonna, E. A.: An autoradiographic study of the rat gingival response to chemical injury, J. Periodontol. **40:**21, 1969.

Wheeler, D. D., Boyarsky, L. L., and Brooks, W. H.: The release of amino acids from nerve during stimulation, J. Cell Physiol. **67:**141, 1966.

White, B., and Shetler, H.: Wound healing: investigation of proteins, glycoproteins, and lipids of experimental wound fluid in dog, Proc. Soc. Exp. Med. **101:**354, 1959.

Williamson, M. B., and Williamson, D. A.: Rate of incorporation of methionine S^{35} into regenerating tissue of experimental wounds, J. Surg. Res. **5:**146, 1965.

Winter, G. D., and Scales, J. T.: Effect of air drying and dressings on the surface of a wound, Nature **197:**91, 1963.

Winter, G. W.: Movement of epidermal cells over the wound surface. Skin, vol. 5, New York, 1964, The Macmillan Co.

Woessner, J. F., Jr.: Biological mechanisms of collagen resorption. In Gould, B. S., editor: Treatise on collagen, vol. 2, part 2, New York, 1968, Academic Press, Inc.

Xeros, N.: Deoxyriboside control and synchronization of mitosis, Nature **194:**682, 1962.

Yoffey, J. M., and Courtice, F. C.: Lymphatics, lymph and lymphoid tissue, London, 1956, Edward Arnold Ltd.

Yoffey, J. M., Sullivan, E. R., and Drinker, C. K.: The lymphatic pathway from the nose and pharynx. The absorption of certain proteins, J. Exp. Med. **68:**941, 1938.

Curettage

Blass, J. L., and Lite, T.: Gingival healing following surgical curettage, N.Y. Dent. J. **25:**127, 1959.

Ewen, S. J.: The ultrasonic wound—some microscopic observations, J. Periodontol. **32:**315, 1961.

Goldman, H. M.: Subgingival curettage: a rationale, J. Periodontol. **19:**54, 1948.

Goldman, H. M.: Curettage by ultrasonic instrument, Oral Surg. **13:**43, 1960.

Kon, S., Novaes, A. B., Ruben, M. P., and Goldman, H. M.: Visualization of microvascularization of the healing periodontal wound. II. Curettage, J. Periodontol. **40:**32, 1969.

Korn, N. A., Schaffer, E. M., and McHugh, R. B.: Experimental assessment of gingivectomy and soft tissue curettage in dogs, J. Periodontol. **36:**96, 1965.

Moskow, B. S.: The response of the gingival sulcus to instrumentation; a histologic investigation. II. Gingival curettage, J. Periodontol. **35:**112, 1964.

Moskow, B. S.: The response of the gingival sulcus to instrumentation; a histologic investigation. I. Scaling procedure, J. Periodontol. **33:**282, 1962.

Nadler, H.: Removal of crevicular epithelium by ultrasonic curettes, J. Periodontol. **33:**220, 1962.

O'Bannon, J. Y.: The gingival tissues before and after scaling the teeth, J. Periodontol. **35:**69, 1964.

Orban, B.: Pocket elimination or reattachment, N.Y. Dent. J. **14:**227, 1948.

Ramfjord, S. P., and Kiester, G.: The gingival sulcus and the periodontal pocket immediately following scaling of teeth, J. Periodontol. **25:**167, 1954.

Ramfjord, S. P., Nissle, R. R., Schick, R. A., and Cooper, H., Jr.: Subgingival curettage versus surgical elimination of periodontal pockets, J. Periodontol. **39:**167, 1968.

Rosling, B., Nyman, S., Lindhe, J., and Jern, B.: The healing potential of the periodontal tissues following different techniques of periodontal surgery, J. Clin. Periodontol. **3:**323, 1976.

Sanderson, A. D.: Gingival curettage by hand and ultrasonic instruments, J. Periodontol. **37:**279, 1966.

Schaffer, E. M., Stende, G., and King, D.: Healing of periodontal tissues following ultrasonic scaling and hand planing, J. Periodontol. **35:**44, 1964.

Spengler, D. E., and Hayward, J. R.: Study of sulcus extension wound healing in dogs, J. Oral Surg. **22:**41, 1964.

Stahl, S. S.: Third annual periodontal symposium, University of Southern California, January, 1977.

Stone, S., Ramfjord, S. P., and Waldron, J.: Scaling and curettage, a radiographic study, J. Periodontol. **37:**415, 1966.

Waerhaug, J.: Microscopic demonstration of tissue reaction incident to removal of subgingival calculus, J. Periodontol. **26:**26, 1955.

Wertheimer, F. W.: A histologic study to determine the effectiveness of the "Berliner epithelial scalpel" in removing the epithelial lining of the periodontal pockets, Northwestern Univ. Bull. **57:**4, 1956.

Yukna, R. A.: A clinical and histologic study of healing following the excisional new attachment procedure in rhesus monkeys, J. Periodontol. **47:**701, 1976.

Yukna, R. A., Bowers, G. M., Lawrence, J. J., and Fedijur, P. F.: A clinical study of healing in humans following excisional new attachment procedure, J. Periodontol. **47:** 696, 1976.

Gingivectomy-gingivoplasty

Bernier, J. L., and Kaplan, H.: The repair of gingival tissues after surgical intervention, J. Am. Dent. Assoc. **35**:697, 1947.

Engler, W. D., Ramfjord, S. P., and Hiniker, J. J.: Healing following simple gingivectomy; a tritiated thymidine radioautographic study. I. Epithelialization, J. Periodontol. **37**:298, 1966.

Fraleigh, C. M.: An evaluation of topical terramycin in post-gingivectomy pack, J. Periodontol. **27**:201, 1956.

Frank, R., Fiore-Bonno, G., Cimmasoni, G., and Ogilvie, A.: Gingival reattachment after surgery in man: an electron microscopic study, J. Periodontol. **43**:597, 1972.

Glickman, I., and Imber, L. R.: Comparison of gingival resection with electrosurgery and periodontal knives — a biometric and histologic study, J. Periodontol. **41**:142, 1970.

Klingsberg, J., and Butcher, E. O.: Epithelial junction in periodontal repair in the rat, J. Periodontol. **34**:315, 1963.

Korn, N. A., Schaffer, E. M., and McHugh, R. B.: Experimental assessment of gingivectomy and soft tissue curettage in dogs, J. Periodontol. **36**:96, 1965.

Listgarten, M. A.: Electron microscopic study of the junction between surgically denuded root surfaces and regenerated periodontal tissues, J. Periodontol. **7**:68, 1972.

Listgarten, M. A., Mao, R., and Robinson, P. J.: Periodontal probing and the relationship of the probe tip to periodontal tissues, J. Periodontol. **47**:511, 1976.

Löe, H., and Sillness, J.: Tissue reactions to a new gingivectomy pack, Oral Surg. **14**:1305, 1961.

Mann, J. B., and Kaplan, H.: Histologic studies of block sections of teeth and investing structures removed at intervals following surgical operations, J. Dent. Res. **20**:281, 1941.

Novaes, A. B., Kon, S., Ruben, M. P., and Goldman, H. M.: Visualization of the microvascularization of the healing periodontal wound. III. Gingivectomy, J. Periodontol. **40**:359, 1969.

Orban, B., and Archer, E. A.: Dynamics of wound healing following elimination of gingival pockets. Am. J. Orthod. **31**:40, 1945.

Persson, P-A.: The healing process in the marginal periodontium after gingivectomy with special regard to the regeneration of the epithelium, Odontol. Tidskr. **67**:593, 1962.

Ramfjord, S. P., and Costich, E. R.: Healing after simple gingivectomy, J. Periodontol. **34**:401, 1963.

Ramfjord, S. P., Ingler, W. O., and Hiniker, J. J.: A radioautographic study of healing following simple gingivectomy. II. The connective tissue, J. Periodontol. **37**:179, 1966.

Rosling, B., Nyman, S., Lindhe, J., and Jern, B.: The healing potential of the periodontal tissues following different techniques of periodontal surgery, J. Clin. Periodontol. **3**:323, 1976.

Stahl, S. S., Witkin, G. J., Heller, A., Brown, R., Jr.: Gingival healing. III. The effects of periodontal dressings on gingivectomy repair, J. Periodontol. **40**:34, 1969; IV. The effects of homecare of gingivectomy repair, J. Periodontol. **40**:264, 1969.

Waerhaug, J.: Depth of incision in gingivectomy, Oral Surg. **8**:707, 1955.

Waerhaug, J.: Gingival pocket; anatomy, pathology, deepening and elimination, Odontol. Tidskr. **60**(suppl.):1952.

Waerhaug, J., and Löe, H.: Tissue reaction to gingivectomy pack, Oral Surg. **10**:923, 1957.

Watanabe, Y., and Sozuki, S.: An experimental study on capillary vascularization in the periodontal tissue following gingivectomy or flap operation, J. Dent. Res. **42**:758, 1963.

Mucogingival surgery

Baer, P. N., and Wertheimer, F. W.: A histologic study of the effects of several periodontal dressings on periosteal-covered and denuded bone, J. Dent. Res. **40**:858, 1961.

Bhaskar, S. N., Cutright, D. E., Beasley, J. D., Perez, B., and Hunsuch, E. E.: Healing under full and partial thickness mucogingival flaps in the miniature swine, J. Periodontol. **41**:675, 1970.

Bhaskar, S. N., Cutright, D. E., Perez, B., and Beasley, J. D.: Full and partial thickness pedicle grafts in miniature swine and man, J. Periodontol. **42**:66, 1971.

Bradley, R.: Histological evaluation of mucogingival surgery, Oral Surg. **12**:1184, 1959.

Carranza, F. A., Jr., and Carraro, J. J.: Effects of removal of periosteum on postoperative result in mucogingival surgery, J. Periodontol. **34**:223, 1963.

Carraro, J. J., Carranza, F. A., Jr., Albano, E. A., and Joly, G. G.: Effect of bone denudation in mucogingival surgery in humans, J. Periodontol. **35**:463, 1964.

Chacker, F. M., and Cohen, D. W.: Regeneration of gingival tissue in non-human primates (abstract), J. Dent. Res. **39**:743, 1960.

Costich, E. R., and Ramfjord, S. P.: Healing after partial denudation of the alveolar process, J. Periodontol. **39**:127, 1968.

Donnenfeld, O. W., Hoag, P. M., and Weissman, D. P.: A clinical study of the effects of osteoplasty, J. Periodontol. **41**:131, 1970.

Giblin, J. M., Levy, S., Staffileno, H., and Gargiulo, A. W.: Healing of re-entry wounds in dogs, J. Periodontol. **37**:238, 1966.

Glickman, I., and Lazansky, J. P.: Reattachment of the marginal gingiva and periodontal membrane in experimental animals, J. Dent. Res. **29**:659, 1950.

Glickman, I., Smulow, J. B., O'Brien, T., and Tannen, R.: Healing of the periodontium following mucogingival surgery, Oral Surg. **16**:530, 1963.

Helburn, R. L., Cohen, D. W., and Chacker, F. M.: Healing of repositioned mucogingival flaps in monkeys, Abstract no. 324, I.A.D.R. Program and abstract of papers, 1963.

Hiatt, W. H., Stallard, R. E., Butler, E. D., and Badgett, B.: Repair following mucoperiosteal flap surgery with full gingival retention, J. Periodontol. **39**:11, 1968.

Kohler, C. A., and Ramfjord, S. P.: Healing of the gingival mucoperiosteal flaps, Oral Surg. **13**:89, 1960.

Kon, S., Novaes, A. B., Ruben, M. P., and Goldman, H. M.: Visualization of the microvascularization of the healing periodontal wound. IV. Mucogingival surgery: full thickness flap, J. Periodontol. **40**:5, 1969.

Kramer, G. M., and Kohn, D. J.: Post-operative care of the infrabony pocket, J. Periodontol. **32**:95, 1961.

Levine, L.: Periodontal flap surgery with gingival fiber retention, J. Periodontol. **43**:91, 1972.

Levine, L., and Stahl, S. S.: Repair following periodontal flap surgery with the retention of gingival fibers, J. Periodontol. **43**:99, 1972.

Marfino, N. R., Organ, B., and Wentz, F. M.: Repair of the dento-gingival junction following surgical intervention, J. Periodontol. **30**:180, 1959.

Melcher, A. H.: Wound healing in monkeys' (Maccaca iris) mandible. Effect of elevating periosteum on the formation of subperiosteal callus, Arch. Oral Biol. **16**:461, 1971.

Melcher, A. H., and Accursi, G. E.: Osteogenic capacity of periosteal and osteoperiosteal flaps elevated from the parietal bone of the rat, Arch. Oral Biol. **16**:573, 1971.

Mörmann, W., Bernimoulin, J. P., and Schmid, M. O.: Fluorescein angiography of gingival autografts, J. Clin. Periodontol. **2**:177, 1975.

Morris, M. L.: Healing of periodontal tissues following surgical detachment; the arrangement of the fibers of the periodontal space, Periodontics **1**:118, 1963.

Morris, M. L.: Healing of human periodontal tissues following surgical detachment from vital teeth, the position of the epithelial attachment, J. Periodontol. **32**:108, 1961.

Morris, M. L.: Healing of human periodontal tissues following surgical detachment and extirpation of vital pulps, J. Periodontol. **31**:23, 1960.

Morris, M. L.: Healing of human periodontal tissues following surgical detachment from nonvital teeth, J. Periodontol. **28**:222, 1957.

Morris, M. L.: Healing of naturally occurring periodontal pockets about vital human teeth, J. Periodontol. **26**:285, 1955.

Morris, M. L.: The removal of pocket and attachment to epithelium in humans; a histological study, J. Periodontol. **25**:7, 1954.

Morris, M. L.: The reattachment of human periodontal tissues following surgical detachment; a clinical and histologic study, J. Periodontol. **24**:220, 1953.

Nevins, L. M.: Environmental control: innovations in the use of the laterally displaced flap, J. Periodontol. **41**:479, 1970.

Novaes, A. B., Kon, S., Ruben, M. P., and Goldman, H. M.: Visualization of microvascularization of the healing periodontal wound. V. Periosteum retention technique of mucogingival surgery, J. Periodontol. **41**:685, 1970.

Ochsenbein, C., and Maynard, J. G.: The problem of attached gingiva in children, J. Dent. Child. **41**:263, 1974.

Parfitt, G., and Mjor, L.: A clinical evaluation of localized gingival recession in children, J. Dent. Child. **31**:257, 1964.

Persson, P-A.: The regeneration of the marginal periodontium after flap operation, Acta Odontol. Scand. **20**:43, 1962.

Pfeifer, J. S.: The reaction of alveolar bone to flap procedures in man, Periodontics **3**:135, 1965.

Pfeifer, J. S.: The growth of gingival tissue over denuded bone, J. Periodontol. **34**:10, 1963.

Pfeifer, J. S., and Doyle, B.: The value of continuous saline rinses in mucoperiosteal flap surgery, J. Periodontol. **37**:326, 1966.

Ruben, M. P., Goldman, H. M., and Janson, W.: Biological considerations in laterally repositioned pedicle flaps and free autogenous gingival grafts in periodontal therapy. In Stahl, S. S., editor: Periodontal surgery—biologic bases and technique, Springfield, Ill., 1975, Charles C Thomas, Publisher, p. 235.

Shaw, J. G.: Treatment of multiple periodontal pockets by extended flap operation, Parodontologie **16**:121, 1962.

Smith, J. H.: The effect of surgically produced foramina on the coverage of exposed bone in mucogingival surgery, Oral Surg. **15**:665, 1962.

Smukler, H.: Laterally positioned mucoperiosteal grafts in the treatment of denuded roots. A clinical and statistical study, J. Periodontol. **47**:590, 1976.

Staffileno, H.: Significant differences and advantages between full thickness and split thickness flaps, J. Periodontol. **45**:421, 1974.

Staffileno, H.: Palatal flap surgery: mucosal flap (split-thick-

ness) and its advantages over the mucoperiosteal flap, J. Periodontol. **40**:547, 1969.

Staffileno, H., Levy, S., and Gargiulo, A.: Histologic study of cellular mobilization and repair following a periosteal retention operation via split thickness mucogingival flap surgery, J. Periodontol. **37**:117, 1966.

Staffileno, H., Wentz, F. M., and Orban, B.: Histologic study of healing of split thickness flap surgery in dogs, J. Periodontol. **33**:56, 1962.

Tavtigian, R.: The height of the facial radicular alveolar crest following apically positioned flap operations, J. Periodontol. **41**:412, 1970.

West, T. L., and Bloom, A.: A histologic study of wound healing following mucogingival surgery (abstract), J. Dent. Res. **40**:675, 1961.

Wilderman, M. N.: Repair after a periosteal retention procedure, J. Periodontol. **34**:487, 1963.

Wilderman, M. N., Pennel, B. M., King, K., and Barron, J. M.: Histogenesis of repair following osseous surgery, J. Periodontol. **41**:551, 1970.

Wilderman, M. N., and Wentz, F. M.: Repair of a dentogingival defect with a pedicle flap, J. Periodontol. **36**:218, 1965.

Wilderman, M. N., Wentz, F. M., and Orban, B.: Histogenesis of repair after mucogingival surgery, J. Periodontol. **33**:283, 1960.

Wright, W. H., and Löe, H.: Tissue reactions incident to osseous surgery via intra-crevicular flap procedures (abstract), Odontol. Tidskr. **73**:625, 1965.

Zander, H. A., and Matherson, D. G.: The effect of osseous surgery on interdental tissue morphology in monkeys, Abstract no. 326, I.A.D.R. Program and abstract of papers, 1962.

Healing after surgical treatment of infrabony pocket

Alderman, N. E.: Sterile plaster of Paris as an implant in the infrabony environment: a preliminary study, J. Periodontol. **40**:11, 1969.

Andreasen, J. O.: Histometric study of the healing of periodontal tissues after surgical injury. II. Healing events of alveolar bone, periodontal ligament and cementum, Odontol. Revy **27**:131, 1976.

Beube, F. E.: A radiographic and histologic study on reattachment, J. Periodontol. **23**:158, 1952.

Beube, F. E.: Study on reattachment of the supporting structures of the teeth, J. Periodontol. **18**:55, 1947.

Carranza, F. A.: Technique for treating infrabony pocket so as to obtain reattachment, Dent. Clin. North Am., p. 75, March, 1960.

Carranza, F. A.: A technique for reattachment, J. Periodontol. **25**:272, 1954.

Cross, W. G.: Reattachment following curettage, Dent. Pract. **7**:38, 1956.

Glickman, I., and Patin, B.: Histologic study of the effect of antiformin on the soft tissue wall of periodontal pockets in human beings, J. Am. Dent. Assoc. **51**:420, 1956.

Goldman, H. M.: A rationale for the treatment of the infrabony pocket, J. Periodontol. **20**:83, 1949.

Jacobs, J. D., and Norton, L. A.: Electrical stimulation of osteogenesis in pathological osseous defects, J. Periodontol. **47**:311, 1976.

Linghorne, W. J.: Studies in the regeneration and reattachment of the supporting structures of the teeth. IV. Regeneration in epithelized pockets following organization of a blood clot, J. Dent. Res. **36**:4, 1957.

Linghorne, W. J., and O'Connell, D. C.: Studies in the regeneration and reattachment of the supporting structures of the teeth. III. Regeneration of epithelized pockets, J. Dent. Res. **34**:164, 1955.

Linghorne, W. J., and O'Connell, D. C.: Studies in the reattachment and regeneration of the supporting structures of the teeth. I. Soft tissue reattachment, J. Dent. Res. **29**:419, 1950.

Morris, M. L.: Healing of human periodontal tissues following surgical detachment and extirpation of vital pulps, J. Periodontol. **31**:23, 1960.

Morris, M. L.: Healing of human periodontal tissues following surgical detachment from non-vital teeth, J. Periodontol. **28**:222, 1957.

Morris, M. L.: Healing of naturally occurring periodontal pockets about vital human teeth, J. Periodontol. **26**:285, 1955.

Morris, M. L.: The reattachment of human periodontal tissue following surgical detachment: a clinical and histologic study, J. Periodontol. **24**:220, 1953.

Orban, B.: Pocket elimination or reattachment, N.Y. State Dent. J. **14**:227, 1948.

Prichard, J.: The infrabony technique as a predictable procedure, J. Periodontol. **28**:202, 1957.

Ramfjord, S. P.: Experimental periodontal reattachment in rhesus monkeys, J. Periodontol. **22**:67, 1958.

Ramfjord, S. P.: Reattachment in periodontal therapy, J. Am. Dent. Assoc. **45**:513, 1952.

Register, A., and Burdick, F.: Accelerated reattachment with cementogenesis to dentin, demineralized in situ. II. Defect repair, J. Periodontol. **47**:497, 1976.

Rockoff, S. C., Rockoff, H. S., and Sackler, A. M.: Reattachment; a case in point, J. Periodontol. **29**:261, 1958.

Schaffer, E. M., and Zander, H. A.: Histologic evidence of periodontal reattachment of pockets, Parodontologie **3**:101, 1953.

Shapiro, M.: A reattachment operation, Dent. Clin. North Am., p. 12, March, 1960.

Skillen, W. G., and Lundquist, G. R.: An experimental study of periodontal membrane reattachment in healthy and pathologic tissues, J. Am. Dent. Assoc. **24**:175, 1937.

Smukler, H., and Tagger, M.: Vital root amputation—a clinical and histologic study, J. Periodontol. **47**:324, 1976.

Stahl, S. S.: The influence of antibiotics on the healing of gingival wounds in rats. III. The influence of pulpal necrosis on gingival reattachment potential, J. Periodontol. **34**:371, 1963.

Stahl, S. S.: The influence of antibiotics on the healing of gingival wounds in rats. II. Reattachment potential of soft and calcified tissues, J. Periodontol. **34**:166, 1963.

Stahl, S. S.: The influence of antibiotics on the healing of gingival wounds in rats. I. Alveolar bone and soft tissue, J. Periodontol. **33**:261, 1962.

Stahl, S., and Persson, P-A.: Mode of reattachment, J. Periodontol. 1962.

Swan, R. H., and Hurt, W. C.: Cervical enamel projections as an etiologic factor in furcation involvement, J. Am. Dent. Assoc. **93**:342, 1976.

Free soft tissue autografts and osseous and marrow autografts

Andreasen, J. O.: Effect of splinting upon periodontal healing after replantation of permanent incisors in monkeys, Acta Odontol. Scand. **33**:313, 1975.

Bjorn, H.: Free transplantation of gingiva propria, Sver. Tandlakarforb. Tidn. **22**:684, 1963.

Bracket, R. C., and Gargiulo, A. W.: Free gingival grafts in humans, J. Periodontol. **41**:581, 1970.

Clemmesen, T.: The early circulation in split skin grafts, Acta Chir. Scand. **127**:1, 1964.

Clemmesen, T.: The early circulation in split skin grafts, Acta Chir. Scand. **124**:11, 1962.

Converse, J. M.: Reconstructive plastic surgery, vol. 1, Philadelphia, 1964, W. B. Saunders Co.

Converse, J. M., Ballantyne, D. L., Rogers, B. O., and Raisbeck, A. P.: Plasmatic circulation in skin grafts, Transpl. Bull. **4**:154, 1957.

Converse, J. M., and Rapaport, F. T.: The vascularization of skin autografts and homografts. An experimental study in man, Ann. Surg. **143**:306, 1956.

Conway, H., Stark, R. B., and Joslin, D.: Observations on the development of circulation in skin grafts. II. The physiologic pattern of early circulation in auto-grafts, Plast. Reconstr. Surg. **8**:312, 1951.

Cushing, M.: Autogenous red marrow grafts: their potential for induction of osteogenesis, J. Periodontol. **40**:492, 1969.

Davis, J. S., and Traut, H. F.: Origin and development of the blood supply of whole-thickness skin grafts, Ann. Surg. **82**:871, 1925.

Edel, A.: Clinical evaluation of free connective tissue grafts used to increase the width of keratinised gingiva, J. Clin. Periodontol. **1**:185, 1974.

Edgerton, M. T., and Edgerton, P. J.: Vascularization of homografts, Transpl. Bull. **2**:98, 1955.

Ellegaard, B., Karring, T., and Löe, H.: The fate of vital and devitalized bone grafts in healing of interradicular lesions, J. Periodont. Res. **10**:88, 1975.

Ewen, S. J.: Bone swaging, J. Periodontol. **36**:57, 1965.

Foman, S.: Cosmetic surgery, Philadelphia, 1960, J. B. Lippincott Co.

Froum, S., Thaler, R., Scopp, I., and Stahl, S. S.: Osseous autografts. II. Histologic responses to osseous coagulum—bone blend grafts, J. Periodontol. **46**:656, 1975.

Gargiulo, A. W., and Arrocha, R.: Histo-clinical evaluation of free gingival grafts, Periodontics **5**:285, 1967.

Gordon, H. P., Sullivan, H. C., and Atkins, J. H.: Free autogenous gingival grafts. II. Supplemental findings—histology of the graft site, Periodontics **6**:130, 1968.

Haggerty, P. C.: The use of free gingival graft to create a healthy environment for full crown preparation, Periodontics **4**:329, 1966.

Halliday, D. G.: The grafting of newly formed autogenous bone in the treatment of osseous defects, J. Periodontol. **40**:511, 1969.

Hawley, C. E., and Staffileno, H.: Clinical evaluation of free gingival grafts in periodontal surgery, J. Periodontol. **41**:105, 1970.

Hiatt, W. H.: The induction of new bone and cementum formation. III. Utilizing bone and marrow allografts in dogs, J. Periodontol. **41**:596, 1970.

Hiatt, W., and Schallhorn, R.: Intraoral transplants of cancellous bone and marrow in periodontal lesions, J. Periodontol. **44**:194, 1973.

Hynes, W.: The early circulation in skin grafts with a consideration of methods to encourage their survival, Br. J. Plast. Surg. **6**:257, 1954.

Janson, W. A., Ruben, M. P., Kramer, G. M., Bloom, A. A., and Turner, H.: Development of the blood supply to split-thickness free gingival autografts, J. Periodontol. **40**:707, 1969.

Johansen, N.: Human block sections in the evaluation of iliac crest grafts. Given at American Academy of Periodontology, spring meeting, New Orleans, May, 1969.

Kazanjian, H., and Converse, J. M.: The surgical treatment of facial injuries, ed. 2, Baltimore, 1959, The Williams & Wilkins Company.

Kromer, H.: Bone homografts, Odontol. Tidskr. **68**:9, 1960.

Levin, M. P., Frisch, J., and Bhaskar, S. N.: Tissue conditioner dressings for free tissue grafts, J. Periodontol. **40**: 271, 1969.

Line, S. E., Polson, A. M., and Zander, H.: Relationship between periodontal injury, selective cell repopulation, and ankylosis, J. Periodontol. **45**:725, 1974.

Matsue, I., Collings, C. K., Zimmerman, E. R., and Vail, W. C.: Microdensitometric analysis of human autogenous alveolar bone implants, J. Periodontol. **41**:489, 1970.

McGregor, I. A.: Fundamental techniques of plastic surgery, ed. 3, Baltimore, 1965, The Williams & Wilkins Company.

Melcher, A.: On the repair potential of periodontal tissues, J. Periodontol. **47**:256, 1976.

Melcher, A., and Accursi, G. E.: Osteogenic capacity of periosteal and osteoperiosteal flaps elevated from parietal bone of the rat, Arch. Oral Biol. **16**:573, 1971.

Morris, M. L.: The implantation of decalcified human dentin and cementum with autogenous bone and marrow into the subcutaneous tissues of the rat, J. Periodontol. **40**:731, 1969.

Morris, M. L.: The implantation of human dentin and cementum with autogenous red marrow into the subcutaneous tissues of the rat, J. Periodontol. **40**:571, 1969.

Morris, M. L.: The implantation of human dentin and cementum with autogenous bone and red marrow into the subcutaneous tissues of the rat, J. Periodontol. **40**:259, 1969.

Nabers, E. L., and O'Leary, T. J.: Autogenous bone transplants in the treatment of osseous defects, J. Periodontol. **36**:5, 1965.

Nabers, J. M.: Free gingival grafts, Periodontics **4**:243, 1966.

Oliver, R. C., Löe, H., and Karring, T.: Microscopic evaluation of the healing and revascularization of free gingival grafts, J. Periodont. Res. **3**:84, 1968.

Pennel, B. M., Tabor, J. C., King, K. O., Towner, J. D., Fritz, B. D., and Higgason, J. D.: Free masticatory mucosa graft, J. Periodontol. **40**:162, 1969.

Robinson, E. R.: Osseous coagulum for bone induction, J. Periodontol. **40**:503, 1969.

Rosling, B., Nyman, S., and Lindhe, J.: Effect of systematic plaque control on bone regeneration in infrabony pockets, J. Clin. Periodontol. **3**:38, 1976.

Ross, R.: Wound healing, Sci. Am. **220**:40, 1969.

Ross, R.: Studies of collagen formation in healing wounds. In Montagna, W., and Billingham, R. E., editors: Advances in biology of skin, New York, 1964, The Macmillan Co.

Ross, S. E., and Cohen, D. W.: The fate of a free osseous tissue autograft, Periodontics **6**:145, 1968.

Schaffer, E. M.: Cartilage transplants into the periosteum of rhesus monkeys, Oral Surg. **9**:1233, 1956.

Schallhorn, R. G.: Postoperative problems associated with iliac transplants, J. Periodontol. **43**:3, 1972.

Schallhorn, R. G.: The use of autogenous hip marrow biopsy implants for bony crater defects, J. Periodontol. **39**:145, 1968.

Schallhorn, R. G.: Eradication of bifurcation defects utilizing frozen autogenous hip marrow implants, Periodont. Abstr. **15**:101, 1967.

Schallhorn, R. G., and Hiatt, W. H.: Human allografts of iliac cancellous bone and marrow in periodontal osseous defects. II. Clinical observations, J. Periodontol. **43**:67, 1972.

Schallhorn, R. G., Hiatt, W. H., and Boyce, W.: Iliac transplants in periodontal therapy, J. Periodontol. **41**:566, 1970.

Schoefl, G. I., and Majno, G.: Regeneration of blood vessels in wound healing. In Montagna, W., and Billingham, R. E., editors: Advances in biology of skin, New York, 1964, The Macmillan Co.

Shulman, L.: Allogenic tooth transplantation, J. Oral Surg. **30**:395, 1972.

Staffileno, H., Jr., and Levy, S.: Histologic and clinical study of mucosal (gingival) transplants in dogs, J. Periodontol. **40**:311, 1969.

Sugarman, E. F.: A clinical and histological study of the attachment of grafted tissue to bone and teeth, J. Periodontol. **40**:381, 1969.

Sullivan, H. C., and Atkins, J. H.: Free autogenous gingival grafts. I. Principles of successful grafting, Periodontics **6**: 121, 1968.

Sullivan, H. C., and Atkins, J. H.: Free autogenous gingival grafts. III. Utilization of grafts in the treatment of gingival recessions, Periodontics **6**:152 1968.

Taylor, A. C., and Lehrfeld, J. W.: Determination of survival time of skin homografts in the rat by observation of vascular changes in the graft, Plast. Reconstr. Surg. **12**:423, 1953.

Waerhaug, J., and Löe, H.: Tissue reaction of gingivectomy pack, Oral Surg. **10**:923, 1957.

Woehrle, R.: Cementum regeneration in replanted teeth with differing pulp treatment, J. Dent. Res. **55**:235, 1976.

24 Gingival curettage

The term "curettage" refers to a procedure of scraping or debriding a tissue or a body cavity. *Gingival curettage is the use of an instrument against the inner side of a pocket in order to scrape and debride the soft tissue wall.* It is a deliberate and systematic approach intended to remove the chronically inflamed wound surface elements.

Subgingival scaling and root planing has been covered in Chapter 17. As has been mentioned previously, when a curet is being used for root planing, some gingival curettage is done inadvertently with the offset blade. This action is incidental and usually incomplete. *Gingival curettage, as we use it in this chapter, refers to a separate procedure of pocket elimination directed specifically at the inner side of the pocket.*

In reality, gingival curettage and root planing usually are used in combination to effect pocket resolution. Some clinicians perform both at one time, whereas others do the curettage as a separate surgical procedure after the scaling and root planing. To perform gingival curettage without careful removal of the subgingival calculus is a useless procedure. Moskow's recent investigations suggest that curettage, when indicated, be performed as a separate and subsequent procedure.

Rationale

The objective of gingival curettage is to debride the soft tissue wall of the pocket for the purpose of converting a chronic ulcerated wound into a surgical wound. This entails the removal of degenerated and diseased tissue elements by scraping so that wound healing may ensue without being retarded or halted by the presence of degenerated tissue elements. Débridement is a rule of all wound treatment. Its basic purpose is to alleviate the necessity for removal and resorption of toxic products by the phagocytic and lytic actions of the body. It is felt by many clinicians that recalcitrant cases of gingival inflammation may resist or yield only partially to the removal of subgingival calculus. With long-standing chronic irritation the epithelial lining, which is degenerated and has deep projections of rete pegs into the underlying corium, does not always heal with the removal of calculus and debris but continues to be affected by a low-grade chronic inflammatory process. To facilitate proper healing this sulcular tissue is removed.

Gingival curettage when used as a method to obtain a healthy gingival attachment is thought to work in one of two ways. Because of the removal of elements that continued to maintain the inflammatory response, currettage creates a surgical wound. The resolution of the inflammation with its concomitant decrease in extra tissue fluid and inflammatory cells causes shrinkage of the gingiva. This decrease in gingival size causes a reduction in pocket depth. Epithelialization of the surface goes on concomitantly with collagenation and resolution of inflammation. In clinical situations where gingival curettage is commonly used, experienced clinicians feel shrinkage is a predictable occurrence.

Indications and contraindications

An understanding of the manner in which pocket elimination occurs and of the rationale behind the use of curettage allows us to predict situations in which we would expect gingival curettage to be of best advantage and also helps us to anticipate situations in which it will not be of much use.

Three considerations are important in the indications and contraindications for gingival curettage. The gingival retracted tissue (pocket) usually surrounds the tooth. The depth of retraction may vary around a given tooth; the total area consists of a buccal wall, a lingual wall, and two proximal walls. The histology of the sulcular diseased tissue is that of a wound. Thus the total area may be considered a wound surface, and it is this wound that is debrided in gingival curettage. The considerations are total wound surface, drainage of the wound, and the amount of shrinkage that will take place during wound healing, namely, epithelialization and collagenation with resolution of inflammation.

The total wound surface area around a mandibular incisor is far less than that around a molar, even if the depth factor is the same. The deeper the pocket, the greater the wound surface, and the wound surface can reach such proportions that epithelialization will not occur. Also drainage is a distinct problem, more in the mandibular, than in the maxillary area, in that gravity works against drainage in the mandibular area. The deeper the pocket, the more hindrance there is to drainage, especially in the mandible. The diseased gingival attachment must be considered a cul-de-sac; its topography works against drainage.

In long-standing chronic inflammation, where the response is characterized by the presence of a large number of collagen fibers along with an inflammatory exudate, shrinkage does not occur so readily. This gingival tissue, which appears clinically to have a firm fibrous consistency, does not respond well to gingival curettage. *In general pockets relatively shallow in nature whose local environment will not prevent drainage and shrinkage are best treated by curettage.* In many instances curettage is performed where the resultant sulcus is likely to remain very deep and where a further surgical procedure is expected to be necessary. Curettage is performed to allow for possible resolution of inflammation to occur so that the tissue will be less edematous and friable during the subsequent surgical procedure.

Gingival curettage is contraindicated in pockets that extend into the alveolar mucosa or have a frenum pulling on the gingival margin. Both these require other surgical procedures that are described in this text. Shrinkage is not common on the lingual aspect of the upper anterior teeth or in the retromolar area because of the thick fibrous nature of this tissue. Shrinkage is also not common in deep, narrow labial pockets. Therefore gingival curettage is of little value in these types of situations. It is also contraindicated in any of the systemic problems that cause gingival enlargement, for example, Dilantin therapy and idiopathic gingival enlargement in children. Nor is it the best method of pocket therapy in a sit-

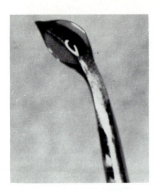

Fig. 24-1. To use a topical anesthetic best, first apply it to external surface. Follow this by dipping curet into a thick glyceriny liquid topical, which will adhere to instrument as shown. Anesthetic fluid can then be carried into pocket.

uation in which the close proximity of root surfaces might interfere with instrumentation.

Technique

Gingival curettage is a definite surgical procedure, and in most cases a local anesthetic will be required. In some cases careful use of a topical anesthetic will suffice if used properly (Fig. 24-1).

With a small sharp curet whose blade is directed against the gingival wall, the diseased sulcular tissue is firmly debrided (Figs. 24-2 and 24-3). Care should be taken not to gouge or tear the tissue. Rather, a smooth débridement of the inner wall should be performed. It will be found that the gingival wall, being unsupported soft tissue, requires some stabilization so that it presents a resistant surface to the curet. This stabilization can be attained by the operator's placing the finger of his left hand on the buccal or lingual surface and directing the curet from within the pocket against the now firmly held gingival wall. Usually the operator can feel the curet in action as a faint ripple against the retaining fingertip. Too great a pressure on the curet blade should be avoided lest the gingival wall be pierced. The curettage procedure is carried on until a firm inner wall is reached. On the interproximal aspect the gingiva will be stabilized by the adjacent tooth, but in the lateral aspect of the papilla it may often be useful to pinch the area from both the buccal and lingual surfaces between the thumb and forefinger to stabilize it before proceeding with the curettage.

If the curet is sharp, only a few deft passages of its blade over the sulcular surface will suffice

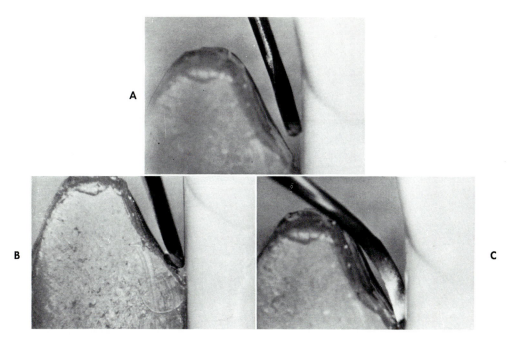

Fig. 24-2. Location of curet in position for, **A,** root planing, **B,** gingival curettage, and, **C,** removal of epithelial attachment.

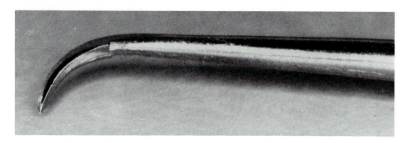

Fig. 24-3. Goldman curet for debriding gingival inflammatory sulcular surface. Instrument is used in a horizontal sweep, engaging tissue and "peeling" it away. Edges are sharp, and blade comes to a point, taking shape of space between tooth and gingival sulcular wall.

to remove the degenerated portion of the wound surface (Fig. 24-4). Attention must be paid to a comprehensive curettage of the entire pocket wall. The lateral aspects of the pocket are just as important as the deepest portions. In addition the curettage should be carried up to the marginal gingiva, even including the margin itself if this area is involved. At this point many therapists irrigate the curetted pocket with warm normal saline solution in a glass-barrel syringe with a lacrimal tip inserted into the pocket. This removes some of the small debris of curettage not removed by the instrument and any calculus and tooth structure that might be present.

The instrument used in subgingival curettage is the curet. Planes and scalers are also used sub-

gingivally, but these are used primarily for subgingival scaling. The instrument head must be small enough to penetrate the orifice of the pocket and go to the very depths of the pocket without excessively distending the gingival wall or tearing it. The attachment base is carefully manipulated; actually the epithelial attachment is removed very quickly in the débridement operation. The actual choice of curet is an item of individual preference. The Goldman no. 12 curet is very effective. Some excellent sets of curets are shown in Figs. 24-5 to 24-8. A useful set, which keeps the number of instruments at a minimum and still adequately reaches all surfaces of the teeth, includes the Gracey nos. 3-4, 11-12, and 13-14. The minimum number of instruments possible is suggested

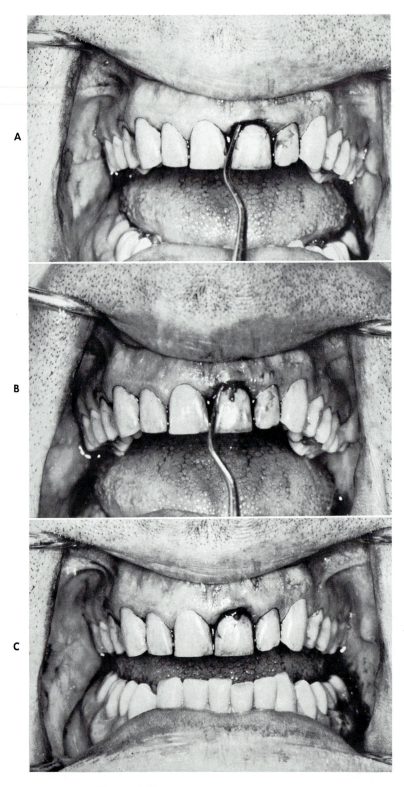

A

B

C

Fig. 24-4. For legend see opposite page.

so that sharpening time can be decreased. Instruments used for curettage must be sharp, since the tissue is removed by cutting rather than tearing. Many clinicians keep a separate set of curets for gingival curettage that they do not use against root surfaces.

Gingival curettage may be performed by ultrasonics. There is experimental evidence to show that effective gingival curettage can be accomplished with the ultrasonic instrument. The mechanism is thought to be both mechanical débridement and heat coagulation. The technique for ultrasonic débridement, when used, is essentially the same as for the hand instrument (Fig. 24-13).

All bleeding should be stopped, and the gingival tissue should be carefully adapted to the tooth and held for a while under pressure. A gauze pad may be utilized for this. It is important to stop hemorrhaging, since if it continues it will cause the gingival tissue to retract from the tooth. If this happens the gingival margin will tend to stand away from the tooth after healing, resulting in poor architectural form. If retraction persists after pressure adaptation, it is wise to suture the interproximal peak in a buccal to lingual direction with 5-0 gut suture, which is thin enough to hold the papillae together and which resorbs quickly.

Immediately after curettage, bleeding from the wound is fairly copious but is easily controlled by a gentle pinching pressure on the gingiva with a gauze sponge for a few minutes. This will also help to readapt the gingival tissues to the tooth surface. After the bleeding has stopped, the operative field may be protected. The covering should not prevent drainage. The essential is to cover the wound until the blood clot is formed. The clot acts as the protective agent.

Postoperative care

Home care of the curetted area immediately postoperatively can be a ticklish problem many times. The area must be cleaned so as to prevent not only accumulation of oral debris, which can interfere with healing, but also traumatization with a toothbrush. A regimen of light cleansing for the first few days, with increasing vigor as the tissues allow, is best. Many clinicians use a modified approach to home care during this period, utilizing cotton swabs, a terry cloth washcloth, and so on. The technique chosen should ensure that the area is cleansed without undue trauma.

Postcurettage pain is usually not a problem and can be dealt with easily by available mild analgesics. If tenderness of the tooth occurs, this can be due to an acute periodontitis that is usually transitory in nature.

The clinical changes of the tissues after curettage have been described by Blass and Lite. Immediately after curettage the marginal gingivae appeared hemorrhagic and blue-red, and blood coagula was present at the margins of the gingiva. One day after curettage the marginal gingivae and a portion of the attached gingiva appeared edematous, swollen, and hemorrhagic, with continued dark bluish red color. In isolated areas slough was present at the gingival margin, and discrete blood clots could still be seen extruding from the sulcus. Two days after curettage the gingival tissue was light bluish red, and edema

Fig. 24-4. Proper instrumentation is an important phase of curettage operative procedure. **A,** Curet entering pocket, distending labial gingiva. Outline of head of instrument is visible on gingiva, causing it to bulge. Greater curvature of blade of instrument is against soft tissue. Note bleeding. Inner portion of gingival tissue, representing sulcular epithelium and subepithelial inflamed granulation tissue, is being removed, a small portion at a time. **B,** Débridement. Instrument used in subgingival curettage is curet. Its head must be small enough so that it penetrates orifice of pocket, going to very depth without excessively distending gingival wall or actually tearing it. Blades of instruments used for curettage should be small and sharp enough to engage and remove easily sections of soft tissue. Curettage procedure illustrated emphasizes correct angulation of head of instrument against gingiva. Blade is engaging inner soft tissue wall in a cutting fashion, and a section of tissue is removed. There is no tearing action whatsoever. Curettage procedure is carried through until a firm inner wall is reached, **C,** Correlation of knowledge from clinical to histologic point of view is of great benefit when one is performing curettage operation. In fact, it is essential to have an understanding of gross pathology of diseased gingiva. Saving material removed by curettage, studying it microscopically, and evaluating clinical results will aid greatly.

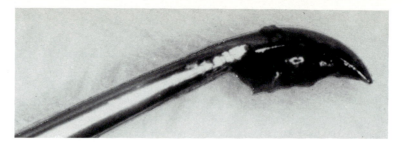

Fig. 24-5. Goldman curet no. 12 with inflammatory tissue that has been removed from gingival sulcular wall adhering to blade. Note amount of tissue; it is soft, friable, and filled with blood. Operator must make sure that wound surface is smooth and clean. Tears and slits should be avoided. This operation consists of converting a chronic inflammatory wound into a surgical wound that is expected to heal.

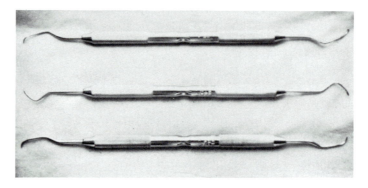

Fig. 24-6. Goldman-Fox curets are generally used for scaling procedure but can be adapted to remove wound surface of sulcular wall. By turning instrument, stroke can be made either horizontally or vertically. Operator must make sure that wound surface is left smooth and completely debrided down to "hard" tissue.

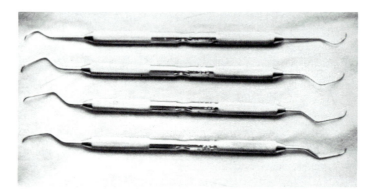

Fig. 24-7. Gracey and Columbia curets also are generally utilized for scaling but can be adapted for curettage.

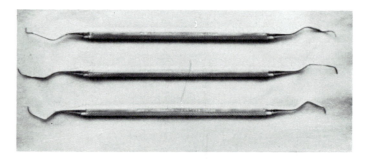

Fig. 24-8. Gracey curets (3-4, 11-12, and 13-14) were designed for scaling procedure but can be utilized for debriding.

and evidence of remaining blood clots were still present. Four days after curettage the gingiva appeared red, and edema and swelling were still evident but were reduced in intensity. By 6 days after curettage the gingival tissue was light red, and the clinical signs of edema were markedly reduced. There was constriction of the marginal gingival tissue with resultant recession evident. At 7 days after curettage the gingival tissue was pink with constriction and recession present. The marginal gingivae were still smooth and glossy. At 8 days the gingivae remained smooth, but signs of healing appeared almost complete. By 9 days the gingivae were pale pink, and the marginal gingivae no longer appeared smooth, indi-

cating the presence of greater surface keratinization. In 10 days normal, well-developed marginal gingivae that were pale pink and resistant to bleeding on palpation were present (Fig. 24-9).

Healing in most cases will be uneventful. If the area has not completely healed clinically in 7 to 10 days, a disturbance in healing should be suspected. This is most commonly due to the presence of local irritants, either calculus that has not been removed or plaque that has recently accumulated. Immediate removal of the irritant will allow the area to progress with normal healing. If a generalized delay in the healing of the entire curetted area occurs, a systemic interference should be suspected.

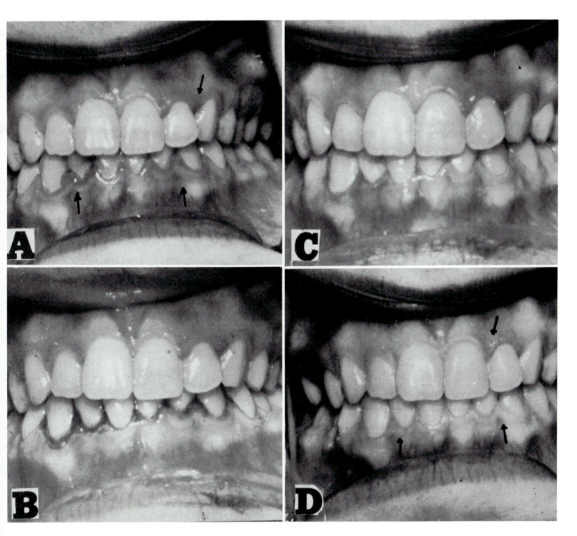

Fig. 24-9. Gingival inflammation in a 19-year-old patient. **A,** Preoperative appearance. Note soft edematous interdental papillae *(arrows).* **B,** Immediately postgingival curettage. **C,** Three weeks later. **D,** Healing 3 months later. Arrows show return of papillae to normal form.

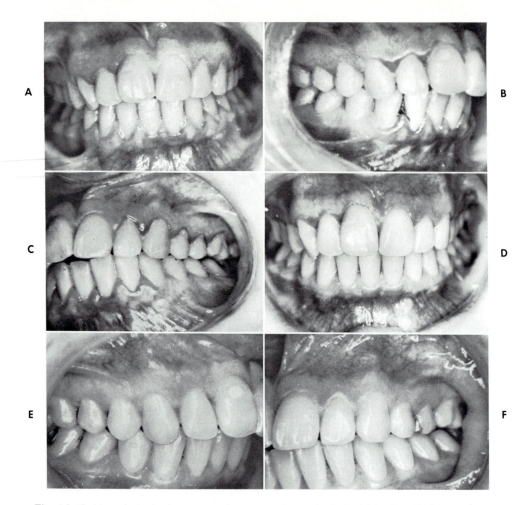

Fig. 24-10. Use of gingival curettage in a case of marginal gingivitis. **A** to **C,** Preoperative. Note all characteristic signs of gingival inflammation. **D** to **F,** Four weeks after completion of root planing and gingival curettage. Note changes in tissue characteristics and resultant architecture.

Fig. 24-11. Curettage procedure is performed in a case of class II occlusion in which habit of mouth breathing was present. Marginal gingival inflammation throughout is evident. In lower jaw gingival margins are bright red in contrast to those in upper jaw; however, on being probed, gingivae bled from all areas. In center photograph curettage was performed for lower anterior gingivae as well as for gingiva around maxillary left lateral incisor. Curettage in this instance consisted of a débridement not only of inner gingival wall but also of gingival margin. Curet was placed flat against gingival margin, and surface was denuded of epithelium with a scraping motion. A covering surgical pack was used for a short time. Curettage was performed around remaining teeth at subsequent visits. Healing was comparatively uneventful, except that it was longer than usual curettage operation. This was due, no doubt, to débridement of gingival margin. Factor of mouth breathing, however, may have played an important role as well. Patient was carefully instructed in oral hygiene program. Gingivae healed and remained healed. Bottom photograph was taken several months after operation. Note character of gingival tissue, especially heavy stippling.

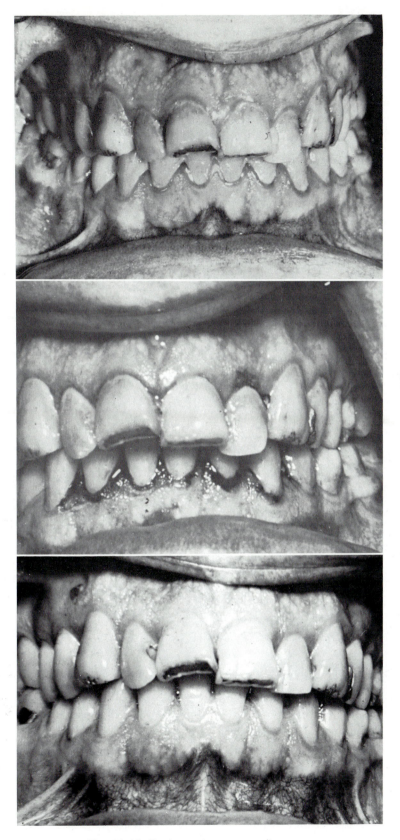

Fig. 24-11. For legend see opposite page.

Bleeding can sometimes occur after the patient has been dismissed. This is due to the opening of a previously clotted vessel and is commonly associated with a remaining piece of calculus. The bleeding area should be located, the local irritant removed if present, and the bleeding controlled with the necessary local measures. Any severe bleeding of a generalized nature should be regarded with suspicion as a systemic involvement.

It is important to evaluate curettage postopera-

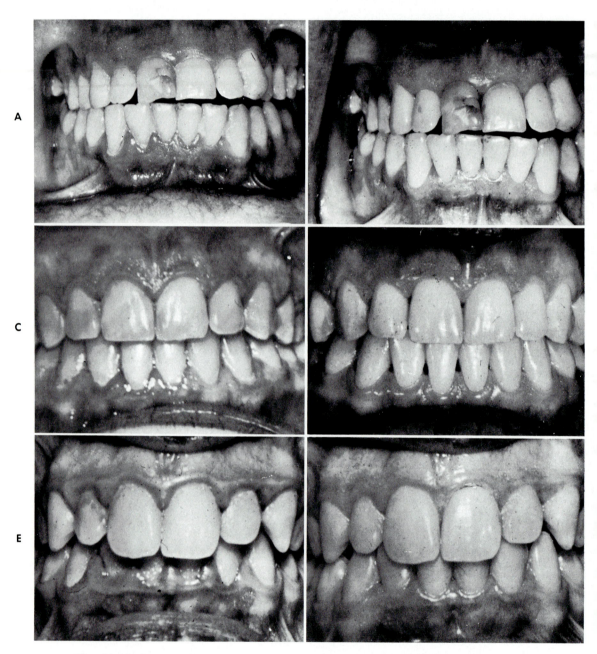

Fig. 24-12. Preoperative and postoperative views of three cases. **A** and **B,** Marginal gingivitis in which gingival tissue was characterized by inflammatory hyperplasia with heavy calculus deposits. **B** and **C,** Similar problem but with early crestal bone loss, characterized by a distinct blunting and cuplike resorption. Subgingival calculus deposits were present, adherent to all surfaces of almost all teeth. **E** and **F,** More severe inflammatory gingival hyperplasia. Rolled, retracted, yet almost friable gingivae could be retracted from tooth surface, accompanied by free bleeding. Note gingival topography after healing.

tively with regard to gingival health. *The external surface of the gingiva, the status of the sulcular lining, the depth of the sulcus, and the contour of the gingiva must all be considered.* The external surface should present all the characteristics of normal gingiva with regard to color, consistency, stippling, tone, and texture (Fig. 24-10). The sulcular lining should be smooth and continuous throughout and should be free of ulceration. Sulci that are ulcerated usually will bleed upon gentle probing. Of interest is O'Bannon's observation in 1964 that sulci over 3 mm deep have ulcerations at their base. The depth of the sulci should be minimal, and a thin well-contoured gingival architecture should be present. Postoperatively, although the gingiva has healed and a shallow sulcus is present, the gingival contour is often poor. The interproximal papillae remain thickened, and the gingival margin enlarged. To correct such a condition gingivoplasty is indicated (Figs. 24-11 and 24-12).

Experimental work

Many aspects of the scaling and curettage procedure have been experimentally investigated in human patients and in animals. A review of this literature is worthwhile to the clinician.

Subgingival scaling and root planing *directed only toward the removal of calculus* has been shown to have concomitant effects upon the soft tissue wall of the pocket. Ramfjord and Kiester, using the Bunting no. 5-6 curet in human patients, reported that thorough *scaling* would tear or split the epithelial attachment. They further reported that in areas of severe inflammation the epithelial lining would be partially or totally removed in the apical third of the pocket. Moskow, studying 266 human gingival biopsy sites in 1926, found also that routine scaling and root planing inadvertently tore and ripped the sulcular epithelium but did not completely remove the epithelial attachment. A partial removal of the sulcular epithelium and a tearing or splitting of the rete pegs occurred. O'Bannon investigated the changes in the soft tissue wall that occurred during scaling with the use of different instruments. He also frequently found splitting and fragmentation of the epithelium and the attachment. There tended to be less epithelial damage when hoes and files were used. It seems therefore as O'Bannon suspected, that the extent of this damage varies greatly with the amount of trauma imposed by the individual operator. Also the angle of instrument placement and many other factors may enter into this. It

is likely that the therapist could increase or decrease this inadvertent effect as he was so inclined. If gingival curettage were being performed at the same time as root planing and subgingival scaling, then the inadvertent removal of the soft tissue side of the pocket would be a desired objective and could be increased. If, however, the clinician wished only to accomplish subgingival scaling and root planing, then careful manipulation and instrument angulation could keep soft tissue destruction to a minimum.

In other studies it has been observed by various investigators that the healthy connective tissue attachment below the pocket in many cases is separated from the tooth during subgingival root planing or curettage. This was noted by Waerhaug in 1955, Moskow in 1962, Ramfjord and Costich in 1963, and O'Bannon in 1964. The clinical significance of this observation is not yet established, nor is it known whether such separation would allow proliferation of the epithelium into the space, thereby creating a deeper pocket than was present originally, or whether this area would reattach during healing. In any respect it seems to indicate judicious and careful use of any instrument subgingivally, with no more force or pressure than is minimally possible.

The ability to completely remove the lining epithelium and the epithelial attachment by the method of gingival curettage has been investigated. Waerhaug curetted the gingival sulci of twelve dog teeth and five human teeth and found that it was not possible to remove successfully the sulcular gingival epithelium by ordinary mechanical means. Sato also found that in human beings curettage of the gingival wall of the pocket was nearly always incomplete. Wertheimer, using Berliner's epithelial scalpel designed to peel out the epithelial linings of pockets, found complete removal of the epithelium in only three of 30 cases. Stone et al. in an autoradiographic study on three adult monkeys in which they did light gingival curettage with the Bunting no. 6-7 curet, with no distinct attempt to remove all the sulcular and attachment epithelium, found lining epithelium and epithelial attachment present most commonly in the bottom part of the sulcus. Conversely, Beube in 1953 performed a biopsy in several cases after curettage and reported that uniform removal of sulcular tissue could be achieved. Morris, using the McCall 2L and 2R curet on fifteen human patients in 1954, operated on the labial pocket of anterior teeth destined for extraction and found that epithelial linings and epithelial attachments up to but not including the gingival margin area were removed in all specimens. Blass and Lite found the sulcular epithelium to be completely removed immediately after curettage on five human patients. In 1964, Moskow, basing his report on 227 human gingival biopsies and two adult dog biopsies, found that gingival curettage as a separate and distinct procedure would if performed diligently remove all the sulcular epithelium and some of the underlying inflamed connective tissue. He found no reason to extend the curettage operation deliberately to ensure complete removal of the epithelial attachment as this structure would be eliminated in a routine operation on the sulcus. When he did find epithelium remaining it was most commonly located at that part of the sulcus approaching the gingival margin.

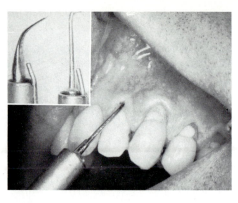

Fig. 24-13. Ultrasonic tips used in curettage (insert). Note placement of the instrument into pocket. Gingivae have been injected with a local anesthetic to make them firm, facilitating débridement.

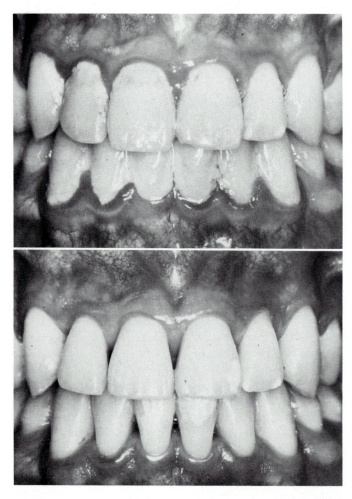

Fig. 24-14. Before and after photographs of a patient with marked inflammatory, edematous gingiva associated with heavy plaque formation and calculus both supragingivally and subgingivally. Teeth were thoroughly scaled, and curettage was performed. Note elimination of gingival inflammation and a healthy postoperative gingival attachment. Of interest is shallow zone of keratinized gingiva preoperatively; note zone postoperatively. If it is deemed inadequate, then a free mucosal graft procedure would be done.

It would seem therefore that a difference of opinion concerning the ability to remove completely the lining epithelium and the epithelial attachment by the technique of gingival curettage exists among the various investigators. These variations of opinion seem to be due to the difficulty inherent in trying to perform controlled investigations of this type. Some variation is due to differences in the depths of the pockets treated, the sites chosen for treatment, the instruments used, and the *thoroughness and capability of the therapist*. From a review of the foregoing articles it appears that *with thorough and diligent soft tissue curettage* under the proper circumstances, removal of the wound surface can be accomplished. The studies infer that to achieve uniform removal of wound surface, the operator must carefully choose the areas in which he will perform curettage and must then be diligent and dedicated to the accomplishment of this objective once he has begun.

The presence of debris and foreign material in the tissues after subgingival instrumentation has been reported experimentally. Ariaudo in 1951, Orban in 1945, Hiatt in 1951, and Barnfield in 1946 all reported the presence of calcified bodies in gingival biopsies. Moskow in 1960 felt that the tears created in the gingival wall during scaling might account for the presence of much of this foreign material in the sulcular tissue seen in post-treatment biopsies. He recommended the use of adequate suction and irrigation during any operation involving gingival tissue. Gibson and Shannon found that during the scaling procedure particles of carbon black that had been placed in the sulcus were introduced deep into the connective tissue. They concluded that bacteria could also gain entry in this manner. The finding of calcified bodies in the gingival tissue after subgingival instrumentation would seem to favor the performance of subgingival scaling and root planing and

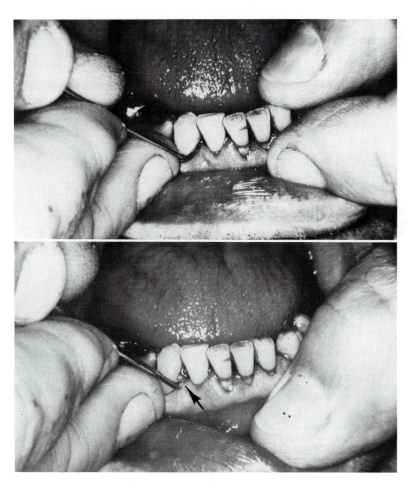

Fig. 24-15. Curettage utilized in initial preparation prior to definitive therapy for management of an osseous defect—osseous crater between lateral incisor and canine.

gingival curettage as separate procedures performed at different times.

The healing rate after curettage has been the subject of experimental investigation. In both animal and human studies epithelization of the sulcus is said to begin about 2 to 3 days after curettage and to be completed between 7 and 10 days after treatment. This time sequence has been reported even when extensive injury to the underlying corium has occurred during curettage. However, the time required for repair of the underlying connective tissue varies. Blass and Lite have described healing of the corium to be almost complete 10 days after curettage. Moskow in 1964 reported the presence of immature collagen fibers below the newly formed lining epithelium 21 days after treatment. Stone et al. have found that connective tissue healing is most active 2 to 3 days after scaling and light curettage. In the latter

study, in which all lining epithelium was not removed due to the light curettage, epithelial regeneration occurred mainly from remaining cells of the epithelial attachment and the sulcular lining. These investigators have also found that a new epithelial attachment may be established as early as 5 days after scaling and curettage. This variation in response of the connective tissue in different studies may be due to the many different variables not controlled in the experiments, or it may be due to a lack of clear-cut standards defining connective tissue repair. Other factors that could account for this variation are the type of patient involved and a difference in the investigator's vigor during curettage.

A few investigations of the amount of pocket reduction that occurs after gingival curettage are present in the literature. Korn et al. compared surgically created pockets in dogs treated by both

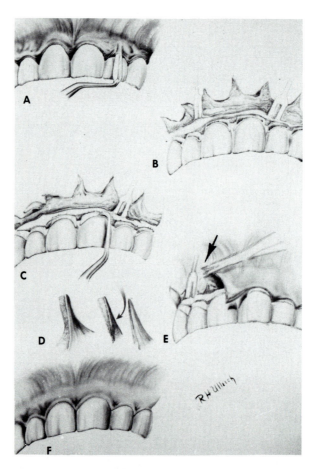

Fig. 24-16. Step-by-step procedure of débridement via flap method. *A,* Inverse incision is made; this is usually performed with a scalpel. *B,* Flap is raised. *C,* Entire tissue above bone is removed, and root surfaces are cleansed. *D* and *E,* Flap is thinned so that upon readaptation it will tautly cover alveolar crestal area. *F,* Healed gingival tissue and gingival attachment.

gingivectomy and gingival curettage. A highly significant degree of pocket reduction was found using gingival curettage. Benjamin in six human patients found the average pocket reduction 1 month after gingival curettage to be 0.9 mm. Ramfjord et al. compared the results of root surface and soft tissue curettage with the surgical elimination of pockets in 32 patients. When checked 1 year after therapy, curettage had reduced mean pocket depth by 1.1 mm. It appears from these investigations that gingival curettage is indeed a valuable tool in the periodontist's armamentarium for healing and for securing an intact gingival attachment.

CURETTAGE WITH ULTRASONIC INSTRUMENT

Débridement using an ultrasonic instrument has been performed now for many years. While the technique is exactly the same as that with a hand instrument, the difference lies in the tip of the instrument of the ultrasonic unit: with reduced water coolant and cavitation, heat is generated. Thus because of the diminished water spray the inner wall is coagulated and then flushed away with the water. The wound surface can be thoroughly debrided in this fashion, leaving a smooth surgical wound (Fig. 24-13).

CURETTAGE IN INITIAL PREPARATION

Curettage may be performed in instances where the operator realizes that the procedure will not meet the objectives of therapy but will prepare the operative site for better handling and management of the gingival tissue when definitive therapy is employed. Deep pockets with marked inflammatory changes and accompanying purulent exudate may be modified by débridement. In these instances the pocket area is flushed and cleansed with an antiseptic prior to débridement. Partial healing will result in that the color and consistency of the tissue exudate and its tendency to bleed will be modified. As a result better tissue management will be possible when osseous therapy is performed, for example, bone implant. Thus the healing that takes place alters the condition of the gingiva and provides significant

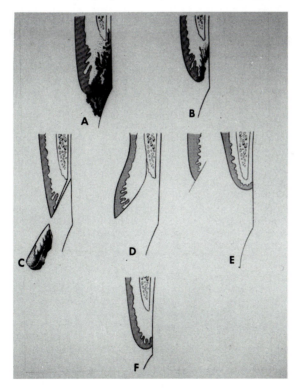

Fig. 24-17. Operative steps of débridement via flap procedure. *A,* Calculus occupying entire pocket; it is removed by scaling. Resultant gingival tissue is seen in *B.* Note that there is still an ulcerated pocket wall. *C,* An inverse bevel is made, and excised section is removed. *D,* Flap is retracted, and tooth surface cleansed. *E* and *F,* Readaptation of flap. In *E* gingival tissue is reduced and tautly placed over bone, whereas in *F* adaptation is more coronal.

changes in the periodontium so that the ultimate gingival treatment plan may be more easily and predictably accomplished (Figs. 24-14 and 24-15).

FLAP CURETTAGE

Unquestionably the most definitive method of removing all the diseased pocket's soft tissue as well as ensuring removal of all deposits on the root surface is by the inverse bevel flap procedure. The inverse beveled incision results in the immediate, total removal of the gingival wound. Reflection of the flap to expose the crest of alveolar bone allows access for complete débridement. After careful root planing and débridement, all areas can be carefully probed and examined and determination made as to the readaptation of

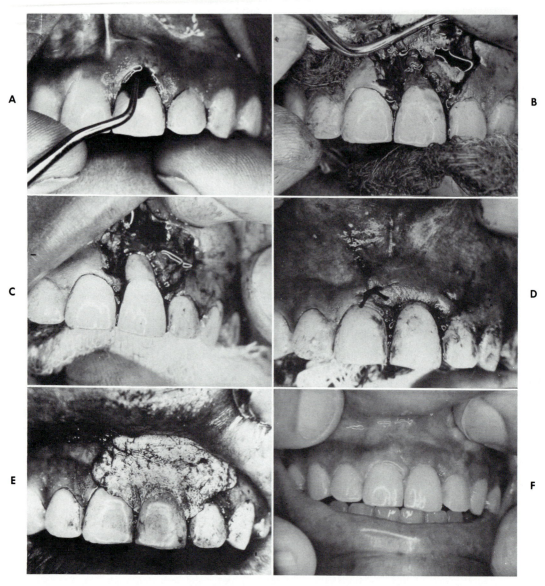

Fig. 24-18. Curettage-debridement procedure via flap method. **A,** Area is probed; detached gingiva is tested for retractability, depth, and lateral extent of detachment. **B,** One marginal and two vertical incisions are made, and flap is raised. Inflammatory tissue covering root surface is visible. Inner wall of flap is studded with inflammatory tissue as well. **C,** Tooth surface is debrided, and all inflammatory tissue is removed from surrounding bone. Inner wall of flap is debrided; all tabs must be removed. Flap is replaced and sutured, **D,** and covered with a periodontal dressing, **E** and **F,** Postoperative healing 10 days later.

the flaps. The gingival flaps are sutured securely with interrupted sutures, and the surgical site is covered with a surgical dressing for 1 week. Usually this is sufficient (Figs. 24-16 to 24-18).

REFERENCES

Aleo, J., DeRenzis, F., and Farber, P.: *In vitro* attachment of human gingival fibroblasts to root surfaces, J. Periodontol. **46:**639, 1975.

Bandt, C. L., Korn, N. A., and Schaffer, E. M.: Bacteremias from ultrasonic and hand instrumentation, J. Periodontol. **35:**214, 1964.

Barkann, L.: A conservative surgical technic for the eradication of a pyorrhea pocket, J. Am. Dent. Assoc. **26:**61, 1939.

Barnfield, W. M.: Pathological calcification of the gingivae, Am. J. Pathol. **22:**1307, 1946.

Bell, D.: Indication and contraindication for subgingival curettage in the treatment of paradentosis, J. Periodontol. **8:**55, 1937.

Benjamin, E. M.: The quantitative comparison of subgingival curettage and gingivectomy in the treatment of periodontitis simplex, J. Periodontol. **27:**144, 1956.

Beube, F. E.: Treatment methods for marginal gingivitis and periodontitis, Tex. Dent. J. **71:**427, 1953.

Beube, F. E.: A study on reattachment of the supporting structures of the teeth, J. Periodontol. **18:**55, 1947.

Bjorndahl, O.: Reattachment and bone regeneration; report of a case, J. Am. Dent. Assoc. **26:**356, 1948.

Blass, J. L., and Lite, T.: Gingival healing following surgical curettage; a histopathologic study, N.Y. Dent. J. **25:**127, 1959.

Borden, S. M.: Histological study of healing following detachment of tissue as is commonly carried out in the vertical incision for the surgical removal of teeth, J. Can. Dent. Assoc. **14:**510, 1948.

Box, H. K.: Studies in periodontal pathology, Toronto, 1924, Canadian Dental Research Foundation.

Chaikin, B. S.: Subgingival curettage, J. Periodontol. **25:**240, 1954.

Ewen, S. J.: Ultrasonic wound — some microscopic observations, J. Periodontol. **33:**315, 1961.

Ewen, S. J.: Ultrasonic surgery in periodontal therapy, N.Y. Dent. J. **25:**189, 1959.

Gibson, W. A., and Shannon, I. L.: Simulation with carbon particles of bacterial infiltration of human gingival tissues, Periodontics **3:**57, 1965.

Goldman, H. M.: Histologic assay of healing following ultrasonic curettage versus hand-instrument curettage, Oral Surg. **14:**925, 1961.

Goldman, H. M.: Curettage by ultrasonic instrument, Oral Surg. **13:**43, 1960.

Goldman, H. M.: Subgingival curettage; a rationale, J. Periodontol. **19:**54, 1948.

Green, G. H., and Sanderson, A. D.: Ultrasonics and periodontal therapy; a review of clinical and biologic effects, J. Periodontol. **36:**232, 1965.

Hiatt, W. H.: Calcified bodies in the gingiva, J. Periodontol. **22:**96, 1951.

Hirschfeld, L.: Subgingival curettage in periodontal therapy, J. Am. Dent. Assoc. **44:**301, 1952.

Ingle, J.: Periodontal curettement in the premaxilla, J. Periodontol. **23:**143, 1952.

Korn, N. A., Schaffer, E. M., and McHugh, R. B.: An experimental assessment of gingivectomy and soft tissue curettage in dogs, J. Periodontol. **36:**96, 1965.

Leonard, H. J.: Raising the line of epithelial attachment and increasing depth of clinical root, J. Periodontol. **21:**221, 1950.

Linghorne, W. J., and O'Connell, D. C.: Studies in the regeneration and reattachment of supporting structures of the teeth. III. Regeneration in epithelized pockets following the organization of a blood clot, J. Dent. Res. **36:**4, 1957.

Linghorne, W. J., and O'Connell, D. C.: Studies in the regeneration and reattachment of supporting structures of the teeth. I. Soft tissue reattachment, J. Dent. Res. **29:**419, 1950.

Marfino, N. R., Orban, B. J., and Wentz, I. M.: Repair of the dento-gingival junction following surgical intervention, J. Periodontol. **30:**180, 1959.

McCall, J. O.: An improved method of inducing reattachment of the gingival tissues in periodontoclasia, Dent. Items Interest **8:**342, 1926.

Morris, M.: The removal of pocket and attachment epithelium in humans; a histological study, J. Periodontol. **25:**7, 1954.

Moskow, B. S.: Response of the gingival sulcus to instrumentation; a histologic investigation. II. Gingival curettage, J. Periodontol. **35:**112, 1964.

Moskow, B. S.: Response of the gingival sulcus to instrumentation; a histologic investigation. I. The scaling procedure, J. Periodontol. **33:**282, 1962.

Moskow, B. S.: Calcifications in gingival biopsies, Dent. Progr. **1:**30, 1960.

Nadler, H.: Removal of crevicular epithelium by ultrasonic curettes, J. Periodontol. **33:**220, 1962.

O'Bannon, J. Y.: The gingival tissues before and after scaling the teeth, J. Periodontol. **35:**69, 1964.

Orban, B.: Gingival inclusions, J. Periodontol. **16:**16, 1945.

Ramfjord, S. P.: Reattachment in periodontal therapy, J. Am. Dent. Assoc. **45:**513, 1952.

Ramfjord, S. P.: Experimental periodontal reattachment in rhesus monkeys, J. Periodontol. **22:**67, 1951.

Ramfjord, S. P., and Costich, E. R.: Healing after simple gingivectomy, J. Periodontol. **34:**401, 1963.

Ramfjord, S. P., Engler, W. O., and Hiniker, J. J.: A radioautographic study of healing following simple gingivectomy. II. The connective tissue, J. Periodontol. **37:**179, 1966.

Ramfjord, S. P., and Kiester, G.: The gingival sulcus and the periodontal pocket immediately following scaling of teeth, J. Periodontol. **25:**167, 1954.

Ramfjord, S. P., Nissle, R. R., Shick, R. A., and Cooper, H., Jr.: Subgingival curettage versus surgical elimination of periodontal pockets, J. Periodontol. **39:**167, 1968.

Register, A. A., and Burdick, F. A.: Accelerated reattachment with cementogenesis to dentin demineralized *in situ*. I. Optimal range, J. Periodontol. **46:**646, 1975.

Ritchey, B., and Orban, B.: The periodontal pocket, J. Periodontol. **23:**199, 1952.

Rosenthal, S. L.: Conservative methods for reduction of the periodontal pocket, Dent. Items Interest **72:**154, 1950.

Rosling, B., et al.: The healing potential of the periodontal tissues following different techniques of periodontal surgery in plaque free dentitions, J. Clin. Periodontol. **3:**233, 1976.

Sanderson, A. D.: Gingival curettage by hand and ultrasonic instruments; a histologic comparison, J. Periodontol. **37:**279, 1966.

Sato, M.: Histopathological study of the healing process after surgical treatment for alveolar pyorrhea, Bull. Tokyo Med. Dent. Univ. **1:**71, 1960.

Schaeffer, E. M., and Zander, H. A.: Histological evidence of reattachment of periodontal pockets, Parodontologic **7:** 101, 1953.

Seibert, J.: Incorporating root planing and gingival curettage into a clinical practice, Continuing Dental Education Series, vol 1, no. 8, Philadelphia, May 1978, University of Pennsylvania Press.

Skillen, W. G., and Lundquist, G. R.: An experimental study of periodontal membrane reattachment in health and pathologic tissues, J. Am. Dent. Assoc. **24:**175, 1937.

Stahl, S. S.: Healing of gingival tissues following various therapeutic regimens; a review of histologic studies, J. Oral Ther. **2:**145, 1965.

Stahl, S. S., and Person, P. P.: Reattachment of epithelium and connective tissue following gingival injury in rats, J. Periodontol. **33:**51, 1962.

Stone, S., Ramfjord, S. P., and Waldron, J.: Scaling and gingival curettage; a radioautographic study, J. Periodontol. **37:**415, 1966.

Stones, H. H.: The reaction and regeneration of cementum in various pathological conditions, Proc. R. Soc. Med. **27:**728, 1934.

Wade, A. B.: Periodontal curettage at operation—method and results, Int. Dent. J. **8:**19, 1958.

Waerhaug, J.: Effect of rough surfaces upon gingival tissue, J. Dent. Res. **35:**323, 1956.

Waerhaug, J.: Microscopic demonstration of tissue reaction incident to removal of subgingival calculus, J. Periodontol. **26:**26, 1955.

Zach, L., and Cohen, G.: The histology of the response to ultrasonic curettage (abstract), J. Dent. Res. **40:**751, 1961.

25 Gingivectomy

Gingivectomy is the surgical procedure designed to resect the detached gingival pocket in inflammatory periodontal disease in such a manner that the remaining gingiva will heal to provide health, function, and aesthetics. The gingival wound is totally excised, leaving a surface surgical wound. The technique is usually restricted to soft tissue removal and reconstruction of the resultant wound surface. *An adequate zone of attached gingiva must be present so that after the excision procedure is performed, sufficient attached gingiva remains.*

Advances in the understanding as well as the recognition of mucogingival and osseous problems have led to the development of highly sophisticated surgical approaches to these problems. It has become obvious that defects in the underlying alveolar bone cannot be treated and corrected or altered predictably by treatment of the soft tissue pocket alone. It also has become apparent that resection of the gingiva down to an irregular osseous base will result in gingival healing in such a fashion as to bridge osseous deformities and eventually resume a parabolic morphology despite the form of the underlying bone. The result in most cases will be the return of detached gingival tissue.

It seems that similar criteria for physiologic morphology of gingiva as espoused by Goldman need also to be applied to alveolar bone when it is affected by periodontal tissue. In light of this it appears that gingivectomy today is best indicated for treatment of suprabony pockets where the underlying alveolar bone has not been topographically affected by the disease process or has such form as to be anatomically acceptable or both.

The objectives of gingivectomy are the elimination of gingival pockets and the creation of physiologic gingival morphology.

The concept of gingivoplasty as an essential aspect of the gingivectomy procedure was introduced by Goldman, who recognized the importance of physiologic tissue form. He felt that morphology of the gingiva postoperatively was closely related to health and prevention of future disease in that cleansibility was essential.

The gingival margins should be thinned, beveled, and adapted tightly to the tooth while extending mesiodistally in a smooth parabolic curve. Whenever possible the gingival margins should be protected by cervical tooth convexities.

The interdental gingiva should be formed by a pyramidal-shaped confluence of the gingival margins of adjacent teeth. The tip of the peak should be located coronally to the adjacent gingival margins, thereby obviating the possibility of reverse marginal architectural form. The interdental soft tissue is ideally formed so as to have a slope of approximately 45 degrees and a linear indentation in an occlusoapical direction forming an interdental sluiceway. In certain instances (i.e., when a diastema is present between two teeth) the interdental form consists of convex tissue surfaces from the buccal to the lingual aspect after healing. These qualities permit ease of cleansing of the interdental areas and provide a measure of protection against the recurrence of gingival inflammation.

Physiologic form necessitates that there be an adequate zone of attached gingiva and that its surface be shaped to allow the passage of foreign substances from the marginal and interdental areas toward the vestibular and lingual fornices. This offers cleansibility to the cervical portion of the tooth. If the margin is thick and irregular, cleansibility is hampered and often impossible.

Indications

Gingivectomy should not be considered an alternative to scaling and curettage or to mucogingival surgical techniques. It is a definitive surgical procedure designed to fulfill certain objectives, as previously noted. Indeed, when utilized where indicated, no other periodontal surgical procedure can as easily and simply produce optimum gingival morphology as can the gingivectomy. It is for this reason that many therapists will frequently utilize gingivoplasty techniques after other surgical techniques that may be required to correct osseous and mucogingival problems.

Discussion of all the following indications for gingivectomy is predicated on the recognition that the underlying alveolar bone must be free from architectural deformities. It should be emphasized, however, that the presence of osseous deformities or architecture that may not be consistent with the therapist's concept of the ideal, in the absence of gingival disease, does not justify osseous surgery. However, the presence of such osseous deformities together with inflammatory periodontal disease now requires that the osseous morphology be examined regarding its possible role in the etiology or as an influencing factor in the pathologic process. The therapist must determine whether osseous deformities such as reverse architecture or heavy osseous ledging have dictated the gingival position and form in such a manner as to make it more susceptible to breakdown by their local etiologic factors. Cleansibility plays an important role in this regard.

Consideration must also be given to the influence that the underlying osseous form may have on the healing of the surgical site and its ability to maintain health. The indications are as follows.

Elimination of tissues disfigured by fibrous enlargement and irregular recession. The reaction of gingival tissue may range from the more acute inflammatory changes of hyperemia, tenderness, and hemorrhage to fibrosis. The fibrotic stage may often follow the initial changes. However, the resistance of the tissues and the type of irritant may be such that the patient is never aware of the initial changes. In more vulnerable areas such as prominent roots, teeth in buccal version, and gingival units with long connective tissue attachments, the results may be recession of the gingival margin.

In areas where fibrotic changes have taken place, gingival margins often are rolled and thickened and interdental papillae are often bulbous and displaced. When these conditions exist and

there are no osseous deformities or potential mucogingival problems and when the etiologic factors have been recognized and controlled or altered, the gingivectomy procedure may be expected to produce excellent results.

Diseased pocket wall. Elimination of the diseased pocket wall is a prime objective of periodontal therapy. When the marginal inflammatory process in periodontal disease causes the destruction of the gingival fibers, the epithelial attachment migrates apically. The result of this process is that the gingival tissue is more or less detached from the tooth, depending on the amount of migration of the epithelial attachment. This detached gingiva (pocket) serves as a repository for plaque, debris, and calculus, since it is extremely difficult for the patient to cleanse this area. Therefore because the plaque cannot be readily controlled in this area, it is chronically inflamed and the destructive process continues. It becomes apparent that the gingival pocket, the result of gingival inflammation, not only enhances its self-perpetuation, but also contributes to continued and further breakdown of the periodontium.

Thus the gingivectomy is an effective and easy means of resecting the gingival pocket in areas free from mucogingival complications and where the underlying alveolar bone does not require therapy.

Width of keratinized tissue. It is important that the gingivectomy be performed in areas having a sufficient width of keratinized tissue so as to leave an adequate band of keratinized tissue after the gingival resection is performed. This means that the primary gingivectomy incision will be negotiated in attached tissue at a level coronal to the mucogingival junction. Thus the base of the pocket should also be distinctly occlusal to this line so as to allow for the beveled primary incision. If the pocket base approaches or is apical to the mucogingival junction, the gingivectomy is contraindicated.

Necrotizing ulcerative gingivitis. One of the protean manifestations of necrotizing ulcerative gingivitis is an irregular pattern of destruction of either or both interdental and marginal gingivae. Interdental soft tissue cratering, reverse gingival architecture in which the interdental gingival crest is at or apical to the adjacent gingival margins, alterations in marginal curvature with loss of the normal parabolic path, soft tissue clefts, and so on may also be prominent when the infectious process has subsided, and partial collagenous and epithelial repair has occurred in the gingiva. This pattern of tissue irregularity is even more noteworthy when the tissue has been subjected to repeated bouts of the disease. It is highly desirable, when the disease is quiescent and relative fibrosis is present, to utilize gingivectomy as a facet of the gingivoplasty operation to create physiologic tissue form. Tissue with self-cleansing and cleansable form (e.g., a clean tooth surface—which is part of a physiologic dentogingival environment) can be a potent factor in the prevention of recurrent disease, often minimizing the strong emotional and somatic influences on the genesis of the lesion.

Fibrous hyperplasia. It is often desirable to resect gingival tissue that is enlarged and distorted because of fibrous hyperplasia. Sustained administration of phenytoin sodium (Dilantin) for the control of convulsive seizures is a fairly common reason for excessive collagen formation in the gingiva, as it is a direct stimulant to fibroblastic activity. An inflammatory component that augments the process is usually found coincidently. The gingivectomy operation, including gingivoplasty, is ideally suited for the elimination of pathologically altered tissue, particularly when the tissue interferes with function (e.g., mastication) and permits lodgment of plaque and debris at the marginal area (thus implementing an inflammatory process), or when it induces oral or facial disfigurement. In gingivectomy, particular attention is given not only to the removal of excess tissue but also to the provision of a physiologic environment by gingivoplasty. Similar measures are necessary in such other gingival enlargements as hereditary diffuse gingivofibromatosis and localized fibrous hyperplasias of irritational origin and in association with operations for the removal of benign gingival tumors.

Altered passive eruption. Gingivectomy may be applicable to cases of altered (retarded) passive eruption. Here, instead of being located at or apical to the axial tooth curvature, the gingival margins fail to recede during tooth eruption to a level apical to the cervical convexity of the tooth crown. In the majority of cases the gingival wall presents evidence of inflammatory disease and concurrently is undesirable cosmetically. It is best resected to the level of the cementoenamel junction when disease is present. It is important that cases of altered passive eruption be carefully probed prior to periodontal surgery. It has been demonstrated that many cases of altered passive eruption exhibit exceptionally heavy buccal plates of alveolar bone. It has been proposed that re-

section of the gingival tissue, without reduction of these heavy osseous plates, may often lead to the regrowth of the gingival tissue.

Osseous configuration of palate. On the palatal and lingual aspects of the teeth, where the osseous configuration is acceptable, with suprabony pocket formation, gingivectomy may be performed. Palatal gingivectomies are easily performed, heal well, and provide acceptable tissue form postoperatively either when the depth of tissue involvement is moderate in the face of adequate alveolar height or when the amount of detachable tissue is slight, concomitant with shallow alveolar height. Much is dependent on the shape of the palatal vault and the height and steepness of the palatal aspect of the alveolar process in relation to the depth of penetration apically of the lesion. The applicability of gingivectomy varies directly with the height of the vault and alveolus and inversely with the depth of the palatal and interdental involvement. Conversely, when the vault is shallowed or when the alveolar height is shortened and the depth of the pockets is relatively great, gingivectomy is contraindicated.

• • •

In summation, the gingivectomy presents an uncomplicated, rapid, and effective means of eradicating suprabony pockets and of functionally reconstructing the remaining attached gingiva. When the incisions at the bases of the pockets do not violate either the area of alveolar mucosa or the attachment at the mucogingival junction, an adequate zone of keratinized tissue should remain.

Desired results

Properly performed, the gingivectomy procedure can produce with minimal effort the most desirable results. Following is a list of gingivectomy's desired results:

1. A thin gingival margin, beveled and adapted tightly to the tooth, should extend mesially and distally in a smooth, parabolic curve.
2. Pyramidally shaped interdental gingiva should be confluent with the gingival margins of adjacent teeth.
3. The tip of the interdental gingival peak should be located coronally to the adjacent gingival margins, eliminating any reverse architecture.
4. The interdental papilla should slope approximately 45 degrees and have a linear indentation to form a sluiceway occlusoapically.

5. The remaining zone of attached gingiva should be—
   a. Adequate
   b. Keratinized
   c. Shaped to allow free passage from the marginal and interdental areas to the vestibule and lingual fornices

It is imperative following gingivectomy that the zone of keratinized gingiva retained be deemed adequate. When the procedure produces a result where any of the following situations arise, then the gingival zone must be considered inadequate:

1. Where the procedure results in the complete loss of keratinized tissue
2. Where tension of the alveolar mucosa causes the apical movement of the free gingival margin
3. Where the original depth of the pocket approaches the mucogingival junction, so that its resection will leave little or no keratinized tissue
4. Where the original pocket depth traverses the mucogingival junction

Contraindications

Gingivectomy, as previously noted, is primarily applicable to pocket elimination when the diseased gingiva presents clinically in the fibrotic phase of the inflammatory process. In this state the tissue is enlarged or distorted and retractable from the tooth surface, yet its consistency is firm. Bleeding may occur upon probing or palpatation, yet the degree of hyperemia is minimal. The clinical evidence of exudation will be slight. If the soft tissue wall of the pocket presents features synonymous with delicacy, friability, flaccidity, and discoloration, gingivectomy is a poor therapeutic choice. Initial well-executed therapy may bring about an attentuation of the inflammatory process, rendering the tissue amenable to resection. If after initial therapy has been performed the depths are moderate or shallow and edematous characteristics are predominant, curettage may be rationally applied.

As stated previously, gingivectomy should not be considered when the pocket bases encroach on the mucogingival junction. Under these circumstances the incision would not only occur in the zone of alveolar mucosa, but would obliterate any remaining attached gingiva. Thus after healing had taken place the new gingival margin could conceivably be composed of alveolar mucosa—a tissue considered unable to adapt successfully to functional demands. Optimum function

requires that the gingiva be dense, firm, thin, and movably attached to underlying structures and have a keratinized epithelial surface. Additionally, the distance from the vestibular fornix to the gingival margin will be shortened, bringing the gingival margin closer to the fornix. Such a relationship contributes to accumulation of plaque and debris marginally and interdentally and to horizontal debris lodgment, with subsequent recurrence of inflammatory disease.

Similarly, gingivectomy should not be relied upon when endosseous defects or anatomic anomalies such as irregular margins and marginal ledging exist. It is important to conserve gingiva in order to allow the treated osseous tissue to be protected during the healing process.

Palatal aspects of maxillary posterior teeth. When the palatal vault is shallow and the depth of periodontal involvement is great, gingivectomy on the palatal aspects of maxillary posterior teeth necessitates starting the initial cut nearer to the midline in order to avoid an inverse cut. In certain second and third molar areas the soft palate could well become the gingival margin. The gingival margin under this condition tends to curl; plaque can readily accumulate because oral hygiene measures are impaired and gingival inflammatory disease can recur.

Interradicular zones. When new attachment or osteoplastic measures are indicated in the interradicular zones, the gingivectomy is contraindicated. It is of prime importance to obtain as much keratinized gingiva as possible for bony protection.

Buccal lesions in mandibular molar areas. When the facial aspects of the alveolar process has a distinct outward flare, tending to form a shelf of bone, in certain cases the lesion *may encroach upon the external oblique ridge* in second molar areas. This situation negates the use of gingivectomy because the new gingival margin would be placed inappropriately in alveolar mucosa. A further deterrent is the fact that the zone of keratinized tissue is often perilously narrow in these areas.

Mandibular retromolar regions. When an incision must be made in movable and delicate mucosa, this tissue often cuts poorly, bleeds profusely, and may be difficult to resect and shape. The use of the distal wedge procedure, as mentioned by Robinson, often simplifies the management of retromolar tissue.

Maxillary retromolar and tuberosity areas. When soft tissue bulk is so great, relative to the depth of periodontal involvement on the distal aspect of the last molar, that its level resectioned would bring about surgical entry into the mucosa of the hamular notch, gingivectomy is contraindicated. The distal wedge procedure utilized in such instances resects the distal pocket wall and reduces tuberosity height and width.

Periodontal clefts. When the apical bases of periodontal clefts are composed of or encroach upon the alveolar mucosa, gingivectomy is contraindicated. Such areas are better managed by laterally positioned flaps, gingival autographs, and double papilla grafts.

Maxillary and mandibular anterior areas. When resection of tissue may lead to unduly long clinical crowns, unsightly and tissueless interdental gingival embrasures, or undesirable exposure of root surfaces or margins of restorations, resection techniques must be combined with other changes to minimize cosmetic or aesthetic disfigurement. Shortening the clinical crown, orthodontics, restorative dentistry, or full coverage of teeth to change spacing may be necessary to camouflage the clinical appearance. Of course if the lip line is low and the teeth do not show, then there is very little problem.

Cases of systemic disease or emotional problems. Diminished patient cooperation and motivation, the possibility of retarded healing, and so on have a direct bearing on the desirability of performing surgical therapy. This holds true for a patient with poorly controlled diabetes mellitus, hyperthyroidism, advanced arteriosclerosis, or a history of coronary insufficiency or thrombosis. Similarly, a patient on a complicating drug regimen (e.g., the anticoagulant dicumarol) or suffering from a hereditary or acquired clotting defect requires special consideration. In a general context these individuals should not be subject to arduous, complicated, or prolonged therapeutic procedures; surely amelioration, control, or cure of the systemic state is a prerequisite to all but emergency treatment.

Initial preparation

The successful application of gingivectomy from a technical standpoint and the stability of functional form in the postoperative corium demand that the incisional and tissue-shaping portions of the procedure be carried out in tissue that is free from overt inflammatory manifestations (hyperemia, exudation, edema, and so on) and is thus in the relatively quiescent, fibrogenic phase of the inflammatory process. To achieve such

qualities one should perform initial therapy in all its facets prior to surgical treatment. Such procedures as scaling—calculus and plaque removal —and tooth surface preparation and smoothing—planing and polishing—should be carried out as fully as possible before subjecting an area to gingival surgery. It has been established that edematous and often hemorrhagic tissue is difficult to handle surgically; such tissue is friable, tearing or shredding during incision, and often bleeds profusely, tending to obscure the surgical site. The results of plastic procedures performed in edematous tissue are difficult to predict and maintain. Facility of surgical performance and stable form are predicated upon execution of the procedure in densely fibrous tissue. Philosophies advocating scaling at the time of surgery, although possibly permitting easier access to calcific deposits, subject nearly all patients to carte blanche surgery. Prescaling in many cases, besides converting the inflammatory process to a clinically less severe one (i.e., reducing edema or erythema) and augmenting fibrogenesis in the tissue, may be sufficient therapy to bring about resolution of the inflammatory process and acquisition of acceptable tissue form, thus negating or minimizing the need for surgical intervention.

Instrumentation

There are many sets of instruments available for the performance of periodontal surgery. All of them should be regarded as simple scalpels, shaped and bent for ready access to comparatively inaccessible regions and formed for maximal cutting efficiency in areas where space is at a premium. Thus retromolar, interproximal, edentulous, lingual, and palatal areas may generally be treated surgically as easily and as efficiently as labial and buccal zones. In addition, special instruments have been devised for preincisional marking of pocket depths, for débridement of tooth and soft tissue surfaces, for dislodgment and removal of incised tissue, and for creation of physiologic tissue form.

It should be emphasized that all cutting instruments be sharpened prior to their sterilization along with the other components of the surgical assembly. Dry heat sterilization is preferred, maintaining a temperature of 177° C for a minimum of 1 hour. For dry heat and other sterilization to be effective all debris and blood must be removed from the instruments either with a scrub brush and cool soapy water or with an ultrasonic instrument cleaning device.

The basic kit for gingivectomy-gingivoplasty should include the following instruments.

Specially formed college pliers for pocket marking. One beak of the college pliers is straight and thin for entrance into the deepened sulcus; the other beak is bent at right angles at its very tip so as to coincide with the first beak when the beaks are compressed. The coincidence of the beaks during pocket marking establishes the depth of the pocket by creating a tissue puncture and thus a bleeding point on the outer aspect of the gingiva, providing a guide for the primary gingivectomy incision. It is imperative that the probing (straight) beak enter the pocket in such a manner that it is related parallel to the tooth. When labial, buccal, or lingual pockets are delineated, this beak must coincide with the direction of the axial surface. Should the beak be inadvertently tipped buccally, a false apically directed bleeding point may be established, guiding the subsequent incision erroneously into intact and attached tissue. Conversely, should the beak be tipped back toward the tooth, an unrealistic coronally displaced bleeding point may be created; thus when the primary incision is made, the pocket wall may not be resected in its entirety, leaving residual depth and diseased tissue. Pocket markers are provided in a set of *right* and *left* instruments. The more popular ones bear the names of their designers, Crane-Kaplan and Goldman-Fox. The Goldman-Fox instruments are considerably more rigid while retaining an exceptional degree of delicacy (Figs. 25-1 and 25-2).

Periodontal probe. The periodontal probe is a dull, thin, narrow calibrated blade used primarily for ascertaining the radicular (or in some instances the coronal) location of the sulcular or pocket base. It is thus an aid to periodontal diagnosis. Conventional pocket markers are often difficult to utilize properly in the interproximal areas; in certain cases the straight beak cannot be placed parallel to the tooth surface to obtain a correct pocket marking. This problem may be overcome by using the periodontal probe as a marker. Its use is quite simple. The probe is utilized in the conventional manner to determine the degree of detachment in a given subgingival area. When the depth has been ascertained from the gingival margin to the base of detachment, this identical measurement is made on the facial (or lingual) aspect of the soft tissue wall; for example, if the pocket measurement is 5 mm, an equivalent zone is delineated on the outer aspect of the gingiva. The tip of the probe is then turned horizontally and used to make

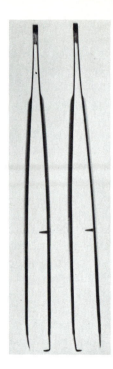

Fig. 25-1. Pocket markers for right and left usage are employed to delineate apical bases of pocket walls, thus furnishing a guide for primary gingivectomy incision. Bent beaks are fine and sharp.

a tissue puncture at a point 5 mm from the gingival margin. The bleeding points, as established by use of the pocket markers and the periodontal probe, are fairly precise guides when linearly connected for the primary gingivectomy incision.

Broad-bladed, rounded scalpels. The shanks of the broad-bladed, rounded scalpels are bent at an angle to allow for access, cutting efficiency, and proper angle of incision on the facial, lingual, and palatal aspects of the dentition. The Goldman-Fox no. 7 instrument has blades at both ends located and angled in such a manner as to facilitate its use on the right and left or buccal and lingual aspects of the teeth.

Narrow-bladed, tapered (spear-shaped) scalpels. The narrow-bladed, tapered scalpels are sharp at the tip bilaterally and are appropriately bent for interproximal and retromolar incision. These scalpels too are double ended, with shanks bent (and thus blade directed) to allow right or left usage. When used for the secondary gingivectomy incision, the spear is directed interdentally at a 45-degree (variable) angle toward the occlusal plane so as to resect interproximal tissue in such a manner that the wound bed has occlusoapical and faciolingual slopes. The Gold-

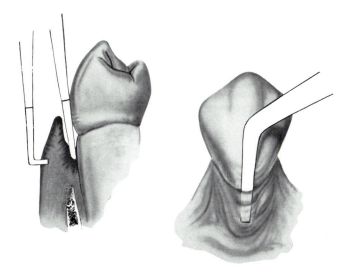

Fig. 25-2. In correct use of pocket marker, probing beak of instrument should be placed parallel to long axis of tooth. This will provide proper orientation for perforating beak to delineate base of pocket. Periodontal probe is also used to locate base of pocket.

man-Fox nos. 8, 9, and 11 satisfy the requirements for interproximal instrumentation.

Surgical handle with detachable and replaceable surgical blades (Bard-Parker no. 15). The small-bladed straight surgical knife is often of value for incision in areas of restricted access such as the buccal aspects of maxillary and mandibular second and third molars when the cheek musculature is full and taut. Blake and Trott have created a special gingivectomy knife handle into which a portion of a Bard-Parker no. 11 blade is placed, while Ramfjord has utilized a special blade (no. 12b) for gingivectomy incisions. The choice of instruments for periodontal procedures is one based on personal preference, experience, requirements in periodontal training, and such intangibles as feel and balance. Of much greater importance than a particular instrument design per se is the ability to use an applicable instrument with facility, efficiency, and accuracy to accomplish a specific objective.

Curets. Curets are included in the surgical kit for removing calculus (and overlying plaque) that may be residual upon coronal and radicular surfaces, for planing irregular or roughened areas of the root so that optically and tactilely smooth surfaces will result, and for removing excess tissue marginally and interdentally. Especially adaptable for these purposes are the Goldman-Fox curets nos. 3 and 21. The no. 21 curet is an instrument with very small, finely tapered, sickle-shaped blades at each end. The blades in cross section are triangular, presenting therefore two cutting edges and a sharp point.

Special hoe-shaped instruments. The hoe-shaped instruments are for dislodging and removing incised tissue. The concave and sharp working edges of the Goldman-Fox no. 10 instrument allow for close adaptation to root and interdental surfaces, thus compressing soft tissue well against the tooth while the final incision and dislodgment are made.

Thin-beaked surgical shears. Thin-beaked shears with serrated cutting surfaces (Goldman-Fox periodontal surgical scissors) are for excising frayed marginal tissues, for freeing incised tissue (especially interdentally) from the underlying wound bed, for providing physiologic curvatures to the gingival margins, for removing granulations from the inner aspect of flaps or semiflaps, and in mucogingival procedures for making mucosal incisions at the mucogingival junction. They may also be utilized as suture scissors. Shears are integral to all surgical instrument assemblies.

Soft tissue rongeur. The soft tissue rongeur is used extensively in gingival surgery, particularly for thinning attached gingiva and removing excessive tissue interproximally, while concomitantly producing the surface topography desirable for maintenance of the tissue in a cleansed state. The rongeur is in reality an adaptation of the cuticle nipper. The periodontal version, however, is provided as a more rigid but finer beaked stainless steel instrument. The device is not new to periodontal therapy, having been used by Kirkland in the 1920s to remove interdental granulations. Its use in gingivoplasty, frenotomy, and muco-gingival surgery is comparatively recent.

Coarse diamond stones. Coarse diamond stones are indicated for gingivoplastic and osteo-plastic procedures. Soft tissue bulk and irregu-larities may be removed so as to thin the tissue and provide a smooth connective tissue wound bed. Such a use on dense, fibrotic tissue not only provides for physiologic form but also permits more rapid and complete epithelization during healing of the gingivectomy wound. It is impor-tant that there be a constant spray of water on the rotating stones during their use. They should be employed with a light brushing movement over the gingival surface. Pressure on the tissue tends to induce irregular tissue removal and fraying of the gingival corium. The most popular diamonds are round (approximately the size of the no. 6 round bur), conical, or doughnut shaped. The doughnut shape is particularly advantageous for use on the buccal, palatal, or lingual gingiva, whereas the conical stones are essentially for the shaping of interdental tissue.

Anesthesia for gingivectomy

Since gingivectomy is performed alone rather than in association with restorative procedures or any grinding on the teeth, adequate and profound anesthesia for soft tissue resection and contouring may be secured through infiltrative anesthetics. Block anesthesia is not a requirement, but may be desirable to reduce the number of needle punc-tures in unanesthetized tissue. After the block, in-tragingival injections may be given to increase tissue rigidity and hemostasis. We prefer (1) in-jections into the vestibular fold or (2) soft tissue anesthetization procured through the injection of minute amounts of local anesthetic into each of the interdental papillae of the surgical area. The in-jections are quite painless, especially if the most anterior (mesial) papilla is anesthetized first; rapid anesthesia will be secured not only in the papillae but also in the marginal and attached gingiva dis-tal to the papilla. One may observe blanching of the tissue as a sign of early anesthesia. The ad-jacent papilla is now entered and is anesthetized along with the marginal gingiva just distal to it. Repeated injections are given, progressing dis-tally. A large measure of anesthesia of the lingual or palatal tissue is concurrently attained; to ensure adequacy of anesthetization, however, similar in-jections are given on lingual (or palatal) gingiva, but these are painless.

The advantages of these techniques are (1) rapid induction of anesthesia, (2) procurement of local ischemia and thus diminished hemorrhage, (3) attainment of an increased measure of tissue rigidity to facilitate tissue incision and shaping, and (4) uncomplicated administration and course of the anesthesia.

Technique
MARKING OF POCKETS

The first task after the induction of anesthesia is to ascertain and demarcate apically the extent of the detachable gingival wall in the operative field. This may be accomplished, as has been sug-gested previously, in two general ways: (1) by the use of pocket markers and (2) by the employment of the periodontal probe. A series of tissue punc-tures (bleeding points) are made in the surface of the attached gingiva, including also the interdental areas, with a minimum of three markings in the gingiva over the facial aspect of each tooth in the operative field. If surgery is to be performed in the lingual gingiva, it will be necessary also to produce markings there. Punctures are made at distofacial, midfacial, and mesiofacial aspects of the teeth. The bleeding points thus marked in a linear series in the tissue denote the apical bases of pathologic sulci and serve as guides, when connected by incision, for the excision of the dis-eased gingival wall.

PRIMARY INCISION

When pocket depths have been clearly marked on the buccal and lingual aspects of the gingiva, one has in effect formed a dotted line, estab-lishing not only the apical bases of a series of pockets but also the occlusal edge of the level of gingival attachment. This will serve as a guide for the resection of the diseased gingival wall. Natu-rally the postsurgical gingival margin will be situated apical to the preoperative one. Some re-growth, creeping in a coronal direction, may occur during healing. If the regenerated tissue is at-tached to the tooth, if the sulcular depth is negli-gible or slight, and if the tissue reflects a state of health with physiologic and aesthetic contour, one may consider the operation a success. Should the postoperative formation of gingiva be such as to demonstrate an inflammatory state and a lack of attachment or adherence to the tooth, the op-erative procedure may be termed a failure (see Fig. 25-3).

To return to the consideration of incision, it should be emphasized, first, that the puncture (bleeding) points represent the *coronal* edge of

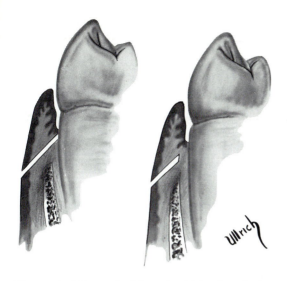

Fig. 25-3. Primary incision should be beveled so as to give a distinct slope to wound bed. Angulation is directly dependent on thickness of gingiva. Note that cut terminates just apical to pocket base subjacent to epithelial attachment. If incision does not terminate at tooth, then gingival tissue will not lift off, but will have to be torn away. This is contraindicted in that it may be difficult to smooth surgical surface, and thus a delay in healing may ensue.

the primary incision, that is, a linear terminus of the resection procedure, and, second, that in order to achieve a thin postoperative gingival margin that blends gracefully into the topography of the surface of attached gingiva it is necessary to make an angled or beveled incision in the tissue. This beveled incision should be made so as to *end* slightly apical to the puncture points; therefore to establish a bevel the angled cut should be made somewhat apical to the bleeding point. *Exactly how far apical the incision is made is largely dependent on the thickness of the tissue to be cut and the anatomic features of the area.* Generally the thicker the tissue, the longer will be the bevel; and the thinner the tissue, the shallower will be the bevel. In one operative field the operator may be required to vary the angulation of the blade as tissue thickness changes over the path of the primary incision. Another factor that may control or modify the length of the bevel is the proximity of the incision to the mucogingival junction. This could place the apical edge of the incision into the alveolar mucosa, inadvertently allowing the mucosa to pull away from its attachment at the mucogingival junction and then to drop toward the vestibular fornix. Rather than unnecessarily violate the alveolar mucosa, the operator should decrease or eliminate the bevel when making the primary incision and establish it later in the procedure by

carefully skiving with the edge of the no. 7 knife, with the soft tissue ronguer, or with rotating diamond stones.

The broad-bladed gingivectomy knife (Goldman-Fox no. 7) is generally used for the initial incision. The knife is drawn through the length of the gingival operative field, while angled in a coronal direction, with deliberate firm steady pressure. If both buccal and lingual aspects are to be operated on, it may be in some instances more expedient to resect first the buccal tissue; this may markedly ease the subsequent removal of lingual tissue because a degree of prior tissue severance will have been obtained in the interdental areas. Of additional importance is a requisite that both the mesial and distal termini of the primary incision be located in uninvolved attached and marginal gingiva at the mesiobuccal or distobuccal line angles of the teeth immediately adjacent to the surgical site. The incision is made similarly on lingual and palatal aspects of the dentition and is begun and terminated at line angles. If this is not done, and the incisions end in interproximal areas, there is a strong likelihood that the form of the interdental gingiva will be irregular, creating a marginal ledge rather than a conical papillary configuration. Imperfect tissue form can contribute to the lodgment of food, debris, and so on in these areas and the return of disease.

Should the terminal point of the incision be an edentulous area, it will usually be necessary to carry the incision from the buccal aspect around and distal (or mesial) to the last tooth, encroaching upon either hard or soft palate, the resultant shelf of fibrotic tissue can be beveled by other means after the initial incision has been completed. It is also possible in cases where a flat palate exists to employ an internally beveled flap rather than the gingivectomy method.

On return to the uncomplicated surgical situation it will be found that the broad-bladed scalpel (no. 7) can cut through the tissue with facility. Because of the rounded nature of its cutting surfaces it glides smoothly over and through irregular tissue without catching when it engages interdental areas or irregular root surfaces. The incision is made in a direct line, guided by the pocket markings and undulating interproximally as much as possible to create vertical spillways in the interdental gingiva. Making the initial cut decisively will obviate the possibility of shredding the tissue. The rigidity of the rounded blade of the no. 7 knife aids materially in producing a smooth incision. Should the primary incision not be adequate to sever the tissue, it is perfectly permissible to repeat the incision by returning the blade to the original track and renegotiating the incision at the original bevel.

Often in the examination it is found that the depth of a pocket around an isolated tooth or even a few teeth may be deeper than the adjacent teeth on both sides, for example, when the pockets on the buccal aspect are relatively shallow in the premolar region but extend apically to a considerable distance on the cuspid and are again shallow on the lateral incisor. In such an instance in the gingivectomy procedure it is necessary that the operator take into consideration not only the physiologic demands but also the aesthetics. It is usually wiser to broaden the initial incision, making it a little more apical in the premolar and lateral incisor regions and blending it into the adjacent tissue so that no ridges will result. If the angulation of the bevel is made as steep as possible, making sure that a buccolingual cone-shaped interproximal tissue is produced, the aesthetic value will be entirely acceptable. However, should the incision be made straight across without any angulation, ledges will result; not only will the appearance be unacceptable, but also the architectural pattern of the gingivae will be nonphysiologic.

Encountered also are situations in which a shallow pocket is found on a labial surface of a tooth, adjacent to which deep pockets on the labial and interproximal surfaces of the neighboring tooth are found. In the effective treatment of this situation by the gingivectomy technique the foregoing principles hold true. Tissue on both sides of the interproximal pocket is removed in order to produce a cone-shaped interproximal papilla. Often in instances such as this the interproximal tissue seemingly regenerates and rises postoperatively, filling the area with firm, healthy tissue. Regardless, the aesthetic value is not unpleasant.

When the roots of adjacent teeth are abnormally close together, it may be difficult to produce physiologic architectural form in marginal and interdental gingiva. Here the mesiodistal width of the interdental gingiva may be concomitantly narrow and even retractable to a level apical to that of the gingival margins of the approximating teeth. Such an undesirable approximation of teeth may be a consequence of the flattening of their proximal contacts because of wear, caries, or imperfect restorations — with their subsequent movement (drifting) together — or it may be a consequence of their rotating in the dental arch, for example, in the contact of the maxillary cuspid

and first premolar, when the cuspid is turned mesially or the premolar is rotated distally or both. In this situation the mesiopalatal line angle of the premolar presents alongside the distopalatal line angle of the cuspid, creating a constricted and shortened gingival embrasure. In making the primary and the subsequent interdental incisions the operator should remove sufficient marginal tissue from the faces of the adjacent teeth in such a manner that parabolic marginal curvatures and conically shaped interdental papillae are created. If this is not done the tip of the interdental tissue will be coincident with or apical to the adjacent gingival margins, producing an environment that can readily accumulate the various gingival irritants.

After the facial aspect of the operative field has been completed, one may now operate on the lingual or palatal side. The lingual or palatal incisions are performed in a fashion similar to those on the labial or buccal side. However, problems in the angulation of the initial incision often exist because of proximity of pocket depth to the palatal vault or to the lingual mucogingival junction. A compromise in which thinning of the resultant gingival margin is performed *after* removal of the unattached pocket wall must often be made. Incisions in the anterior portion of the palate may be complicated by the presence and configuration of the rugae. Rugae may have to be incised or reduced in height in order to eliminate diseased tissue and to secure proper tissue architecture.

SECONDARY INCISIONS

If one continually recognizes the fundamental objectives of gingivectomy (i.e., the removal of the pocket wall at its maximum occlusoapical dimension and the concurrent establishment of physiologic tissue form), the performance of the procedure can be rational, effective, and facile. Thus when the therapist now proceeds to make the secondary incisions — the interdental cuts — not only should he angle them so as to give physiologic slope to the tissues, but he should also resect interdental gingiva to the apical base of the diseased tissue. This means, first, that the interdental resection of tissue along the proximal aspects of the contiguous teeth will be made apical to the epithelial attachments bilaterally at the junction of detachable and attached tissues and, second, if an interdental tissue crater is present, the cut(s) will resect one or both of the soft tissue walls of the pathologic col so as to eradicate the defect and produce either a sloping or a convex form to the interproximal gingiva. In either case the stage is set for the replacement of the original defective col epithelium by ingrowing keratinizing epithelium of the adjacent attached gingiva.

The interdental incisions are most efficiently made with the spear-shaped knife, Goldman-Fox no. 11. The blade is narrow, with two sharp sides converging to a point; entrance into the interproximal areas may be gained in most instances with ease. The incision should be made at a bevel generally at an angle 45 degrees to the face of the attached gingiva, pointed occlusally while directed interdentally. The stab is initiated on the face of attached gingiva at the primary incisional line. The penetration of the tissue should be performed decisively and with a sawing type of motion, embodying also bilateral movements so that the proximal surfaces of the teeth are reached. When this has been accomplished the interdental soft tissue will have been connected to the marginal tissues in such a manner that a strip of gingiva can be released and subsequently discarded. The reward for careful incision is easy and clean tissue removal, with a minimum of tissue tags and irregular margins.

REMOVAL OF EXCISED TISSUE

The instrument most applicable to the actual removal of the incised gingiva is the Goldman-Fox no. 10, a twin-ended device, with sharp, concave blades that can be applied and fitted to the radicular and proximal surfaces of the teeth by compressing the incised gingiva against the teeth. By so doing the therapist can, with a concomitant vigorous but controlled pulling movement, sharply detach the tissue. Other instruments that can be used include the sickle scaler (Goldman-Fox no. 1) or curets (Goldman-Fox no. 3, 4, or 21).

When the therapist has dislodged and removed the gingival tissue mass on the facial, lingual, and interdental aspects of the teeth, it becomes most desirable thoroughly to inspect the wound bed. Irregular or rough gingival margins should be given smooth convexities. Tabs of tissue should be removed so as to promote uncomplicated healing. *Marginal zones should be probed to ascertain if there is a residual pocket wall;* if so, resection should be repeated in these isolated areas. Bevels of tissue should be examined and corrected, if necessary, for length and for the elimination of ledges at the primary incisional line. The wound bed, if ragged, should be made perfectly smooth.

REMOVAL OF TISSUE TAGS

Tissue tags are easily removed with sharp curets, fine surgical scissors (Goldman-Fox or iris) or soft tissue rongeurs (nippers). The tissue shred may be raised from the wound with an aspirator tip, if one is available, so that it stands out at right angles to the wound surface; it may then be more easily sheared off at its base.

Débridement of interdental tissue may be additionally accomplished by utilizing a twisted length of dental tape as a soft tissue saw or rasp. The tape is passed interproximally and then in tight adaptation to the tissue is moved mesiodistally, while maintaining a buccolingual bevel. Small sections or particles of tissue can be excised in this fashion, producing a smooth interproximal wound surface.

CORRECTION OF CONTOUR

Even when gingivectomy has been performed with angled primary and interdental incisions, resulting in a beveled relationship between the remaining attached gingiva and the wound bed, with sloping interproximal tissue form, a certain degree of finishing is required so as to provide the attributes constituting physiologic contour. Although the operator may have made his incisions skillfully and meticulously, it is not always possible to secure the requisite surface morphology in the original incisions for gingival resection. These characteristics include the following:

1. *Smooth, free flowing blend of the wound edge with the contiguous gingival surface.* This may require not only skiving of the tissue junction to obviate an angular relationship but also in certain cases thinning of the adjacent gingiva, extending the wound somewhat apically. This is particularly true when gingiva has a decided faciolingual thickness. This finishing or plastic procedure may be accomplished by use of the soft tissue nipper and the edge of the no. 7 blade in an abrading manner.

2. *Parabolic curvatures mesiodistally of gingival margins.* Well-curved marginal form is particularly necessary so as to form pyramidally shaped interdental papillae at the confluence of the gingival margins of adjacent teeth. Such morphology not only improves the functional environment but also promotes an aesthetic appearance. The convexities can be produced and accentuated by using the no. 3 curet as a cutting instrument or by appropriately excising the marginal tissue with scissors or soft tissue rongeurs. The tissue margin may be concomitantly thinned.

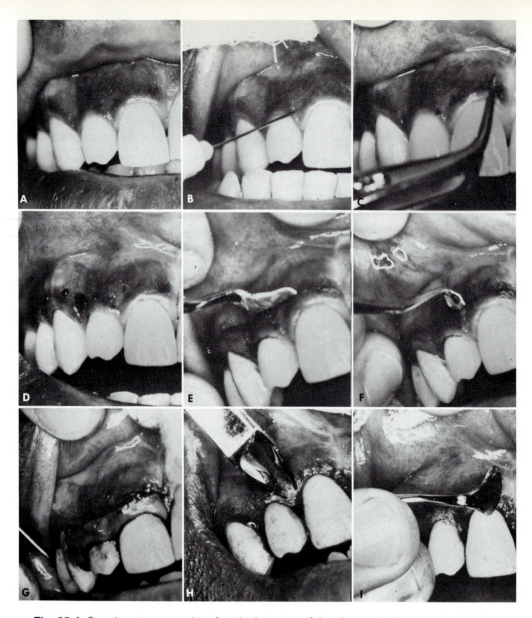

Fig. 25-4. Step-by-step procedure for gingivectomy. A local anesthetic has been injected into mucogingival area, resulting in anesthesia of area. Anesthetic fluid is also injected into palatal area corresponding to mucogingival site. **A,** Before anesthetic. **B,** Injection of anesthetic into buccal peaks; this is also done in palatal peaks. By doing so, tissue becomes firmer and thus easier to contour. **C,** Pocket marking is then performed. Beaks of pocket marker must be parallel to root surface. Markings are made on mesial, central marginal, and distal aspects. **D,** Markings are then surveyed to ascertain relative levels of resultant gingival margins after resection of tissue. **E,** Initial cut is made; knife is held at an angle of approximately 45 degrees. It is made on a continuous line guided by markings. Cut starts apical to markings, since it must end slightly apical to them. Cut must be made firmly and extend down to teeth. **F,** Interdental cut is then made. Knife (no. 11 Goldman-Fox) is inserted into primary incision and extended interdentally as far as possible. **G,** If cuts are complete, tissue will lift off easily. Surgical surface is then inspected carefully. Teeth are dried to see if any calculus is present and scaled if necessary. Gingival topography usually needs further correction, and tissue tabs must be removed. For this, nippers, **H,** scraping with Goldman-Fox no. 7 knife, **I,** and a curet, **J,** are useful. Resultant surface should be smooth and clean, **K** and **M.** Use of dental tape will release any loosened tissue. Gingival margin should be thin and beveled. Interdental tissue should be pyramidally shaped. Operator must probe each margin to ascertain that *all* detached tissue has been removed. Same procedure is performed on palatal aspect. **T,** Interdental tissue must be left smooth. **N** to **S,** Step-by-step procedures for palatal aspect. Use of a diamond stone to shape gingival tissue is seen in **Q.** Interdental sluiceways are easily produced by this method. **L** and **U,** Gingival area is then covered with a Coe-pack periodontal dressing.

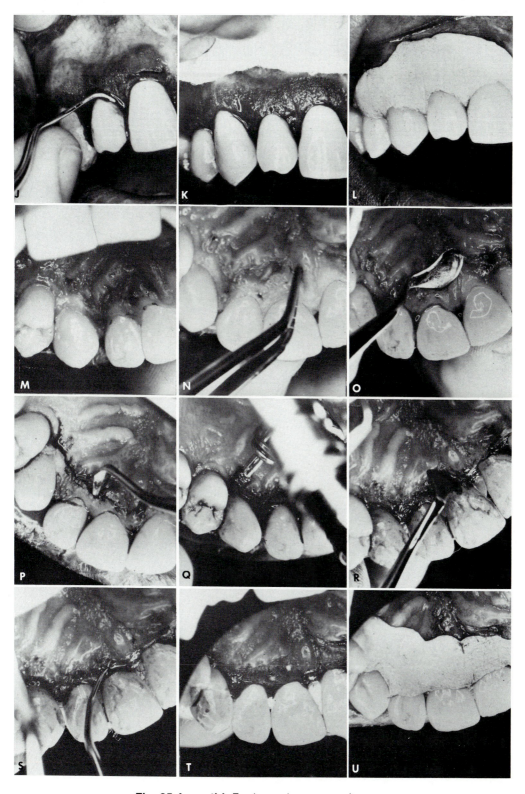

Fig. 25-4, cont'd. For legend see opposite page.

Continued.

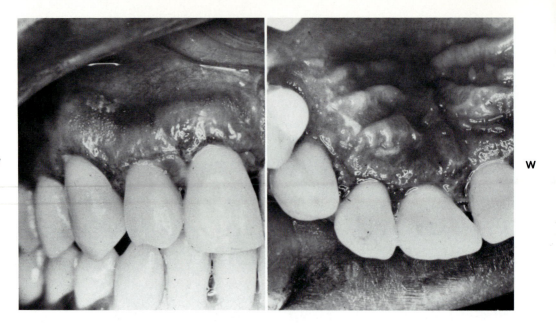

Fig. 25-4, cont'd. V and **W,** Appearance of the gingival tissue 1 week postoperatively.

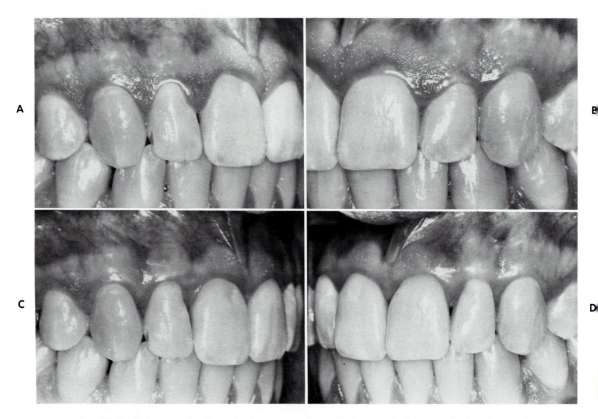

Fig. 25-5. Before and after gingivectomy. **A** and **B,** Gingival hyperplasia. **C** and **D,** Acceptable gingival topography has been achieved postoperatively. There is an adequate band of keratinized gingiva.

3. *Conically shaped interdental papillae with sluiceways directed axially.* Much of the production of papillary form is accomplished by skillfully uniting and blending facial (or lingual) marginal curvatures. The hemiconically shaped surface depression in the papillary face is best made by employing the soft tissue rongeur as an excisional instrument; if applied to the tissue with firm pressure while making the excision, the jaws (blades) will tend to remove a V-shaped area of tissue. In constricted areas one may find it necessary to use the rotary diamonds (with water spray) to accomplish these objectives.

4. *Deflecting soft tissue contours in interradicular areas.* The requisite form is comparable to that established in the interdental tissues. Accessibility is often difficult, particularly when the vestibular fold is shallow, the cheek musculature taut, the lingual alveolar height short, or the tongue an interfering factor. In such instances rotary abrasives—for example, round or conically shaped coarse diamonds (Fox)—may be used to advantage to attain the desired form (Figs. 25-4 to 25-8).

Areas requiring special surgical considerations
MANAGEMENT OF RETROMOLAR AREAS

Individualized attention must be given to the excision of gingival tissue in maxillary and mandibular retromolar areas. Often a flap of dense gingiva rests against the distal surface of the maxillary second molar, rising coronally to a level approximating that of the marginal ridge of the tooth; the pocket depth tends to be rather deep, including not only the full height of the crown but also an additional extension onto the radicular surface of the tooth. This dentogingival relationship is seen especially when the third molar is embedded or in a state of incomplete eruption. If the third molar has been removed in the presence of such bulky and fibrotic gingiva, without concurrent excision of excessive tissue, pocket depth may be even greater. Not infrequently a bony defect is also present, ruling out the applicability of gingivectomy to the lesion. However, if there is no osseous defect, gingival resection may be in order. The excision of the retromolar pad should be performed in such a manner that a well-festooned saddle area is formed, the prime objectives being the excision of the pocket wall and the creation of morphology that will allow proper placement of the toothbrush and other hygienic aids at the distopalatal, distal, and distobuccal cervical zones. The saddle is so shaped that the buccal and palatal gingiva converge toward the crest of the alveolar ridge; thus the occlusal aspect is convex and conically rounded. The mesiodistal form of the saddle should present a gradual slope, extending from the distocervical aspect of the tooth to the posterior edge of the tuberosity; at minimum this should be a level configuration. It will therefore be necessary, in performing the gingivectomy, to blend the cut made for the excision of the pad with both the buccal and palatal initial (primary) incisions; additional and concurrent gingivoplastic measures are indicated. If in planning the surgery the therapist should note that the incision encroaches on the mucosa at the hamular notch, it would be wiser to utilize a double flap (palatal and buccal) approach,

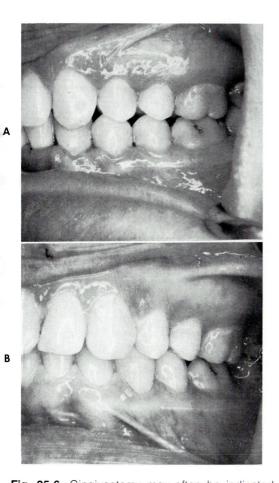

A

B

Fig. 25-6. Gingivectomy may often be indicated after resolution of acute phase of necrotizing ulcerative gingivitis. **A,** Soon after initial therapy and débridement of tissue. Gingiva is fibrotic and irregular in form. **B,** Same area 11 months after surgical procedure. Gingiva is in a state of good health made possible in large measure by surgical improvement of tissue form.

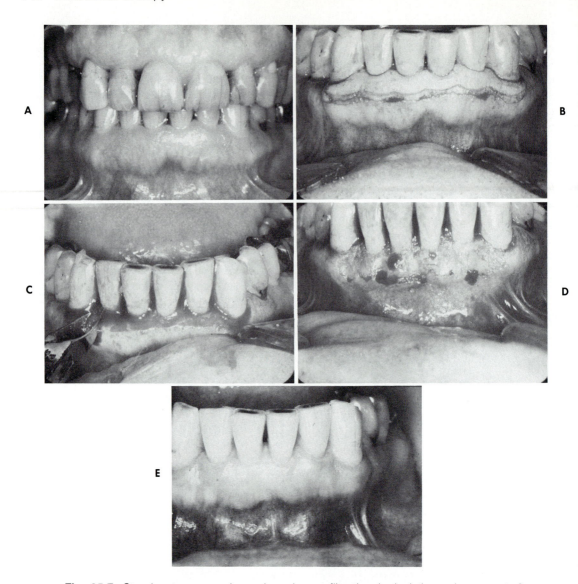

Fig. 25-7. Step-by-step procedure where heavy fibrotic gingival tissue is present. **A,** Therapist must be sure that typography is due to soft tissue and not to osseous thickness. This can be determined by needling tissue. **B,** Pockets were outlined and initial incision made. **C,** Notice how tissue is thinned out. **D,** Postoperative architecture. **E,** Results of therapy.

with submucous resection of excess gingival corium, and replacement of the flaps against the underlying alveolar process.

The management of the lesion involving the tissue distal to the mandibular second (or third) molar is often most difficult. Should the character of the tissue be that of alveolar mucosa—soft, movable, displaceable, and friable—it is extremely difficult to excise, tending to shred and tear rather than to cut smoothly. The sequelae may include hemorrhage, postoperative edema and pain, retarded healing, and failure of complete elimina-

tion of the pocket. If the preoperative character of the tissue is mucosal, the therapist should utilize a wedge type of excision, forming twin flaps that may then be collapsed against the distal bone to eliminate the distal involvement. However, if the tissue is firm, a gingivectomy approach may be employed (providing that a bony defect is not present); during the tissue excision the blade of the no. 7 knife should be placed horizontally, with the heel facing anteriorly, thus easing the resection of tissue to the very base of the pocket. The deeper the distal pocket, the farther distally the beginning

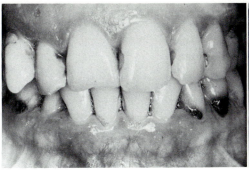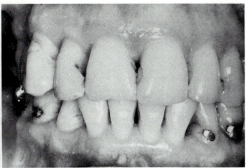

Fig. 25-8. Management of relatively deep pockets in anterior segment of dentition by gingivectomy. Question is often asked if elimination of deep pockets would not be disfiguring. In this instance gingival resection was performed but camouflaged. Considerations were as follows: (1) whether patient shows teeth and gingiva, (2) spacing of teeth, (3) root form, (4) occlusion, and (5) age of patient. Each is significant in diagnosis and treatment planning. In this case gingival resection in maxilla can be noted by landmarks on teeth. Maxillary right lateral incisor has a mesial discoloration. It can be seen in before and after photographs. Viewer can now realize how much gingiva has been removed; yet this is not apparent in after photographs because occlusion and age of patient allowed cutting of incisal edge of tooth, thereby reducing clinical crown length. Note gingival form postoperatively. Patient was unaware that so much of gingival tissue had been removed.

of the incision should be located. The objectives are pocket elimination and an essentially level retromolar crestal form.

If osseous defects are present distal to the last molar, the wedge flap operation is indicated.

MANAGEMENT OF EDENTULOUS AREAS

Surgical handling of an edentulous area alongside or interposed between sites of edentulous involvement requires the removal (and physiologically oriented shaping) of gingival tissue in the saddle area so as to eliminate the pockets adjacent to the teeth that abut the edentulous zone. Thus the primary (initial) gingivectomy incisions are extended so as to traverse the saddle area linearly at a superoinferior level, connecting the pocket markings of the teeth that adjoin the mesial and distal aspects of the saddle. In order that the crest of the edentulous area be conically convex rather than flat, the surgical blade must be angulated at a bevel when buccal and linguopalatal primary incisions are made. The same angulations are maintained during the secondary (similar to interdental) incisions adjacent to the teeth, thus releasing the gingiva at the pocket bases. When gingivectomy is adeptly performed over the ridge, the tissue may actually be removed in one piece. The form of the saddle is now perfected, assuring smooth convex shape buccolingually, level mesiodistal crest and complete pocket elimination, tab

removal, and gingivoplasty alongside the contiguous teeth.

COMPLICATIONS OF FRENA, MUSCLE ATTACHMENTS, AND RUGAE

Not uncommonly frena are located in the path of the initial gingivectomy incision, since the pocket bases often lie at or apical to the attachments of the frena. This situation is especially prevalent in the maxillary anterior region. When required, the primary incision should be made so as to traverse the frenum; after the labial gingival resection is completed, the frenum is then released, using nippers or scissors, from its gingival base. In this way the frenum attachment is actually positioned apically rather than being excised completely. Interfering muscle attachments and mandibular frena are managed similarly. If it should be necessary to detach the mandibular lingual frenum, care must be taken to avoid accidental entrance into the mucosa of the floor of the mouth; postoperative sequelae of pain, edema, and hematoma are often associated with surgery at the lingual fornix area.

The rugae may serve as interferences to the establishment of proper surface contour of the palatal gingiva, when the initial incision is performed. When required, the rugae should be flattened or removed by locating the beginning of the incision posterior to the rise of the rugae. This of course broadens the wound base produced by the primary incision; however, proper tissue contour is achieved. Healing is generally uneventful; epithelization may appear somewhat retarded clinically because of the wider exposure of gingival corium.

MANAGEMENT OF NARROW AND BROAD EMBRASURE AREAS

The size and shape of gingival embrasures are important considerations in the etiology of periodontal disease and in the prognosis after therapy. Variations in embrasure form should therefore be recognized during the periodontal examination. When the clinical crowns of adjacent teeth are long, and their roots are close together, the gingival embrasures are short and narrow. The long proximal relationship of the teeth minimizes the protective effect of dental contacts to the subjacent tissues, allowing the interproximal accumulation of irritative substances such as bacterial plaque and fibrous food debris. Dislodgment of these materials by routine oral hygiene measures is especially difficult; there is a tendency therefore toward constant and progressive inflammatory involvement of the gingiva. Such an environment is also a hindrance to the attainment of proper architectural form of the interdental gingiva during the gingivectomy operation. If this tissue cannot be shaped into a papillary form, with deflecting surface contours, and if the adjacent gingival margins cannot be made thin and parabolically curved mesiodistally, the interdental area may not be cleansed effectively, and renewal of gingival disease will occur. Special attention must be given to such a situation at the time of gingivectomy by the following methods:

1. The marginal curvatures of the gingiva of adjacent teeth must be accentuated so as to form a distinct peak to the interdental tissue at the point of confluence of the gingival margins. The margins must be made very thin.

2. The buccal and linguopalatal faces of the interdental papillae must be contoured so as to have definite sluiceways that will allow for egress of food materials from the interdental area.

3. The embrasure must be widened and shaped by planing the root surfaces of the teeth with heavy scalers and by grinding the teeth, if necessary, at the cementoenamel junctions and the sulci. The modified areas of the teeth should then be smoothed and polished with linen strips, rubber and pumice rotary discs and points, and so on. Dentinal desensitization may be additionally necessary.

When the embrasures are wide, problems of postoperative aesthetics and interdental cleansing may arise. It is important in designing the tissue during surgery to make sure that the interdental tissue is cone shaped; it is additionally advisable to avoid sloping the tissue either to the buccal or lingual aspect so as to maintain buccal and lingual convexities to the tissue. The conical form of the tissue facilitates self-cleansing and enhances the efficiency of oral hygiene measures. Application of the toothbrush from the buccal and lingual aspects will permit ready sanitation of the exposed proximal surfaces of the teeth, the proximobuccal and proximolingual line angles, and the interdental soft tissue cone.

MANAGEMENT OF MANDIBULAR LINGUAL AREAS

Gingival tissues requiring resection at the lingual aspect of mandibular incisors that are in linguoversion present a problem of access not only for removal of the pocket wall but also for plastic reshaping of the wound bed. The primary incision for gingival resection may of necessity be negotiated without marginal or interdental bevels; the requisite tissue contours are formed as a later step in the surgical procedure. Resection of tissue and placement of physiologic form may be secured in selected instances by using the electrosurgical instrument.

CONTROL OF BLEEDING

Hemorrhage is rarely a problem of magnitude at or after the time of gingivectomy. Hemorrhage may be minimized by judicious handling of the tissues at the time of surgery, avoiding tissue trauma, laceration, excessive probing, and so on. Bleeding may and should be stopped by tamponing and by pressure with gauze squares against the wound. The pressure should be firm and protracted, extending for a time sufficient to assure hemostasis. The surgical dressing should not be placed while bleeding is in progress. If after a few minutes of pressure small or punctate areas of bleeding persist, they may usually be quickly controlled by the topical application of Oxycel (oxidized cellulose gauze type), Gelfoam, or Gelfoam and thrombin. If it is evident that bleeding is arterial, the vessel will have to be tied, usually by placing the suture around a segment of tissue through which the artery passes. If catgut suture material is employed, it will not be necessary to interfere further. If appropriate care is given to the tissues at the time of surgery to obviate bleeding, one can expect little or no postoperative bleeding sequelae. Additionally, most surgical dressings contain agents, particularly tannic acid, as aids to continued hemostasis.

Of significance for the control of postoperative bleeding is a secure and rigid surgical dressing. If the dressing is poorly adherent to the teeth and tissues and thus is movable, it may tend to promote hemorrhage by inducing abrasion of the wound. The surgical dressing should be locked tightly into interdental embrasures when it is placed so as to attain and maintain intimate and strong contact between the dressing and the tissue.

APPLICATION OF THE SURGICAL DRESSING

It is customary to protect the surgical site until wound healing has progressed to an epithelized state. Recognizing that the rate of epithelial migration over the forming gingival corium varies between 0.5 and 1 mm per day, one may quickly estimate, barring postoperative complications, the period for which a dressing is required. In calculating the time one should allow for an initial lag period of 24 to 36 hours prior to the commencement of epithelization; for example, a wound with a 4 mm occlusoapical dimension will cover in 5 to 9 days. If both buccal and lingual gingivectomies are performed, one should realize that epithelization will commence from both the lingual and buccal peripheries of the wound. Very often areas of palatal surgery are quite wide because of the necessity either to thin the tissue adjacent to the primary incision or to begin the incision substantially apical to the pocket base because the palatal tissue is thick; epithelization of such areas may therefore require a more protracted period.

Coe-Pak consists of two pastes, one a zinc oxide combined with an oil for plasticity, and a gum for cohesiveness, to which is added a fungicide. The other paste contains light cocoanut fatty acids thickened with a resin and chlorothymol as a bacteriostatic. The material sets up by soap formation between the zinc oxides and the fatty acids. The pastes are mixed together, which sets. Once a technique of managing the tacking material has been acquired, it is easy to use.

The Baer-Sumner formula utilizes a surface-acting antibiotic, bacitracin, apparently to minimize the potential for wound infection. The incorporation of tetracyclines or penicillin is strongly discouraged because of the dual danger of possible sensitization of the patient to the drug and encouragement of monilial overgrowth beneath and in association with the dressing. *Candida albicans,*

a yeastlike fungus unaffected by the antibiotics, behaves as an opportunist, overgrowing when bacterial elements of the oral flora are depressed in number and activity by the drugs. Infection by the fungus is responsible for formation of off-white, curdy masses on the tissue surface. These membranes, consisting of necrotic epithelium and twisted strands of the fungi, are detachable from the tissue, leaving exposed a raw, bleeding gingival corium. Topically applied antibiotics are rarely if ever indicated in periodontal therapeutics. When needed, they are best administered orally or parenterally.

Modern day surgical dressings are formulated primarily for bland, unobtrusive wound protection. These include among their qualities several attributes essential to easy handling by the dentist, comfort for the patient, and protection to the wound and oral mucous membranes.

When the periodontal dressing has been properly placed, the cervical portions of the teeth, the interdental areas, the wound surface, and a narrow zone of uninvolved tissue peripheral to the wound will all have been covered. The borders of the dressing will have been formed to a thin roll at the linguopalatal peripheries. A more rounded edge is desirable at the labiobuccal vestibular fornices when these zones are included. The intimate interdental application of the pack may be improved by compressing firmly with the smooth sides of closed cotton pliers. Buccal, lingual, and palatal compression is accomplished by finger pressure while the peripheries of the dressing can be shaped by guided lip, cheek, and tongue muscle trimming.

When surgery is performed distal to the terminal tooth in the dental arch, pack placement and retention are helped greatly if lingual, distal, and buccal sites are covered, using a U-shaped pencil of the dressing. The closed end of the U is placed about the distal aspect of the most posterior tooth.

Isolated teeth should be circumscribed with the dressing material to prevent pack displacement. If the tooth crown does not have adequate cervical convexities, even a hardened dressing will tend to slip from position. To cope with such a problem the operator may do the following: He may select an oversized copper band; festoon the gingival periphery so as to conform to the undulations of the margins of the gingiva; trim the band at its occlusal aspect so as to prevent any occlusal interference; scissors snip the gingival edge of the band at several points about its periphery and then bend the edge outward in a haphazard manner (this will provide a retentive area for the periodontal dressing); and fill the band with the softened dressing, placing it over the tooth as one would take a tube impression (however, he must not force the band against the gingiva). The copper band may now be surrounded with a strip of dressing and be brought in apposition to the wound. The dressing should be muscle trimmed.

In all instances, particularly during the period of hardening, the adaptation and retention of the dressing may be improved if the dressing is covered with a well-adapted (thick) shield of adhesive periodontal foil. The tinfoil is closely applied so as to cover the lingual, occlusal, and facial surfaces of the dressing, but it should terminate several millimeters short of the margins of the pack to prevent impingement of the edges of the foil upon the lingual and alveolar mucosa. Most operators prefer to round off the corners of the square of foil to decrease the tendency for tongue, cheek, and mucosal irritation. Appropriate instructions for postoperative care should be presented to the patient prior to his dismissal. These include the following:

1. A soft dietary regimen should be followed, and the opposite side of the dentition should be utilized for mastication. Sticky, harsh, hard, brittle, crumbly, spicy, or highly seasoned foods should be avoided. The diet should be nutritive and bland, with nonirritative consistency. Meats should be tender, in small morsels or chopped. Eggs, milk, cool or tepid soups, custards, cottage cheese, and so on may be ideally included; there is no need for a Sippy diet.

2. Bleeding is rarely a postoperative problem. If it does occur and is of consequence, the patient should be advised to return to the office for treatment of the complication.

3. Pain generally is of minor degree in the postoperative period and may be controlled with the common analgesics: aspirin, 10 grains every 4 hours; aspirin compound; and so on. If pain is more severe, the nonnarcotic analogues of codeine may be advantageously prescribed (Darvon compound, 65 mg [one capsule] every 1 to 6 hours). Narcotic agents are rarely needed.

4. Postoperative edema, when present in facial tissues, may be controlled with topically applied cold compresses. There is a greater need for this measure if mucogingival surgical procedures have been performed along with gingivectomy.

5. If the periodontal dressing or a portion thereof is detached and lost, a thin layer of white petrolatum (Vaseline) may be applied over the wound as a protective until such time that return to the office for replacement of the pack is possible.

6. Oral hygiene measures are to be maintained with diligence in the unoperated areas of the dentition. If a mucinous film should form over the dressing, it may be brushed off with the toothbrush and warm water. Thus oral sanitation is preserved.

7. Return for dressing change or removal should be in 1 week.

CHANGE OF DRESSING

The periodontal dressing is generally removed or replaced 1 week after the surgical procedure. It is particularly important to remove the entire dressing, with a minimal amount of manipulation, since the tissues are often tender and friable. The teeth and tissues should be thoroughly inspected. Residual particles of dressing must be found and removed so as to prevent their impaction into the wound when a new dressing is applied over them. The sequelae of accidental lodgment of foreign substances within the tissues include inflammatory hyperplasias, gingival abscesses, foreign body reactions (giant cell granulomas), and impaired wound healing, particularly epithelization. A whitish surface coagulum, possibly consisting of mucinous plaque, materia alba, desquamated epithelial cells, and so on is often found under the dressing; it should be gently removed with a warm water spray or a moist swab. Particles of dressing adherent to tooth surfaces should be removed; the ultrasonic tooth cleaning device is often efficacious for this purpose. If small tissue tags are present, they may usually be quickly and painlessly removed with a sharp curet; if pain is evident or anticipated, it may be wiser to apply a topical anesthetic agent (lidocaine ointment [Xylocaine]) on the area prior to removal of the tissue. Actually pain should be of little consequence in these zones as the neural supply at 7 days has usually not regenerated.

A new dressing is now applied. It should be soft so that light pressure is required to adapt it to position. The dressing may be tamped to the teeth and tissue with broad finger pressure and with the ancillary use of the patient's cheek, lips, and tongue. If performed quickly and efficiently, there is little discomfort for the patient. If the tissues are highly sensitive a topical anesthetic agent may be used.

Bleeding areas if present may be eliminated by applying a hemostatic agent on the tissues before placement of the surgical cement. Oxycel (gauze type) is an appropriate substance for punctate hemorrhage control.

In nearly all instances there is no further requirement for a dressing after a 10- to 14-day postoperative period. The patient may now proceed onto a normal dietary and oral hygiene regimen, being careful, however, to avoid those foods and measures that are conducive to topical irritation and abrasion.

Conditions frequently observed 1 week after operation

The following conditions are frequently observed 1 week after operation.

1. *Granulation tissues*. Small, red, beadlike protuberances from the cut gingival surfaces in the interproximal spaces and on the labial or lingual surfaces can be seen. These masses consist of granulation tissues, usually arising from the gingiva close to the tooth surface where calculus has not completely been removed or resulting from pack movement during healing that has initiated an alteration in the usual sequence of healing. These areas do not undergo normal organization and are a consideration for future, recurrent pocket depth. It is important to remove not only the detached granulation tissue, but also the etiologic factor (calculus) at this time with sharp scalers and curets in a highly visible field of operation.

2. *Calculus*. It is important that all root surfaces be checked for small fragments of calculus inadvertently left during the surgical procedure. Explorers and visual examination should be instituted. Oftentimes deposits are similar to root surface color, and the junction of gingiva and root is a common location at which to find them. Gently directed warm air is an excellent aid.

3. *Sensitivity to thermal change and exploration*. Following surgical intervention and pack removal, patients will experience increased root surface sensitivity and reactions to thermal change. This is usually a fleeting condition. However, the use of desensitizing agents such as fluoride paste, Thermodent, Sensodyne, or desensitizing rinses might have to be judiciously introduced.

4. *Alterations in root surface*. Carious softening at or below the cementoenamel junction is a common source of discomfort. These areas usually require careful excavation and restoration.

REFERENCES

Ambrose, J. A., and Detamore, R. J.: Correlation of histologic and clinical findings in periodontal treatment; effect of scaling on reduction of gingival inflammation prior to surgery, J. Periodontol. **31**:238, 1960.

Ariaudo, A. A.: Symposium on the surgical approach to the periodontal problem; procedure for gingivectomy, J. Periodontol. **28**:62, 1957.

Baer, P., Goldman, H. M., and Scigliano, H.: Studies on a bacitracin periodontal dressing, Oral Surg. **11**:712, 1958.

Berdon, J. K.: Blood loss during gingival surgery, J. Periodontol. **36**:12, 1965.

Bernier, J. L., and Kaplan, H.: The repair of gingival tissue after surgical intervention, J. Am. Dent. Assoc. **35**:697, 1947.

Blake, G. C.: Universal gingivectomy knife using Bard-Parker blades, Br. Dent. J. **89**:226, 1950.

Blanquie, R. H.: Preoperative procedures and postoperative expedients in periodontal surgery, J. Periodontol. **25**:167, 1954.

Bradin, M.: Precautions and hazards in periodontal surgery, J. Periodontol. **33**:154, 1962.

Caffesse, R. G.: Cicatrizacion periodontal experimental, Rev. Asoc. Odontol. Argent. **59**:5, 1970.

Carranza, F. A., and Cabrini, R. L.: The healing of oral wounds, Periodontics **1**:70, 1963.

Caucino, L. M., and Palazuelos, H. R.: Anestesia general de Corta duracion en odontologia, Rev. Asoc. Odontol. Argent. **59**:11, 1970.

Coolidge, E. D.: Elimination of the periodontal pocket in the treatment of pyorrhea, J. Am. Dent. Assoc. **25**:1627, 1938.

Cowan, A.: A technique for gingivectomy, Dent. Pract. Dent. Rec. **9**:128, 1958.

Donnenfeld, O. W., and Glickman, I.: A biometric study of the effects of gingivectomy, J. Periodontol. **37**:5, 1966.

Engler, W., Ramfjord, S., and Hiniker, J.: Healing following simple gingivectomy; a tritiated thymidine radioautographic study. I. Epithelialization, J. Periodontol. **37**:298, 1966.

Ewen, S. J., and Pasternak, R.: Periodontal surgery—an adjunct to orthodontic treatment, Periodontics **2**:162, 1964.

Fox, L.: Rotating abrasives in the management of periodontal hard and soft tissues, Oral Surg. **3**:1134, 1955.

Gilson, C. M.: Surgical treatment of periodontal disease, J. Am. Dent. Assoc. **44**:733, 1952.

Glickman, I., and Imber, L. R.: Comparison of gingival resection with electrosurgery and periodontal knives. A biometric and histologic study, J. Periodontol. **41**:142, 1970.

Goldman, H. M.: Gingivectomy, Oral Surg. **4**:1136, 1951.

Goldman, H. M.: Development of physiologic gingival contours by gingivoplasty, Oral Surg. **3**:879, 1950.

Goldman, H. M.: Gingivectomy; indications, contraindications and method, Am. J. Orthod. **32**:323, 1946.

Gottsegen, R.: Should teeth be scaled prior to surgery? J. Periodontol. **32**:301, 1961.

Grant, D. A.: Experimental periodontal surgery: sequestration of alveolar bone, J. Periodontol. **38**:409, 1967.

Grillo, H. C.: Derivation of fibroblasts in the healing wound, Arch. Surg. **88**:218, 1964.

Hiatt, W. H., Stallard, R. E., Kramer, G. M., and Grant, D. A.: Is the simple gingivectomy obsolete? Periodontol. Abstr. **13**:62, 1965.

Kalis, P. J.: Gingivectomy, its use and abuse, Dent. Dig. **77**:5, 1971.

Kaplan, H., and Milobsky, L.: A surgical procedure for periodontal pocket technique, Oral Surg. **4**:546, 1951.

Kirkland, O.: Modified flap operation in surgical treatment of periodontoclasia, J. Am. Dent. Assoc. **19**:1918, 1932.

Korn, N. A., Schaffer, E. M., and McHugh, R. B.: An experimental assessment of gingivectomy and soft tissue curettage in dogs, J. Periodontol. **36**:96, 1965.

Löe, H.: Chemical gingivectomy; effect of potassium hydroxide on periodontal tissues, Acta Odontol. Scand. **19**:517, 1961.

MacDonald, R. A.: Origin of fibroblasts in experimental healing wounds, Surgery **46**:376, 1959.

Manne, M. S., and Standish, S. M.: Use of oral exfoliative cytology in the evaluation of gingivectomy healing, J. Periodontol. **36**:27, 1965.

McHugh, W. D., and Persson, P. A.: Fluorescence microscopy of healing gingival epithelium, Acta Odontol. Scand. **16**:205, 1958.

McIvor, J., and Wengraf, A.: Blood loss in periodontal surgery, Dent. Pract. Dent. Rec. **16**:448, 1966.

Mittleman, H., Toto, P., Sicher, H., and Wentz, F.: Healing in human attached gingiva, Periodontics **2**:106, 1964.

Orban, B.: Surgical gingivectomy, J. Am. Dent. Assoc. **32**:701, 1945.

Orban, B., and Archer, E.: Dynamics of wound healing following elimination of periodontal pockets, J. Oral Surg. **31**:40, 1945.

Pennel, B. M., King, K. O., Wilderman, M. N., and Barron, J. M.: Repair of the alveolar process following osseous surgery, J. Periodontol. **38**:426, 1967.

Persson, P-A.: The healing process in the marginal periodontium after gingivectomy with special regard to the regeneration of epithelium, Dent. Pract. Dent. Rec. **11**:427, 1961.

Pfeifer, J. S.: The growth of gingiva over denuded bone, J. Periodontol. **34**:10, 1963.

Powell, R. N., and Alexander, A. G.: The treatment of periodontal disease, Br. Dent. J. **119**:522, 1965.

Prichard, J.: Changing concepts in periodontal therapy, Tex. Dent. J. **79**:4, 1961.

Prichard, J.: Gingivoplasty, gingivectomy and osseous surgery, J. Periodontol. **32**:275, 1961.

Ramfjord, S.: Gingivectomy; its place in periodontal therapy, J. Periodontol. **23**:30, 1952.

Ramfjord, S., and Costich, E. R.: Gingivectomy; its place in periodontal therapy, J. Periodontol. **34**:401, 1963.

Ramfjord, S., Engler, W., and Hiniker, J.: A radioautographic study of healing following simple gingivectomy. II. The connective tissue, J. Periodontol. **37**:179, 1966.

Rateitschak, K. H., Graf, H., and Guldener, P.: Periodontal pack without eugenol, J. Periodontol. **35**:290, 1964.

Robinson, R. E.: The distal wedge operation, Periodontics **4**:256, 1966.

Ruben, M. P., and Goldman, H. M.: Current concepts of periodontal therapy, Periodontics **1**:7, 1963.

Sandin, G.: Periodontal surgery and grinding of tooth surfaces using rotating instruments, Sven. Tandlak. Tidskr. **57**:345, 1965.

Schoefe, G. I., and Majno, G.: Regeneration of blood vessels in wound healing. In Montagna, W., and Billingham, R. E., editors: Advances in biology of skin; vol. 5, Wound healing, New York, 1964, The Macmillan Co.

Shapiro, M.: Acceleration of gingival wound healing in nonepileptic patients receiving diphenylhydantoin sodium, Parodontologie **13**:56, 1959.

Stahl, S. S., Soberman, A., and DeCesare, A.: Gingival healing. V. The effects of antibiotics administered during the early stages of repair, J. Periodontol. **40**:521, 1969.

Stahl, S. S., Witkin, G. J., Heller, A., and Brown, R., Jr.: Gingival healing. IV. The effects of home care on gingivectomy repair, J. Periodontol. **40**:264, 1969.

Swenson, H.: Success or failure in periodontal surgery, J. Am. Dent. Assoc. **67**:193, 1963.

Toto, P. D., and Abati, A.: The histogenesis of granulation tissue, Oral Surg. **16**:218, 1963.

Trotter, P. A.: Gingivectomy, Br. Dent. J. **90**:18, 1951.

Viziam, C., Matoltsky, A., and Mescon, H.: Epithelialization of small wounds, J. Invest. Dermatol. **43**:499, 1964.

Wade, A. B.: Where gingivectomy fails, J. Periodontol. **25**:189, 1954.

Waerhaug, J.: Depth of incision in gingivectomy, Oral Surg. **8**:707, 1955.

Waerhaug, J., and Löe, H.: Tissue reaction to gingivectomy pack, Oral Surg. **8**:707, 1955.

Ward, A. W.: The surgical eradication of pyorrhea, J. Am. Dent. Assoc. **15**:2146, 1928.

Zamet, J. S.: Initial preparation of gingival tissues prior to surgery, Dent. Pract. Dent. Rec. **17**:115. 1966.

Zentler, A.: Suppurative gingivitis with alveolar involvement: a new surgical procedure, J.A.M.A. **71**:1530, 1918.

Ziezel, W.: Pyorrhea extermination; gingivectomy, Dent. Cosmos **63**:352, 1921.

26 Reconstructive mucogingival surgery

Reconstructive mucogingival surgery enhances the success of periodontal treatment by encompassing plastic surgery procedures that correct, restore, transplant, transform, and preserve the tissues of the mucogingival complex. It restores the destroyed or diseased mucogingival complex or transplants tissue to establish a healthy mucogingival relationship.

The mucogingival complex is composed of the mucogingival junction and its relation to the attached gingiva, the alveolar mucosa, the associated muscles, the frena, and the depth of the vestibule. Mucogingival surgery incorporates plastic surgery procedures that correct the mucogingival complex affected by periodontal disease (Friedman, 1962, 1957). The terms "reconstructive surgery" and "mucogingival surgery" are very similar and will be used interchangeably throughout this chapter.

The irreversible destructive process of advancing periodontal disease leaves defects that must be corrected if the periodontium is to survive. Reconstructive mucogingival surgery can be successful in altering this destructive process and in reestablishing the structures of the mucogingival complex so that they can withstand the functional demands required of them.

Recently acquired knowledge concerning the origin of granulation tissue (Karring et al., 1975) and its ability to predict resultant keratinized gingiva has brought into clearer focus the rationale of current surgical procedures. Further study has shown that the characteristics of keratinized gingiva and nonkeratinized alveolar mucosa are genetically determined and are not the result of functional adaptation to environmental stimuli (Karring et al., 1971). Carefully designed mucogingival surgery can reconstruct a *new* healthy gingival attachment since the differentiation of keratinized gingival epithelium is determined by inductive stimuli from the underlying connective tissue (Karring et al., 1974, 1972).

The time lag has narrowed between refinement in mucogingival surgery and the animal and human research that support its clinical success. Greater predictability of postsurgical results can be realized when more discriminating observations are made of the preoperative marginal tissue morphology and of whether pockets are present and extend beyond the mucogingival junction.

When there is an *insufficient* margin of gingiva, either a *partial-thickness apically positioned pedicle graft* or a *free soft tissue autograft* should be chosen. Either method will establish an adequate zone of attached gingiva without creating a deformity at the dentogingival junction. When there is no margin of gingiva the use of a *pedicle graft* with a *mature epithelialized surface* or a *free soft tissue autograft* is suggested (Fagan, 1975).

The planning and description of the clinical procedures will be discussed, emphasizing the importance of basic biologic knowledge.

HISTORICAL REVIEW

In the past quarter century emphasis has been placed on control of the inflammatory process that has extended into the alveolar mucosa beyond the boundary of the attached gingiva. In an effort to eliminate pockets with this morphology the usual resection techniques, when used, have resulted in margins of alveolar mucosa, which create an environment prone to breakdown in the following manner (Goldman and Cohen, 1953).

1. Margins of alveolar mucosa are retractable when incised and heal slowly postoperatively. The tissues are fragile, noncornified, and less endowed structurally to withstand the effect of physiologic forces and oral hygiene procedures.
2. With or without a shallow vestibular fornix the close proximity of muscle attachments

and frena creates tensional pull, retraction of the mucosal margin, pocket formation, initiation of an inflammatory process, proliferation of the junctional epithelium, and renewed extension of the pathologic process.

Hirschfeld in 1939 showed evidence that the abnormal attachment of the labial frenum near the gingival margin of the tooth played an important part in the recession, in the pocket formation, and in the inflamed condition of the gingival flap, which could be drawn away from the tooth by a pull on the lip. Treatment consisted of partial resection of the frenum, which was then sutured apically.

Goldman first introduced three specific problems that involved the interrelation between the gingiva and the mucosal structures (Goldman, 1953). The first problem dealt with periodontal pockets that extended beyond the gingiva or traversed the gingiva and ended in the alveolar mucosa. The second problem dealt with an abnormal frenum pull that dissipated its tension on the gingival margin and caused retraction of the margin. The third problem involved the functional orientation of a shallow vestibular fornix. He solved these problems by surgical procedures that eliminated the frenum pull and increased the depth of the vestibular fornix. This surgical endeavor initiated the era of mucogingival surgery

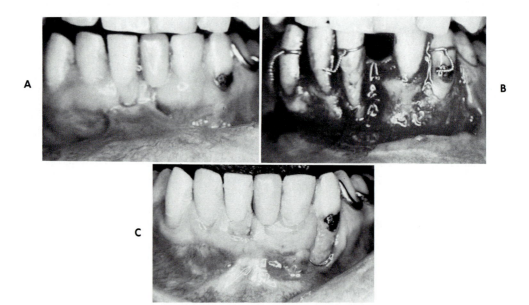

Fig. 26-1. Hazards of complete denudation. **A,** Preoperative view. Severe recession of mandibular right central incisor, absence of gingiva, and broad frenum pull at margin. Note level of gingival margin on left canine. **B,** Complete denudation procedure. **C,** Mandibular canine area did not heal. Large sequestrum was removed, resulting in a severe anatomic defect in this area.

that has motivated other clinicians to develop numerous refinements. From these basic corrective procedures clinicians have modified, remodified, and enhanced an entire spectrum of surgical designs (Ariaudo and Tyrell, 1960, 1957; Becker, 1967; Bjorn, 1963; Formicola et al., 1976) in an effort to create stable, predictable procedures that would result in an intact, healthy gingival unit, free of local environmental influences, with optimal preservation of the periodontium.

In the exploration for surgical variations the pendulum moved from *complete denudation procedures* (Goldman et al., 1956; Carranza and Carraro, 1963; Bohannan, 1963, 1962; Chacker and Cohen, 1960; Pfeifer, 1963) to the current consistent use of periodontal flap techniques and periosteal retention approaches. Unfortunately the earlier clinical procedure, that is, bone denudation, was not preceded by wound healing studies in the laboratory. Postoperative results at a clinical level brought disappointing findings (Fig. 26-1).

Many investigators explored wound healing in dogs, monkeys, and human beings. They offered evidence that demanded reappraisal of our surgical designs (Arnold and Hatchett, 1962; Fagan, 1975). Through these studies it was found that the use of flap procedures in the correction of soft tissue and osseous lesions caused the least trauma to the supporting structures, particularly the vulnerable marginal radicular bone. Cohen and Chacker (1960), Friedman and Levine (1964), Helburn et al. (1963), Pfeifer (1971, 1963), Staffileno and Levy (1969), Staffileno et al. (1966), Wilderman (1964), and Wilderman et al. (1960) substantiated the fact that complete denudation procedures caused anatomic deformities that were irreversible, whereas the procedures that protected the highly responsive vestibular bone produced a functional repair without anatomic deformity. It was also determined that the interproximal bone, when exposed, was initially resorbed and then completely re-formed to its original height (Wilderman et al., 1960).

Currently those procedures are utilized that postsurgically leave a protective covering to this vulnerable tissue and if at all possible do not leave the radicular bone denuded subsequent to surgery. Concern should be for the maximum conservation of attached gingiva, since its sacrifice precipitates a series of surgical maneuvers to restore an intact functional gingival unit.

Nabers (1957, 1954) first recognized the need for the retention of attached gingiva. He designed his technique for repositioning and conserving attached gingiva to minimize the magnitude of the surgical trauma. Another modification of this approach by Ariaudo and Tyrell (1960) introduced two vertical incisions that made the flap easier to manipulate. They placed the flap apical to the marginal bone, thus endangering the tissue that was left denuded. The zone of attached gingiva was increased because new gingiva was created coronal to the apically positioned gingiva.

Friedman (1964, 1962, 1957) called attention to the error of removing and discarding attached gingiva and then creating new gingiva through traumatic surgical procedures. He proposed the term "apically repositioned flap" to describe the repositioning of the attached gingiva as conceived by Nabers. The entire tissue complex of gingiva, alveolar mucosa, submucosa, mucogingival junction, and base of the vestibule was repositioned apically. He pointed out that the vestibular deepening did not become more shallow during the healing process because the flap was composed of mature tissues and structures that when shifted apically in toto would not change in their relationship.

Clinical research has appeared in the literature dealing with the wound healing of pedicle grafts and free soft tissue autografts. The treatises of Janson et al. (1969), Sullivan et al. (1971), and Sullivan and Atkins (1968) on these procedures have provided the basis for their routine use plus their imaginative and successful modifications. Much has been learned about the conversion of submucosal tissue into an immobile collagenous recipient bed, the control of the vestibular fornix, and the functional gingival attachment at this site. Technique modifications to cover denuded roots using pedicle (Corn, 1972; Grupe and Warren, 1956; Staffileno, 1964) or free grafts (Corn, 1972; Mlinek, et al., 1973; Sullivan and Atkins, 1968) rely on maximum adjacent connective tissue recipient beds for repair and revascularization.

Through the evolution of these plastic surgery procedures, developed with the objective of establishing a healthy intact gingival attachment, much has been learned about the manipulation of these delicate tissue structures and the reparative response to this manipulation. It is evident that the indiscriminate detachment of connective tissue from the dental and osseous structures results in anatomic deformities that could have been prevented. The basic design of our reconstructive repairs should be planned with the optimal conservation of these structures in mind. The information gained through wound healing studies obligates us to design our procedures to avoid the violation of these biologic attachments.

OBJECTIVES

1. To eliminate pocket defects that approach or traverse the mucogingival junction
2. To permit access to the underlying alveolar process, and to correct osseous deformities when there is sufficient or insufficient attached gingiva
3. To create an adequate zone of attached gingiva
4. To eliminate unaesthetic gingival clefts
5. To eliminate gingival recession
6. To relieve the pull of frena and muscle attachments on the gingival margin

SCOPE
Pocket deformities involving the mucogingival junction

The uncontrolled inflammation within a pocket involving the mucogingival junction causes a perpetuation of the periodontal disease in this area, resulting in the resorption of the thin, radicular, alveolar crest, cratering, reverse architecture, furcation involvement, ledging, and infrabony defects when the alveolar process is thick. Plaque removal cannot be achieved, and pocket depth increases. Gingival resection techniques cannot be considered because marginal tissue of the alveolar mucosa will result. Detached gingiva associated with a pocket must be transformed into functional gingiva with a shallow sulcus and sufficient width of attached gingiva to permit ease of plaque removal and gingival health.

The gingival attachment to the tooth may be considered as (1) a barrier by the epithelium and (2) an adherence factor from the gingival fiber apparatus. One function of attached gingiva is to serve as a buffer for the gingival margin against the pull of skeletal muscle fibers (muscles of facial expression) located within the alveolar mucosa. If the band of attached gingiva is wide enough, it will prevent any retraction of the marginal gingiva during the movement of the alveolar mucosa (adherence of the gingival margin). The fiber apparatus of the gingiva is most important in holding the gingiva closely adapted to the tooth. The gingival fiber apparatus is housed in the attached gingiva; hence the need for an adequate zone of attached gingiva.

It may be noted that major importance has not been placed on the indications for deepening of the vestibular fornix. Much of the early literature was devoted to this as an objective. If the band of the gingiva is sufficient, the depth of the vestibular fornix is not of primary importance and should not be changed for this reason alone. A minimal zone of attached gingiva may be present and should not be changed if no evidence of disease is observed.

Often mucogingival surgery is performed in conjunction with procedures for the correction of underlying osseous and anatomic deformities. The mucogingival complex is retained. Osseous, furcation, and root deformities are readily accessible for corrective procedures with full-thickness mucogingival flaps. Definitive pocket elimination with minimal sulcular depth can be accomplished. Often new retention and osseous regeneration procedures also are completed by this approach.

Mucogingival deformities

Gingival recession and clefts: surgical correction. Gingival recession and clefts cause local tissue problems that are associated with little or no gingiva. Frequently retraction of the gingival margin is associated with a shallow vestibular fornix and protracted retention of food debris, plaque, and resultant calculus. If the pull of the frena and muscle attachments on the gingival margin are detected early enough, gingival defects can be avoided (Corn, 1968; Kopczyk and Saxe, 1974; Vincent et al., 1976). The inadequate zone of attached gingiva permits the retraction or blanching of the gingival margin with the potential for bone loss and subsequent recession. Recession will be more severe if the alveolar profile is pronounced with thin overlying alveolar support.

Aside from the control of progressive destruction related to such local environmental problems, patients are concerned about the unaesthetic root exposure, which can be corrected by the following therapeutic methods:

1. Connective tissue attachment (reattachment) to the denuded root via a pedicle or a free soft tissue autograft
2. Increased zone of attached gingiva below the receded area via a pedicle or a free soft tissue autograft

Frenum pull. The close proximity of the frenum to the gingival margin has the potential of causing retraction of the gingival margin. When the pull of the frenum causes blanching and retraction of the gingival margin, surgical correction should be performed. Otherwise plaque retention and toothbrush irritation will cause periodontal breakdown. When indicated, this procedure should be completed prior to orthodontic treatment (see discussion on Frenotomy and Frenectomy).

Absent or inadequate zones of attached gingiva. The gingiva functions as a protective mechanism for the attachment apparatus, maintaining a seal for the underlying tissues against debris and organisms in the oral cavity. When the gingiva becomes affected to a point beyond its ability to maintain the seal, inflammation spreads into the deeper structures. The absence or inadequate zones of attached gingiva cannot withstand the mechanical and masticatory irritational forces or the stress of muscle retraction. The connective tissue seal is disrupted, and periodontal disease progresses.

How much gingiva is required? Some clinicians indicate that 3 mm is an adequate width of gingiva. Others strive for more (Grant et al., 1972). It is difficult to apply a mathematic rule to this biologic phenomenon. Nevertheless, the zone of attached gingiva should be broad enough to prevent marginal retraction during facial movements (Friedman, 1962). Lang and Löe (1972) in their clinical studies suggest that 2 mm of keratinized gingiva (corresponding to 1 mm of attached gingiva) is adequate to maintain gingival health. Bowers (1963) studied the width of attached gingiva in 160 human subjects from 3 to 35 years of age and concluded that less than 1 mm of attached gingiva could maintain a clinically healthy state. However, emphasis was placed on the need for meticulous oral hygiene to prevent inflammation and pocket formation. He stated further that some attached gingiva is required since alveolar mucosa is not acceptable at the soft tissue margin.

GENERAL PRINCIPLES IN PLANNING SURGERY

Evaluation of the tissue morphology will dictate the surgical technique selected for the involved area and should encompass the following information:

1. Whenever possible an adequate width of mature gingiva should be retained and preserved to avoid needless traumatic surgery to recreate that which has been destroyed.

2. It has been shown that gingival health is compatible with very narrow gingiva (Bowers, 1963), and it has been suggested that 2 mm of keratinized gingiva (corresponding to 1 mm of attached gingiva) is adequate (Lang and Löe, 1972). Attached gingiva is sufficient if it prevents tension on the gingival margin. This is particularly significant in children anticipating orthodontic

therapy. A free soft tissue autograft should be performed prior to tooth movement if there is insufficient keratinized tissue (Maynard and Ochsenbein, 1975).

3. The physiologic requirements for the width of the attached gingiva are most critical for the teeth that will have full-coverage restorations.

4. New attached gingiva can replace marginal alveolar mucosa provided that the connective tissue of the graft is genetically coded to produce dense collagen fibers. It is the connective tissue of a free soft tissue autograft that provides this source of granulation tissue. The granulation tissue proliferating from the periodontal ligament, residual periosteal connective tissue, bone marrow spaces, and adjacent gingiva can induce the formation of keratinized gingival epithelium.

5. The connective tissue of pedicle grafts from varying donor sites provides the granulation tissue, which maintains keratinized gingival epithelium. The mucogingival complex can be changed in a stable way without the risk of wounds healing by secondary intention.

6. Primary intention closures should be selected over broad-based secondary intention healing wounds.

7. The use of full-thickness mucoperiosteal flaps should be avoided when roots are prominent (as in the mandibular incisor, canine, premolar, and rotated molar areas). Indiscriminate dissection of long connective tissue attachments may result in needless anatomic deformities.

8. When an osseous defect requires correction the surgical design must protect these tissues at the completion of the procedure. The risk of the permanent loss of alveolar bone height is reduced in the presence of thick cortical bone, for example, when the external oblique ridge is in close proximity to the area of the second and third mandibular molars.

9. All full-thickness grafts should be sutured securely so that the gingival margin covers the crest of the alveolar bone or is between 1 and 2 mm coronal to it. To preserve the aesthetics of the anterior teeth (especially in preparation for full-coverage restorations) the gingival margin may be positioned on the root 2 mm from the alveolar crest (see discussion on Palatal region).

10. Areas of inadequate attached gingiva involving the mucogingival junction can be functionally repaired without an anatomic defect. Depending upon the availability of donor tissue, a pedicle graft for an isolated tooth, or a free soft tissue autograft or a multiple interdental papilla graft for a segment of the arch, can increase the width of the attached gingiva. The gingival collar can be preserved, and the graft immobilized adjacent and apical to it. A better opportunity for "creeping attachment" is provided if the recipient bed is extended to the periphery of the tissue margin (Goldman et al., 1976).

11. Aesthetic correction of denuded roots can be successful if there are no interproximal defects and no pocket formation and if the tissue fills the interdental space. The connective tissue recipient bed adjacent to the avascular recipient site provides the scaffolding and primary attachment during the repair of a laterally positioned flap. This interdental connective tissue bed is the source of plasmatic circulation initially and of collateral circulation for a free graft attachment to a root (Sullivan and Atkins, 1968).

12. Knowing what not to do surgically is more important than the technical knowledge of the procedure itself.

13. The simplest technique should be chosen to eliminate the defect left by the disease and to avoid needless trauma, prolonged healing, undue discomfort, and permanent damage to the periodontium.

14. Complete hemostasis must be accomplished, and close adaptation of the flaps to the underlying tissue is mandatory to avoid dead spaces and submucosal or subperiosteal hemorrhage.

15. Resolution of postsurgical inflammation and edema is usually complete in 1 week. Patients are comfortable by this time. Initial healing has progressed so that suture removal and dressing changes are optimal 7 to 10 days postsurgically. Earlier suture removal may cause unnecessary patient discomfort, flap instability, and iatrogenic displacement.

CONSIDERATIONS PRIOR TO SURGERY

The active involvement of a person in his own health is the essence of any successful therapy. The importance of attitude toward *total health* is demonstrated by the dentist's recording blood pressure and recommending a complete physical examination with blood studies. As the relationship develops between dentist and patient, nutritional counseling (Nizel, 1972) and new health habits, for example, elimination of smoking, can be suggested. Sessions in patient education teach, emphasize, reinforce, and motivate a commitment for bacterial plaque control, fluoride therapy, and control of sucrose (Corn et al., 1976, 1968; Corn and Marks, 1969).

SCALING AND ROOT PLANING

Prior to mucogingival surgery, scaling and root planing are imperative. Sufficient time must be allowed for the tissues to heal and mature before the need for surgical intervention is determined. Removal of calculus and bacterial plaque are advantageous particularly when the mucogingival junction and alveolar mucosa are involved. Many times the reduction and localization of the inflammation by presurgical scaling changes the quality of the tissue, making it easier to incise and reflect. It may eliminate the need for surgery entirely

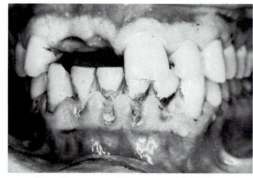
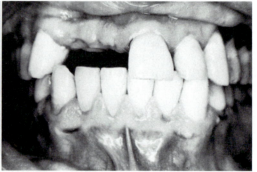

A

B

Fig. 26-2. A, Calculus deposits on mandibular incisors. If surgery were to be performed and calculus removed, mucogingival surgery would be necessary since bases of pockets are in mucosa. Note narrow zone of gingiva. **B,** Same case 1 week after scaling. Note reduction in gingival inflammation. Gingival margins on central incisors have moved coronally, providing more gingiva. This is advantageous if an internal beveled incision with an apically positioned flap is necessary. (From Corn, H. C.: Dent. Clin. North Am., p. 79, March 1964.)

(Fig. 26-2). Reducing inflammation may confine the surgical technique to a more limited area. This happens frequently in isolated areas of recession and gingival clefts where the use of a laterally positioned graft had been planned.

Gaining a wider band of gingiva is another benefit of presurgical scaling. After the deposits are removed from the tooth surfaces, the coronal movement of the gingival margin makes this possible. When reattachment occurs, and this is not predictable, it is similar to creeping attachment where the gingiva attaches to the tooth surface postsurgically. Surgery may not be necessary (Fig. 26-3). When the tissue is neither attached nor adapted to the tooth following scaling, the resultant wider band of gingiva facilitates certain flap procedures in which as much gingiva as possible is desirable.

Root planing is completed with the débridement of all accretions and irregularities from the root surface. Air drying of the roots improves the detection of residual calculus, although instrumentation should be performed in a wet field.

IATROGENIC DENTISTRY

No periodontal procedure, surgical or otherwise, offers much hope for success in the presence of local etiologic factors iatrogenically induced, some of which are as follows:

1. Open or loose contact areas
2. Inadequate embrasures
3. Deficient or overextended margins
4. High restorations
5. Poor or overcontoured crowns
6. Poorly designed pontics
7. Inadequate or ill-fitting removable prostheses

A comprehensive discussion of these etiologic factors is found in Chapter 4.

SOFT TISSUE CURETTAGE

Reconstruction of the gingival unit and the attachment apparatus can occur if chronic inflammation and its associated osseous deformities are treated. The pocket epithelium, epithelial attachment, granulomatous tissue beneath the connective tissue, and transseptal fibers must be removed. Their removal can be accomplished by a closed procedure (when horizontal bone loss is present) or by open flap curettage performed with a knife and curet (when infrabony pockets are present).

Soft tissue curettage is beneficial before and during orthodontic procedures. When the periodontium is free of inflammation it permits remarkable reconstruction of the attachment apparatus (repair of bony defects), elimination of pockets, and an increased width of attached gingiva (Fig. 26-4).

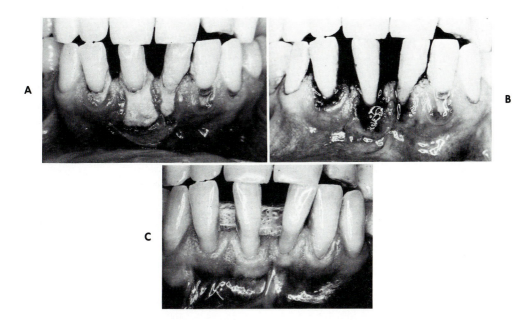

Fig. 26-3. A, Heavy calculus deposits on mandibular central incisors. Pocket wall is everted with retraction of lip. **B,** Appearance of area immediately after root scaling and planing. **C,** Six months postoperatively. Creeping attachment has occurred. No further soft tissue treatment is indicated.

ORTHODONTIC CONSIDERATIONS

There are well-accepted principles of occlusion that determine the need for orthodontic therapy. Considerations that are critical are the buccolingual landmarks, tooth prominence in the arch, poor axial inclinations, uneven cementoenamel junction relationships, crowding, a deep overbite, and posterior bite collapse (see Chapter 30). Often upon completion of orthodontics, planned osseous and mucogingival surgery will be obviated. Adult orthodontics is discussed in Chapter 21.

OCCLUSAL ADJUSTMENT AND STABILIZATION

The relative influence of the inflammatory and traumatic factors on periodontal healing has been clarified. Now there appears to be a biologic basis for initial therapy in the management of occlusal periodontitis (Lindhe and Svanberg, 1974; Kantor et al., 1976; Meitner, 1975). The objective of initial treatment should be to utilize and maximize the innate healing potential at this time. To achieve this, inflammatory and traumatic factors should be removed. Following occlusal adjustment, sufficient time should elapse to allow repair of the marginal and attachment apparatus lesions. If mobilities remain, the use of stabilization prior to extensive mucogingival surgery is suggested.

PATIENT CARE

The relationship of much trust and little fear between a person and his dentist is developed through empathy, respect, and personal warmth. The involvement of a ''caring'' staff provides an atmosphere of reduced tension and anxiety for a person anticipating a dental experience. The relationship will grow when the staff is genuine and open about the procedures that are necessary. Concern for a person's comfort must assume the highest priority. All procedures should be explained and updated, all questions answered, and fears allayed.

Patient management during surgery is unique in that the procedure is usually longer than other surgical procedures requiring local anesthetics. The use of sedatives or tranquilizers the evening before surgery reduces anxiety, allows a restful sleep, and enables a calm patient to arrive for surgery. Longer acting narcotics in combination with sedatives or tranquilizers and antisialagogues (if needed) provide elevation of pain threshold, sedation and drying of oral tissues through reduction of salivary flow, and slight amnesia. They may be administered orally, intramuscularly, or intravenously. The route of administration depends upon the training and experience of the dentist. Nitrous oxide as an inhalation sedation (analgesic) offers another alternative for control of patient apprehension.

Prior to periodontal surgery the blood pressure and pulse rate should be recorded. For high-risk patients with a history of rheumatic fever or congenital heart disease or for those with prosthetic cardiac valves, antibiotics are used routinely. They also are administered to patients receiving extensive osseous surgery and grafts. Antibiotics are usually not taken for more than 5 days. Ross et al. (1976) in their comprehensive review list systemic disorders that affect periodontal surgery planning.

Extensive procedures, especially in the mandibular posterior and retromolar areas, cause more postoperative discomfort and pain. This is due to the edema within the loose connective tissue rather than to the actual surgical event. The use of steroids in decreasing frequency over a 6-day period allows for almost complete comfort with a minimum of analgesics required. There are medical contraindications to the use of steroids that must be considered and discussed with the patient's physician before they are prescribed.

Adequate nutrition must be maintained following periodontal surgery. Periodontal dressings, exposed injured tissue, and soreness prevent many patients from eating and drinking properly. This denies the body adequate nutrient levels and increases dehydration at a time when optimum tissue healing is desired. Complete postoperative instructions, including a soft diet with possible supplementation and ample fluid intake, contribute to optimum healing (Nizel, 1972).

Perhaps the best way to evaluate a patient's postoperative status is to phone personally about 3 to 4 hours after surgery. Inquire about the response to the procedure, and discuss questions or instructions that were not clear. This conversation reinforces the ''caring'' relationship between the dentist and the patient. Psychologically the dentist's concern is a great morale booster for the patient. It sustains an involvement in the patient's well-being and can be a dynamic aid to recovery.

INSTRUMENTS

Instruments used for various periodontal surgical procedures are shown in Fig. 26-5. Trays are set up and sterilized for the surgical procedures. If special instruments are needed in addi-

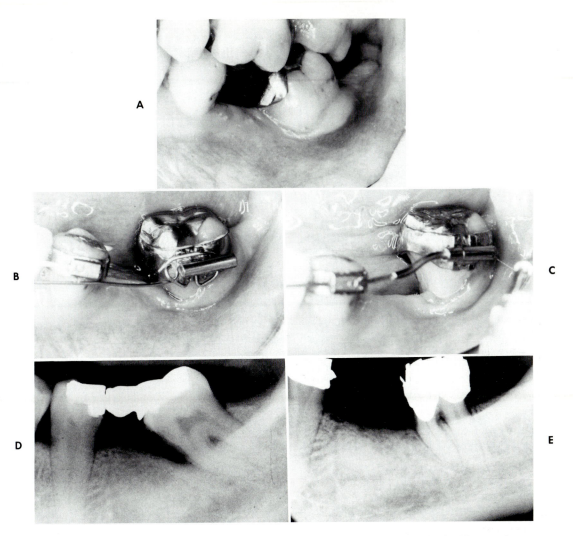

Fig. 26-4. Curettage and molar uprighting. **A,** Minimal gingiva at mesiogingival line angle. A 9 mm infrabony pocket is present. Inlay margin at gingiva. **B,** Use of a Broussard uprighting attachment. **C,** Uprighting completed. Molar in retention. Sulcular wall increased width of attached gingiva present at margin. Infrabony pocket has been eliminated after 5 months. **D,** Preoperative radiograph (after tooth movement). **E,** Six months after provisional stabilization.

tion to those on the tray, they are arranged on a second tray. The special instruments are stored individually in transparent heat-resistant sterile bags. They are readily available when required.

The dental assistant's tray should contain the following instruments:

1. Mirror
2. Cotton applicators for presurgical preparation
3. Equipment for administering local anesthesia
4. Sponges dampened with an antiseptic solution for cleansing perioral tissues and instruments
5. Periosteal elevator
6. Cheek retractors
7. Suction tips for dependable evacuation system
8. Supply of 2″ × 2″ gauze sponges
9. Local anesthesia
10. Surgical blades
11. Suture material

TYPES OF INCISIONS

Many patients with normal appearing gingiva can have gross changes in the underlying bone. Periodontal disease cannot be diagnosed by the mere observation of the soft tissue, and patho-

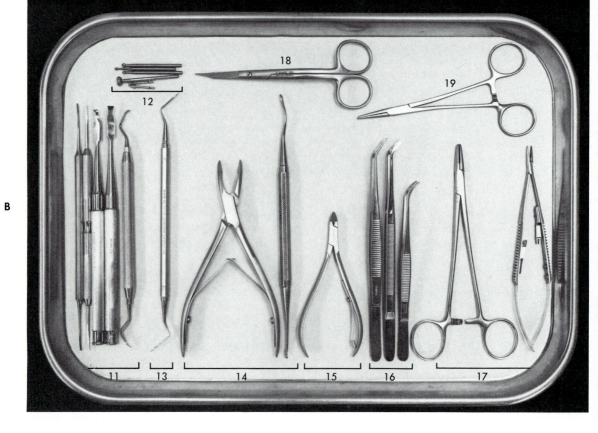

A

B

Fig. 26-5. A, *1,* Mirrors, at least two large ones. Explorers, double-ended combination of no. 23 and 17 explorers, and double-ended cowhorn explorer for examination of furcation areas. *2,* Probe, thin Williams probe or Michigan type and Crane-Kaplan pocket markers. *3,* Knife, double-ended broad blade nondisposable knife. Examples are Goldman-Fox no. 7, Kirkland no. 14/15, and Buck no. 3/4. These knives may be used in various types of initial incisions, particularly in techniques that are basically involved in removal or dissection of soft tissues. Blades are angled for ease of access and sharpened on all sides, allowing operator to utilize a push or pull motion with any surface of blade. Major disadvantage is necessity of maintaining a refined surgical edge. Knife usually requires sharpening after each use. *4,* Knife, double ended with a thin, pointed blade that is sharp on both edges. Examples are Goldman-Fox no. 11, Buck no. 5/6, and Sanders no. 4/5. These knives may be used to free interproximal tissue after initial incision, to thin and scallop flaps, or to make initial apically directed incisions during mucogingival surgery. Knives must also be sharpened to a fine surgical edge. The Orban nos. 1 and 2 are well designed for resection of mandibular lingual interproximal tissue. *5,* Disposable surgical blades with nondisposable Bard-Parker handles, nos. 11, 12, 12B, and 15. No. 11 blade is long and pointed. It has one cutting edge and is useful in delicate sulcular incisions. Nos. 12 and 12B are curved "hawk-beak" blades. No. 12 blade is sharp on both surfaces of curve and may be used in a push or pull motion. No. 15 is most commonly used blade. It is traditionally shaped surgical scalpel blade. Disposable blades are usually very sharp and are packaged as sterile. Disadvantages are limited shapes available and angulation of blade to handle, which makes access to many areas difficult. *6,* Special blade handles, to overcome access problem, particularly in partial-thickness dissections of edentulous area of retromolar and tuberosity area. Examples are Blake handle (ash), and beaver handle. Blake handle can use usual disposable surgical blades and provides a 360-degree angle rotation for all areas of mouth. Two handles with blades are provided on surgical trays to enable access either buccally or lingually. Beaver handle (no. 3 KD) has a variety of stainless steel replaceable blades that can be used in gingivectomy and flap procedures. Castroviejo blade breaker is a handle that uses disposable razor blades. It is particularly useful for delicate graft dissections. *7,* Periosteal elevators, two are used on surgical tray. Examples are Prichard no. 3 and Allen no. 9 or Goldman-Fox. Goldman-Fox has sharp edges to aid in reflection of more delicate flaps. *8,* Instruments of various shapes, for gross removal of hard deposits, granulation tissue, and tissue that remains attached to teeth following initial incision and reflection. Examples are Prichard nos. 41 and 42 (large curet), Goldman-Fox no. 10 (large surgical hoe), and Goldman-Fox no. 1 (Star) (large scaler). *9,* Instruments for definitive root planing and removal of remaining tissue fragments, curets. Examples are Goldman-Fox nos. 2, 3, and 4; Columbia nos. 2R, 2L, 13, and 14; and Gracey nos. 7, 8, 11, 12, 13, and 14. *10,* Stones, for sharpening curets. Examples are flat Arkansas no. 4 or Ivory no. 68 and Norton MB no. 4. **B,** Instruments that should be available for osseous and gingival reduction and contouring. *11,* Chisels, examples are Wedelstaedt (Hu-Friedy) nos. 41 and 42, Schumacher no. 401 and Star nos. 1 and 2. These are narrow-ended, side-cutting enamel chisels used for elimination of osseous craters and removal of interproximal hemiseptums. Ochsenbein nos. 1 and 2 are excellent for removal of bone because of their shape and angulation. Rhodes chisel no. 36/37, used for distal interproximal and radicular bony margin correction. Instrument is designed so that correct parabolic curve to osseous morphology can be achieved. Rhodes no. 38/39 is used on mesial surfaces. *12,* Burs and diamonds, for ultraspeed or slow-speed handpieces. Gingivoplasty diamonds, F-1, cone-shaped; F-2 (Star), small round; F-3 (Star), large doughnut nos. 8, 10, and 12, round surgical burs. *13,* Interproximal file, Buck no. 11/12 (safe-sided). *14,* Rongeurs, Useful in gross osseous reduction for obtaining osseous material for grafting. Examples are Cohen-Brenman (premier 5½ inch no. 4A) with small angled beak. Spoon curet, Miller no. 8 (Hu-Friedy) is ideal for developing correct osseous contour. *15,* Tissue nippers, used for removing elastic connective tissue fibers and for gingivoplasty. *16,* Pliers, serrated cotton pliers, Corn suture pliers, and tissue forceps (Hu-Friedy no. 34). *17,* Needle holder, diamond-jawed 6 inch Crile-Wood, designed for plastic surgery. It grasps very positively with minimum pressure to prevent flattening of small needles used in many periodontal surgical procedures. Castroviejo, small, delicate instrument that releases upon continuous closure and lends itself to more delicate suturing. *18,* Scissors, Goldman-Fox, fine tissue scissors excellent for tissue tag removal; LaGrange (Banditt no. 905), double-curved scissors excellent in areas of difficult access. *19,* Mosquito hemostat, straight or curved 5 inch hemostat.

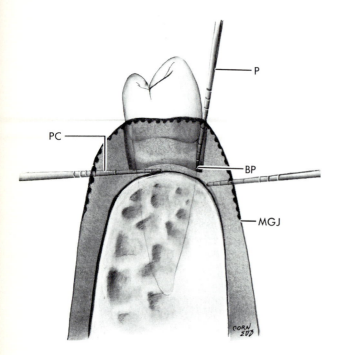

Fig. 26-6. Use of a probe to measure pocket depth, and "sounding" to locate alveolar crest. Vertical probe, *P,* approaches base of pocket, *BP.* Horizontally sounding through soft tissue, probe can locate crest, *PC.* There is sufficient attached gingiva apical to crest and base of pocket as delineated by mucogingival junction, *MGJ.*

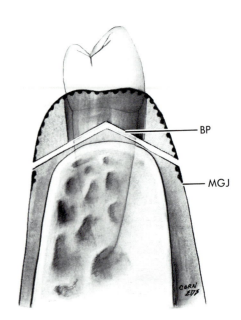

Fig. 26-7. Coronally directed incision. A suprabony pocket, *BP,* can be eliminated if the osseous morphology is not thick and if there will be sufficient gingiva coronal to the mucogingival junction, *MGJ,* following surgery. Outlines of gingivectomy incisions are illustrated.

logic conditions can be easily overlooked. It is incumbent upon the dentist to explore accurately the periodontal architecture during the initial soft and hard tissue débridement stages. Following débridement and after sufficient healing has occurred, precise observation may alter the original prognosis and the surgical treatment plan (Dahlberg, 1969; Ross et al., 1976).

Periodontal probe: planning the incision

The periodontal probe is used conventionally to measure pocket depth. Before the design of the surgical incision is planned, it is necessary to evaluate the topography of the soft tissue pockets and the defects of the underlying osseous morphology. The degree of detachment around the tooth is recorded in six different areas. The depths that approximate the mucogingival junction are noted. The approximation of the pocket depth to the mucogingival junction determines the design of the incision. The incision must be planned either to salvage the masticatory mucosa that is present or to prepare a bed so that soft tissue grafts

can reestablish a functional gingival attachment.

The periodontal probe is used also as a sounding technique (see Chapter 12) and is described in detail by Tibbetts (1976). Properly used, the probe penetrates at right angles to the soft tissue and locates the level of the alveolar crest (Fig. 26-6). If the pocket depth recording is *coronal* to the horizontal sounding of the alveolar crest, a resectional technique can be planned (Fig. 26-7). Conversely, when the recording is *apical,* an inverse bevel incision (apically positioned graft) should be planned.

Coronally directed incision

The coronally directed incision (Kopczyk and Young, 1976) also is referred to as a gingivectomy or an external beveled incision. Primarily it is used for the removal of excess gingiva when no osseous defects or thick bony ledging is present. Unless a sufficient band of attached gingiva is present to ensure an adequate band of attached gingiva after surgery, the coronally directed incision should not be used (Fig. 26-7).

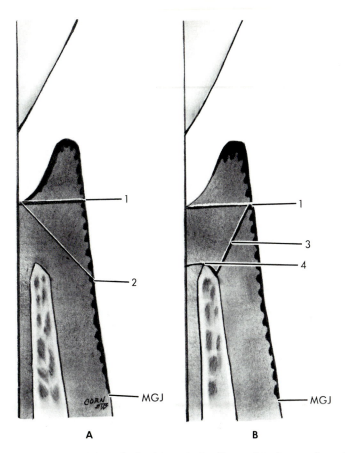

A   **B**

Fig. 26-8. Right-angled incision. **A,** Incision, *1,* is directed to base of pocket. If there is sufficient attached gingiva as indicated by mucogingival junction, *MGJ,* and if underlying bone is not thick, *gingivoplasty* (with a no. 7 Goldman-Fox knife or diamond stones) can shape tissue, *2.* **B,** To contour, thin, or gain access to underlying bone, a secondary incision, *3,* is required. All connective tissue coronal to crest, *4,* is removed to visualize interproximal area.

Right-angled incision

The right-angled incision (Kopczyk and Young, 1976) is used diagnostically to explore underlying bone and is utilized only when there is a wide band of attached gingiva. The base of the periodontal pocket must be far enough (coronally) from the mucogingival junction to allow an adequate zone of attached gingiva to remain after surgery. The incision is directed horizontally into the gingival tissue at the base of the pocket. The incised tissue is removed. The operator can determine if the underlying osseous structures require reshaping to provide the acceptable soft tissue contours. If reshaping is not required, the proper contour can be obtained by a gingivoplasty. A gingivoplasty using diamond stones is substituted often for the coronally directed second incision. However, when reshaping is necessary

a flap may be elevated to gain access to the underlying bone and to achieve physiologic architecture in bone and soft tissue. A second incision is required (directed either coronally or apically) to contour, thin, or gain access to the underlying structures (Fig. 26-8).

Apically directed incision

Because of its versatility the apically directed incision (Kopczyk and Young, 1976) is used to correct osseous deformities and for pocket elimination. The surgical knife is placed against the soft tissue with the cutting edge directed apically. Altering the entry point of this incision can accomplish different surgical needs. Fig. 26-9 shows different locations of the incisions as follows:

1. In releasing a papilla (Fig. 26-9, *A*).
2. Within the gingival crevice (sulcular in-

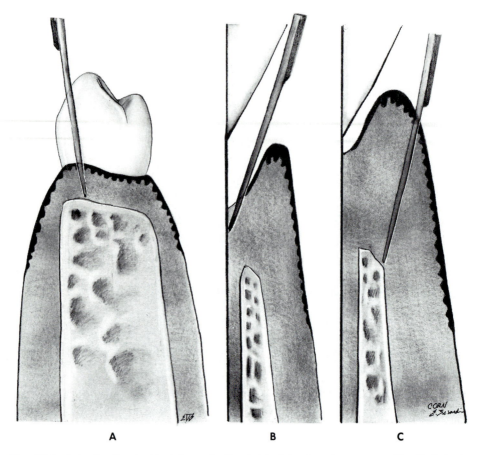

Fig. 26-9. Apically directed incisions. **A,** Crestal incision to release a papilla. **B,** Sulcular incision retains maximum amount of gingiva. It allows retention of connective tissue attachment to tooth when combined with a partial-thickness graft that will retain a periosteal cover for thin radicular bone. **C,** Inverse bevel incision to gain access to underlying osseous tissue and permit removal of inflamed crevicular tissue.

cision) when the tissue is very thin, when all the gingival tissue is needed, or when the marginal tissue is alveolar mucosa. The sulcular incision may retain a portion of the epithelial sulcular wall (Fig. 26-9, *B*).

3. Within the gingiva for thinning it internally and for removing inflamed crevicular tissue. The incision is frequently called an "inverse bevel incision" or an "internal gingivectomy" (Fig. 26-9, *C*).

The apically directed incision cannot be used when an alveolar dehiscence or fenestration is present.

Partial-thickness incision

When there is need for a partial-thickness flap the partial-thickness incision is employed. The incision is located within the lamina propria of the gingiva and the loose connective tissue of the alveolar mucosa. Partial-thickness incisions can be directed either coronally or apically, based upon the purpose of the procedure. The apically directed incision is particularly difficult when it is used to increase the width of attached gingiva, because there are no tissue planes to follow. The soft tissue (with little or no attached gingiva) is usually very thin in the area where the incision is indicated. The partial-thickness coronally directed incision is initiated in the alveolar mucosa (through a releasing incision) and continues to the margin (Fig. 26-10). It allows visualization of the path of the incision and overcomes the problem of tissue friability. The palatal flap approach uses the coronally directed partial-thickness incision to establish the final thickness of the primary flap as it is reflected.

The apically directed partial-thickness flap is used as a means of thinning the bulky tissues of the retromolar and tuberosity areas. Here the incisions are apically directed, gradually sloping to thin the gingiva from the margin of the initial

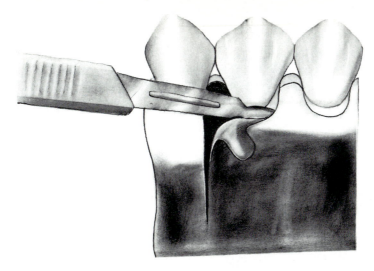

Fig. 26-10. Partial-thickness coronally directed incision is initiated in mucosa (through a releasing incision) and is seen terminating at gingival margin.

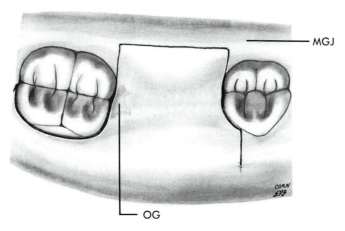

Fig. 26-11. Linear partial-thickness incision outline for preparation of a flap for protection of recipient site of osseous graft, *OG*.

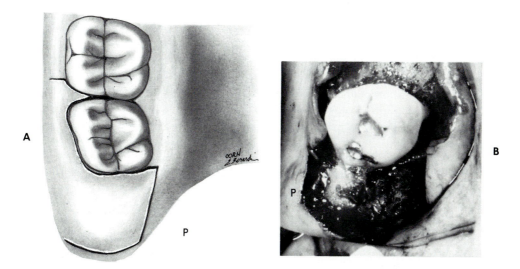

Fig. 26-12. A, Tuberosity linear incision outline to provide access to osseous graft donor site. **B,** Exposure of maxillary sinus can be protected by the incisional design. (Courtesy Dr. Peter A. Rubelman, North Miami Beach, Fla.)

incision to the bone. The flap allows for the retention of mature external tissue and minimizes pocket recurrence.

A linear partial-thickness incision (Corn, 1964) is ideal to prepare a flap for the protection of a donor or recipient site of an osseous graft. The incision is directed along the lingual mucogingival junction of an edentulous area, allowing a flap to be reflected (Fig. 26-11). The area is treated, and then the flap is repositioned and sutured to its original position. Similarly, the linear incision allows access to the tuberosity, which serves as the best intraoral source of osseous donor tissue (Tibbetts and Ochsenbein, 1976) (Fig. 26-12). It affords protection to this site and to an inadvertent maxillary sinus communication, should this occur (Ochsenbein and Ross, in press).

A modification of the partial-thickness incision is used to prepare a bed for free soft tissue autografts. When minimal gingiva is present, the incision is initiated coronal to the mucogingival junction. This incision line serves as a guide for the subsequent dissection. Most of this dissection is directed coronally within the alveolar mucosa. It can be performed with ease.

Releasing incisions

Vertical incision. A vertical incision is often used for access and flap mobility since it can avoid dehiscences or fenestrations and yet ensure maximum postsurgical bone coverage (Dahlberg, 1969). A short incision over an interdental space or over a furcation will increase the linear length of the flap and allow better flap placement, elimination of dead spaces, and better final tissue contour. A vertical incision is usually along a line angle rather than interproximally or directly over radicular surfaces. This allows the elevation and adaptation of the flap for the protection of the root prominence. The vertical incision is especially helpful when a flap must be positioned apically without tension at the extremity of the flap. The incision begins at the gingival margin, traverses the mucogingival junction, and terminates in the alveolar mucosa.

As a rule no releasing incision should be made on the lingual surfaces. Access to underlying structures can be increased by extending the apically directed incision mesially or distally. A flap with no releasing incision is called an "envelope flap." When one equates the arc of the tissue covering the alveolar process to a circle, it is obvious that the tissue must be stretched to a greater circumference to gain access to the facial

surfaces. A vertical incision can relieve the mechanical tension that often disrupts circulation and tears the tissue. In contrast, the lingual tissue tends to drape itself toward the center of the circle, negating the need for a releasing incision to obtain access (Dahlberg, 1969; Kopczyk and Young, 1976). In the lingual tissue of the retromolar area, occasionally additional access is required for flap placement. A vertical incision is used but should extend only to the mucogingival junction so that no tissue spaces are endangered. Dahlberg speaks of this as follows:

On the lingual aspect of the mandible there is a thin and fragile tissue complex. Since the incision and flap are on the inside of a curve, except in the second and third molar areas, adequate access can usually be obtained by extending the flap mesially. Three complications may occur with vertical incisions extending into the mucosa in the mandibular lingual region:

a. A vertical incision opens into the sublingual space and, if beyond the mylohyoid muscle, into the submandibular space. In the second molar area, infection can extend rather directly into the lateral pharyngeal space. We thereby open a number of potential tissue spaces other than the subperiosteal space that is opened with the full-thickness mucogingival flap usually employed in this location.

b. A vertical incision in the second molar area or distally frequently involves unnecessary hemorrhage due to the vascularity of the area.

c. A vertical incision frequently gapes widely and heals slowly over dense bone on the lingual surface. This gaping is probably due to the elastic fibers in the mucosa and the frequently lengthened mesial-distal distance following interdental osseous grooving. If these incisions extend only to the mucogingival line in this lingual area, they generally afford adequate release without opening into the spaces previously discussed. [Dahlberg, 1969]

The vertical incision is used on the palate (even though the palate is on the inside of a curve) to thin a partial-thickness flap and remove the bulk of the underlying connective tissue. Usually the buccal flaps (envelope flaps) in both arches can be handled without vertical incisions and still provide adequate access and positioning in the average case.

Cutback incision. A modification of a releasing incision to gain mobility is the cutback incision (Corn, 1964). It is used to reduce tissue tension when a flap is to be positioned laterally (see discussion on Edentulous Area Pedicle Graft).

Supplemental releasing incisions. Occasionally a full-thickness flap will have limited mobility because of the periosteum. A supplemental releasing incision through the periosteum from the inside of the flap will free it (Dahlberg, 1969; Ochsenbein, 1963, 1960). This is required in a coronally positioned graft procedure (Bernimoulin et al., 1975).

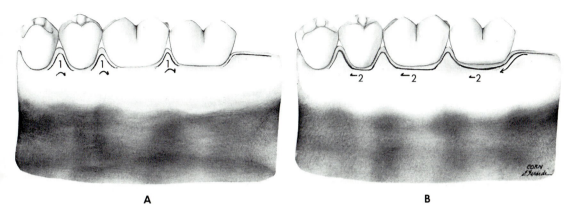

A

B

Fig. 26-13. Use of a scalloped incision on *lingual* aspect is difficult to execute. This two-step procedure simplifies flap design. **A,** Step 1. Papillae incision, *1,* is initiated antero-posterior to bone. **B,** Step 2. Incision, *2,* beginning posteriorly extends to alveolar crest and courses anteriorly, connecting all freed papillae. This develops a uniform scalloped incision outline for a full-thickness flap.

SWAGED NEEDLE AND SUTURE MATERIAL SELECTION*

Black silk

4-0	Swaged	⅜ circle	Reverse cutting	FS-2 needle	(2766)
4-0	Swaged	½ circle	Reverse cutting	J-1 needle	(734)
4-0	Swaged	⅜ circle	Reverse cutting	P-3 needle	(641)
6-0	Swaged	½ circle	Reverse cutting	PS-4 needle	1685

Ethibond (Dacron with polybutylate)†

4-0	Swaged	½ circle	Reverse cutting	P5-4 needle	B695
4-0	Swaged	⅜ circle	Reverse cutting	P5-2 needle	B682
5-0	Swaged	⅜ circle	Reverse cutting	P5-3 needle	B681

Plain gut

| 4-0 | Swaged | ⅜ circle | Reverse cutting | FS-2 needle | H821 |
| 5-0 | Swaged | ⅜ circle | Reverse cutting | P-3 needle | 686 |

Mersilene

| 5-0 | Swaged | ⅜ circle | Reverse cutting | F5-3 | R670 |
| 6-0 | Swaged | ⅜ circle | Reverse cutting | G-1 | R780 |

Vicryl (absorbable)

| 5-0 | Swaged | ⅜ circle | Reverse cutting | F5-3 | V388 |

Dermilon (monofilament nylon)‡

| 4-0 | Swaged | ⅜ circle | Reverse cutting | CE-4 | 1756-31 |

*Ethicon, Inc., Sommerville, N.J.
†Allows for ease of passage through tissue.
‡Manufactured by Davis-Geck, Pearl River, N.Y.

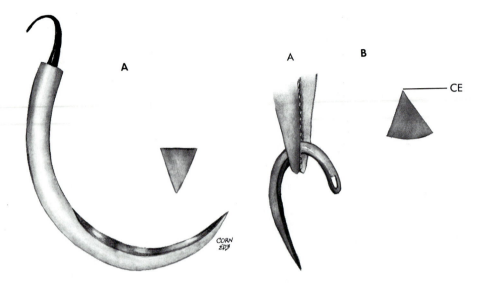

Fig. 26-14. Needles. **A,** Atraumatic reverse cutting needle. Inner curve of needle is flat with cutting edge on outer surface of curve (see insert). Eyed needle can have a reverse cutting edge, *A,* or **B,** a cutting needle has a cutting edge, *CE,* on inner curve.

Scalloped incision

The design of the primary incision varies; it may be either straight or scalloped. A straight line incision usually requires less dissection time than a scalloped incision. However a scalloped incision provides more primary coverage of bone during the immediate postsurgical period and perhaps less pain and faster healing. Extreme care should be exercised in the postsurgical positioning of the flap to avoid the formation of soft tissue craters and malalignment of the tissue to its interproximal position. Though these can occur with either incision, they seem less likely to occur with the scalloped incision.

The scalloped incision is advantageous in allowing a change in the surgical design to be made should unexpected clinical findings occur. The papillae can be used to cover autogenous bone grafts where new attachment procedures were planned. Salvaging the papillae allows the use of multiple interdental papillae grafts without causing another donor site wound.

There are occasions where limited access on the mandibular lingual surface hinders the delicate execution of a scalloped flap. A two-step procedure simplifies the retention of the papillae so that the proper realignment of the flap can be accomplished (Fig. 26-13).

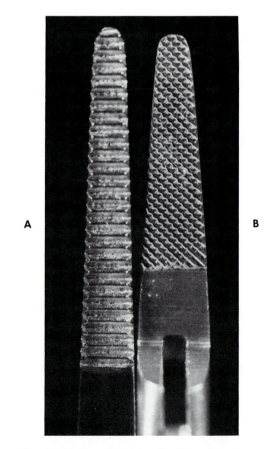

Fig. 26-15. Needle holder, **B,** differs from hemostat, **A,** in crosshatch pattern on jaws that enables better control with use of needle.

SUTURES AND SUTURING

The most popular method of tissue coaptation is suturing (Dahlberg, 1969; Glickman, 1972; Kopczyk and Young, 1976; Morris, 1965). In recent years there has been considerable interest in the area of tissue adhesives (Bhaskar et al., 1966; Binnie and Forrest, 1974; Forrest, 1974; Frisch and Bhaskar, 1968; Miller et al., 1974). However, these cyanoacrylates have been used only on an experimental basis.

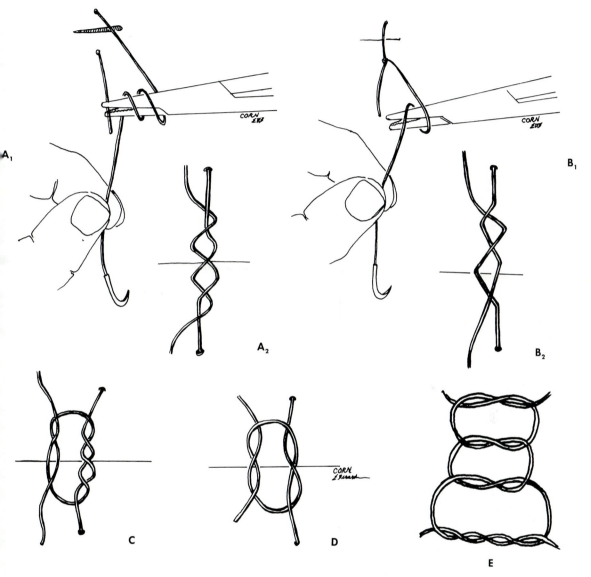

Fig. 26-16. Surgical and square knots. **A₁,** For surgical knot, hold needle end of suture material and wrap suture *under* needle holder for two turns. Pick up short end of suture and tighten knot over incision by crossing needle holder over incision. **A₂,** Number of loops that will appear. **B₁,** To complete surgical knot, suture is wrapped *over* needle holder for one single turn and tied again to short end. This time needle end of suture material is crossed over incision, and needle holder stays on same side. **B₂** illustrates second portion of surgical tie. **C,** Final arrangement of surgical knot (combination of **A₂** + **B₂**). For square knot, instead of two turns of the suture material as in **A,** hold needle end of suture material and wrap suture *over* needle holder for only one turn. To complete square knot, **B,** suture is wrapped *under* needle holder for one single turn. **D,** Arrangement of square knot. **E,** Standard synthetic knot-tying technique consists of double-looped surgeon's throw with a square knot on top.

BASIC CONSIDERATIONS AND GUIDELINES

1. Use the smallest and least reactive suture material compatible with the surgical problem (Halsted, 1913).
2. Leave a minimum of suture material under the flap.
3. Keep the sutures close to the tissues to avoid entanglement in the dressing.
4. Remove the sutures as soon as they are not necessary, usually 5 to 7 days, at most 10 days.

BASIC MATERIALS

1. 4-0 to 6-0 black braided silk
2. A curved needle with a reverse cutting edge and a swaged attachment to the silk strand
3. Ethibond, Mersilene, and Dermilon, which are finer, more inert materials, and smaller needles are preferred for delicate pedicle and gingival grafts
4. Needle holder
5. Suture scissors

Kopczyk and Young (1976) state that "silk is the most popular suturing material. It is neither digested nor absorbed during the wound healing process. Black silk is used so that it can be seen easily against the color of the oral tissues. Silk is easy to handle, easy to tie, and relatively inexpensive when compared to the synthetic materials."

There are two disadvantages in using silk. It must be removed postoperatively, as it does not resorb, and it is made of many strands of material that can permit passage of fluid and bacteria into the surgical wound.

A selection of swaged needles and suture materials is presented on p. 811.

Suturing needles vary in shape, cutting edge, and attachment to the suturing material. An atraumatic, disposable, eyeless needle is best (Fig. 26-14). The needle is usually swaged to the suture strand. This eyeless attachment produces a smooth unbroken surface from the needle tip to the end of the suturing material. Since the needle end and suture material are approximately the same diameter, tissue drag and rough areas are minimized, and tissue trauma is reduced. Threading is eliminated, and each suture strand has a new sharp needle. The cutting edge of the needle can be varied according to the intended use of the needle. A reverse cutting edge is best for suturing flaps and is used to minimize inadvertent tissue tears. A cutting edge needle simplifies penetration into tough tissues.

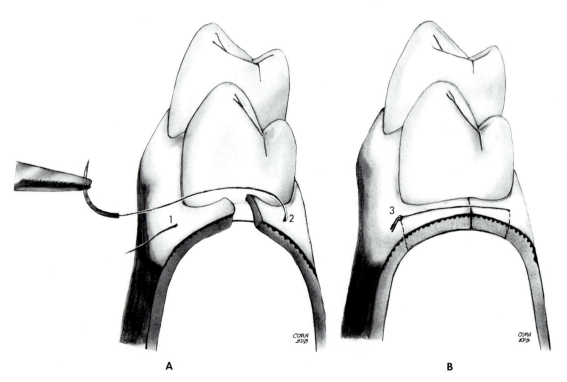

A **B**

Fig. 26-17. Interrupted suture. **A,** Suture enters attached gingiva, *1,* penetrates buccal flap, enters connective tissue side of lingual flap, and exits through lingual attached gingiva, *2.* **B,** Knot is completed on buccal flap, *3.*

Needle holders are instruments that hold the suturing needle in a predetermined position. When a hemostat is used for this purpose the needle tends to turn with the pressure. The needle holder differs from the hemostat because of the cross-hatch pattern on the jaws, which allows for better control of the needle (Fig. 26-15).

The knot (Kopczyk and Young, 1976) is the most critical step in the tying of sutures. To be successful the knot should be small to minimize tissue reaction, should not slip, and should not break easily. A surgical knot or the square knot fulfills these requirements (Fig. 26-16). A double square knot is necessary when using Ethiflex or Tevdek.

The suture scissors is used to cut the sutures after tying. The scissors should be closed when it is placed in the mouth, then opened cautiously when cutting the suture.

TYPES OF SUTURES

Interrupted suture. The interrupted suture is the simplest suture used in periodontics (Fig. 26-17). It is used when (1) tissue positioning is not critical, (2) both sides of the incision require the same amount of tension, (3) one side of the incision is firmly fixed, and (4) the suture is attached directly to the underlying periosteum. Tuberosity reduction, pedicles, or grafts are usually indications for use of the interrupted suture.

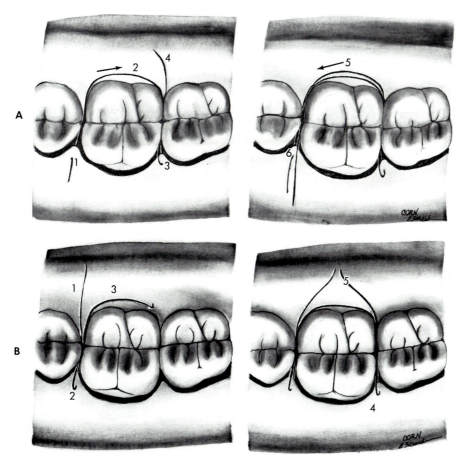

Fig. 26-18. Sling suture. **A,** Buccal tie. Suture material does not enter lingual gingiva but courses in direction of arrows. Needle enters at *1* and exits under contact above tissue around lingual *(2)*. Needle is brought to buccal and enters mature gingiva at *3,* returning under contact *(4).* Suture courses distally on lingual *(5)* and is tied finally, *6,* at original point of entry, *1.* **B,** Lingual tie. Needle enters lingual embrasure, leaving a tail of suture, *1.* Gingiva is entered on buccal flap, *2,* and needle goes under contact point but above lingual intact gingiva. Suture material courses around lingual flap of molar, *3,* and enters embrasure in direction of arrow. Needle passes again under contact area but over intact lingual gingiva. Tissue is entered again at *4* with a similar entry to lingual flap and is tied at *5.*

It should not be chosen for mobile flaps on both the buccal and lingual surfaces. Use here can result in one side's being too high and the other side's being too low, with improper tension on one or both sides.

Sling suture. The sling suture described by Morris (1965) and Dahlberg (1969) allows precise positioning of a flap around individual teeth when various teeth require that the flap be at different levels. Most often it is used on the buccal surface in the posterior regions. It can be tied on either the buccal or lingual side (Fig. 26-18). (For other modifications of the sling suture see the discussions on Multiple Interdental Papilla Graft and Double Papilla Graft.)

Continuous sling suture. The continuous sling suture is timesaving, particularly on the lingual surface in both arches. It can be initiated with a loose loop, allowing easy access for the scissors at the time of removal of the sutures. As the suture is continued around the teeth it is tied upon itself (Fig. 26-19).

A modification of the continuous sling suture is the continuous locked suture. It distributes tension throughout the incision line and is fast and easy to use. It is used in long edentulous areas, particularly the retromolar and tuberosity areas, and is suitable in suturing double papilla and pedicle grafts (Figs. 26-20 and 26-21).

Mattress sutures. There are several types of mattress sutures that leave a minimum of suture material under a flap. Wherever mattress sutures are used, single interrupted sutures are placed on the proximal ends of incisions for strength and stability. Some types of mattress sutures are as follows:

1. Simple mattress sutures (Fig. 26-22).
2. Crossed mattress sutures—used to coapt larger areas of the incision (Fig. 26-23).
3. Horizontal mattress (continuous) sutures—used to control the position of the papilla and adapt the flaps interdentally (Fig. 26-24).
4. Vertical sutures—used to keep suture material from under the flap margin. They are advantageous when the wick effect of the sutures is undesirable, as in bone grafts. They are most satisfactory when placed within the attached gingiva to contour the tissue to the underlying bone (Fig. 26-25).

Anchor suture. The anchor suture described by Morris (1965) allows delicate positioning of a single papilla when it is undesirable to tie into tissue on the lingual or on the adjacent embrasures (Fig. 26-26).

Figure eight suture. With the figure eight suture on the distal side of the terminal molars, the incised tissue can be approximated quickly

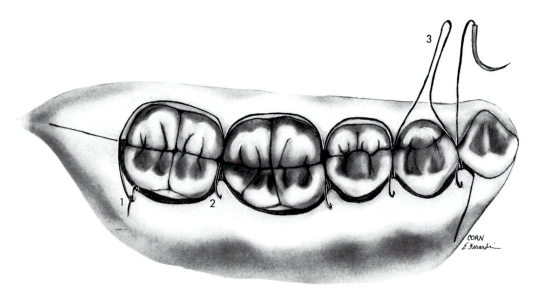

Fig. 26-19. Continuous sling suture. A loose loop of no. 4-0 black silk suture material is tied within mesiodistal width of terminal molar, *1*. This facilitates suture removal. Suture is wrapped around molar and enters buccal embrasure over gingival flap; needle passes through gingiva, *2*, to lingual flap. This process continues until a loose lingual loop, *3*, is left, to which final surgical knot is tied.

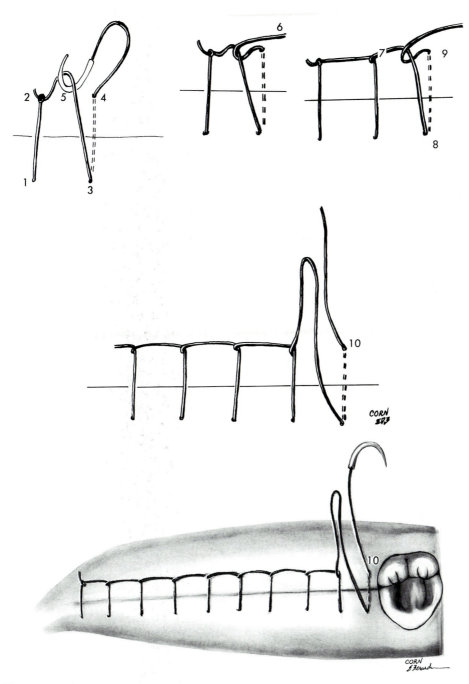

Fig. 26-20. Continuous locked suture. Needle enters tissue, *1*, and exits on opposite side of incision, *2*, where a knot is tied. At approximately the same distance from incision needle enters at *3*, exits at *4*, goes under diagonal loop at *5*, is pulled taut at *6*, and is completed at *7*. This process continues through *8* and *9*, until final tie occurs at *10*.

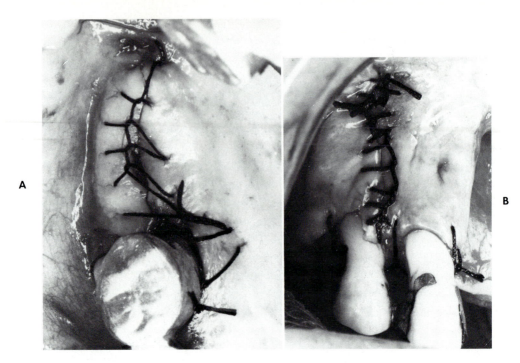

Fig. 26-21. A, Continuous locked suture of tuberosity area. **B,** Double pedicle graft.

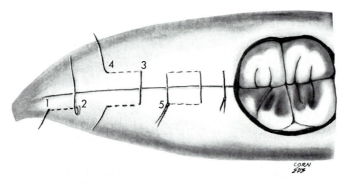

Fig. 26-22. Simple mattress suture. Suture needle penetrates tissue approximately ¼ inch but must be within attached gingiva, *1.* Pass needle and suture through tissue parallel to incision and exit at *2.* Suture passes over incision and enters tissue at *3,* exits at *4,* and is tied at original point of entry, *5.*

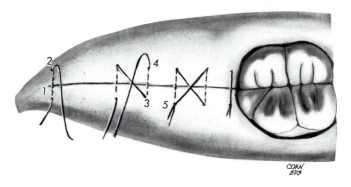

Fig. 26-23. Cross-mattress suture. This suture ensures complete coaptation of incision and also is used to maintain pressure over an area.

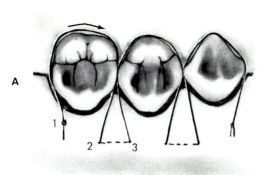 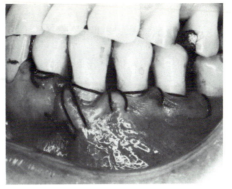

Fig. 26-24. Horizontal mattress suture. **A,** Demonstration of technique. An interrupted suture, *1*, adapts flap to alveolar crest. Suture is draped around tooth and enters buccal embrasure. Suture needle enters gingiva, *2*, and exits through inner aspect of flap, *3*. Suture then adapts papilla to underlying osseous contour between two premolars. This type of suture can be continuous and can be used to stabilize a series of papillae in a similar manner. **B,** Clinical case.

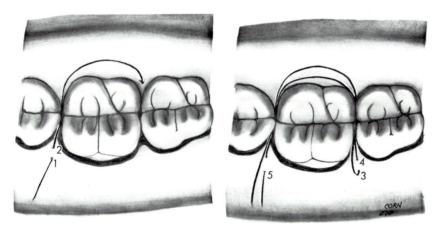

Fig. 26-25. Vertical mattress suture. Design keeps amount of suture material that is under flap to minimum. It also prevents suture material from being under incision interdentally. Final knot is at *5*; initial suture needle entered tissue at *1*, and exits vertically approximately 3 mm from tip of papilla *(2)*. Suture passes around lingual under contact to enter tissue on buccal at *3* and vertically exists on buccal *(4)*. Suture again passes under contact around lingual and distal to final knot at *5*.

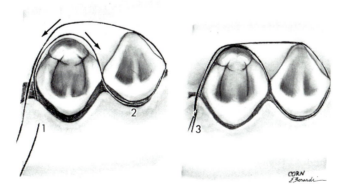

Fig. 26-26. Anchor suture. Needle enters buccal gingiva, *1*. Suture is wrapped around first premolar on lingual aspect and follows arrow to labial aspect of canine, *2*. Suture is wrapped around canine and first premolar on lingual side and is tied on buccal side, *3*, at original needle entry, *1*.

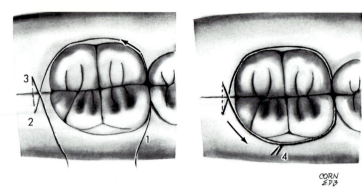

Fig. 26-27. Figure eight suture. Suture needle enters embrasure from buccal aspect, *1*. Suture is brought to distal edentulous area where needle enters buccal flap *(2)* and exits on lingual side of incision *(3)*. It is tied on buccal aspect at *4*.

and tightly, especially when complete closure for a bone graft is needed (Fig. 26-27).

For practicing suturing techniques a model is available (Kuba et al., 1972).

TISSUE ADHESIVES

The tissue adhesive IBC (isobutyl cyanoacrylate, Johnson & Johnson Co.) has been used experimentally to replace or augment the sutures used in periodontal surgery (Bhaskar et al., 1966; Binnie and Forrest, 1974; Forrest, 1962; Frisch and Bhaskar, 1968; Miller et al., 1974; Morris, 1965; Nizel, 1972). In some procedures, such as the free soft tissue autograft, utilization of IBC can eliminate the need for sutures. However, in the United States IBC is not available to the profession, and at this time there is no acceptable substitute for this material.

PERIODONTAL DRESSINGS

Advancement in the area of mucogingival and osseous surgery has included the introduction of surgical dressings that exclude eugenol from the formula. Eugenol has been implicated as an irritant to osseous tissues. Studies using the noneugenol dressing in mucogingival surgery indicate that proliferation of granulation tissue seems to be more rapid (Baer et al., 1964, 1960). Several types of semimixed or completely premixed dressings have become available, lessening the burden on the dentist or his assistant who previously had to spatulate the dressing material. Frisch et al. (1967) have reported research that takes exception to the implication that eugenol dressings act as greater irritants.

FLAPS AND GRAFTS

In periodontal surgery a flap is a segment of gingiva, mucosa, or both that has been partially detached surgically from the underlying tissues to provide visibility and accessibility necessary for treatment.

There are two basic flap designs. A *full-thickness flap* is one in which the entire tissue complex, including the periosteum, is elevated (mucoperiosteal flap). A *partial-thickness flap* is one in which only a portion of the tissue complex (primary flap) is raised, while the periosteum and connective tissue fibers remain attached to the root or the alveolar process or both. The incision is directed within the lamina propria of the gingiva and the submucosa of the alveolar mucosa (Fig. 26-28). Both major types of flaps may be divided according to surface morphology into (1) mucogingival flaps, (2) mucosal flaps, and (3) gingival flaps (Fig. 26-29).

The term "split-thickness flap" as described by Staffileno et al. (1966) is synonymous with the term "partial-thickness flap." Because partial thickness defines the design of the flap more aptly, its use is suggested. The full-thickness flap is used mainly for gaining access to underlying bone. The partial-thickness flap is used for gingival autograft recipient sites and to avoid exposing fenestrations and dehiscences. A *graft* is tissue transferred from one site and used to replace damaged structures in another area. Gingiva, oral mucosa, bone, and bone marrow are the tissues usually used as grafts. The area from which a graft is obtained is called the "donor site." Grafts that remain attached to the donor site by a base or pedicle are known as pedicle grafts. Tissue that is completely removed from one location and transferred to another without retaining connection with the donor site is known as a *gingival autograft*. Grafts are classified according to *source: autologous grafts* (autografts) are tissues obtained from the same individual; *homolo-*

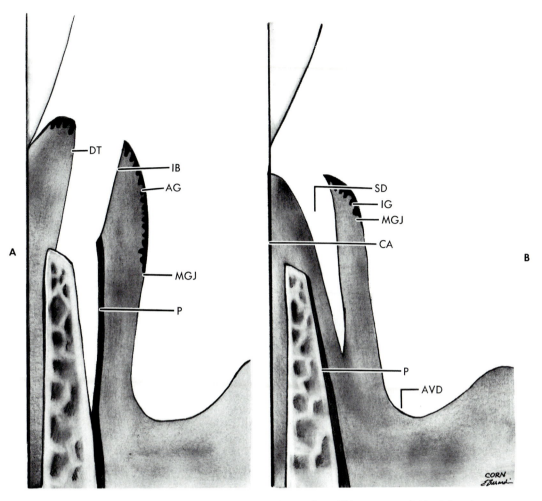

Fig. 26-28. Classification of flaps. **A,** Full-thickness flap. This mucoperiosteal flap leaves bone exposed since periosteum, *P,* is elevated with flap. This procedure is used most often when there is sufficient attached gingiva, *AG,* from tip of tissue margin to mucogingival junction, *MGJ.* Inverse beveled incision, *IB,* is directed toward crest, leaving pocket tissue that will be discarded, *DT.* **B,** Partial-thickness flap. This flap is best performed with adequate vestibular depth, *AVD.* A general requirement is insufficient gingiva, *IG,* from tip of tissue margin to mucogingival junction, *MGJ.* Sharp dissection, *SD,* leaves periosteum, *P,* and connective tissue covering bone, and an attempt is made to salvage collagenous attachment, *CA,* to tooth. This flap design is frequently used to increase width of gingiva.

gous grafts (homografts) are tissues obtained from different individuals of the same species; *heterologous grafts* are tissues obtained from another species. The term "graft" as used throughout this text will describe the entire *procedure* (Formicola, et al., 1976) of moving tissue from one location to another to improve periodontal form and function, while the term "flap" will be used to describe *morphology* of the tissue components involved.

Many of the surgical techniques are described in the literature by the flap design. Gage (1967) suggested the more apt descriptive term "posi-

tioned" flap instead of "repositioned" flap. To be more consistent with plastic surgery terminology, in this chapter grafts will describe the *surgical procedures;* for example, the terms "pedicle graft" and "positioned flap" (graft) will be interchangeable because they refer to the same procedure.

Grafts are used to reconstruct the gingival attachment, increase the width of attached gingiva, or transfer gingiva for covering denuded roots. An outline for selection of a graft is provided, and then the reconstructive procedures are described in detail.

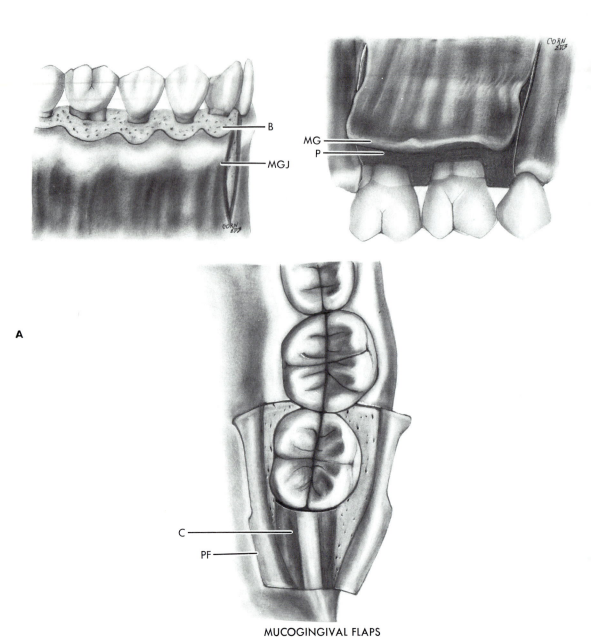

MUCOGINGIVAL FLAPS

Fig. 26-29. Subdivision of full-thickness and partial-thickness flaps. **A,** Full-thickness mucogingival flap. This flap is included in design of apically positioned graft. Gingiva is preserved, allowing for exposure of osseous tissue, *B,* for therapy. *MGJ,* mucogingival junction (top left). Partial-thickness mucogingival flap. Increase width of attached gingiva. Partial-thickness mucogingival flap has minimal gingiva, *MG,* present. Periosteum, *P,* is retained as recipient bed or source of granulation tissue for genetically coded gingiva (top right). Retromolar area. A partial-thickness primary flap, *PF,* is prepared in retromolar area. Beveled incision leaves bulk of retromolar connective tissue, *C,* to be removed (bottom).

I. *Preservation and retention of gingiva*
  A. Full-thickness apically positioned graft*
  B. Partial-thickness apically positioned graft*
  C. Full-thickness repositioned graft*
II. *Increasing width of attached gingiva*
  A. Frenotomy and frenectomy (nongraft technique)
  B. Partial-thickness apically positioned graft*
  C. Multiple interdental papilla graft*
  D. Free soft tissue autograft
  E. Edentulous area pedicle graft*
  F. Oblique rotated graft*
  G. Double papilla graft
III. *Reconstruction of anatomic deformities and gingival clefts*
  A. Laterally positioned graft*
  B. Double papilla graft*
  C. Free soft tissue autograft (bridging)
  D. Coronally repositioning graft*

RECONSTRUCTIVE PROCEDURES
Preservation and retention of gingiva
FULL-THICKNESS APICALLY POSITIONED GRAFT (FLAP) (Donnenfeld, 1964; Friedman, 1962; Friedman et al., 1964)

INDICATIONS

1. To eliminate pocket defects where the base of the pocket approaches or traverses the mucogingival junction
2. To eliminate pocket defects in conjunction with osseous corrective surgery
3. To establish functional attached gingiva

PRECAUTIONS

1. There must be sufficient width of gingival tissue to reestablish the desired mucogingival complex.
2. There must be no fenestrations, bony dehiscences, or thin radicular bone at the reflected site.

If there is any suspicion of the above, the partial-thickness flap approach should be used instead.

Whenever an adequate band of functional or nonfunctional gingiva exists and there is reasonable assurance that no fenestrations or dehiscences are present, a full-thickness flap approach should be used. The distinction must be made between prominent root position and prominent alveolar housing. In prominent root position prudent judgment may dictate the use of a partial-thickness dissection so that the connective tissue attachment can be maintained at its most coronal level. Thus the interproximal osseous defects can be architecturally corrected, and final radicular configurations can be planned. However, when the alveolar housing is prominent, a full-thickness

*Pedicle grafts.

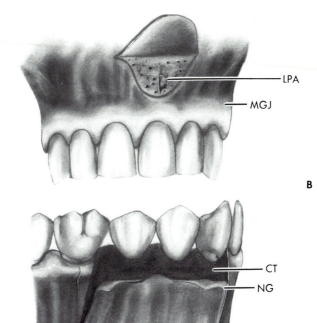

B

MUCOSAL FLAPS

Fig. 26-29, cont'd. B, Full-thickness mucosal flap. It is used for access to lateral periodontal abscesses, *LPA,* and endodontic therapy. *MGJ,* mucogingival junction (top). Partial-thickness mucosal flap. Lacking gingiva, *NG,* there is risk of crestal bone loss and an anatomic defect by leaving connective tissue, *CT,* exposed. A graft must be used (bottom).   *Continued.*

flap does not endanger the radicular support to the tooth, and osseous corrections can be made accordingly.

Several modifications in procedure have occurred since C. Nabers described gingival repositioning (Nabers, 1954). He later described an oblique internal incision from the gingival margin to the alveolar crest to aid in the reflection of the flap (Nabers, 1957). Friedman has described in great detail the rationale for this method. He correlates the clinical procedures with the healing studies when he describes the precise location of the flap and its stabilization with sutures. The formation of a new gingival fiber apparatus occurs within a 14-day period, and the mesenchymal cells of the periodontal ligament and marrow spaces are thought to provide the source of basic repair tissue in the healing of these wounds. It takes 7 to 10 days for the flap to attach to the underlying alveolar process, and it seems advisable to keep the sutures in place for 7 to 10 days (Friedman, 1964, 1962).

The apically positioned graft has provided the clinician with a method of fulfilling many of the objectives of mucogingival surgery with a minimum of tissue trauma and with less postoperative pain. It permits the operator to preserve and retain the functional or nonfunctional gingiva and to establish adequate attached gingiva on a predictable basis.

The technique (Fig. 26-30) consists of removing the inner wound portion of the gingival wall while preserving the outer mature, keratinized, attached gingiva. This is accomplished by an internal beveled incision that extends from the gingival margin to the alveolar crest, reducing the thickness of the gingival flap. The incision is made through the entire mesiodistal length of

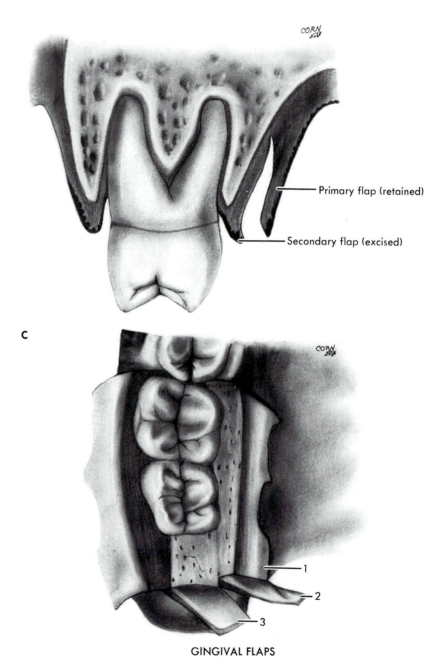

— Primary flap (retained)

— Secondary flap (excised)

C

1
2
3

GINGIVAL FLAPS

Fig. 26-29, cont'd. C, Gingival flap; palate (top). Primarily a partial-thickness flap (primary flap) is retained, and underlying secondary flap is excised. This enables access to osseous tissues. Tuberosity (bottom). Management of tuberosity also uses a partial-thickness primary flap, *1*. It provides access to continuation of palatal tissue removal, *2*, and dense fibrous connective tissue of tuberosity, *3*.

tissue being treated (Fig. 26-30, *A*). Nabers (1957) has described an internal incision that permits scalloping of the margin of the flap. The inner portion of the gingiva (the pocket) is removed from the tooth side of the wound with a spear-shaped interproximal knife, and the inflamed tissue is discarded. At this point the operator may decide to use vertical releasing incisions to facilitate flap reflection and to permit access to the underlying attachment apparatus (Fig. 26-30, *B*). In certain cases a vertical releasing incision may not be required. The envelope flap is then reflected with a periosteal elevator to visualize the alveolar process (Fig. 26-31). The bone con-

tours are corrected by osseous surgery techniques, and the flap is replaced to cover the alveolar crest and sutured (Fig. 26-30, *C* and *D*). Several suturing techniques that permit precise relocation of the flap are available. Dahlberg's modification (1969) of continuous suturing is rapid and prevents displacement of the flap (Fig. 26-19). An assistant usually is required to hold the flap in its proper position when the suture is being tied by the operator (a periosteal elevator held at the margin prevents coronal displacement of the flap). It may be necessary to utilize several sutures, especially at the vertical incisions, to ensure the proper stabilization of the flap (Fig. 26-30,

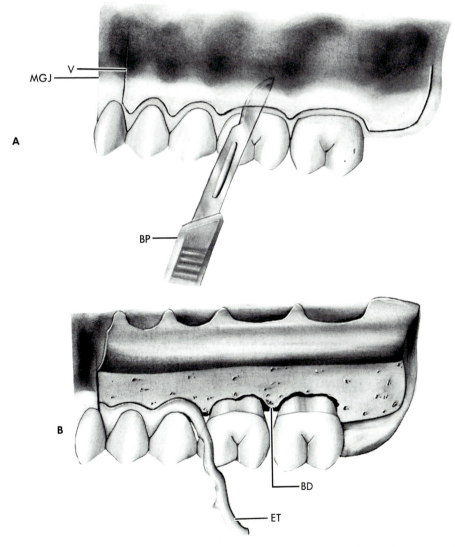

Fig. 26-30. Apically positioned graft (flap). **A,** Pockets extend beyond mucogingival junction, *MGJ.* A scalloped inverse beveled incision extends from fall-off of tuberosity to distal aspect of canine. Incision with a Bard-Parker blade *(BP)* extends to crest, allowing a mucoperiosteal flap to be elevated. A vertical, *V,* incision may be necessary to gain access to underlying bone. **B,** Pocket epithelial tissue, *ET,* is excised, exposing bone defects, *BD.*

Continued.

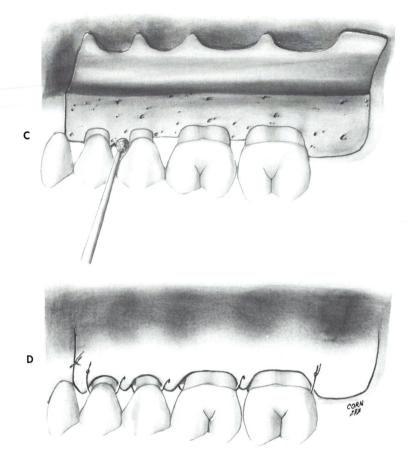

Fig. 26-30, cont'd. C, Completion of osseous surgery. **D,** Continuous sling suture positions flap above crest. Interrupted suture coapts tissue at vertical incision.

D). The use of the full-thickness apically positioned graft should not permit compromise in the continued optimal goal of physiologic gingival form (Fig. 26-31), which may be achieved with facility by the simple expediency of the gingivoplasty procedure (Fig. 26-32).

PARTIAL-THICKNESS APICALLY POSITIONED GRAFT (FLAP)

INDICATIONS
1. To eliminate pocket defects where the base of the pocket approaches or traverses the mucogingival junction
2. To avoid exposing fenestrations, bony dehiscences or thin radicular bone at the reflected site
3. To increase the width of attached gingiva in conjunction with pocket elimination (see discussion on Increasing Width of Attached Gingiva)
4. To treat suprabony defects by marginal dis-

placement, and infrabony defects by regeneration

PRECAUTIONS
1. Adequate vestibular depth is required.
2. There must be an absence of bony ledges or exostoses requiring osseous resection.

There are inherent dangers in the promiscuous use of full-thickness flaps when fenestrations and dehiscences are present. The elevation of the flap in search of the radicular alveolar crest can destroy an intact long connective tissue attachment to the tooth, resulting in an anatomic defect.

Early in the experience with the full-thickness flap approach therapists learned that unless careful appraisal of the tooth position and osseous morphology were made, anatomic defects could be observed, that is, fenestrations and dehiscences. One cannot deny that the repositioning of the flap could and would permit healing and attachment of the flap to tooth and bone in most instances (Rosling et al., 1976). However, re-entry procedures as reported by Bohannan (1963,

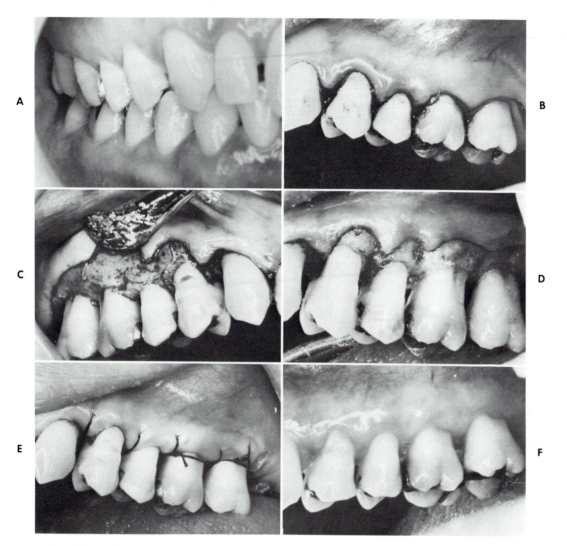

Fig. 26-31. Furcation management with apically positioned graft. **A,** Pockets extending to mucogingival junction and heavy alveolar architecture require use of apically positioned graft (flap) technique. Pockets range from 5 to 8 mm in this quadrant. Buccal furca of first and second molars can be probed. **B,** Flap procedures in quadrant surgery combine many disciplines. Management of tuberosity combined with scalloped incision into crevicular space has been carried out. Ulcerated sulcular lining is left attached to tooth so that undersurface of flap is connective tissue. When combined with tuberosity procedure, incision for buccal flap initiates at fall-off of tuberosity, extending anteriorly along buccal incline of tuberosity and retaining mucogingival complex. Anteriorly it is not necessary to make a vertical incision because disparity in alveolar height is not too severe (mirror view). **C,** Reflection of mucogingival flap with forward extension into crevicular area of canine allows for ample access. Note furcation involvements and buccal ledging in second molar area. **D,** Elimination of osseous defects has been completed. **E,** Continuous suturing technique allows margin of gingiva to be positioned over crest and approximately 1 mm on roots of teeth. A vertical incision distal to second molar allows for complete coaptation of thin tuberosity tissue (mirror view). **F,** Two-year postoperative result. Observe close similarity of gingival contour to corrected osseous morphology as seen in **D** (mirrow view).

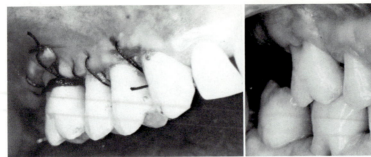
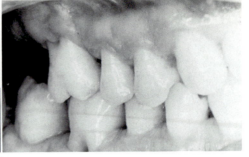

Fig. 26-32. A, Apically positioned flap with one vertical incision on mesial aspect of maxillary right first molar to compensate for varying levels of marginal bone. **B,** Nine months after surgical intervention. Note gingival form that has developed in furcation area and blending of gingiva with differing osseous heights. Gingivoplasty was performed at second dressing change.

1962), Levine (1972), and Goldman and Cohen (1968) have shown areas of fenestrations becoming dehiscences. If one could avoid detaching the connective tissue attachment to the tooth and yet make the necessary osseous corrections interproximally, this would be a more favorable solution to the problem (Fig. 26-33). The concept of retention of the gingiva has been shown to be most biologically acceptable to the periodontium. However, if one could improve one's judgment to anticipate osseous morphologic defects, discrete areas of further destruction might be avoided. All the techniques in mucogingival surgery should be directed toward the optimal conservation of the periodontium so that no radicular bone is lost. It is realized now that raising a full-thickness mucoperiosteal flap is not without hazard.

Before an apically positioned flap is utilized, certain clinical findings should be examined. Using a diagnostic probe (Tibbetts, 1969) one can determine whether the thickness of the tissue morphology is due to thick bone and thin overlying gingiva or to thick gingiva and thin underlying bone. Of course there may be thin and minimal gingiva and thin underlying bone present as well. If the latter situation exists, one must be cautious of a fenestration or dehiscence and of the anatomic defects that might result (Fig. 26-34). In the presence of thin gingiva and thick underlying bone there need not be concern with the elevation of a full-thickness flap. However, a partial-thickness flap should be prepared when there is concern about destroying the long connective tissue attachment to a tooth and finding the thin radicular bone at a far more apical level.

Increased knowledge about the pathogenesis of furcation involvements has modified the approach to the elimination of disease in these areas

(Basaraba, 1969). The method to deal with distal furcation problems of the maxillary first molar may be the resection of the distobuccal root (Corn and Marks, 1969). When the no. 17 explorer can completely enter the distal furca, an osseous defect is found interproximally (see discussions on Special problems: furcation management). Another prominent use of this surgical flap design is for increasing the width of the attached gingiva without exposing marginal bone when minimal nonfunctional gingiva is present (see discussions on Increasing Width of Attached Gingiva and Multiple Interdental Papilla Grafts).

REPOSITIONED (REPLACED) GRAFT

There has been confusion in the terminology related to the repositioned flap (Kirkland, 1932; Klavan, 1970; Morris, 1965; Wade, 1966; Zentler, 1918). The Nomenclature Committee of the American Academy of Periodontology states in its glossary that a flap may be "positioned" apically, but if put back in its original location it is "repositioned" or "replaced."

The repositioned graft was described by Morris (1965) as an "unrepositioned flap." He recently clarified that the repositioned graft is not the same as the Widman flap. The Widman procedure ends in the exact place as the apically positioned flap (Widman, 1917). The philosophic basis of these latter techniques denies the possibility of connective tissue reattachment to the root, whereas the repositioned graft depends on it (Morris, 1976).

Zamet (1975) compared curettage, replaced flaps, and apically repositioned flap procedures in a 4-month trial. All procedures reduced pocket depth. The apically repositioned grafts were the most successful. Despite failure to improve tissue

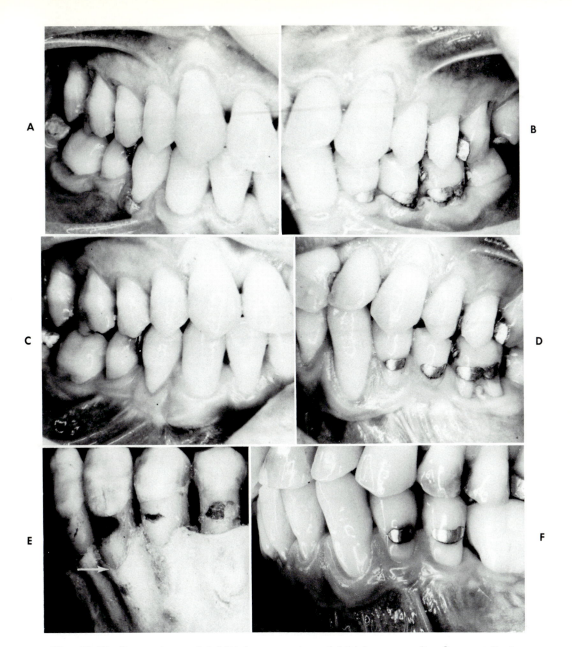

Fig. 26-33. Comparison of full-thickness and partial-thickness grafts. Same patient; opposite sides treated differently. This case demonstrates possible hazard of full-thickness apically positioned flap. **A** and **B,** Preoperative view. Pockets involve alveolar mucosa. Pocket depth on left canine is 3 mm. Note frena attachments at marginal area and minimal zone of attached gingiva. **C,** Mandibular right side results after molars and second premolar were treated by full-thickness apically positioned flap. First premolar and canine were treated by vestibular extension (periosteal retention) and periosteal separation. Gingival margin remained at high coronal level, and frenum pull is ineffective. **D,** Mandibular left side after full-thickness flap was elevated and long connective tissue attachment to canine and first premolar were destroyed in exposure of marginal bone. This unnecessary search for crest created an anatomic defect as margin of flap was positioned covering crest. If a partial-thickness flap had been used as on left side, margin of flap could have been positioned at most coronal level of connective tissue attachment. This would have avoided anatomic and aesthetic defect. **E,** Great disparity in alveolar margin height (canine–first premolar area of a human mandible specimen). Canine is in prominent position in arch. Note fenestrations through radicular alveolar process. Specimen is similar to osseous anatomy observed here. **F,** Twelve years after surgery. Pockets remain eliminated; anatomic defect is still obvious. Destroyed connective tissue attachment to root of tooth has not been repaired. (**A** to **D** from Corn, H. C.: Dent. Clin. North Am., p. 79, March 1964.)

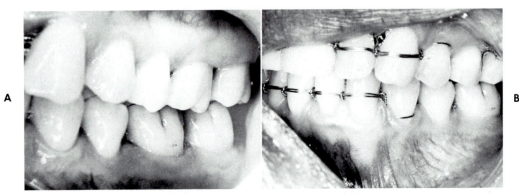

Fig. 26-34. Partial-thickness apically positioned graft to increase width of gingiva and yet enable correction of underlying osseous marginal defects. **A,** Pretreatment view of mandibular left side. Canine and premolars are prominently positioned in arch. Fenestrations and dehiscences are suspected. **B,** Absence of adequate gingiva is seen on mandibular left canine and first and second premolars. Muscle pull creates marginal tension (blanching) on canine and first premolar. **C,** Interproximal papillae are separated by dissection in apicocoronal direction using no. 15 Bard-Parker blade. **D,** A vertical incision is made at most anterior terminus of surgical area. A Bard-Parker no. 15 blade is placed in alveolar mucosa and dissects tissue in an apicocoronal direction directed to gingival margin so that sulcular epithelium remains intact adjacent to tooth. In this way, most coronal connective tissue fiber attachment to root of tooth is not destroyed. **E,** Partial-thickness mucogingival flap is raised, exposing irregular osseous margins. To successfully achieve an increased gingival width, it is necessary to remove all loose connective tissue and muscle fibers in submucosa, converting it in morphology so that it resembles lamina propria. This immovably bound-down tissue will repair so that gingiva is formed. **F,** Continuous suturing technique enable draping of mucogingival flap. Exposed osseous tissue in molar area is completely covered. Vertical incision at distal line angle of left central incisor expedites draping of flap. **G,** Postsurgical appearance after 20 days shows granulating areas arising from connective tissue bed left exposed by surgical procedure. Gingivoplasty is carried out in 20 days to blend retained gingival tissue with newly formed gingival margin. Osseous form achieved in molar area allows for flat gingival margin corresponding with form outline of cementoenamel junction. **H,** One year after surgery. **I,** Two-year healed result.

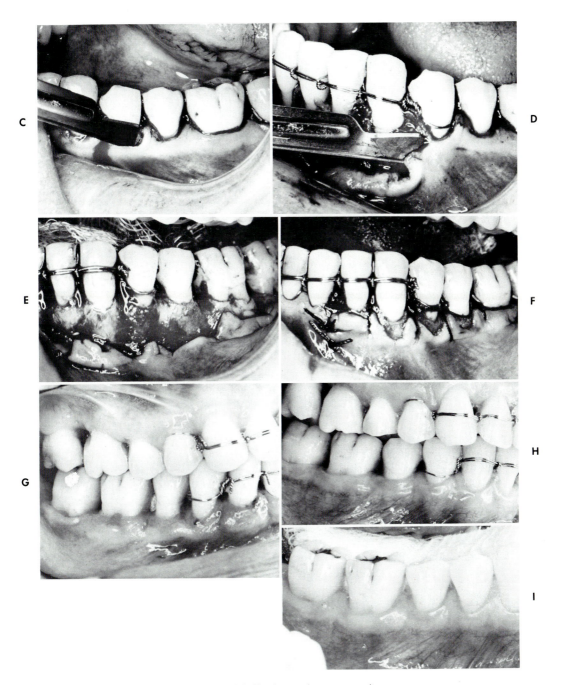

Fig. 26-34, cont'd. For legend see opposite page.

contour, replaced flap procedures showed an equal degree of success in maintaining plaque control when compared to apically repositioned flaps. Replaced flap procedures were also the only group to show improved gingival health over the 4-month postoperative period with lower gingival indexes. It would seem that good healing followed by a high standard of oral hygiene may overcome the presence of gingival and marginal osseous deformities (Fig. 26-35).

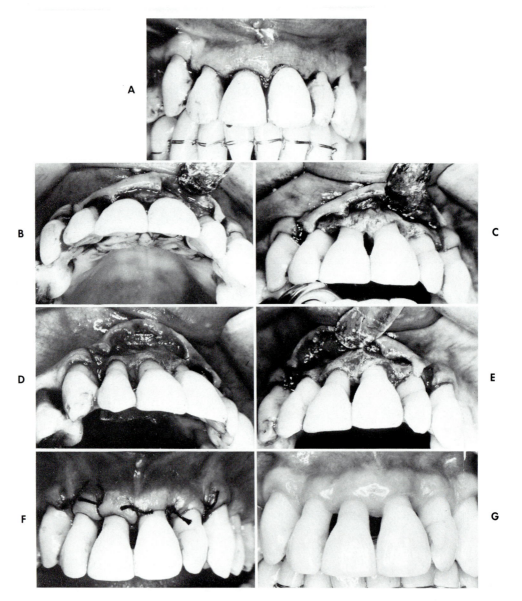

Fig. 26-35. Repositioned graft procedure. **A,** Following sulcular curettage, a scalloped sulcular incision is executed down to bone from a vertical incision on mesial aspect of maxillary right canine to a vertical incision on mesial aspect of left canine. **B,** Incisal view. Note thinness of full-thickness flap, looking into mesial defect of right central incisor. **C,** Elevation of full-thickness flap. Note osseous defects on mesial and distal aspects of right central incisor and distal aspect of left central incisor. **D** and **E,** Minor marginal osseous corrections are made. Autogenous bone implants are firmly positioned in prepared defects. **F,** Interrupted sutures are used to adapt facial and lingual flaps closely to teeth and to position them as coronally as tissues will permit. **G,** Healing 3 years later. Osseous implants have been partially successful. Sulcular depth is not more than 2 mm. Flaps did not remain as coronally positioned as orginally.

Increasing width of attached gingiva
FRENOTOMY AND FRENECTOMY (Bressman, 1973; Corn, 1961; Friedman, 1957; Gottsegen, 1954; Hirschfeld, 1939)

INDICATIONS

1. To eliminate tension on and retraction of the gingival margin that has been caused by the frenum during lip movements. If left untreated it may cause—
   a. Distention of the orifice of the sulcus or pocket, leading to debris accumulation
   b. An increase in the severity of the pocket, impairing healing
2. To eliminate a well-developed frenum that penetrates the gingival papilla to its origin on the incisive papilla. The coronally attached frenum may lead to a midline diastema and prevent mesial drift, which usually closes this space.
3. To facilitate orthodontic treatment. A thick frenum resists orthodontic forces, and its wedging action can be responsible for slight spacing of the maxillary central incisors following orthodontic therapy.
4. To eliminate a frenum that makes it difficult or impossible to use a toothbrush effectively in the area.
5. To control recession of facial gingiva when combined with more sophisticated periodontal surgery, for example, to eliminate periodontal pockets and increase attached gingiva and depth of vestibular trough.

A *frenotomy* is defined as a procedure that severs the frenum by excising it from its apex toward its base. A *frenectomy* simply involves the excision of the frenum, including its attachment to underlying bone (Friedman, 1957). Frenotomy and frenectomy are *localized* procedures that increase the width of attached gingiva.

In addition to maintaining space between the central incisors, the frenum has been implicated in creating an area of food impaction, poor oral hygiene (due to difficulty in toothbrushing), re-

sultant inflammation, and periodontal destruction (Gottsegen, 1954; Hirschfeld, 1939).

Frena are sickle-shaped folds normally found in the maxillary and mandibular alveolar mucosa, in the canine premolar area, and between the central incisors. Closely associated with the frena is the location of the mucogingival junction, a boundary that separates the gingiva from the alveolar mucosa. These folds contain (between two layers of the mucous membrane) a variable amount of loose connective tissue with elastic and dense collagen fibers, fat cells, and occasionally acini of mucous-producing salivary glands (Henry et al., 1976).

Disagreement exists concerning the histologic morphology of these frenum relating to the presence or absence of muscle. It has been stated that muscle fibers are found in the maxillary frenum (Archer, 1966; Bisnoff, 1944; Glickman, 1972; Gottsegen, 1954; Knox and Young, 1962). Yet this has not been accompanied by histologic material. In contradiction, several articles and current texts state that no muscle is present (Kopczyk and Saxe, 1974; Dewel, 1964; Shirazy, 1938; Sicher, 1970; Taylor, 1939). Henry et al. (1976), using fresh biopsy and autopsy specimens, found no muscle fibers present. To describe more accurately the location of the origin of the frenum, a morphologic-functional classification of labial frenum attachments has been described as follows (Placek et al., 1974):

1. *Mucosal* attachment refers to an attachment of the frenum to the mucogingival junction.
2. *Gingival* attachment refers to an attachment of the frenum within the attached gingiva.
3. *Papillary* attachment refers to an attachment of the frenum within the papilla.
4. *Papilla-penetrating* attachment refers to an attachment of the frenum passing through the papilla while inserting into attached gingiva (of the palate).

The prevalence of individual types of labial frenum attachments is shown in the box below.

PERCENTAGE OF TYPES OF ATTACHMENT		
	Maxillary midline area	**Mandibular midline area**
Mucosal attachment	46.5	92.1
Gingival attachment	34.3	6.5
Papillary attachment	3.1	0.7
Papilla-penetrating attachment	16.1	1.2

PERCENTAGE OF PULL SYNDROME		
	Maxillary midline area	Mandibular midline area
Mucosal attachment	4.5	6.5
Gingival attachment	53.4	76.2
Papillary attachment	100	100
Papilla-penetrating attachment	84.0	100

Only disease-free periodontiums were included in the study. The mucosal and gingival frenum attachments were prevalent in the maxillary anterior area; the mucosal frenum attachment was prevalent in the mandibular anterior area. A detaching movement of the marginal gingiva transferred from the lip by the frenum has been termed the "pull syndrome" (Placek et al., 1974). This retraction of the gingival margin has been indicted as an etiologic factor in the pathogenesis of periodontal disease. The "tension test" is another term used to describe the movement or displacement of marginal gingiva when tension is applied to the lower lip in an outward, downward, and lateral direction (Glickman, 1964; Kopczyk and Saxe, 1974; Vincent et al., 1976). The pull syndrome occurs in various percentages in different types of attachments (see boxed material). It is of interest to note that the presence of the pull syndrome in the mucosal attachments can be observed only where there is a narrow strip of attached gingiva. As the functional display of the frenum, the pull syndrome appeared regularly in papillary and papilla-penetrating types and in most gingival types of the frenum in both jaws. Gaberthuel and Mormann (1978) use an angiographic tension test to determine if gingival ischemia is caused by frenum over tension.

The condition of the midline papilla is another factor that has been evaluated. All changes in color and shape are considered pathologic. In the maxillary anterior area pathologic changes were observed in the papillary frenum attachments (45.5%) and mandible midline area; the papillary, gingival, and papilla-penetrating attachments were 83.3%, 71.4%, and 50%, respectively. Lower rates of periodontal disease resistance were noted in the papillary frenum attachments when pathologically involved papilla were observed (Placek et al., 1974).

Ideally the mucogingival junction is separated from the free gingival margin by several millimeters of dense connective tissue that is covered by keratinized epithelium—the attached gingiva

(Corn, 1960); 46.5% and 92.1% in the maxillary and mandibular midline areas, respectively. Unfortunately this ideal relationship is not always found. A high maxillary midline attachment of the frenum coronally on the alveolar wall is not infrequent. In these instances the mucogingival junction and the alveolar mucosa extend marginally between the gingiva as well.

As the frenum extends toward the marginal gingiva, there is a concomitant shallowing of the vestibular fornix. These boundaries are a constant threat to the integrity of the periodontium. In the mandibular anterior area and in the maxillary canine area the muscles of facial expression (i.e., the incisive muscles and the mental muscle) have their origin relatively close to the alveolar border. The action of the mental muscle elevates the skin of the chin and turns the lower lip outward. Since its origin extends to a level higher than that of the vestibule, this muscle—and to a lesser extent the incisive muscles—cause the vestibule to become shallow.

Frena may be long, thin, and delicate in form or they may be short, broad, and inseparably associated with the aforementioned musculature. Therapeutic management is greatly influenced by the extent of the associated periodontal disease.

The wound that results from a frenectomy is triangular in shape. It is bound on two sides by attached gingiva (fixed tissue). The gingiva, which comprises two sides of the triangle, provides one source of the granulation tissue. The other source of this tissue is the exposed bone that occurs as all the tissue is removed. A clinical observation (not yet reported by wound healing studies) suggests that when the bone is not exposed by the removal of periosteum, gingiva will also regenerate. However, all the loose connective tissue, elastic fibers, and fatty tissue elements must be removed, leaving the dense collagen fibers over the periosteum. This immovable base upon which new granulation tissue can form results in new attached gingiva.

The frenectomy is a limited partial-thickness

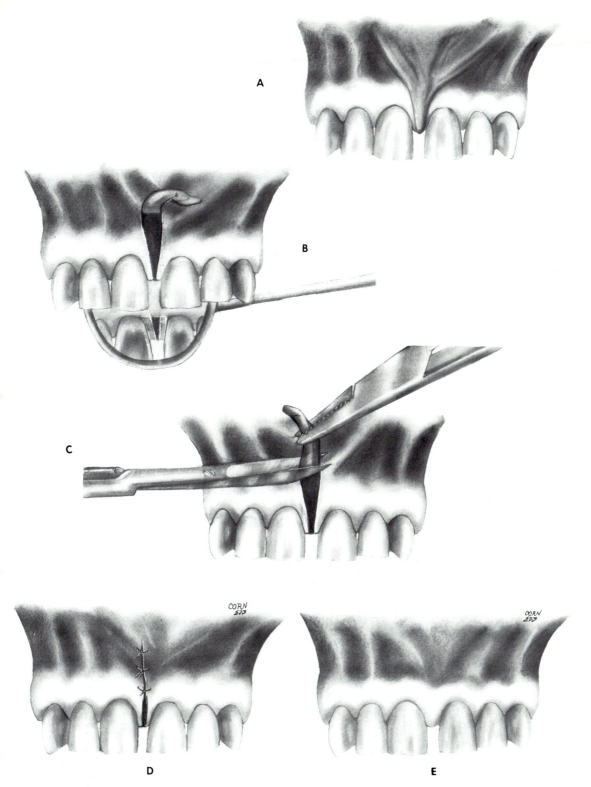

Fig. 26-36. Frenectomy. **A,** Frenum originating at incisive papilla on palate. Note vertical component of mucogingival junction. **B,** Horizontal palatal incision and two parallel vertical incisions release frenum, which retracts to labial vestibule. Gingiva on proximal surface of incisors remains undisturbed. **C,** Excision of frenum. **D,** Suturing. **E,** Uniform width of attached gingiva in midline.

mucosal flap. Seldom is the management of the frenum performed as a single procedure. It is usually combined with other aspects of periodontal surgery. Frenectomy in the maxillary midline is also a simple procedure and takes a few moments to perform. The vestibule in the maxillary anterior area is usually of sufficient depth, but it shallows out precipitously to the gingival margin where the frenum is attached. Therefore release and removal of the frenum are all that is necessary since blending of this area with the adjacent vestibular tissue is achieved automatically.

The frenectomy procedure as follows:

1. Following the administration of local anesthesia the frenum is held with slight tension by a mosquito hemostat. The frenum originates (at its tip) at the incisive papilla, extends between the gingival collar of the central incisors, and inserts into the lip (Fig. 26-36, *A*).

2. With the frenum under tension, two parallel vertical incisions (utilizing a no. 15 Bard-Parker blade) are made from the palatal aspect of the tip of the papilla through the interdental mucogingival junction. A collar of gingiva is left attached to the central incisors while the palatal fibers of the frenum retract labially (Fig. 26-36, *B*). The paral-

lel vertical incisions are extended labially into the vestibular fornix. If the papillary area of the frenum is enlarged, it will create the impression that the gingival collar is absent. With the edge of the scalpel blade the papilla of the frenum is displaced toward the midline. Then the incision can be made lateral to the gingival collar. The incisions penetrate the periosteum to the bone.

3. The two vertical incisions are connected on the palate by a horizontal incision extending toward the mesiolingual line angles of the central incisors. This will release the entire frenum, which has its insertion in the alveolar mucosa and lip (Fig. 26-36, *B*).

4. With a fine periodontal scissors the frenum is excised (Fig. 26-36).

5. If a gradual blending of vestibular tissue is required, an incision parallel to the mucogingival junction is made (Fig. 26-40).

6. All the loose connective fibers extending to the base of the dense collagenous tissue should be removed. It may be necessary to expose the bone.

7. Once hemostasis is obtained the wound is sutured with 4-0 black silk or gut suture (Fig. 26-36, *D*).

8. Periodontal dressing is placed to cover the

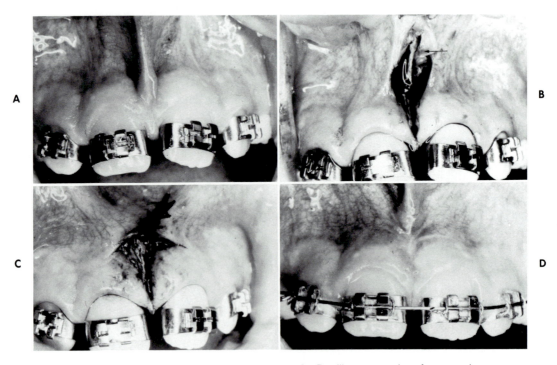

Fig. 26-37. Orthodontic need for frenectomy. **A,** Papilla-penetrating frenum obscures presence of free gingival collars on mesial aspect of central incisors. **B,** Vertical incisions release frenum and reveal mesial marginal gingiva of central incisors. *Arrow* shows insertion of frenum prior to excision. **C,** Horizontal releasing incision and suturing. Note gingival collar present. **D,** Two-month postoperative healing. Midline attached gingiva.

gingiva and the palatal interdental tissues. No dressing is needed on the sutured areas. The dressing and silk sutures are removed in 10 days. Frequently no further dressing is required. Keratinized gingiva will be delineated by 1 month (Fig. 26-36, *E*).

The following example clearly demonstrates how the frenum can be a major etiologic factor. A 5-year-old girl with a space between the maxillary central incisors had a strongly developed frenum (papilla-penetrating attachment). It was felt that the frenum prevented the mesial drift

and contact of these two teeth, exerting tension on the marginal gingiva, which could be a contributing factor toward future periodontal disease. There was also concern for the aesthetics and a desire to allow natural closure of this space (Fig. 26-37).

There are occasions when orthodontists move teeth against a prominent frenum to overpower its wedging effect. However, slight spacing occurs when the bands are removed. A better approach is to eliminate the frenum initially and follow with orthodontic treatment (Fig. 26-38).

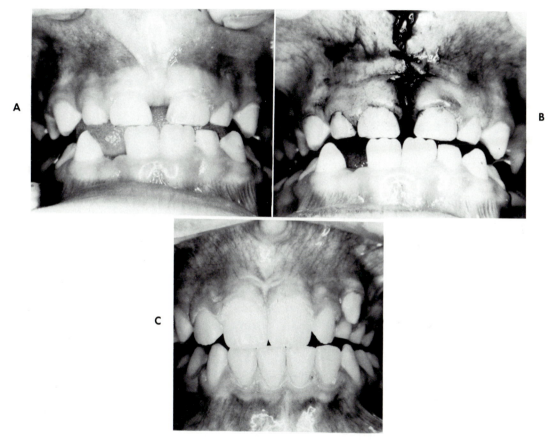

Fig. 26-38. Maxillary midline frenectomy. **A,** A 5-year-old child. **B,** Diastema between maxillary central incisors; strongly developed frenum connects with incisive papilla. Frenum prevents mesial contact of these teeth and exerts tension on marginal gingiva. **B,** Frenectomy extends to include palatal fibers of frenum. Two vertical parallel incisions are made along mucogingival junction coursing interdentally. These incisions extend labially from palatal aspect of papilla tip through alveolar mucosa and periosteum to osseous tissue. Care must be exercised to preserve delicate gingival collar on mesial surface of each central incisor, thus avoiding a postoperative midline defect. These incisions are connected on palate by a horizontal incision immediately adjacent to incisors. Released frenum is excised and sutured. **C,** Six years later. Influence of frenum has been eliminated. Incisors are in proper relationship. Normal physiologic mesial movement of teeth enables closure of space. (From Corn, H. C.: Dent. Clin. North Am., p. 79, March 1964.)

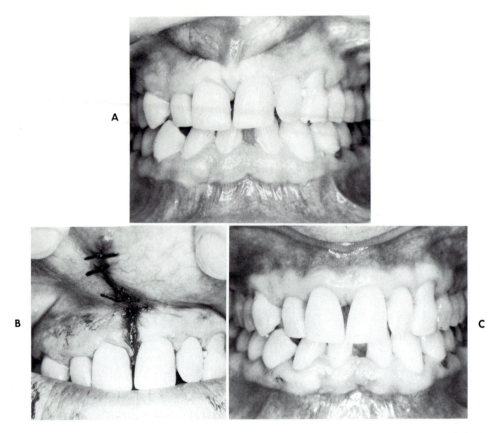

Fig. 26-39. Adult maxillary midline frenectomy. **A,** Prominent frenum attached to marginal gingiva, a primary etiologic factor in pocket formation. Frenum was bruised during oral physiotherapy. **B,** Frenectomy. Delicate gingival collar is preserved interdentally, avoiding a midline defect that could affect speech. **C,** Healing of subsequent gingivectomy. Frenum has been eliminated. (From Corn, H. C.: Dent. Clin. North Am., p. 79, March 1964.)

There is controversy as to the proper timing of a frenectomy in the maxillary midline diastemas in children. Some feel that it should be done at an early age, especially if there are hereditary and aesthetic problems (Corn, 1961). Others feel that the frenectomy should be considered after the eruption of the permanent canines because not infrequently the frenum atrophies as the central incisors approximate each other (Bressman, 1973; Hirschfeld and Geiger, 1966; West, 1968).

In an adult, when the maxillary midline frenum is attached to the interdental marginal gingiva, it must be corrected. It is usually managed at the time of pocket elimination. This is shown by the following example. When a patient complained of bruising the frenum while brushing his teeth, a frenectomy was performed. Coupled with the relief gained after plaque control, the patient was amenable to complete periodontal therapy. Subsequently a maxillary gingivectomy was per-

formed. Details of the technique (Fig. 26-39) are similar to those described in Fig. 26-36.

The inadvertent or indiscriminate excision of a maxillary midline frenum can be fraught with disappointment. The patient's concern for improving the aesthetics of the two narrow central incisors requires restorative dentistry. The improvement in appearance created by the new crowns (Fig. 26-40) would be negated by any increase of the midline space.

When the frenum is at the mandibular midline, the diagnostic decisions that must be made can be very provocative. They are dependent upon the size and dimension of the frenum, the extent of the vestibular depth, and the existence of gingiva. When there is a simple thin frenum problem with an adequate vestibular fornix, the management is similar to that of the maxillary frenum. Fig. 26-41 illustrates the effect of the frenum pull, the recession on the right central incisor, and the

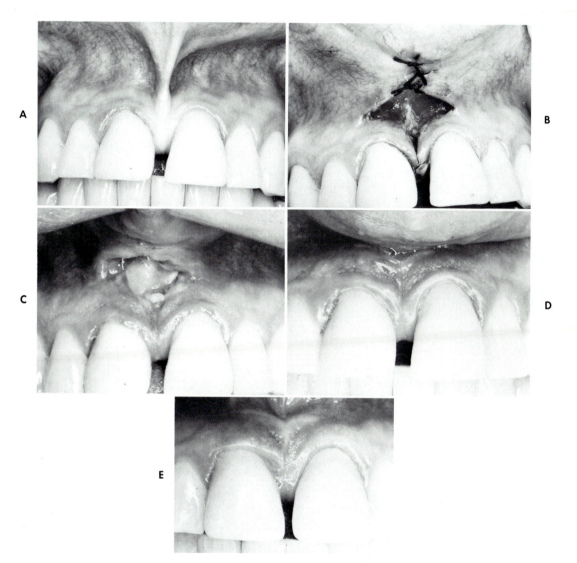

Fig. 26-40. Frenectomy technique. **A,** Preoperative view. Congenital diastema between central incisors created aesthetic problem. Anomalous incisors have been restored with provisional crowns. Heavy midline frenum extends interproximally with origin in median papillae on palate. Usual frenectomy would result in further midline defect. Surgeon should design incision to follow mucogingival junction interproximally, allowing thin gingival collar to remain. **B,** Frenectomy complete. Alveolar mucosa of frenum extending interdentally to its origin at median papilla has been released and removed, enabling gingival collar to relax and approximate itself. A horizontal incision is frequently necessary with broad frena to relax vestibular area. **C,** Frenum removed. Wound on alveolar process side of vestibule will repair by secondary intention (10 days after surgery). **D,** Eight-week postsurgical response. Mucogingival junction has its normal configuration. Attached gingiva extends from tip of papillae toward vestibular area that is stippled. **E,** Two-year response after final restorations. (Restorative dentistry procedures courtesy Donald Trachtenberg, Philadelphia.)

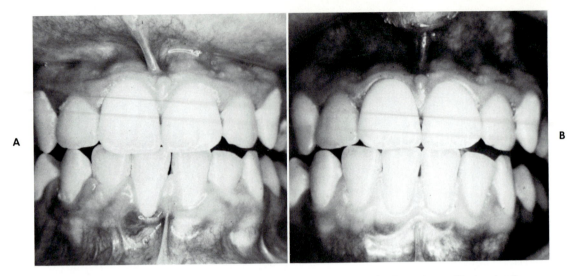

Fig. 26-41. Mandibular midline frenectomy. **A,** In presence of adequate vestibular depth, a thin frenum can be treated by frenectomy. Note effect of frenum pull, recession of right central incisor, and inadequate oral physiotherapy of area. **B,** Two years after soft tissue curettage, root planing, and frenectomy. Note creeping attachment. Effect of frenum has been negated, and gingival margin is at its normal location.

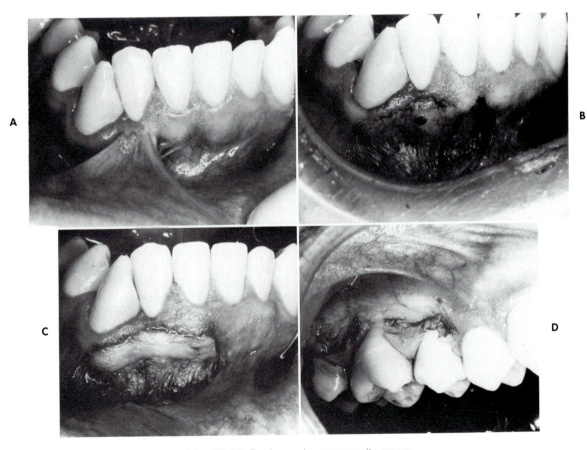

Fig. 26-42. For legend see opposite page.

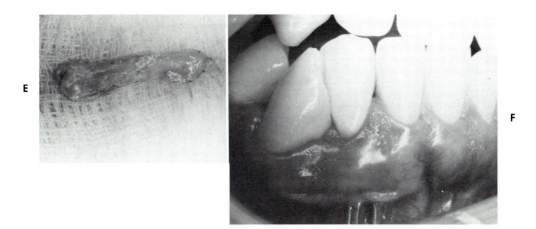

Fig. 26-42. Broad coronally positioned frenum resulting from automobile accident. **A,** Localized shallow vestibule. Broad frenum is attached to gingival margin. **B,** Preparation of recipient site. **C,** Free soft tissue using experimental cyanoacrylate instead of sutures. **D,** Donor site of graft (maxillary buccal attached gingivae). **E,** Undersurface of donor tissue. **F,** Increase in vestibular depth created by new attached gingiva, correcting retraction of gingival margin.

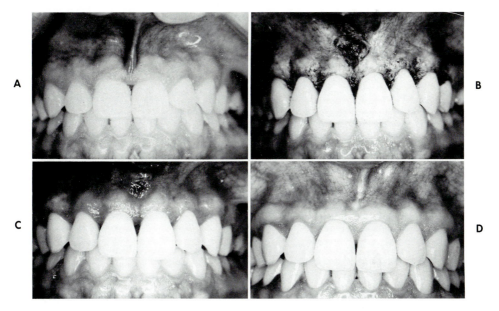

Fig. 26-43. Frenotomy. **A,** Preoperative view. Gingival hyperplasia with soft tissue crater in midline area involving frenum. **B,** Initially gingivectomy is performed. Then incision is made into frenum at apex of triangle at mucogingival junction. Immovable connective tissue remains, covering interproximal osseous tissue. Gentle pressure against base of triangular wound blends prepared area with adjacent tissues. Dressing placed on wound is changed weekly. **C,** Two weeks after surgery. **D,** One year later.

inability of adequate plaque control for the area. Repeated attempts at resolving the inflammation and improving the plaque control in the area failed. Soft tissue curettage and a frenectomy were performed. The 2-year result is seen in Fig. 26-41, *B*.

Factors complicating the elimination of an aberrant frenum pull in the mandibular incisor area are (1) absence or minimal attached gingiva, (2) pockets extending into the alveolar mucosa, and (3) an associated shallow vestibular fornix. Gingivectomy and simple frenectomy will not correct these problems. Because of the origin of the musculature on the alveolar process and the mobility of the lips, the partial-thickness apically positioned graft cannot be used, since it is technically unmanageable. This area remains unique. The above circumstances may occur, and increasing the width of the gingiva requires a greater understanding of surgical anatomy and tissue response for an appropriate repair. The solution can be managed most effectively by the use of the free soft tissue autograft (see discussions on Free soft tissue autograft and Laterally positioned graft).

The technique of frenotomy is illustrated in Fig. 26-43.

PARTIAL-THICKNESS APICALLY POSITIONED GRAFT

PREREQUISITES
1. Bony ledges or exostoses that require osseous resection must be absent.
2. Radicular bone must be of normal thickness.
3. Vestibular depth must be adequate.

INDICATIONS
1. To eliminate pocket defects where the base of the pocket approaches or traverses the mucogingival junction
2. To increase the width of attached gingiva when minimum attached gingiva is present
3. To avoid exposing fenestrations, bony dehiscences, or thin radicular bone

PRECAUTIONS
1. Exposure of the periosteum on the thin alveolar process without subsequent flap coverage results in loss of the marginal radicular bone (Ramfjord and Costich, 1968).
2. If the area of surgery is not going to be covered by an epithelialized flap, as thick as possible a layer of connective tissue should be left covering the periosteum (Ramfjord and Costich, 1968).

Meticulous presurgical diagnosis is a prerequisite for selecting the partial-thickness apically positioned graft to increase the width of the attached gingiva. Formerly it was felt that when a free gingival margin or a dentogingival junction of alveolar mucosa was present, it qualified for the use of this procedure. However, the procedure has shown disappointing results and even complete failure. Lately, more discriminating investigation has prompted a different approach. When gingiva rather than alveolar mucosa is present preoperatively at the dentogingival junction, the partial-thickness apically positioned graft can provide adequate results without deformity at the dentogingival junction (Fagan, 1975; Staffileno, 1974, 1973).

Karring et al. (1971) showed that the characteristics of keratinized gingiva and nonkeratinized alveolar mucosa are genetically determined and are not the result of functional adaptation to environmental stimuli. It was suggested that granulation tissue proliferating from gingival connective tissue and periodontal ligament possesses the ability to induce the formation of keratinized gingival epithelium.

The differentiation of keratinized gingival epithelium is determined by inductive stimuli from underlying connective tissue. These results lend support to the idea that success or failure in extending the width of keratinized gingiva by surgical means rests with the origin of granulation tissue (Karring et al., 1974, 1972).

Granulation tissue proliferating from the supra-alveolar connective tissue or from the periodontal ligament will lead to keratinized epithelium (Levine and Stahl, 1972). The distinct transition between keratinized and nonkeratinized epithelium invariably and exactly corresponds to the junction between elastic and nonelastic tissues (Karring et al., 1971). Granulation tissue originates from supracrestal connective tissue, residual periosteal connective tissue, periodontal ligament, bone marrow spaces, adjacent gingiva, and alveolar mucosa (Karring et al., 1975). This is in agreement with previous reports on the origin of granulation tissue following mucogingival surgery (Arnold and Hatchett, 1962; Pfeifer, 1963; Wilderman, 1963, 1960; Smith, 1970). It seems justified to conclude that the postsurgical location of the mucogingival junction is determined by the extent to which the various sources of granulation tissue contribute to the regeneration of the connective tissue of the wound (Karring et al., 1975). It appears that the use of a partial-thickness apically positioned graft can achieve an increased width of attached gingiva provided that at least minimum attached gingiva is present preoperatively (Janson et al., 1969; Fagan, 1975). Fagan (1975) suggested that the lamina propria present preoperatively may have acted in two ways to influence the following results obtained:

1. An adequate thickness of connective tissue may have remained after the reflection of the partial-thickness flap, affording maximum protection to the underlying radicular bone and preventing recession due to bone loss (Friedman, 1962; Ramfjord and Costich, 1968; Wilderman, 1964, 1963). This requirement is greater when the marginal bone is thin.

2. The original lamina propria may have determined the type of epithelium that would develop subsequently (Billingham and Silvers, 1967; Slavkin, 1970; Soehren et al., 1973).

Fagan (1975) compared the repair of the preoperative mucosal and gingival margins by testing the partial-thickness apically positioned graft approach with the results obtained using the free soft tissue autograft. He concluded that where the area consisted of *alveolar mucosa* (soft tissue margin at the dentogingival junction), a statistically significant ($P < 0.05$) difference was found in the amount of attached gingiva present in 12 weeks. The *autograft* produces the *greatest* attached gingiva when there is an alveolar mucosal margin present. However, when gingiva formed the preoperative tissue margin, no significant difference in the amount of attached gingiva was found 12 weeks postoperatively. The results of this study indicate that the presence of gingiva at the dentogingival margin preoperatively may have influenced both the postoperative amount of attached gingiva and the degree of recession when comparing the two grafts.

Before the decision to utilize a partial-thickness flap design is made, the resulting postoperative recession or anatomic defect must be considered. Loss of marginal radicular bone with this procedure has been demonstrated by Wood et al. (1972) and Ramfjord and Costich (1968). The thickness and structure of the labial and buccal bone may be important factors in determining the amount of bone loss during healing. With a thin labial alveolar plate the risk of bone loss is usually extensive. It allows a considerable portion of the marginal area of the wound to be covered with granulation tissue from the periodontal ligament space.

When a mucosal margin is present preoperatively and the thin underlying labial plate is covered with periosteum, information (Fagan, 1975) suggests that the loss of bone will cause an anatomic defect (recession) to the planned mucogingival junction (base of the prepared bed). Without an increase in gingival width the results can be disappointing, and an even greater defect may result. Under these circumstances it is suggested that the prepared periosteal bed be covered by a mature epithelialized surface (i.e., a multiple interdental papilla graft or a free soft tissue autograft) (Hiatt et al., 1968).

When at least minimal gingiva is present at the margin, the partial-thickness dissection can provide the therapist with the following alternatives:

1. Following the preparation of the recipient site the original supracrestal connective tissue attached to the tooth and the original lamina propria remain. The alveolar mucosa has been prepared by creating an immobile bed of tissue over the bone. Upon this bed the original epithelialized gingival margin of the graft is positioned. A prerequisite for this approach is a thick connective tissue covering a normal thickness and structure of radicular bone.

2. When the recipient site is composed of a thin connective tissue periosteal bed, thin radicular bone, or both, there is a risk of resorption of the bone coronal to the apically positioned gingival margin. Under these circumstances the entire prepared bed should be covered by a graft. This will prevent an anatomic defect and still increase the width of attached gingiva.

The contradictory reports on the efficacy of the partial-thickness apically positioned flap may be due to the differences between the preoperative soft tissue margin at the dentogingival junction and the thickness of bone in various regions of the jaw rather than to the surgical procedure itself. Where indicated, the preparation of the graft bed should preserve as much as possible of the attachment to the root (supracrestal connective tissue) and the connective tissue (lamina propria) covering the alveolar crest.

Frequently asked questions are as follows: "Does the collagenous attachment to the root and the thin, periosteal covering of the alveolar process survive? Does not granulation tissue develop from the open marrow spaces of the resorbing exposed crestal bone?'' Novaes et al. (1976) studied these problems in dogs. After partial-thickness flap surgery and removal of most of the outer half to two thirds of the vessels that furnished nutrition to the area, only the vasculature of the dentogingival junction and some of the periosteal vessels remained. Very little progenitor tissue remained to give rise to the rebuilding of the vast vascularized area that was surgically destroyed. The perfusion of carbon suspension via the carotid arteries showed surprisingly rapid vasoprolifera-tion, which (after 48 hours) was already abundant. It was obvious that there was no necrosis of the connective tissue and that it survives.

Several components contribute to the new gingi-val unit: (1) the granulation tissue from the supra-crestal connective tissue and the original lamina propria, (2) the granulomatous tissue from the smooth, firmly bound-down immovable base that was alveolar mucosa; all loose elastic connective tissue and muscle fibers must be stripped away (using nippers), (3) the retained gingival margin of the apically positioned flap, which is placed upon the properly prepared bed, and (4) the ad-jacent gingiva. The zone of attached gingiva thus can be increased without an anatomic defect. The architectual form of the gingiva is not compro-mised. Slight surface irregularities are corrected to obtain conceptual physiologic gingival form (Goldman, 1950), which is achieved by subse-quent gingivoplasty during healing.

When there is doubt as to whether the elevation of a full-thickness flap will expose a fenestration or dehiscence, a *partial-thickness graft design* should be selected. This is applicable even when

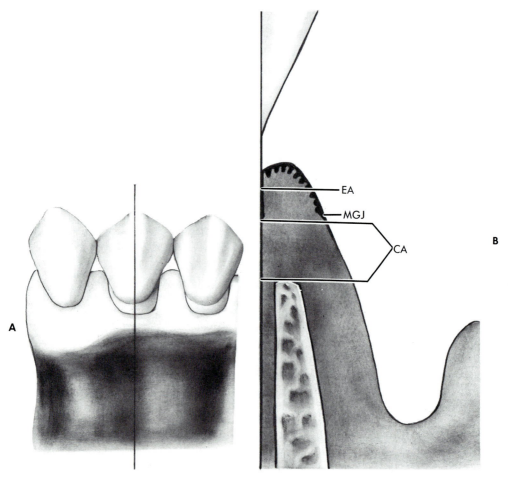

Fig. 26-44. Partial-thickness apically positioned graft technique. **A,** Minimal attached gingiva on first and second premolars. Cross-sectional views are through middle of first premolar. **B,** Junctional epithelium, *EA.* There is a long connective tissue attachment to tooth, *CA. MGJ,* Mucogingival junction.

adequate gingiva is present for retention and apical positioning. This procedure is most frequently indicated in the maxillary and mandibular premolar and canine area and in the mandibular anterior area (Pustigioni et al., 1975).

In Fig. 26-44 there is only a free gingival margin present. If one were to use the typical apically positioned flap approach, an incision would be made into the sulcular area down to the crest of the bone and a full-thickness flap would be elevated, destroying the connective tissue attachment to the tooth. In an effort to create gingiva the margin of the flap would be positioned at the alveolar crest or apical to the crest (far removed from its original attachment to the tooth). An anatomic defect would thus be created. The margin of the gingiva is attached to the cementum at the arrow in Fig. 26-44, *B*. When no radicu-

lar osseous corrections are necessary but interproximal osseous defects require therapy, the partial-thickness apically positioned flap should be used. An anatomic deformity would be avoided, while the zone of attachment would be increased.

PROCEDURE (Fig. 26-44)

1. After curetting the sulcular epithelium (Fig. 26-38, *C*) dissect the interdental papilla from their connective tissue bed using an appropriate blade (Bard-Parker no. 15). This is accomplished easily by reversing the direction of the blade apicocoronally and entering the mesial border of each papilla, then undermining the tissue until it is completely free. This will maintain the scalloped form of the flap margin.

2. Make a vertical incision from the gingival margin into the vestibular fornix at each end of

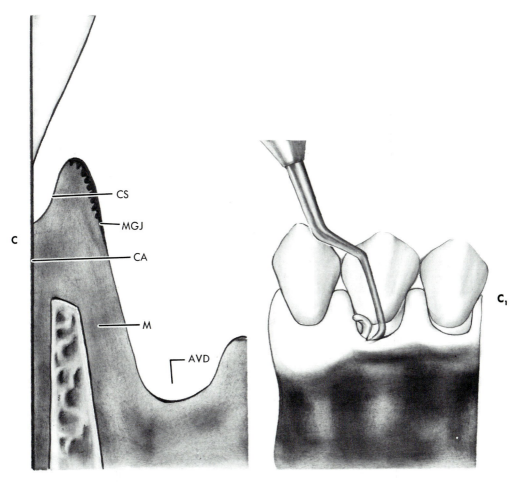

Fig. 26-44, cont'd. C, Curettage of sulcular epithelium, *CS,* prepares a connective tissue surface of sulcular wall. There is sufficient vertical height of alveolar mucosa, *M,* resulting in adequate vestibular depth, *AVD.* **C₁,** Curet removing wall of sulcus with a horizontal sweeping stroke on buccal surface.

Continued.

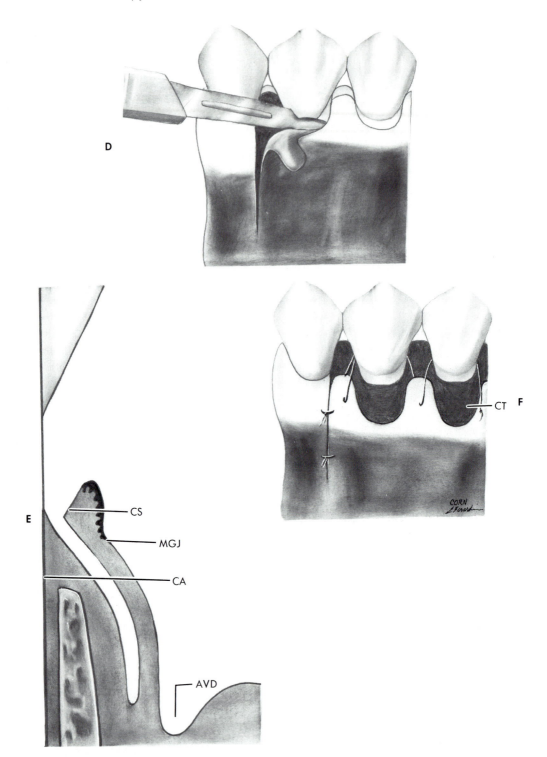

Fig. 26-44, cont'd. D, Papillae are initially incised and blended with sulcular wall. This is best achieved by an anteroposterior and an apicocoronal separation of papillae. Vertical incision provides access for apicocoronal partial-thickness dissection of alveolar mucosa, joining sulcular dissection and papillary dissection. **E,** Connective tissue attachment, *CA,* to root remains. An immovable connective tissue base must be created on periosteal surface. A connective tissue surface, *CS,* lines inner surface of flap. **F,** Continuous sling suture controls margin of graft and exposes prepared connective tissue, *CT,* bed for granulation tissue, which will create attached gingiva.

the operative field. The incisions should be placed to include the entire papilla of the anterior and posterior borders of the operative area. Avoid an interproximal vertical incision as this will prevent correction of interproximal osseous deformities and may result in notching of the interdental papillae. The incision should penetrate *to* but not *through* the periosteum (Fig. 26-44, *D*).

3. At the anterior vertical incision, insert the no. 15 Bard-Parker blade and reverse the direction of the cutting edge, dissecting the flap in an apicocoronal direction. Slight tension on the flap eases the dissection as the blade courses through the submucosa and lamina propria and frees the flap as the incision ends at the edge of the gingival margin. Be sure to dissect the flap far enough into the fornix to provide space for the apical positioning of the graft without "buckling" (Fig. 26-44, *E*).

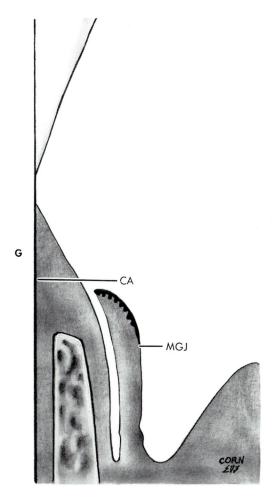

Fig. 26-44, cont'd. G, New gingiva will be formed from connective tissue attachment, *CA,* to root of tooth to mucogingival junction, *MGJ.*

4. Remove the inner wall of the periodontal pockets from the teeth. If the sulcus is shallow it can remain undisturbed. *Do not* remove the connective tissue attached to the root and covering the crest. Avoid exposing fenestrations, bony dehiscences, or thin radicular bone.

5. Scale and root plane the root surfaces until free of all deposits. Air drying of the roots may enable detection of residual calculus and irregularities. However, instrumentation should be performed in a wet field.

6. Complete preparation of the recipient bed. With nippers remove all elastic connective tissue apical to the lamina propria so that an immovable bed can be provided for the apically positioned mucogingival flap. CAUTION: if the marginal connective tissue is thin and if the radicular bone is suspected of being thin, use a multiple interdental papilla graft or a free soft tissue autograft.

7. Position graft flap(s) so that the gingival flap margin plus the exposed connective tissue coronal to flap(s) will provide an increased width of attached gingiva (measure from the coronal edge of the connective tissue to the mucogingival junction of the flap). The location of the flap margin can be moved 1 to 2 mm further apically from the exposed connective tissue if more attached gingiva is required (Fig. 26-44, *F* and *G*).

8. Stabilize the graft with 4-0 black suture in a continuous sling suture. The tips of the papillae should align with the interdental areas, and the gingival margin of the flap should be draped as described above. If there has been a lingual flap raised, suspend the facial and lingual tissues independent of each other.

9. Apply digital pressure to the tissues with moistened gauze sponges for 1 to 2 minutes. Reinspect for correct tissue position.

10. Apply periodontal dressing for 10 days. Redress as necessary.

11. If tissue irregularity remains following healing, a gingivoplasty is in order.

• • •

Critical reevaluation is required to ensure the fulfillment of the treatment objectives.

The importance of the partial-thickness flap design is vividly demonstrated in Fig. 26-33. Careful reevaluation for the routine use of full-thickness flaps is necessary. On the right side there was a frenum problem complicated by pockets extending into the mucosa. A partial-thickness dissection was used, and the level of the connective tissue attachment to the tooth was not changed. The zone of attached gingiva could be increased without creating an anatomic defect. On the left side nonfunctional gingiva was present, with pockets extending into the mucosa. A full-thickness flap was raised in search of the margin of the bone. This occurred during the time when positioning of the margin of the flap at the crest of the bone was the concern. Fig. 26-33, *D* shows the level of the cementoenamel junction and the level where a connective tissue attachment to the tooth had been. Unfortunately the bone was distant apically to these measurements. Unnecessary destruction of the connective tissue attachment to the tooth was obvious. It prompted modification of the surgical design to avoid the exposure of the radicular surface of the teeth. The therapist must decide whether a partial-thickness graft or a full-thickness graft is preferable to avoid the anxiety and disappointment of less than optimal surgical results. Such planning will allow consistent predictability of the postoperative responses (Figs. 26-45 and 26-46).

Procedures for pocket elimination and for increasing attached gingiva can involve areas of possible fenestrations, dehiscences, or long connective tissue attachments. It must be understood that the connective tissue bed in the partial-thickness apically positioned graft technique heals by secondary intention and heals more slowly than when covered with a free soft tissue or pedicle graft. To control the position of the graft, periosteal sutures may be used (Kramer et al., 1970).

MULTIPLE INTERDENTAL PAPILLA GRAFTS

INDICATIONS

1. To create a new zone of attached gingiva
2. To increase the width of attached gingiva where there is an absence of gingiva or where inadequate gingiva is present
3. To avoid the exposure of deformities such as an absence of radicular bone, a thin radicular plate of bone, or a dehiscence or a fenestration on the radicular surface, particularly where there are prominently positioned teeth (Roth, 1965)
4. To permit interproximal osseous surgery and occasional vestibular osseous surgery and yet allow the marginal bone to be covered

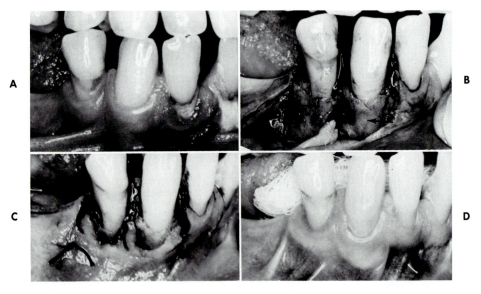

Fig. 26-45. Safeguards through partial-thickness graft design. **A,** Heavy calculus on right mandibular lateral and central incisors. Minimal gingiva on canine and first premolar. First premolar shows evidence of toothbrush abrasion. Pockets extend beyond free gingival margin into mucosa. There is adequate vestibular depth. **B,** Note safety of partial-thickness flap design through connective tissue attachment to teeth. Dehiscence on first premolar (connective tissue remains attached to tooth) and connective tissue covered fenestration approximately 1 mm from alveolar margin *(arrows)*. **C,** Apical positioning of flap leaves connective tissue exposed. Delicate connective tissue attachment remains viable, enabling new gingiva to form. Although thin, this undisturbed connective tissue attachment has great potential for repair. **D,** One year after surgery. Note increase in gingiva. Gingival margin is at most coronal level of connective tissue attachment.

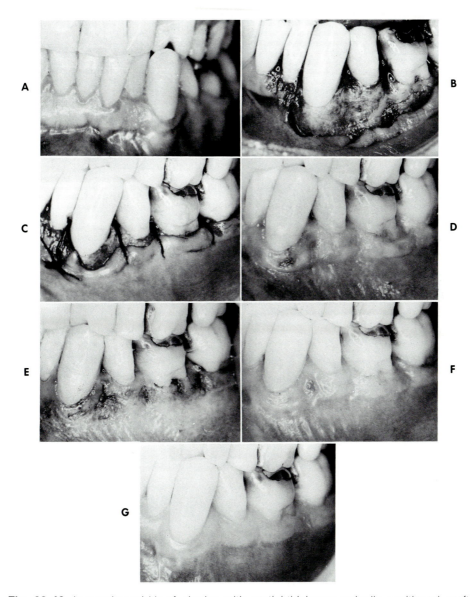

Fig. 26-46. Increasing width of gingiva with partial-thickness apically positioned graft. **A,** Minimal attached gingiva. Mandibular canine tooth is in prominent position and in crossbite relationship with maxillary lateral incisor. If full-thickness flap were raised to locate alveolar margin, level of bone might be remote from its normal location and result in an anatomic defect. **B,** With partial-thickness dissection principle (vertical incision directing scalpel from apical to coronal direction) perforation of flap can be avoided. Osseous problem on molar is corrected after flap is raised but connective tissue remains on premolar and canine. Periosteal separation determines thickness of adjacent connective tissue. **C,** Flap is positioned over radicular surface of molar. Connective tissue remains exposed on canine premolar area. **D,** Attached gingiva forms coronal to margin of flap in premolar canine area. Gingivoplasty obtains ideal physiologic gingival form after 20-day healing period. Residual thickened gingiva should be thinned after flap is repositioned in this manner. My preference is not to allow gingiva to bridge over thickened area, increasing sulcular depth, but to thin surface epithelium for desired form. **E,** Tissue immediately after gingivoplasty. **F,** Dressing removal after 30 days. **G,** Four years after surgery. Gingival dimension is increased.

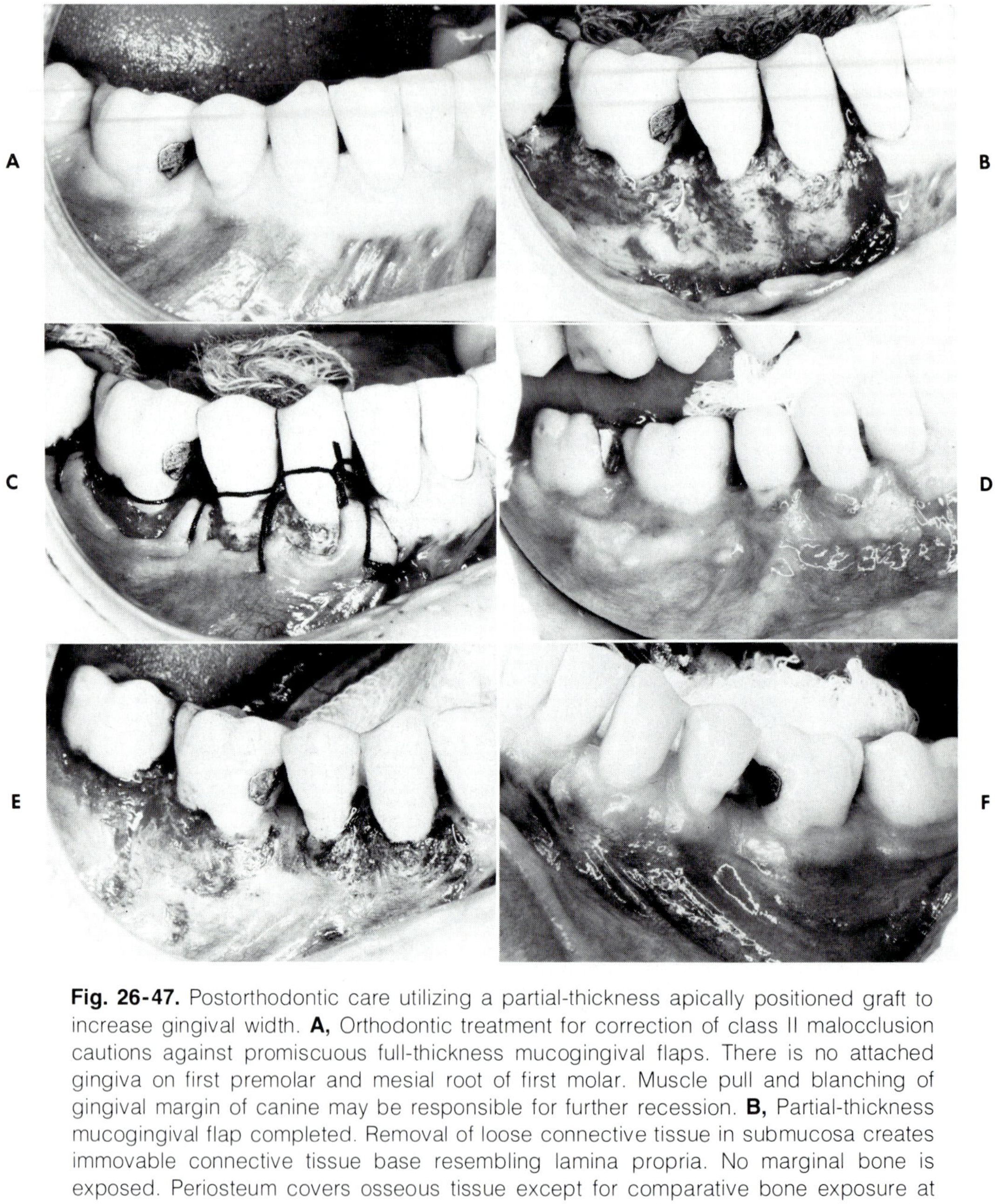

Fig. 26-47. Postorthodontic care utilizing a partial-thickness apically positioned graft to increase gingival width. **A,** Orthodontic treatment for correction of class II malocclusion cautions against promiscuous full-thickness mucogingival flaps. There is no attached gingiva on first premolar and mesial root of first molar. Muscle pull and blanching of gingival margin of canine may be responsible for further recession. **B,** Partial-thickness mucogingival flap completed. Removal of loose connective tissue in submucosa creates immovable connective tissue base resembling lamina propria. No marginal bone is exposed. Periosteum covers osseous tissue except for comparative bone exposure at apical area of molar. **C,** With suspensory continuous suturing technique mucogingival flap is draped so that approximately 2 mm of connective tissue–covered bone is exposed. Attached gingiva will proliferate from connective tissue bed. It is not necessary to expose alveolar margin to gain attached gingiva. **D,** After 20 days epithelialized granulation tissue (developed from connective tissue bed) can be differentiated from mature retained flap. **E,** Gingivoplasty removes irregular margin of retained flap and blends both tissues. **F,** One year after surgery. Adequate width of gingival tissue remains. Muscle pull on canine has been dissipated, and all pockets eliminated. Interestingly, connective tissue attachment on root of tooth has been preserved at most coronal level (mirror view).

with the epithelialized interdental papilla

5. To avoid anatomic defects (recession) beyond the original dentogingival junction

PRECAUTIONS

1. The interdental papilla must have sufficient length (at least 3 mm) and sufficient width at the mucogingival junction (at least 3 mm).
2. The shallower the vestibule, the greater the length of papilla required.

When the surface morphology of several teeth have 1 mm or less of gingiva and the probe penetrates to and beyond the mucogingival junction, multiple interdental papilla grafts are warranted. Formerly the solution to such circumstances was to excise the alveolar mucosa. A large expanse of bone was exposed and eventually covered by proliferating granulation tissue that originated from the periodontal ligament spaces or from the exposed marrow spaces. Subsequent wound healing studies (Bohannan, 1963, 1962; Carranza

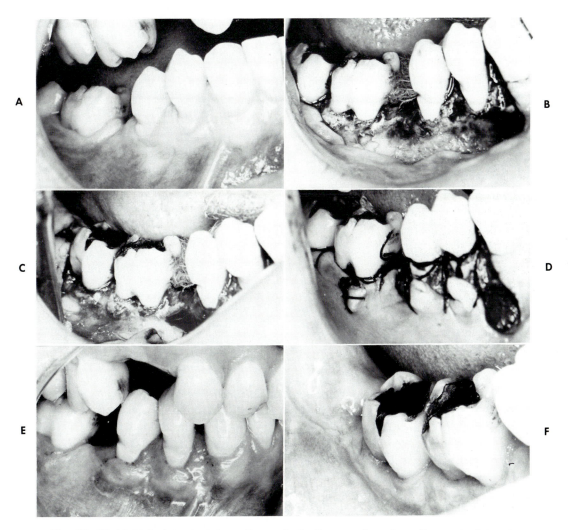

Fig. 26-48. Multiple interdental papilla graft. **A,** Preoperative view. Severe toothbrush abrasion on mandibular premolars, and collar of free gingiva on second premolar. Wide zone of interdental gingiva. **B,** Partial-thickness primary flap and interdental papillae have been preserved. Recipient site prepared with an immovable connective tissue base and connective tissue attachment to root of intact tooth. **C,** Partial-thickness dissection extends to distal aspect of third molar as shown by incision into periosteum exposing bone for comparison. **D,** Partial-thickness flap moved laterally, distally, and apically so that interdental gingiva rests on radicular surface of involved teeth. Continuous suspensory sutures permit draping and control of papillae. **E** and **F,** Twenty-day healing response illustrates valuable role of retained interdental gingiva. Functional attached gingiva extends to retromolar area. Gingivoplasty improves tissue contour.

Continued.

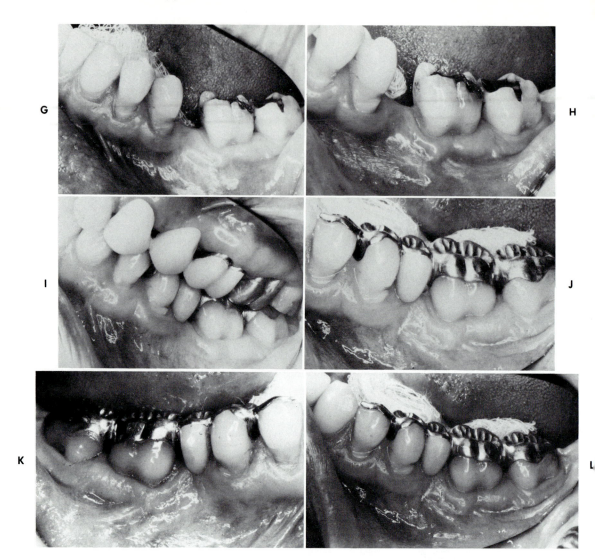

Fig. 26-48, cont'd. G and **H,** Ten-month healed response shows functional attached gingiva (mirrow view) and gingival contours managing furcation areas. **I** and **J,** Two-year result. **K** and **L,** Nine-year result. Toothbrush abrasion has increased but functional gingiva remains.

and Carraro, 1963; Chacker and Cohen, 1960; Clark, 1963; Costich and Ramfjord, 1968; Karring, 1975; Pfeifer, 1963; Wilderman, 1964, and 1963) showed that this approach was destructive to the radicular bone and resulted in an anatomic defect. A logical modification of the surgery led to the preservation of as much of the biologic attachment to the tooth and root as possible. Lacking gingiva, the underlying connective tissue consists of loose connective tissue that genetically produces granulation tissue. It will evolve first as connective tissue and subsequently as alveolar mucosa. In addition, when this type of recipient bed is left exposed, a severe inflammatory reaction occurs. There is a greater

likelihood of bone resorption although it will be less than when a denudation procedure is used.

Hattler (1967) improved the healing response by using the interdental gingiva. The multiple interdental papillae graft is moved laterally so that the interdental papillae rest upon the radicular connective tissue or bone. This tissue provides the mature epithelialized flap, which will create a new zone of attached gingiva and increase the width of the attached gingiva. It protects the delicate radicular bone, moves the mucogingival complex apically, removes the marginal frena pull, and increases the depth of the vestibular fornix (Fig. 26-48).

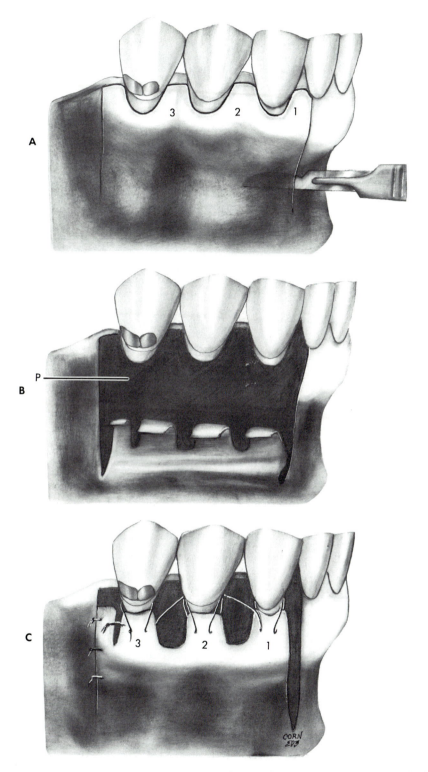

Fig. 26-49. Multiple interdental papilla graft technique; inadequate attached gingiva. **A,** Papillae, *1, 2, 3,* are undetermined initially, and partial-thickness dissection is initiated within alveolar mucosa and directed coronally toward margin of gingiva. Tension on alveolar mucosa facilitates release of dissected flap. **B,** Preparation of periosteal bed, *P.* An immovable bed results. **C,** Papillae, *1, 2, 3,* are moved to radicular surface of alveolar process to cover connective tissue bed and 1 mm of root.

Continued.

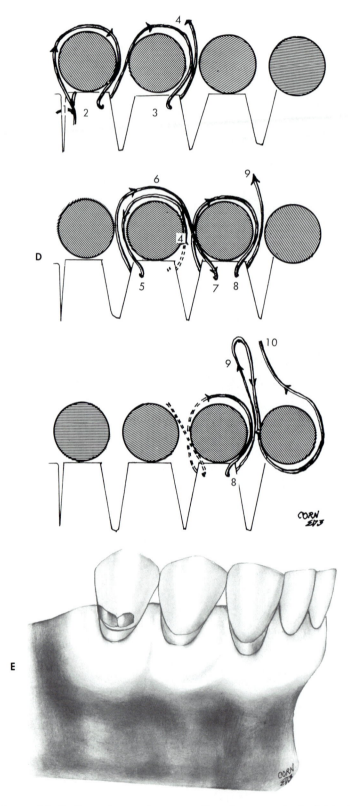

Fig. 26-49, cont'd. D, Steps in suturing are self-explanatory. An individual knot is tied at *1* and is finally completed by a knot formed by tying *9* and *10*. **E,** New functional gingiva is created. A gingivoplasty is often required to obtain this surface blending.

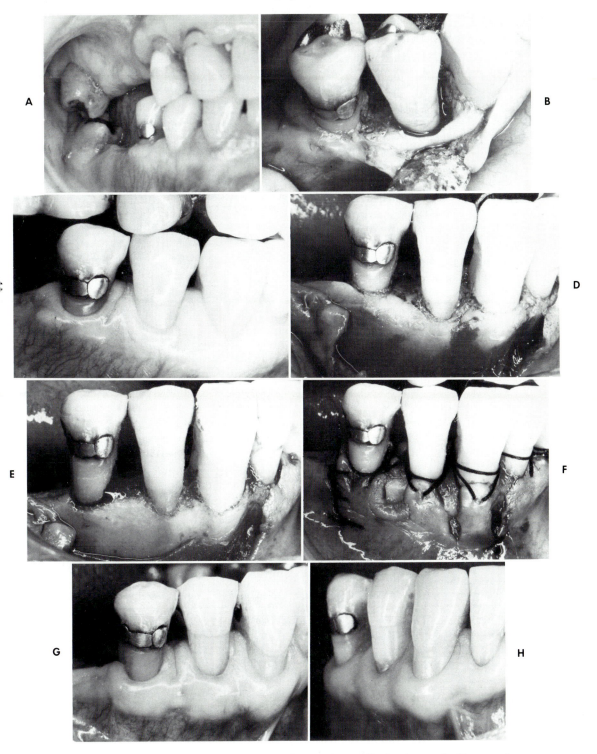

Fig. 26-50. Multiple interdental papilla graft covering radicular bone. **A,** Preoperative view. **B,** Gingival flap during initial treatment that attempts new attachment. **C,** Nine-month appearance; time of reconstructive surgery reentry. **D,** Bone fill. **E,** Following osteoplasty. **F,** Interdental papillae covering radicular alveolar crest. **G** and **H,** Preventive maintenance visit 8 months later.

TECHNIQUE (Fig. 26-49)

1. All or most of the interdental papillae are preserved, depending upon the length of the interdental tissue. A partial-thickness dissection of the interdental papillae is carried out in an antero-posterior direction using a no. 12 or no. 15 Bard-Parker blade. The papillae are thinned and detached from the underlying connective tissue with an undermining dissection.

2. At the anterior terminus of the surgical area a vertical incision is initiated from the distal line angle of the lateral incisor. The entire mesiodistal width of the papilla is preserved. The Bard-Parker blade is inserted through the vertical incision (within the alveolar mucosa), and the dissection is continued in an apicocoronal direction, releasing the papillae. The dissection progresses posteriorly, releasing the flap as the dissection is directed within the free gingival margin. Tension on the alveolar mucosa facilitates the partial-thickness dissection and the release of the graft (Fig. 26-49, *A*).

3. All the loose elastic connective tissue and muscle fibers are removed from the periosteum (Fig. 26-49, *B*). An immovable bed is created 4 to 5 mm from the refined connective tissue margin with nippers.

4. The root planing is completed. All root irregularities are removed, and any tooth accretions that may have been overlooked are checked by air drying.

5. The graft is positioned so that the interdental papillae lie over the radicular surface of the alveolus. The suturing technique is described in Fig. 26-49, *C* and *D*.

6. Periodontal dressing is placed to protect the exposed connective tissue and to maintain the position of the graft. All other postoperative procedures are the same as those previously described.

An added advantage of the multiple interdental papillae graft is the ability to alter the surgical management of an area when unexpected marginal osseous corrections are required. The technique provides a mature epithelialized pedicle, which covers the exposed bone (Fig. 26-50). The availability of this grafting approach negates the need for a free graft, particularly when abundant interdental tissue is available.

FREE SOFT TISSUE AUTOGRAFTS (GINGIVAL GRAFTS) (Dordick et al., 1976; Hawley and Staffileno, 1970; Soehren et al., 1973; Sullivan and Atkins, 1968)

INDICATIONS

1. To increase the width of attached gingiva associated (1) with (or without) a shallow vestibular fornix (Sternlicht, 1975), (2) with a frenum involvement (Ward, 1974), and (3) with prominent tooth position (possibility of fenestration or dehiscence) (Dordick et al., 1976; Vandersall, 1974)
2. To create a new zone of attached gingiva (Pennel et al., 1969)
3. To correct a genetically scanty zone of attached gingiva in which the remaining gingiva is "free" marginal tissue and not attached (Soehren, et al., 1973)
4. For correction where the alveolar crest is thin in facial to lingual dimension and there

Table 17. Comparison of periosteal retention procedure requirements

Partial-thickness apically positioned graft	Multiple interdental papilla graft*	Free soft tissue autograft (apical to mucogingival junction)
Adequate vestibular fornix	Shallow or adequate vestibular fornix	Shallow or adequate vestibular fornix
Minimum attached gingiva	Little or no attached gingiva Gingival papilla should have sufficient length (at least 3 mm) and sufficient width (at least 3 mm) at mucogingival junction	Little or no attached gingiva
Interproximal pockets	Interproximal pockets	Occasional interproximal pockets; gingivectomy needed
May need interproximal osseous surgery	May need interproximal osseous surgery	No osseous correction needed
No vestibular osseous surgery needed.	May need vestibular osseous surgery	No osseous correction needed

*Hattler procedure.

are prominent root surfaces in the jaw (Maynard and Ochsenbein, 1975)

Björn's (1963) transplantation of gingiva demonstrated the value of grafts to periodontal therapy. In the past decade the use of the free soft tissue autograft has been a monumental, innovative surgical discipline in mucogingival surgery. Introduction of the free soft tissue grafts in American literature was by King and Pennel in 1964. Cowan in 1965 utilized a mucosal graft to reduce vestibular shallowing after an extension procedure. J. Nabers (1966) used a gingival graft to increase the zone of attached gingiva for a full-crown preparation.

Prior to the use of gingival grafts, anatomic corrections were limited by other mucogingival techniques:

1. *Lack of adequate donor tissue.* double papilla graft and lateral positioned graft cannot be used.
2. *Shallow vestibular fornix.* partial-thickness apically positioned graft cannot be used, and vestibular extension and periosteal separation techniques are too traumatic and are outmoded.
3. *Thin marginal bone and prominent tooth position* (possibility of fenestration and dehiscence (Clarke and Bueltmann, 1971; Corn, 1962; Robinson and Agnew, 1963) combined with a shallow vestibular fornix). Partial-thickness apically positioned graft cannot be used, and vestibular extension and periosteal separation techniques are too traumatic and are outmoded.
4. *Single or multiple areas of recession with a shallow vestibular fornix.* Double papillae graft, lateral positioned graft, and partial-thickness apically positioned graft cannot be used, and vestibular extension and periosteal separation techniques are too traumatic and are obsolete (Clarke, 1971; Corn, 1962; Robinson and Agnew, 1963).
5. *Prominent external oblique ridge.* Pedicle

grafts are not available, and denudation is too traumatic and is obsolete (Costich and Ramfjord, 1968; Carranza and Carraro, 1963).

The three most frequently used periosteal retention procedures are compared in Table 17. Sources of granulation tissue are found in Table 18.

Principles of gingival grafting. In gingival grafting a *free soft tissue graft* is a portion of the masticatory mucosa that is completely detached from its original site and is transferred to another site. The area from which the free soft tissue graft is taken is known as the *donor site,* and the site upon which the graft is placed is known as the *recipient site.* *Autografts* are those grafts taken from one part of an individual and used on another part of that same individual. In contrast to a *pedicle graft,* which maintains its vascularity, the free graft's vascular connections are severed. It is this loss of nutritional supply that makes gingival grafting an exacting procedure. Strict attention to the basic principles of grafting is essential for optimal success.

A *partial-thickness free soft tissue graft* contains not only epithelium but also a greater or lesser amount of the lamina propria. A *full-thickness free soft tissue graft* contains all the layers of both the epithelium and the lamina propria but not the structures of the submucosa. Any glandular structure should be excluded as it would act as a barrier preventing plasmatic diffusion and circulation from reaching the graft.

Regardless of the type of graft, specific requirements are necessary for the success of transplants.

Donor site

Source of tissue. An acceptable donor tissue is characterized by a keratinized or parakeratinized epithelium and a dense lamina propria. Basically, the areas that are available are (1) the edentulous ridge tissue, (2) the attached gingiva, (3) the palatal mucosa (most frequently used), and

Table 18. Source of granulation tissue for keratinized gingiva

Partial-thickness apically positioned graft	Multiple interdental papilla graft	Free soft tissue autograft (apical to mucogingival junction)
Supracrestal connective tissue	Connective tissue of papilla	Connective tissue of free autograft
Original lamina propria	Supracrestal connective tissue	Supracrestal connective tissue
Periodontal ligament	Periodontal ligament	Periodontal ligament
Displaced original gingiva		

(4) the interdental papilla (Fig. 26-51). Any of these sources is suitable if a sufficient amount of tissue is available. Meticulous care in the surgical approach is desirable, but overcomplication of technique and selection of donor tissue should not discourage their use for they are a most predictable adjunct of surgery. When gingiva is resected it should be considered for use in combined procedures if indications for a free soft tissue autograft apply (Megarbane, 1975; Sandalli, 1974). Edel (1974) has used free connective tissue grafts as donor tissue. Yukna et al. (1977) also have used freeze-dried skin allografts.

The palate has certain anatomic limitations. With the exception of the gingival region the palate is composed of submucosa. In the posterior palate the greater palatine vessels must be avoided, and dissection should exclude the glandular tissue. In the anterior palate, fatty tissue is present in the submucosa. If the graft includes

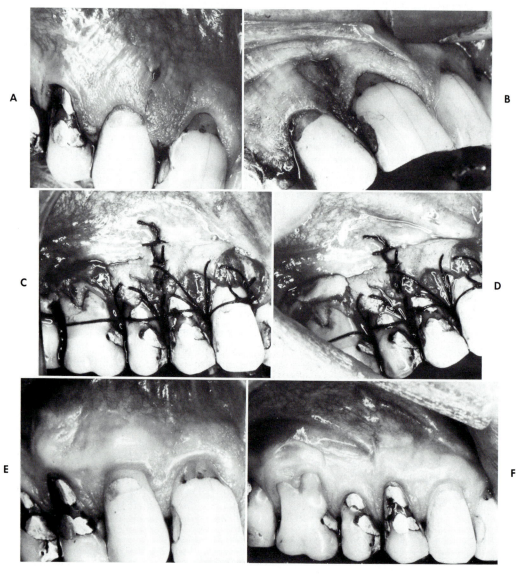

Fig. 26-51. Interdental papilla as donor site. **A,** Incision outline of interdental papilla that will be used as free graft on mesial aspect of maxillary right first molar. **B,** Following removal of partial-thickness gingival graft. **C,** Multiple interdental papilla graft positioned on radicular surface of roots and sutured in preparation for recipient bed on first molar. Positioning of tissue permitted a double papilla graft on first premolar. **D,** Free graft in position. No sutures were used. **E** and **F,** Six-month postoperative results prior to fixed restorative dentistry.

components of the submucosa, necrosis can occur. Diffusion of the plasmatic fluids for the recipient bed to the lamina propria and the epithelium of the graft is blocked. After the donor tissue has been removed, it should be examined. The fat and glandular tissue should be removed with a scalpel.

Classification of free grafts. Barsky et al. (1964) classified grafts into full-thickness and partial-thickness grafts. A *full-thickness graft* consists of the entire lamina propria, whereas *partial-thickness grafts* contain only a portion of it. Partial-thickness grafts are further divided into thin (epithelium and connective tissue ridges), intermediate, and thick according to the thickness of the lamina propria. If a portion of a graft is too thin (a graft of epithelium without the original lamina propria), it will slough off and be replaced by adjacent contiguous tissues. The new mucogingival junction will be established where the original

lamina propria remains (Soehren et al., 1973). Most frequently full-thickness or intermediate and thick partial-thickness grafts are removed (Fig. 26-52).

Characteristics of donor tissue. The thickness of a graft will determine its behavior during healing as well as its ultimate characteristics. Gingival grafts undergo less primary contraction. Davis states that primary contraction causes the vessels of the tissue to collapse, delaying the graft's revascularization (Davis and Kitlowski, 1931). Sullivan and Atkins (1968) confirm these findings with gingival grafts. Secondary contraction is caused by cicatrization of the tissue that unites the graft to its base. The effect of this cicatrization on the graft is dependent upon the rigidity of the recipient bed and the thickness of the graft's lamina propria. A thick graft on a rigid bed offers maximum resistance to scarring and thus will

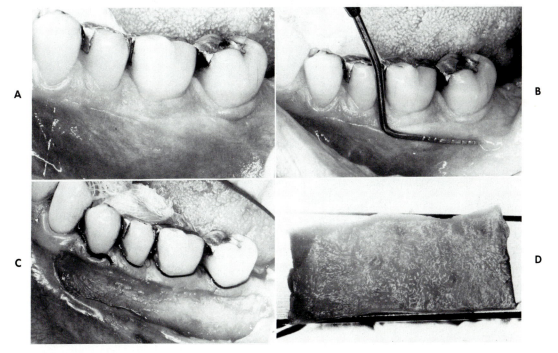

Fig. 26-52. Soft tissue autograft to correct inadequate gingiva complicated by buccal molar alveolar ledges. This procedure was combined with lingual osseous surgery and pocket elimination in retromolar area. **A,** Preoperative appearance of operative site. There is inadequate gingiva from first premolar to terminal molar. **B,** Probe moves alveolar mucosal margin to mucogingival junction that extends to free gingival margin in molar area. **C,** Incision for recipient bed is made coronal to mucogingival junction within free gingiva. Dissection is parallel to alveolar process. All muscle fibers and loose connective tissue are removed. Immovable connective tissue bed (resembling lamina propria) is prepared at recipient site. Osteoplasty is required to eliminate ledge of bone, thus removing periosteum from midportion of first molar to distal aspect of second molar. **D,** Partial-thickness graft for recipient site is 60 mm long. To avoid two wounds, one graft 30 mm × 10 mm is taken from one source.

Continued.

undergo little contraction. As Sullivan and Atkins (1968) state: ''The graft's thickness also dictates its resistance to functional stress. . . . The thickness of the graft's lamina propria is directly related to the graft's ability to resist the stresses of mastication and toothbrushing. Thus, a thicker graft is indicated in areas where greater functional demands are anticipated.''

Survival of the graft. Graft survival also is related to the graft's thickness. This is due primarily to the manner in which the different tissue components receive their nourishment and the time required by the graft's thickness to vascularize. Epithelium, lacking blood vessels, normally exchanges metabolites and waste products by diffusion. Lamina propria, however, requires a direct vascular system for its metabolism and therefore has a more acute need for vascularization than epithelium. When the lamina propria is transplanted, a diffusion system similar to that normally used by epithelium will maintain both the graft's epithelium and the lamina propria for approximately 3 days until circulation is restored. Thus graft survival is enhanced by decreasing the amount of lamina propria in the graft. Therefore the thinner graft can be maintained more easily by diffusion and is easier to vascularize.

The difficulty in maintaining and vascularizing

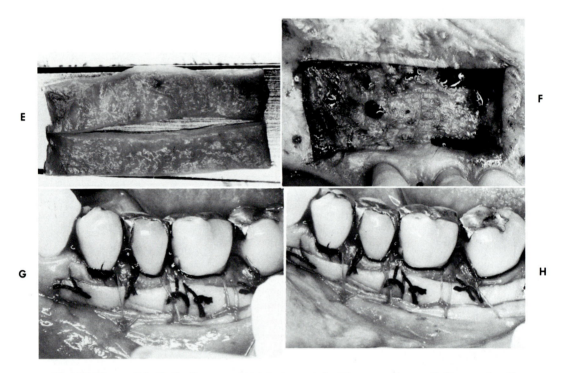

Fig. 26-52, cont'd. E, Graft separated into two grafts 30 mm × 5 mm. **F,** Donor site. **G** and **H,** Buccal portion of interdental papillae preserved and intact, enabling graft to be stabilized to this tissue. Osseous defects have been ramped on lingual aspect, enabling pockets to be eliminated. This combination approach allows preservation of gingival margin, which supplies nutrition to adjacent free graft and provides collateral circulation from vestibular mucosa and underlying connective tissue bed. Coronal margin of grafted area is sutured to interdental gingiva with no. 4-0 black silk suture. Mucosal margin is approximated to free graft by no. 4-0 gut pressure suture fixed to interproximal papillae. Apical portion of free graft is not sutured to alveolar mucosa. Movement of cheek using pressure suture allows free soft tissue autograft to remain passive. There is no ''dead'' space or bleeding at completion of procedure. **I,** Appearance of grafted area in relation to retromolar area. **J** and **K,** Healing at suture removal 10 days later. Although bone was exposed in molar area, diffusion of plasmatic fluid from gingival margin retromolar area, mucosal tissue, and adjacent connective tissue bed enables graft to survive. **L,** Palatal tissue at other donor site heals in 20 days. **M** and **N,** Six-month postoperative view illustrates increase in gingival attachment at operative site. **O** and **P,** One-year postoperative view after gingivoplasty. Enamel projections seen on molars.

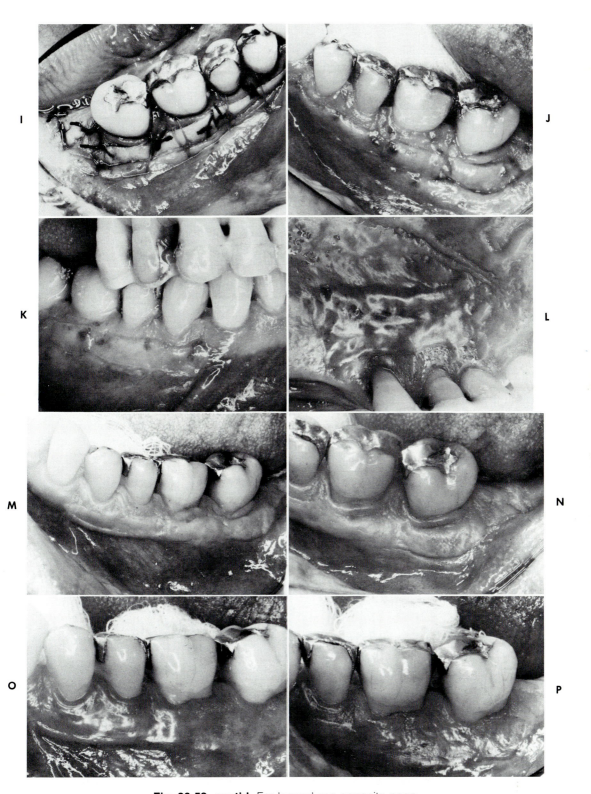

Fig. 26-52, cont'd. For legend see opposite page.

the thicker graft is illustrated by the number of thick grafts that have desquamated their superficial layers 1 week following surgery. Though the desquamated appearance of the graft may make it appear hopeless, it will reepithelialize from the remaining epithelial cells in its rete ridges. However, if the vascularization is further delayed, necrosis and loss of the graft will be unavoidable (Sullivan and Atkins, 1968).

Recipient site

Viability of new graft. The most important factor to consider in the selection of a recipient bed is its capability to maintain the viability of the new graft. A tissue bed capable of forming rapid granulation tissue has the potential of capillary outgrowth to vascularize the graft. On a bed incapable of forming capillary outgrowth, the graft will not survive. Until the host's blood vessels invade the grafted tissue, the graft is dependent upon diffusion of tissue fluids.

Sullivan and Atkins describe the stages of a graft "take" as follows:

The stages of a graft "take" are plasmic (plasmatic) circulation, vascularization, and organic union. Prior to reestablishment of vascularization (24-48 hours), the graft is solely dependent upon diffusion from its host bed. This diffusion is called plasmic (plasmatic) circulation and occurs most efficiently through the fibrin clot. . . .

The next step is the reestablishment of vascularization in the graft. Capillary proliferation begins at the end of the first day, and by the second

or third day some capillaries have extended into the graft and others have anastomosed or penetrated the graft's vasculature. Although circulation is noted in the graft on the third day, . . . an adequate blood supply does not appear to be present until about the eighth day. . . .

Concurrent with vascularization, organic connective tissue union is developing between the graft and its bed. This begins on the fourth or fifth day and a fibrous attachment is "complete" by the tenth day. [Sullivan and Atkins, 1968]

Sullivan and Atkins (1968) and Janson et al. (1969) have further evaluated the oral revascularization of full-thickness gingival grafts (see outline below). Brackett and Gargiulo (1970), in their human studies, suggest that total repair is accomplished by the eighth day.

  I. *Revascularization of partial-thickness gingival grafts*
    A. Stage of plasmatic circulation
      1. Complete—0 to 30 hours
      2. Partial—0 hours to 6 days
    B. Stage of revascularization: 30 hours to 9 days
    C. Stage of vascular reorganization: 9 to 28 days

Preparation of recipient bed. The usual bed for a free graft is a site that is within the area of the alveolar mucosa. If the vestibular fornix is shallow, requiring a vestibular extension procedure, the clinician must remove all the loose elastic connective tissue components of the submucosa within the vertical increase of the alveolar profile. This dissection on the alveolar process side of the wound to the immobile periosteum

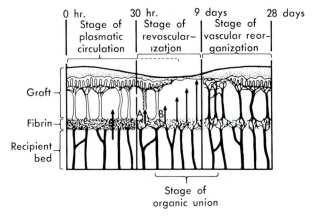

Fig. 26-53. Stages of a graft "take." During stage of plasmatic circulation (0 to 30 hours) graft lives by diffusion from bed. Stage of revascularization (30 hours to 9 days) begins as capillaries from bed anastomose with graft's vasculature, *A.* Slower but primary mode of revascularization is by capillary invasion of graft's connective tissue, *B,* with capillaries reaching epithelium in 8 or 9 days. Stage of vascular reorganization begins at this time and vascularity returns to normal by twenty-eighth day. Stage of organic union begins after 4 days as fibrin clot begins to organize into connective tissue, and by tenth day initial fibrous attachment is present.

should leave a smooth surface. Particular care should be taken to remove the muscle fibers in the interradicular depressions. To avoid mobility of the healed graft, some clinicians (Dordeck et al., 1976) expose the bone at the recipient site, and others create foramina through the cortical bone (Smith, 1962). Periosteal separation (Corn, 1962). has little effect on dimensional stability of grafts (Zingale, 1974). The mucosal margin should be sufficiently displaced to allow the passive placement of the donor tissue.

In contrast to the vestibular involvement (in the absence of attached gingiva with ample dimension in a vertical direction) similar bed preparation is required. However, the apical mucosal margin is no threat to the graft. The tendency for too much displacement should be avoided (Egli et al., 1975). An attempt should be made to relate the mucosal edge in juxtaposition to the graft. The failure to remove sufficient loose alveolar tissue and muscle fibers on the recipient bed results in graft mobility.

Hemostasis. Hemostasis in the recipient area is essential. The possibility of even the slightest bleeding must be avoided. A free graft on a nonbleeding recipient bed enhances graft survival. The preparation of the recipient site in the surgical procedure is the initial step to allow time for control of bleeding and hemostasis. Further control of capillary oozing usually can be controlled by moist saline packs and application of pressure. If the graft is placed on a bleeding recipient bed or if postoperative seepage occurs, a hematoma will form that will separate the graft from its bed. The tissue will become necrotic since neither rapid capillary penetration nor nutritional diffusion can occur through the hematoma.

Positioning of the graft. Following hemostasis, the properly prepared donor tissue is transferred to the prepared bed. The positioning of the graft depends on the goals of the surgical procedure. If only increased functional gingiva is required, especially in preparation for restorative dentistry (Haggerty, 1966), a graft of 4 or 5 mm is placed on a rigid connective tissue bed (Fig. 26-54).

Increasing the gingival width in an area with a shallow vestibular fornix (particularly with the heavy musculature of the mandibular anterior area) may require the use of periosteal separation at the apical border of the increased vertical height to the alveolar process side of the wound. This separation should be at least 4 mm from the coronal connective tissue margin of the surgical area. The separation should expose 2 or 3 mm of the

bone. Under these circumstances the donor tissue should be positioned between the connective tissue margin and the periosteal separation (Corn, 1962; Robinson and Agnew, 1963).

Immobilization of graft. Barsky et al. (1964) state that primary tissue contact, that is, actual contact between the cut surface of the graft and the recipient bed, is essential so that vascular sprouts can grow up from below into the graft without having to traverse a dead space. A graft properly immobilized (Dordick et al., 1976) and in contact with a rigid bed will undergo rapid vascularization. If the graft is mobile, the ingrowing capillaries will be torn. The tearing results in bleeding and hematoma formation that endanger graft survival.

The steps in immobilization include (1) suturing, (2) the formation of the fibrin clot, and (3) the dressing. In *suturing* the graft is stretched to conform to the recipient bed. Stark (1962) states that this tension counteracts primary contraction and aids vascularization by reopening the graft's collapsed vessels.

The graft should be immobilized as atraumatically as possible with as few sutures as practical. This prevents unnecessary damage to the graft's vasculature. The sutures should not be tied too tightly, since this will prevent revascularization and subsequent necrosis. Each suture puncture causes a localized hematoma at the site, reducing the graft "take." With a 4-0 or 5-0 black silk suture material on a reverse cutting needle guided frequently by a notched tissue pliers the graft is sutured into the fixed interdental gingiva.

As the graft is stretched, it is tied to the fixed periosteum or attached gingiva at its lateral borders. The apical border is not sutured to the underlying connective tissue, since the dressing will adapt the graft in this area. To avoid the possibility of shearing and tearing the ingrowing capillaries, the graft should not be sutured at its apical border to the mucosal margin of the flap. Otherwise the graft can be displaced by facial movement. Frequently, when vestibular depth is not a problem, the mucosal margin of the flap is brought into juxtaposition to the graft by draping the flap with a pressure suture tied above the graft into the fixed attached gingiva (Fig. 26-55).

In the second or third molar area the vestibule is shallow and the vestibular extension results in the mucosal margin contracting toward the cheek. Although ample area for proper graft placement is prepared, a pouch develops and the cut connective tissue of the mucosal margin overlaps

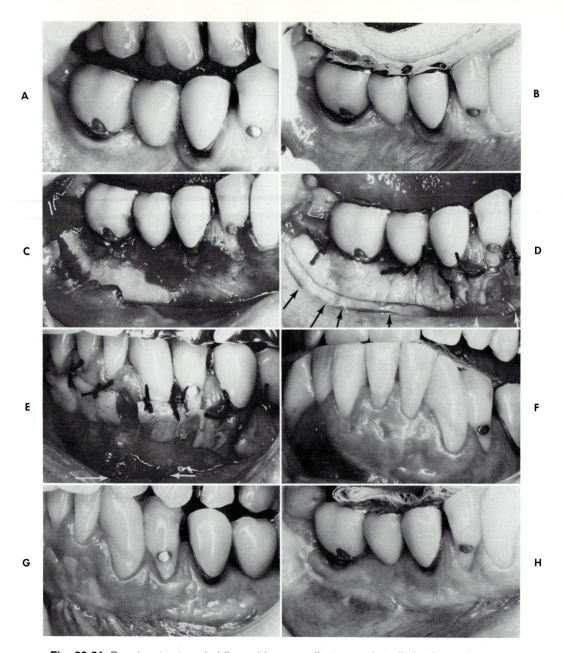

Fig. 26-54. Prominent external oblique ridge complicates pocket elimination and creates attached gingiva on mandibular second molar. Surgical site extends to right central incisor. Shallow vestibular fornix is level with gingival margins posteriorly. **A** and **B,** Preoperative views show free gingival margins, recession, and shallow vestibular fornix in mirror view of mandibular left side. **C,** Partial-thickness dissection of recipient site is completed. Free gingiva has been removed on second molar and second premolar. Incision was initiated coronal to mucogingival junction within free gingiva on first premolar and canine. Furcation involvement and prominent external oblique ridge requires osseous correction; therefore denuded marginal bone can be seen. Nutritional source for free graft on denuded bone comes from interdental connective tissue, connective tissue lateral borders, and apical mucosal margin. Connective tissue bed from second premolar anteriorly is source of revascularization of gingival grafts. **D** and **E,** Molar gingival graft is placed to cover root and is sutured interdentally. Mucosal margin is sutured to cheek musculature at base of extended vestibule. Absorbable reconstituted collagen suture is used (arrows). This prevents shallowing of vestibular fornix and avoids movement of graft. Three small grafts are used to provide attached gingiva in the remaining surgical area. **F** to **H,** Twelve-week grafting result is successful. Necrosis occurred on avascular molar mesial root; however, vestibular depth has been increased with a functional gingival attachment.

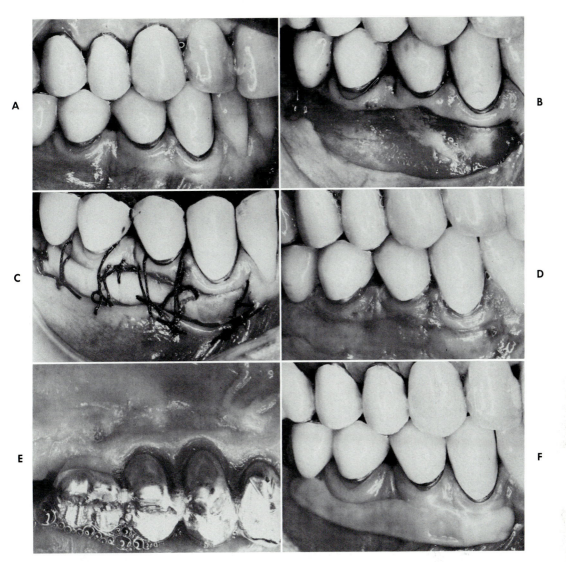

Fig. 26-55. Free soft tissue autograft prevents continued recession on abutment teeth and avoids need for bridge replacement. **A,** Preoperative view clearly shows blanching effect of frenum pull on mandibular right canine. Probe extends beyond mucogingival junction on premolars and recession exposes margin of abutment crowns. **B,** Marginal incision outlining graft site is coronal to mucogingival junction and within free gingiva. It extends distally along alveolar ridge. Recipient bed has been prepared so that all muscle fibers and loose connective tissues have been removed. There is no mobility to recipient bed. Muscle on canine is released. **C,** A 40 mm. free soft tissue autograft is sutured interproximally at its coronal border and vestibular mucosa is approximated to vestibular border of free graft but is not sutured to it. Pressure suture gains security by attachment to interproximal gingiva. There is no tension on free graft and movement of cheek allows the graft to remain passive. There are no "dead" spaces. **D,** Ten-day healing view. **E,** Twenty-day healing view of donor site. **F,** Six months subsequent to placement of graft, tension on frenum pull has been eliminated and adequate functional gingiva has been established. A common observation subsequent to gingivoplasty procedures is that placement of a free graft, in an alveolar mucosa environment by very nature of dimension of attached gingiva in relationship to thinness of alveolar mucosa, develops an apical rolled border. This biologic bandage placed within alveolar mucosal profile has a thickness that is dissimilar to thinness of alveolar mucosa and repair tissue becomes rolled at its apical border. (Restorative dentistry by Leonard W. Cohen, Levittown, Pa.)

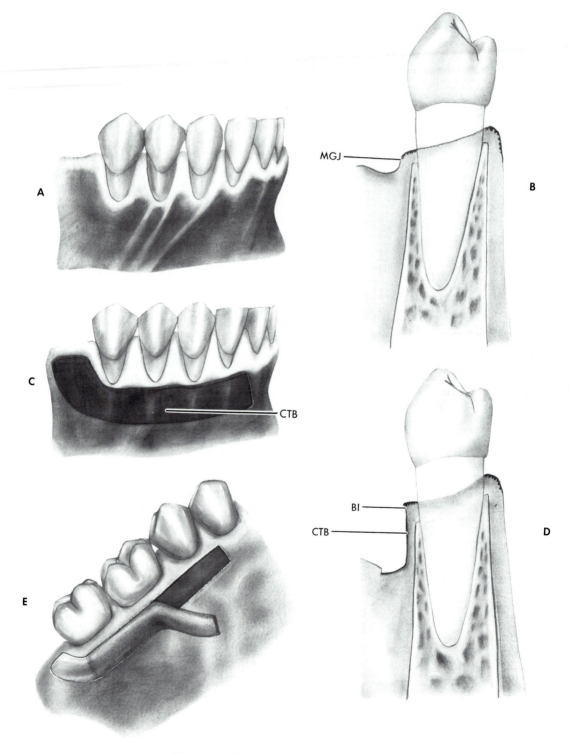

Fig. 26-56. For legend see opposite page.

the epithelium of the graft. Attempts to displace the pouch with dressing have failed, and the graft is invaginated within the resulting shallowed vestibule. This can be overcome by the usual suturing of the graft to marginal and lateral areas and the stretching and suturing of the mucosal margin of the flap at the base of the vestibule to the cheek musculature. It eliminates the possibility of pouching and entrapment of the graft within the contracting margin of the wound. Suture removal is difficult deep within the vestibular cheek border, so absorbable reconstituted collagen suture is used here (Fig. 26-56).

In *formation of the fibrin clot,* pressure is applied to the graft for at least 5 minutes to displace the blood underneath after the graft has been sutured at the nonbleeding bed. Irregularities on the subsurface of the donor tissue or indentations on the recipient bed prevent total blood displacement. It is within these indentations that localized pooling of blood occurs, resulting in hematoma formation between the graft and the recipient bed. Leaving the apical margin unsutured and using sections of grafts containing even vertical slits at their apical border appears to have overcome this problem. When both connective tissue surfaces are free of surface irregularity and can be closely approximated, blood displacement can occur and rapid revascularization follows.

Fomon (1960) explains that while pressure displaces the blood under the graft, plasma is converted to fibrin. This fibrin clot anchors the graft to its bed, allows rapid penetration by the capillaries, and acts as a matrix through which metabolites and waste products diffuse. This principle enabled Tabor and Pennel (1967) to demonstrate successful grafting without the need for periodontal dressing. Eating with care and controlled facial movements did not impede repair.

I feel that no protective covering is neces-

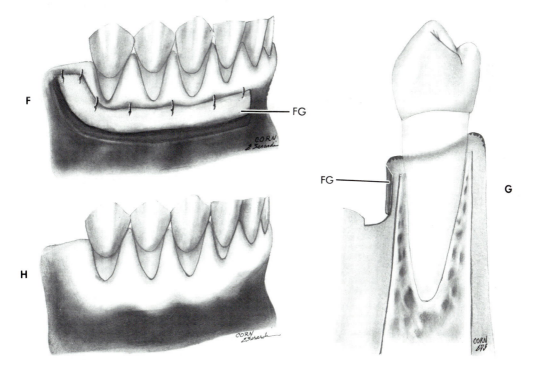

Fig. 26-56. Free soft tissue autograft. **A,** Shallow vestibular fornix with associated frena problems and inadequate gingiva. No pockets are present interproximally. Continuing recession is of concern to patient. **B,** Mucogingival junction, *MGJ,* is confluent with vestibule. **C,** Incision is initiated coronal to mucogingival junction and extended into alveolar mucosa to increase vertical height of vestibule. Connective tissue bed, *CTB,* is free of loose connective tissue and muscle fibers. **D,** A beveled incision, *BI,* and prepared connective tissue bed, *CTB,* provide surface upon which donor tissue is placed. **E,** Linear outline of recipient bed is transferred to donor site. An intermediate-thickness graft (about ¾ mm thick) is removed. **F,** Free soft tissue autograft, *FG,* is sutured with either no. 4-0 or 5-0 black silk suture. **G,** Beveled graft blends into recipient bed. **H,** New functional attached gingiva is present. Gingival margin is not affected by tensional pull on vestibule.

sary between the graft and the periodontal dressing unless bridging is planned. A modification of the Baer-Sumner dressing is used to immobilize and maintain positive pressure on the graft. There should be no displacing forces or tension on the graft when the dressing is in place. In accordance with wound healing the dressing and suture removal occurs in 10 days when organic connective tissue union is complete. Frequently no further dressing is required. Generally, soft tissue auto-

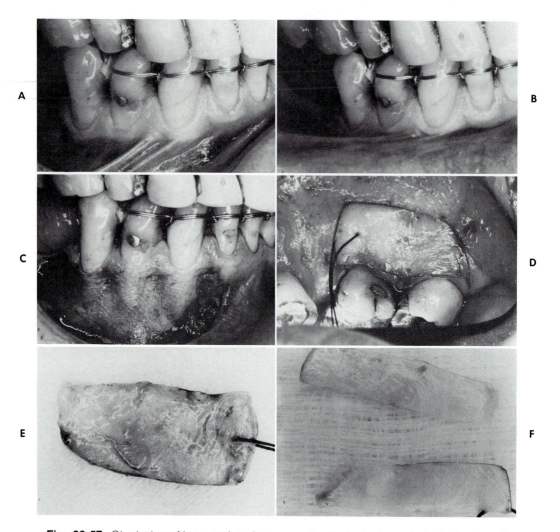

Fig. 26-57. Gingival grafting used to increase attached gingiva, eliminate frena pull, and increase depth of vestibular fornix. **A** and **B,** Preoperative views show prominent frena on right mandibular canine, absence of attached gingiva, and true depth of vestibular fornix. **C,** Preparation of recipient bed initiates from free gingival margin and includes edentulous ridge distal to second premolar. Upon completion, bed is immobile. Interdental depressions are free from muscle fibers and elastic connective tissue, leaving periosteum covering bone. Isolated areas of exposed bone can be seen at recipient site. **D,** Length of graft requires more donor tissue than available from one site. A graft twice as wide as necessary is outlined and cut lengthwise to provide gingival length needed. Suture through anterior portion of graft provides tension and facilitates uniform dissection. **E** and **F,** Graft is removed and cut in two lengthwise. **G,** Handling and initial suturing of graft are expedited by notched surgical pliers. **H,** No. 4-0 reconstituted collagen suture is used to stabilize graft interdentally and control vestibular extension. Two grafts are not sutured at their apical border. **I,** Six-month postoperative view shows increased attached gingiva provided by gingival grafts. Edentulous area has been prepared for a cantilevered pontic. (In conjunction with Manuel H. Marks, Levittown, Pa., and Leonard Juros, Willingboro, N.J.)

graft procedures are performed in conjunction with quadrant surgery. Under these circumstances an additional dressing is placed for 10 days to protect the graft, since plaque control procedures are difficult with an adjacent dressing. If periosteal vertical mattress sutures are used in adjacent grafts, adhesive foil covering the sutures prevents the dressing from entangling the sutures and disturbing the outcome of the grafts.

Asepsis. The importance of asepsis should be obvious. The oral cavity, with its unusually rich vascular supply and its local tissues that are immune to the resident bacterial flora, should be protected from foreign bacteria, particularly when subjected to surgery.

Antibiotics. The use of antibiotics offers additional protection against secondary infections. Surgical vigilance should not be relaxed. A slight infection is enough to jeopardize the success of the graft.

Surgical technique (Fig. 26-57). The general preoperative considerations applicable are described in the discussion on the Partial-Thickness Apically Positioned Graft. The procedure for preparation of the recipient site is presented below.

Initial preparation. A disease control program is successfully completed (Corn et al., 1976, 1969, 1968) and the patient is able to demonstrate continued plaque control on a sustained, reinforced basis prior to surgery. Prescaling and root planing remove local irritants. Frequently a cleft almost

obliterates the zone of attached gingiva. With repair, creeping attachment occurs and surgery is no longer necessary. The value of initial preparation cannot be overemphasized.

Incisions. The following considerations must be taken into account in making incisions.

1. *Shallow vestibular fornix.* Where there is a shallow vestibular fornix it is essential that the vestibular extension provide ample height to the vertical alveolar profile to allow room for the placement of the donor tissue. Sufficient mesiodistal extension will facilitate the vestibular deepening when necessary. Oblique relaxing incisions also provide additional room.

a. *Alveolar mucosal marginal tissue and shallow crevice.* A vertical incision is made at the anterior terminus of the operative site using a no. 15 Bard-Parker blade. The blade is placed into the submucosa, tension is applied to the lip or cheek, and the mucosal flap is dissected free as the blade passes through the tissue in an apicocoronal direction. The method does not obstruct the clinician's vision as he directs the blade to the alveolar mucosal margin, attempting to preserve the most coronal connective tissue fiber attachment to the root of the tooth. The sulcular epithelium must be removed subsequently if reattachment to the root is the clinical goal (Fig. 26-58).

b. *Free gingival marginal tissue and shallow crevice.* The dissection begins with a horizontal

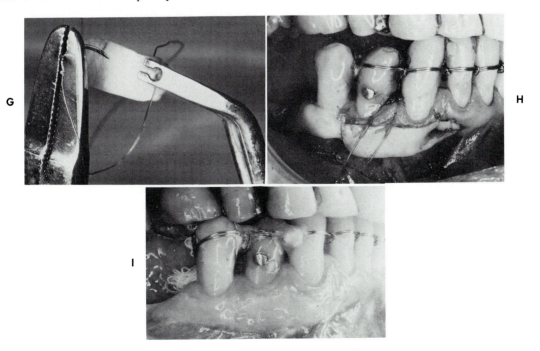

Fig. 26-57, cont'd. For legend see opposite page.

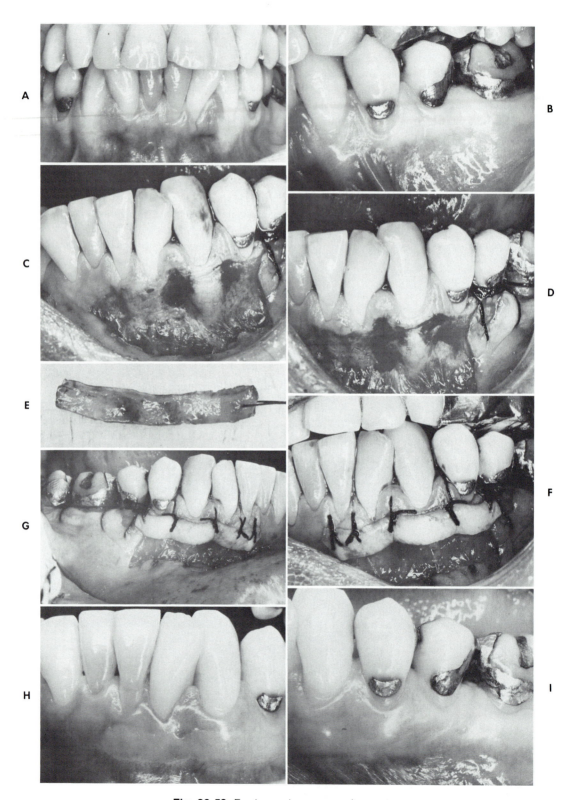

Fig. 26-58. For legend see opposite page.

incision coronal to the mucogingival junction, is beveled within the free gingiva (Soehren et al., 1973), and extends the entire length of the operative area. A vertical incision follows, and, with tension on the flap as it is dissected, the no. 15 Bard-Parker blade is directed close to the alveolar profile as it courses through the submucosa in an apicocoronal direction. Here the blade is targeted to the previous initial incision. Tension on the flap facilitates the blending of both incisions. (Fig. 26-59).

c. *Pockets extending beyond the mucogingival junction.* The incision initiates at the mucogingival junction and extends mesiodistally parallel to the alveolus. The mesiodistal extremities of the incision should allow ample vestibular extension. If labial or buccal pockets exist with intact interdental gingiva, pocket elimination is required (Goldman et al., 1976).

2. *Adequate vestibular depth.* The principles apply as just described, but unnecessary connective tissue exposure should be avoided. Only a recipient site that is adequate to receive the requirements of the graft should be exposed if increased functional gingiva is the objective (Fig. 26-53).

Connective tissue bed. To obtain functional gingiva all the loose connective tissue and muscle fibers are sharply dissected down to the periosteum with surgical nippers. The remaining thin layer of soft tissue forms a rigid base resembling lamina propria that allows for immobilization of

the graft and reduces the graft's postoperative contraction as suggested by Fomon (1960). Osteoplasty occasionally may be necessary in adjacent areas to correct minimal osseous defects that are not in the direct recipient bed. Large areas with osseous defects, particularly in the mandibular second and third molar area, requiring osteoplasty must have four sources perimetrically for successful bridging: (1) the intact periosteum lateral to the denuded bone anteriorly, (2) the intact periosteum lateral to the denuded bone posteriorly, (3) the connective tissue of the gingival collar coronally, and (4) the mucosal margin with close approximation but not sutured at this apical border. They all contribute to the diffusion system that is required (Fig. 26-52).

The prepared surfaces of the recipient site should be smooth to prevent blood pooling and ultimate clot formation. For example, in areas of irregularities when teeth are prominent in the arch, giving a washboard effect to the alveolar surface, muscle fibers must be removed from these interdental indentations. Special care is required to make the graft conform to the undulating alveolar surface to effect a successful "take" (Fig. 26-59). Inadvertent exposure of fenestrations or dehiscences has not presented a problem (Dordick et al., 1976).

This bed preparation allows ample time for hemostasis of the recipient bed, and it minimizes the time interval between the procurement of the graft and its placement. A warm moist gauze

---

Fig. 26-58. Value of free soft tissue autografts when teeth are prominently positioned in arch. Risk of dehiscence and fenestration is present. **A** and **B,** Preparative views. Gingival clefts involve mandibular left central and lateral incisors. Left canine and first premolar are in prominent position, suggestive of possible fenestration or dehiscence. Although frenum attachment is between canine and first premolar, there is blanching radiating to each of these teeth, implicating tensional pull of this frenum. **C** and **D,** Partial-thickness dissection initiated coronal to mucogingival junction within free gingiva. After removal of loose connective tissue and muscle fibers at recipient site, fenestration is observed through periosteum on left central incisor. Similarly, canine appears involved. Second premolar is treated with partial-thickness apically positioned flap. Note pooling of blood in alveolar indentations between teeth. **E,** Size of soft tissue autograft shown. **F,** A 4 mm soft tissue autograft is sutured to interproximal papillae at its coronal margin. Graft is not sutured at its vestibular border; however, mucosal margin of flap is sutured to underlying connective tissue at base of vestibule with 4-0 gut suture. Adaptation of graft to alveolar indentation. **G,** Mirror view of completed surgical procedure. **H** and **I,** Six-month postsurgical result. Marginal clefts have almost disappeared, functional gingiva is present, and muscle pull has been dissipated. Note that response to partial-thickness apically positioned graft on second premolar is equally successful; however, rate of healing is much slower. Gingivoplasty was performed after 20 days to blend repairing tissue. It is anticipated that creeping attachment will occur.

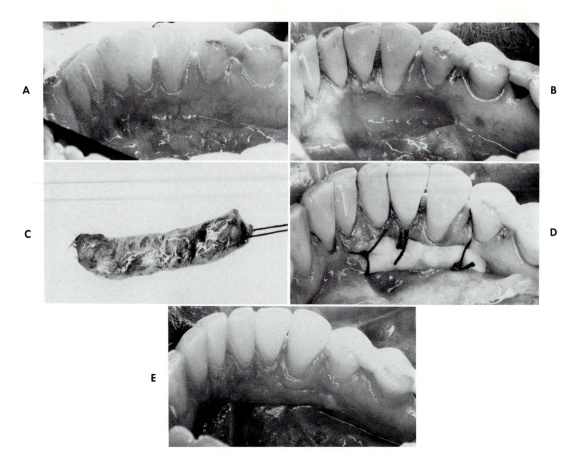

Fig. 26-59. Lingual free soft tissue autograft. **A,** Preoperative view shows absence of attached gingiva on mandibular left central and lateral incisors. **B,** Dissection initiating within free gingiva allows a collar of residual gingiva to remain. Loose elastic connective tissue of submucosa is removed until immovable lamina propria–like base is established. Adequate vestibular depth developed at recipient site. **C,** Undersurface of palatal free graft is seen. Glandular tissue must be removed, leaving smooth surface and avoiding "dead" space. Original tension suture remains until immobilized at recipient bed. **D,** Interrupted no. 4-0 black silk suture secures graft at coronal margin and at lateral borders. Apical area is not sutured. **E,** Survival of free graft and increased attached gingiva after 6 months.

sponge dipped in normal saline solution and placed over the bed will ensure control of bleeding while the donor tissue is being placed.

• • •

The procedure for preparation of the donor site is presented below:

Site selection. Although the interdental papilla and the edentulous ridge tissue can provide donor tissue, large grafts are taken from palatal mucosa.

Design of donor tissue. Experience has taught that relatively straight line incisions at the recipient site should be planned. This will eliminate the need for a tinfoil template, which is time consuming. A periodontal probe is used to mea-

sure the linear length of the recipient site at its coronal margin. The width of the graft varies in width from 3 to 4 mm to 8 to 9 mm in selected areas when attachment to the root is the objective. The measurements are transferred to the palatal gingival margin following the administration of local anesthesia. They are also recorded on the patient's chart. The incision is kept a short distance from the margin and plotted with puncture marks using the probe. For example, if a long graft of 60 × 4 mm is required and insufficient rugae-free palatal mucosa is available, a graft outline of 30 × 8 mm is removed and then cut lengthwise (Fig. 26-46). Barsky et al. (1964) warn that trauma will cause damage to the tissue's vessels

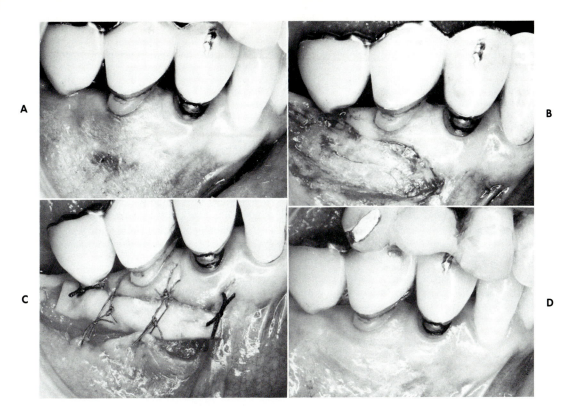

Fig. 26-60. Free soft tissue autograft used to provide adequate gingiva for abutment tooth and prepare edentulous area for reception of pontic. **A,** Preoperative view. Alveolar mucosa is in close proximity to thin free gingiva margin on mandibular second premolar. Mucogingival junction extends to crest of edentulous area. **B,** Partial-thickness dissection coronal to mucogingival junction. Outline extends beyond crest of ridge in pontic area that was formerly alveolar mucosa. All loose connective tissue has been removed and immovable bound-down connective tissue recipient bed has been prepared. **C,** Free soft tissue autograft is sutured to remaining gingiva at its coronal margin. Vestibular area is not sutured to free graft at its base, but there is a pressure suture overlaying graft and gaining fixation with marginal gingiva. No. 5-0 Ethiflex suture is used. **D,** Four-month postgraft result shows that abutment second premolar has adequate functional gingiva, crevicular depth is less than 2 mm, and pontic area has masticatory mucosa for a pontic contact.

that will delay the graft's vascularization. Atraumatic removal of donor tissue is the most important phase in donor site preparation. As the donor tissue outline is cut, the coronal and mesiovertical incisions permit a beveled margin with a no. 15 Bard-Parker blade. The graft tissue is kept under tension with a 4-0 black silk traction suture as removal occurs. A partial-thickness intermediate graft generally is the goal when it is desirable to cover large avascular areas. These are approximately 0.75 mm thick. Thicker grafts to 1.25 mm are used where greater functional stress is present.

In removing the donor tissue, every effort is made to create a smooth subsurface. After removal the graft is examined for glandular tissue,

subsurface irregularities, and thickness. Correction of these properties can be made with a scalpel blade while the graft is held in a gauze sponge moistened with normal saline solution. To minimize trauma and dehydration the graft is placed on the previously prepared recipient bed as soon as possible. If delay is necessary because of inadequate hemostasis, the graft is wrapped in a gauze sponge moistened with normal saline solution.

Position of the graft. When aesthetics is not a concern, the goal of the grafting is to attain attached gingiva around a defect, especially if minimal gingiva is present on the lingual of the mandibular incisors (Fig. 26-60).

Immobilization of the graft. The graft should be placed with a minimal number of sutures. It should be in direct contact with the recipient bed and passively held in position without subsurface "dead space" and without tension at the suture areas. Facial movements should not shear the graft from the ingrowth of new capillaries (Fig. 26-61).

Postoperative care. There has been some previous mention of postoperative care in the discussion on Principles of Gingival Grafting. Other considerations are as follows.

Recipient site. Following dressing placement the patient is instructed to avoid its displacement by eating a soft diet and minimizing facial movements. Bleeding or dislodging of the dressing should be reported immediately. Organic union develops around the tenth day so it is preferable not to disturb the dressing until that time. Care must be taken to avoid injury to the graft during suture removal. A moist cotton swab is used to debride the surgical site. Epithelialization is usually complete, although thicker graft areas may have epithelial desquamation and require a dressing (any zinc oxide–eugenol dressing) for an additional 10 days. After dressing removal, plaque control is reinstituted. The patient is instructed to use a disclosing agent frequently as a guide to plaque control effectiveness. A Perio-Aid is used to remove plaque at the necks of the teeth. The area of the graft must be cleaned atraumatically in a coronal direction for a 1- to 2-week period with moist cotton applicators. Where functional gingiva has been restored the cautious use of an intracrevicular brushing technique can be instituted. However, where bridging has occurred and attachment covering a denuded root has been successful, a prescribed technique of brushing should be taught.

Donor site. The postoperative response at this site is generally unremarkable. Occasional bleeding is controlled with local anesthesia and pres-

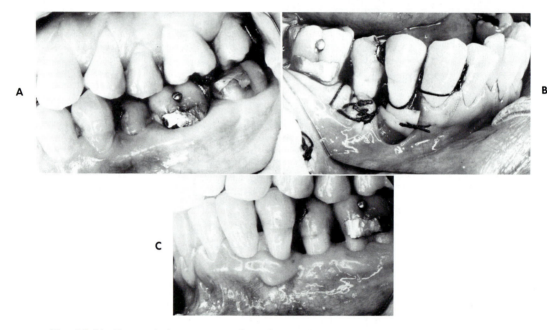

Fig. 26-61. Free soft tissue autograft replaces alveolar mucosal margin in conjunction with double papillae-flap procedure. **A,** Preoperative view. Prominently positioned left first premolar in which there is absence of functional attached gingiva. Mandibular second premolar appears to have adequate gingiva but subsequent to plaque control, root scaling, root planing, and soft tissue curettage inadequate gingiva was present. **B,** Double papillae procedure was used to gain gingival width required for second premolar and a free soft tissue autograft provides gingival source on first premolar. Underlying connective tissue bed has been prepared by partial-thickness dissection removing all loose connective tissue fibers and has immovable base upon which free soft tissue autograft is placed (mirrow view). **C,** Eight months subsequent to surgical procedure, free soft tissue autograft and double papillae procedures have been successful in providing adequate functional gingiva.

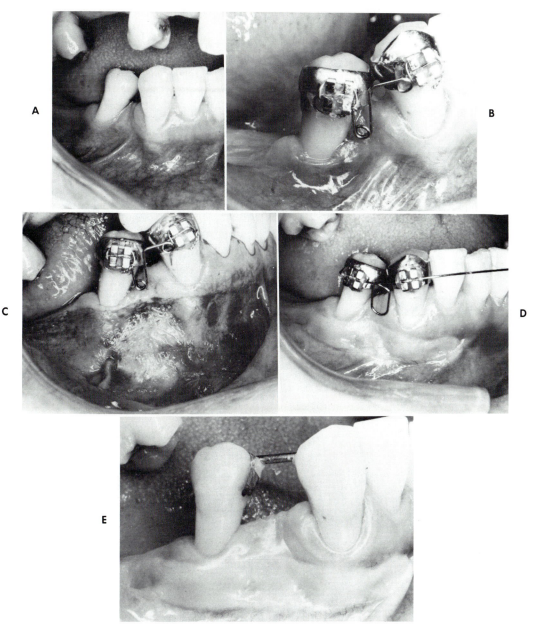

Fig. 26-62. Free soft tissue autograft to repair pontic area of edentulous donor site used for a laterally positioned pedicle graft. **A,** Preoperative view. Recession on maxillary second premolar with no functional gingiva. Pedicle graft from edentulous area of pontic will be donor tissue. **B,** Absorbable gut suture used to attach pedicle graft over exposed root surface previously prepared for graft. Wide V-shaped donor site left gingival defect at pontic area. **C,** Free soft tissue autograft sutured to pontic area to avoid food retention and maintain profile of edentulous mucosa. **D,** Palatal donor site for graft used in edentulous area. **E,** Six-month repaired site shows elimination of gingival cleft. Functional attached gingiva on second premolar cannot be probed more than 1 mm. Complete repair in edentulous area by free soft tissue autograft. (Restorative dentistry by Leonard W. Cohen, Levittown, Pa.)

sure. Traumatic and postoperative patient discomfort is negligible. Since the grafts are taken from the marginal area, the application of the usual periodontal dressing provides ample protection. No stent is necessary. The thinner grafts are sufficiently healed in 10 days, requiring no further care. Thicker grafts are healed in 20 days. The thicker grafts may require gingivoplasty procedures at the recipient site upon complete healing.

The use of pedicle grafts with their blood supply should not be overlooked as donor tissue to ideally correct gingival clefts and areas of recession. An edentulous area pedicle graft can repair a gingival cleft if the adjacent alveolar crests are normal and no pockets are present. Occasionally a donor site has a fixed bridge in place, and the use of a pedicle graft would leave a defect in relation to a pontic. The edentulous area can be

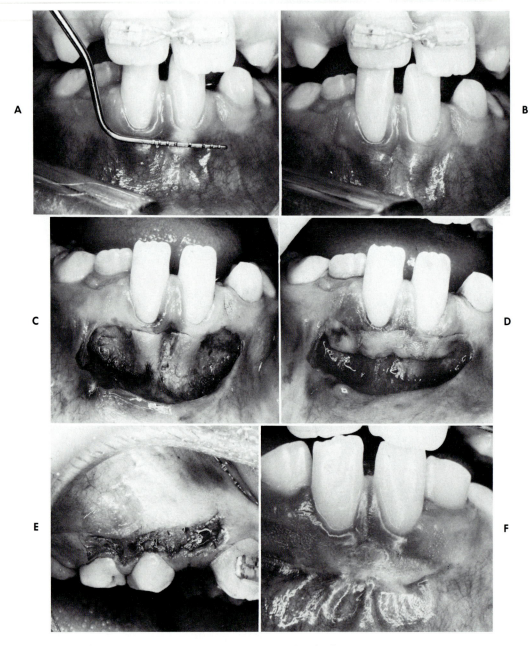

Fig. 26-63. Preorthodontic need for gingiva in child. **A,** Only free gingiva present on right central incisor. **B,** Probe verifies need for a graft. **C,** Preparation of recipient bed. **D,** Gingival graft in position. **E,** Maxillary buccal attached gingiva is source of donor tissue. **F,** New gingiva one year later.

repaired by a free graft (Fig. 26-62). However, for multiple recipient site problems, gingival graft principles are available. Future wound healing will reveal the nature of this attachment.

Summary. The use of the gingival graft has made available methods for managing cases that could otherwise present hazardous sequelae. A patient (Fig. 26-63) undergoing orthodontic therapy requires functional gingiva to prevent bone loss and recession (Maynard and Ochsenbein, 1975). Deficient margins of restorations cause gingival loss and recession. The gingival graft prevents continued destruction (Fig. 26-64).

Free grafts can be positioned over bone denuded as a result of osteoplasty procedures and can survive (Dordick et al., 1976). The viability of the graft is maintained initially by the plasmatic circulation provided perimetrically on all aspects of the grafted site. The intact periosteum that is lateral to the denuded bone, the connective tissue of the free gingival collar that is coronal, and the mucosal margin that is in juxtaposition (although not sutured at this apical border) contribute to

the diffusion system. They maintain the graft's epithelium and lamina propria for approximately 3 days until the circulation is restored (Fig. 26-46).

Gingival grafts increase the width of existing gingiva or replace an alveolar mucosal margin with an immobile, keratinized marginal tissue. This may be desired for restorative purposes (Fig. 26-56), to eliminate a frenum or muscle pull (Fig. 26-59), or to facilitate disease control procedures.

The complexities of a shallow vestibular fornix require special consideration. An increase in the vestibular fornix alone is not an indication for mucogingival surgery. The decision to deepen a vestibule is made when additional vertical height is needed at the recipient site for the placement and immobilization of a graft. The preparation of the recipient bed along with the vestibular extension enables the clinician to increase the width of the existing gingiva and to deepen the vestibule in a single procedure. There is concern for premature shallowing of the vestibule prior to complete stabilization of the graft during healing. It is overcome by the mesial and distal extension

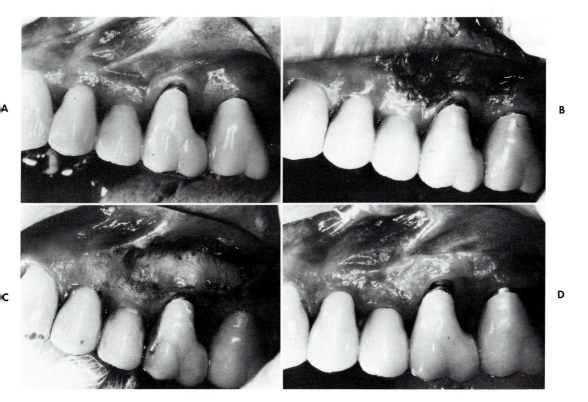

Fig. 26-64. Recession revealing defective crown margin. No attached gingiva is present. **A,** Gingival graft necessary to control further recession. **B,** Preparation of recipient bed. **C,** Graft in position. **D,** Three-year postoperative response. No further recession is evident.

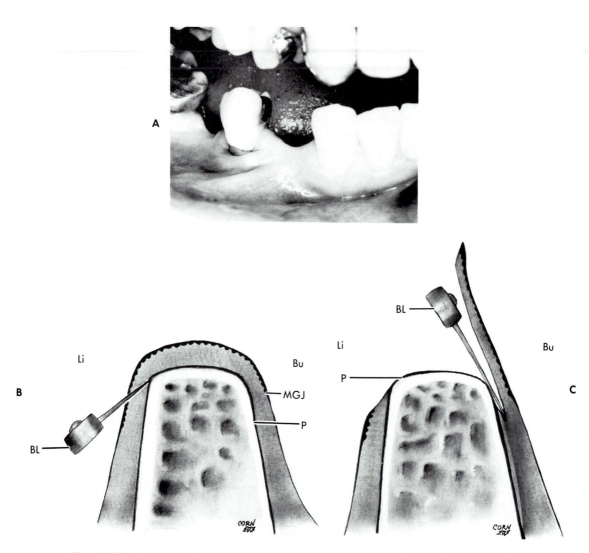

Fig. 26-65. Double pedicle grafts used to restore gingival unit and deepen vestibular fornix. Donor source is lingual aspect of edentulous ridge. *BL,* Bard-Parker blade; *P,* periosteum; *Li,* lingual aspect; *Bu,* buccal aspect; *MGJ,* mucogingival junction. **A,** Pretreatment view of mandibular right second premolar. Shows alveolar mucosal margin and close relationship with vestibular fornix. Pocket depth 6 mm on radicular surface. **B,** Pedicle grafts offer opportunity to increase gingival dimension equivalent to width of available masticatory mucosa from mucogingival junction on lingual aspect of edentulous ridge over crest to terminus of gingiva on buccal surface. Because of the angulation of the no. 15 Bard-Parker blade, *BL,* on the Blake handle, a partial-thickness dissection of the entire masticatory edentulous tissue is possible. **C,** Periosteum is not included with the graft so that mobility of the pedicle grafts can be increased.

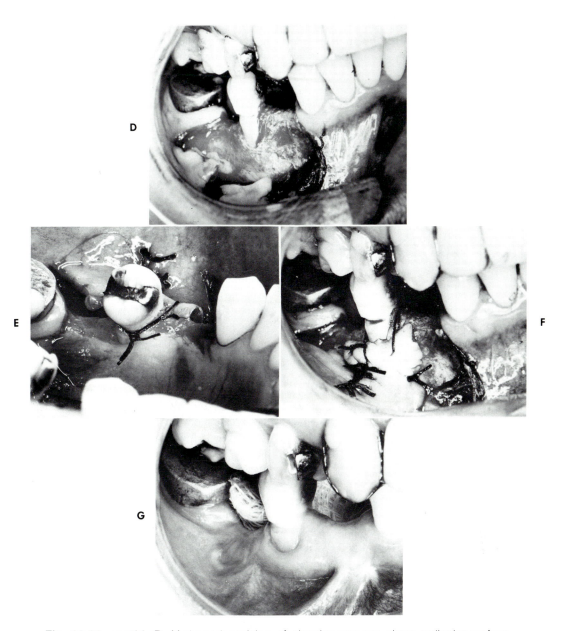

Fig. 26-65, cont'd. D, V-shaped excision of alveolar mucosa along radicular surface of second premolar. Two pedicle grafts have been released from their attachment on edentulous area. Distance between each pedicle graft represents excised mucosal tissue at recipient site. Loose connective tissue fibers of alveolar mucosa are dissected from periosteum creating immobile bed resembling lamina propria. **E,** Both pedicle grafts are suspended and sutured on lingual surface. The donor site sources can be seen from the lingual view. **F,** Margin of the donor tissue covers connective tissue attachment on root of tooth and a portion of exposed cementum. Vestibular fornix has been deepened. Interrupted sutures at midradicular area join both pedicles. **G,** One year after surgery. Pedicle graft technique has controlled vestibular depth and restored gingival attachment.

of the operative site over a wide area (Fig. 26-59) or the incorporation of a periosteal separation principle at the apical border of the free graft with oblique relaxing incisions at the terminus of the extension procedure. Incorporation is performed when there is a limited area of vertical alveolar height available for graft placement.

The use of the free soft tissue autograft has provided additional dimension to the therapeutic management of marginal problems. In an arch where only free gingival margins are present, large segments have been treated successfully by preserving the gingival height and replacing the adjacent alveolar mucosa with large gingival grafts. The preparation of the recipient bed incorporates the principles of vestibular extension (stripping) and periosteal separation that have become obsolete as pure surgical procedures. The use of free full-thickness or partial-thickness soft tissue autografts as a "biologic dressing" has minimized patient discomfort, and healing is rapid.

EDENTULOUS AREA PEDICLE GRAFT
(PARTIAL THICKNESS) (Corn, 1964; Robinson, 1964)

INDICATIONS
1. To increase the width of attached gingiva using edentulous area masticatory mucosa
2. To create new attached gingiva
3. To correct gingival recession provided adjacent interproximal osseous height is normal

PRECAUTIONS
1. The depth of the vestibule should be sufficient or should be dissected to create sufficient vertical rise to the alveolar relocation of the graft; otherwise it is possible that the graft cannot be positioned at the recipient site.
2. The length of the graft should be no greater than three times its width or survival of the graft may be threatened.

The use of pedicle grafts has expanded the application of mucogingival surgery by providing a new perspective in the manipulation of tissues (Bhaskar et al., 1971, 1970; Corn, 1964; Robinson, 1964). A favorable permanent change is often observed in the mucogingival complex. In the absence of gingiva and with a shallow vestibular fornix even a limited area can be involved to establish the objectives discussed in this chapter. An important facet for this tissue change is the preparation of the immovable connective tissue bed at the recipient site (Fig. 26-65).

The edentulous area pedicle graft combines a graft of masticatory mucosa and alveolar mucosa. Compared to skin grafts, the pedicle graft in the oral cavity is unique. The distal portion, which resembles gingiva, consists of keratinized epithelium and dense inelastic connective tissue of the lamina propria. The proximal portion (the alveolar mucosa) is composed of a thin, nonkeratinized epithelium, a thin lamina propria, and a thick submucosal layer. It reflects into the cheek at its base.

The procedure utilizes a graft of tissue from the edentulous ridge area. It is a partial-thickness flap dissected from the periosteum and connective tissue while remaining attached to the osseous tissue at the donor site. The pedicle gains its blood supply from the small supraperiosteal blood vessels and is not dependent upon the underlying periosteum for its viability. Therefore it is most essential that the base of the pedicle be of sufficient width so that it will not compromise the circulation of the terminal portion of the flap.

Once mobilized, the graft can be positioned at the appropriately prepared recipient site. The attachment of the graft at its new location has been equally successful whether placed over a collagenous attachment to the tooth or at the margin of the alveolar process. Regardless of the preparation of the recipient site the pedicle graft is positioned not only laterally but apically as well. Success of the surgical technique in graft transplantation is dependent upon *asepsis, hemostasis,* and *immobilization of the graft.*

Surgical procedure. The description of the pedicle graft procedure will be discussed in relation to (1) a suitable surgical design, (2) the preparation of the pedicle graft at the donor site, (3) the preparation of the recipient site, and (4) the proper atraumatic surgical technique in its transplantation.

Suitable surgical design (Fig. 26-66). The design of the pedicle graft relies principally on the utilization of available masticatory mucosa on the edentulous alveolar ridge. Compare the absence of attached gingiva on the mesial root of the mandibular left first molar with the abundant reserve of gingivalike tissue on the saddle area of the second premolar region (Fig. 26-66). Because of recession the marginal tissue of alveolar mucosa on the mesial root is confluent with the mucogingival junction. The probe shows that the base of the pocket extends well into the alveolar mucosa. In addition, exploration reveals that there are slight osseous defects in the furcation and on the mesial and distal alveolar margins of this tooth.

With a Bard-Parker no. 15 blade (Fig. 26-66) an incision is made along the alveolar crest distomesially in its course and occlusoapically in direction. The incision with the scalpel is not through the inelastic periosteum but in the corium of the connective tissue, thereby creating a partial-thickness flap. The ridge remains covered by the periosteum and connective tissue. Fig. 26-66, *B* shows the direction of the scalpel on the buccal

incline of the alveolar ridge, leaving the periosteum intact. Here there is adequate gingiva on the buccal aspect of the ridge as delineated by the mucogingival junction.

There are circumstances in which the mucogingival junction is located near the alveolar crest, leaving inadequate gingiva for use as a donor. The design of the incision as described in Fig. 26-66 would result in failure. Modification of the surgical design would be necessary. The marginal incision would have to originate along

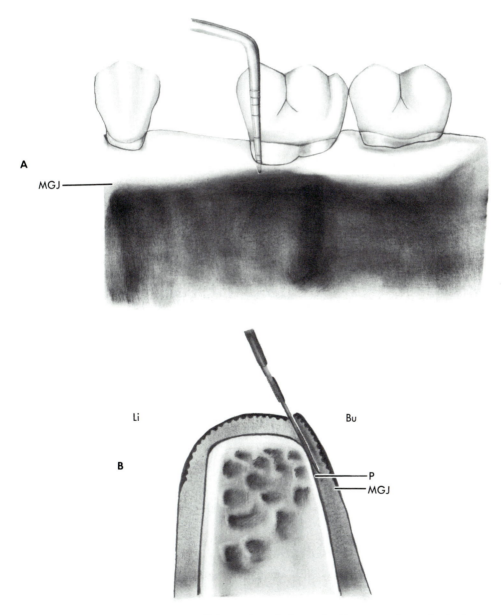

Fig. 26-66. Edentulous area pedicle graft technique. **A,** Absence of attached gingiva on mesial root of first molar. Probe extends beyond mucogingival junction, *MGJ.* **B,** Buccolingual view of edentulous ridge. Angulation of no. 15 scalpel blade. Periosteum, *P,* remains intact.

Continued.

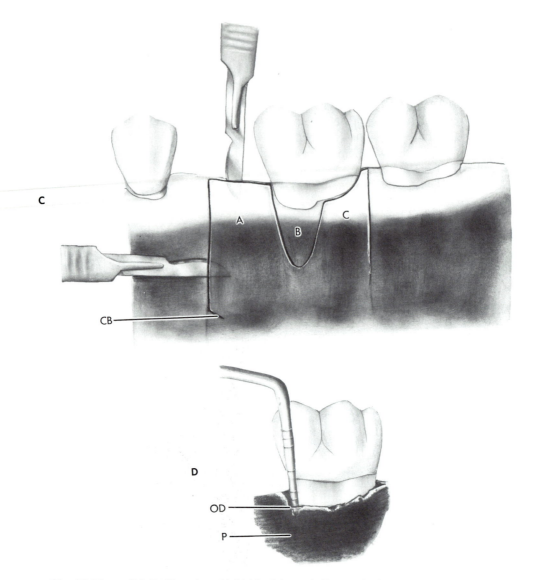

Fig. 26-66, cont'd. C, Direction of initial incisions. *A,* Donor site from which pedicle graft is obtained. *B,* Mucosal wedge of tissue at recipient site where this tissue will be excised. *C,* Tissue managed as apically positioned graft. Note paths of oblique incisions. *CB,* Cutback incisions. Apicocoronal path of scalpel releases donor tissue. **D,** Osseous defect, *OD,* can be probed while periosteum, *P,* covers osseous tissue. Pedicle grafts have been reflected.

the lingual aspect of the edentulous ridge in order to create a suitable morphologic tissue complex as a graft (Fig. 26-65).

Preparation of pedicle graft at donor site. The tissue at the donor site must be delicately dissected (Fig. 26-66, *C*). The width of the pedicle graft at its free border should be at least as wide as the defect to be corrected and preferably wider. The vertical incisions to elevate the flap are planned so that the base of the pedicle is broader than its margin. This is achieved by two oblique incisions starting from the crestal area. The ver-

tical incision proximal to the molar extends into the mucosa and terminates at a midposition over the mesial root. The other vertical incision courses apically and diagonally into the mucosa toward the first premolar. Tissue forceps held at the crestal free margin facilitates the elevation of the flap.

The critical area is at the mucogingival junction. To avoid perforating the thin tissue at this location, the direction of the dissection should be changed (Fig. 26-66, *C*). The Bard-Parker blade is inserted into the submucosa through the two

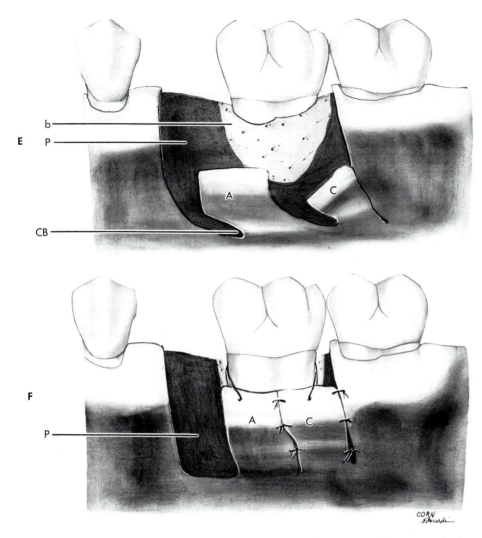

Fig. 26-66, cont'd. E, After osseous correction, *b.* **F,** Completion. Pedicle graft, *A,* has been positioned horizontally and apically at margin, covering alveolar process. *C,* Apically positioned graft. Sling suture is tied on lingual surface.

vertical incisions, undermining the flap. The path of the dissection is now coronal to the mucogingival junction. Paralleling the plane of the alveolar process, this incision and the original incision that started at the alveolar crest meet in the area of the mucogingival junction, and the pedicle graft is free. Connective tissue and periosteum remain attached to the alveolar process.

The flap that is now freely movable cannot be accurately positioned at its future recipient site without a cutback incision extending the oblique incision adjacent to the first premolar. The cutback

incision is extended in the direction to which the pedicle is to be moved. With the base of the pedicle in alveolar mucosa free from the immovable underlying periosteum and with the cutback incision the graft can be positioned with greater facility.

Preparation of recipient site. The removal of the alveolar mucosal wedge of tissue at the recipient site is accomplished by a diagonal incision in the furcation area, creating a wedge-shaped form as it joins the oblique incision previously executed (Fig. 26-66, *C*). The wedge is cut at its apex, is held by the tissue forceps, and is removed by the scalpel blade moving in a coronal direction. At this time the periosteum remains attached to the bone at the recipient site until probing determines the degree of osseous defects (Fig. 26-66, *D*).

Because the furcation and the distal surface of the first molar require osseous correction, the gingiva over the distal root can be managed as an apically positioned flap. Either a mucoperiosteal flap or a partial-thickness flap can be raised. The latter approach is used here prior to osseous exposure. In Fig. 26-66, *D*, to avoid the unneccessary exposure of a dehiscence or fenestration of bone, a mucoperiosteal flap is not elevated initially to gain access to the osseous deformities in Fig. 26-66, *B* and *C*.

When sounding through the periosteum ensures

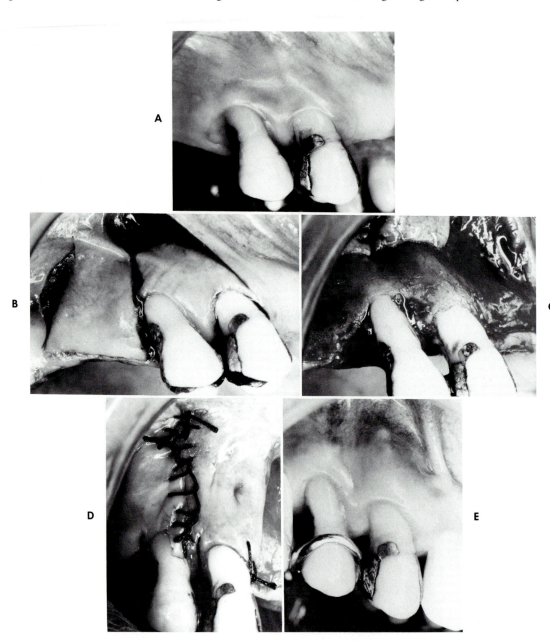

Fig. 26-67. Double edentulous area pedicle grafts for maxillary premolars. **A,** Absence of gingiva on maxillary premolars. **B,** V-shaped incision includes marginal tissue of both teeth. Note incision outline of distal pedicle donor site. **C,** Connective tissue bed is prepared. **D,** Mesial and distal pedicle grafts are sutured with vertical continuous locked suturing. **E,** Eighteen-month postsurgical result.

the nonexistence of these defects, the periosteum can be reflected. If a dehiscence or fenestration is suspected, osteoplasty may be performed through the soft tissue, avoiding the radicular surface of the alveolar process.

Proper atraumatic surgical technique in transplantation. After osteoplasty (Fig. 26-66, *E*) only the osseous tissue requiring contouring has been exposed. The pedicle graft is easily positioned over the mesial root of the first molar,

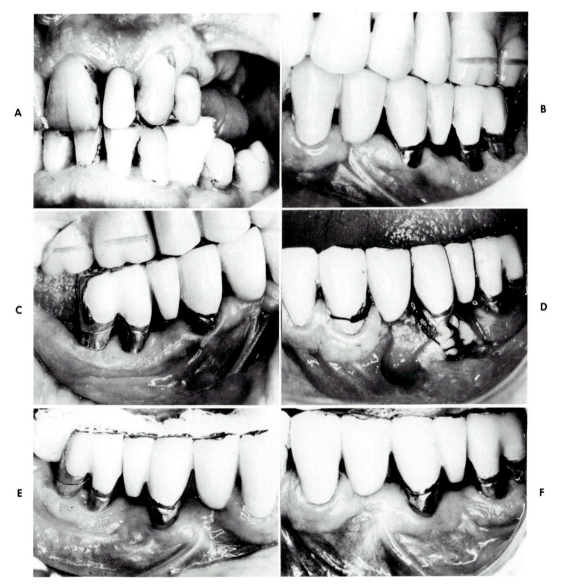

Fig. 26-68. Double pedicle grafts to repair gingival attachments involving restorative dentistry. **A,** Initial view of mandibular left second premolar illustrating adequate functional gingival attachment. **B,** Following restorative dentistry, gingival attachment is not present and vestibular fornix movement retracts gingival margin. Alveolar mucosal margin can be probed to 2 mm. **C,** Effect of frenum pull in area of second premolar further supports retraction of alveolar mucosal margin with extension of frenum to this margin (mirror view). **D,** Partial-thickness pedicle grafts taken from adjacent edentulous area supply donor tissue to eliminate muscle pull and restore healthy gingival attachment. **E,** Successful pedicle graft procedure with six-month result (mirror view). **F,** One year result. Creeping of gingival attachment coronally can be seen. Probe extends 1 mm into crevice. (Restorative dentistry by Herman Press, Fairless Hills, Pa.)

replacing the mucosal wedge of tissue at the recipient site. Note that the free edge of the graft is to be located at the alveolar margin. The flap is not twisted or under tension if the cutback incision has been adequate.

The pedicle graft and the apically positioned flap are approximated as shown in Fig. 26-66, *F*. No. 4-0 black silk suture with a reverse cutting needle (Atraloc, Ethicon, Inc., New Brunswick, N.J.) is used. This needle avoids tearing the deli-

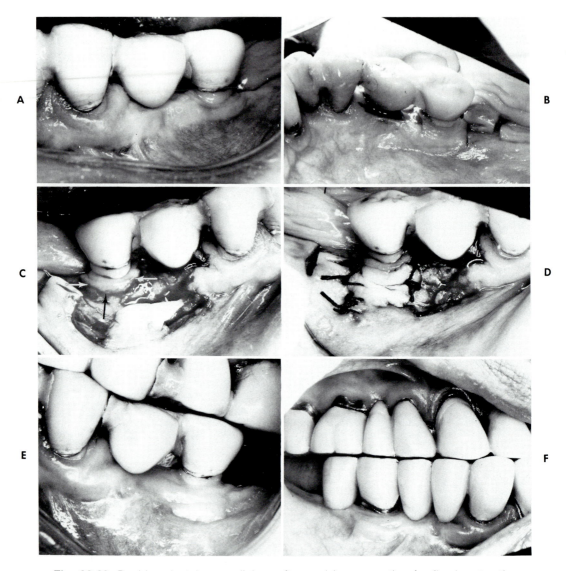

Fig. 26-69. Double edentulous pedicle grafts used in preparation for fixed restorative dentistry. **A,** Provisional splint in place. Inadequate functional gingival attachment on mandibular second premolar. **B,** Pedicle grafts taken from lingual edentulous areas to increase linear length of pedicle grafts that will be utilized at recipient site. **C,** Remaining gingival attachment of second premolar was not disturbed *(arrow)*. Incision was directed just coronal to mucogingival junction with a bevel sufficient to adapt double pedicle grafts on radicular surface of second premolar. **D,** Mesial pedicle graft provides bulk of gingiva positioned at retained gingival collar. Distal pedicle graft increases edentulous pontic area and vestibular depth so that vestibular depth can be blended with anterior area (mirrow view). **E,** Thirty-day repair of double pedicle grafts demonstrates increase of gingival width in premolar area and the creation of a masticatory base for future cantilevered pontic. **F,** Six months later. Adequate gingival attachment in second premolar area has been accomplished. No gingivoplasty has yet been performed (mirror view). (Restorative dentistry by Stanley Lipkowitz, Fairless Hills, Pa.)

cate tissues. The pedicle graft and the apically positioned flap are sutured at the furcation. The flap is sutured to the fixed tissue of the second molar. Hemorrhage must be under complete control at the completion of the procedure. Light

pressure adapts the pedicle graft to the recipient site so that no dead space develops where blood can accumulate. This prevents an unfavorable response. The position of the graft must be stabilized by the suturing technique, and periosteal

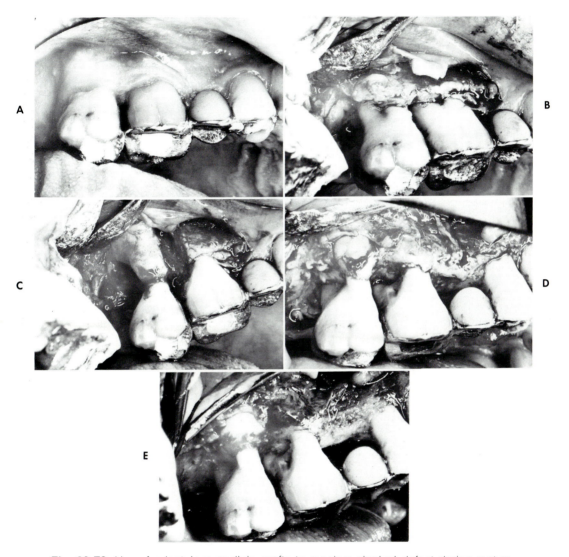

Fig. 26-70. Use of edentulous pedicle grafts to repair a gingival defect during root resections. **A,** Pretreatment view of maxillary left first and second molar-subsequent to endodontic treatment and in preparation for distobuccal root resections of both teeth (mirror view). **B,** Partial-thickness mucogingival flap is elevated. Distal osseous defect is exposed on second molar. Distobuccal root of first molar is in close proximity to second molar mesiobuccal root. Explorer can enter buccal furcae. **C,** Removal of distobuccal roots expedited by removal of buccal plates, enabling access to distal alveolar crest on mesiobuccal roots. Partial-thickness dissection protects these roots. **D,** Nine-month reentry procedure allows for complete repair of buccal alveolus. Some correction of defects on distal aspect of mesiobuccal roots of both molars. Reverse osseus architecture on mesiobuccal radicular roots requires correction. **E,** Osseous correction completed. Craters in edentulous and tuberosity areas eliminated. Utilization of pedicle graft from mesial edentulous area to first molar will replace gingival unit on mesiobuccal of first molar.

Continued.

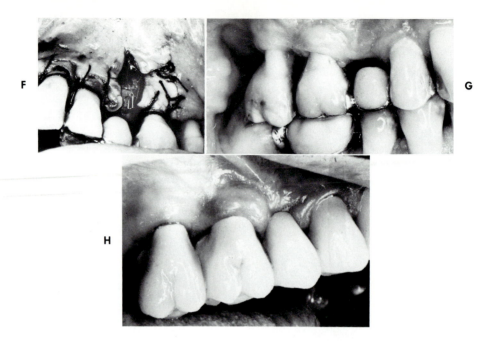

Fig. 26-70, cont'd. F, Pedicle graft from edentulous area supplies attached gingiva for mesiobuccal root of first molar. Individual sutures coapt pedicle graft with main flap. A cutback incision passively positions pedicle so that margin is horizontal to alveolar crest and is coronal to it on root. **G,** Healed area after distobuccal root resections and pedicle graft. Six-month postoperative mirror view. **H,** Eighteen months after surgery. Ceramco fixed bridge in position with pedicle grafts serving as attached gingival unit. Design of molar crowns permits easy access for bacterial plaque control. (mirror view). (Restorative dentistry by Daniel Isaacson, University of Pennsylvania School of Dental Medicine.)

sutures may be required (Kramer et al., 1970). It must be immobilized at the recipient area without undue tension or torsion on the pedicle. The periodontal dressing properly placed and set aids in this objective (Fig. 26-67).

Postsurgical pain is mild. The sutures are removed and the dressing changed in 10 days. By the third or fourth week healing has usually progressed sufficiently so that no further dressing is necessary.

The use of edentulous area pedicle grafts broadens the surgical design selection to repair gingival units and protect the marginal environment after restorative dentistry (Fig. 26-68). After periodontal surgery the resultant attached gingiva may be too minimal to risk detachment caused by restorative procedures. The edentulous pedicle grafts are successful in widening the zone of attached gingiva when approximated to the retained minimal gingival collars (Fig. 26-69). Frequently advanced periodontal therapy requires the resection of distobuccal roots and the restoration of the gingival unit prior to fixed prosthesis (Fig.

26-70). These delicate grafts are easily handled and sutured with specially designed notched surgical pliers, which are perforated so that suture material can be passed through the tissue held with this instrument.

Donor tissue may be needed as a graft for an anterior and a posterior tooth adjacent to an edentulous area. If the width of the donor site is insufficient to supply gingiva to both teeth at the same time (Fig. 26-71), the reserve of tissue on the ridge may be used again following healing and tissue maturation.

OBLIQUE ROTATED GRAFT (Pennel et al., 1965)

INDICATIONS

1. To increase the width of attached gingiva while retaining the gingival margin of tissue (Fig. 26-72)
2. To increase the width of attached gingiva along with pocket elimination (Fig. 26-73)

PRECAUTIONS. Although this procedure is indicated when a shallow vestibular fornix is present, there must be sufficient width and height to the

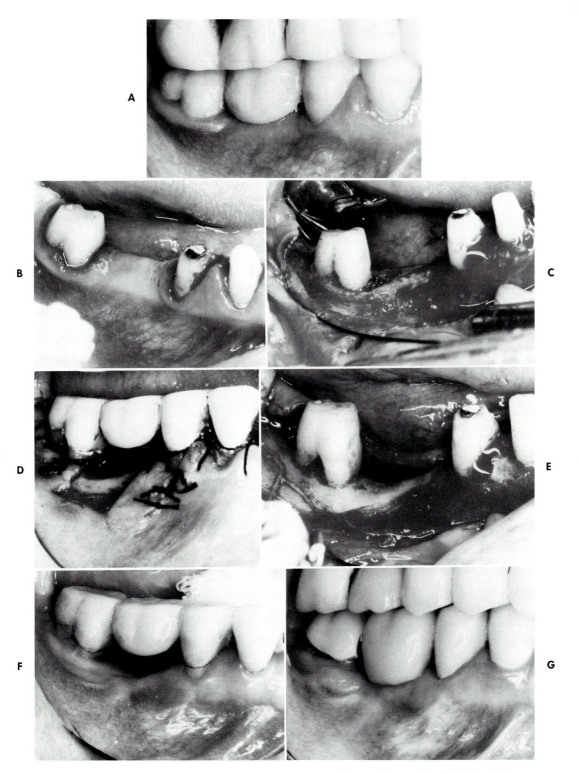

Fig. 26-71. Single donor site for edentulous area double pedicle grafts. **A,** Minimal gingiva on mandibular second premolar and molar. **B,** Removal of provisional splint prior to surgery. **C,** Mesial infrabony defect. **D,** Osteoplasty. **E,** Pedicle grafts from edentulous area sutured on radicular surface of molar and premolar. **F,** Healing 2 months later. **G,** Periodontal maintenance visit 2 years later. (In conjunction with Manuel H. Marks, Levittown, Pa., and Leonard Abrams, Philadelphia, Pa.)

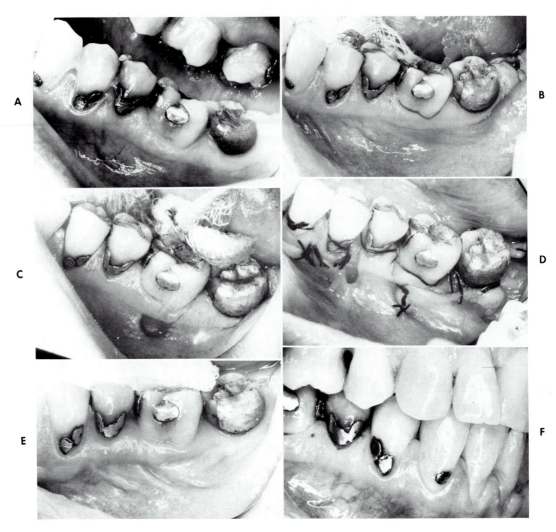

Fig. 26-72. Oblique rotated papilla grafts restore lost gingival attachments. **A,** Pockets extend beyond mucogingival junction on buccal aspect of canine and first premolar and distal root of first molar (mirror view, right side). **B,** Entire retromolar area prepared for elevation by incision along lingual aspect of retromolar pad and approximately 10 mm distal to terminal molar. Partial-thickness dissection prepares thin mucogingival retromolar area (mirror view). **C,** Gingival collar covering distal root of mandibular first molar left intact. Triangular area of alveolar mucosa is excised apical to it. A fine oblique incision along distal line angle of first molar connects with entire papilla. This will be used to replace alveolar mucosa (mirror view). **D,** Entire flap (from papilla between two molars, gingival margin of second molar, and retromolar area masticatory mucosa) is used. Allows oblique rotated papilla to gain gingiva over distal root of first molar. Retromolar gingiva increases gingival width of second molar. A suspensory suture supports distal portion of flap. Interrupted sutures coapt mesial portion of flap. **E,** Six-month response shows functional gingiva restored to molar teeth. No gingivoplasty performed. **F,** Presurgical view of canine and first premolar area that lacks adequate attached gingiva. Probe extends 2 mm through each mucogingival junction.

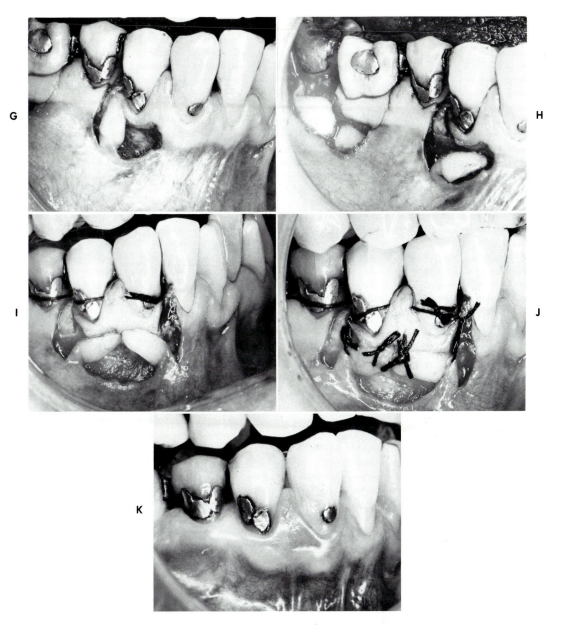

Fig. 26-72, cont'd. G, Papilla distal to first premolar prepared by partial-thickness dissection. Incision initiating slightly coronal to mucogingival junction prepares recipient bed. Loose connective tissue fibers have been removed. Immovable connective tissue bed remains. **H,** Partial-thickness papilla has been rotated to recipient site on first premolar. Partial-thickness flap involving papilla between first and second molars has been elevated. **I,** Partial-thickness dissection allows mesial papilla to cover recipient site for deficient attached gingiva of right canine. Free gingival collars preserved on both teeth. Oblique rotation of these papillae will increase gingival dimension. **J,** Rotated papillae are sutured in their correct position; free gingiva are contacted with interrupted sutures. **K,** Eight months later repaired rotated papilla grafts are viewed. Base of crevice does not approach mucogingival junction.

interdental papillae for use as a rotated graft. Pennel et al. (1965) described these circumstances: "Gingival clefts or denuded root surfaces involving two adjacent teeth present a special situation that often requires some form of mucogingival surgery. Deformities of this type are most frequently located in the mandibular anterior region involving the labial periodontium of the central incisors. The lesion is characterized by gingival recession, little or no attached gingiva, a shallow vestibule, and chronic marginal inflammation. This may be further complicated by the presence of periodontal pockets and an aberrant frenal attachment." Successful management of this type of deformity can be achieved by utilizing an oblique rotating flap operation, which is a modification of the horizontally positioned graft.

Surgical technique. After initial treatment Pennel et al. (1965) state that the incisions are made into the attached gingiva and alveolar mucosa lateral to the lesion. The flaps (papillae) are elevated by using sharp dissection. The periosteum and some connective tissue are retained intentionally over the bone. This will reduce the amount of crestal bone lost from the donor site. If the labial bone is prominent, careful dissection also is necessary to prevent perforating tissue at the mucogingival junction.

A horizontal incision is made coronal to the free gingival margin of the recipient area so that free gingiva, alveolar mucosa, or both can be separated from the underlying periosteum by sharp dissection. As separation occurs the alveolar mucosa draws apically and exposes a zone of periosteum sufficient in size to receive the

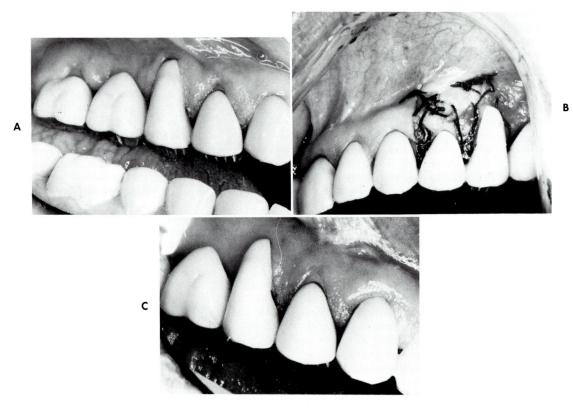

Fig. 26-73. Oblique rotated flap used to form a double papilla positioned flap and edentulous area pedicle graft for correction of shallow vestibular fornix and absence of gingiva. Procedure planned in preparation for restorative dentistry. **A,** Toothbrush abrasion and root caries caused severe recession on maxillary second premolar and recession on first premolar. Pockets extend beyond mucogingival junction. **B,** Double papilla–type flap procedures used to replace gingiva on first premolar. Edentulous pedicle graft deepens vestibule in area of pontic and second premolar. Interdental papilla distal to first premolar is incised. Anterior two thirds can be rotated obliquely to form a double papilla. Posterior third provides gradual apical transition with edentulous area pedicle graft. **C,** Four months after surgery. Increase in gingival attachment and vestibular depth sustained. Fixed restorative dentistry to be completed. (In conjunction with Leonard Juros, Willingboro, N.J.)

flaps. All the loose connective tissue and muscle fibers must be removed to prepare a rigid base for the flaps; otherwise the resultant attached gingiva will be mobile.

The two flaps of mature gingiva are rotated distally or mesially as required and moved apically into a horizontal position. The edges of the flaps are approximated and sutured to each other and to the underlying tissue. Occasionally minor trimming is necessary to improve the approximation. This positions attached gingiva over the exposed marginal periosteum that was previously covered by alveolar mucosa.

Difficulty in placing and suturing the flaps is decreased by the selection of adequate widths of tissue to manipulate because the flap size decreases when reflected. The use of atraumatic needles aids in decreasing the incidence of tissue margin tear.

This graft technique is versatile and can be adapted in all areas of the mouth. If there is ade-

quate vestibular depth the gingival collar can be left undisturbed. The oblique rotated papillae can be approximated apical to these margins to increase the attached gingiva (Fig. 26-73). The oblique rotated papillae graft can be combined with multiple interdental papillae grafts, particularly when the gingival margin is retained intact (Fig. 26-74).

In a localized area involving the maxillary left premolars, a single papilla is obliquely rotated and sutured to an apically and laterally positioned papilla (double papillae approach). The second molar was treated by an obliquely rotated edentulous pedicle graft.

DOUBLE PAPILLA GRAFT (Cohen, 1964; Cohen and Ross, 1968)

INDICATIONS
1. To increase width of attached gingiva with or without *interproximal pocket elimination* (Fig. 26-73)

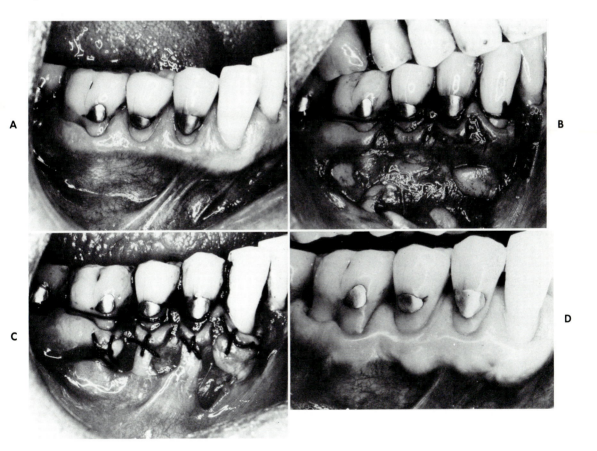

Fig. 26-74. Oblique rotated papilla grafts combined with multiple interdental papilla grafts. **A,** Pockets extend beyond mucogingival junction from mesial aspect of molar to canine. **B,** Partial-thickness dissection of recipient bed. Interdental papillae are retained as part of graft. Gingival collars are retained. **C,** Oblique rotated grafts on molar and canine. Interdental papillae increased width of attached gingiva on premolars. **D,** Three-year result.

2. To increase width of attached gingiva while retaining gingival margin of tissue (Fig. 26-74)
3. To provide sufficient width to pedicle graft donor tissue to minimize exposure of underlying periodontium (Fig. 26-74)
4. To eliminate frenum pull upon marginal tissues (Fig. 26-73)

PRECAUTIONS
1. Sufficient vertical height to alveolar profile must be created by partial-thickness dissection to permit crestal coverage by this graft.
2. Elevation and mobilization of graft must allow passive positioning at recipient site. Any tensional positioning will cause subsequent retraction of graft.

The use of the double papilla graft provides an additional dimension to the sources of gingival tissue available for correcting inadequate gingival attachments. The interdental tissues are most frequently masticatory gingiva, therefore providing a consistent donor source for these grafts. This approach is used in conjunction with other procedures in this chapter.

The interdental crestal bone height is not permanently affected by this approach, adding safety to the technique. The interdental septa of bone is thicker than the radicular bone, lessening the chance for a defect to occur at the donor site. The availability of a greater amount of interdental gingiva (in comparison to that of buccal and labial surfaces of the teeth) encourages the selection of this donor tissue.

The objective in this procedure is not the aesthetic and anatomic correction of a denuded root but the reconstruction of the gingival tissue, thus restoring function and preventing further mucogingival complications in the area.

The technique, when used to increase only the width of attached gingiva without attempting root coverage, differs from its original design (Cohen, 1964; Cohen and Ross, 1968). There is very little risk of failure. Predictability of success is observed when the technique is performed on the lingual surface (Fig. 26-97).

In preparation of the donor site and recipient site and in mobilization of the graft at the recipient site, the basic surgical discipline is similar to those used in other pedicle grafts. The two papillae are ''lapped'' upon each other at the midradicular location when covering a denuded root. This is not necessary when the two papillae are placed on a previously prepared connective tissue bed. Instead the tissues are approximated as a butt joint and are sutured at the midradicular area of the alveolus. To obtain sufficient width to the double papilla, the initial incision is horizontal within the papilla. When both flaps are joined in this manner, a wide linear gingival margin is created. This margin can be positioned coronal to the crest or can be placed submarginally to a retained gingival collar (Fig. 26-74). A further advantage to this approach is that interdental pocket elimination in no way interferes with the grafting objectives.

Reconstruction of anatomic deformities and gingival clefts

LATERALLY POSITIONED GRAFT (Corn, 1968; Grupe, 1966; Grupe and Warren, 1956; Staffileno, 1964)

INDICATIONS
Indications include aesthetic and functional correction of the following gingival clefts and recession:
1. Those where the zone of attached gingiva is almost obliterated
2. Those with deep periodontal pockets that require surgical elimination or that traverse the zone of attached gingiva and terminate in the zone of alveolar mucosa
3. Those with deep periodontal pockets that require surgical elimination and not only extend beyond the mucogingival junction but also are in an area with a shallow vestibular trough
4. Those with associated aberrant frena and muscle attachments at or near the gingival margins or into the soft tissue wall of a periodontal pocket

PRECAUTIONS
1. Shallow clinical sulcus depth should be present interproximally adjacent to the facial surface of the root to be grafted.
2. The crest of the interproximal bone should have normal or near-normal relationship to the cementoenamel junction.
3. Only minimal cervical erosion or abrasion is acceptable.
4. No lingual or palatal pockets should be present.
5. Root prominence must be reduced within the plane of the adjacent alveolar process. However, root planing should not be excessive.

Reconstructive procedures in mucogingival surgery were introduced by Grupe and Warren in 1956 when they described their pedicle grafting procedure. Initially these techniques were designed to relocate gingiva from a donor site in close proximity to an isolated defect. Many modifications of this basic approach have been developed and have become more sophisticated as our knowledge of tissue response and wound healing has increased.

The laterally positioned graft has been referred to as the "sliding flap operation." It has been used in treating a single denuded tooth that has an adjacent gingival area that can serve as a donor site. It may be the only receded area in the dentition, and it is more frequently found on the buccal and labial surfaces than on the lingual surface. The gingival margin, which consists of alveolar mucosa, becomes retracted from the lodgment of food because all the attached gingiva usually is lost.

Grupe and Warren (1956) have advocated the repair of these gingival defects by a sliding flap operation. The results of their procedure as outlined have not been totally satisfactory because (1) marginal changes at the donor site have resulted in recession in this area, (2) the radicular bone when left exposed at the donor site has resulted in osseous resorption with an anatomic deformity, (3) incompletely described technical details have resulted in less than optimal results in the level of gingival attachment at the recipient site, (4) the frenum involvement associated with a cleft has necessitated careful maneuvering, and (5) confusion has occurred in the incisional design to compensate for a cleft with a contiguous shallow vestibular fornix. The mode of healing is not clear because of the lack of human histologic material repaired with this technique.

It has been speculated that the cut gingival fibers of the donor tissue become reinserted into the new cementum formed at the recipient site when healing occurs. Most likely the attachment of the flap on the tooth consists of tissue proliferating from the exposed periodontal ligament and connective tissue of the flap. Sullivan et al. (1971 a and b) have reported on human wound healing of the laterally positioned flap, observing a connective tissue attachment to the root of the tooth, although primarily there is a long epithelial attachment.

A pilot study by Pfeifer and Heller (1971) shows that in a partial-thickness laterally positioned flap a close epithelial adaptation to the root surface is present, but there is no connective tissue attachment. Further research is necessary. Care in the design of the lateral flap must be emphasized. If marginal sulcular epithelium is a part of the relocated flap, the long epithelial attachment would be expected. An attempt should be made to place the margin of the flap on the enamel so that the connective tissue portion of the flap can be approximated to the cementoenamel junction.

Corn (1973) and Staffileno (1964) have detailed a modification of the laterally or horizontally positioned flap, raising a partial-thickness flap via sharp dissection and leaving periosteum and connective tissue on the alveolar process of the donor site. The versatility of this approach is consistent with current wound healing principles.

On the other hand, Goldman and Smukler (1978) have observed that clinically, full-thickness flaps, including a stimulated periosteum and flaps with new bone that has formed, are better attached to the root surfaces than partial-thickness flaps. The grafts are thicker, and the sulcular area cannot be probed to any degree even with a thin stainless steel strip.

The pedicle graft is based on the transposition of a full periosteal flap previously stimulated over a denuded root and prepared to receive the graft. Root surface preparation, in light of present-day knowledge, requires the careful cleansing of plaque from the tooth surface and tooth structure, which has been altered by inflammatory exudates, bacteria from plaque, and oral fluids. Another important factor is the exposed periodontal ligament resulting from the lateral incisions made around the denuded portion extending to the alveolar bone. This exposure liberates reparative tissues from the periodontal ligament, which is capable of migrating over the root surface. Periosteal tissue is included in the pedicle graft, and this tissue may also participate in the formation of an attachment to the tooth surface. This periosteal tissue in the donor area is stimulated 17 to 24 days before operation. Research has shown that numerous osteoblasts and new bone formation are present on the surface of the pedicle.

Preoperative considerations

Elimination or control of etiologic factors. The etiologic factors must be controlled or eliminated before the laterally positioned graft procedure can be considered (Fig. 26-75).

Determination of extent of tissue destruction (hard and soft). If too much support has been lost on all other surfaces of the tooth, a graft may not be warranted. A key consideration in the choice of a graft is whether the height of bone interproximally can be properly related to the

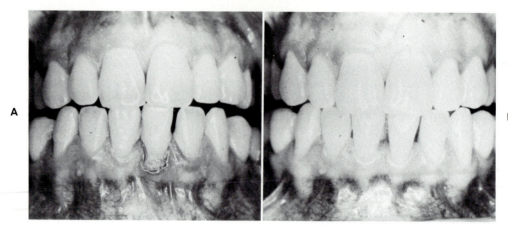

Fig. 26-75. Gingival cleft. No surgery was performed. This was a case of unusual creeping attachment. **A,** Gingival cleft almost obliterates zone of attached gingiva on mandibular left central incisor. **B,** Ten-year result. Root scaling and root planing removed all local etiologic factors. Creeping attachment has occurred. Sulcular depth is 1 mm (From Corn, H. C.: Dent. Clin. North Am., p. 79, March 1964.)

cementoenamel junction so that the graft can attach at that location.

Position of tooth. The position of the tooth should allow the greatest curvature of the root to be within the boundaries of the alveolar housing. Hiatt (1966) has stated that a tooth in too prominent a position in the arch has less chance for a successful graft when draped in this position. The root should be planed judiciously so that the radicular surface is within the alveolar border.

Stabilization of mobile tooth. When the mobility of the tooth is too great the prognosis is poor.

Availability of sufficient donor tissue. Enough tissue must be available for relocation on the cemental surface of the recipient site. The procedure should not be contemplated if there is an absence of adjacent gingiva either interproximally

or on the radicular surface. When gingiva is available, it must be a healthy gingival unit with minimal sulcular depth. If inflammation with minimal depth is present, prescaling should correct the condition in preparation for surgery. The apicocoronal width of the gingiva should be adequate and fairly thick. Although gingiva with sufficient thickness is preferable since it is easier to dissect and manipulate, thin gingiva may be used in preparation for a partial-thickness flap. Greater care is necessary to avoid soft tissue perforations.

Preferability of donor site with normal alveolar height and radicular bone thickness. When there is a choice as to the selection of one donor site over another, the one with the suspected best alveolar support should be chosen. In Fig. 26-76 all the teeth were prominently positioned in the

Fig. 26-76. Laterally positioned graft with adequate vestibular fornix. **A,** Preoperative view. Gingival recession on mandibular right central incisor. Teeth in prominent position in arch. Gingiva is thin. **B,** Results after 6 months of periodontal maintenance. Periodic root scaling and root planing have not increased gingival dimension. Note washboard effect of alveolar process after resolution of inflammation. **C,** Partial-thickness laterally positioned flap procedure performed. Tissue at donor site (including labial half of interproximal papillae) raised. Connective tissue and periosteum cover bone. Distal oblique incision at mesial side of canine avoids greater convexity of root but enters alveolar mucosa in angular direction, creating a base wider than margin. V-shaped incision can be seen at recipient site. Note connective tissue mesial margin on right central incisor prepared to receive graft. **D,** Graft sutured on enamel below height of contour coronal to cementoenamel junction. **E,** Appearance of tissue at suture removal 14 days later. Graft appears successful. **F,** Five-year result. Probe reveals minimal sulcular depth. Note wrinkling of tissue under pressure. **G,** Appearance of graft at 5-year recall visit. **H,** Appearance after 9 years.

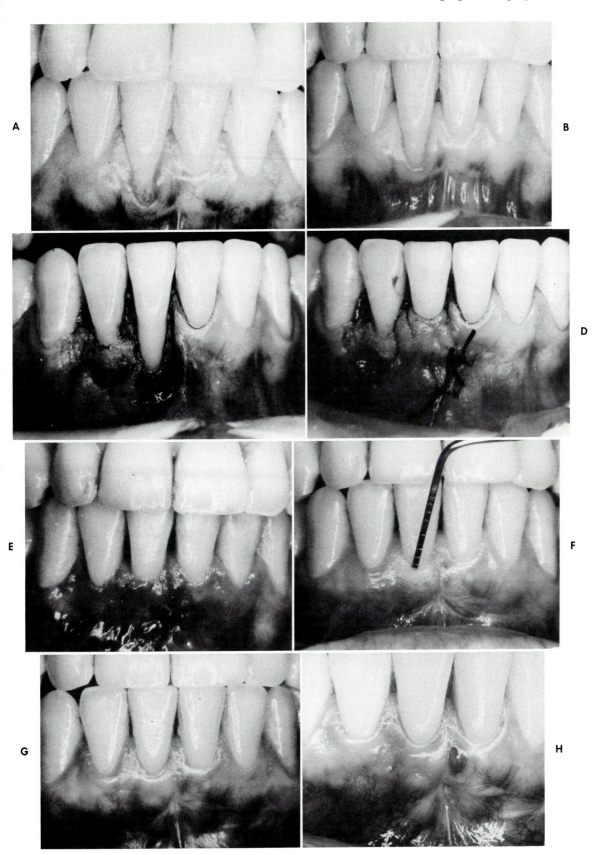

Fig. 26-76. For legend see opposite page.

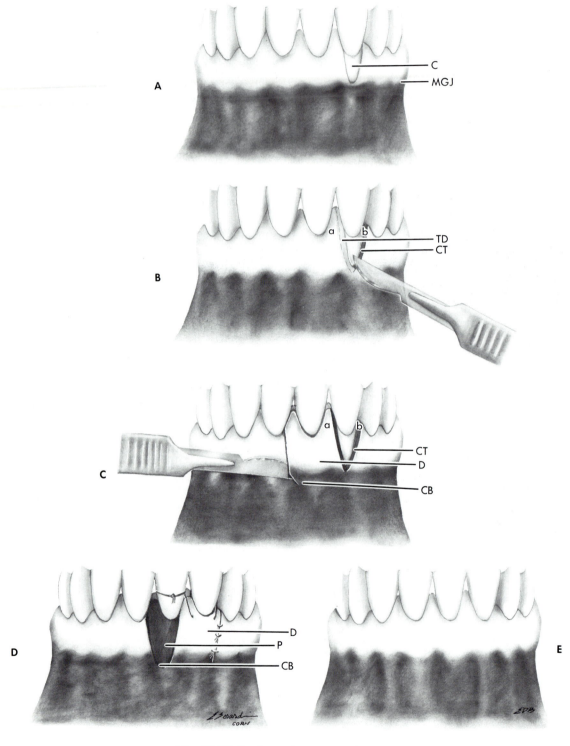

Fig. 26-77. For legend see opposite page.

arch and minimal radicular bone (if any) was present. However, by employing the partial-thickness flap design, the connective tissue attachment to the tooth and bone remained intact. A successful attachment of the graft to the recipient tooth occurred. Concern for a thin alveolar process is reduced by using a partial-thickness flap design. When a dehiscence or a fenestration is present, the use of a full-thickness flap will invite failure. One defect is exchanged for another.

Preparation of recipient site

Initial preparation. A disease control program is successfully completed and the patient is able to demonstrate continued plaque control on a sustained reinforced basis. Prior to surgery, prescaling and root planing remove local irritants. Frequently a cleft almost obliterates the zone of attached gingiva. Creeping attachment occurs during repair, and surgery is no longer necessary (Goldman et al., 1964). The value of initial preparation cannot be overemphasized (Fig. 26-71).

V-shaped incision. The V-shaped incision into the soft tissue adjacent to the cleft provides a narrow fresh soft tissue wound (Fig. 26-77). There are three local environmental factors that modify the design of the initial V-shaped incision.

1. Deep periodontal pockets extending into the mucosa, in the presence of an adequate vestibular fornix, permit the apex of the V-shaped incision to terminate on the midradicular surface of the tooth at the level of the alveolar margin (Fig. 26-76).

2. Associated frena involvements require that the V-shaped incision be modified to include the entire frenum, even if the extension of the incisions goes into the labial side of the vestibule (Fig. 26-78). If a frenum causes retraction and recession of the gingival margin, there are occasions when reattachment occurs following scaling and root planing procedures. Under these circumstances the V-shaped incision can be made apical to the free gingival margin (Fig. 26-79).

3. Deep periodontal pockets extending into the mucosa in the presence of a shallow vestibular fornix require that the V-shaped incision enter the shallow fornix, incising the musculature until the osseous structures are in contact. The subsequent preparation of this site and the donor site are more involved here. To prepare a proper recipient bed the operator must strip away the muscle fibers from both these sites to develop a smooth rise to the alveolar process side of the wound (Fig. 26-59). The portion of the V-shaped incision that is most distant from the donor tissue should include at least half the interproximal papillae. The graft, when positioned at the recipient site, will thus have a broader connective tissue base upon which to repair (Fig. 26-58, *C*). The remaining portion of the papilla is left undisturbed. If the graft just covers the root structure defect, it may separate at this junction, and an angular cleft may recur.

Root and osseous preparation. All the granulation tissue and soft tissue within the borders of the V-shaped incision are removed, exposing the osseous support to the tooth. Any osseous defects are corrected. The root of the tooth is planed until smooth. All the soft structures are removed, particularly at the cementoenamel junction. If the tooth is in a prominent position in

---

Fig. 26-77. Laterally positioned graft. **A,** Preoperative view. Severe gingival recession with cleft, *C*, extending into alveolar mucosa of mandibular left lateral incisor. Gingiva is inadequate for a laterally positioned graft. There is adequate depth to vestibular fornix. Prescaling was performed. *MGJ,* mucogingival junction. **B,** V-shaped incision into soft tissue adjacent to cleft provides fresh soft tissue wound, *CT.* Tissue to be discarded, *TD,* at donor site outlined. Incision terminates on midradicular area of alveolar process at base of pocket, exposing periosteum. All granulation tissue was removed, and root carefully planed. Width of papilla at *a* should fit at *b.* **C,** At donor site, *D,* width of graft should be one and one-half times measurement of defect. Oblique incision and scalloped marginal incision are connected. Direction of scalpel changes when instrument is inserted into oblique incision remote from recipient wound. There is dissection in apicocoronal direction. To avoid tension on partial-thickness graft, cutback incision, *CB,* may be necessary. Papilla at *a* will cover connective tissue, *CT,* at *b.* **D,** Laterally positioned graft, *D,* placed on enamel below height of contour coronal to cementoenamel junction. Suturing on labial aspect of central incisor prevents graft from slipping apically. Precise dissection provides donor bed covered with connective tissue and periosteum, *P,* protecting underlying highly reactive radicular bone. **E,** Repair of recession with combination of connective and epithelial tissue attachment to root.

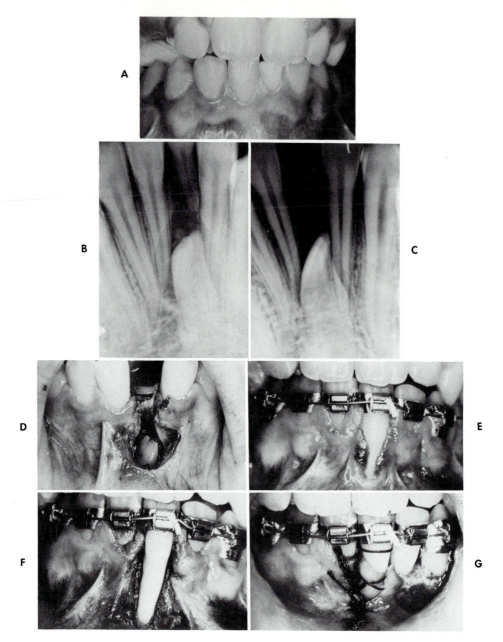

Fig. 26-78. Laterally positioned graft with aberrant frena. **A,** A 9-year-old boy with retained deciduous left central incisor. **B,** Preoperative radiograph of retained deciduous incisor and impacted permanent incisor. **C,** Orthodontist extracts deciduous tooth and utilizes space maintainer. One year later tooth has erupted slowly. **D,** Opening in alveolar process to enable orthodontist to place band on lateral incisor and bring tooth into proper position. Incisor is in vestibular area, not under crest of ridge. **E,** Orthodontic treatment completed when boy was 12 years old. Apparently oral surgery that was necessary to expose tooth destroyed alveolar process. Note double frena adjacent to severe gingival cleft. **F,** Oblique incisions extend into mucosa to include frena. Granulation tissue has been removed. Tooth has been root planed. **G,** Partial-thickness graft placed on enamel of central incisor just below height of contour. Sutures firmly coapt graft to fixed tissue at midline. Graft has been moved great distance. Cutback incision is necessary to relieve tension on tissue. **H,** One year following surgery. Note slight recession exposing root and minimal pocket depth. Gingival form and contour are greatly improved. Orthodontic retention period was extended to permit stability to mandibular anterior segment. Five-year appearance is essentially the same. **I,** Nine-year appearance. (In conjunction with Irving Kraut, Trenton, N.J.)

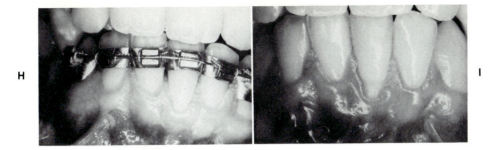

Fig. 26-78, cont'd. For legend see opposite page.

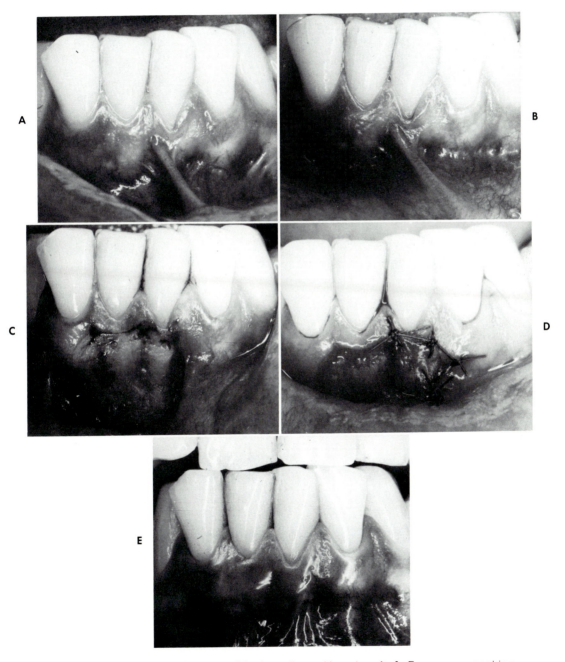

Fig. 26-79. Correction of frenum pull by laterally positioned graft. **A,** Frenum encroaching upon free gingiva. Retraction of gingiva allows calculus and plaque accumulation. **B,** Close-up. **C,** Excision of frenum and dissection of donor tissue, leaving collar of gingiva on both central incisors. **D,** Graft sutured in place. **E,** Nine months later.

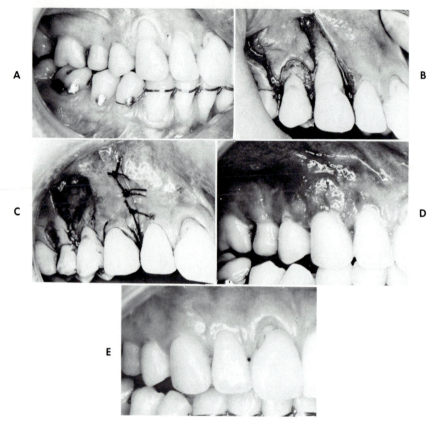

Fig. 26-80. Laterally positioned graft on maxillary anterior teeth demonstrating cutback incision. **A,** Preoperative view. Severe cleft on maxillary right canine. Tooth is in prominent position in arch. Note caries on mesiolabial line angle at cementoenamel junction. **B,** Partial-thickness flap raised. Note V-shaped preparation of recipient site. Root surface planed to try to bring it within confines of alveolar housing. Graft cannot be moved distance required without tension. Cutback incision is made in direction that graft is moved *(arrow).* **C,** Graft sutured on enamel. Cutback incision allows great mobility of graft as seen by size of donor bed. Alveolar process at donor bed protected by connective tissue and periosteum over radicular surface of first premolar. **D,** Ten-day postoperative appearance of graft is suggestive of soft tissue attachment to canine root. Careless dressing replacement invites failure. **E,** Repair of defect after 6 months.

the arch, it is root planed to reduce this prominence to within the boundaries of the alveolar housing. However, the root should not be excessively planed (Fig. 26-80).

Aesthetically the success of a lateral positioned graft is dependent upon the anatomy of the radicular root surface following root planing and the level of the interproximal crestal bone height. If the interdental alveolar crest is normal in its relationship to the cementoenamel junction, the gingival margin of the graft will remain on the enamel above the cementoenamel junction (Fig. 26-76). However, if the interproximal bone loss is significant, the attachment of the graft to the tooth will be dictated by this relationship (Fig. 26-81).

Preparation of donor site
Design of the graft

1. The width of the donor tissue should be at least one and one-half times the measurement of the defect to allow sufficient connective tissue support for the graft. Greater connective tissue bed support is required when there is greater width of the denuded root mesiodistally. A wider graft placed on a larger connective tissue surface offers the best opportunity for attachment (Fig. 26-82). The epithelium is removed from the distal margin of the recipient bed to provide this greater surface area.

2. An oblique incision is made at the line

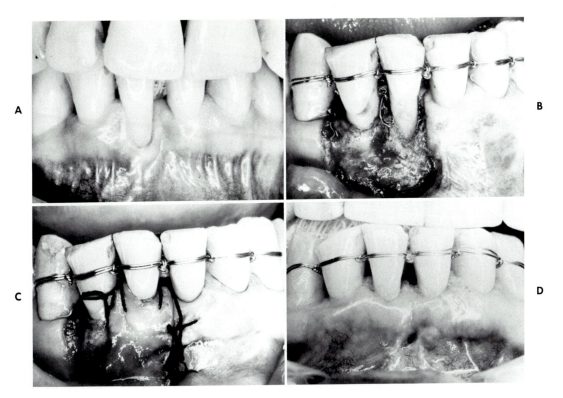

Fig. 26-81. Interdental bone loss limits reconstruction of gingiva. **A,** Recession on right central incisor complicated by a cleft and a frenum involvement. Interproximal bone loss limits level to which laterally positioned graft can be placed. **B,** Preparation of recipient bed. **C,** Laterally positioned graft in position. **D,** Maximum coronal level of gingiva that can be expected after 1 year.

angle of the distal extremity of the donor flap. The incision should not encroach upon the gingival margin of the greater convexity of the involved tooth. The incision extends into the alveolar mucosa and should outline a graft that is wider at its base than at its margin.

3. A Bard-Parker no. 15 scalpel should dissect carefully the interproximal papilla from its lingual portion.

4. A scalloped marginal incision into the gingival margin includes the tips of the papillae and connects with the oblique incisions (Fig. 26-76).

5. The direction of the scalpel blade is changed when the instrument is inserted into the oblique incision remote from the recipient wound (Fig. 26-77). While dissecting close to the periosteum in an apicocoronal direction, the operator directs the blade to the gingival margin, creating a partial-thickness mucogingival flap. The dissection is directed to the most coronally attached gingival fiber, therefore not affecting the level of the connective tissue attachment.

Mobilization of graft

1. The flap is gently raised from its underlying attachment. If there is adequate depth to the vestibule, usually there is no problem in mobilizing the flap toward its recipient site. This allows a uniform smoothness and contour of the alveolar process side of the wound. It also eliminates resistance to the proper adaptation of the laterally positioned flap at its new recipient site.

2. The flap should be so mobile that it can be positioned at its new location without tension. The extremities of the flap should rest passively on a connective tissue base.

3. If there is tension on the flap (as it is tested at the recipient site) a cutback incision will offer additional mobility to the graft (Fig. 26-80).

Remaining donor bed. Precise dissection of the partial-thickness mucogingival flap provides a donor bed that is covered with connective tissue

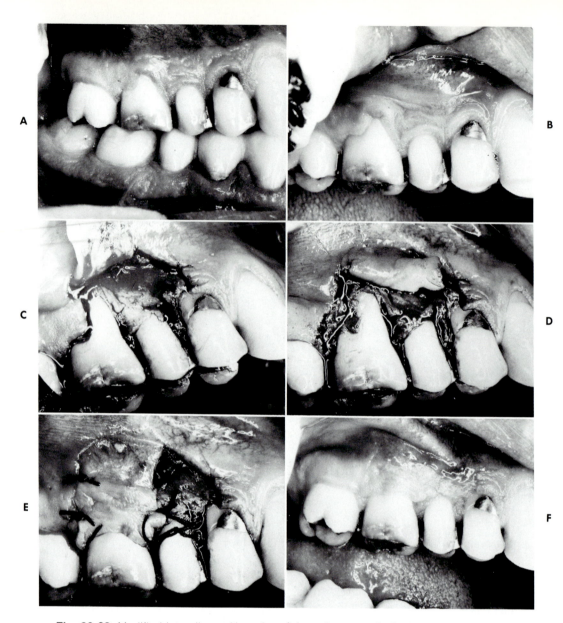

Fig. 26-82. Modified laterally positioned graft in molar area. **A,** Gingival cleft present on mesiobuccal root of maxillary right first molar. Minimum zone of attached gingiva is present. Probe just approaches mucogingival junction. **B,** Two years after holding period pocket depth extends beyond mucogingival junction. Two radiating clefts are present. **C,** Partial-thickness flap elevated over donor premolar site. Dissection leaves crevicular epithelium attached on second premolar to avoid anatomic and aesthetic defects. Mesiobuccal root of first molar has been root planed. Narrow V-shaped preparation of recipient site. **D,** Preparation of connective tissue bed on either side of recipient site ensures primary intention healing, minimal risk of detachment, and an optimal opportunity for repair on root. Epithelium removed over distobuccal root to mesial line angle of second molar. **E,** Large flap requires cutback incision in its mesial aspect. This allows flap (covering defect on root and connective tissue bed) to remain in position passively and eliminates "dead" space and tension on graft. Suspensory sutures are tied on buccal aspect of second premolar. Distal vertical incision is sutured by interrupted sutures. Size of recipient site (including connective tissue bed approximating mesial of second molar) is equivalent to resultant connective tissue bed at donor site. **F,** Twelve months after treatment. Area successfully repaired by laterally positioned graft. Probe does not extend beyond 1 mm over mesiobuccal root of first molar. Gingivoplasty has not been performed (mirror view).

and periosteum, protecting the underlying highly reactive radicular bone. There is a continuity of this connective tissue attachment with the cut gingival fibers remaining attached to the tooth. This ensures the repair of the dentogingival junction to its original height without an anatomic deformity. The alveolar bone is protected, avoiding the formation of a dehiscence or fenestration (Nabers, et al., 1960; Roth, 1965; Stahl et al., 1963). The therapist must be prepared for unforeseen complications during surgery. When a partial-thickness flap is raised at a donor site where a long connective tissue attachment to the labial root surface is present, a severe anatomic defect might result if this area were left exposed. *A solution is to place a free soft tissue autograft on the connective tissue bed.* This avoids a severe cleft formation, and adjacent areas of deficient gingiva

can be managed at the same time (Irwin, 1977). Fig. 26-83 illustrates this situation, showing the design of the laterally positioned graft.

Relocation of graft at recipient site

Objective. The objective of the laterally positioned flap is the restoration of gingival form, contour, and function while aesthetically repairing the area.

Flap position. The flap should cover the entire defect, and the lateral margins of the flap should rest on a connective tissue base to expedite repair. The margin of the flap, with its intact sulcular lining, should be placed high on the enamel below the height of contour and coronal to the cemento-enamel junction.

Suturing. No. 5-0 black silk suture is used to fix the graft securely in this position (Fig. 26-80). An individual continuous suture may support the

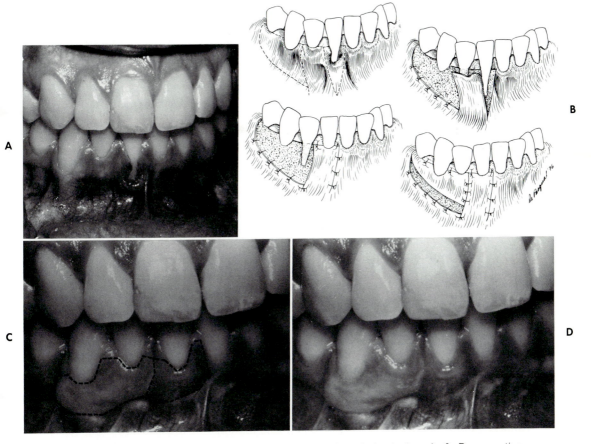

Fig. 26-83. Combined use of laterally positioned graft and gingival graft. **A,** Preoperative view of acute mucogingival defect. **B,** Dotted lines demonstrate incisions for combined pedicle and gingival graft procedure. Pedicle graft is elevated and then positioned and sutured. Gingival graft is positioned to cover denuded surface of lateral incisor. **C,** Outline of areas covered by pedicle graft and gingival graft. **D,** A 24-month postoperative view illustrates stability of combined surgical repair. (From Irwin, R. K.: J. Periodontal **48:**38, 1977.)

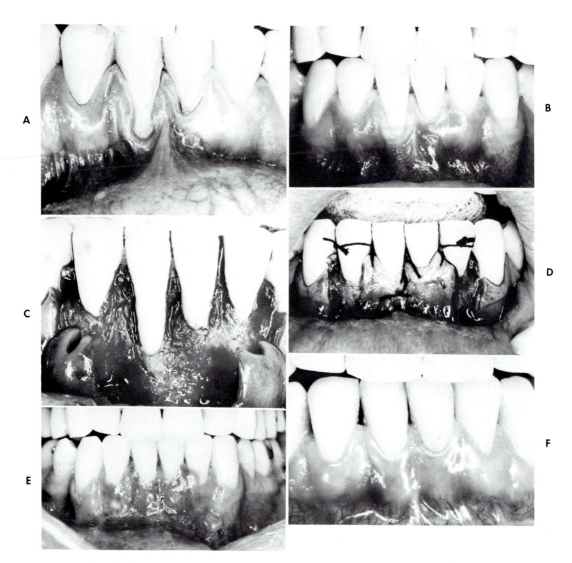

Fig. 26-84. Double lateral positioned graft. **A,** Preoperative view shows gingival cleft on mandibular right central incisor and shallow cleft on left central incisor. Absence of functional attached gingiva and shallow vestibular fornix is complicated by high frenum attachment. **B,** Following disease control instruction, root scaling, root planing, and soft tissue curettage, absence of gingiva is observed. Extension of frenum between incisors extends coronally to level of cementoenamel junction. **C,** Partial-thickness flaps of donor tissue from lateral incisors have been elevated. Frenum has been excised. Connective tissue covering alveolar process has been prepared to resemble lamina propria. Dissection of donor tissue leaves sulcular wall remaining on lateral incisors. Definitve root planing on central incisors is carried out to remove only softened tooth structure. **D,** Double lateral positioned flaps are placed on enamel of tooth below height of contour and sutured at midline area. Flaps are suspended by suturing technique that prevents apical slipping of grafted flaps at recipient site. Connective tissue attachment and sulcular walls remain attached at donor site. **E,** Fourteen-day postsurgical view shows that donor graft sites are repairing without aesthetic defect. Recipient site grafts appear attached coronal to cementoenamel junction. **F,** Six months later. Note repair of gingival clefts and elimination of frenum pull. Donor sites are completely repaired. Gingival margin is coronal to cementoenamel junction. Disease control must be reinforced.

graft circumferentially, while individual sutures coapt the oblique line of the incision. A sag in the suture can occur, which will allow the flap to slip apically. By placing the suture around an adjacent tooth and tying it on the labial surface, subsequent movement of the graft will be avoided. The position of the graft should be tested so that the flap does not slide down on the root, obviously committing the graft to an apical position at the outset (Figs. 26-77 and 26-84).

Dressing. The control of hemorrhage and the close adaptation of the graft to the tooth to prevent dead space should precede the placement of a noneugenol dressing.

1. The dressing should be placed in an apicocoronal direction so that it will not be displaced toward the root.
2. Initially the dressing should be placed at the donor site graft to support this newly located graft. By gentle pressure the dressing can be blended toward the recipient site.
3. The dressing should adapt the graft passively to the root surface without tension.
4. A bulky dressing, particularly in the vestibular fornix, should be avoided. It may stretch the graft and displace it apically.
5. Before the dressing is finally adapted, be certain that the graft is still properly positioned. If not, the dressing should be removed and the graft resutured.
6. The patient must be warned against extending the lip to inspect the graft or dressing.
7. If the dressing become displaced inadvertently, the patient must be cautioned to see that it is replaced between visits.

Postoperative considerations

Medication. The usual postsurgical drugs are prescribed. The dressing is changed in 10 days when the sutures are removed. The dressing is replaced at 10-day intervals for 1 month. Healing is uneventful, and pain is minimal.

Dressing. Although success appears certain, iatrogenic abuse of dressing replacement can detach the graft and allow its displacement with repair at a more apical level. The dressing must be soft when applied.

Recession. Necrosis of a graft is uncommon. However, slight recession (though infrequent) may occur (Moskow et al., 1965). Placement of the flap high on the enamel will reduce postsurgical root exposure. Recession is less than an optimal result. However, if the pockets have been eliminated and an adequate band of attached gingiva exists, a great service has been provided

for the patient (McFall, 1967; Patur and Glickman, 1958).

Plaque control instructions. Once the dressing has been removed, gentle massage applied in a coronal direction with a gauze sponge is recommended. The modified Stillman method of brushing with a soft bristle multituft toothbrush can be instituted subsequently. The technique of directing the bristles into the sulcular space should be avoided.

DOUBLE PAPILLA GRAFT (Cohen, 1964; Cohen and Ross, 1968)

INDICATIONS

1. To repair gingival recession and clefts
2. To reconstruct the gingival attachment to the exposed root surfaces
3. To avoid exposing adjacent fenestrations or dehiscences on radicular surfaces of the donor site
4. To avoid anatomic defects on adjacent donor sites
5. To provide adequate sources of donor tissue when adjacent radicular donor sites are devoid of gingiva
6. To provide adequate sources of donor tissue when pockets are present on the labial or lingual surfaces of the approximating teeth

PRECAUTIONS

1. If the coaptation of the two papilla provides a graft that is too narrow, angular clefts can occur.
2. Interproximal pockets should not be present.
3. The interdental bone height determines the degree of root coverage that is possible.
4. The length of the V-shaped incision should be kept to a minimum and yet fulfill the objective of radicular surface pocket elimination. Then the likelihood of failure is minimized.

In the design of this procedure Cohen (1964) and Cohen and Ross (1968) take the necessary gingiva from both interdental papillae bordering the defect. These papillae are brought together to cover the recipient site. The amount of underlying tissue exposed is restricted to the interdental areas (Fig. 26-85). Here again, Goldman believes that a stimulated periosteal pedicle serves in a better fashion than the partial-thickness flap.

This procedure has one advantage over the laterally positioned graft. The length of interdental gingiva is greater than that of the radicular surface. The bone is much thicker in the interdental area than on the labial surface. Healing studies performed on interdental tissues show complete repair in this site, whereas the labial plate may not be completely restored to the original height after exposure (Staffileno et al., 1966; Wilderman, 1964; Wilderman and Wentz; 1965). The two papilla are sutured together to form a flap; this flap is then sutured to the tooth. Fig. 26-81 describes the technique.

Isolated areas in the maxillary and the mandibular premolar areas are successfully treated by a double papilla graft (Fig. 26-82) (see discussion on Increasing width of gingiva: double papilla). The lingual anterior recession, which results in

an absence of attached gingiva, and the mucogingival complications are solved by utilizing the delicate papilla adjacent to a cleft. The loss of interdental bone prevents the coverage of the root. The success of this procedure has encouraged further clinical testing and modifications (see Fig. 26-97).

Modifications in technique

1. Nos. 5-0 and 6-0 suture material are used for delicately coapting the two papillae into a well-supported graft. It is positioned on the enamel of the crown below the height of contour coronal to the cementoenamel junction. An individual

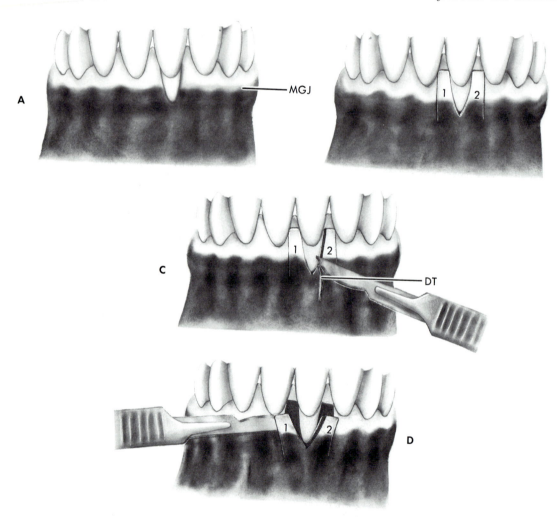

Fig. 26-85. Double papilla graft. **A,** Cleft on mandibular left central incisor extends deep beyond mucogingival junction, *MGJ*. **B,** Outline of V-shaped incisions and identification of papillae, *1* and *2*, to be grafted. To design straight margin (when both papillae are sutured together), a horizontal partial-thickness incision, providing sufficent attached gingiva, is completed interdentally. **C,** A beveled incision of papilla, *2*, prepares connective tissue bed on mesial aspect of this papilla so that undersurface of connective tissue of papilla, *1*, can be overlapping, *2*. Beveled incision creates connective tissue bed after discarded tissue, *DT* is removed. **D,** Partial-thickness flap is prepared at *1* by using no. 15 Bard-Parker blade directed in apicocoronal direction.

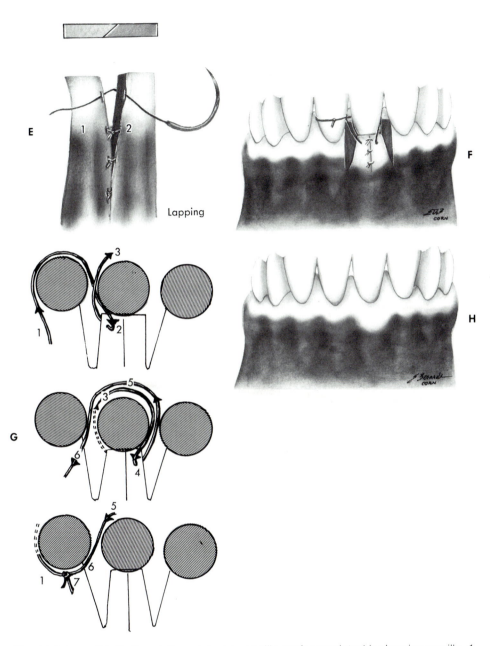

Fig. 26-85, cont'd. E, Coaptation of double papilla graft completed by *lapping* papilla, *1,* over beveled papilla, *2.* Black silk suture (no. 5-0) with atraumatic needle was used. **F,** Double papilla graft should be of sufficient width to cover prepared denuded root and adjacent connective tissue. Margin should be positioned on enamel below height of contour, allowing most coronal connective tissue attachment at cementoenamel junction. By tying suture on labial of right central incisor, graft will not slip apically. **G,** Suturing technique is carried out as follows. On distal aspect of right central incisor, suture material is passed from labial aspect, *1,* progressing along path of suture material as shown by arrows and numbers. Eventual return of suture material to mesiolabial aspect of right central incisor completes surgical knot, *1* and *7.* Compare with **F. H,** Cleft is repaired. Ideally it should not be probed beyond cementoenamel junction.

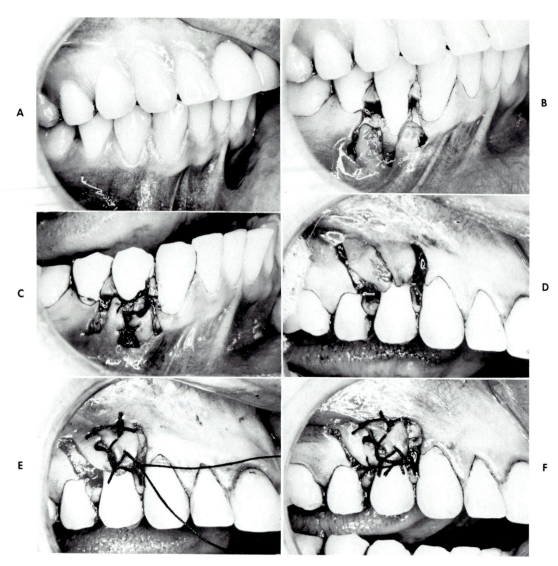

Fig. 26-86. Double papilla graft procedure. **A,** Preoperative view shows gingival clefts on maxillary and mandibular first premolars. There are adequate gingival papillae adjacent to clefts for donor tissue. **B,** Horizontal incision creates vertical length to each papilla adjacent to mandibular cleft. Failure in double papilla procedure is often due to separation of joined papilla at midline. This can be avoided by removing epithelium from connective tissue layer on one papilla. The joined papilla can then create a "lapped" flap. Preparation of roots is similar to laterally positioned flap. V-shaped preparation of recipient site should extend well into vestibular area. Terminal vertical incisions of papilla can extend just beyond mucogingival junction. **C,** Lapped flaps are sutured on buccal surface of first premolar with margin of double papilla positioned on enamel below height of contour. Flaps are joined by interrupted sutures. Suspensory suture at margin is designed to bring papilla together and is tied on buccal surface. **D,** Root surface has been planed. Distal papilla has connective tissue exposed in preparation for overlapping of mesial papilla. Note small connective tissue wounds resulting from this technique. **E,** Lower length of suture will be a component for suturing double papilla on buccal surface. **F,** Maxillary double papilla are sutured so that marginal tension brings papillae together rather than separates them. **G,** Ten-day dressing change. Flaps involving both teeth have not been displaced apically. **H,** Appearance of grafted sites immediately after suture removal. **I,** Eight-month postoperative result shows that a functional gingival unit has been established with gingival margins on crown.

sling suture through the attached interdental papillae prevents apical movement of the graft. A successful graft provides an aesthetically pleasing result (Fig. 26-86).

2. The readily available interdental papillae, when combined into one flap, may not be of sufficient width to cover a large defect. Use of the partial-thickness flap dissection increases the latitude of applicability for this procedure. The size of each component of the flap can be increased to include part of the marginal gingiva. Since the remaining connective tissue and periosteum protect the radicular bone from resorption, the therapist need not hesitate to create a double papillae of the correct measurement (Fig. 26-86).

3. Aside from the aesthetic benefits, there are mucogingival problems that require an increase in the width of attached gingiva in a uniform pattern. Use of the partial-thickness double papillae combined with other plastic surgery procedures facilitate these corrective measures (see Fig. 26-

98). Under these circumstances it is desirable to relate the new dentogingival junction to the connective tissue–covered alveolar process rather than to the cementoenamel junction. No clinical or histologic evidence is available to prove that grafts with new attachments at the cementoenamel junction will also allow successful restorative results over a long range of time.

4. Kramer and Kohn (1966) suggested the removal of the outer epithelium from a portion of one of the papillae to provide a lapped flap. This modification, adapting two connective tissue surfaces, helps to prevent inadvertent nonunion of the flaps over the midradicular surface (Fig. 26-86).

5. I have suggested placing the suture around an adjacent tooth. This individual continuous suture may support the graft circumferentially when it is finally tied on the labial surface of the adjacent tooth (Fig. 26-85). Another procedure demonstrating the use of this suturing technique is seen in Figs. 26-76, 26-82, and 26-84.

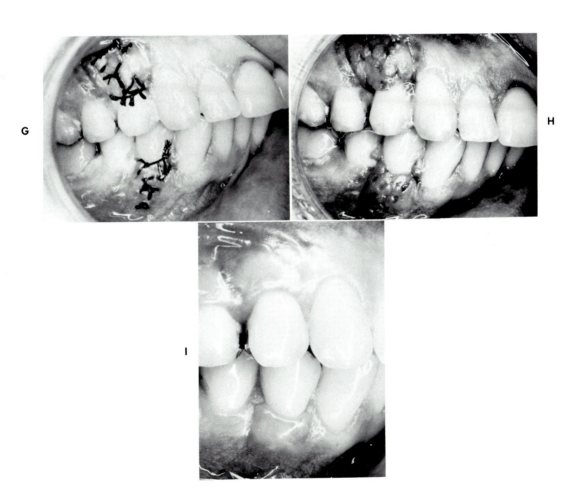

Fig. 26-86, cont'd. For legend see opposite page.

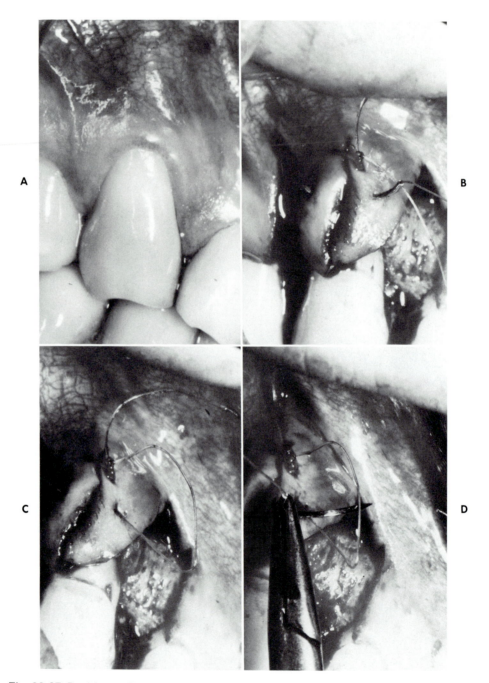

Fig. 26-87. Double papilla graft with continuous locked suturing technique. **A,** Preoperative view of mucogingival problem. **B,** Surgical knot (absorbable collagen suture) is completed at apical end of double papilla. Suture enters beveled papillae. **C,** Suture is passed through second papilla, and a loop remains. **D,** Needle is passed under loop.

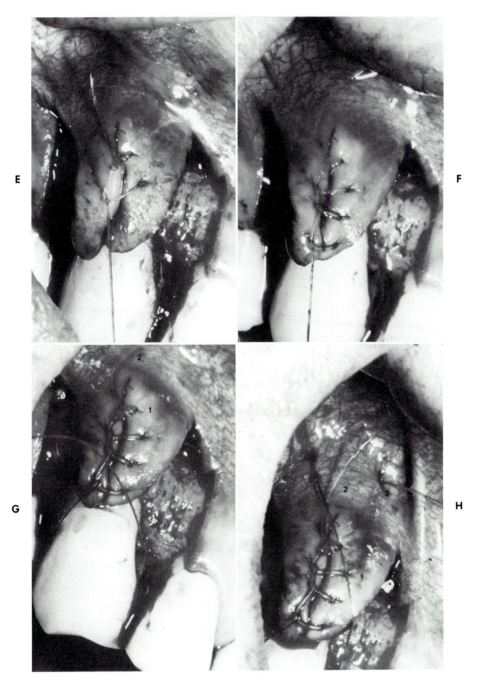

Fig. 26-87, cont'd. E, Completion of first step of continuous locked suture. **F,** Completion of coaptation of tissue. **G,** To stabilize flap on radicular surface of root, suture material is passed around distal aspect of canine and exits on mesial aspect. Original surgical knot is at *1* with its tail at *2*. **H,** Suture crosses and adapts flap to tooth with a periosteal vestibular suture going from distal aspect to exit at mesial aspect, *3*. Original suture extension is at *2*.

Continued.

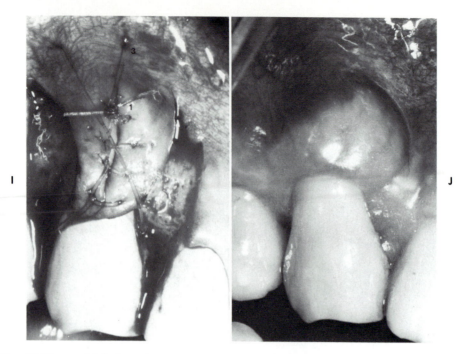

Fig. 26-87, cont'd. I, Completion of stabilization of graft and its suturing at original surgical knot, *1.* Loose end of suture, *2,* is tied to suture from *3* and is completed at *1.* **J,** Successful graft. (Courtesy Dr. Peter Rubelman, North Miami Beach, Fla.)

6. Rubelman is credited for a unique modification of the continuous locked suturing technique. He adapts the suture material obliquely over the graft, enhancing its contact and stability against the root (Fig. 26-87).

There are clinical situations where a combination of the double papilla graft and the laterally positioned graft and a free soft tissue autograft offer the correct surgical solution.

The double papilla graft has been used to evaluate the effect of a muscle pull on the marginal gingiva. As suspected, inadvertent dehiscences can be avoided by leaving the connective tissue attachment to the root of the tooth (Fig. 26-73). Fig. 26-74 shows a 17-year documentation of periodontal disease that implicates an insidious muscle effect that had been repaired by a single papilla graft (see discussion on Anatomic Considerations in Reconstructive Mucogingival Surgery).

FREE SOFT TISSUE AUTOGRAFTS:
BRIDGING PRINCIPLE (Sullivan and Atkins, 1968; Livingston, 1975; Mlinck et al., 1973)

INDICATIONS
1. Functional correction of gingival clefts (recession), creating an intact gingival attachment (Fig. 26-88).
2. Aesthetic correction of root exposure

PRECAUTIONS
1. If the width of the exposed cemental surface is greater than 3 mm and the depth of the exposed root surface in an apical direction is greater than 3 mm, limited aesthetic correction should be anticipated (Mlinek et al., 1973).
2. Sufficient interdental connective tissue bed height must be available coronal to the cementoenamel junction to achieve ideal cemental coverage.
3. The graft should be of sufficient length to cover at least 3 mm of connective tissue bed apical to the exposed root.

The refinement of this technique has enabled the graft to attach to the tooth surface coronally to the cementoenamel junction. The principle of bridging included within the surgical design and incorporating the potential of collateral circulation has increased the predictability of correcting a gingival cleft with aesthetic gingival attachment to an avascular tooth surface.

The clinical impression of attachment using gingival grafts to correct exposed roots (that have resulted from recession, cleft formation, and pocket elimination) have been of great interest (Fig. 26-89). Sullivan and Atkins (1968) have carefully defined the principles involved, the precautions, and the limitations for success. The need for

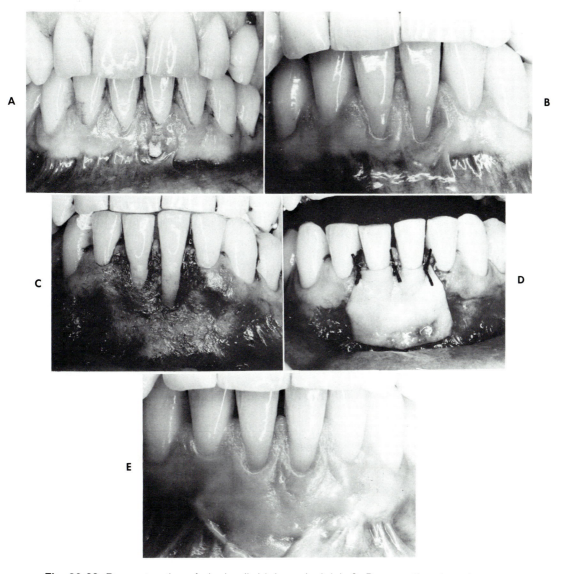

Fig. 26-88. Reconstruction of gingiva (bridging principle). **A,** Preoperative view of severe recession and pocket formation beyond mucogingival junction on mandibular left central incisor. Right central incisor has pocket formation into mucosa. **B,** Following initial hygienic phase of treatment, minimal creeping attachment has occurred. **C,** Recipient site prior to graft placement. Note level of connective tissue preparation interdentally. **D,** Placement of graft. Inadequate collateral circulation exists marginally. **E,** Three-year postoperative view. There has been a functional correction of gingival cleft, creating an intact gingival attachment.

adequate plasmatic diffusion and collateral circulation has been stressed.

The revascularized intraoral graft has great reparative capabilities. In Fig. 26-90 grafts of intermediate partial-thickness were positioned coronally on the root. After a 2-year period they showed creeping attachment to the cementoenamel junction, and after 6 years still could not be probed beyond 2 mm (Matter and Cimasoni, 1976).

Surgical technique for "bridging." The general principles applicable are described in the discussion on the Laterally Positioned Graft. Correction of gingival clefts (recession) for improved aesthetics and preparation of recipient site are described as follows.

Connective tissue bed and root preparation. Considerations are similar for the general preparation of the connective tissue bed as for other gingival grafts. However, the connective

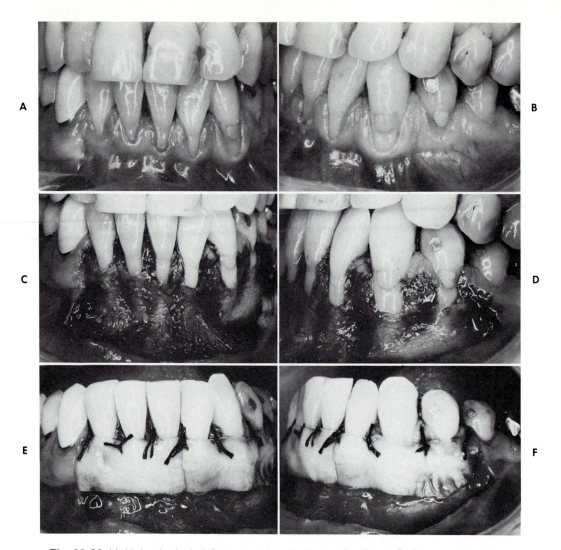

Fig. 26-89. Multiple gingival clefts treated by gingival grafts. **A** and **B,** Preoperative views. Note gingival clefts on six teeth extending from mandibular right lateral incisor to left first premolar. All labial pockets extend beyond mucogingival junction and are associated with a shallow vestibular fornix. **C** and **D,** Partial-thickness dissection extending parallel to alveolus deepens vestibule. Marginal gingivoplasty removes labial pocket walls and preserves interproximal height to papillae, yet outer epithelium is removed. Connective tissue interdental bed is prepared coronal to labial cementoenamel junction, and exposed root surfaces are carefully but not excessively planed. Loose connective tissue and muscle fibers are removed from recipient bed, particularly in undulating interradicular area. Pooling of blood can be seen in interradicular area. Immobile recipient bed is prepared. **E** and **F,** Two intermediate-thickness free gingival grafts (9 mm wide) are sutured interdentally to connective tissue papillae bed. Effort is made to attach grafts to most coronal level of cementum. Apical border of grafts and mucosal margin of vestibular fornix are not sutured. To avoid risk of embedding suture material in noneugenol dressing, aluminum foil is used between grafts and dressing. This enables close adaptation of grafts to undulating alveolar profile, avoiding "dead" spaces. **G** and **H,** Ten days later. Suture removal shows varying degrees of "take" to avascular roots. Vertical necrosis appears on right lateral incisor. Right and left central incisors appear to be surviving to cementoenamel junction. There is incomplete epithelialization on lateral incisor and necrosis of graft margin on left canine and first premolar. All teeth have significant "take" on avascular roots. **I,** Preventive maintenance visit 12 months later. **J,** Crevicular measurements are 2 mm or less. **K,** Creeping attachment at varying levels on six teeth. It is anticipated that additional coronal creeping attachment will occur. **L** to **N,** Six-year results show that further creeping attachment has occurred.

tissue bed margins should extend apically from the borders of the recession. The epithelium may be removed to the tip of the interdental papillae as well as the adjacent attached gingiva. With a nippers the sulcular epithelium is removed, eliminating any pockets. Additional root exposure should be kept to a minimum. This bed will provide a vascular area around the recession from which collateral circulation can develop.

Careful root planing follows to remove softened tooth structure and to avoid overmanipulation of the roots. Effort is expended not to destroy the

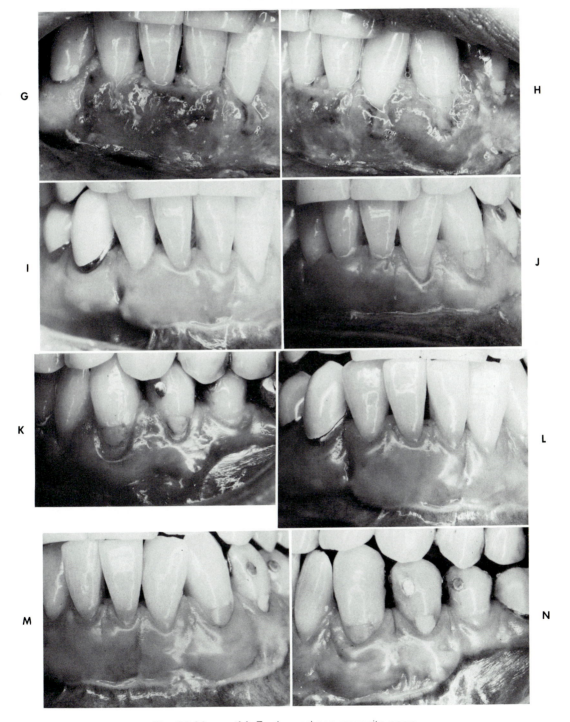

Fig. 26-89, cont'd. For legend see opposite page.

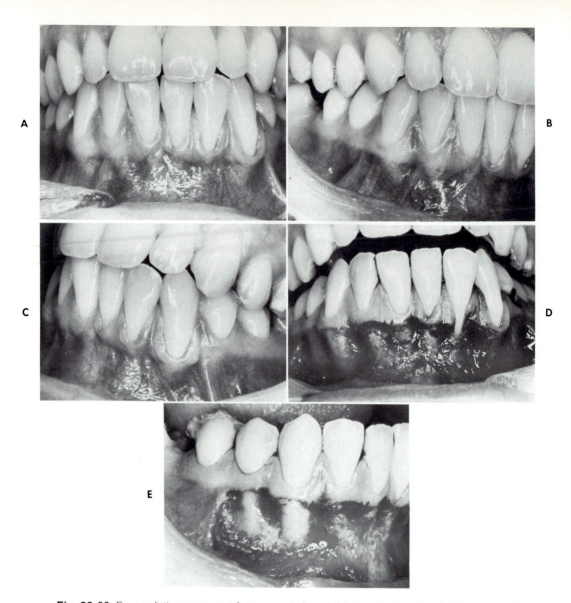

Fig. 26-90. Free soft tissue autograft to correct deep labial pocket and to eliminate muscle pull on marginal gingiva that will result in creeping attachment. **A** to **C,** Preoperative views. Recession present on mandibular left central, lateral, and canine. Only free gingiva remains in these areas. Rolled marginal gingiva is effect of muscle pull. Nonfunctional gingiva exists from right first premolar to left first premolar. There is blanching of gingival margin from muscle pull on right canine. **D** to **F,** Incision initiated coronal to mucogingival junction within free gingiva. Dissection is parallel with alveolar process, deepening vestibule. Muscle fibers and loose connective tissue are removed, and immovable connective tissue bed prepared. Pocket of 5 mm is removed on labial of lateral incisor (as evidenced by severe cleft). Root surface is planed to remove only softened tooth structure. **G** to **I,** Two free soft tissue autografts sutured in juxtaposition to free gingival margin and interdentally. No. 4-0 black silk suture used at marginal area. No. 4-0 gut suture fixes mucosal margin to underlying periosteum at newly established vestibular depth. Length of free graft increased in left lateral incisor area for bridging and attachment to root. Additional apicocoronal length ensures against necrosis of graft on avascular root. If necrosis should occur, a functional gingival attachment could survive on connective tissue recipient bed, slightly coronal to it. Amount of collateral circulation at apical area of denuded root determines amount of root surface covered by graft. **J** to **L,** Three months after surgery. Left lateral incisor root appears to be successfully covered by graft. Cleft on original gingival margin of left central incisor has almost been eliminated. Rolled gingival margin on left canine is no longer present. All pockets have been eliminated, and functional attached gingiva is present.

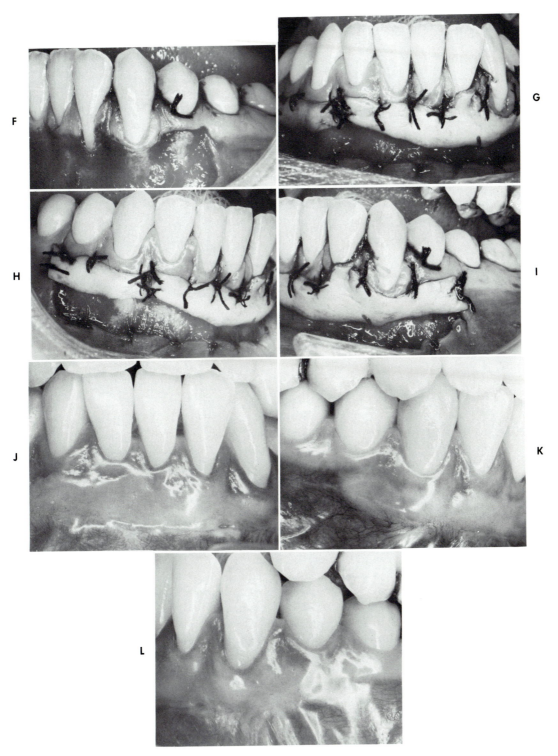

Fig. 26-90, cont'd. For legend see opposite page.

Continued.

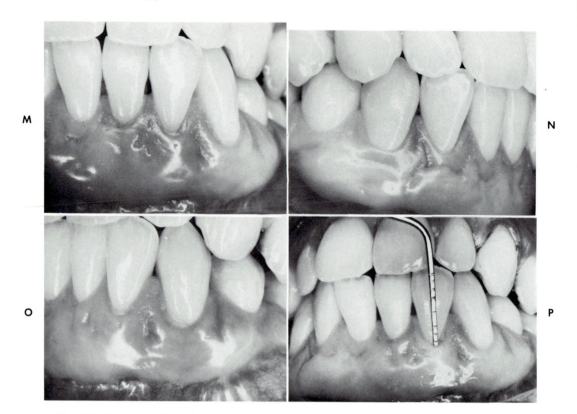

Fig. 26-90, cont'd. M to **O,** Two years after surgery. With excellent plaque control, gingival graft has survived. Creeping attachment has occurred on left central and lateral incisors and canine. Rolled gingival margins have disappeared. Free graft provided increased attached gingiva and negated effect of muscle pull at marginal area. **P,** Crevicular depth is less than 1 mm on left central incisor where root was exposed 5 mm.

connective tissue attachment at the apical and lateral borders of the cleft.

The lower margin of the bed should be placed several millimeters apical to the apex of the recession. If necrosis should occur over the avascular area, an adequate vascular bed apical to the denuded root will remain. It will provide ample functional attached gingiva around the margins of the recession. When a "take" occurs, the clinical impression suggests that reattachment to the cementum may exist. Human wound-healing research must substantiate this (Fig. 26-89).

Bridging phenomenon. If root coverage is planned to correct gingival recession, collateral circulation is critical for a successful "take" on the avascular tooth structure. It may necessitate the removal of the epithelium to the tip of the adjacent interdental papillae. These vascular areas give rise to capillaries that link with the graft's original vessels to form a network of collateral circulation over the avascular area (Fig. 26-90).

Graft survival over the avascular region ensues

and is known as the "phenomenon of bridging" (Figs. 26-91 and 26-92). McGregor (1962) concludes that the amount of bridging is strictly limited by the width of the defect and the vascularity of the recipient bed and the donor tissue.

Approximately 70% root coverage can be expected if the width of the exposed surface is less than 3 mm and the depth of the lesion in an apical direction is 3 mm or less (Mlinek et al., 1973). Sullivan and Atkins (1968) have classified gingival recession into four general morphologic categories according to depth and width: (1) the deep wide recession, (2) the shallow wide recession, (3) the deep narrow recession, and (4) the shallow narrow recession (Fig. 26-92). Sullivan and Atkins further explain that "a common factor in grafting over any denuded root surface is that a limited amount (1 or 2 mm) of new tissue will take over the apical end of the avascular area if the surgical procedure is performed correctly. This take is related to the presence of collateral circulation from the three vascular borders at the

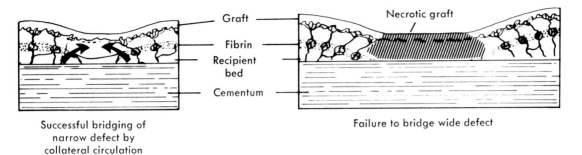

Fig. 26-91. Phenomenon of bridging avascular areas. Collateral circulation *(arrows)* arises from vascular bed and maintains tissue over avascular area. Note importance of width of avascular area upon graft survival. (From Sullivan, H. C., and Atkins, J. H.: Periodontics **6:**152, 1968.)

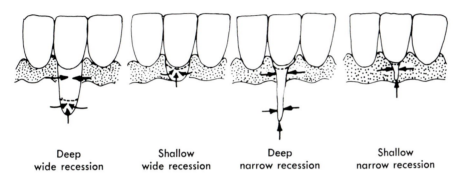

Fig. 26-92. Four classes of gingival recession. Amount of bridging that can be anticipated is represented by areas apical to dotted lines. Note arrows representing three-point collateral circulation at apex of each recession and two-point circulation in coronal regions of two deep recessions. (From Sullivan, H. C., and Atkins, J. H.: Periodontics **6:**152, 1968.)

mesial, distal, and apical margins of the recession." In contrast, two-point collateral circulation (from the mesial and distal vascular margins in the coronal region, particularly in deep wide recession) is not usually sufficient to maintain the graft tissues over the coronal avascular area.

This classification is a subjective clinical guide to postsurgical expectation. The deep narrow, shallow narrow, and shallow wide gingival clefts may respond to initial root scaling, root planing, and soft tissue curettage. Success is achieved by creeping attachment (Figs. 26-89 and 26-90). Failing here, three-point collateral circulation is probable, and root coverage can be accomplished for both types of shallow clefts. Theoretically, two-point collateral circulation will successfully bridge the deep narrow cleft. However, for this situation and particularly in the attempted grafting of deep wide recession areas, the length of the graft must be sufficient to cover at least 3 mm of the connective tissue bed apically to the exposed

root. This is necessary to ensure a functional gingival attachment if the root coverage should fail. The sulcular epithelium must be carefully removed in these circumstances. Further care must be exerted in these circumstances. Further care must be exerted to avoid excessive tissue removal, since that may produce an increased avascular area with a reduced amount of bridging (Fig. 26-89).

If maximum bridging is planned, a thinner graft should be designed. It will survive longer without circulation. This graft must maintain its viability by diffusion until collateral circulation has developed. A thicker graft is indicated when there is a need for functional gingiva around the recession and when root coverage is not the surgical goal.

The clinical impression of organic reattachment has not been substantiated by wound-healing studies. Further research is required.

Positioning of graft. With improved aesthetics

as a consideration for correction of recession, the attempt at root coverage requires careful details (see discussion on Bridging Phenomenon). If the interproximal papillae fill the embrasure space and can be prepared properly, the graft can be positioned on the enamel below the height of contour maximizing "reattachment" opportunity at the most coronal level of the cementum. The coronal margin always should be placed at the level of the marginal tissue on the adjacent teeth. Overcompensation for the graft's coronal position, lacking any adjacent vascular supply, may yield greater necrosis than anticipated. The vertical width of the graft must cover at least 3 mm of the connective tissue bed, ensuring increased attached gingiva at the apical border if bridging should fail (Fig. 26-89).

Immobilization of graft. With 4-0 or 5-0 black silk suture material on a reverse cutting needle the graft is sutured into the fixed interdental gingiva. When root coverage is attempted, caution is advised to avoid encroachment upon the collateral circulation at the marginal area. Since each suture puncture causes a localized hematoma at the site, reducing the graft "take," the suture placement should be away from the avascular root. A modification of the Baer-Sumner dressing is used to immobilize and maintain positive pressure on the graft (Baer et al., 1960).

The attachment to an avascular surface is tenuous, and the suture entrapment within the dressing can result in detachment from the root surface at the 10-day dressing change. Thin tinfoil is used under the dressing. This foil permits pressure that is necessary for the close approximation of the healing tissue to the alveolar indentations (Fig. 26-89). The sutures are removed in 10 days and followed by a dressing replacement.

Care following dressing removal. Review of plaque-control procedures will alert the patient to the danger of intracrevicular brushing. Initially a gauze sponge should be used to debride the area along with a Perio-Aid to carefully cleanse the tooth surface. As further healing occurs, the modified Stillman toothbrushing method is added.

CORONALLY POSITIONED GRAFT (Bernimoulen et al., 1975; Caffesse et al., 1978; Harvey, 1965)

INDICATIONS
1. For recession associated with an inadequate width of keratinized gingiva on facial aspect of tooth
2. For root sensitivity and recession, and unacceptable aesthetics caused by recession

3. For recession and continued retraction of marginal tissue due to tensional pull of a frenum
4. For multiple areas of gingival recession

PRECAUTIONS
1. Shallow clinical sulcus depth should be present interproximally adjacent to the facial surface of the root to be grafted.
2. The crest of the interproximal bone should have a normal or near-normal relationship to the cementoenamel junction.
3. Only minimal cervical erosion or abrasion is acceptable.
4. Abnormally shaped gingiva should be recontoured before positioning the graft coronally.
5. No lingual or palatal pockets should be present.
6. The graft must be mobilized from the underlying bound-down periosteum using either a partial-thickness dissection (Maynard, 1977) or a full-thickness flap. The periosteum must be separated by undermining incisions (Fig. 26-72) with a full-thickness flap (Bernimoulin et al., 1975).
7. Root prominence must be reduced within the plane of the adjacent alveolar process. However, root planing should not be excessive.
8. Adequate time must be allowed for healing and development of a blood supply before moving the autogenous graft. Six weeks is generally sufficient (Maynard, 1977). Two months also has been suggested (Bernimoulin et al., 1975).

Inconsistent results in the correction of recession have precipitated the study and use of the coronally positioned graft. In utilizing this graft, two methods have been employed to correct the anatomic defect:
1. By the coronal movement of the existent mucogingival complex, which has unsatisfactory limitations (minimal gingiva may be available) (Brustein, 1970; Restrepo, 1973; Sumner, 1969).
2. By initial creation of gingival width by a gingival graft, followed by a secondary procedure moving the complex coronally Bernimoulin et al., 1975; Maynard, 1977).

Harvey in 1970 noted the shallowing of the vestibular depth by coronal movement of the existing mucogingival complex and resorted to creation of a gingival graft to overcome this shortcoming and benefit from the increased width of the marginal gingiva.

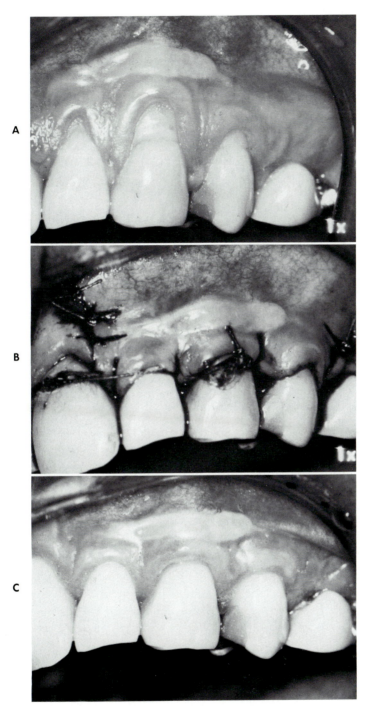

Fig. 26-93. Coronally positioned graft involving three teeth. **A,** Preoperative view showing gingival graft in place. Varying degrees of toothbrush abrasion are obvious. **B,** Surgical procedure is completed to cover exposed roots of maxillary left lateral incisor, canine, and first premolar. **C,** Postoperative result 1 year later. (Courtesy J. P. Bernimoulin, Zurich, Switzerland.)

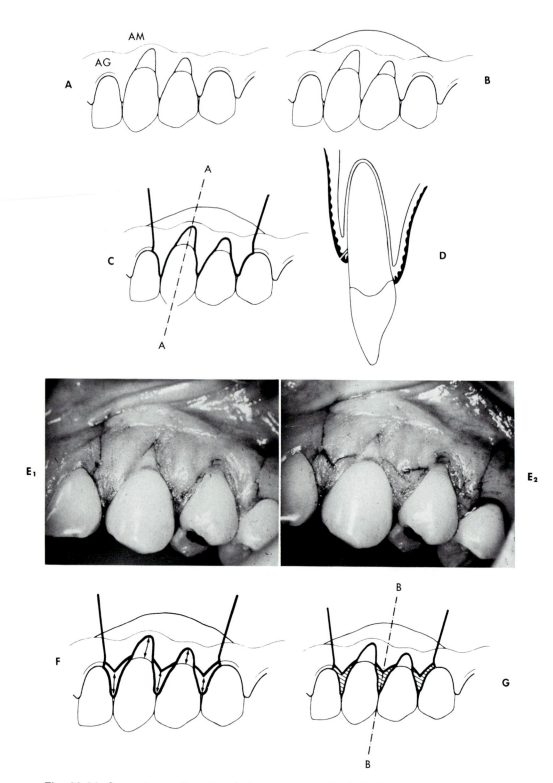

Fig. 26-94. Coronally positioned graft (surgical procedure). **A,** Two teeth exhibiting gingival recession. Note small width of attached gingiva, *AG,* at recession sites, *AM,* Alveolar mucosa. **B,** Attached gingiva has been widened by a free soft tissue autograft. **C,** Schema of initial incisions. **D,** Cross-sectional drawing of marginal incision. Clinical view of vertical incisions, **E₁,** and of horizontal incisions, **E₂. F,** Schema and clinical view of papillary incisions.

There is no doubt that we are dealing with a new reconstructive approach to the restoration of lost gingiva (Restrepo, 1973). Bernimoulin et al. (1975) were impressed with Harvey's 8 years of clinical experience with the combination of free soft tissue autograft and subsequent coronal positioning of the graft.

The clinical data of the Bernimoulin (1975)

study included 41 teeth with measurements at 1, 6, and 12 months postoperatively. Failure to reduce the magnitude of recession was low; only two sites showed no reduction. Of 12 canines involved, six showed a 100% reduction of recession while the remaining six had reductions of 60% to 83%. The 12-month postoperative results permitted evaluation of the relapse tendency.

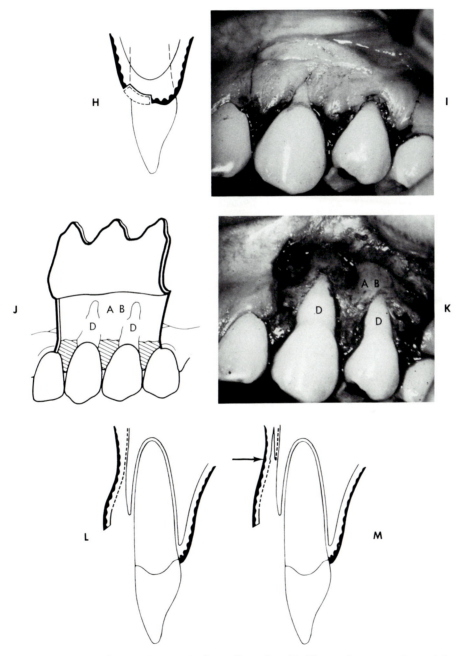

Fig. 26-94, cont'd. G to **I,** Removal of papillae. **J** to **K,** Elevated mucoperiosteal flap exposing alveolar bone, *AB,* and dehiscences, *D,* on two roots. **L** and **M,** Schema of graft elevation and horizontal periosteal incision *(arrow).*

Continued.

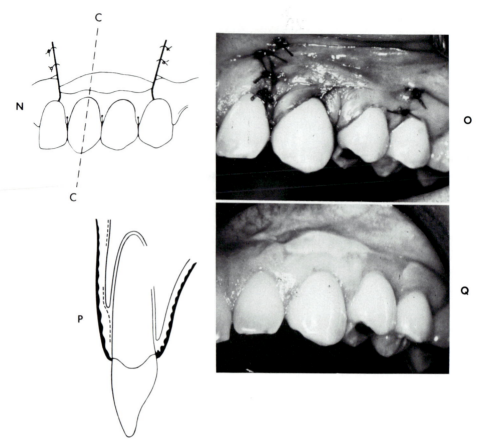

Fig. 26-94, cont'd. N and **O,** Coronally positioned graft. Lateral sutures are in place and new papilla tips are sutured in desired position. **P** and **Q,** One-year postoperative result. (From Bernimoulin, J. P., Lüscher, B., and Mühlemann, H. R.: J. Clin. Periodont. **2:**1, 1975.)

There were no significant differences between reattachment values at 1, 6, and 12 months post-operatively. Results show that the coronally positioned graft performed on more than one tooth consistently resulted in a significant reduction of recession (Fig. 26-93).

Technique (after Bernimoulin) (Fig. 26-94). The primary procedure increases the width of gingiva with a free soft tissue autograft (Fig. 26-94, *A* and *B*). The secondary procedure is as follows:

1. The facial and lingual aspects are anesthetized using lidocaine (Xylocaine) with 1:50,000 epinephrine. Lingual anesthesia is administered through the mesial and distal papilla adjacent to the involved teeth.
2. Two vertical paramarginal incisions are made bordering the papillae adjacent to the recession area. They are connected with a reverse bevel scalloped incision along the gingival margin (Fig. 26-94, *C* to *E*). Care

is required to avoid incisions that will result in a graft with the apical border narrower than the marginal area. The effect will create a space between the fixed borders of the adjacent tissue and the graft.

3. Care is taken to create new papillae that will fit their future locations (Fig. 26-94, *F*). The recession is measured from the soft tissue margin to 1 mm coronal to the cementoenamel junction. This determines the distance that the graft is to move coronally. It also decides where the incisions from the papillary margin should be made.
4. With an opthalmic scissors or nippers, a thin layer of the remaining papillary gingiva is removed (Fig. 26-94, *G* to *I*).
5. A mucoperiosteal flap is elevated to expose root surfaces and alveolar bone dehiscences. With curettes the denuded root surfaces are planed gently (Fig. 26-94, *J* and *K*).
6. To facilitate the coronal displacement of the

graft, its base is separated from the periosteum with undermining incisions (Fig. 26-94, *L* and *M*).

7. The graft is then pulled and positioned coronally and sutured in the desired position, 1 mm coronal to the cementoenamel junction. The lateral borders of the flap are sutured first in a direction diagonal to the adjacent attached gingiva using 5-0 gut and a P-3 needle (Ethicon 686); then papillary sling sutures are placed (Fig. 26-94, *N* and *O*).

8. The graft is firmly adapted to its recipient bed with gauze and finger pressure, for several minutes to promote adhesion.

9. Bernimoulin (1975) does not use periodontal dressing, although others use a dressing for 10 days (Maynard, 1977; Restrepo, 1973; Sumner, 1969).

Healing is uneventful (Fig. 26-94, *P*). No probing should be attempted for at least 1 month. All patients are instructed in improved oral hygiene. Special emphasis is placed on the Stillman brushing technique to avoid horizontal toothbrush abrasive movements. The reattachment results are stable as reported for at least 4 years (Maynard, 1977).

ANATOMIC CONSIDERATIONS IN RECONSTRUCTIVE MUCOGINGIVAL SURGERY

A dentist must understand the anatomic structures (Clarke and Bueltmann, 1971; Dahlberg, 1969; Hunt, 1976; Kopczyk and Young, 1976) that will be entered surgically and be aware of possible problems that may occur in the surgical venture (Kopczyk, and Young, 1976).

Alveolar process

In the maxillary and mandibular anterior area, the mandibular premolar area, and the maxillary first molar region the cortical plate of the alveolar process is often quite thin. The greater the prominence of a tooth, the more likely that radicular bone deformities will be present. The isolated areas where the root is denuded of bone and where the root surface is covered only by periosteum and overlying gingiva, but where the marginal bone is intact are called "fenestrations." When the denuded areas extend to the margin they are called "dehiscences." Deformities of the alveolar process can complicate mucogingival surgery. The use of the partial-thickness flap design prevents additional anatomic deformities or their exposure.

Mandible
ANTERIOR FACIAL REGION

Mental protuberance. In and near the midline the anterior surface of the body of the mandible is elevated to a triangular prominence or mental protuberance. Only with severe loss of the alveolar process would there be some limitation in the surgery (e.g., when the bony chin is encroached upon). Even when there is extreme alveolar process loss it is the musculature inserting into the lip and not the body of the mandible, that gives the impression that one is approaching the chin. In this area the muscles of facial expression (i.e., the incisive and mental muscles) have their origin relatively close to the alveolar border. The action of the mental muscle elevates the skin and turns the lip outward. Since its origin extends to a level higher than that of the vestibule, the mental muscle and to a lesser extent the incisive muscles cause the vestibule to become shallow. Careful dissection has proved that an acceptable gingival environment can be developed (Fig. 26-89).

Frenum pull. From time to time evidence appears showing the continued inflammatory effect of marginal retraction by a frenum pull. Recession occurs when the mucosal margin or detached gingiva have lost their underlying osseous support. Some label this concept as speculative and question its rationale. The following two cases substantiate this concept.

CASE 1

An 18-year-old girl had a frenum pull extending to the gingival margin that blanched under tension. The gingival margin was at its normal position on the enamel. To relieve the marginal frenum pull and examine the possible effects on the alveolar margin, the radicular area was prepared for a double papilla-positioned graft. The partial-thickness dissection left the most coronal connective tissue fiber attachment to the root of the tooth. A dehiscence at the location of the muscle pull origin could be seen through this delicate connective tissue attachment. I felt that this area would result in recession if left untreated (Fig. 26-95).

CASE 2

The natural history of periodontal disease can be followed in a 17-year case history showing changes in a mandibular left first premolar. In 1954 a vestibular extension procedure combined with a gingivoplasty was performed as a gingival replacement to treat recession on the mandibular left central incisor. Creeping attachment to the cementoenamel junction occurred on the incisor over 6 years. The cheek retraction now showed

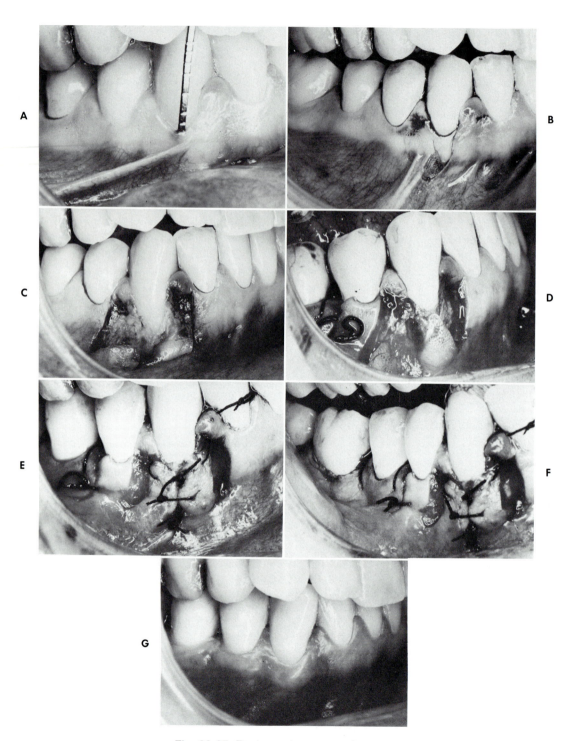

Fig. 26-95. For legend see opposite page.

significant recession and the presence of a frenum pull on the first premolar. In 12 years, recession had progressed to cause patient discomfort. Attached gingiva had been lost, and the frenum pull blanched the gingival margin. A 6 mm pocket was present on the radicular surface. Other etiologic factors were present but the effect of the frenum pull could not be excluded. Fig. 26-96 includes a 5-year postoperative result.

Smukler (1976) has conducted a clinical study and has substantiated the success of the laterally positioned papilla (pedicle) graft; 80% of the grafted tissue endured very well over a 9-month period.

Jaw height. The development of the alveolar process height obviously varies with the physical characteristics of each individual. The interrelationship between tooth size, height of the alveolar process, and the extent of chronic destructive periodontal disease determines the limit of the therapeutic efforts. For pedicle grafts or free soft tissue autografts to succeed, adequate alveolar process height must be established by partial-thickness dissections. Inadequate alveolar process height occurs less frequently in the maxilla.

ANTERIOR LINGUAL REGION: GENIAL TUBERCLES

The geniohyoid and the genioglossus muscles originate at the level of the genial tubercles. When the tubercles (upon which these muscles attach) are unusually large or high, they can cause concern in mucogingival surgery. As alveolar process destruction encroaches upon these anatomic landmarks, the muscle fibers lose their direct attachment to the bone and gain an indirect fibrous attachment through the remnants of the periosteum. The choices for surgery in this area are (1) the elevation of a full thickness flap positioning the gingiva over the alveolar crest, (2) a partial-thickness dissection of loose connective tissue and muscle fibers to increase the width of the attached gingiva using a double papilla-positioned graft (Fig. 26-97), and (3) a gingival graft (Fig. 26-65). Fortunately, deep osseous defects and osseous resorption rarely approximate these tubercles, since they could prevent lingual osseous recontouring during periodontal surgery.

POSTERIOR FACIAL REGION

External oblique ridge (second and third molar relationships). When there is an absence of gingiva in the mandibular second and third molar area, complicated by the anatomic limitations of the external oblique ridge, it is difficult to establish an adequate zone of attached gingiva. Complete denudation and the double flap approach have shown unsatisfactory results with painfully slow wound healing.

The space between the mucosal lining of the tooth and the external oblique ridge (with its associated trough) is filled with loose, textured submucous tissue and muscle attachments. The mobility of the cheek necessitates this loose attachment. It permits flexibility of the cheek for a considerable distance. Surgical entry into this area requires considerable extension of the incisions to allow the cheek to drape into the submucosal area.

The use of pedicle grafts from the edentulous

Fig. 26-95. Effect of a muscle frenum pull extending to free gingiva, and its correction by double papilla graft technique. **A,** Preoperative view. Absence of attached gingiva, extension of crevice to mucogingival junction, and a marginal muscle pull. Probe reveals shallow crevicular depth. **B,** Narrow V-shaped relaxing incision releases muscle pull. At donor site, alveolar mucosa must be resected. With abundance of interdental gingiva, horizontal incisions are initiated in papillary area. **C,** Partial-thickness flaps of donor tissues have been reflected. Appearance of recipient site is examined after resection of covering alveolar mucosa. There is delicate connective tissue attachment on root of tooth and a definite marginal dehiscence that suggests influence of muscle or frenum pull. **D,** Epithelium is removed on distal surface of mesial papilla. It is placed at radicular surface of canine to test its tensional release. Retained sulcular wall is observed above graft. **E,** Distal papilla is lapped over mesial papilla. It is joined at midradicular area of canine and sutured on enamel below height of contour. Careful suturing of double papilla flap without tension enables suspension of flap with a labial suture on lateral incisor. Suturing technique must not create force that will separate graft. **F,** Double papilla approach can be combined with apically positioned flap in other areas. **G,** Six-month healed result. Connective tissue attachment on root of tooth is preserved, muscle pull is eliminated, and functional gingival unit is established.

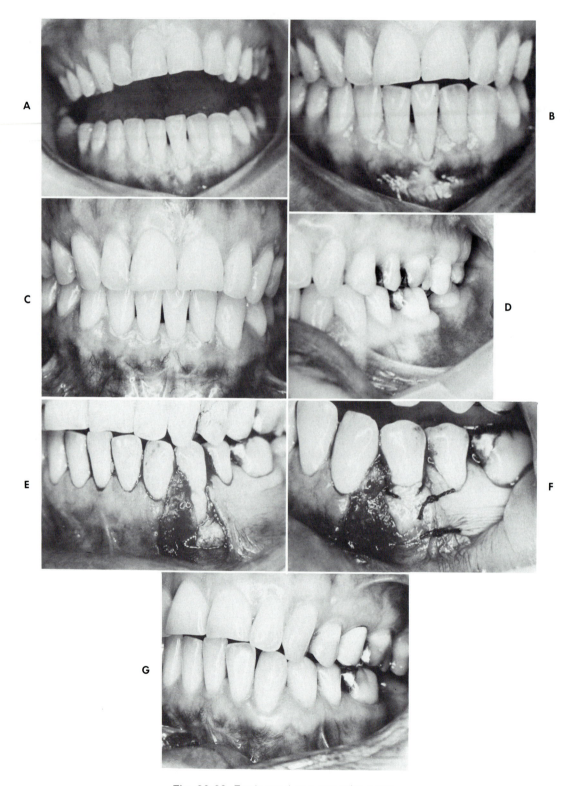

Fig. 26-96. For legend see opposite page.

area beyond the terminal tooth and the interdental papillae has greatly reduced wound dimension and minimized trauma. More important, these grafts provide mature gingiva at their terminus for adaptation to the corrected osseous morphology. After many years of clinical repair this mature tissue has not demonstrated significant shrinkage or contracture (Fig. 26-98). Aside from establishing an intact gingival unit in this manner, grafts can provide protective covering for therapeutic management of osseous defects.

Mental foramen. The neurovascular structures exiting from the mental foramen may present a problem in mucogingival surgery. The mental foramen opening is located halfway between the alveolar crest and the lower border of the mandible, usually between the first and second premolars. A mucogingival lesion may dictate that the mucogingival junction be located apically to gain attached gingiva or to deepen the vestibule in preparation for a free soft tissue or pedicle graft. Often variations in the location of the foramen are found. Elevating a full-thickness mucoperiosteal flap will allow direct visualization of these neurovascular structures. After a partial-thickness flap is initiated and the vestibule is deepened safely by sharp dissection, further extension of the vestibule may be needed. It should be accomplished by blunt dissection (pressure with a moist gauze sponge). As the loose areolar connective tissue is moved apically, the mental structures can be seen more readily. Traumatizing or severing the mental nerve can result in temporary or permanent paresthesia of the lip and gingiva.

Severing the mental artery is less significant since adequate collateral circulation exists. However, hemorrhage control is an immediate necessity (Fig. 26-99).

POSTERIOR LINGUAL REGION

Mylohyoid ridge and lingual nerve. The mylohyoid ridge anatomy may present difficulties in this area. Severe bone loss on the lingual surface of the molars creating wide bony ledges, infrabony defects, and inconsistent osseous margins requires a full-thickness mucoperiosteal flap for correction.

On the internal aspect of the body of the mandible the prominent mylohyoid ridge passes down and forward from the ramus distal to the third molar. It gradually terminates by fading into the inferior portion of the alveolar process in the premolar region. The mylohyoid ridge is the origin of the mylohyoid muscle, which forms the floor of the mouth. The mylohyoid ridge can vary in form (blunt, markedly elevated, or spiked). Severe bone loss on the lingual surfaces of the molar due to inadequate oral hygiene creates wide bony ledges, infrabony defects, and inconsistent osseous margins. Lingual infrabony pockets often can extend into the bifurcations of the molars (Tibbetts et al., 1976). With this understanding of the relationship of the mylohyoid ridge and the periodontal osseous defects, the other structures related to this area are of interest.

During periodontal surgery on the lingual aspect of the mandible, the major precaution is to avoid incising the superficial structures that lie just under the thin mucosa. The lingual nerve is easily

---

Fig. 26-96. Implication of a prolonged frenum pull corrected by single papillary graft procedure. Shown are severe etiologic factors in natural history of periodontal disease. **A,** In 1954 a gingival cleft resulting in a compensatory hyperkeratosis of gingival margin was observed on mandibular left central incisor. Gingival margin of left first premolar appeared normal. **B,** Mandibular anterior area was treated by vestibular extension and gingivoplasty. Scarification was seen 1 month postsurgically. Note width of attached gingiva on left first premolar as outlined by mucogingival junction. **C,** Six-year creeping attachment resulted on mandibular left central incisor. Significant recession and existence of a frenum pull were observed on first premolar. **D,** Twelve years later recession progressed to cause discomfort. Note direct visual influence of frenum pull, causing blanching of gingival margin. Probe extends 6 mm into pocket. **E,** V-shaped incision removing frenum pull has been completed. Partial-thickness papillary graft has been positioned at recipient site. Initially, careful root planing removed softened dentinal structures. Note severe buccal bone loss. **F,** Papillary graft was sutured passively at level of cervical abrasion and stabilized by interrupted sutures. Speculation would indicate operation of a combination of etiologic factors: toothbrush abrasion, lateral tongue thrusting, and secondary influence of frenum pull. **G,** Seventeen years later, 5 years after surgery. Crevicular depth is less than 2 mm. Influence of frenum is dissipated as evidenced by fine frenum now located interproximally.

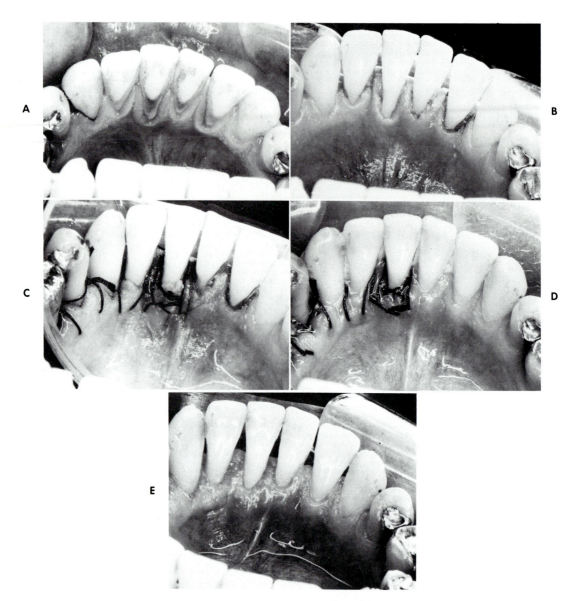

Fig. 26-97. Lingual double papilla graft. **A,** Prescaling view of gingival cleft on mandibular right central incisor. **B,** After plaque control, root scaling, root planing, and soft tissue curettage. **C,** Mucoperiosteal flap has treated lingual area extending from right lateral incisor to second molar. Continuous suturing has properly positioned flap 1 mm coronal to alveolar crest. Delicate papillae contiguous to right central incisor are overlapped and sutured to cover radicular lingual surface. Suspensory suture supports double papilla graft. **D,** Ten days after treatment, prior to removal of sutures. **E,** Repair of double papilla 4 months after surgery.

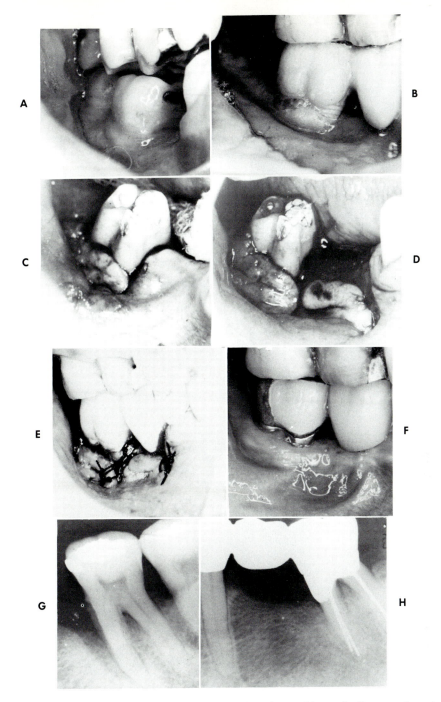

Fig. 26-98. Solution for external oblique second molar problem. **A,** Preoperative view. Free gingival margin on mandibular second molar. Note that vestibule extends to alveolar ridge in first molar area. **B,** Provisional splint was constructed. After several root scaling and root planing visits, gingival environment was inconsistent with sound periodontal preparation of tooth. Final restoration was delayed until intact gingival unit was developed. **C,** Pedicle graft of sufficient length was prepared from edentulous third molar area. Vestibular trough required deepening to permit space for relocated graft. Following these preparations a severe rise of alveolar mucosa at edentulous crest resulted. **D,** Partial-thickness graft has been moved apically at edentulous area of first molar. This creates environment of gingiva for pontic and a uniform level for mucogingival junction. **E,** Provisional splint has been replaced; pedicle grafts have been sutured; adequate zone of gingiva has been relocated. **F,** Optimal gingival health 12 years after surgery. **G,** Preoperative roentgenogram. Note deep radiolucency on mesial aspect of second molar. Pocket depth is 10 mm. **H,** Twelve-year recall visit. Endodontics and root planing have created this roentgenographic result. No osseous therapy or surgery was necessary. (In conjunction with Manual H. Marks, Levittown, Pa., and Arnold Weisgold, Philadelphia.)

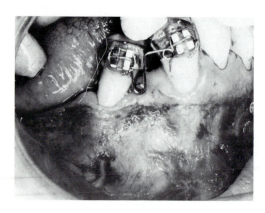

Fig. 26-99. Blunt dissection exposes mental foramen structures and avoids paresthesia.

damaged as it lies very close to the mucosal surface in the region of the second and third molars. The submandibular gland and duct and the lingual artery (although on the oral surface of the mylohyoid muscle) are less likely to be violated because of their deeper position. However, all of these structures are relatively safe from trauma if full-thickness mucoperiosteal flaps are used with blunt rather than sharp dissection. The elevation of the intact periosteum with the lingual flap avoids entry into the deeper structures and fascial planes as well as possible extension of infection (Fig. 26-100).

The full-thickness mucoperiosteal flap allows for proper flap retraction, good visibility, and good hemostasis. Vertical releasing incisions dis-

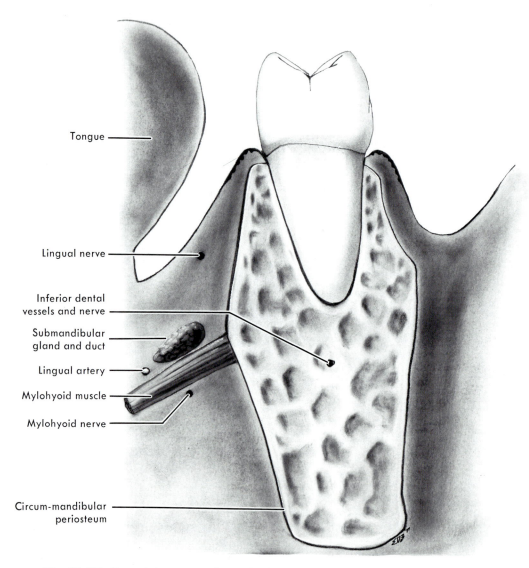

Tongue

Lingual nerve

Inferior dental vessels and nerve

Submandibular gland and duct

Lingual artery

Mylohyoid muscle

Mylohyoid nerve

Circum-mandibular periosteum

Fig. 26-100. Essential anatomy of mandibular lingual region; section through mandibular second molar.

tal to the molars should not extend beyond the mucogingival junction. Incisions into the mucosa are likely to involve branches of the sublingual artery. Hunt (1976) stresses four main problems in this area: (1) hemorrhage and postoperative hematoma, (2) nerve trauma, (3) trauma to the submandibular gland, and (4) infection. With these precautions in mind the elimination of the osseous defects and the reduction of the mylohyoid ridge are necessary to achieve ideal osseous contour.

Lingual tori. The most common location of mandibular tori is along the lingual aspect of the mandible, superior to the mylohyoid muscle, in the region of the canines and premolars. Lingual tori should be removed when associated with pocket depth. Complications may arise in flap elevation. The tissue is thin and tends to tear unless the elevation is cautious. Finger pressure should be used on the external surface of the gingiva to guide the periosteal elevator (Kopczyk and Young, 1976).

RETROMOLAR REGION: PTERYGOMANDIBULAR SPACE

The anterior wall of the pterygomandibular space is readily identified in the oral cavity as that part of oral mucosa between the elevations formed by a portion of the tendon of the temporal muscle and the pterygomandibular raphe. Those tendons of the temporal muscle that insert along the anterior border of the mandibular ramus form a prominent palpable ridge. The pterygomandibular raphe is formed by the attachment of the buccinator muscle to the superior pharyngeal constrictor muscle and lies immediately in front of the anterior border of the medial pterygoid muscle.

The pterygomandibular space is found between the ramus of the mandible and the pterygoid muscles. The fascial space is of particular significance as it contains the inferior alveolar artery and veins, the lingual nerve, and the inferior alveolar nerve. The space is bounded medially by the medial pterygoid muscle and laterally by the medial surface of the mandibular ramus (Clarke and Bueltmann, 1971). This space is entered when administering inferior alveolar nerve block anesthesia.

Surgical procedures in the retromolar area can encroach upon the pterygomandibular raphe and enter the pterygomandibular space. Aseptic technique must prevail to avoid infection spreading into this space or the deeper structures. Similarly, control of hemorrhage is essential to avoid the danger of a hematoma. Otherwise, because of their posterior position within the space, the structures are relatively difficult to injure (Hunt, 1976).

Maxilla
ANTERIOR FACIAL REGION (MUSCLES AND FRENA)

The alveolar process of the maxilla is the origin of several muscles. The attachment rarely limits the attempt for vestibular extension with flap procedures. The maxillary midline frenum has been extensively studied (see discussion on Frenotomy and Frenectomy).

POSTERIOR FACIAL REGION: ZYGOMATICOALVEOLAR RIDGE

The anterolateral surface of the maxillary body forms the skeleton of the anterior part of the cheek. The posterior surface is bounded by a bony ridge that begins at the tip of the zygomatic process, continues in a concave arc laterally and inferiorly in the direction of the socket of the first molar, and disappears at the base of the alveolar process. This bony crest is the zygomaticoalveolar ridge. When the jaw height is minimal and recession occurs, access to the molar areas becomes limited. Frequently there is insufficient space to establish a zone of attached gingiva before approaching the concavity of the molar surface. This is true especially with the second and third molars. Free soft tissue autografts are useful in this situation (Fig. 26-101).

PALATAL REGION

An understanding of the neurovascular structures that involve the foramen of the palate is necessary prior to palatal surgery. The greater palatine artery supplies the mucous membranes and the glands of the hard palate as well as the gingiva of the palatal surfaces of the maxillary alveolar process. It arises in the pterygopalatine fossa, descends through the pterygopalatine canal, and enters the oral cavity via the greater (or anterior) palatine foramen. This opening is situated at the angle formed by the intersection of the alveolar process and the horizontal portion of the palatine bone. It lies approximately 3 to 4 mm in front of the posterior border of the hard palate. After passing through the foramen the greater palatine artery turns anteriorly and courses forward in the submucosa of the hard palate, occupying a position in the groove found between the base of the alveolar process and the horizontal palatine process of the maxilla. The terminal por-

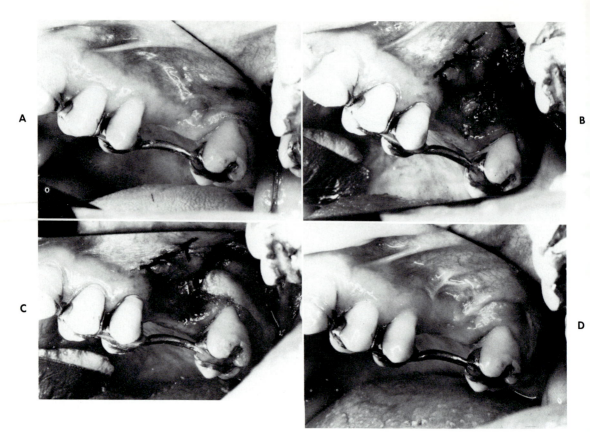

Fig. 26-101. Shallow maxillary vestibular fornix encroaching upon zygomaticoalveolar ridge. **A,** Recession on mesiobuccal root of second molar results in a free gingival margin and a shallow vestibular fornix. Buccinator muscle that limits depth of fornix approaches zygomaticoalveolar ridge. **B,** Partial-thickness connective tissue recipient bed preparation. Edentulous ridge vestibular depth is blended to deepened vestibule. **C,** Placement of gingival graft. **D,** One year after surgery. (In conjunction with Manuel H. Marks, Levittown, Pa.)

tion of the greater palatine artery, upon reaching the incisive foramen, becomes the nasopalatine artery and ascends through the incisive canal to the nasal cavity. The incisive foramen is located immediately behind the maxillary central incisors (Clarke, 1971).

The greater palatine nerve (a branch of the pterygopalatine nerve) enters the oral cavity (the greater palatine foramen), accompanying the greater palatine artery in its forward course along the palate. Another branch of the pterygopalatine nerve is characterized by its great length as it courses down and forward along the nasal septum, traverses the nasopalatine canal, and enters the oral cavity via the incisive foramen. The greater palatine nerve supplies the mucosa of the hard palate distal to the maxillary canine teeth; the nasopalatine nerve supplies the mucosa of the hard palate anterior to the maxillary canine teeth (Clarke, 1971).

Flap procedures of the anterior palate often sever nerves and vessels of the incisive foramen. Bleeding usually is not a problem because the vessels are so small. Paresthesia resulting from nerve damage is temporary. Unless a partial-thickness flap is required, severing these structures can be avoided by careful elevation of full-thickness flaps.

When the partial-thickness flap procedure is used in the posterior part of the palate, the neurovascular contents of the greater palatine foramen should be avoided. Fortunately, the greater palatine foramen is a safe distance from the bony crest and usually is not encountered. However, with advanced periodontal disease and a shallow palatal vault, greater care must be exercised to avoid these structures. If the tuberosity is flat with deep pockets distal to the terminal molar, a palatal vertical incision may be necessary and should be kept within the vertical height of the alveolar process. Terminal vessels are severed, and bleeding can be controlled easily by applying pressure with the retracting elevator, using a vaso-constrictor in the local anesthesia, or tying the vessel with absorbable sutures.

LOCATION OF GRAFT MARGIN

Should the flap be positioned at the crest, apical to the crest 1 or 2 mm coronal to the crest on the root, or as high coronally to the cementoenamel junction as the tissues will allow?

APICALLY POSITIONED GRAFT

With the use of the apically positioned full-thickness graft, Friedman (1962) originally felt that the radicular bone should be protected and that the margin of the graft should be placed to "just cover" the alveolar crest. Friedman and Levine (1964) modified their incision to create a scalloped margin of the graft that is "sutured so that the marginal bone and approximately 1 or 2 mm of cementum are covered." This is applicable to situations where a wide zone of gingiva (4 to 6 mm) is present. It is their most used apically repositioned graft. This is the most common graft used.

We know that when the gingival margin is placed to cover the crest, a biologic width of gingival fibers must form so that there is an increase in the gingival width by at least 1 mm beyond the existent measurement of the retained gingiva. With this in mind, the rationale of placing the flap 1 or 2 mm on the root (as advocated by Friedman and Levine) is sound. They reasoned that since a biologic width of gingiva coronal to the crest was obtained, why not protect this area and expedite repair. It was sound planning, provided that the width of salvaged gingiva was sufficient to compensate for any changes that might occur.

Holmes and Strem (1976) were the first to study the position of the flap on the root immediately after interrupted interproximal sutures were used with the apically positioned graft procedure. Root coverage was about 2 mm from the flap margin to the crest of the alveolar process. There was no correlation between the amount of root covered by the flap margin immediately following surgery and the residual crevicular depth on healing.

When only 1 or 2 mm of gingiva is available and is positioned on a cemental surface, any marginal necrosis, injury, or loss of gingiva will result in failure and a recurrence of sulcular depth into the mucosa. Another contraindication against

placement of a minimal width of gingiva on the root is that the approximate 2 mm of gingival width may be insufficient to dissipate the muscle and frenum pull. Although attachment and healing occur interproximally, transient marginal pull may interfere with close adaptation and healing. In addition, if the radicular bone is thin (with or without a fenestration or dehiscence), the mere elevation of a full-thickness flap has been shown to result in bone loss (clinically in human patients). If the thin gingival band remains unattached or becomes detached, pocket depth can recur.

Where the gingival margin will be placed will depend upon the amount of gingiva available. If 2 or 3 mm of gingiva is present, all the gingiva is retained and the pocket wall is debrided. A partial-thickness flap is raised; interproximal osseous corrections are made; any reverse connective tissue architecture is corrected to the conceptual form using a curet; and the gingival margin of the flap is placed apically so that 1 or 2 mm of the connective tissue attachment over the tooth or bone is left uncovered. From this original gingival connective tissue bed, new gingiva will form. If the radicular surface should require osseous correction, the marginal bone should not be left exposed but should be covered by some type of pedicle graft. If a pedicle graft is not available the flap should cover the bone. Later a free soft tissue autograft can increase the attached gingiva.

MULTIPLE INTERDENTAL PAPILLA GRAFT

The presence of 0.5 to 1 mm of gingiva or an alveolar mucosal margin requires a more critical surgical diagnosis. Consideration has to include the need for interproximal osseous correction, the thickness of the marginal bone, and the depth of the vestibule.

Generally with little or no gingiva the marginal bone is thin and is complicated frequently by fenestrations and dehiscences. There may be a relatively shallow vestibule with interproximal osseous defects that require correction. If a partial-thickness flap dissection were employed, the periosteum would be exposed, resulting in bone loss, anatomic defects, and lack of gingiva. A better choice would be the use of the multiple interdental papilla graft. It would provide a keratinized epithelial surface and avoid the above hazards. The length and width of the papilla should be at least 3 mm, placed between 1 and 2 mm coronal to the alveolar crest.

If there is little or no attached gingiva with no

interproximal defects and a shallow vestibule, a free soft tissue autograft is preferred. Accordingly, it should be placed to cover the root. With normal interproximal bone height, anatomic defects of the root can be covered by either graft. Root deformity, root caries, availability of donor tissue, and collateral circulation will influence the success of the correction.

PALATAL GRAFT

The gingiva is scalloped so that 1 or 2 mm of the palatal crest is covered.

LATERALLY POSITIONED GRAFT

Grupe describes this graft, which covers the exposed root surface, implying that the gingival margin is at the cementoenamel junction (Grupe and Warren, 1956). Technical problems involve the depth of the gingival sulcus, the movement of the flap after suturing, and the slight apical displacement of the flap in applying the dressing. Under normal circumstances the gingival margin should be located on the enamel below the height of contour and coronal to the cementoenamel junction. The graft positioned in this manner compensates for the inherent problems. The aesthetic result is optimal.

DOUBLE PAPILLA POSITIONED GRAFT

The double papilla positioned graft is placed to improve the aesthetics, as in the laterally positioned graft. However, if the restorative dentistry must involve this area, the margin of the flap is placed at the connective tissue attachment to the tooth or between 1 and 2 mm on the root, covering the free exposed marginal bone.

EDENTULOUS AREA PEDICLE GRAFT

The margin of this partial-thickness mucogingival graft is moved laterally and apically. It is placed between 1 and 2 mm on the root to cover the crestal margin of the bone or at the connective tissue attachment to the tooth. If the edentulous alveolar crest is near the normal cementoenamel junction level, the position of the pedicle graft on the root of the tooth can be related to the adjacent supporting tissue (Fig. 26-79). Without this supporting tissue the grafts will fail. If the free gingival collar can be preserved, increased attached gingiva can be obtained by approximating the pedicle graft to the retained free gingiva. In this manner limited donor tissue can be effective (Fig. 26-73).

FREE SOFT TISSUE GRAFT

When a functional repair of increased attached gingiva is desired, the major portion of the graft must be placed on a rigid connective tissue bed attached to the bone and the tooth. This is the source from which early vascularization is derived.

When an aesthetic correction is desirable to repair a denuded root, the principles of bridging must be followed carefully. The type of recession will dictate the degree of graft attachment to the root. The free graft may be placed on the cementum or it may even cover the cementoenamel junction. This will be dependent upon the height of the adjacent interdental papillae and the amount of cementum that is exposed. The collateral circulation is developed from the adjacent mesial and distal recipient beds and the apical connective tissue site. It can provide the vascularization necessary for the graft to "take" to the coronal edge of the cementum. In the deep wide type of recession, it is most difficult to develop complete bridging to cover the root. Approximately 70% root coverage can be expected if the width of the exposed cemental surface is less than 3 mm and the depth of the lesion in an apical direction is 3 mm or less (Mlinek et al., 1973).

If necrosis does occur on the avascular root, the length of the graft should be sufficient to provide at least 3 mm of apical connective tissue coverage so that a functional gingival attachment will survive. Clinical success has been experienced with exposed bone as part of the recipient bed (Dordick et al., 1976). This depends upon whether the perimeter of the graft can supply sufficient plasmatic diffusion to maintain its viability until capillaries from the host bed revascularize the graft. Under most circumstances, 1 or 2 mm of the denuded root can be covered by the free graft because of the three-point collateral circulation that develops at the apical portion of the exposed root.

CORONALLY POSITIONED GRAFT

A two-stage procedure has been the most consistent method of gaining increased gingival width and correcting unaesthetic areas of recession. It is suggested that the margin of the graft be placed 1 mm on the enamel coronal to the cementoenamel junction (Bernimoulin, 1975).

SUMMARY

Accomplishment of the therapeutic objectives in reconstructive mucogingival surgery is dependent upon initial incision planning, flap design, and tissue placement by effective suturing. Collectively, the technique revisions rely upon genetic coding, the origins of tissues, and the biologic repair principles of using keratinized tissues to cover operative sites.

The laterally positioned graft takes advantage of increased connective tissue support adjacent to the avascular denuded root. This has improved the consistency of successful attachment to denuded roots. Similarly, the principles of collateral circulation utilizing the free soft tissue autograft have improved the aesthetic repair of teeth with recession. The retention of marginal free gingiva has maintained the most coronal connective tissue attachment to the roots of teeth, while pedicle grafts positioned adjacent to these margins have restored functional gingiva.

The range in mucogingival surgery design is limited only by the imaginative planning of the clinician. It is not unreasonable to expect the clinical testing of creative surgical designs directed toward the increased longevity of an intact functional periodontium. Overly ambitious efforts that violate biologic principles should be condemned. Experience and introspective evaluation offer promise that needless surgery will be avoided.

Rather than categorize all treatment to satisfy a limited surgical capability, the accomplished periodontist should select the appropriate surgical design to correct the morphologic and topographic defects present, to minimize trauma, and to be considerate of patient comfort.

ACKNOWLEDGMENT

Appreciation is expressed to Ms. Elissa Berardi, University of Pennsylvania School of Dental Medicine, for the illustrations and to Mr. David Sullivan, Director of Photography, University of Pennsylvania School of Dental Medicine, for his artistic reproduction of photographs.

REFERENCES

Abrams, L., and Coslet, J. G.: Occlusal adjustment by selective grinding. In Goldman, H. M., and Cohen, D. W., editors: Periodontal therapy, ed. 5, St. Louis, 1973, The C. V. Mosby Co., p. 547.

Archer, W. H.: Oral surgery, ed. 4, St. Louis, 1966, The C. V. Mosby Co., p. 249.

Ariaudo, A., and Tyrrell, H.: Elimination of pockets extending to or beyond the mucogingival junction, Dent. Clin. North Am., p. 67, March, 1960.

Ariaudo, A., and Tyrrell, H.: Repositioning and increasing the zone of attached gingiva, J. Periodontol. **28:**106, 1957.

Arnold, N., and Hatchett, G.: A comparative investigation of two mucogingival surgical methods, J. Periodontol. **33:**129, 1962.

Baer, P. N., Sumner, C. F., and Miller, G.: Periodontal dressings, Dent. Clin. North Am. **13:**181, 1969.

Baer, P. N., Sumner, C. F., and Scigliano, J.: Studies on a hydrogenated fat–zinc bacitracin periodontal dressing, Oral Surg. **13:**494, 1960.

Barsky, A. J., Kahn, S., and Simon, B. E.: Principles and practice of plastic surgery, ed. 2, New York, 1964, McGraw-Hill Book Company.

Basaraba, N.: Root amputation and tooth hemisection, Dent. Clin. North Am. **13:**121, 1969.

Becker, N. G.: A free gingival graft utilizing a pre-suturing technique, Periodontics **5:**194, 1967.

Bernimoulin, J. P., Luscher, B., and Muhlemann, H. R.: Coronally repositioned periodontal flap, J. Clin. Periodontol. **2:**1, 1975.

Bhaskar, S. N., editor: Orban's oral history and embryology, ed. 8, St. Louis, 1976, The C. V. Mosby Co.

Bhaskar, S. N., Cutright, D. E., Bienvenidao, P., and Beasley, J. D.: Full and partial thickness pedicle grafts in miniature swine and man, J. Periodontol. **42:**66, 1971.

Bhaskar, S. N., Cutright, D. E., Beasley, J. D., Perez, B., and Hunsuck, E. E.: Healing under full and partial thickness mucogingival flaps in the miniature swine, J. Periodontol. **41:**675, 1970.

Bhaskar, S. N., Frisch, J., Margetis, P. M., and Leonard, F.: Oral surgery — oral pathology conference no. 18, Walter Reed Army Medical Center. Application of a new chemical adhesive in periodontic and oral surgery, Oral Surg. **22:**526, 1966.

Bhaskar, S. N., Jacoway, J. R., Margetis, P. M., Leonard, F., and Pani, K. G.: Oral tissue response to chemical adhesives (cyanoacrylates), Oral Surg. **22:**394, 1966.

Bjorn, H.: Free transplantation of gingiva propria, Sven. Tandlak. Tidskr. **22:**684, 1963.

Billingham, R. E., and Silvers, W. K.: Studies on the conservation of epidermal specificities of skin and certain mucosas in adult mammals, J. Exp. Med. **125:**429, 1967.

Binnie, W. H., and Forrest, J. O.: A study of tissue response to cyanoacrylate adhesive in periodontal surgery, J. Periodontol. **45:**619, 1974.

Bisnoff, H. L., The labile frenum, Dent. Outlook **31:**146, 1944.

Bohannan, H.: Studies in the alteration of the vestibular depth. III. Vestibular incision, J. Periodontol. **34:**209, 1963.

Bohannan, H.: Studies in the alteration of the vestibular depth. II. Periosteum retention, J. Periodontol. **33:**354, 1962.

Bohannan, H.: Studies in the alteration of the vestibular depth. I. Complete denudation, J. Periodontol. **33:**120, 1962.

Bowers, G.: A study of the width of attached gingiva, J. Periodontol. **34:**201, 1963.

Brackett, R. C., and Gargiulo, A. W.: Free gingival grafts in humans, J. Periodontol. **41:**581, 1970.

Bressman, E.: The importance of the frenum pull in periodontal disease. In Ward, H. L., editor: A periodontal point of view, Springfield, Ill., 1973, Charles C Thomas, Publisher, p. 323.

Brustein, D.: Cosmetic periodontics: coronally repositioned pedicle graft, Dent. Surv. **46:**22, 1970.

Caffesse, R. G., and Guinard, E.: Treatment of localized gingival recessions. I. Lateral sliding flap. II. Coronally repositioned flap with a free gingival graft. III. Lateral sliding and coronally repositioned flaps. J. Periodontol. **49:**351, 357, 457, 1978.

Carranza, F. A., Jr., and Carraro, J. J.: Effect of removal of periosteum on postoperative results of mucogingival surgery, J. Periodontol. **34:**223, 1963.

Chacker, F. M., and Cohen, D. W.: Regeneration of gingival tissues in non-human primates (abstract), J. Dent. Res. **39:**743, 1960.

Clark, J.: Mucogingival surgical techniques; an appraisal, J. Periodontol. **34:**158, 1963.

Clarke, M. A., and Bueltmann, K. W.: Anatomical considerations in periodontal surgery, J. Periodontol. **42:**610, 1971.

Cohen, D. W., and Ross, S. D.: The double papillae repositioned flap in periodontal therapy, J. Periodontol. **39:**65, 1968.

Corn, H.: Mucogingival surgery and associated problems. In Goldman, H. M., and Cohen, D. W., editors: Periodontal therapy, ed. 5, St. Louis, 1973, The C. V. Mosby Co., p. 716.

Corn, H.: Edentulous area pedicle grafts in mucogingival surgery, Periodontics **2:**229, 1964.

Corn, H.: Periosteal separation — its clinical significance, J. Periodontol. **33:**140, 1962.

Corn, H.: Technique for repositioning the frenum in periodontal problems, Dent. Clin. North Am., p. 79, March, 1961.

Corn, H., and Marks, M. H.: The role of the dental assistant in oral hygiene instruction, Dent. Assist. **38:**12, 1969.

Corn, H., and Marks, M. H.: Strategic extractions in periodontal therapy, Dent. Clin. North Am. **13:**817, 1969.

Corn, H., Marks, M. H., and Corn, B. M.: Educating the patient in effective plaque control, vol. 2. In Clark, J. W., editor: Clinical dentistry, New York, 1976, Harper & Row, Publishers.

Corn, H., Marks, M. H., and Coslet, J. G.: Oral hygiene instructions, your insurance for healthy teeth and gums, Philadelphia, 1968, University of Pennsylvania Press.

Costich, E. R., and Ramfjord, S. P.: Healing after partial denudation of the alveolar process, J. Periodontol. **39:**127, 1968.

Cowan, A.: Sulcus deepening incorporating mucosal graft, J. Periodontol. **36:**188, 1965.

Dahlberg, W. H.: Incisions and suturing: some basic considerations about each in periodontal flap surgery, Dent. Clin. North Am. **13:**149, 1969.

Davis, J. S., and Kitlowski, E. A.: The immediate contraction of cutaneous grafts and its cause, Arch. Surg. **23:**954, 1931.

Dewel, B. F.: Normal and abnormal labial frenum differentiation, J. Am. Dent. Assoc. **33:**318, 1964.

Donnenfeld, O., Marks, R., and Glickman, I.: The apically repositioned flap — a clinical study, J. Periodontol. **35:**381, 1964.

Dordick, B., Coslet, J. G., and Seibert, J. S.: Clinical evaluation of free autogenous gingival grafts placed on alveolar bone. II. Coverage of non-pathologic dehiscences and fenestrations, J. Periodontol. **47:**568, 1976.

Dordick, B., Coslet, J. G., and Seibert, J. S.: Clinical evaluation of free autogenous gingival grafts placed on alveolar bone. I. Clinical predictability, J. Periodontol. **47:**559, 1976.

Edel, A.: Clinical evaluation of free connective tissue grafts used to increase the width of keratinized gingiva, J. Clin. Periodontol. **1**(4):185, 1974.

Egli, U., Vollmer, W. H., and Rateitschak, R. H.: Followup studies of free gingival grafts, J. Clin. Periodontol. **2**(2):98, 1975.

Fagan, F.: Clinical comparison of the free soft tissue autograft and partial thickness apically positioned flap — preoperative

gingival or mucosal margins, J. Periodontol. **46:**586, 1975.

Fagan, F., and Freeman, E.: Clinical comparison of the free gingival graft and partial thickness apically positioned flap, J. Periodontol. **45:**3, 1974.

Fomon, S.: Cosmetic surgery, Philadelphia, 1960, J. B. Lippincott Co.

Formicola, A. J., Simon, B., and Pennel, B.: Non-pocket mucogingival deformities, vol. 3. In Clark, J. W., editor: Clinical dentistry, New York, 1976, Harper & Row, Publishers.

Forrest, J. O.: The use of cyanoacrylates in periodontal surgery, J. Periodontol. **45:**225, 1974.

Friedman, N.: Mucogingival surgery, the apically repositioned flap, J. Periodontol. **33:**328, 1962.

Friedman, N.: Mucogingival surgery, Tex. Dent. J. **75:**358, 1957.

Friedman, N., and Levine, L.: Mucogingival surgery, current status, J. Periodontol. **35:**5, 1964; Dent. Clin. North Am., p. 63, March, 1964.

Frisch, J., and Bhaskar, S. N.: Free mucosal graft with tissue adhesives — report of 17 cases, J. Periodontol. **39:**190, 1968.

Frisch, J., and Bhaskar, S. N.: Tissue response to eugenol-containing periodontal dressing, J. Periodontol. **38:**402, 1967.

Gaberthull, T. W., and Mormann, W.: The angrographic tension test in mucogingival surgery, J. Periodont. **49:**385, 1978.

Gage, R. W., II.: Personal communication, Ft. Lauderdale, Florida, 1967.

Gargiulo, A., and Arrocha, E.: Histochemical evaluations of free gingival grafts, Periodontics **5:**285, 1967.

Geiger, A., and Hirschfeld, L.: Minor tooth movement in general practice, ed. 3, St. Louis, 1974, The C. V. Mosby Co.

Glickman, I.: Clinical periodontology, ed. 4, Philadelphia, 1972, W. B. Saunders Co., pp. 719, 728.

Goldman, H. M.: The Development of physiologic contours by gingivoplasty, Oral Surg. **3:**879, 1950.

Goldman, H. M., and Cohen, D. W., editors: Periodontal therapy, ed. 4, St. Louis, 1964, The C. V. Mosby Co.

Goldman, H. M., and Cohen, D. W., editors: Periodontal therapy, ed. 5, St. Louis, 1968, The C. V. Mosby Co.

Goldman, H. M., and Cohen, D. W.: Periodontia, ed. 4, St. Louis, 1957, The C. V. Mosby Co.

Goldman, H. M., Isenberg, G., and Shuman, A.: The gingival autograft and gingivectomy, J. Periodontol. **47:**586, 1976.

Goldman, H. M., and Smukler, H.: Controlled surgical stimulation of periosteum, J. Periodontol. **49:**518, 1978.

Gottsegen, R.: Frenum position and vestibular depth in relation to gingival health, Oral Surg. **7:**1069, 1954.

Grant, D. A., Stern, I. B., and Everett, F. G.: Orban's periodontics, ed. 4, St. Louis, 1972, The C. V. Mosby Co., p. 7.

Grupe, H. E.: Modified technique for the sliding flap operation, J. Periodontol. **37:**491, 1966.

Grupe, H. E., and Warren, R. F.: Repair of gingival defects by a sliding flap operation, J. Periodontol. **27:**290, 1956.

Haggerty, P. G.: The use of a free gingival graft to create a healthy environment for full crown preparation, case history, Periodontics **4:**329, 1966.

Halsted, W. S.: Ligature and suture material, J.A.M.A. **60:** 1119, 1913.

Harvey, P. M.: Surgical reconstruction of the gingiva. II. Procedures, N.Z. Dent. J. **66:**42, 1970.

Harvey, P. M.: Management of advanced periodontitis. I.

Preliminary report of a method of surgical reconstruction, N. Z. Dent. J. **61:**180, 1965.

Hattler, A. B.: Mucogingival surgery — Utilization of interdental gingiva as attached gingiva by surgical displacement, Periodontics **5:**126, 1967.

Hawley, C. E., and Staffileno, H.: Clinical evaluation of free gingival grafts in periodontal surgery, J. Periodontol. **41:**105, 1970.

Helburn, R. L., Cohen, D. W., and Chacker, F. M.: Healing of repositioned mucogingival flaps in monkeys, Abstract no. 324, I.A.D.R. Program and abstract of papers, 1963.

Henry, S. W., Levin, M. P., and Tsaknis, P. J.: Histologic features of the superior labial frenum, J. Periodontol. **47:**25, 1976.

Hiatt, W. H.: Regeneration via flap operation and the pulpal periodontal lesion, Periodontics **4:**205, 1966.

Hiatt, W. H., Stallard, R. E., Butler, E. D., and Badgett, B.: Repair following mucoperiosteal flap surgery with full gingival retention, J. Periodontol. **39:**11, 1968.

Hirschfeld, I.: The toothbrush; its use and abuse, J. Am. Dent. Assoc. **26:**1237, 1939.

Holmes, C. H., and Strem, B. E.: Location of flap margin after suturing, J. Periodontol. **47:**674, 1976.

Hunt, P. R.: Safety aspects of mandibular lingual surgery, J. Periodontol. **47:**224, 1976.

Irwin, R. K.: Combined use of the gingival graft and rotated pedicle procedures; case reports, J. Periodontol. **48:**38, 1977.

Janson, W. A., Ruben, M. P., Kramer, G. M., Bloom, A. A., and Turner, H.: Development of the blood supply to split-thickness free gingival autografts, J. Periodontol. **40:**707, 1969.

Kantor, M., Polson, A. M., and Zander, A. A.: Alveolar bone regeneration after removal of inflammatory and traumatic factors, J. Periodontol. **47:**687, 1976.

Karring, T., Cumming, B. R., Oliver, R. C., and Löe, H.: The origin of granulation tissue and its impact on postoperative results of mucogingival surgery, J. Periodontol. **46:**577, 1975.

Karring, T., Lang, N. P., and Löe, H.: Role of connective tissue in determining epithelial specificity, J. Dent. Res. **51:**1303, 1972.

Karring, T., Lang, N. P., and Löe, H.: The role of gingival connective tissue in determining epithelial differentiation, J. Periodont. Res. **10:**1, 1974.

Karring, T., Ostergaard, E., and Löe, H.: Conservation of tissue specificity after heterotopic transplantation of gingiva and alveolar mucosa, J. Periodont. Res. **6:**282, 1971.

King, K., and Pennel, B. M.: Evaluation of attempts to increase the width of attached gingiva. Presented to the Philadelphia Society of Periodontology, 1964.

Kirkland, O.: Modified flap operation in surgical treatments of periodontoclasia, J. Am. Dent. Assoc. **19:**1918, 1932.

Klavan, B.: The replaced graft, J. Periodontol. **41:**406, 1970.

Knox, L. R., and Young, H. C.: Histological studies of the labial frenum, I.A.D.R. Program and abstract of Papers, 1962.

Kopczyk, R. A., and Saxe, S. F.: Clinical signs of gingival inadequacy: the tension test, J. Dent. Child. **41:**22, 1974.

Kopczyk, R. A., and Young, L. L.: Principles of periodontal surgery, vol. 3. In Clark, J. W., editor: Clinical dentistry, New York, 1976, Harper & Row, Publishers.

Kramer, G. M., and Kohn, J. D.: A classification of periodontal surgery; an approach based on tissue coverage, Periodontics **4:**80, 1966.

Kramer, G. M., Nevins, M., and Kohn, J. D.: The utilization of periosteal suturing in periodontal surgical procedures, J. Periodontol. **41:**457, 1970.

Kuba, S. K., Hoag, P. M., and Rosenfeld, L. O.: A model for the demonstration of suturing technics, J. Periodontol. **43:**573, 1972.

Lange, N. P., and Löe, H.: The relationship between the width of keratinized gingiva and gingival health, J. Periodontol. **43:**623, 1972.

Levine, H. L.: Periodontal flap surgery with gingival fiber retention, J. Periodontol. **43:**91, 1972.

Levine, H. L., and Stahl, S. S.: Repair following periodontal flap surgery with the retention of gingival fibers: J. Periodontol. **43:**99, 1972.

Lindhe, J., and Svanberg, G.: Influence of trauma from occlusion on progression of experimental periodontitis in beagle dog, J. Clin. Periodont. **1:**3, 1974.

Livingston, H. L.: Total coverage of multiple and adjacent denuded root surfaces with a free gingival autograft, a case report, J. Periodontol. **46:**209, 1975.

Matter, J., and Cimasoni, G.: Creeping attachment after free gingival grafts, J. Periodontol. **47:**574, 1976.

Maynard, J. G., Jr.: Coronal positioning of a previously placed autogenous gingival graft, J. Periodontol. **48:**151, 1977.

Maynard, J. G., Jr., and Ochsenbein, C.: Mucogingival problems — prevalence and therapy in children, J. Periodontol. **46:**543, 1975.

McFall, W. T., Jr.: The laterally repositioned flap — criteria for success, Periodontics **5:**89, 1967.

McGregor, I. A.: Fundamental techniques of plastic surgery, ed. 2, Baltimore, 1962, The Williams & Wilkins Company.

Megarbane, J.: A new approach for gingival grafting. Maximizing attached gingiva and minimizing surgical trauma, J. Periodontol. **46:**217, 1975.

Melcher, S. W.: Codestructive factors of marginal periodontitis and repetitive mechanical injury, J. Dent. Res. (special issue C) **54:**78-85, 1975.

Miller, G. M., Dannenbaum, R., and Cohen, D. W.: A preliminary histologic study of the wound healing of mucogingival flaps when secured with the cyanoacrylate tissue adhesives, J. Periodontol. **45:**608, 1974.

Mlinek, A., Smukler, H., and Buchner, A.: The use of free gingival grafts for the coverage of denuded roots, J. Periodontol. **44:**248, 1973.

Morris, M. L.: Short communications — flap terminology, J. Periodontol. **47:**543, 1976.

Morris, M. L.: Suturing technique in periodontal surgery, Periodontics **3:**84, 1965.

Morris, M. L.: The unrepositioned mucoperiosteal flap, periodontics **3:**147, 1965.

Moskow, B. S., and Bressman, E.: Localized gingival recession, Dent. Radiogr. Photogr. **38:**3, 1965.

Nabers, C. L.: When is gingival repositioning an indicated procedure? Periodont. Abstr. **5:**93, 1957.

Nabers, C. L.: Repositioning the attached gingiva, J. Periodontol. **25:**38, 1954.

Nabers, C. L., Spear, G. R., and Beckham, L. C.: Alveolar dehiscence, Tex. Dent. J. **78:**4, 1960.

Nabers, J.: Extension of the vestibular fornix utilizing a gingival graft, Periodontics **4:**77, 1966.

Nizel, A. E.: Nutrition in preventive dentistry: science and practice, Philadelphia, 1972, W. B. Saunders Co.

Novaes, A. B., Kon, S., Ruben, M. P., and Novaes, A. B., Jr.: Rebuilding of microvascularization following surgical gingival elimination by split flap study by perfusion and diaphanization, J. Periodontol. **47:**217, 1976.

Ochsenbein, C.: The double flap procedure, Periodontics **1:** 17, 1963.

Ochsenbein, C.: Newer concepts of mucogingival surgery, J. Periodontol. **31:**75, 1960.

Ochsenbein, C., and Ross, S.: The tuberosity pedicle flap, J. Periodontol. In press.

Oliver, R. C., Löe, H., and Karring, T.: Microscopic evaluation of the healing and revascularization of free gingival grafts, J. Periodontol. Res. **3:**84, 1968.

Patur, B., and Glickman, I.: Gingival pedicle flaps for covering root surfaces denuded by chronic destructive periodontal disease — a clinical experiment, J. Periodontol. **29:**51, 1958.

Pennel, B. M., Higgason, J. D., Towner, J. D., King, K. O., Fritz, B. D., and Sadler, F. F.: Retention of periosteum in mucogingival surgery, J. Periodontol. **36:**39, 1965.

Pennel, B. M., Higgason, J. D., Towner, J. D., King, K. O., Fritz, B. D., and Sadler, J. F.: Oblique rotated flap, J. Periodontol. **36:**305, 1965.

Pennel, B. M., Tabor, J. C., King, K. O., Justin, D. T., Fritz, B. D., and Higgason, J. D.: Free masticatory mucosa graft, J. Periodontol. **40:**162, 1969.

Pfeifer, J. S.: The reaction of alveolar bone to flap procedures in man, Periodontics **3:**135, 1965.

Pfeifer, J. S.: The growth of gingival tissue over denuded bone, J. Periodontol. **34:**10, 1963.

Pfeifer, J. S., and Heller, R.: Histologic evaluation of full and partial thickness laterally repositioned flaps — a pilot study, J. Periodontol. **42:**331, 1971.

Placek, M., Skach, M., and Mrklas, L.: Significance of the labial frenum attachment in periodontal disease in man. II. I. J. Periodontol. **45:**891, 1974.

Placek, M., Skach, M., and Mrklas, L.: Significance of the labial frenum attachment in periodontal disease in Man. II. J. Periodontol. **45:**895, 1974.

Pustigioni, F. E., Kon, S., Novaes, A. B., and Ruben, M. P.: Split thickness flap, apically replaced with protected linear periosteal fenestration, J. Periodontol. **46:**742, 1975.

Ramfjord, S. P., and Costich, E. R.: Healing after exposure of periosteum on the alveolar process, J. Periodontol. **39:** 199, 1968.

Ramfjord, S. P., Knowles, J. W., Nissle, R. R., Burgett, F. G., and Shick, R. A.: Results following three modalities of periodontal therapy, J. Periodontol. **46:**522, 1975.

Ramfjord, S. P., and Nissle, R. R.: The modified Widman flap, J. Periodontol. **45:**601, 1974.

Rosling, B., Nyman, S., Lindhe, J., and Jern, B.: The healing potential of periodontal tissues following different techniques of periodontal surgery in plaque-free dentitions. A two year clinical study, J. Clin. Periodontol. **3:**233, 1976.

Ross, J. R., Miller, P. D., Sconyers, J., and Kimmelman, J. R.: Presurgical considerations in clinical dentistry. In Clark, J. W., editor: vol. 3, New York, 1976, Harper & Row, Publishers, p. 12.

Restrepo, O. J.: Coronally repositioned flap — report of four cases, J. Periodontol. **44:**564, 1973.

Robinson, R. E.: Utilizing an edentulous area as a donor site in the lateral repositioned flap, Periodontics **2:**79, 1964.

Robinson, R. E., and Agnew, R. G.: Periosteal fenestration at the mucogingival line, J. Periodontol. **34:**503, 1963.

Roth, H.: Some speculation as to predictable fenestrations prior to mucogingival surgery; a preliminary report, Periodontics **3:**29, 1965.

Sandalli, P.: A new method in gingival graft, J. Periodontol. **45:**595, 1974.

Shirazy, E.: Frenum labii superioris, J. Am. Dent. Assoc. **25:**761, 1938.

Sicher, H., and DuBrul, E. L.: Oral anatomy, ed. 6, St. Louis, 1975, The C. V. Mosby Co.

Slavkin, H. C.: Epithelial-mesenchymal interactions related to periodontal disease, J. Periodontol. **41:**373, 1970.

Smith, J. H.: The effect of surgically produced foramina on the coverage of exposed bone in mucogingival surgery, Oral Surg. **15:**665, 1962.

Smith, R. N.: A study of intertransplantation of gingiva, Oral Surg. **29:**169, 1970.

Smukler, H.: Laterally positioned mucoperiosteal pedicle grafts in treatment of denuded roots — a classical and statistical study, J. Periodontol. **47:**590, 1976.

Soehren, S. E., Allen, A. L., Cutright, D. E., and Seibert, J. S.: Clinical and histologic studies of donor tissues utilized for free grafts of masticatory mucosa, J. Periodontol. **44:** 727, 1973.

Staffileno, H.: Significant differences and advantages between the full thickness and split thickness flaps, J. Periodontol. **45:**421, 1974.

Staffileno, H.: Significant differences and advantages between the full thickness and split thickness flaps, In Ward, H. L., editor: A periodontal point of view, Springfield, Ill., 1973, Charles C Thomas, Publisher.

Staffileno, H.: Management of gingival recession and root exposure problems associated with periodontal disease, Dent. Clin. North Am., p. 111, March, 1964.

Staffileno, H., Jr., and Levy, S.: Histologic and clinical study of mucosal (gingival) transplants in dogs, J. Periodontol. **40:**5, 1969.

Staffileno, H., Levy, S., and Gargiulo, A.: Histologic study of cellular mobilization and repair following a periosteal retention operation via split thickness mucogingival flap surgery, J. Periodontol. **37:**117, 1966.

Stahl, S. S., Cantor, M., and Ziwig, E.: Fenestrations of the labial alveolar plate in human skulls, Periodontics **1:**99, 1963.

Stark, R. B.: Plastic surgery, New York, 1962, Harper & Row, Publishers.

Sternlicht, H. C.: A Contiguous mucosal graft, J. Periodontol. **46:**221, 1975.

Sullivan, H. C., and Atkins, J. H.: Free autogenous gingival grafts. I. Principles of successful grafting, Periodontics **6:** 127, 1968.

Sullivan, H. C., and Atkins, J. H.: Free autogenous gingival grafts. III. Utilization of grafts in the treatment of gingival recessions, Periodontics **6:**152, 1968.

Sullivan, H. C., Carmen, D., and Dinner, D.: Histologic evaluation of the laterally positioned flap, Abstract no. 467, I.A.D.R. Program and Abstract of Papers, p. 169, 1971a.

Sullivan, H. C., Dinner, D., and Carmen, D.: Clinical evaluation of the laterally positioned flap, Abstract no. 466, I.A.D.R. Program and Abstract of Papers, p. 169, 1971b.

Sumner, C. F.: Surgical repair of recession on the maxillary cuspid; incisally repositioning the gingival tissues, J. Periodontol. **40:**55, 1969.

Tabor, J., and Pennel, B. M.: Lecture presented to American Society of Periodontists, Colorado Springs, Colo., 1967.

Taylor, J. E.: Clinical observations relating to the normal and abnormal frenum labii superioris, Am. J. Orthod. and Oral Surg. **25:**646, 1939.

Tibbetts, L. S.: Use of diagnostic probes for detection of periodontal disease, J. Am. Dent. Assoc. **78:**551, 1969.

Tibbetts, L. S., Ochsenbein, C., and Loughlin, D. M.: Rationale for the lingual approach to mandibular osseous surgery, Dent. Clin. North Am. **20**(1):61-78, 1976.

Tibbetts, L. S.: The initial incision in pocket surgery, vol. 3. In Clark, J. W., editor: Clinical dentistry, New York, 1976, Harper & Row, Publishers.

Tibbetts, L. S., and Ochsenbein, C.: Management of problems in the posterior maxilla, vol. 3. In Clark, J. W., editor: Clinical dentistry, New York, 1976, Harper & Row, Publishers.

Vandersall, D. C.: Management of gingival recession and a surgical dehiscence with a soft tissue autograft; four year observation, J. Periodontol. **45:**274, 1974.

Vincent, J. W., Mochen, J. B., Levin, M. P.: Assessment of attached gingiva using the tension test and clinical measurement, J. Periodontol. **47:**412, 1976.

Wade, A. B.: The flap operation, J. Periodontol. **37:**95, 1966.

Ward, V. J.: A clinical assessment of the use of the free gingival graft for correcting localized recession associated with frena pull, J. Periodontol. **45:**78, 1974.

West, E. E.: Diastema, a cause for concern, Dent. Clin. North Am., p. 431, July, 1968.

Widman, L.: The operative treatment of alveolar pyorrhea, Br. Dent. J. **37:**105, 1917.

Wilderman, M. M.: Periosteal retention; repair, J. Periodontol. **34:**487, 1963.

Wilderman, M. M.: Exposure of the bone in periodontal surgery, Dent. Clin. North Am., p. 23, March, 1964.

Wilderman, M. M., and Wentz, F. M.: Repair of a dentogingival defect with a pedicle graft, J. Periodontol. **36:**218, 1965.

Wilderman, M. M., Wentz, F. M., and Orban, B. J.: Histogenesis of repair after mucogingival surgery, J. Periodontol. **31:**283, 1960.

Wood, D. L., Hoag, P. M., Donnenfeld, O. W., and Rosenfeld, L. D.: Alveolar crest reduction following full and partial thickness flaps, J. Periodontol. **43:**141, 1972.

Yukna, R. A., Tow, H. D., Carroll, P. B., Vernino, A. R., and Bright, R. W.: Evaluation of the use of freeze-dried skin allografts in the treatment of human mucogingival problems, J. Periodontol. **48:**187, 1977.

Zamet, J. S.: A comparative clinical study of three periodontal surgical techniques, J. Clin. Periodont. **2**(2):87, 1975.

Zentler, A.: Suppurative gingivitis—with alveolar involvement, J.A.M.A. **71:**1530, 1918.

Zingale, J. A.: Observations on free gingival autografts, J. Periodontol. **45:**748, 1974.

27 Surgical management of osseous deformity and defects

Bacterial plaque has been implicated as the major etiologic agent in the initiation and progression of inflammatory periodontal disease. Deviations from normal form and function within the masticatory apparatus that favor the accumulation and retention of bacterial plaque aid in perpetuating the disease process and contributing to the loss of the attachment apparatus. In attempting to eliminate or control the disease process clinicians have traditionally focused their therapeutic efforts toward eradication of the deformities produced within the periodontium. This in turn has led to the wide acceptance of an objective of therapy that states that periodontal pockets should be eliminated and physiologic architectural form should be established and maintained in the hard and soft tissues that invest the teeth.

Health care administrators, government agencies, consumer interest groups, and providers of dental insurance have questioned many of our traditional modes of dental practice. The effectiveness of periodontal therapy has been challenged,

and organized dentistry has been called upon to defend its position that periodontal disease can be controlled. Recent clinical studies by Ramfjord et al. (1975, 1973, 1968), Nyman et al. (1975), and Lindhe et al. (1975) have forced researchers, clinicians, and educators to reexamine the efficacy of many of our accepted surgical and nonsurgical treatment procedures. Data gained from longitudinal clinical studies in animals and humans (Axelsson and Lindhe, 1974; Löe et al., 1965; Nyman et al., 1975; Saxe et al., 1967; Suomi et al., 1971, 1969; Theilade et al., 1966) indicates that maintenance or continuing loss of the attachment apparatus is directly related to the level of plaque control that is attained and maintained in the periodontium. Maintenance, *or net gain,* in the level of connective tissue attachment was found in cases where the indices of inflammatory periodontal disease (Plaque Index, Gingival Index) approached zero regardless of the surgical technique that was used in treatment (Nyman et al., 1975). These studies have provoked considerable discussion in periodontal circles and have called attention to the need for a reevaluation of the aims, objectives, and rationale for employment of many of our periodontal procedures.

Nyman et al. (1975) compared the following surgical procedures in a closely controlled test group to gain data on the most effective means of treating periodontal pockets:

1. Gingivectomy
2. Open flap curettage with repositioned flaps (Widman procedure)
3. Open flap curettage with repositioned flaps plus osseous resection
4. Apically positioned flaps
5. Apically positioned flaps plus osseous resection

A net gain of attachment apparatus was noted in the interdental areas treated via open flap curettage in the test group that maintained excellent plaque control. Those in the test group treated by apically positioned flaps and osseous resection demonstrated comparable long-term stability of the attachment apparatus but an overall net loss of connective tissue attachment corresponding to the amount of bone sacrificed by osseous resection. The test groups maintained the levels of their connective tissue attachment over the 2-year period of the clinical experiment. The patients in the control group who were seen at 6-month intervals for maintenance therapy experienced a return to their preoperative levels of plaque and inflammation and a re-formation of their periodontal pockets with a corresponding loss of attachment levels *regardless of the surgical* modality employed to eliminate the pockets. Amsterdam (1974) and Lindhe (1975) have demonstrated that the connective tissue attachment level can be maintained even in advanced cases of periodontal disease if the etiologic factors of plaque and trauma (primary and secondary occlusal trauma) are adequately controlled.

This chapter will devote itself to discussion and illustration of the various surgical procedures most commonly used to eliminate osseous deformities within the periodontium. They will be described and illustrated in a step-by-step fashion to aid the student and practitioner in gaining a better understanding of the procedures employed. It has been observed all too frequently that the neophyte in mastering a new procedure tends to lose sight of the philosophy or rationale for its employment, and the procedure becomes an end unto itself. At the risk of being repetitive, let it be stated that the techniques in and by themselves are of little value unless they are employed in the proper *sequence* in overall therapy and within the context that *inflammation* (plaque) must be controlled in the im-

mediate and long-term posttreatment phases of therapy.

MORPHOLOGY OF THE PERIODONTIUM

Knowledge of the morphology and physiology of the healthy periodontium is a prerequisite for rational osseous therapy. Ideal gingival architecture consists of knife-edged gingival margins that are tightly adapted to the teeth and interdental papillae that fill the interproximal spaces to the contact areas of the teeth. In most areas of the mouth the gingiva and alveolar crest follow the same architectural pattern. The marginal bone normally is thin at its junction with the tooth, and the interdental septa project coronally in relation to the marginal bone on the facial and lingual surfaces, imparting a scalloped configuration in the surface contours. Interdental osseous grooves are more prominent in the anterior segment of the dental arches. Their presence in the molar areas depends on the prominence of the roots of the teeth and the anatomy of adjacent bony structures. Ritchey and Orban (1953) called attention to the fact that the crests of interdental septa derive their form from the proximal shape of the teeth and the configuration and relationship of the cemento-enamel junctions of the adjacent teeth. In the incisor region the interdental septa tend to be prominent and convex in form, whereas in the molar areas the curvature is considerably less, and they tend to be broad and flat (Figs. 27-1 and 27-2). O'Connor and Biggs (1964) studied the facial-lingual interproximal bone contours in 118 skulls obtained from India. They noted that the percentage of convex bony interproximal areas was lowest

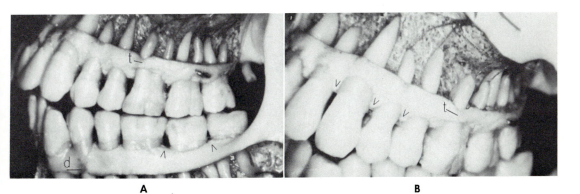

A   B

Fig. 27-1. Normal osseous morphology. **A,** Skull specimen, flat interdental septa in molar areas *(arrows).* Thin, *t,* cortical bone covering prominent mesial root, maxillary first molar. Dehiscence, *d,* of alveolus, prominent root of mandibular canine. **B,** Convex interdental septa in anterior areas *(arrows).* Dentoalveolar margins follow contours of cementoenamel junction.

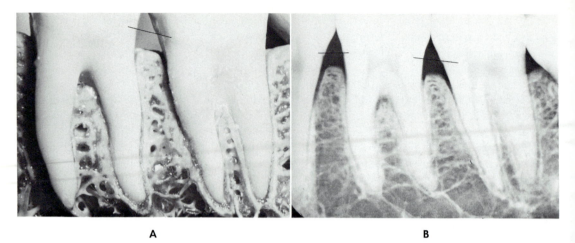

Fig. 27-2. A, Dissected dry skull specimen, normal architecture, contour of osseous crest in harmony with configuration of cementoenamel junction, and horizontal relationship of cementoenamel junction of adjacent teeth. **B,** Roentgenogram of specimen. Note relationship of osseous crest to cementoenamel junctions.

mesial to the third molars and that the percentage of convexities increased rapidly until it was the dominant configuration from the mesial of the second premolar to the incisors.

It is important that the student be familiar with the many factors that determine the topography of the alveolar bone and contiguous alveolar process. Individuals will vary considerably from what may be considered ideal form; however, this topography may be harmonious and normal for the individual patient. The following factors govern the topography of the periodontium:

1. The orthodontic alignment of the dental arches in relation to the basal bone
2. Tooth size in relationship to arch size, such as small teeth in large arches or large teeth in small or V-shaped arches
3. The shape of the anatomic crowns of the teeth
4. Cervical enamel projections or enamel pearls
5. Prominent position of the teeth within the dental arches, as in buccoversion or linguoversion
6. Prominent position of the roots of the teeth and dehiscence or fenestration, as commonly observed on the mesial roots and buccal surfaces of first molars
7. A mesial, distal, buccal, or lingual tilt of the teeth
8. Partially erupted or impacted teeth, and extruded or overerupted teeth
9. Rotated teeth

10. Relationship of the mylohyoid line or ridge, external oblique line or ridge, and zygomaticoalveolar crest to the dentoalveolar margins
11. Exostoses or tori
12. Closed embrasures due to unrestored cavities and mesial drift of the teeth

In many patients the relationship of the underlying bone to the gingiva is consistent, and the bone is thin and tapered at its junction with the tooth. However, many patients have been observed in whom the bony margin is thick or beaded and the overlying gingiva meets the tooth in a thin margin with a shallow healthy crevice. Such a disparity is compatible with periodontal health and is discovered by chance when a flap is created for surgical exposure of an area. Large bony protuberances or exostoses may be present that create broad, flat, shelflike gingival margins. Careful probing of such areas often discloses a normal attachment apparatus and shallow gingival crevice. Fig. 27-3 shows such contours in a healthy 85-year-old patient. These cases seemingly violate established concepts of ideal form and function. We must never lose sight of the fact that our goal in therapy is elimination of the periodontal pocket and establishment of a shallow sulcus. We do not prophylactically operate on an area to prevent future disease or to create an ideal form in the periodontium simply because the existing topography of the tissues varies with our idea of normal. These areas are operated on if a bony defect exists between the tooth and exostosis (Fig. 27-4) or to gain

A B

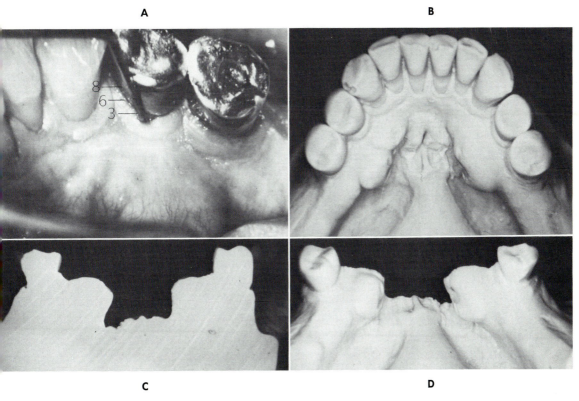

C D

Fig. 27-3. A, Large lingual tori and flat gingival contours, 85-year-old man. Thin Michigan probe used to chart crevicular depth. Average depth 1.5 to 2 mm, crevice healthy and tightly adapted to teeth. **B,** Diagnostic cast of mandibular arch. **C** and **D,** Cast ground to show profile of gingival contours and relationship to tori.

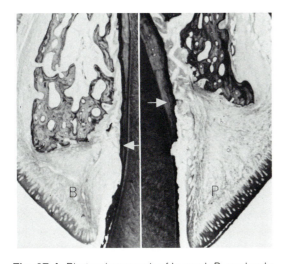

Fig. 27-4. Photomicrograph of buccal, *B,* and palatal, *P,* dentoalveolar contours. Osseous defects exist between tooth and exostosis, or beaded marginal bone. Arrows indicate base of pockets. (Courtesy Dr. B. Orban.)

space for the path of insertion of a partial denture framework.

The location of the initial osseous lesion in inflammatory periodontal disease is usually in the interdental area (Akiyoshi and Mori, 1967; Goldman, 1957; Weinmann, 1941). The interdental septa are broad and relatively flat in a buccolingual dimension in the posterior segments of the dental arches, and incipient to moderate bone loss rapidly creates interdental craters in the col area under the contacts of the teeth. It usually requires a greater degree of bone loss to create comparable craters in the anterior segments of the dental arches since incipient bone resorption produces a gradual blunting of the conical septum. As the inflammatory process extends apically its intensity will vary depending upon the local anatomy of the teeth and tissues and the presence of traumatic occlusal forces exerted upon the teeth (Kantor et al., 1976; Lindhe and Svanberg, 1974; Polson, 1974; Polson et al., 1976a and b, 1974). In the study of bone behavior in periodontal disease it is found that the bone may not be affected at all, as is seen in an early gingivitis, or that the bone may be resorbed but retains for the most part its architectural topography, or that ridges, ledges, and irregular topography at the crestal areas are seen, or that osseous defects are present. In regard to the first two instances, no bone interference is necessary, whereas in the case of ledges, ridges, and irregular topography, bone correction is necessary to achieve gingival topography that permits self-cleansing and easier patient care.

The osseous deformities that are produced will assume a wide variety of shapes and volumetric loss of supporting bone. The morphology of osseous defects and their classification is of more than passing academic interest since the majority of our therapeutic approaches in therapy and the potential for repair of the osseous defects and formation of new attachment to the teeth are equated to the number of bony walls remaining around the teeth (Goldman and Cohen, 1958).

CLASSIFICATION OF OSSEOUS DEFECTS

  I. *Three osseous walls*
     A. Proximal, buccal, and lingual walls
     B. Buccal, mesial, and distal walls
     C. Lingual, mesial, and distal walls
 II. *Two osseous walls*
     A. Buccal and lingual (crater) walls
     B. Buccal and proximal walls
     C. Lingual and proximal walls
III. *One osseous wall*
     A. Proximal wall
     B. Buccal wall
     C. Lingual wall
 IV. *Combination*
     A. Three walls plus two walls
     B. Three walls plus two walls plus one wall

THERAPEUTIC PROCEDURES AND GOALS

Osseous defects may be eliminated by a number of methods. A list of currently employed procedures would include—

1. Osseous resection
2. Tooth movement
3. Reconstructive (new attachment) procedures
4. Root resection, hemisection, and trisection
5. Extraction

Our overall goal in therapy is to restore the dentogingival unit to health in the most *conservative* manner possible. Procedures that maximize the potential for repair of the attachment at more coronal levels on the roots of the teeth are preferred over those that eliminate the osseous defects by resection procedures. Depending upon the morphology of the osseous defects, the quantity and quality (marrow-cortical ratio) of the bone composing the walls of the osseous defects and the orthodontic-occlusal relationships that exist, osseous defects may be treated by single-stage or multistage procedures.

Osseous resection has been the procedure of choice of most periodontists to eliminate osseous defects that are not suitable to be treated by new attachment procedures. The technique permits great versatility and can be used to manage a wide variety of osseous deformities. It is relatively easy to execute, wound healing is rapid, and the results are definitive and predictable. The single-stage nature of the procedure makes it attractive to both therapist and patient. Osseous resection is limited to defects whose base is located 3 to 5 mm from the cementoenamel junction of the teeth. In cases where the roots of the teeth are long the limits of practicality may be raised to 7 mm from the cementoenamel junction. The removal of supporting bone in defects greater than 7 mm becomes self-defeating because of the excessive loss of attachment apparatus that is incurred in eliminating the defects.

New attachment procedures, stimulated periosteum, osseous autografts, and allografts are employed in the treatment of extensive (large volume) defects that are not amenable for treatment by osseous resection. They have as their goal the reconstruction of the attachment apparatus—bone, cementum, and periodontal ligament. If they are less than 100% effective in gaining "bone fill" and a new attachment to the general level of the osseous crest, they frequently reduce the severity of the defect and change its morphology into one that may be eliminated by a second-stage osseous resection procedure. Also, during the last decade we have come to appreciate the contribution that orthodontic tooth movement can make in the management of osseous defects. Tooth movement can greatly alter the topography of the alveolar crest and osseous deformities. Orthodontic therapy, like root planing and curettage, is a part of initial preparation. *The time and effort expended during initial therapy to set up a case for definitive pocket elimination therapy greatly reduces the complexity and extent of the surgery required to eliminate the remaining osseous defects.*

In managing cases of advanced periodontal disease the survival of the dental arch becomes of greater importance than the individual teeth that make up the dental arch. The extraction of teeth or roots of molar teeth with a hopeless prognosis is oftentimes more conservative therapy than attempts at treatment that would sacrifice large amounts of support from adjacent teeth.

In treating the advanced case of periodontal disease we frequently combine all the above forms of therapy in proper sequence and stages in an attempt to achieve our goal of pocket elimination with maximum conservation of the attachment apparatus. Before we begin a discussion of osseous resection and new attachment techniques we must consider the evaluation of the surgical site, for the choice of surgical maneuver is usually based upon the assessment of the topography of this site.

EVALUATION OF SURGICAL SITE

The clinician should acquire a detailed knowledge of the location and topography of all osseous defects during the initial documentation of a case. A comparison of the pocket depths recorded during the probing examination with full dentition radiographs of *diagnostic value* will usually give the clinician a fairly accurate assessment of the bony topography. Probing is a painful experience for many patients, and frequently the clinician cannot fully explore the depths of deep pockets during the initial examination. Later in the sequence of treatment, during the root planing–curettage phase of initial preparation, the full extent of the pockets may be explored when the patient is anesthetized for this stage of therapy. The attachment level may be sounded with probes and curets, and it is not uncommon to discover that the osseous defects enter further into furcation areas or involve more surfaces of the teeth and to a greater extent than originally recorded.

The thickness and relationship of the mucogingival complex of tissues and adjacent anatomic structures must be considered as the surgical site is examined (Fig. 27-5). The following factors should be reviewed by the clinician during the evaluation of the surgical area as an aid in selecting the most conservative mode of therapy to meet the surgical objectives that have been established for the case (Rosenberg and Ross, 1976):

1. Crown-root-bone relationships
2. Relationship of mucogingival tissues
3. Depth and width (mm³) of the osseous defects
4. Number of osseous walls surrounding the osseous defects
5. Type of bone (cortical plate or cancellous) making up the osseous walls
6. Tooth mobility
7. Tooth vitality
8. Root anatomy; dimension of root trunk of multirooted teeth
9. Axial inclination of the tooth
10. Prominence of tooth position and alveolar housing
11. Root proximity
12. Bone loss in furcation areas
13. Dimensions of interdental septum in mesiodistal and buccolingual directions
14. Width of interradicular septum of multirooted teeth
15. Anatomic structures (external oblique ridge, tori, maxillary sinus, mental foramen and so on)

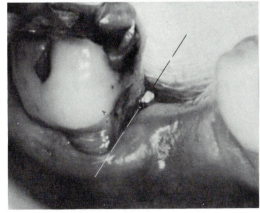
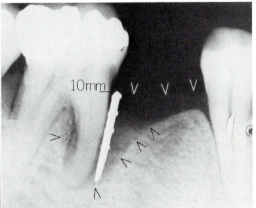

A   **B**

Fig. 27-5. A, Combination (three walls plus two walls plus one wall) osseous defect. Calibrated Hirschfeld silver point, 10 mm, in pocket and level with gingival margin. **B,** Roentgenogram discloses depth and contour of pocket in respect to bone outline *(black arrows)* and soft tissue contours *(white arrows)*.

ELIMINATION OF OSSEOUS DEFECTS BY OSSEOUS RESECTION

The terms ''osteoplasty'' and ''ostectomy'' have been offered to define the type and extent of bone recontouring that is to be accomplished (Friedman, 1955). Osteoplasty involves the reshaping of the bony structures that support the alveolus. Ostectomy is used to imply the actual removal of the alveolus, the bony portion of the attachment apparatus that directly supports the root. It becomes difficult at times to define where ostectomy procedures terminate and osteoplasty begins, or vice versa. The essential point to be remembered is that ostectomy removes bony support and changes the crown-root-bone relationship. Such a change may be of minor consequence in many circumstances and a small price to pay to achieve the final objectives of therapy, or it may be of such magnitude that it would threaten retention of the teeth in question or severely weaken the support of adjacent teeth. Hence there is a need to consider the indications and contraindications for osseous resection procedures.

INDICATIONS

1. To eliminate osseous defects that are not suitable for attempts at treatment to gain a new attachment apparatus. Such infrabony pockets (defects) usually have a shallow or wide aspect to their topography. The volume of missing or destroyed periodontium is great in proportion to the remaining bony walls of the defect, or the remaining walls are composed of thin cortical plates of bone. These factors can be grouped as the ''quantity and quality factor'' of remaining osseous tissue.

2. To eliminate shallow to moderately deep osseous defects about stable teeth with long, large, well-formed roots. Such teeth have a favorable crown-root-bone-relationship and can withstand the loss of moderate amounts of support without untoward clinical effects.

3. To eliminate ledging, inconsistent bony margins, lipping of the crestal bone, exostoses, tori, and so on that may interfere with the management of the soft tissue portion of the lesion. Bony aberrations that interfere with placement and stabilization of the overlying tissue flap must be reshaped if desired contours are to be produced in the healed soft tissue portion of the treated lesion so that the host is able to cleanse the teeth without interference because of unfavorable soft tissue–osseous tissue topography.

4. To alter soft tissue–osseous tissue topography adjacent to incipient or moderate furcation involvement areas to facilitate cleansing of the area and lessening of the tendency for plaque accumulation.

5. To alter osseous contours adjacent to (1) root resection areas; (2) hemisections; (3) fractured crowns or roots and other such problems associated with periodontic-endodontic lesions; (4) traumatic fractures; or (5) deep-seated caries. While osseous resection procedures are accomplished for recontouring saddle areas, tuberosities, and so on they are not germane to the specific topic under consideration and will not be considered further other than this brief mention of their existence.

CONTRAINDICATIONS TO BONE RESECTION

1. Osseous defects whose overall topography would facilitate attempts at treatment to gain a new attachment apparatus. Such pockets associated with these defects have narrow, deeper conformations and a more favorable ratio between the volume of the periodontium to be regenerated and the surface area present in the surrounding bony walls. Also the osseous walls of the pocket have ample cancellous bone and marrow spaces lateral to them that are capable of furnishing the progenitor cells necessary to effect regeneration of bone, collagen fibers, and cementum.

2. Osseous defects of large volume and dimension, which if treated by osseous recontouring to produce physiologic contours at more apical levels would necessitate the removal of excessive amounts of bone and irreparably weaken the support of the tooth or teeth in the area.

3. Infrabony pockets and associated osseous defects of shallow depth or dimension about mobile teeth with short, cone-shaped roots. Such teeth have an unfavorable crown-root-bone relationship and cannot withstand the loss of minimal to moderate support without untoward clinical effects.

4. Osseous defects, which if considered as a separate entity could be treated by osseous resection, but whose adjacent soft tissues do not permit successful treatment to be accomplished. This is frequently experienced in infrabony defects distal to second and third molars in which the contiguous soft tissue is loose elastic alveolar mucosa, the contents of the hamular notch area, and so on. Since both the osseous lesion and soft tissue lesion must be treated, it is not infrequent that the attendant mucogingival problem dictates the course of therapy to be followed, if any, and assumes a position of greater importance in therapy than the underlying osseous portion of the pocket.

5. Where the underlying osseous structures have produced lipping, exostoses, and so on and a resulting flat or shelflike gingival topography, but where no pockets exist. *Prophylactic recontouring of the periodontal tissues in the absence of disease to produce "ideal" form within the tissues is neither indicated nor condoned.*

ADVANTAGES OF THE PROCEDURE

Dependability and promptness. Dependability and promptness are best considered as a unit, for in many ways they are inseparable and one becomes a function of the other. If the problems incurred from altered osseous topography in relation to postoperative cleansibility are to be overcome (slight to moderately deep infrabony defects, inconsistent marginal ridges of bone, bony ledges, exostoses, and so on in and about teeth that have ample root structure remaining invested in bone and no unmanageable mucogingival problems) then correction can be made with dispatch and assurance in a relatively simple one-step procedure. The procedure is dependable, for one has visual assurance that the pockets have been eliminated and the desired contours produced. Nothing is left to chance in the hope that the defects will fill with bone and new attachment to the roots will take place. This obviates the possibility that future second-stage reentry procedures may become a necessity to eliminate residual portions of osseous defects that did not completely "fill" where new attachment procedures were done. Promptness becomes important when a succession of procedures must be completed, each in its turn, to treat a complicated case. If the waiting time between steps can be shortened, the advantages that can be accrued in lessening the total time necessary to treat a case become obvious. Many patients cannot afford to make themselves available for protracted treatment or remain in one location for long periods of time for a variety of legitimate reasons. Availability for treatment therefore becomes an important criteria in case treatment planning, and procedures that can shorten the time required for treatment may have a direct bearing on how a case must be treated.

Simplicity. The skill level and training required to raise a surgical flap and contour osseous tissues to the desired degree fall well within the treatment capabilities of the general practitioner who is interested in treating periodontal disease. The skills required to accomplish the mechanics of the procedures can be mastered without undue difficulty. As a matter of daily routine third-year dental students accomplish osseous resection procedures. The students become reasonably adept at performing the technical phases of the surgery after operating on a small number of cases. *The difficulty and challenge lies in the area of treatment planning and in understanding the anatomic and biologic limitations of treatment* as well as in one's personal limitations in skill and experience.

Elimination of additional surgical sites. If infrabony defects are to be treated by the use of stimulated periosteum autogenous donor bone, secondary oral or extraoral (iliac crest) surgical procedures must be carried out to secure the required donor material. This poses problems with requirements for an additional surgical site, additional time for treatment, additional discomfort, and usually additional expense for the patient. If treatment can be accomplished successfully by osseous resection techniques, the advantages to be gained are apparent and deserving of our most serious attention. Overtreatment of relatively uncomplicated cases in no way can be justified.

DISADVANTAGES OF THE PROCEDURE

Sacrifice of attachment apparatus. Regardless of how one wishes to approach or view the subject of osseous resection procedures or how one attempts to camouflage basic facts in an attempt to justify a rationale for the procedure, one clear and unescapable fact remains—in some instances nonsupporting bone is removed, but in most instances attachment apparatus is intentionally sacrificed. In these latter instances the bony portion of the alveolus into which the principal fibers of the periodontal ligament insert is removed, and the amount of root structure embedded into a supporting socket is lessened. If this fact and its ramifications are clearly understood and if one can place this knowledge in perspective to the total oral cavity, its total degree of disease, and total plan for optimum therapeutic results, one can then weigh relative values and the price that must be paid in terms of sacrifice of periodontium required to gain the goals of comprehensive therapy. Retention and function in health of the dental arch are more important than survival of the individual component parts thereof. *Although resection techniques are negative, or subtraction, procedures, when used intelligently in an integrated plan of treatment they can have positive and salutary effects upon the longevity of the dentition and its remaining supporting tissues by providing a topography in the periodontium that facilitates ready access for plaque control by the patient.*

PROCEDURE

Documentation and initial preparation. If meticulous attention is devoted to the prerequisites of (1) documentation, (2) coaching of the patient to master a program for effective cleansing, (3) thorough root preparation, (4) securing of proper tooth form and alignment, and (5) control of occlusal habits and periodontal trauma, one can approach the surgical procedure fully informed of the problems to be surmounted.

Flap design and management. By knowing the amount and distribution of gingiva in the area of the surgical site and the probable conformation of the infrabony pockets to be exposed, a surgical incision can be made and a flap of proper geometric configuration can be raised. The relative merits of full-thickness, partial-thickness, or combination full-thickness–partial-thickness flaps are presented in Chapter 26. Of paramount importance is the location of the mucogingival junction and the width of the zone of attached gingiva that surrounds the infrabony pocket. The design of the flap, how it is raised from the bone, how much it is reflected, how it is handled during the retraction phase of surgery, and how and where it is placed for stabilization during the initial stages of wound repair all reflect on how well the soft tissue component of the infrabony pocket will be resolved.

Basic differences in flap design. At the termination of the osseous resection procedure the infrabony pockets will have been eliminated by the contouring of the bone. This usually leaves a physiologically contoured, bleeding, bony surface upon which the flap will be placed. The flap therefore can be thinned in the marginal area and made to follow the contours carved into the bone. It covers the bone in veneerlike fashion, and the margin of the flap is preferably placed at the dento-osseous margin. Since the thinned flap has a minimum amount of connective tissue under the incised keratinized epithelium of the gingiva, its minimal biologic thickness will place the oral surface of the flap approximately 1 to 1.5 mm above the bony margin next to the planed root of the tooth. In the early stages of wound healing granulation tissue originating from the periodontal ligament space will join with the repairing connective tissue surface of the flap to produce a new dentogingival junction. *If the flap is displaced too far coronally, especially in the interdental areas, it is likely that the flap-tooth interface will be covered by epithelium, resulting in a healed sulcus of greater depth than desired.* If one is to err in approximating the flap during the suturing procedure at the termination of surgery, it is better to place the flap *slightly* shy of the dento-osseous margin. The granulation tissue from the periodontal ligament will quickly fill the void, and the chances for attaining a shallow sulcus postoperatively are improved.

An exception to this general rule of flap management can be made in areas where several millimeters of bone have been removed by ostectomy to produce the desired contours in the bone. The bone that is removed via ostectomy exposes root structure (cementum) that *has not* been exposed in the pocket. This cementum is vital, and the periodontal ligament fibers are torn as this bone is removed. It is important that this area of the root not be planed with curets, for to do so would destroy the severed collagen fibers embedded in the cementum. If the cut edge of the connective tissue of the flap is approximated against these fibers remaining in the root it is possible to have the flap *reattach* to the teeth (Garret, 1975; Levine and Stahl, 1972; Stahl, 1977; Stahl, 1975).

A different set of circumstances exists when one is treating osseous defects in an attempt to gain a new attachment. In this situation one hopes to gain new bone, cementum, and fiber apparatus to fill the former osseous defect. In an attempt to cover these defects at the termination of this type of procedure one needs a flap that will fit back against the circumference of the teeth to seal the healing osseous wound from the plaque and fluids of the oral cavity. If the flap is thinned excessively it may be difficult if not impossible to obtain adequate adaptation of the flap to the circumference of the teeth, particularly adjacent to concave root surfaces. A sulcular incision is usually used when attempting new attachment procedures. This may produce undesirable soft tissue contours and unwanted soft tissue depth in attaining the objectives of elimination of the infrabony portion of the pocket. A second-stage flap procedure is usually required in these instances 9 to 12 months later to eliminate any residual osseous defects that did not fill or to remodel and perform definitive mucogingival surgery to obtain the desired soft tissue contours and shallow sulci.

Keeping the above basic differences of flap design in mind, the clinician can select a path of incision that will best suit the requirements and objectives of the surgical procedure to be accomplished. Additional consideration must be given to the fixed areas of masticatory mucosa that cannot be apically positioned by freely sliding the tissues along the periosteum-bone interface. The connective tissue of the palate, tuberosity, and retromolar area is attached to the underlying osseous surface. It can be maneuvered by undermining it, thereby permitting movement of the wound margin, but it will not slide over the bony surface like a full-thickness mucoperiosteal flap.

A general rule that can be followed is to remove a wedge of tissue in these areas equal to half the pocket depth. Fig. 26-38 illustrates the rationale for this type of incision and shows how the margin of the flap will adapt to the dento-osseous margin at the finish of the surgical procedure. It is better to design a flap with thoughts in mind of how to *close* the wound rather than of how to gain entrance to the surgical site. It is more conservative to make a second or third incision to remove excessive flap tissue to shorten the flap during closure of the wound than to find that excessive amounts of soft tissue were resected during creation of the flap, resulting in incomplete closure and exposed connective tissue. When this happens wound healing is delayed and painful compared to areas where complete wound closure was obtained.

INSPECTION OF OSSEOUS DEFECTS

Once the flap or flaps have been raised and the surgical site debrided of all granulomatous tissue, the preoperative assessment of the nature and extent of the infrabony pockets can be confirmed or revised. There is no substitute for direct visual inspection of the surgical site while exploring the contours of the bony surface with a probe or curet. When the exact surface topography of the area has been established the amount of osteoplasty and ostectomy necessary to eliminate the infrabony pockets can be determined.

SELECTION OF SURFACES TO BE RESECTED

If the bone can be contoured in a buccal or lingual direction and harmonious contours produced by confining the majority of the surgery to a single side of the arch, less supporting bone (ostectomy) will be removed. If ostectomy is carried out on both sides of the dental arch more supporting bone will of necessity be sacrificed (Fig. 27-6). In the maxillary arch the palatal approach may be indicated for a variety of reasons and may prove to be a more conservative approach than entry from the more accessible buccal surface. The reader is referred to an excellent discussion by Ochsenbein and Bohannan on the merits of the palatal approach for osseous resection (1964, 1963).

It is difficult to photograph many of the steps in

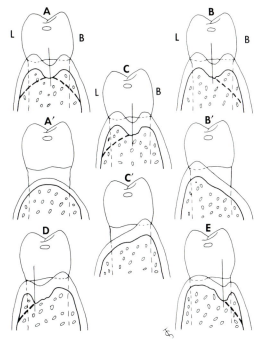

Fig. 27-6. A, Two-wall (crater) osseous defect, centrally located. If base of crater is selected as location for crest of interdental septa in healed case, ostectomy is required on both buccal and lingual surfaces. **A′,** Postoperative contour. **B,** Buccal approach, buccal surface ostectomy and osteoplasty. **B′,** Postoperative contour. **C,** Lingual surface approach, lingual ostectomy-osteoplasty. **C′,** Postoperative contours. **D,** Lingual approach indicated for defects located to lingual or palatal side of alveolar process. **E,** Buccal approach indicated for defects located on buccal side of alveolar process.

the actual sequence of osseous surgery in patients because of problems of instrument angulation, hemorrhage, inadequate lighting, and shadows that obscure areas of interest for the reader and clinician. Drawings can be of help to illustrate specific points in therapy, but they frequently lack depth and realism. A dentoform (Precision Anatomics, 9524 West Pico Boulevard, Los Angeles, Calif. 90035) is commercially available that realistically duplicates the osseous defects found in patients with moderate to advanced states of periodontal disease. While clinicians may have individual preferences in selection of hand instruments, the basic principles underlying their use remain identical, and the following illustrations have been produced with that thought in mind.

TECHNIQUE

Osteoplasty. Osteoplasty is usually accomplished first with rotary instruments to remove the

Text continued on p. 964.

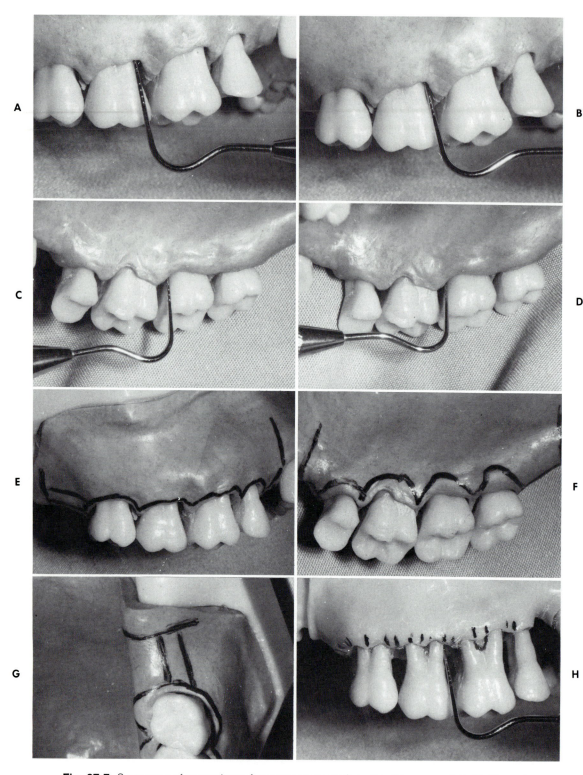

Fig. 27-7. Sequence of procedures for osseous resection, maxillary area. **A** to **D,** Buccal and palatal views of periodontal dentoform with probe in defect on mesial aspect of second molar. Note differences in depth readings as probe is passed from axial corner of tooth into depth of osseous crater. **E** to **G,** Outline of paths of incision on vinyl-simulated gingival covering. **H,** Probe in depth of two-wall craters.

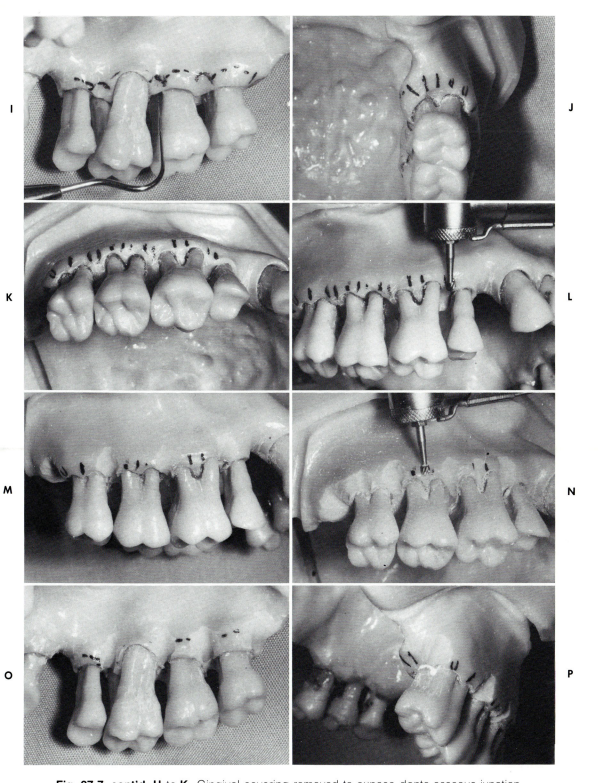

Fig. 27-7, cont'd. H to **K,** Gingival covering removed to expose dento-osseous junction and osseous defects. Probe in depth of two-wall craters. Site of initial osseous resection marked on bone with pen. Note defect, class II furca, entering mesial aspect of second molar. **L** to **N,** Initial osteoplasty in interdental areas performed using bur to remove buccal and palatal bony walls of defects. **O** to **Q,** Reversal of architectural form is accentuated as base of crater becomes crest of new interdental septum. Sharp bony peaks of bone that remain on axial corners of teeth must be removed.

Continued.

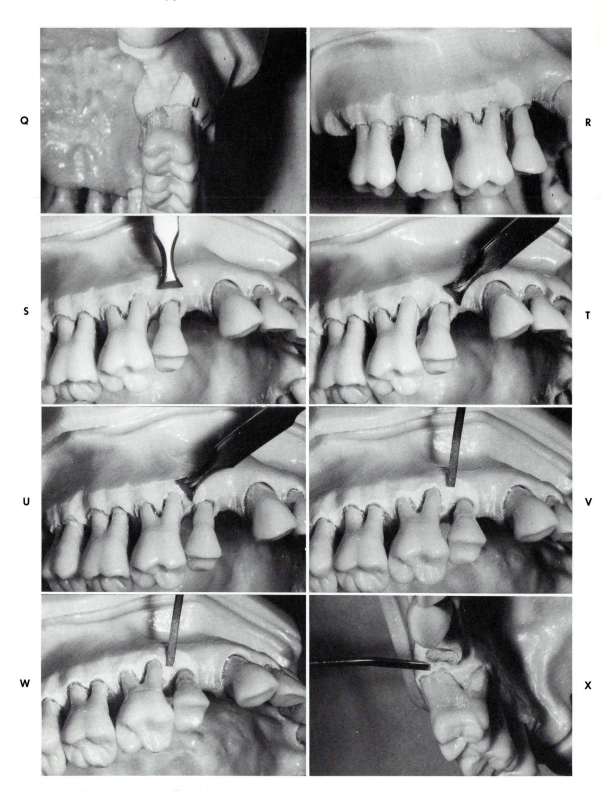

Fig. 27-7, cont'd. R, Initial ostectomy has been accomplished to remove reverse architecture. Compare topography with **H, M,** and **N. S** to **U,** Ochsenbein chisel used to remove buccal supporting bone (ostectomy). **V** and **W,** Use of smaller Wedelstaedt chisel to blend contour on axial corners to a smooth rise into interdental areas. **X,** Premolar removed to permit buccopalatal view of convex osseous crest being created on mesial aspect of molar. Scratch marks on teeth are marks left from root planing of simulated calculus. Note in **P** that calculus has not been removed on unoperated contralateral side of dentoform.

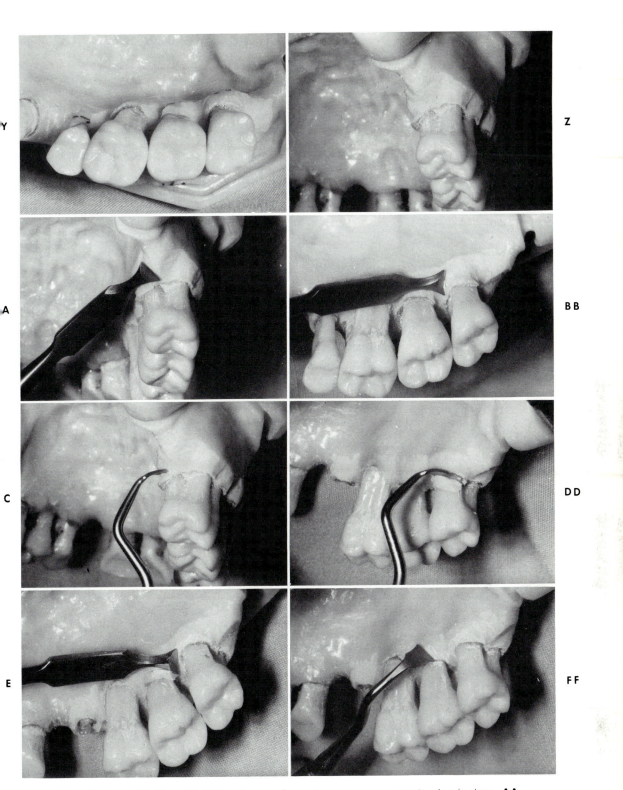

Fig. 27-7, cont'd. Y and **Z,** Note changes in contour as gross recontouring is done. **AA,** Ochsenbein chisel designed so that side of instrument may be used on axial corners with a pull stroke where access limited for normal push stroke. **BB,** Push stroke for ostectomy on mesioaxial corner. **CC** and **DD,** Use of no. 36/37 Rhodes back action chisel to remove bone on axial corner of tooth with a pull stroke after creating a fracture line in bone with Ochsenbein chisel as shown in **EE. FF,** Use of Rhodes chisel to start blending and smoothing of osseous surface after initial gross reduction of bone is completed.

Continued.

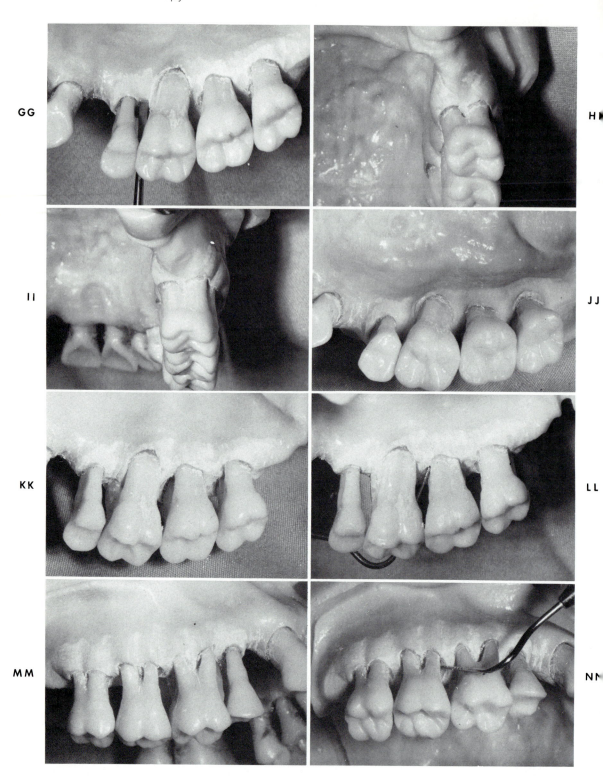

GG

HH

II

JJ

KK

LL

MM

NN

Fig. 27-7, cont'd. GG, Wedelstaedt chisel used to blend contour of crest from buccal to palatal side adjacent to tooth to ensure smooth flow of contour. **HH** to **JJ,** Final smoothing and blending of contours. Compare with preoperative contour in **I** to **L. KK** to **NN,** Various views of remaining portion of crater that enters mesial furcation of second molar. Too much bone would have to be sacrificed to completely remove remainder of defect, thereby weakening support of both molars. Clinical decision made to resect mesiobuccal root of second molar.

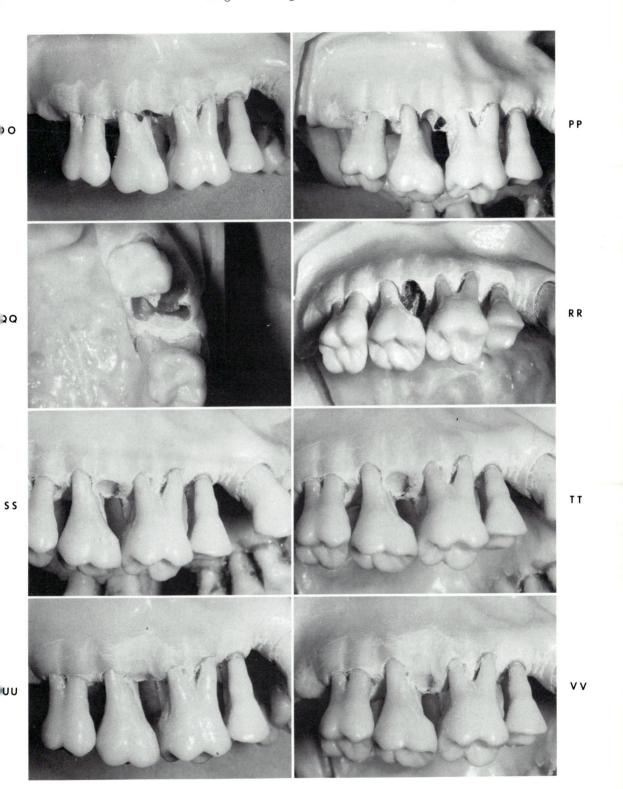

Fig. 27-7, cont'd. OO and **RR,** Mesiobuccal root resected. Remainder of crater that could not be removed shaded to contrast with bone on rim of socket. Tooth removed in **QQ** for better view of extent of base of osseous defect. **SS** and **TT,** Simulated initial socket healing to show marked gain in width of embrasure attained by removal of root. **UU** and **VV,** Remodeling attained by complete healing of socket-ridge area or contour produced by second-stage osteoplasty procedure.

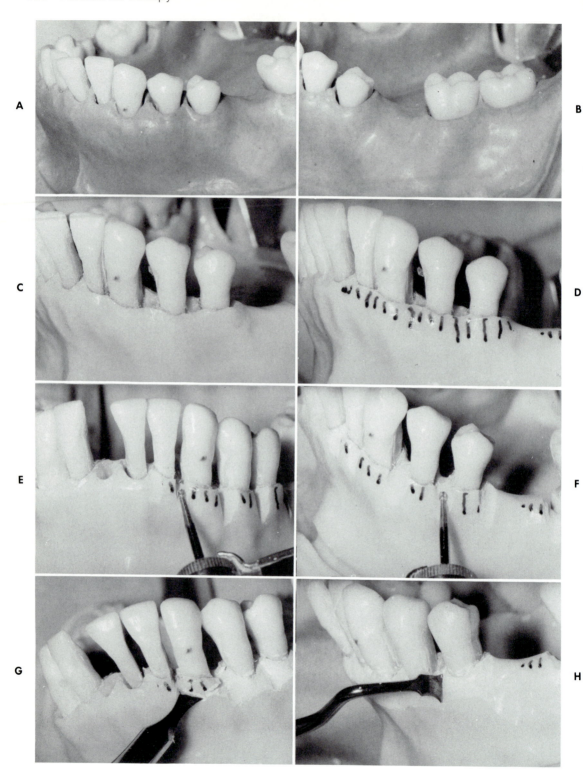

Fig. 27-8. Sequence of procedure for osseous resection, mandibular quadrant. **A** and **B,** Preoperative view with simulated gingiva in place. **C,** Buccal view of two-wall craters in canine area. **D,** Outline of bone to be removed in initial gross reduction of lateral walls of defects. **E** and **F,** Use of bur for ramping into craters from buccal aspect (osteoplasty). **G,** Ochsenbein chisel used to create split in bone on radicular surface where bone is thin. Care is taken not to nick root of tooth (ostectomy).

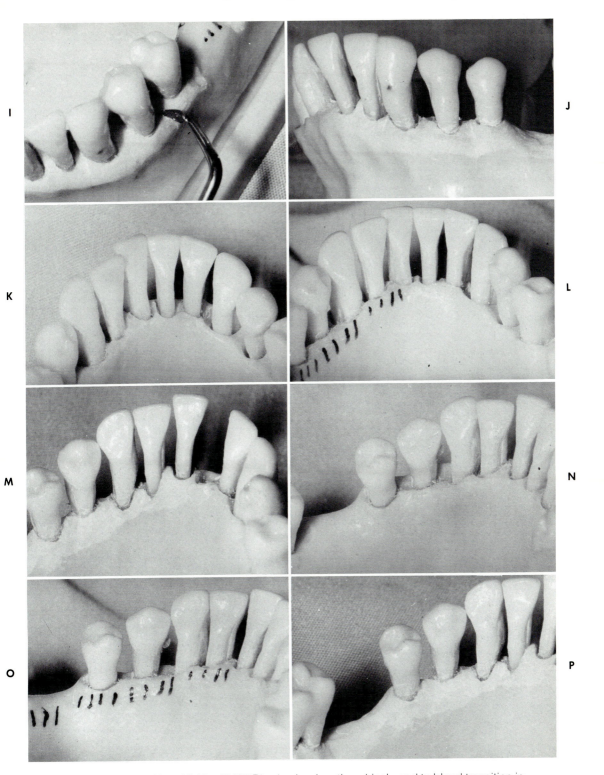

Fig. 27-8, cont'd. H and **I,** No. 36/37 Rhodes back action chisel used to blend transition in contour from ramped interdental areas around axial corners to convex radicular surfaces. **J,** Initial osseous resection completed on buccal side. Lingual surface not operated on as yet. **K** and **L,** Lingual view of area to be resected in incisor area. **M,** Concavities of craters turned into convexities by osteoplasty and ostectomy procedures. Right central incisor removed to show "normal" interdental crest unaffected by bone loss in **E** and **M. N** to **P,** Lingual view of osseous reduction in premolar area.

Continued.

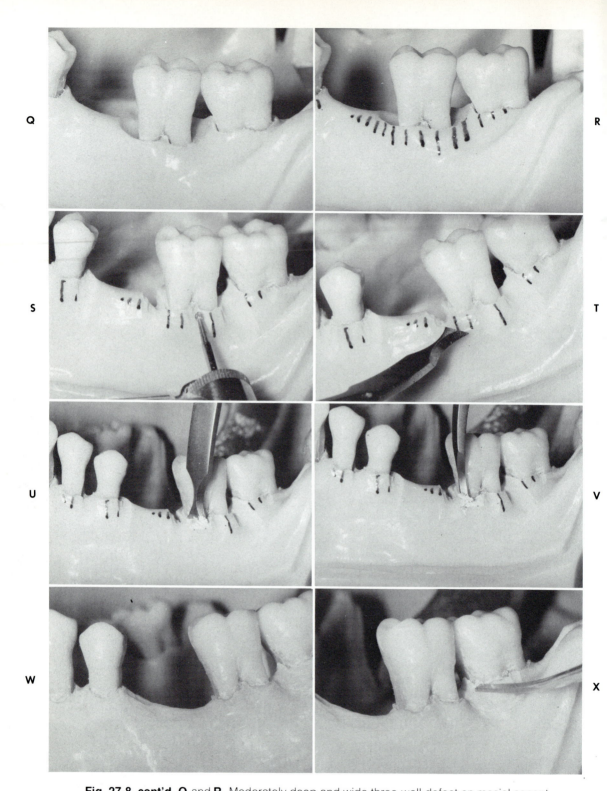

Fig. 27-8, cont'd. Q and **R,** Moderately deep and wide three-wall defect on mesial aspect of second molar and similar defect on distal aspect of same tooth, producing a "hemiseptum" on mesial aspect of third molar. Base of defect on mesial aspect of second molar will determine extent to which edentulous ridge area will have to be reduced to produce a blending of contours and mesial rise approaching mesial aspect of molar. **S,** Start of buccal osteoplasty with bur to reach bottom of craters by removing lateral bony walls. **T,** Ochsenbein chisel being used to create split in bone for ostectomy. **U** and **V,** Ochsenbein chisel held against tooth. While pressed apically against bone it is rotated somewhat like a screwdriver to peel off buccoaxial radicular segment of bone that has previously been delineated via split produced by perpendicular application of the chisel. Note bone peeling off. **W,** Buccal view of contoured ridge area to saddle shape with coronal rise to mesial aspect of second molar. Hemiseptum must be reduced on mesial aspect of third molar.

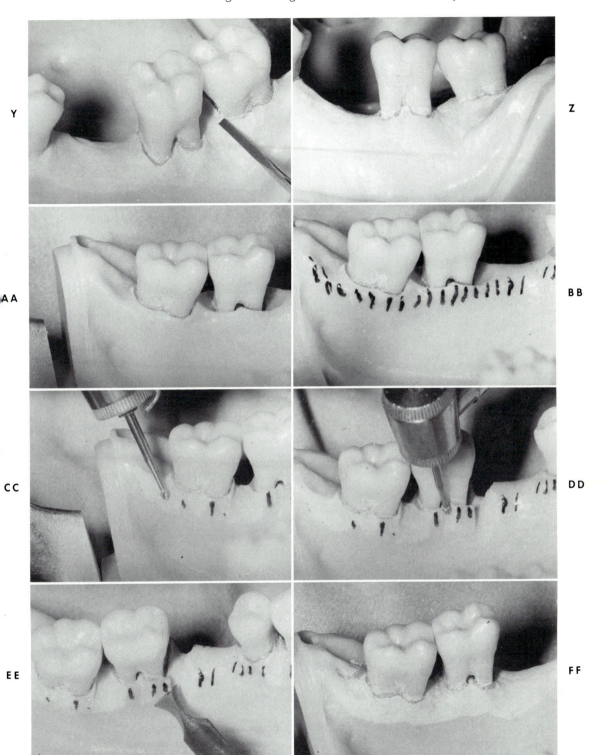

Fig. 27-8, cont'd. X and **Y,** Wedelstaedt chisel used to lower crest on mesial aspect of third molar. **Z,** Final adjustment of interdental osseous profile to be done after completion of lingual resection. **AA** and **BB,** Note lingual shelf created by mylohyoid ridge. Contour drops off into a concavity immediately below shelflike projection. **CC** to **EE,** Resection of lingual lateral walls of defects and contouring of ridge area. **FF,** Views of recontoured lingual and retromolar area. Note blending of contours in harmony with contiguous anatomy of jaw and ascending ramus.

Continued.

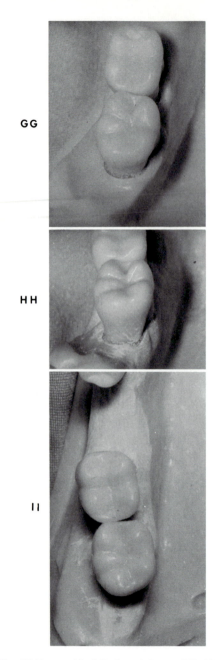

GG

HH

II

Fig. 27-8, cont'd. GG, See **AA** and **BB. HH** and **II,** See **FF.**

buccal and oral (lingual-palatal) walls of the crater and any tori or exostoses that may be included in the surgical site (Figs. 27-7, *H* to *R*; 27-8, *E* and *F*; 27-9, *D*). To eliminate the reversal of architectural form in the bony topography the walls of the defects in the interdental areas must be removed to permit the base of the crater or combination defect to be reshaped to form the crest of the interdental septum. The depth of the interdental defect governs the amount of bone that must be removed

laterally to it to turn the concavity in the crestal surface into a convexity. A carbide bur or diamond point of suitable size is preferred for the bulk removal of bone and general rough shaping of the area. If rotating instruments are used, copious amounts of water or isotonic saline must be used to irrigate the area and prevent overheating of the bone as it is cut. Studies in animals on the effects of high-speed cutting of bone using diamonds and carbide burs have shown the carbide burs to generate less heat and drying at the point of application to the bone. They induced less peripheral trauma and osseous remodeling than diamonds used under identical conditions (Boyne, 1966; Costich et al., 1964; Hall, 1965; Moss, 1964; Spatz, 1965). Great care must be exercised in using rotating instruments close to tooth surfaces. A minor slip in the confined area of the surgical site can produce unwanted damage to root surfaces literally in the blink of an eye. It is good surgical practice to limit the cutting with a bur to short bursts of speed with frequent stops for evacuation of the irrigating solution. If the patient is informed ahead of time that frequent stops will be made, there will be less of a tendency for him to want to swallow. Unexpected muscle action on the part of an anesthetized patient, whose tissues are wet and slippery, can produce tissue laceration or tooth damage as mentioned. Frequent stops for irrigation, evacuation, and assessment of the surgical site also help to prevent unintentional overcutting of the bone. A variety of rongeurs and surgical chisels with special angulations and tip sizes that also can be used for the bulk of removal of bone in maxillary and mandibular locations are readily available through dental instrument manufacturers.

It is good surgical practice to pause and reprobe the interdental defects after the initial gross reduction of the lateral walls of the craters. At this point the amount of concavity remaining can be assessed and the relationship of the base of the defects to the bone levels on the buccal and oral surfaces and furcations can be studied. It is not unusual to discover additional granulomatous tissue remaining in the depths of the defects that must be removed to reach the base of the defects. Since further osteoplasty of the lateral slopes of the defects demands that greater amounts of supporting bone will have to be removed (ostectomy) on the buccal and oral surfaces to create a rise of the osseous contour in the interdental areas, decisions must be made for each area as to the extent that further osseous reduction is warranted. The question that must be resolved for each case and area is whether or not the gain that is to be achieved by the removal of bone to eliminate the defects is worth the price that must be paid in the sacrifice of supporting bone. If the osseous defects are no deeper (from the cementoenamel junction) than 3 to 5 mm, they usually can be completely removed by osteoplasty and ostectomy procedures. If the defects are deep-

er than this, one may have to leave some residual depth and reversal of architectural form as an elective compromise in therapy as a point of diminishing returns is reached and it is decided that it is neither practical nor warranted to remove further amounts of healthy supporting bone. This very situation was reached on this dentoform in the de-

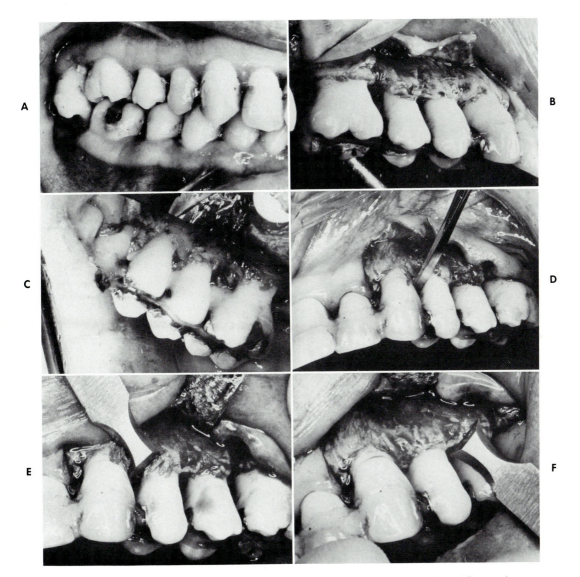

Fig. 27-9. Combined procedure using a partial-thickness apically positioned flap on buccal aspect and a partial-thickness palatal gingival flap utilized in the correction of moderate osseous defects. **A,** Pretreatment, buccal view. **B,** There is cratering on distal of the maxillary left molar and between premolars and molars (mirror view). **C,** Palatal exposure showing irregular osseous defects as well as granulation tissue invading mesial furca of first molar. Teeth are in secondary occlusal trauma and have been stabilized by means of intracoronal amalgam wire-and-acrylic A splint. **D,** A no. 401 Wedelstadt chisel is used to eliminate interdental craters. **E** and **F,** Ochsenbein chisel, because of its unusual design, enables correction of distal line angle of canine, interproximal rise between canine and first premolar, and radicular elliptical form on mesial aspect of first premolar. This chisel can cleave off irregular osseous margins.

Continued.

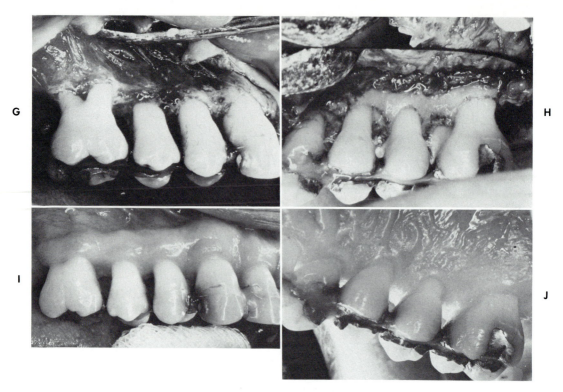

Fig. 27-9, cont'd. G, Completion of osseous surgery with elimination of all defects. Elastic connective tissue of submucosa has been removed, and an immobile base remains. **H,** Correction of palatal defects. Note mesial furca of molar has correct osseous configuration permitting an interproximal gingival rise and thus avoids return of interproximal pocket formation. **I** and **J,** One year after surgery, all pockets are eliminated. (Courtesy Dr. Herman Corn and Dr. Manuel H. Marks, Levittown, Pa.)

fect on the mesial of the maxillary second molar (Fig. 27-7, *KK* to *RR*). To completely eliminate the residual defect entering the mesial furcation of the molar it was elected to resect the mesial buccal root of the molar. The rationale for this decision appears later in the chapter.

Ostectomy. Ostectomy is accomplished next to produce a coronal rise in the bony profile from the buccal and oral surfaces of the teeth into the interdental areas (Figs. 27-7, *S* to *X* and *AA* to *GG*; 27-8, *G*; 27-9, *D* to *F*; 27-10, *B*, *C*, *G*, and *I*). At this point the clinician is attempting to produce a scalloped architectural form that is normal or physiologic for the particular case being treated at a more apical level surrounding the teeth. The existing reversal of normal architectural form is accentuated at the termination of the initial osteoplastic reshaping of the lateral walls of the defects (Figs. 27-7, *M* to *P;* 27-8, *F* and *S*). The bone rises abruptly on the buccal and oral surfaces, and a sharp peak or spine of bone usually remains on the axial corners of the teeth. If the bone is thick on the buccal and oral surfaces it is usually easier to thin

the bone with rotary instruments before proceeding to remove it from the root surfaces with chisels (Fig. 27-7, *N* and *R*). Hand instruments such as Ochsenbein chisels nos. 1 and 2, Wedelstaedt chisels, and Rhodes back action chisels nos. 36 and 37 are excellent for removing bone adjacent to the root surfaces. The angulation of these instruments permits the working tip of the instrument to engage the bone on the mesial and distal axial line angles of the teeth.

Bone may be cut with chisels in a manner similar to wood. While this may not be perfectly correct from a biologic standpoint, clinically it will split and splinter along seams similar to the grain in wood. If the chisel is applied in a perpendicular manner to the osseous surface, a horizontal split can be introduced in the bone at the level the new dento-osseous margin is to be established (Fig. 27-7, *S* to *U*, *AA* and *BB*). The key to the technique is to control the force applied to the chisel and lighten the thrust and pressure applied to the instrument once bone is felt or observed to give. Brute force and gross move-

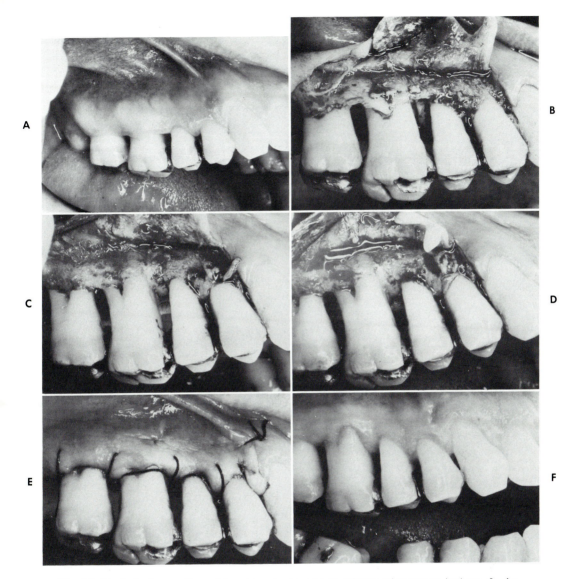

Fig. 27-10. Apically positioned flap to gain access to advanced osseous lesions. **A,** Appearance of tissue after plaque control, root scaling, root planing, and soft tissue curettage. Interproximal cratering is obvious. Crater exists distal to second molar. **B,** Elevation of a partial-thickness mucogingival flap to distal aspect of mesiobuccal root of first molar and full-thickness mucogingival flap posterior to this. Osseous defects are readily seen involving second premolar and molars. Distal furcations cannot be probed. **C,** Ostectomy and osteoplasty procedures correct osseous defects. Removal of radicular bone on mesial aspect eliminates reverse osseous architecture and class I furcation involvements result. Partial-thickness dissection on mesiobuccal root of first molar prevents exposure of a fenestration. **D,** Elimination of infrabony defects between second premolar and first molar has been carried out. **E,** Continuous sutures close surgical site and permit close adaptation of mucogingival flap to underlying osseous tissue. Gingival margin is positioned on roots 1 mm coronal to alveolar crest. Vertical incision at distal line angle of canine facilitates crestal positioning of flap. Coaptation of tuberosity tissue is achieved by interrupted sutures. **F,** One-year postoperative view shows preservation of gingival unit with functional attached gingiva. Gingival margin remains in close approximation to correct osseous form. (Courtesy Dr. Herman Corn, Levittown, Pa.)

ments are not desirable as they permit the point of the chisel to travel through the bone and strike the cemental surface with sufficient force to gouge or nick the root surface. Once a horizontal split is made the chisel can be applied parallel to the root surface in an apical direction, and starting at the osseous margin it can be rotated in a man-

ner one would use with a screwdriver (Fig. 27-8, *U* and *V*). This action permits bulk removal of bone as it is peeled off apically to the predetermined split and guards against overcutting and damage to the root. The degree to which the bone must be contoured is dependent on the amount of bone lost (height and width) and the contour

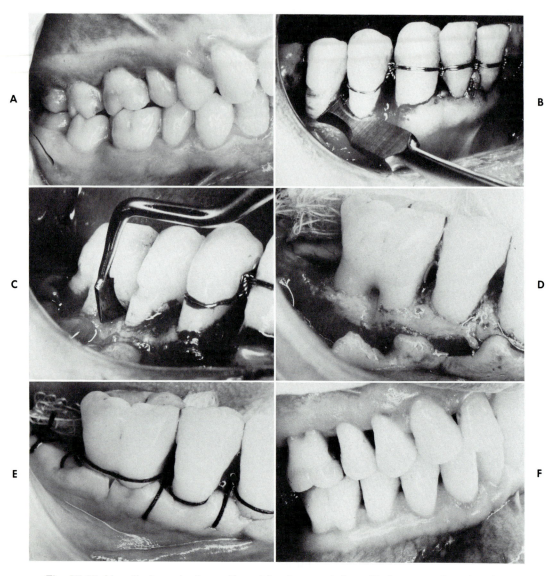

Fig. 27-11. Mandibular apically positioned flap in association with the correction of underlying osseous defects. **A,** Pretreatment view. **B,** Example of use of Ochsenbein chisel to create correct osseous morphology. **C,** Hartzell no. 36/37 (Rhodes) chisel creates level interdental osseous crest. **D,** Reflection of full-thickness mucogingival flap shows corrected osseous form. Note alveolar margin in molar area is designed to relate in profile with cementoenamel junction area. There is purposeful effort to avoid interradicular osseous rise that would cause a soft tissue management problem in this area. Class I furca form is grooved to eliminate ledge at margin. **E,** Continuous suturing enables flap to be positioned 1 mm coronal to alveolar crest. A vertical groove in furca area helps to avoid proliferating granulation tissue and thickened gingival form. **F,** Postoperative 1-year view showing repair of apically positioned flap with functional gingival unit established.

of the adjacent unaffected bone. Smaller chisels such as the Wedelstaedt, Ochsenbein, and Hartzell chisels, contra-angled operative chisels, and rotating instruments may be used to ramp the bone into constricted interdental or interradicular areas (Figs. 27-7, *O* to *X* and *GG;* 27-13, *D;* 27-11, *C, G,* and *I*).

Blending of osseous contours. The final shape of the surgically altered osseous surface begins to emerge as the bone is removed during ostec-

tomy. It is usually found at this stage of the procedure that additional bone must be removed in the interdental areas—buccally and orally at the most apical extensions of the surgical site—to produce a gradual blending of the contours from the basal bone to the dento-osseous margin. It is not unusual to have to reflect the flaps further from the osseous surface to permit a gradual blending of the osseous contours. This in turn usually requires the additional removal of marginal

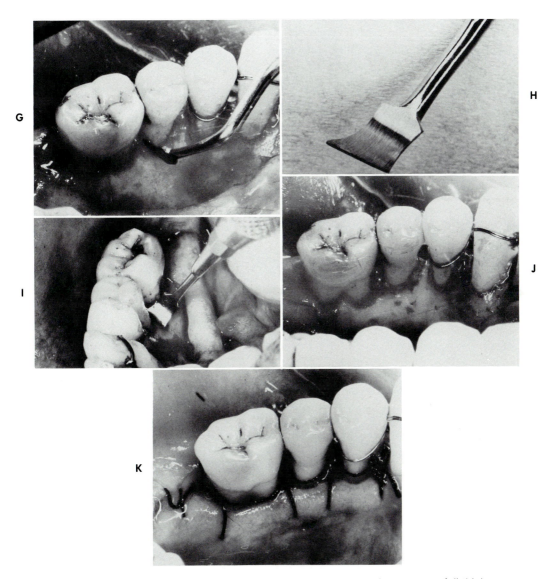

Fig. 27-11, cont'd. G, Lingual view of exposed osseous area subsequent to full-thickness mucogingival flap shows correction of osseous irregularities developing interproximal osseous rise to septal tissue using no. 36/37 Hartzell osseous chisel designed by Rhodes. **H,** Close-up view of Rhodes osseous chisel. **I,** Anteroposterior view showing angulation design of Hartzell instrument creating a natural interproximal rise to interdental bone. **J,** Completed osseous surgery to correct interproximal defect as well as correct osseous marginal irregularities. **K,** Complete closure of surgical site distal to terminal molar is seen. (Courtesy Dr. Herman Corn, Levittown, Pa.)

bone as the final contouring is completed and the osseous surface made smooth.

Anatomic limitations and considerations. In the maxillary arch the dimension and extension of the maxillary sinus must be kept in mind as the bone is reduced. This anatomic area may force one to accept a compromise in therapy lest one perforate into the sinus in an attempt to completely remove an osseous defect. The divergence of the roots of maxillary molars and proximity of

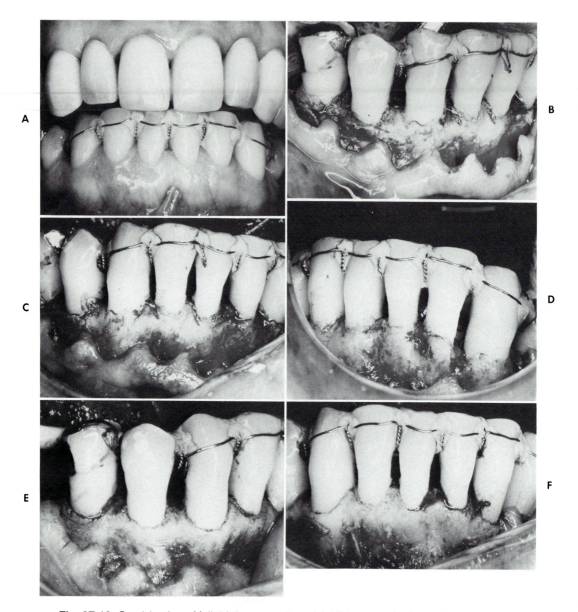

Fig. 27-12. Combination of full-thickness and partial-thickness apically positioned flaps. **A,** In mandibular anterior and premolar areas, purpose of procedure is to eliminate pockets extending beyond mucogingival junction and to correct osseous defects. **B,** Scalloped mucogingival flap reflected revealing partial-thickness dissection involving mandibular right premolars and full-thickness reflection exposing irregular osseous margin of right canine and incisors. **C,** Exposure of right lateral incisor and central incisor area. **D,** Irregular osseous defects involving left central incisor, lateral incisor, and canine. **E** to **G,** Osseous corrections are completed. Note interproximal rise of bone peaking at crest with flat osseous planes at peak of crest to interproximal line angles involving adjacent teeth. Elliptical form is related to cementoenamel junction profile. Osseous corrections can be made directly through connective tissue.

the location of furcation areas usually requires a palatal approach for the resection of craters in the maxillary posterior area. The root trunk (cementoenamel junction to furcation) for maxillary molars extends 3 to 6 mm apical to the cemento-

enamel junction. The buccal furcation is usually located 3 to 4 mm apical to the cementoenamel junction, and the proximal furcations are located slightly more apically at 4 to 6 mm from the cementoenamel junction. If one were to remove

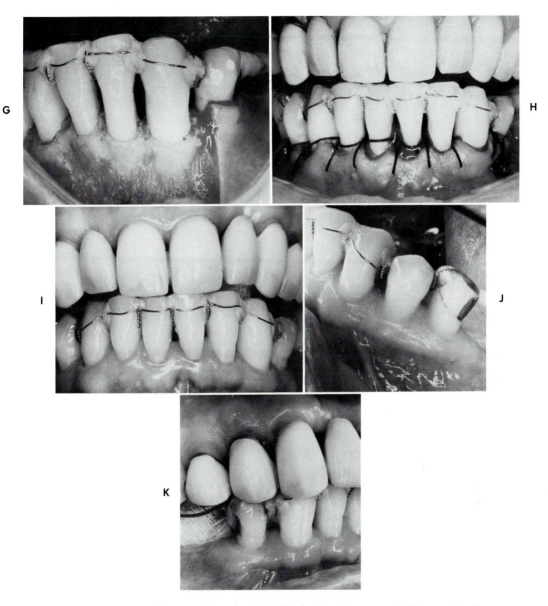

Fig. 27-12, cont'd. H, Closure of surgical site. Vertical incision at mesial line angle of mandibular left first premolar permits draping of apically positioned flap to cover crests and approximately 1 mm coronal to crest on root. Preserved gingiva is positioned in relationship to alveolar crest where bone has been exposed and only is draped apically where there is a connective tissue attachment covering alveolus. Note canine and first premolar area. **I** to **K,** Four-month postoperative view of completed surgical site demonstrating gingival form and its relationship with corrected underlying osseous tissue (posterior are mirror views). (Courtesy Dr. Herman Corn, Levittown, Pa., and Dr. Leonard Juros, Willingboro, N.J.)

the buccal wall of a crater by using a buccal approach for the osseous resection, the buccal furcation could needlessly be exposed with loss of the thin bone supporting the buccal roots. As bone is removed on the buccal surfaces the distance between converging roots (distobuccal first molar–mesiobuccal second molar) narrows, thereby reducing the width of the interdental area and creating a less favorable environment for the interdental papilla. Removal of the lingual wall of the crater has less of a tendency to involve the proximal furcations and turns the topography of the palatal root into a premolar one (Figs. 27-7, *JJ* and *KK;* 27-9, *H* and *J*). The palatal approach increases the distance (mesiodistally) between the palatal roots of adjacent teeth, permits greater access to the defect, space for an interdental papilla, and more convenient access for plaque control.

In the mandibular arch the mylohyoid ridge frequently presents as a shelf of bone extending lingually in a horizontal direction. As one extends the flap further apically, the contour drops off precipitously into an undercut as the contour cuts back upon itself (Fig. 27-8, *BB* to *II*). A long bevel must be produced in the bone in this area so that the contours may be blended and the flap readapted to the bone in a smooth tapering profile from the floor of the mouth to the dento-osseous margin.

Instrumentation of the teeth. Once bone has been contoured final attention should be directed to the teeth. The area should be irrigated thoroughly, preferably with isotonic saline, and blotted with 2- by 2-inch gauze pads, and the roots should be given a final inspection for calcareous deposits. Any remaining deposits should be removed, and the roots smoothed. Periodontists attempt to get roots as smooth as possible and frequently will not close a surgical site until they have reinstrumented all teeth in the surgical area as a final check. Due thought should be given to areas where bone was freshly removed from the roots by ostectomy procedures. These were normal areas free of periodontal disease. Bone was removed from these sites solely for the purpose of attaining physiologic contours in the marginal bone. The cementum in these areas contains the embedded remnants of torn fiber bundles. If the cut edge of the surgical flap can be positioned and stabilized against this surface, the chances for repair by reattachment during healing are heightened. If one root planes these areas out of habit just to make sure they are smooth, the freshly cut fibers and cementoid-cemental surface will be traumatized and healing will have to occur via formation of a new attachment to the tooth.

Closure of the surgical site. Once the clinician is satisfied that the teeth have been prepared and the bone has been contoured to the desired degree, the flap is readied for closure. Soft tissue tags or uneven margins are trimmed from the underside of the flap, and the area is irrigated thoroughly to ensure that debris will not be entrapped beneath the flap. The flap is positioned against the bone, and its ability to adapt to the contours of the bone and teeth is carefully studied. It may require further thinning for it to cover the bone as an even veneer. It should be free of tensional displacing forces from the adjacent mucogingival complex of tissues, permitting it to rest passively against bone and teeth. If it remains under displacing tensional forces, additional releasing incisions or extensions of existing releasing incisions must be made to ensure accurate placement and stabilization of the flaps by the restraining sutures (Fig. 27-10, *E*). If a tug-of-war ensues between the restraining sutures and the pull of the surrounding musculature, the muscles will invariably win, sutures will tear, and the flap will be displaced to a point where the forces are neutralized.

Any combination of suture material and suture configuration that will maintain the flap at the dento-osseous margin or slightly coronal to it is acceptable (see Chapter 26). It is usually advisable to suture lingual or palatal flaps independently of buccal flaps to ensure better adaptation and more accurate placement. Every effort is made to protect the vulnerable thin bone covering radicular surfaces, as wound healing studies have shown this area may be resorbed with partial repair or no repair if left exposed. However, it is not at all unusual for the opposite to occur and the flap be pulled too far coronally.

All too frequently the time and effort expended upon the contouring of the underlying bone are negated by inattention or careless manipulation of the flap during closure of the surgical site. If the flap is sutured too tightly and pulled too far coronally by the tension of the sutures it cannot adapt to the undulating contours that have been festooned into the bone. The voids created fill initially with a fibrinous clot, and later granulation tissue and fibrous connective tissue replace the clot, filling the concave contours so painstakingly produced during the osseous portion of the surgery.

While these events are occurring below the flap, a similar set of circumstances may occur in the marginal and papillary area of the flap. The coronally displaced papillary portion of the flap is not supported by the contoured interdental bone, and the fingerlike projections of soft tissue collapse to re-form interdental craters, producing unwanted depth and reverse gingival architecture. The importance of well-planned and skillfully executed flap management cannot be overemphasized. Occasionally, despite all efforts to ensure an even adaptation of flaps, they will heal with uneven margins and unwanted thickness. This is particularly the case with palatal flaps, which can be exceedingly difficult to thin and contour to the degree desired. If they are permitted to remain in this fashion, unwanted depth will return as the tissues in the surgical site mature and reach their biologic thickness. Infrabony defects no longer exist in the healing surgical site, and a gingivoplasty can be done to thin the soft tissues and revise the architectural form should this occur. If a gingivoplasty is done at the time of removal of the second dressing (usually 14 to 21 days), the minor corrections necessary can be accomplished quickly and simply. Wound healing studies have shown the connective tissues to be most reactive 14 to 28 days after initial wounding. By timing the second-stage corrective gingivoplasty to coincide with maximum reparative activity in the connective tissues, rapid repair is noted with little additional discomfort to the patient. It is usually necessary to keep the wound covered for another 5 to 7 days, but the touch-up procedure pays handsome dividends in the contours produced in the healed surgical site.

Dressing the wound and postoperative care. The surgical dressing serves several purposes:

1. It aids in displacing or holding flaps in an apical direction to the position governed by the restraining suspension sutures.
2. It aids in positioning the marginal area of the flap tightly against the underlying osseous surface. This aids in hemorrhage control, preventing unwanted pooling of blood and fibrin under the flap and assures the clinician that the flap is adapted as closely as possible to the undulating contours of the bone and teeth.
3. It obliterates interdental spaces in the cervical areas of the teeth that would trap food and plaque during the initial period of healing when the wound is too tender to permit mechanical cleansing.
4. It stabilizes the flap against movements of muscle pull, tongue pressure, and displacing pressures or trauma that would occur during mastication if the wound were left uncovered.

The dressing should be mixed to a moderately firm consistency so that it will have sufficient body to resist displacing forces and to perform as listed above. It should not be mixed so firmly that upon application it will displace a flap from its intended area of stabilization or tear sutures from their points of anchorage.

The introduction of semimixed and premixed dressing materials has simplified problems associated with time necessary for mixing and the mess created during preparation and spatulation in the work area. The previous controversies over the irritating properties of eugenol-containing dressings have abated now that bone is no longer left exposed in our mucogingival procedures. The cyanoacrylate tissue adhesives continue to remain classified for use in experimental studies and have not been cleared by the Food and Drug Administration for unrestricted clinical use as of this writing. The choice of dressing materials at this point is probably governed more by individual preferences for handling characteristics and convenience in mixing and storage than it is for its content of eugenol or specific components.

The first dressing is usually changed 7 to 10 days after the surgical procedure, at which time the sutures are removed. Lilly (1968) and Lilly et al. (1972, 1969, 1968) have shown that monofilament sutures are less irritating than multiple-filament suture materials, which tend to act as an absorbent wick, thereby promoting a greater inflammatory reaction in the connective tissues. Hiatt's study on flap retraction (1968) would appear to indicate that sutures can be removed at this time without undue concern that the flap may be displaced. It is frequently observed that the sutures are loose at this time and have ceased to serve in a restraining or retentive capacity and are serving only to retain debris. Their removal appears to hasten wound healing. The surgical site is irrigated, cleansed, and dressed for a second 7- to 10-day period, after which the wound is left uncovered and routine cleansing procedures are resumed in a cautious, gentle manner.

Wound healing studies have shown there is sufficient epithelial healing and initial connective tissue healing to permit the wound to remain uncovered after 14 to 20 days. The timing of dressing changes in clinical practice is no doubt related as much to convenience in scheduling appointments as it is to the biologic events in wound healing.

Studies by Ramfjord (1966) and others have called attention to the need for meticulous plaque control during the first 2 months of wound healing. Newly formed collagen, in contrast to mature collagen, is readily degraded in the presence of plaque and the inflammatory response that it provokes in the host. The first few months after surgery become a critical period in wound healing, and patients must be made aware of the necessity for extra thoroughness in their program of personal plaque control in order for wound healing to be carried to completion.

MAINTENANCE OF SURGICALLY ALTERED OSSEOUS TOPOGRAPHY

Cohen (1959) called attention to the fact that the morphology of the interdental gingiva consists of a buccal and a lingual peak connected by a col or depression. He demonstrated that the col and interdental soft tissue morphology was related to interproximal tooth contours and contact relationships.

Zander and Matherson conducted a study in two young adult rhesus monkeys to determine the effects of osteoplasty and ostectomy on interdental tissue morphology. They found that:

After osseous reduction and reshaping to produce a buccolingual peak in the bone interdentally, the animals were sacrificed after six months. The tissues were then processed for histological studies. Three dimensional wax and plexiglass reconstructions were made from these sections at 20x. The osteoplastic procedure had no significant influence on the morphology of the interdental tissues. The histology, morphology and dimensions of the interdental col were similar in operative and control areas. Reduction of bone height did not produce any significant alterations in the mandibular interdental area and the results were similar to those noted with osteoplasty alone. However, in the maxilla there is a trend toward disappearance of the col as evidenced by the closer approximation of buccal and palatal peaks. In two interdental areas, between the two premolars and first and second molar, the buccal peak was eliminated. A wax reconstruction of the areas showed the palatal peak closely associated with an enamel space. These observations lead us to believe that the morphology of the interdental gingiva is much more influenced by adjoining tooth surfaces than by the shape of the underlying bone. [Zander and Matherson, 1963]

In a clinical study of 24 osseous defects in humans Patur and Glickman (1962) reflected mucoperiosteal flaps from the alveolar processes, removed granulomatous tissue from the bone, root planed the teeth, and made rubber base impressions of the osseous contours before the flaps were replaced and sutured. In addition to detailed clinical measurements they used a film positioning device to permit accurate comparisons to be made of standardized radiographs taken during treatment. They reoperated on the cases 5 to 12 months later, repeating the procedure to evaluate healing in one-, two-, and three-wall infrabony pockets. They found slight resorption and remodeling of the alveolar crest and stated that "the extent of natural recontouring of the bone which will occur in individual cases cannot be predicted."

Matherson and Zander (1963) undertook a study to determine the extent of alveolar process maintenance following osteoplasty and ostectomy in three young adult rhesus monkeys. One procedure consisted of reducing crestal height 1 to 2 mm and recontouring the interdental and radicular areas buccally and lingually. Another procedure was interdental osteoplasty with no bone reduction. In both procedures an effort was made to create a buccolingual peak in the interdental bone. After 6 months the bone was studied macroscopically and microscopically and was observed to have maintained the experimentally produced reduction and contour. Microscopic study of their material indicated a similar rate of bone deposition and osteoblastic activity in the operated and control areas, indicating that the bone will not return to its original morphology. Their work would indicate that we are justified in reshaping crestal bone.

There are a variety of clinical situations in which it is not advisable to remove bone via osseous resective techniques to eliminate the osseous deformities existing within the periodontium (see discussions on Indications and Contraindications). This leads us into the topic of new attachment procedures that have as their objective the reconstruction of the lost units of the periodontium — bone, periodontal ligament fibers, and cementum.

NEW ATTACHMENT PROCEDURES (RECONSTRUCTIVE-REPARATIVE OSSEOUS PROCEDURES)

If one were to state the ultimate goal of all periodontal therapy, it would be the total prevention of periodontal destruction coupled with the ability to reconstruct the attachment apparatus back to a normal relationship with the cemento-enamel junction. For many decades periodontists have sought to effect a reattachment of the tissues surrounding periodontal pockets to the roots of the teeth. It is unfortunate that the term "reattachment" was introduced into our dental vocabulary and literature, for once we have a periodontal pocket, whether it be infrabony or suprabony, we sustain a *net loss* of the attachment apparatus— bone, periodontal ligament fibers, and cementum. If we are to be successful in our therapeutic endeavors and eliminate periodontal pockets, *new* bone, periodontal ligament fibers, and cementum will be required. The term "new attachment" is preferable to "reattachment," for it more clearly portrays the cellular kinetics and sequence of events that take place in wound healing to bring about the coronal migration of the base of a pocket and its conversion into a healthy sulcus.

It would be best at this point if we defined the terms "repair" and "regeneration" and used them in their classic rather than clinical sense to avoid confusion and misunderstanding. Melcher offers an excellent description of these processes:

Descriptions of wound healing use the terms regeneration and repair to describe the processes by which defects in tissues or organs are "made good." Gillman (1961) has underlined the importance of understanding that restoration of lost tissue may be achieved by two distinct processes. In the one, the architecture and function of the lost tissue is completely renewed, and for this process he reserves the term regeneration. In the other, continuity of the disrupted tissues is restored by new tissues which do not replicate the structure and function of the lost tissue. He calls this process repair. This distinction is important, for it implies that not all tissues can regenerate themselves after injury, and that their capacity to do so varies with type of injury, and from tissue to tissue. There is also variations between species. To quote two extreme examples: following amputation, the salamander will regenerate a new limb with all its complicated arrangement of tissues; by contrast, man cannot replace even a small amount of lost central nervous tissue. So, in considering the healing of a wound, it is not only necessary to assess the capacity of the organism to fill the defect with new tissue, but it is also important to observe how this is done, to what extent the new tissue is able to carry out the functions of the old, and finally whether, with the passage of time, repair may be followed by regeneration as may occur to some extent in wounds of muscle.

[Melcher, A. H., and Bowen, W. H.: Biology of the Periodontium, London, 1969, Academic Press, Inc. Copyright by Academic Press, Inc. Used by permission]

It would appear that many of our attempts at effecting a new attachment in the treatment of periodontal pockets result in a repair of the lost tissue units rather than regeneration. This is particularly the case with cementum (Stahl, 1977).

A question frequently asked by students is, "Why not attempt to gain a new attachment in the treatment of all osseous defects rather than resort to the use of osseous resection for the treatment of shallow to moderately deep defects?" The question is an excellent one and calls attention to the need to consider the morphology of the defects and the cellular kinetics involved in wound healing. One may expect in a chapter devoted to the treatment of osseous defects to have it stated that bone is indeed the key tissue and the cornerstone for success in rebuilding the periodontium. The periodontal literature would aid in creating this impression, for in past years attention has been focused on bone-fill procedures and procedures in which the primary aim was *bone* grafting and the elimination of *bony* defects. While one cannot discount the importance of bone, it is the cementum that is needed, on a timely and predictable basis *early* in wound healing, for repair or regeneration to occur. The majority of the animal and human studies that have been reported are in general agreement that the first appearance of new cementum occurs at approximately the twenty-first day in wound healing. (Goldman studies show cementum being laid down on the tooth surface as early as 10 days.) The lag phase in the formation of cementum is critical, for if the regenerating epithelial cells are not impeded by contact inhibition in the maturing connective tissue of the fibrous callus and migrate into the organizing clot and apically along the root surface, they will win the "race" and prevent collagen fibers from attaching into cementum more coronally along the root in the healing wound.

Research emphasis has shifted to a quest for greater understanding of the nature and role of cementum and cementogenesis in the pathogenesis and treatment of periodontal disease in the later half of this decade (Aleo et al., 1974; Garrett, 1975; Selvig, 1965; Stahl, 1975; Zander, 1958). Once we gain a greater understanding of the factors that influence the rate of cementogenesis and learn how to successfully modulate the cell populations involved in the healing infrabony or suprabony pocket, we will be in a position to attempt new attachment procedures on all types and classes of osseous defects. Until such time as that becomes a reality the morphology of the osseous defects will continue to influence our modes of therapy and prognosis for success in gaining new attachment.

Morphologic requirements for repair in three-wall osseous defects

Prichard (1968) has focused attention on the significance of the number of bony walls that surround an osseous defect and their importance in new attachment procedures and has stated that "only one type of osseous deformity can be eliminated by a new growth of bone, and that is a cavity 'inside or within bone,' an intrabony defect." Confusion exists over the terminology that has been used to describe pockets or cavities "within" bone. "Subcrestal" is too general a term, and "intra-alveolar" is not accurate, since an osseous defect extends into the alveolar process beyond the cribriform plate of the alveolus. The term "infrabony" signifies a defect "below" the bone, but is not specific as to the number of walls that surround the defect and is not anatomically correct for defects occurring within the maxilla. The word "intrabony," meaning "inside or within," is descriptive of the location of the pocket, but it too is not completely accurate from the anatomic standpoint of a three-wall defect occurring next to a tooth. Since the tooth is the fourth wall of such a defect, the defect is not completely "inside" bone. It would appear that the number of bony walls surrounding an osseous defect will have to be stated until more descriptive terms are adopted.

The number of bony walls that surround an osseous defect, the quantity factor, and the type of bone that exists within the bony walls, the quality factor, have a direct bearing on the prognosis and treatment of osseous defects. In order for an osseous defect to fill in, to be repaired, bone must be regenerated from the periodontal ligament tissue and the viable bony surfaces that surround the defect. Bone remodels, resorbs, or rebuilds only on the surface of existing viable bone. Bone cannot expand and grow by interstitial growth in a manner similar to cartilage. New bone is produced from within the marrow spaces of the bone surrounding an osseous defect. The nature of the bone bordering osseous defects is important, since thin cortical bone has proportionately less marrow than

cancellous bone and therefore offers less potential for bone regeneration.

Deep, narrow, three-wall infrabony defects, because of their special morphology, will heal by a repair of bone, connective tissue fibers, and cementum when the irritants are removed and the chronic inflammation in bone is converted to a freshly prepared, acutely inflamed surgical wound. A favorable ratio exists in narrow three-wall defects between the surface area of the bone surrounding the defect (mm^2) and the volume of the defect (mm^3) that must be restored to effect repair. The bony walls provide the undifferentiated mesenchymal cells from the marrow spaces and endosteal tissues for the generation of new bone, fibroblasts, and interstitial connective tissues. The mesenchymal cells within the periodontal ligament also participate in the reparative process, and it has been speculated that the layer of ecto-mesenchymal cells and their derivatives on the cemental side of the periodontal ligament space are the requisite cells for cementum regeneration (Freeman and Ten Cate, 1971; Stahl, 1977; Ten Cate, 1975).

Most osseous defects are combination-type defects with three walls at the base and two walls or one wall at the orifice. The three-wall portion at the base of the defect will respond to treatment attempts to gain a new attachment. The wide sloping portion of the defect near the orifice will not completely repair. The volume of periodontium destroyed is too great in proportion to the surface area of bone remaining, which must function as the reservoir of reparative cells.

Bone and cementum are formed at much slower rates than the epithelial covering overlying the infrabony pockets. All too frequently the soft tissues of the flaps over the defects collapse into the orifice of the defects and occupy the space where it is desired to gain new bone and cementum. Epithelium will invade the blood clot formed in the osseous defect and pass apically until it reaches young granulation tissue growing into the clot from the periphery of the wound. Granulation tissue inhibits further apical migration of the epithelium by a phenomenon known as *contact inhibition*. If the rapidly growing epithelium quickly establishes a new junctional epithelial attachment to the root it will hinder the formation of new cementum and a cemental attachment coronal to the level of the epithelium. This is why it is so difficult to gain 100% bone fill and a new attachment to the level of the osseous crest in wide, large volume osseous defects.

Ellegaard et al. (1974, 1973b) have developed a technique for epithelial retardation by covering treated osseous defects with a free gingival graft in lieu of the conventional flap approach. Since free grafts slough their epithelium during the first 1 to 5 days in wound healing and require an additional 5 to 7 days to regain their surface epithelium, the connective tissues in the healing osseous defect are provided a 12- to 14-day head start in the race toward healing. Register (1973) and Register and Burdick (1976, 1975) have sought to speed the rate at which cementum will form by decalcifying the surface of the root in the area of the pocket with citric acid. Unfortunately, our knowledge of the factors and cellular processes that influence cementogenesis are most meager at this time. Once we learn how to influence and modulate the rates of cellular formation among bone, cementum, and epithelium we can alter our technical procedures to increase the potential for attaining complete or total new attachment on a predictable basis.

Surgical preparation of osseous defects for new attachment therapy

While there are many methods advocated for attaining new attachment in infrabony defects, the preparation of the tooth surface, contents of the defect, and surrounding bony walls of infrabony pockets are similar for almost all the surgical techniques in use today. The infrabony pocket must be cleaned out thoroughly, and the root surface planed to a hard, smooth, surface. These two requirements are common to all the procedures to be mentioned and have a biologic basis for inclusion in our surgical techniques. It is important that one be familiar with the histopathologic changes that take place in the tissues surrounding infrabony pockets, for periodontal surgery is designed to reverse the pathologic changes in the tissues and promote regeneration of the attachment apparatus.

In health the marrow spaces of the alveolar process and contiguous supporting bone contain a fatty type of marrow. Hematopoietic marrow is not normally found in the jaws, and it differs considerably in form and function from the fatty marrow of the alveolar process. A comparison of the two types of marrow is shown in Fig. 27-13. Changes take place in the marrow during destructive periodontal disease. The cellular events that accompany chronic inflammation convert the fatty marrow to a fibrous type of marrow. Fibroblasts, blood vessels, and inflammatory cells change the characteristics of the cancellous bone bordering the periodontal pocket. Collagen fibers produced within the marrow spaces adjacent to the lesion unite with those of neighboring marrow spaces as the bone is resorbed to form an altered transseptal covering for the bony defect. The direction of these fiber bundles differs markedly from the orientation of unaffected transseptal fibers (Fig. 27-14). The soft tissue contents and altered transseptal fibers must be enucleated during curettage of the defect. The granulomatous tissue and altered transseptal fibers are difficult to remove as these tissues are firmly anchored in partially resorbed cul-de-sac areas of the crestal fibrous marrow. Novice clinicians usually make two errors in attempting to remove this tissue; they will use a small curet instead of a larger one to enucleate these firmly anchored tissues and shred the tissue instead of scooping it free from the bony surface. If a large curet is used firmly against the bony walls of the pocket the fibers are more easily dislodged and a bleeding bony surface remains. Smaller curets are used to open into the periodontal ligament space and smaller recesses of the pocket once the bulk of the granulomatous tissue has been removed. These fiber bundles of mature collagen must be removed to convert the chronic lesion into a surgical wound capable of undergoing complete repair.

If the bony walls of the defects appear dense or sclerotic after the soft tissue contents of the pockets have been removed, they can be pierced with small sharp curets or burs to make intramarrow penetrations. The openings created into the surrounding normal marrow speed the sequence of events in healing, for they provide access pathways for new capillaries, fibroblasts, and basic mesenchymal cells to enter into the wound site. The timing of the entry of required cell populations is most critical at this point in wound healing. If the dense bony walls have to be breached by the slower physiologic process of undermining (rear) resorption, the establishment of an early capillary circulation and formation of a fibrous callus will be delayed. The major role of the blood clot in wound healing is to control hemorrhage. Its role as a scaffold to support granulation tissue growing in from the periphery of the wound has been overstated. The contraction of the clot early in the stages of wound healing permits the overlying gingival flaps to collapse to some extent into the orifice of the defect. The epithelium from the cut edges of the flaps burrows into the clot and extends apically until it reaches healthy granulation tissue (Bernier and

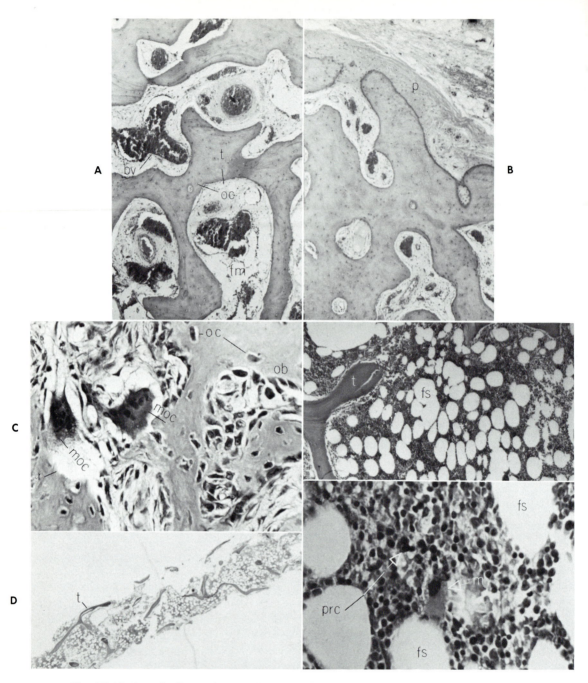

Fig. 27-13. A to **C,** Photomicrographs, cancellous bone, human jaw specimen. **A,** Fatty marrow spaces, *fm;* blood vessels, *bv;* and trabeculae, *t,* of normal cancellous bone. Vital osteocytes, *oc,* in lacunae. **B,** Margin of cancellous bone with periosteum, *p,* covering surface. **C,** Higher power showing plump osteocytes, *oc,* in lacunae; osteoblasts, *ob,* lining trabecular surface; multinucleated osteoclasts, *moc,* with brush borders in resorption bay, *r.* **D** to **F,** Photomicrographs, normal hematopoietic marrow specimen obtained from posterosuperior iliac crest (human). **D,** Low power of marrow core. Note high ratio of cellular material to cancellous bone. This accounts for relatively radiolucent appearance of newly implanted marrow noted on posttreatment roentgenograms. **E,** Fat spaces, *fs,* among precursor cells of white blood cell and red blood cell lines. Trabecula, *t,* of cancellous bone. **F,** High-power view of primitive reticular cells, *prc,* in stroma of marrow. Large megakaryocyte, *m,* at arrow. There is abundant evidence that least differentiated marrow cells can form bone as readily as they can form marrow cells. Note marked difference between two different types of bone marrow.

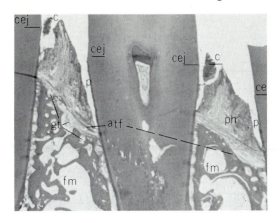

Fig. 27-14. Photomicrograph, mandibular second premolar. Mesial tilt to teeth with cementoenamel junctions, *cej,* located at different levels in relationship to horizontal plane. Calculus, *c,* in pockets, *p;* space of pocket an artifact created in histologic processing. Altered transseptal fibers, *atf,* covering osseous defects. Fatty marrow, *fm,* converted into a fibrous, edematous marrow with granulation tissue, *gt,* adjacent to inflammatory infiltrate of pockets. Pseudoepitheliomatous hyperplasia, *ph,* of sulcular epithelium extending into gingival corium.

Kaplan, 1947; Orban and Archer, 1945). Fig. 27-15 shows epithelial cells invading a blood clot situated between the cut edge of a flap and the root of a tooth. It is advantageous therefore to have the clot quickly invaded by young granulation tissue and resorbed and replaced by a healthy fibrous callus as rapidly as possible.

The oral cavity presents many obstacles that work against the successful accomplishment of reconstructive procedures. We cannot close the wound in tissue layers and immobilize the surgical site as would an orthopedic surgeon. It is almost impossible to obtain a "watertight" seal of the flaps over the osseous defects when the wound is closed via sutures at the termination of the surgical procedure. The fibrous callus must be protected from infection for it to mature and have the collagen matrix converted into calcified cancellous bone.

It is deemed advisable by most clinicians to utilize a suitable antibiotic regimen on a prophylactic basis for the first 7 to 10 days of wound healing to prevent contamination and infection

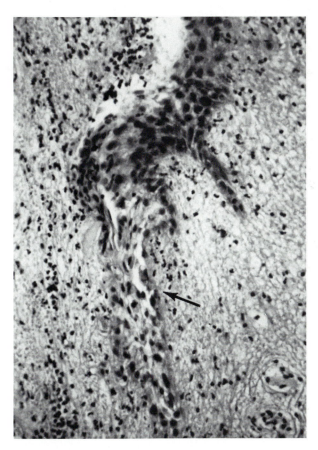

Fig. 27-15. Photomicrograph of epithelium *(arrow)* invading blood clot early in wound healing. (Courtesy Dr. B. Ellegaard, Arhus, Denmark.)

within the surgical site. Comparison studies in animals and humans have shown that healing is accelerated during the first postoperative week if antibiotics are used (Ariaudo, 1969; Stahl, 1963).

The tooth wall of the infrabony pocket must be prepared with the same meticulous attention to detail as that devoted to the osseous walls. We have learned more about the nature of the root surface in periodontal pockets both before and after instrumentation from studies using the scanning electron microscope. Selvig (1966, 1965) and Sottosanti (1976) have shown calculus embedded in the pitted root surface of extracted teeth that were associated with deep periodontal pockets. The root surface adjacent to infrabony pockets must be *thoroughly planed* to remove the calculus from the pitted tooth surface plus the contaminated

surface layer of the cementum. Aleo et al. (1975, 1974) have demonstrated the diseased nature of the root surface in teeth associated with periodontal pockets. They incubated the roots of healthy teeth and those with periodontal disease in a cell culture of human gingival fibroblasts. The fibroblasts would grow and attach to the roots of the healthy teeth, but a cell-free zone was observed adjacent to the roots associated with periodontal pockets. If the roots of the periodontally involved teeth were thoroughly planed or if they were treated with phenol-water to extract absorbed endotoxin, fibroblasts would grow and attach to the roots in the same manner as with healthy roots.

Studies such as this show that the root surface must be adequately prepared if it is to participate

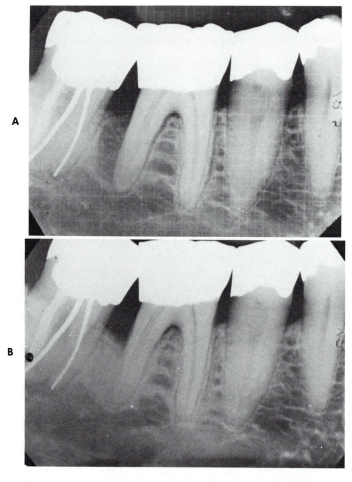

Fig. 27-16. A, Preoperative radiograph. Large-volume three-wall infrabony pocket on distal aspect of first molar was treated by open flap curettage and replaced flap. **B,** Radiograph 1 year later showing new attachment to level of osseous crest. (Courtesy Dr. D. Walter Cohen, Philadelphia.)

in the dynamic events of wound healing. If the root surface is not rendered biologically acceptable, the cementoblasts that most probably originate from the mesenchymal precursor cells on the root side of the periodontal ligament space (Stahl, 1977; Ten Cate, 1975) will be prevented from adhering to the root surface and a true new attachment will not be attained. Scaling will not suffice to render the root surface biologically acceptable. It requires meticulous and methodical planing with a curet to remove the diseased cemental surface. One of the advantages of the open-flap approach for the reconstructive treatment of infrabony defects is that it provides the mechanical and visual access necessary to assure the clinician that the root surfaces have been adequately prepared to participate in wound healing. There is probably

no other procedure in dentistry that is more demanding and taxing of one's skill, patience, and perseverance than thorough root planing. Until such time as tissue-compatible chemical agents can be employed to render the root surface biologically acceptable, sharp curets, patience, and old-fashioned elbow grease must be employed.

Once the basic steps in the preparation of the root surfaces and bony walls of the infrabony pockets have been completed as discussed above, the surgical site is thoroughly irrigated and inspected and the flaps are made ready for closure in the same manner as if one were eliminating the osseous defects by osseous resection. It is at this point in new attachment therapy that we reach a point of departure in surgical technique and rationale of procedure as to how to best attain

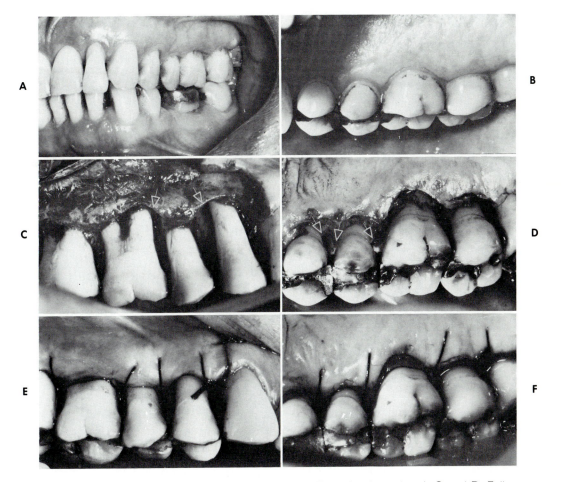

Fig. 27-17. A and **B,** Preoperative views, left side (**B** to **J,** mirror views). **C** and **D,** Full-thickness mucoperiosteal flaps reflected for access to perform root planing and open flap curettage. Note uneven marginal contour of bone on buccal aspect and three-walled infrabony defects *(arrows).* On palatal side bone is not involved. Osseous defects slope apically and to buccal aspect once probe is passed toward midpoint of interdental area. **E** and **F,** Flaps are replaced to former positions (repositioned) at termination of open flap curettage in an attempt to gain maximum bone coverage and repair in three-wall defects.

Continued.

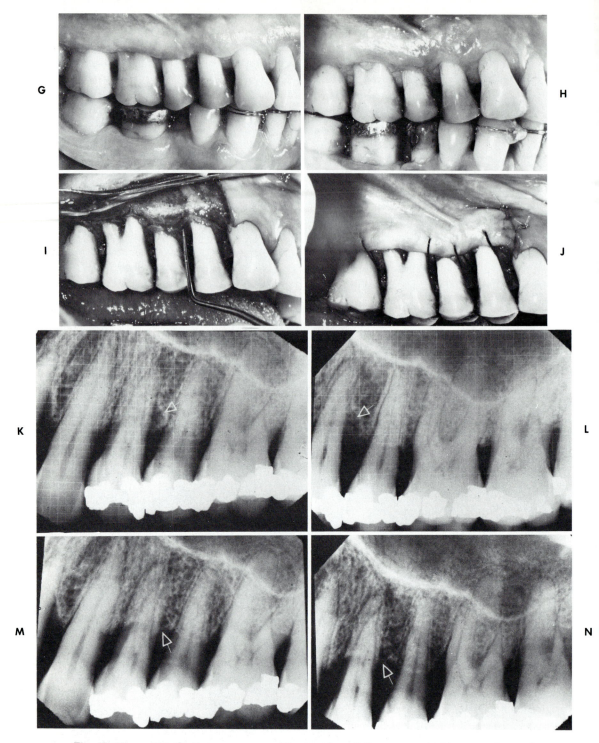

Fig. 27-17, cont'd. G, Note reverse architecture in soft tissues created by use of repositioned flap and acceptance of reverse osseous architecture 4 months after surgery. **H,** Note change of contours due to bone remodeling and soft tissue proliferation 13 months after surgery. At this point probing reveals minimal pocket depth. **I,** Area reentered at 13 months to show new attachment attained on distal aspect of first premolar and mesial aspect of molar. Probe is resting on bone, having pierced connective tissue covering bone to depth of 1 mm (compare with **C**). **J,** Minor osteoplasty performed and flap apically positioned at the dento-osseous margin. **K** and **L,** Preoperative radiographs. Arrows indicate infrabony defect on distobuccal aspect of first premolar. **M** and **N,** Radiographs taken 9 months after surgery indicate repair taking place on first premolar (arrows).

the desired end result of a new attachment apparatus. The clinician may elect to—

1. Close the flaps over the prepared osseous defects and attempt to gain bone fill and new attachment to the roots by the sequence of events normal to wound healing in bone. The rationale for this approach in therapy is based upon the favorable morphology found in three-wall osseous defects and a favorable ratio between the surface area of the surrounding bony walls and the volume of the periodontium to be restored (Figs. 27-16 and 27-17).

2. Close the flaps over the prepared osseous defects that have been filled with an implant of stimulated periosteum, fresh or frozen autogenous bone, or frozen or freeze-dried bone allografts, or various biodegradable or nondegradable synthetic allograft materials (Fig. 27-18). The rationale for this approach in therapy is based upon attaining one or more of the following objectives:

a. Promoting rapid osteogenesis
b. Promoting rapid cementogenesis
c. Eliminating large blood clots that must be resorbed and replaced by bone matrix (fibrous callus)
d. Supporting the soft tissue "walls" of the osseous defects—the "roof" of large volume three-wall defects or lateral walls of combination two-wall and one-wall defects
e. Providing a biologically acceptable scaffold

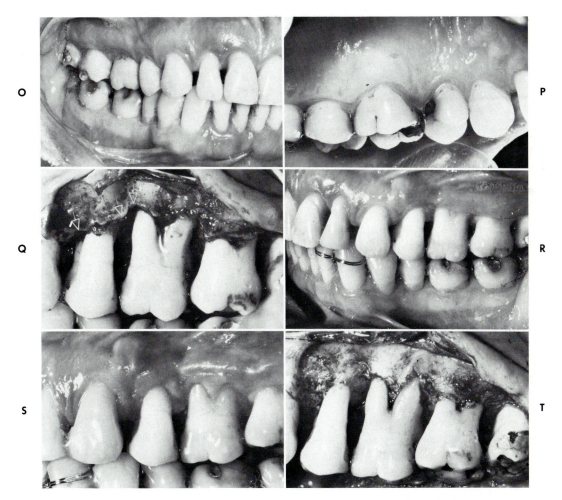

Fig. 27-17, cont'd. O and **P,** Preoperative views, right side (**P** to **T,** mirror views). **Q,** Uneven marginal contour of bone and infrabony defects on mesial aspect of premolar and first molar similar to left side *(arrows).* Open flap curettage, root planing, and repositioned flap same as on left side. **R,** Four months after surgery. **S,** Thirteen months after surgery. Former infrabony defects cannot be probed more than 3 mm. **T,** Area reentered to show new attachment attained and extent of osseous remodeling (compare with **Q**). Flap apically positioned at dento-osseous margin to attain shallow sulcus depth.

Continued.

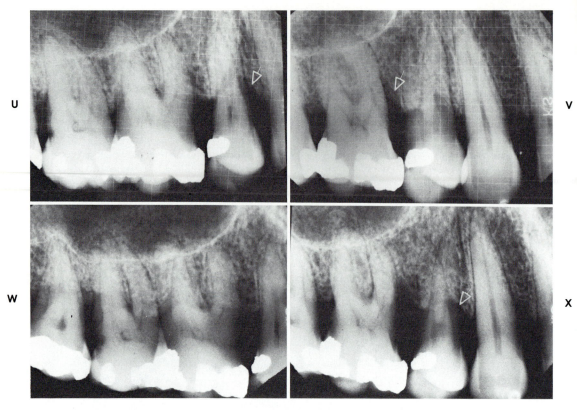

Fig. 27-17, cont'd. U and **V,** Preoperative radiographs indicate osseous defects on buccal aspect *(arrows).* **W** and **X,** Repair on mesial aspect of premolar 9 months after surgery *(arrow).*

for new granulation tissue (bone matrix–fibrous callus) to grow upon from the lateral walls of the defects

f. Blocking epithelial downgrowth via contact inhibition

3. Eliminate the osseous defects in selected cases by surgically moving the osseous walls of the pockets into contact with the teeth and closing the flaps over the area of the former defects. The rationale for this technique is based on the premise that a greenstick fracture can be created in the bone and the bone stabilized against the tooth as a contiguous autograft (bone swage technique, Ewen, 1965; Ross et al., 1966). The sequence of events in wound healing are technically similar to that of a narrow three-wall infrabony pocket as mentioned in 1 above (Figs. 27-19 and 27-20).

4. Resect the gingival portion of the flaps that would normally reside over the osseous defect or defects, regardless of whether or not they have been implanted with bone or bone substitutes, and utilize free autogenous gingival grafts (masticatory mucosa) to cover the osseous defects (Ellegaard et al. 1974, 1973). The rationale for this technique, as previously mentioned, is to retard

epithelial migration into the area of the healing infrabony segment of the pocket (Fig. 27-21).

It is not the intent of this text to cover the full range of experimental work in bone grafting and reconstructive periodontal procedures that are being conducted and reported upon in this country and abroad. Many of the procedures advocated require further research and study to determine if they are clinically safe, valid, and practical for use in a private practice or clinical setting. A brief discussion of the rationale and some of the techniques that have been advocated for bone grafting will be presented next.

Free or contiguous grafts

The donor material utilized in periodontal new attachment procedures varies as to source of the donor material and the nature of its placement into the osseous defect. Grafts may be free, taken from another area of the mouth or body, and placed into the osseous defect. If the bony wall adjacent to or surrounding a defect is bent or malleted into the space of the defect, the procedure is classified as a contiguous autogenous graft. In theory a greenstick fracture is made at the base of

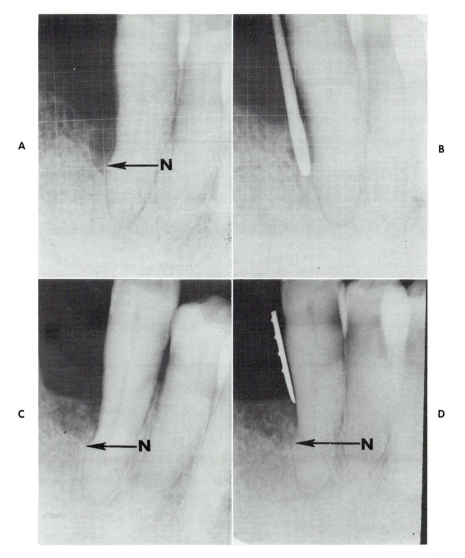

Fig. 27-18. A, Preoperative radiograph of lesion in mesial surface of mandibular left premolar. *N,* Notch on tooth. A Fixott-Everett grid has been used in this film. **B,** Preoperative radiograph with a periodontal probe in infrabony lesion. Base of the pocket is apical to notch in tooth. **C,** Radiograph 8 months postoperatively. *N,* Original notch on tooth. **D,** A Hirschfeld silver point in position and radiograph 8 months postoperatively. *N,* Original notch on tooth.

Continued.

the bony wall or hemisepta, and the bone is not separated from its blood supply in the contiguous autograft (Figs. 27-19 and 27-20).

Free grafts may be autogenous or allogenic (homogenous) and may be further subclassified by the type of donor bone such as cortical bone, cancellous bone with fatty, yellow marrow, or cancellous bone with hematopoietic, red marrow (Fig. 27-13). Autogenous grafts are presently the most suitable for use in humans. Goldman has demonstrated the use of stimulated periosteum for free grafts in the treatment of osseous defects. The interdental area is stimulated by piercing through the gingiva against the bone at a 45-degree angle 17 to 21 days prior to harvesting the stimulated tissue. Microscopic examination of this tissue shows new bone formation and numerous osteoblasts. The implant in animal experimentation hooks up to the bone surface by vascular connections, thus allowing the implant material to remain viable. Hematopoietic marrow also appears to offer great potential for regeneration of new attachment tissues. The ratio of pluripotential mesenchymal cells to trabecular bone is very favorable in he-

Text continued on p. 991.

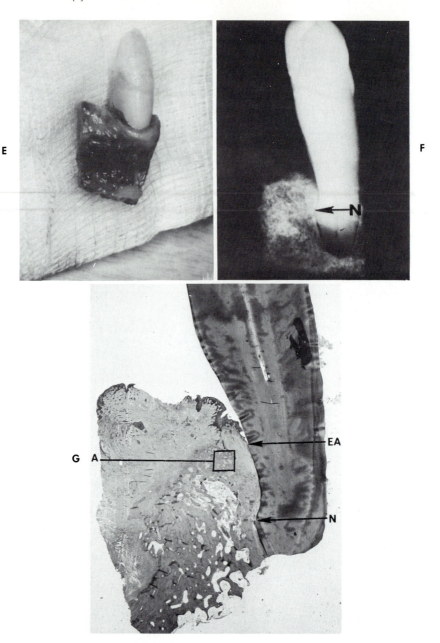

Fig. 27-18, cont'd. E, Specimen at time of removal consists of tooth and its periodontium. Eight months postoperatively. **F,** Radiograph of specimen after removal. **G,** Photomicrograph of specimen. *EA,* Epithelial attachment; *N,* notch in root; *A,* autograft at the alveolar crest which is seen in higher magnification in **H** and **I.** Hematoxylin and eosin. **H,** Higher magnification of box labeled *A* in **G.** Osseous tissue autograft *A* is being remodeled and new bone deposited on it. Pores with missing osteocytes are seen in autograft. *R,* Resorptive line; *NB,* new bone; *OB,* osteoblasts; *FT,* fibrous tissue. **I,** Another area from insert *A* of **G** in higher magnification showing remodeling of autograft at alveolar crest site. *O,* Osteoblasts; *A,* autograft; *NB,* new bone; *R,* resorptive line; *FT,* fibrous tissue. **J,** Higher power of section seen in **G.** This area is coronal to notch and demonstrates new attachment. *D,* Dentin; *C,* cellular cementum; *at,* artifact; *PL,* periodontal ligament; *A,* osseous tissue autograft; *NB,* new bone. **K,** Higher power of section seen in **G.** This area is more coronal than site in **J.** Empty spaces in autograft are evident with osteocytes missing. *D,* Dentin; *CC,* cellular cementum; *PL,* periodontal ligament; *NB,* new bone; *A,* osseous tissue autograft. New attachment is clearly seen. (**G** 4×; **H** to **K** 90×.) (From Ross, S. E., and Cohen, D. W.: Periodontics **6:**145, 1968.)

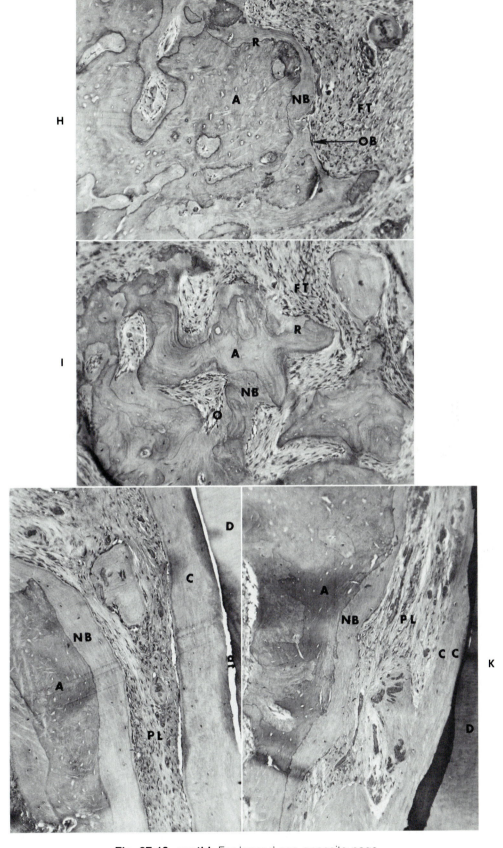

Fig. 27-18, cont'd. For legend see opposite page.

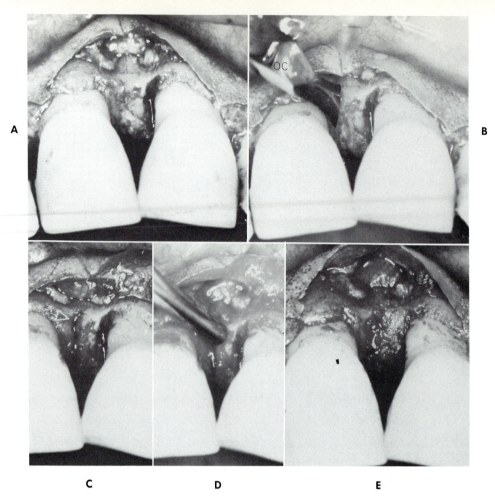

Fig. 27-19. Contiguous autograft procedure. **A,** Sloping osseous defect mesial of incisor. **B,** Ochsenbein chisel used to make lateral releasing cut in bone. **C,** Releasing cut completed. **D,** Surgical chisel modified as "bone swaging" instrument, to displace segment of bone against tooth. **E,** Contiguous segment of bone positioned against tooth to eliminate osseous defect. (Courtesy Col P. Boegel and Lt Col C. Hawley, U.S. Army Dental Corps.)

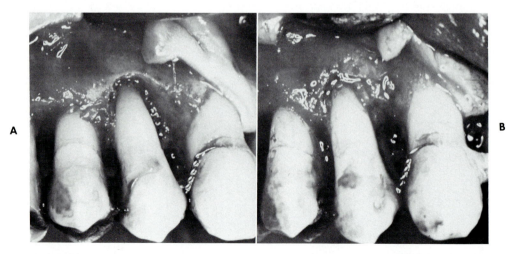

Fig. 27-20. A, Wide, sloping osseous defect first maxillary premolar. Note circumferential wire-and-acrylic splint. **B,** Buccal and mesial rim of osseous defect displaced against root surface as a contiguous autograft to eliminate osseous defect. (Courtesy Lt Col C. Hawley, U.S. Army Dental Corps.)

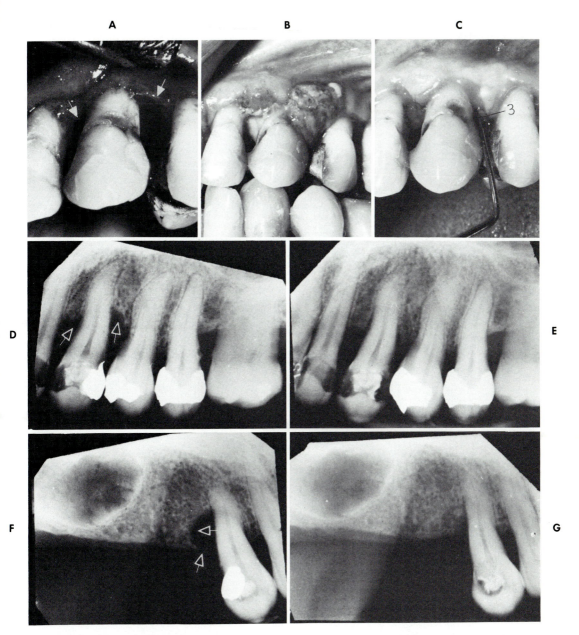

Fig. 27-21. Variations in management of osseous defects in same patient. **A,** Shallow, wide three-wall defects on mesial and distal aspects of canine *(arrows).* Defects filled with bone chips from molar region. Margin of buccal and palatal flaps cut back, and orifice of defects covered with free graft of palatal masticatory mucosa in an attempt to retard proliferation of epithelium. **B,** Appearance of connective tissue of free graft 7 days after surgery. Note loss of epithelial covering. **C,** Defect being probed 3 months after surgery. **D,** Preoperative radiograph. Arrows are at three-wall defects. **E,** Note degree of new attachment and leveling of osseous crest 6 months after implant. **F,** Opposite side before treatment. Note wide circumferential defect 9 mm deep on distal and palatal surfaces *(arrows).* It was treated by aggressive root planing and curettage (no flap). **G,** Six months after treatment defect measures 4 mm and radiograph indicates considerable bone repair and new attachment.

Continued.

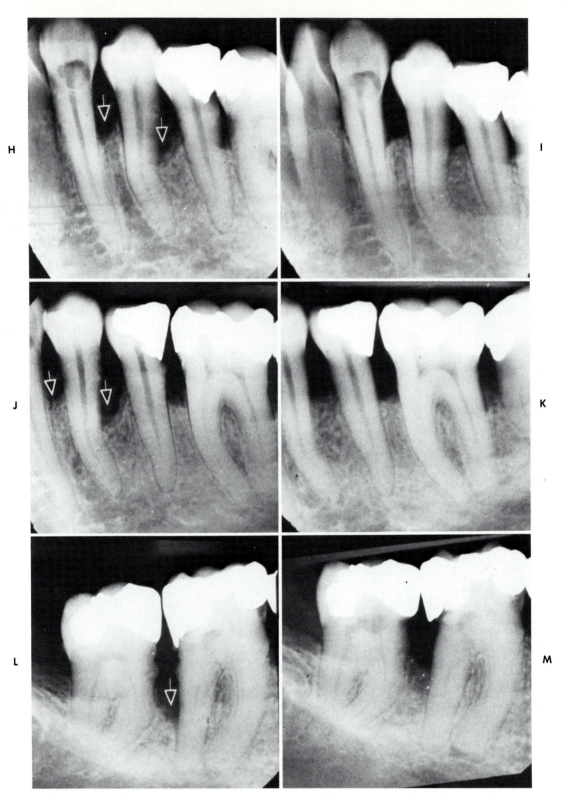

Fig. 27-21, cont'd. H and **J,** Pretreatment radiographs of three-wall defects on distal aspects of canine and first premolar *(arrows)*. Note calculus on roots. Defects were treated by open flap curettage, root planing, bone chip implants from distal aspect of second molar and crests of hemisepta, and replaced flaps. **I** and **K,** Note leveling of osseous crests and new attachment attained 6 months after treatment. **L,** Three-wall defect on distal aspect of molar on right side treated by open flap curettage, root planing, and replaced flaps (no implant) *(arrow)*. Note heavy calculus deposits on roots. **M,** New attachment attained to level of osseous crest. Note amalgam filings or particles created during root planing and incorporated into repaired area of former defect 6 months after treatment.

matopoietic marrow. The large number of viable cells that are implanted into the osseous defect may be responsible for the rapid osteogenic repair observed when red marrow grafts are used. The work of Boyne (1970, 1969, 1968), Schallhorn (1972, 1968, 1967), Schallhorn et al. (1970), Schallhorn and Hiatt (1972), Hiatt et al. (1971), and others appears to substantiate this theory.

Boyne and Yeager (1969) have evaluated the osteogenic potential of frozen marrow to stimulate and support osseous proliferation when placed on supracortical sites in the mandibles of dogs and rhesus monkeys. Their work indicates that there is no difference between the osteogenic potential of properly prepared frozen marrow and that of freshly obtained marrow to form new bone when it is placed in a suitable osseous environment. The probability of cellular survival in bone transplantation and storage has produced much controversy and received much attention in the orthopedic literature. Many investigators doubt that the cells survive after being transplanted or remain viable after programmed storage and that it may be the bone matrix that is responsible for the osteogenic potential of the graft material. Other investigators feel that it may be the death or lysis of the implanted cellular material that acts as the inductive stimulus for osteogenesis; however, the exact mechanism remains unknown (Burwell, 1964).

Cancellous bone is thought to be superior to cortical bone because of the greater surface area available to the blood supply and repair cells at the recipient site. Large pieces of bone used as grafts are remodeled at an extremely slow rate. In 1968 Ross and Cohen reported on the fate of a free osseous tissue autograft that was removed in block section for histologic study of the events that took place after therapy. The autograft had undergone partial resorption and was actively being remodeled 8 months after the surgical procedure. New alveolar bone was deposited on the autograft, and new cellular cementum was deposited on the dentin as well as on the acellular cementum (Fig. 27-18). Although the specimen was removed 8 months after treatment, the site was quite active as far as further healing was concerned. Their report suggested that osseous tissue autografts may still be actively remodeled for up to 2 years after transplantation. In a similar case reported by Hawley and Miller (1975), areas of the transplanted bone were observed in the site of the repaired osseous defect 30 months after the bone graft procedure (Fig. 27-22).

It is doubted by many that implanted cancellous bone possesses much of an osteogenic-inducing factor. Osteocytes within implanted cancellous bone do not survive. Their vascular supply is severed during the procedures required to obtain the donor bone. Boyne, in a review of the literature on the cryopreservation of bone, summed up the problem quite succinctly when he stated:

> The very nature of bone matrix limits cell osteocytic nutrition by diffusion to an estimated maximum distance of 0.2 mm under the best of environmental circumstances. It is felt, then, that unless an adequate circulatory system can be reestablished with the host shortly after transplantation, most or all of the graft cells, whether they are of an autogenous or homogenous source, will die. [Boyne, 1968]

The donor bone becomes nonvital and is slowly resorbed and replaced during healing of the wound. Nonvital bone should not be confused with necrotic bone (Figs. 27-18 and 27-22).

Stallard and Hiatt (1968) have observed new bone and cementum formation around mineralized fragments incorporated in a mucoperiosteal flap. They concluded that bone, cementum, and dentin particles that remain in the wound after periodontal flap surgery induce new bone and cementum formation in the vicinity of the implanted particles. Their findings support the earlier work of Ramfjord (1951), Schaffer (1958, 1957), Schaffer and Packer (1962), Schreiber et al. (1959), and Schreiber (1964). Although hematopoietic marrow and cancellous bone from the alveolar process are thought to be the most desirable donor materials, this evidence suggests that other mineralized tissues stimulate bone formation.

Many clinicians have noted that when large bone chips are used in graft procedures, they have a tendency to sequestrate during healing and maturation of the surgical site. Robinson (1970, 1969) has developed a technique employing small particles of cortical bone, and cancellous bone if available, as the donor material. The small bone particles or ''bone dust'' created by grinding with rotary instruments are mixed with extravasated blood from the area of surgery and formed into an osseous coagulum for use as donor material.

The mechanism of repair after bone graft procedures and implants of calcified material is not fully understood. The cells, cellular constituents, or other factors that stimulate osteogenesis and repair of the attachment apparatus have not been identified. Many theories have been proposed to explain the events observed during healing. To date, scientific evidence to support them has not

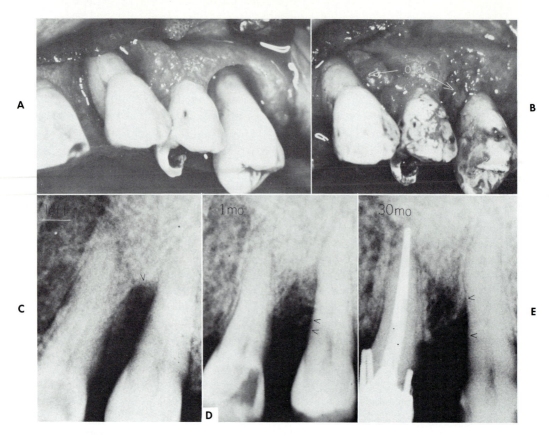

Fig. 27-22. A, Circumferential osseous defect second premolar, combination osseous defect canine, 32-year-old woman. Periodontal diagnosis of periodontitis and occlusal trauma. **B,** Canine treated by a combination contiguous osseous autograft and free osseous tissue autograft, *ota.* Defect on premolar filled with donor bone removed from edentulous ridge distal to second premolar, Jan. 17, 1968. **C,** Preoperative roentgenogram. Arrow is at base of defect. **D,** One month after treatment. **E,** Thirty months after treatment. Note radiographic evidence of repair and angle of osseous crest *(arrows).*

been presented. This area of clinical endeavor continues to offer exciting possibilities for further research.

Autogenous bone graft procedures

Autogenous bone grafts may be divided into three types, depending on the histologic nature of the donor material: (1) those in which cortical or cancellous bone with fatty marrow is used as the donor material, (2) stimulated periosteum comprising new bone and numerous osteoblasts, and (3) those in which cancellous bone with hematopoietic marrow is utilized as donor material. Cancellous bone with fatty marrow is secured from any area in the patient's mouth requiring ostectomy or osteoplasty or from areas intentionally operated on to provide bone. Stimulated periosteum is obtained 17 to 21 days after stimulation by split flap technique in an interdental area in the maxilla or edentulous areas of the maxilla. Hematopoietic marrow may be obtained from an extraoral source such as the ilium. If hematopoietic marrow is to be used, it must be frozen prior to the grafting procedure. If the tuberosity is used, trephines or rongeurs are used to obtain the cancellous bone. If the ilium is used, marrow cores are obtained by a punch biopsy technique or a surgical cutdown procedure. When an extraoral source such as the ilium is used, an orthopedic surgeon or hematologist obtains the donor bone marrow for the dentist.

The wall of an osseous defect may be surgically positioned against the root of the tooth as a contiguous osseous autograft. Healing tooth sockets and edentulous ridges also may be utilized as donor sites. Small bone chips are secured by rongeurs, chisels, trephines, or by making a series of bur holes through the cortical plate into the underlying cancellous bone. If tori or exostoses are re-

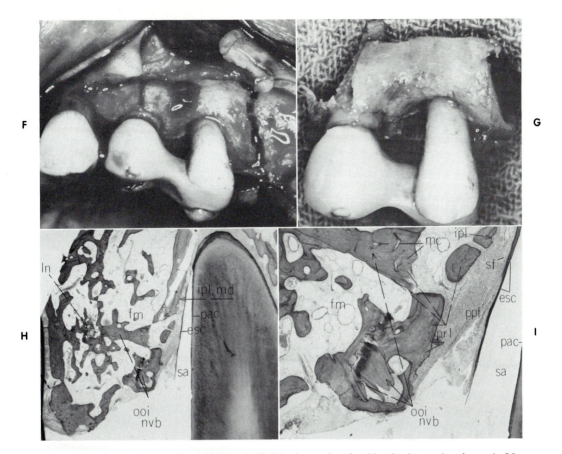

Fig. 27-22, cont'd. F, Tooth removed in block section for histologic study of repair 30 months after osseous tissue autograft procedure. **G,** Specimen of tooth and bone, contiguous gingival tissues not removed for study, retained for flap closure over surgical site. **H,** Photomicrograph, low-power view. Separation artifact, *sa,* incurred during processing of tissue. Original osseous implant, *ooi,* nonvital bone, *nvb,* surrounded by fatty marrow, *fm.* Irregular periodontal ligament, *ipl,* indicating mesial drift, *md,* of tooth. Eosinophilic cellular secondary cementum, *esc,* separated from primary acellular cementum, *pac.* Lymphatic nodule, *ln,* adjacent to implanted bone. **I,** Higher power. Parallel resting lines, *prl,* and new bone deposition noted on original osseous implant that is still being remodeled 30 months after graft procedure. Marrow channels, *mc,* can be seen in center portion of nonvital original graft. Parallel principal fibers, *ppf,* covering osseous crest assume a functional orientation to cemental surface further apically. Sharpey's fibers, *sf,* inserting into cementum. Histologic evidence would indicate that a functional attachment apparatus had formed in the area of former osseous defect. (Courtesy Lt Col C. Hawley, U.S. Army Dental Corps.)

duced by osteoplasty procedures, the small particles of bone may be collected and used as donor material (osseous coagulum).

Free osseous tissue autograft procedure

The osseous defect, or recipient site, is prepared in the same manner regardless of the type of donor material that is placed into the space of the defect. The various methods for securing donor material are presented separately at the end of this discussion in more detailed form.

Prior to the surgical procedure, initial preparation of the dentition is completed to provide an optimum environment for repair in the periodontium. Teeth with slight to moderate mobility patterns have been successfully treated without splinting as part of initial preparation; however, teeth with moderate to severe mobility patterns should be splinted. Occlusion is adjusted to eliminate any fremitus through functional range of jaw movements. Occlusal habit appliances are constructed when indicated to mitigate nonfunctional occlusal forces.

The graft procedure is carried out using local anesthesia. Systemic antibiotic coverage is usually started the day prior to the procedure and continued for at least 7 to 10 days, as previously discussed. Access to the operative site is usually obtained by using full-thickness flaps. Care must be exercised to conserve gingival tissue so that complete closure of the flap can be secured over the graft area. The root surfaces bordering the osseous defect are planed to remove any remaining concretions and softened root surface. All soft tissue is removed from the osseous defect, and any additional root planing necessary is carried out. The periodontal ligament space adjacent to the defect is carefully inspected to ensure that all granulomatous tissue and altered transseptal fibers have been removed. In chronic defects the osseous lining may be sclerotic and relatively avascular. To improve vascularity and healing potential, intramarrow penetrations may be made through the sclerotic lining into the underlying cancellous bone.

The osseous defect is thoroughly irrigated and inspected prior to inserting the donor material. Hemorrhage must be stopped to ensure adequate visibility prior to placement of the donor material. Suction must cease in the area of the osseous defect as the donor material is placed into the defect. Careless suctioning of the surgical site by an inattentive assistant can bring an abrupt end to the graft procedure. The osseous defects should not be overfiled. Any donor bone and attendant cellular elements exposed to the environment of the oral cavity will become necrotic above the area where they are not protected by the fibrin seal of the clot. The osteoclastic response marshaled to resorb the exposed necrotic bone may well endanger the contiguous cemental and dentinal surfaces to unwanted resorption and delayed repair.

The flap or flaps are readapted and sutured to obtain complete closure over the implant area. Surgical or dry foil and periodontal dressing are usually placed over the operative site. If the flap can be positioned tightly against the tooth and adequately stabilized by sutures, periodontal dressing may not be necessary. Although the dressing aids in protecting the surgical area, it also encourages accumulation of debris and hinders drainage of tissue fluids. The sutures and dressing, if used, are usually removed 7 to 10 days postoperatively. Many clinicians prefer to use absorbable suture materials to avoid manipulation of the flaps in the immediate postoperative period. Protective dressings may be maintained with periodic changes up

to 3 weeks, depending on the design of the surgical flap and degree of seal obtained over the implant area.

Roentgenograms taken to monitor the healing response should be exposed with less radiation during the first few months after surgery. The implanted donor bone becomes more radiolucent during the first to third month after treatment as the calcified material in the graft is remodeled during wound healing. The graft area appears to reach its maximum degree of radiopacity 8 months to 1 year after treatment. The treated area is not probed with force for 3 to 4 months after surgery.

Donor material

Oral sources. The following oral sources may serve as suitable locations for collection of donor material. As the donor bone is removed, it is placed into a sterile dappen dish or other suitable container for temporary storage prior to placement in the prepared osseous defects.

Bone removed during ostectomy-osteoplasty procedures. Cancellous bone is preferred over cortical bone for grafting purposes. End-cutting rongeurs, which bite off small segments of bone, offer a convenient means of securing pieces of bone. Bone chips and small particles of bone created with hand chisels may be used. The coronal peak of a ''hemiseptum'' (usually more or less than half the interdental septum) may be cut off and turned into the defect. If this is done the cancellous portion is placed into the depth of the defect and the cortical portion positioned nearest to the oral surface (Fig. 27-21).

Stimulated periosteum. This tissue has great bone production potential since it consists of new bone formation surrounded by numerous osteoblasts. One disadvantage is that a prior sitting is necessary to stimulate an interdental area in the maxilla 17 to 21 days prior to the surgical procedure. The method of procuring the tissue is to raise a split flap, followed by scoring the outline of the tissue to be removed down into the bone surface. The tissue is then removed as a strip with a chisel. The chisel engages the bone, lifting up as much of the surface bone as possible. Actually only spicules of old bone together with new proliferate of new bone are secured. The outer portion of the split flap is returned and sutured. Healing is uneventful.

Bone fragments obtained from healing extraction sockets. Immature bone and attendant cellular elements are felt by many clinicians to offer excellent healing potential if secured 6 to 8 weeks after

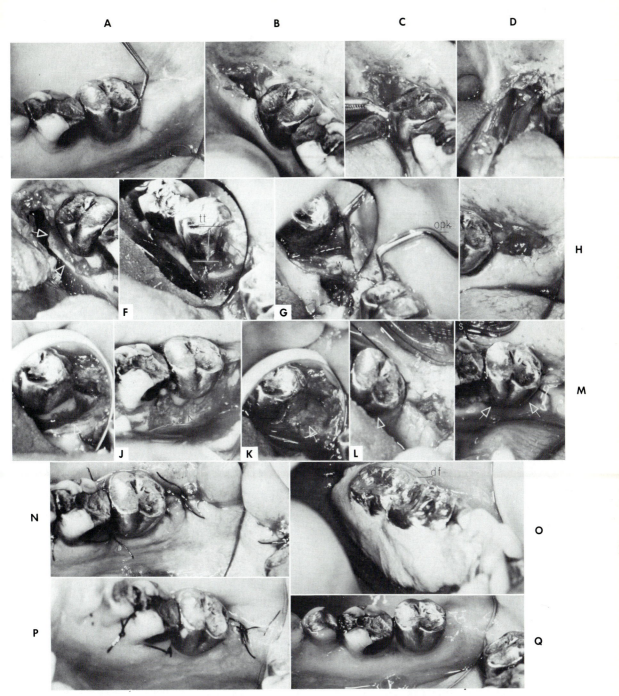

Fig. 27-23. A, Osseous defect distal and lingual, mandibular second molar (mirror view). **B,** Distal wedge of tissue removed, flap extended to buccal and lingual surfaces. **C** and **D,** Reflection and undermining of flap. **E,** Rim of osseous defect *(arrows).* **F,** Note thickness of gingival tissue, *tt,* in retromolar area over distal surface osseous defect. **G,** Orban periodontal knife, *opk,* no. 12, used to remove wedge of tissue, *w.* **H** and **I,** Flap thinned, roots planed, and soft tissue enucleated from osseous defects. **J** and **K,** Osseous coagulum, *oc,* used to fill osseous defects on lingual and distal surfaces *(arrows).* **L** and **M,** Initial suture to close flap. Note, after completion of first knot, suture, *s,* tied around tooth to pull flap tightly against distal of molar. **N,** Secondary sutures in place. Flap approximates tooth surface tightly making a good seal over implanted osseous coagulum. **O,** Dry foil, *df,* placed over surgical site, with periodontal dressing over dry foil. **P,** One week after surgery. **Q,** Two weeks after surgery, rapid wound healing. (Courtesy Dr. R. E. Robinson, San Mateo, Calif.)

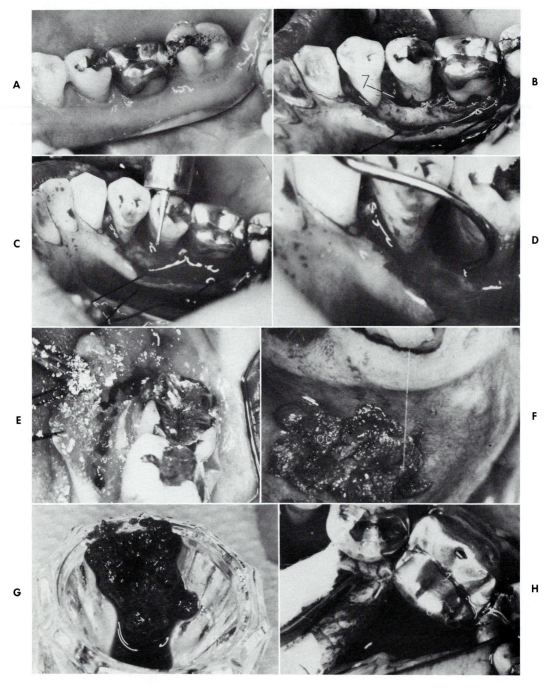

Fig. 27-24. Osseous coagulum technique. **A,** Mirror view of lingual aspect of mandible. A 7 mm pocket exists between first and second premolar. **B,** Flap retracted, osseous defect exposed. **C,** Small round bur used to make intramarrow penetrations. Note resultant hemorrhage. **D,** Use of a stainless steel cow-horn explorer for decortication. **E,** Example of bone dust created by grinding with a rotary instrument. **F,** Bone dust coated with blood, now an osseous coagulum, *oc.* **G,** Temporary storage of osseous coagulum in a sterile dappen dish. **H,** Example of utilization of sterile gauze for packing and drying of osseous coagulum.

tooth extraction. Coordination is necessary in planning treatment to ensure proper timing of the extractions in relation to the anticipated date for the graft procedures. The bone is removed from healing sockets with end-cutting rongeurs or large curets after a flap is made.

Bone removed through fenestrations made in cortical plate of edentulous ridges. An opening or fenestration in the cortical bone can be made by connecting a series of small bur holes. Some rotary trephines produce too small a plug of bone in proportion to the area of bone disturbed in obtaining donor material. The underlying cancellous bone of the alveolar process is usually difficult to remove with curets because of its dense, highly calcified nature. Therefore it must be cut out in pieces.

Tuberosity area. A flap may be made over the

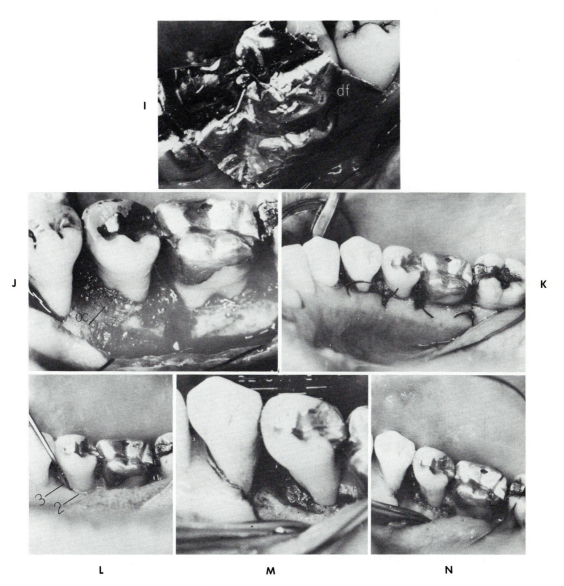

Fig. 27-24, cont'd. I, Example of the placement of dry foil, *df,* over an operated area. **J,** Placement of osseous coagulum, *oc,* into 7 mm osseous defect. **K,** Area sutured. Note excess of osseous coagulum above margin of flap. **L,** Three months after treatment. Crevice depth 2 to 3 mm. **M,** Upon reentry new attachment can be noted. Note pebbly appearance of new bone in contrast to remaining original bone. **N,** Osteoplasty accomplished at 3 months after treatment to reduce residual defect and create better contours for plaque removal procedures. New attachment area not subjected to osteoplasty procedures. (Courtesy Dr. R. E. Robinson, San Mateo, Calif.)

tuberosity area for access to the underlying cancellous bone, either as part of treatment in a maxillary quadrant or as a separate procedure to secure donor bone. The bone is best removed with end-cutting rongeurs. Because of limited visual and mechanical access and the extension of the maxillary antrum into this location, the tuberosity is a difficult area from which to secure donor bone. The cancellous bone contained within the tuberosity is usually composed of fatty marrow.

Osseous coagulum. Bone may be removed with rotary instruments from the lingual ridge adjacent to molar teeth, from exostoses, and from the alveolar process during the contouring of osseous defects adjacent to teeth. If these areas are not available, bone can be obtained from the lingual surface of the mandible, the palatal surface of the maxilla, or the distal area of terminal teeth or edentulous ridges. Robinson (1970, 1969) has perfected a technique of making an osseous coagulum from bone particles formed during cutting of bone with a no. 6 or a no. 8 carbide bur at speeds between 5,000 to 30,000 rpm. The bone dust mixes with blood and becomes a coagulum. Sharp burs must be used with this procedure because a coolant

cannot be used. The coagulum is collected and saved for implanting into the defects (Figs. 27-23 and 27-24).

Vision of the surgical site is limited in this technique, since irrigation and suction must be reduced or cease during creation of the coagulum. Hutchinson (1973) has developed a modification of the coagulum technique that allows irrigation (saline) and suction to be used during creation of the coagulum. A sterile in-line filter (150 ml filter unit, Falcon Plastics, Los Angeles, Calif.) is adapted by a T valve to the suction apparatus. The T valve permits selective use of the in-line filter to evacuate the bone dust and hemorrhage as it is created. Irrigation can be used that improves visibility and acts as a coolant. The coagulum is conveniently collected on the filter screen until ready for use. When sufficient coagulum has been collected, the filter is opened and the coagulum removed from the filter with a suitable instrument (Fig. 27-25).

Contiguous autograft. The wall of the defect may be surgically displaced into the space of the defect as a contiguous autograft. Technically these are not free grafts. Thin bony walls are bent or malleted into contact with the root surface adjacent

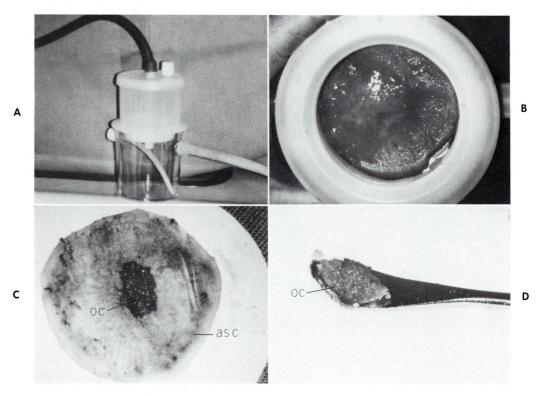

Fig. 27-25. A, Gas-sterilized, 150 ml filter units used to collect osseous coagulum. **B,** Opened unit, osseous coagulum resting on filter. **C,** Sterile amalgam squeeze cloth, *asc,* used as filter. **D,** Osseous coagulum, *oc,* scooped off filter for transfer to surgical site. (Courtesy Dr. R. Hutchinson, Charleston, S.C.)

to the defect. Undermining or releasing cuts are made in the bone lateral to the area that is to be placed against the tooth. The bony wall is then forcefully moved into apposition with the tooth to obliterate the defect. In theory a greenstick fracture is created, and the bone is incompletely fractured at its base. In practice it is found that the dense cancellous bone and cortical plate firmly resist attempts at displacement. Heavy pressure is usually required to move the bone; the attempted greenstick fracture usually becomes a complete fracture, and the contiguous graft becomes a free graft. Surgical elevators can be modified for use as "bone swaging" instruments. Despite the difficulties occasionally encountered in displacing bone against teeth, excellent results are obtainable with this technique (Figs. 27-19 and 27-20).

Bone-blending technique. The pieces of bone removed during osteoplasty-ostectomy, or with rongeurs or trephines, are usually too large to be implanted directly into the osseous defects. They must be broken into smaller pieces to aid in inserting them into the confines of the bony defects, and to prevent sequestration. Clinical research appears to indicate that bone particles in the range of 50 to 100 μm may be the most advantageous to use as bone implants (Rivault et al., 1971). It is most difficult to attempt to crush the bone that has been collected with sharp chisels or rongeurs in or over a sterile dappen dish or other suitable container. The dense bone resists cutting, and pieces skid

from under the chisel or fly from the surgical tray, reducing the amount available for implantation. Diem et al. (1972) have developed a technique for bone blending using a sterile capsule and a pestle that is usually used for mixing amalgam in mechanical mixers. The capsule and pestle must be new ones that have not been contaminated with mercury or traces of amalgam. The bone pieces or chips are placed into the sterile capsule, and an assistant places the capsule in a mechanical mixer and crushes the bone in short bursts to avoid heat buildup. The bone is then scooped from the opened capsule with a suitable instrument and emerges in a pastelike consistency (Figs. 27-26 and 27-27). The small particle size and pastelike consistency provide the clinician with an implant material that is convenient to handle and place into the osseous defects. The defects may be overfilled with the blended bone, and any observed to be remaining above the sutured flaps is easily wiped away because of its consistency and small particle size.

Extraoral sources. If the osseous defects are isolated and of minimal size, sufficient donor material can frequently be obtained from within the oral cavity by one of the above listed procedures. The volume of donor material required for treatment increases proportionately with the severity and distribution of periodontal destruction. The requirement for donor material frequently exceeds amounts that can be obtained from oral sources, and extraoral sources must be utilized.

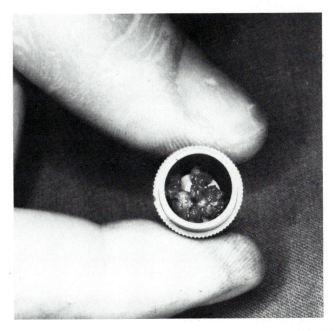

Fig. 27-26. Bone blend technique. Bone chips placed into sterile Wig-L-Bug capsule. Pestle not shown. (Courtesy Dr. C. Diem, U.S. Navy Dental Corps.)

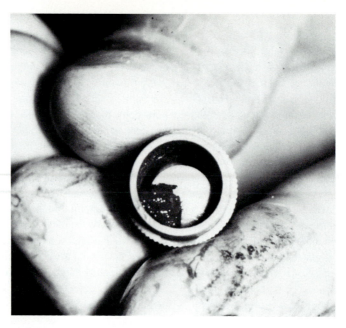

Fig. 27-27. Appearance of bone after reduction to smaller size particles after a few seconds in Wig-L-Bug. (Courtesy Dr. C. Diem, U.S. Navy Dental Corps.)

Orthopedic, plastic, and maxillofacial surgeons routinely utilize the ilium as a donor site to obtain large quantities of bone marrow for use in reconstructive surgery. The anterior superior iliac crest or posterior superior iliac crest contains large quantities of marrow that may be easily and safely removed. In order to obtain large quantities of bone marrow from these sites in the ilium, a cutdown procedure is necessary. The procedure may be done with the patient under local anesthesia and heavy sedation or under general anesthetic. The skin is incised in the appropriate area, and the muscles overlying the periosteal surface are dissected to expose the bone. Chisels are used to remove a portion of cortical bone to expose the marrow of the iliac bone. Large quantities (many cubic centimeters) of hematopoietic marrow are then scooped out for storage in a suitable container and medium. The surgical wound is closed by layers.

Two problems arise if this type of procedure is utilized to gain donor bone. First, the donor marrow and cancellous bone must be frozen before it is implanted into the recipient site. Minimal essential medium (MEM) is the most commonly used medium for freezing and storage of the donor material (Schallhorn, 1967; Schallhorn and Hiatt, 1972; Schallhorn et al., 1970). Clinical experience in animals (Ellegaard et al., 1973) and humans (Burnette, 1972; Dragoo and Sullivan, 1973 a and b; Schallhorn, 1972; Seibert, 1973) has shown that if hematopoietic marrow is implanted in the fresh state it will cause root resorption and ankylosis to occur in the majority of the cases so treated. It is not known whether the rapid growth of new bone within 5 days after implantation by the surviving reticular cells of the graft (Barkin and Newman, 1972; Bhaskar et al., 1970) prevents cementogenesis, if it is from an odontoclastic induction mechanism triggered by the graft, or if a cementoblastic inhibiting mechanism induced by the hematopoietic marrow is responsible for the resorption and ankylosis observed (Ellegaard et al., 1973a). Fig. 27-28 is typical of the root resorption and ankylosis observed in such cases. It is not fully understood how freezing alters the cellular kinetics involved or promotes cementogenesis, but it appears to alter the turnover time of the implant and delay production of new bone to permit the lead time necessary for cementum to form (21 days) to protect the roots (Barkin and Newman, 1972; Bierly et al., 1975; Line et al., 1974; Sottosanti and Bierly, 1975).

The ilium and the surrounding musculature are very tender for several days after this procedure. The patient is usually confined to bed for 3 days after the procedure to obtain donor bone. Walking and bending are difficult for the patient to accomplish for 7 to 10 days after surgery. The great advantage to this procedure is the large quantity of bone marrow that can be obtained through use of a relatively uncomplicated general surgical procedure. Many patients prefer a single procedure to

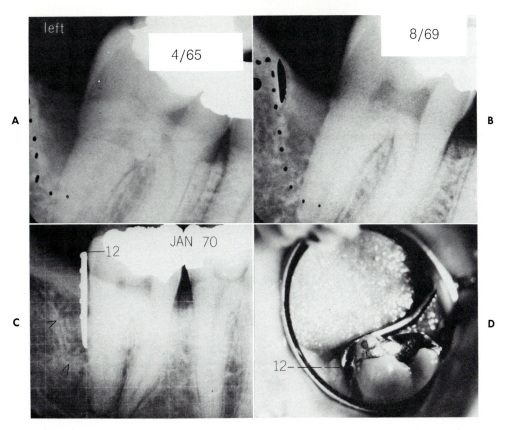

Fig. 27-28. A and **B,** Deep, wide, chronic osseous defect on distal aspect of mandibular second molar. Defect extends to lingual and buccal surfaces but does not enter interradicular area. Previous history (15 years) of surgical extraction of impacted third molars. **C,** Pretreatment roentgenogram with 12 mm Hirschfeld point flush with gingival margin. **D,** Full length of probe in pocket.

Continued.

obtain all the donor bone needed rather than repeated procedures to obtain smaller amounts by punch biopsy technique.

Hematologists use a punch biopsy technique to remove bone marrow from the posterior superior iliac crest for marrow studies. This procedure is accomplished on an outpatient basis and is relatively simple compared to a surgical cutdown procedure. The skin over the operative site is cleansed with antiseptics. The skin and periosteum over the posterior superior iliac crest are anesthetized by local infiltration with lidocaine (Xylocaine). A small (4 to 5 mm) incision is made in the skin, and a Westerman-Jensen bone biopsy needle is used to pierce the cortical plate of the iliac crest. Once the biopsy needle has pierced the cortical plate of the bone, the stylus that obliterates the lumen of the needle is withdrawn while the tubular shaft remains in position. The longer cutting portion is then inserted through the shaft of the needle and advanced into the medullary portion of the bone.

The shaft is advanced around the cutting portion of the needle to grasp the plug of marrow contained between the blades of the cutting stylus. Both portions of the needle are removed as a unit with a twisting motion to deliver the core of bone marrow (Fig. 27-29).

By changing the angle of insertion of the needle, five to six marrow cores can be removed through the same entrance incision. The marrow cores are temporarily stored in Hank's medium or minimal essential medium prior to freezing. Isotonic saline may cause cellular changes, and for this reason it is the least desirable solution to be used as a temporary storage medium. The cores must be placed in an appropriate medium and frozen. The skin incision is not sutured in the hip biopsy technique. A pressure dressing of 2- by 2-inch gauze and adhesive tape is placed over the skin wound. The patient is ambulatory immediately after the procedure and able to resume normal activities. The area over the iliac crest is tender for several days, but the

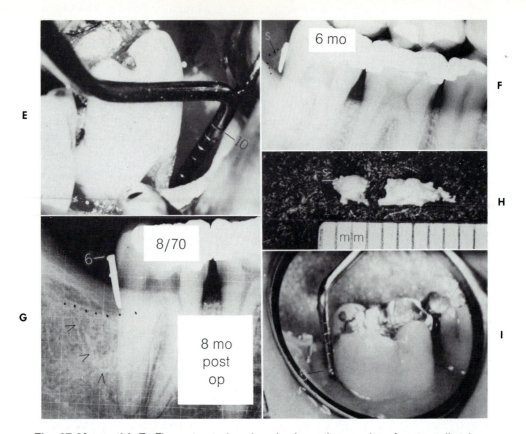

Fig. 27-28, cont'd. E, Flap retracted and probe is resting on rim of surrounding bone. Cubic dimensions of osseous defect are very large. Hip marrow and cancellous bone implanted to rim of defect. **F,** Six months after treatment, flap retracted from distal surface of molar, exposing coronal portion of implanted marrow and cancellous bone. Sequestrum, *s,* can be seen distal to calibrated point. **G,** Eight months after treatment, pieces of nonvital bone were curetted out of pocket. Arrows mark former distal wall of defect. **H,** Note degree of osseous repair 8 months after treatment. Coronal end of calibrated point extended 1 mm above gingival margin. **I,** Probe in position 8 months after treatment. Ascending ramus curves upward immediately behind tooth creating soft tissue depth. **J,** Reexamination at 23 months after treatment disclosed cavity below gingival margin on distal surface extending into pulp chamber. Resorption cavity can be seen at *r.* Root was notched, *n,* at base of former pocket during root planing. Tooth was decalcified for histologic study. **K,** Low-power view; mesiodistal section, showing resorption cavity and obliteration of pulp chamber and root canal, *rc,* in distal root. It would appear that tooth and pulp contents were resorbed during initial phases of healing and only bone was formed, effecting an ankylosis instead of a new attachment apparatus of bone, periodontal ligament, and cementum. **L,** Medium-power view from area *a* in **K.** Chronic inflammatory response in reparative phase. Note lamellar bone, *lb,* in former resorptive bays of dentin, *d.* Odontoclastic cells, *o,* resorbing dentin and bone. **M,** Higher power of area in **L.** Multinucleated odontoclasts in lacunae against lamellar bone, *lb,* and dentin, *d.* Osteocytes can be seen in bone. A slight inflammatory, *si,* response was observed in marrow spaces of the bone. **N,** High-power view of area *b* in **K.** Root canal and dentinal walls replaced with lamellar bone. A small number of inflammatory cells can be seen in marrow spaces of bone. **O,** High-power view of root surface–graft interface area, *c,* in **K.** Notch corresponds to base of former pocket. Cellular cementum has formed on root planed surface. Periodontal ligament fibers were severed during extraction and a separation artifact, *sa,* can be seen. Why a functional repair was effected in one area, the deeper or more apical area, and a marked resorption and ankylosis in the crestal area remains unanswered at present. It would appear bone formed too fast, or before cementum could be deposited, in crestal area of implant. Chronic irritation from plaque was active in crestal area, causing a reactive response in bone deposited within tooth. (Courtesy Lt Col D. Spano, U.S. Army Dental Corps.)

patient is not incapacitated. The degree of general discomfort and postoperative soreness appears to be proportional to the number of marrow cores secured.

The advantages of this technique are (1) simplicity of procedure and (2) the procedure may be repeated as necessary, alternating right and left sides of the hip. The major disadvantage lies in the relatively small amount of bone that can be obtained. Sufficient marrow can be obtained during a single procedure for treatment of several isolated defects, but not for multiple, extensive defects.

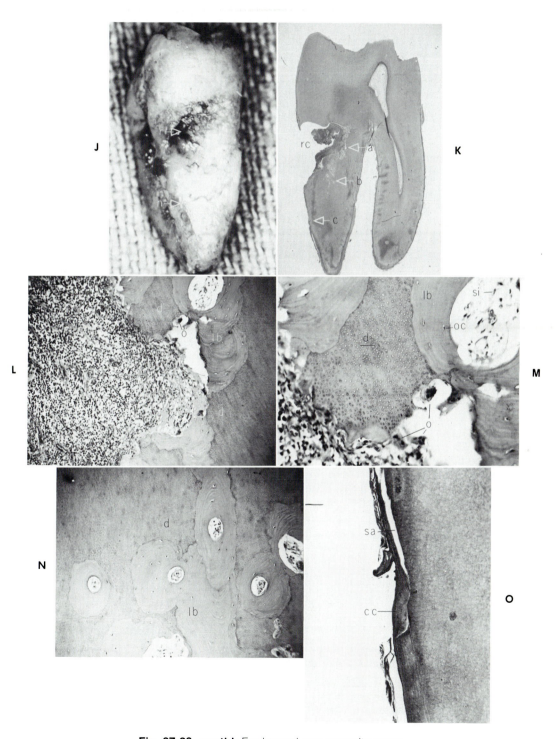

Fig. 27-28, cont'd. For legend see opposite page.

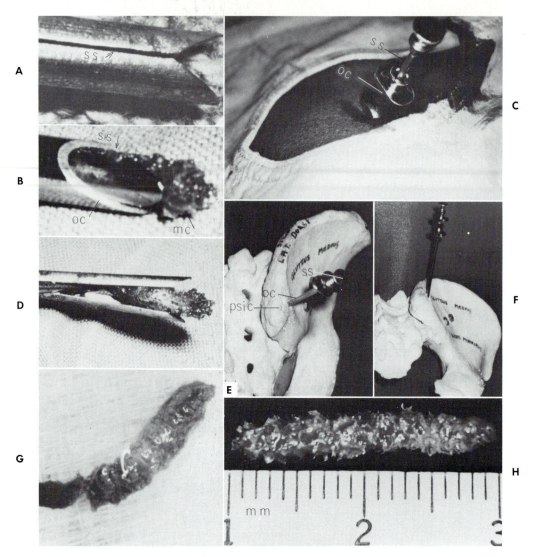

Fig. 27-29. Punch biopsy technique for hip marrow. **A,** Split stylet, *ss,* that is passed through outer cannula to penetrate into marrow. **B,** Split stylet in outer cannula, *oc,* of Westerman-Jensen needle. Marrow core, *mc,* pressed within lumen of split stylet. **C,** Needle assembly in position. After cortical plate is punctured, solid stylus is withdrawn, and split stylet, which extends ½ inch past end of outer cannula, is inserted to cut a core of marrow. Outer cannula, *oc,* then advanced to crimp marrow within beaks of split stylet. Assembly then removed as a unit with a twisting motion to free core of marrow. **D,** Typical core of hip marrow. **E** and **F,** Position of needle in relationship to posterior superior iliac crest, *psic.* **G,** Marrow core in temporary storage container. **H,** Larger than average core, 2 cm. Note trabeculae and cellular material.

Bone allografts and synthetic implant materials

The treatment of combination-type infrabony defects could be greatly simplified if other extraoral sources of donor material could be obtained without resorting to secondary surgical procedures elsewhere on the patient in sites such as the ilium to obtain the required autogenous donor material for implantation. This has led researchers to other sources in their search for a safe, nonantigenic, effective, readily available implant material that would induce or promote osteogenesis and cementogenesis. If such a material or materials could be found, it would bring the era of reconstructive periodontal surgery closer to reality and permit these procedures to be done on a routine outpatient basis in dental offices. Schallhorn and Hiatt (1972) have shown promising results obtained with frozen bone allografts obtained from fresh cadavers or from patients declared legally dead who were maintained on heart-lung machines while legal consent was awaited to obtain donor organs and bone that could be used as suitable donor material. Mellonig et al. (1976) and Freeman and Turnbull (1977) have done similar work using freeze-dried (lyophilized) bone obtained from the Tissue Bank at the National Naval Medical Center, Bethesda, Maryland. If the many problems involved with this source of allograft material can be overcome and the medical centers of our nation can process this type of donor bone in a safe and reasonably inexpensive form, this method of treating osseous deformities may become a practical reality.

A second promising area of research centers around the development of synthetic biodegradable implant materials of a ceramic or ceramiclike nature. By controlling particle size, pore size, and the binders used in the material it is hoped that a material can be found that will act as a supporting scaffolding for the overlying flaps and granulation tissue growing into the material whose turnover rate will be in synchronization with the formation of new bone and cementum. The advantages to be gained from the development of a safe, effective, nonantigenic, and inexpensive material that would have a long shelf life are quite obvious. Until such time as these techniques are proven and readily available, we must fall back on the use of donor materials and techniques currently available to us.

SUMMARY

It must not be assumed that every periodontal problem has a solution in therapy. There are many situations in which our methods are as yet ineffective, and a compromise in goals has to be accepted or the teeth extracted. There is a range of anatomic variation and osseous destruction in which we can maneuver. That range is constantly being extended, but only on the basis of a rational approach to therapy. Reconstructive periodontal surgical techniques that employ all the principles of mucogingival and osseous surgery offer the greatest potential for extending the longevity of teeth affected with advanced periodontal disease. Reconstructive periodontal surgery, as with other plastic surgery procedures, is carried out in stages to reconstruct the attachment apparatus and gingival unit of the periodontium to satisfy the basic objectives of periodontal therapy (see Chapter 28 for special problems in osseous and mucogingival surgery).

REFERENCES

Akiyoshi, M., and Mori, K.: Marginal periodontitis: a histological study of the incipient stage, J. Periodontol. **38:**45, 1967.

Aleo, J. J., DeRenzis, F. A., and Farber, P. A.: In vitro attachment of human gingival fibroblasts to root surfaces, J. Periodontol. **46:**639, 1975.

Aleo, J. J., De Renzis, F. A., Farber, P. A., and Varboncoeur, A. P.: The presence and biologic activity of cementum-bound endotoxin, J. Periodontol. **45:**672, 1974.

Amsterdam, M.: Periodontal prosthesis, twenty-five years in retrospect, Alpha Omegan, scientific issue, December, 1974.

Ariaudo, A. A.: The efficacy of antibiotics in periodontal surgery: a controlled study with lincomycin and placebo in 68 patients, J. Periodontol. **40:**150, 1969.

Axelsson, P., and Lindhe, J.: The effect of a preventive programme on dental plaque, gingivitis and caries in schoolchildren. Results after one and two years, J. Clin. Periodontol. **1:**126, 1974.

Barkin, M., and Newman, M.: Ultrastructure of bone marrow prior to and after programmed freezing, J. Oral Surg. **33:**341, 1972.

Bernier, J. L., and Kaplan, H.: The repair of gingival tissue after surgical intervention, J. Am. Dent. Assoc. **35:**697, 1947.

Bhaskar, S. A., Cutright, D. E., and Boyers, R. E.: Autogenous bone marrow transplants in the rat, J. Oral Surg. **29:**472, 1970.

Bierly, J. A., Sottosanti, J. S., Costley, J. M., and Cherrick, H. M.: An evaluation of the osteogenic potential of marrow, J. Periodontol. **46:**277, 1975.

Boyne, P. J.: Autogenous cancellous bone and marrow transplants, Clin. Orthop. **73:**199, 1970.

Boyne, P. J.: Restoration of osseous defects in maxillofacial casualties, J. Am. Dent. Assoc. **78:**767, 1969.

Boyne, P. J.: Proceedings of the second cryopreservation conference; review of the literature on cryopreservation of bone, Cryobiology **4:**341, 1968.

Boyne, P. J.: Histologic response of bone to sectioning by high-speed rotary instruments, J. Dent. Res. **45:**270, 1966.

Boyne, P. J., and Yeager, J. E.: An evaluation of the osteogenic potential of frozen marrow, Oral Surg. **28:**764, 1969.

Burnette, E. W.: Fate on an iliac crest graft, J. Periodontol. **43:**88, 1972.

Burwell, R. G.: Studies in the transplantation of bone, J. Bone Joint Surg. **46B:**110, 1964.

Cohen, B.: Morphological factors in the pathogenesis of periodontal disease, Br. Dent. J. **107:**31, 1959.

Costich, E. R., Youngblood, J. P., and Walden, J. M.: A study of the effects of high-speed rotary instrument on bone repair in dogs, Oral Surg. **17:**563, 1964.

Diem, C. R., Bowers, G. M., and Moffitt, W. C.: Bone blending: a technique for osseous implants, J. Periodontol. **43:**295, 1972.

Dragoo, M. R., and Sullivan, H. C.: A clinical and histologic evaluation of autogeneous iliac bone grafts in humans. I Wound healing 2 to 8 months, J. Periodontol. **44:**599, 1973a.

Dragoo, M. R., and Sullivan, H. C.: A clinical and histologic evaluation of autogeneous iliac bone grafts in humans. II. External root resorption, J. Periodontol. **44:**614, 1973b.

Ellegaard, B., Karring, T., Listgarten, M., and Löe, H.: New attachment after treatment of interradicular lesions, J. Periodontol. **44:**209, 1973a.

Ellegaard, B., Karring, T., and Löe, H.: New periodontal

attachment procedure based on retardation of epithelial migration, J. Clin. Periodontol. **1**:75, 1974.

Ellegaard, B., Karring, T., and Löe, H.: New attachment attempts based on prevention of epithelial downgrowth, I.A.D.R. Abstracts, p. 156, 1973b.

Ewen, S. J.: Bone swaging, J. Periodontol. **36**:57, 1965.

Freeman, E., and Ten Cate, A. R.: Development of the periodontium: an electron microscopic study, J. Periodontol. **42**:387, 1971.

Freeman, E., and Turnbull, R. S.: Short communication—histological evaluation of freeze-dried fine particle bone allografts. Preliminary observations, J. Periodontol. **48**:288, 1977.

Friedman, N.: Periodontal osseous surgery: osteoplasty and ostectomy, J. Periodontol. **26**:257, 1955.

Garrett, J. S.: Cementum in periodontal disease, Periodont. Abstr. **23**:6, 1975.

Goldman, H. M.: Extension of exudate into supportive structures of the teeth in marginal periodontitis, J. Periodontol. **28**:175, 1957.

Goldman, H. M., and Cohen, D. W., editors: Periodontal therapy, ed. 5, St. Louis, 1973, The C. V. Mosby Co.

Goldman, H. M., and Cohen, D. W.: The infrabony pocket; classification and treatment, J. Periodontol. **29**:272, 1958.

Hall, R. M.: The effect of high-speed bone cutting without the use of water coolant, Oral Surg. **20**:150, 1965.

Hawley, C. E., and Miller, G.: A histological examination of a healed free osseous autograft: case report, J. Periodontol. **56**:289, 1975.

Hiatt, W. H., Stallard, R. E., Butler, E. D., and Badgett, B.: Repair following mucoperiosteal flap surgery with full gingival retention, J. Periodontol. **39**:11, 1968.

Hiatt, W. H., and Schallhorn, R. G.: Human allografts of iliac cancellous bone and marrow in periodontal osseous defects. I. Rationale and methodology, J. Periodontol. **42**:642, 1971.

Hutchinson, R. A.: Utilization of an osseous coagulum collection filter, J. Periodontol. **44**:688, 1973.

Kantor, M., Polson, A. M., and Zander, H. A.: Alveolar bone regeneration after removal of inflammatory and traumatic factors, J. Periodontol. **47**:687, 1976.

Levine, L., and Stahl, S. S.: Repair following periodontal flap surgery with the retention of gingival fibers, J. Periodontol. **43**:99, 1972.

Lilly, G. E.: Reaction of oral tissues to suture materials, Oral Surg. **26**:128, 1968.

Lilly, G. E., Armstrong, J. H., Salem, J. E., and Cutcher, J. L.: Reaction of oral tissues to suture materials. II. Oral Surg. **26**:592, 1968.

Lilly, G. E., Cutcher, J. L., Jones, J. C., and Armstrong, J. H.: Reaction of oral tissues to suture materials, IV. Oral Surg. **33**:152, 1972.

Lilly, G. E., Salem, J. E., Armstrong, J. H., and Cutcher, J. L.: Reaction of oral tissues to suture materials, III. Oral Surg. **28**:432, 1969.

Lindhe, J., and Nyman, S.: The effect of plaque control and surgical pocket elimination on the establishment and maintenance of periodontal health. A longitudinal study of periodontal therapy in cases of advanced disease, J. Clin. Periodontol. **2**:67, 1975.

Lindhe, J., and Svanberg, G.: Influence of trauma from occlusion on progression of experimental periodontitis in the beagle dog, J. Clin. Periodontol. **1**:3, 1974.

Line, S. E., Polson, A. M., and Zander, H. A.: Relationship between periodontal injury, selective cell repopulation and ankylosis, J. Periodontol. **45**:725, 1974.

Löe, H., Theilade, E., and Jensen, S. B.: Experimental gingivitis in man, J. Periodontol. **36**:177, 1965.

Matherson, D. G., and Zander, H. A.: An evaluation of osseous surgery in monkeys, Abstract no. 325, I.A.D.R. Program and abstract of papers, 1963.

Melcher, A. H., and Bowen, W. H.: Biology of the periodontium, New York, 1969, Academic Press, Inc., p. 499.

Mellonig, J. T., Bowers, G. M., Bright, R. W., and Lawrence, J. J.: Clinical evaluation of freeze-dried bone allografts in periodontal osseous defects, J. Periodontol. **47**:125, 1976.

Moss, R. W.: Histopathologic reaction of bone to surgical cutting, Oral Surg. **17**:405, 1964.

Nyman, S., Bengt, R., and Lindhe, J.: Effect of professional tooth cleaning on healing after periodontal surgery, J. Clin. Periodontol. **2**:80, 1975.

Nyman, S., and Lindhe, J.: Considerations in the treatment of patients with multiple teeth with furcation involvement, J. Clin. Periodontol. **3**:4, 1976a.

Nyman, S., and Lindhe, J.: Prosthetic rehabilitation of patients with advanced periodontal disease, J. Clin. Periodontol. **3**:135, 1976b.

Ochsenbein, C., and Bohannan, H. M.: Palatal approach to osseous surgery. II. Clinical application, J. Periodontol. **35**:54, 1964.

Ochsenbein, C., and Bohannan, H. M.: Palatal approach to osseous surgery. I. Rationale, J. Periodontal. **34**:60, 1963.

O'Connor, T. W., and Biggs, N. L.: Interproximal bony contours, J. Periodontol. **35**:326, 1964.

Orban, B., and Archer, E. A.: Dynamics of wound healing following elimination of gingival pockets, Am. J. Orthod. and Oral Surg. **31**:40, 1945.

Patur, B., and Glickman, I.: Clinical and roentgenographic evaluation of the post-treatment healing of infrabony pockets, J. Periodontol. **33**:164, 1962.

Polson, A. M.: Trauma and progression of marginal periodontitis in squirrel monkeys. II. Co-destructive factors of periodontitis and mechanically produced injury, J. Periodont. Res. **9**:108, 1974.

Polson, A. M., Kennedy, J. E., and Zander, H. A.: Trauma and progression of marginal periodontitis in squirrel monkeys. I. Co-destructive factors of periodontitis and thermally produced injury, J. Periodont. Res. **9**:100, 1974.

Polson, A. M., Meitner, S. W., and Zander, H. A.: Trauma and progression of marginal periodontitis in squirrel monkeys. III. Adaptation of interproximal alveolar bone to repetitive injury, J. Periodont. Res. **11**:279, 1976a.

Polson, A. M., Meitner, S. W., and Zander, H. A.: Trauma and progression of marginal periodontitis in squirrel monkeys. IV. Reversibility of bone loss due to trauma alone and trauma superimposed upon periodontitis, J. Periodont. Res. **11**:290, 1976b.

Prichard, J. F.: Advanced periodontal disease; surgical and prosthetic management, Philadelphia, 1965, W. B. Saunders Co.

Ramfjord, S. P.: Experimental periodontal reattachment in rhesus monkeys, J. Periodontol. **22**:67, 1951.

Ramfjord, S. P., Ingler, W. O., and Hiniker, J. J.: A radioautographic study of healing following simple gingivectomy. II. The connective tissue, J. Periodontol. **37**:179, 1966.

Ramfjord, S. P., Knowles, J. W., Nissle, R. R., Burgett, F. G., and Shick, R. A.: Results following three modalities of periodontal therapy, J. Periodontol. **46**:522, 1975.

Ramfjord, S. P., Knowles, J. W., Nissle, R. R., Shick, R. A., and Burgett, F. G.: Longitudinal study of periodontal therapy, J. Periodontol. **44:**66, 1973.

Ramfjord, S. P., Nissle, R. R., Shick, R. A., and Cooper, H., Jr.: Subgingival curettage versus surgical elimination of periodontal pockets, J. Periodontol. **39:**167, 1968.

Register, A. A.: Bone and cementum induction by dentin, demineralized in situ, J. Periodontol. **44:**49, 1973.

Register, A. A., and Burdick, F. A.: Accelerated reattachment with cementogenesis to dentin, demineralized in situ. II. Defect repair, J. Periodontol **47:**497, 1976.

Register, A. A., and Burdick, F. A.: Accelerated reattachment with cementogenesis to dentin, demineralized in situ. I. Optimum range, J. Periodontol. **46:**646, 1975.

Ritchey, B., and Orban, B.: The crest of the interdental alveolar septa, J. Periodontol. **24:**75, 1953.

Rivault, A. F., Toto, P. D., Levy S., and Gargivlo, A. W.: Autogenous bone grafts: osseous coagulum and osseous retrograde procedures in primates, J. Periodontol. **42:**787, 1971.

Robinson, R. E.: The osseous coagulum for bone induction technique; a review, J. Calif. Dent. Assoc. **46:**18, 1970.

Robinson, R. E.: Osseous coagulum for bone induction, J. Periodontol. **40:**503, 1969.

Rosenberg, M., and Ross, S. E.: Management of osseous defects. In Clark, J. W., editor: Clinical dentistry, periodontal and oral surgery, vol. 3, New York, 1976, Harper & Row, Publishers.

Ross, S. E., and Cohen, D. W.: The fate of a free osseous tissue autograft, a clinical and histologic case report, Periodontics **6:**145, 1968.

Ross, S. E., Malamed, E. H., and Amsterdam, M.: The contiguous autogenous transplant—its rationale, indications and technique, Periodontics **4:**246, 1966.

Saxe, S. R., Greene, J. C., Bohannan, H. M., and Vermillion, J. R.: Oral debris, calculus and periodontal disease in the beagle dog, Periodontics **5:**217, 1967.

Schaffer, E. M.: Cartilage grafts in human periodontal pockets, J. Periodontol. **29:**176, 1958.

Schaffer, E. M.: Cementum and dentin implants in a dog and a rhesus monkey, J. Periodontol. **28:**125, 1957.

Schaffer, E. M., and Packer, M. W.: Bone regeneration: cartilage and tooth grafts in periodontal pockets, Dent. Clin. North Am., p. 459, January, 1962.

Schallhorn, R. G.: Postoperative problems associated with iliac transplants, J. Periodontol. **43:**3, 1972.

Schallhorn, R. G.: The use of autogenous hip marrow biopsy implants for bony crater defects, J. Periodontol. **39:**145, 1968.

Schallhorn, R. G.: Eradication of bifurcation defects utilizing frozen autogenous hip marrow implants, Periodont. Abstr. **15:**101, 1967.

Schallhorn, R. G., and Hiatt, W. H.: Human allografts of iliac cancellous bone and marrow in periodontal osseous defects. II. Clinical observations, J. Periodontol. **43:**67, 1972.

Schallhorn, R. G., Hiatt, W. H., and Boyce, W.: Iliac transplants in periodontal therapy, J. Periodontol. **41:**566, 1970.

Schreiber, H. R.: Management of vertical bone resorption in periodontal disease, Oral Surg. **17:**161, 1964.

Schreiber, H. R., Harder, E. W., and Thompson, L. B.: Cartilage and bone grafts in suprabony pockets in dogs, J. Periodontol. **30:**291, 1959.

Seibert, J. S.: Surgical management of osseous defects. In Goldman, H. M., and Cohen, D. W., editors: Periodontal therapy, ed. 5, St. Louis, 1973, The C. V. Mosby Co.

Selvig, K. A.: Ultrastructural changes in cementum and adjacent connective tissue in periodontal disease, Acta Odontol. Scand. **23:**459, 1966.

Selvig, K. A.: The fine structure of human cementum, Acta Odontol. Scand. **27:**423, 1965.

Sottosanti, J. S.: A new look at diseased cementum using the scanning electron microscope. Presentation, sixty-second annual meeting, American Academy of Periodontology, November 18, 1976, San Francisco.

Sottosanti, J. S., and Bierly, J. A.: The storage of bone marrow and its relation to periodontal grafting procedures, J. Periodontol. **46:**162, 1975.

Spatz, S.: Early reaction in bone following the use of burs rotating at conventional and ultra speeds, Oral Surg. **19:**808, 1965.

Stahl, S. S.: Healing following simulated fiber retention procedures in rats, J. Periodontol. **48:**67, 1977.

Stahl, S. S.: The nature of healthy and diseased root surfaces, J. Periodontol. **46:**156, 1975.

Stahl, S. S.: The influence of antibiotics on the healing of gingival wounds in rats. III. The influence of pulpal necrosis on gingival reattachment potential, J. Periodontol. **34:**371, 1963.

Stahl, S. S.: The influence of antibiotics on the healing of gingival wounds in rats. I. Alveolar bone and soft tissue, J. Periodontol. **33:**261, 1962.

Stallard, R. E., and Hiatt, W. M.: The induction of new bone and cementum formation. I. Retention of mineralized fragments within the flap, J. Periodontol. **39:**273, 1968.

Suomi, J. D., Greene, J. C., Vermillion, J. R., Chang, J. J., and Leatherwood, E. C.: The effect of controlled oral hygiene procedures on the progression of periodontal disease in adults: Results after two years, J. Periodontol. **40:**416, 1969.

Suomi, J. D., Greene, J. C., Vermillion, J. R., Doyle, J., Chang, J. J., and Leatherwood, E. C.: The effect of controlled oral hygiene procedures on the progression of periodontal disease in adults: Results after third and final year, J. Periodontol. **42:**152, 1971.

Ten Cate, A. R.: Formation of supporting bone in association with periodontal ligament organization in the mouse, Arch. Oral Biol. **20:**137, 1975.

Theilade, E., Wright, W. H., Borglum-Jensen, S., and Löe, H.: Experimental gingivitis in man. II. A longitudinal clinical and bacteriological investigation, J. Periodont. Res. **1:**1, 1966.

Wagenberg, B. D., and Langer, B.: Management of osseous lesions: a case report, Perio. Case Reports **1:**7, 1979.

Weinmann, J. P.: Progress of gingival inflammation into the supporting structures of the teeth, J. Periodontol. **12:**71, 1941.

Zander, H. A.: Continuous cementum apposition, J. Dent. Res. **37:**1035, 1958.

Zander, H. A., and Matherson, D. G.: The effect of osseous surgery on interdental tissue morphology in monkeys. Abstract no. 326, I.A.D.R. Program and abstract of papers, 1963.

28 Special problems in periodontal therapy

Part I

In a text of this kind it is inevitable that techniques of case management be grouped in broad classes of standard methods. Although this has advantages in clarity and unity, it loses somewhat in specificity. It is the specific case in its infinite variations that we shall now consider; that is not to say that standard methods do not apply in these cases. On the contrary, all the variations to follow are based on standard methods. It is the variation and blending of these methods that we describe here.

The possibility for clinical variation is infinite. It would be impossible to consider every conceivable variation from the standard indication. What is intended here is the consideration of some of the more common ones, and by the process of discussion of clinical requirements and clinical resourcefulness enough of the broad principles will be established to enable the reader to use the same methods of reasoning to solve other cases when they are presented. The purpose here is not a simple list of solutions for problems, but rather a method of case consideration and solution. There is no intent to present a formula; the promotion of clinical acuity is the aim.

In all efforts of this kind a focal point of orientation is sometimes helpful. In this instance the requirements of physiologic architecture and essentials of correct form are offered as the cornerstones of management. Since cleansability—constant removal of plaque accumulation—is the chief goal. The key in these problem areas is to recapture the essentials of correct form so that the teeth may be completely cleansed without hindrance. This is not exactly a duplication of ideal contour. It is reshaping of the tissues to function in the changed environment caused by disease. We are dealing with diseased tissue in an unphysiologic environment. Correction and palliation of these deformities are our immediate objectives. The survival of the dentition in health is our goal.

FAULTY TOOTH ANATOMY

The interdependence of tooth form and gingival health has been well established. For many years the marginal ridge and general occlusal anatomy have been alluded to as etiologic factors of considerable importance in certain patterns of periodontal breakdown. The principles of occlusal anatomy have been discussed too widely in the literature to merit further treatment as a special problem. The aspect of tooth form that has not been so thoroughly reported, however, is the relation of the general overall anatomy of the tooth itself to the health of the gingival tissues. The buccal and lingual contours, the occlusal embrasure patterns, the interproximal embrasures, and the cervical anatomy all have powerful influences on the gingival margin because the form of these features

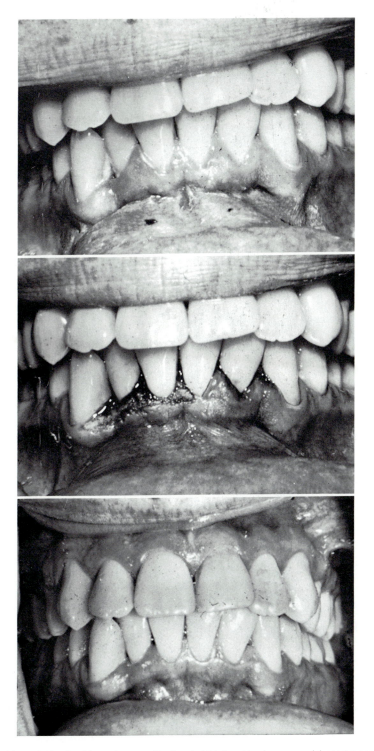

Fig. 28-1. Altered gingival form in mandibular right lateral incisor-cuspid area as a result of positioning of teeth. Therapy consisted of curettage and gingivoplasty for this area. Note postoperative results in bottom photograph. Alveolar crest topography was acceptable.

qualifies the course, direction, and quality of the forces brought to bear on the gingiva in function. These are the features that will be discussed briefly, with remedial measures offered for their correction when they are unphysiologic.

INTERPROXIMAL EMBRASURE

The problem of the poorly shaped interproximal embrasure is almost always the result of the shape of the crowns of the teeth and the proximity of the roots. It is a well-established principle that the closer together adjacent roots are, the higher will be the interproximal tissue between them; conversely, the farther apart these adjacent roots, the flatter will be the interdental tissue. This principle unfortunately is often violated so that in restorations requiring multiple abutments the interproximal embrasure is obliterated either by bulky solder joints or by crown contour itself. This results in alterations of the col area as well as in peaks of the

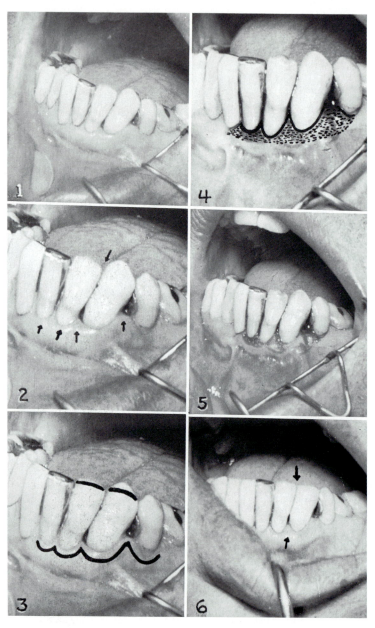

Fig. 28-2. Elimination of gingival crater between mandibular lateral incisor and cuspid. Note contouring procedure and grinding of teeth. Note also postoperative gingival architecture in 6.

interdental tissue. Thus there is frequently established a proliferating tissue in the form of an ugly, hyperemic, crater-shaped mass that perverts the function of the interdental tissue and behaves as an entrapping device (Fig. 28-1).

It is well known that to restore in exact dimension the enamel reduced or removed in crown preparation is practically impossible. These encroachments usually occur because of too great a bulk interproximally in the casting. They occur also in cases in which multiple porcelain jacket crowns on gold thimble preparations require a cervical solder joint. For this reason the latter is usually not suitable as a restoration in which interdental tissue form is a factor. As for bulky crown castings, these are particularly difficult to avoid in the lower anterior teeth. The teeth are small, and the roots are rather close together, which makes the

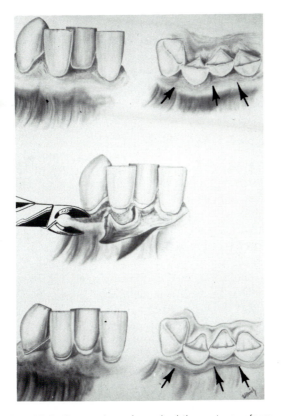

Fig. 28-3. Contouring of surgical tissue to conform to malalignment of teeth. Gingival inflammation is controlled by scaling and curettage. Retractable gingival tissue is resected, and wound surface is contoured with nippers. Sluiceways are made interdentally. Depressions are made to conform to interdental osseous structure. If necessary, because of bone topography, contouring of bone may be performed; if this is done, then flap procedure is necessary.

removal of enough tooth material to provide embrasure room a real problem. Unfortunately this problem has no other practical solution. It should be stated clearly, however, that conservation of tooth material in these situations is false conservatism because the life of the restoration and the very retention of the teeth themselves are jeopardized. Embrasure patterns must be preserved at all costs, and these must be maintained carefully by the patient through home oral physiotherapy (Figs. 28-2 and 28-3).

Incision of the peak in cases of constricted embrasures accomplishes nothing, since the peaks will inevitably regrow. Solution of this problem is inextricably bound up in correct form in prosthetic reconstruction.

OCCLUSAL EMBRASURE

The occlusal embrasures are an important factor in the health of the gingival tissues cervical to them.

This is one area that can be constricted either by artificial or by natural means. No great explanation is required to describe an inlay or crown with a broad, flat contact extending too far buccally and lingually. These imperfections unfortunately are seen often. Contact point wear will create a similar situation in the natural tooth.

The remedy for this is easy and obvious. Reshaping the area on both adjoining teeth, both buccal and lingual, so that there is a flaring embrasure pattern and a narrow contact area is necessary. These remedial measures are particularly important in areas where gingivectomy or osteoplasty has been performed. Since in posterior regions the buccolingual dimension of the alveolar process is great, there is a tendency for flat, shelflike contours interproximally, even when proper osteoplastic contouring has been done. When this occurs, it will be wise to examine the occlusal embrasure pattern involved.

Particular care of these areas must be taken when the buccolingual dimension of the posterior teeth is reduced. The reshaping of the crowns in narrowing leaves the occlusal embrasures smaller than ever proportionately so that the teeth are inadvertently squared off to broad, flat contacts. It is therefore of utmost importance to extend the reshaping procedures to the occlusal embrasures.

LONG CONTACT POINT WITH APPROXIMATING ROOTS

The variations in tooth alignment are infinite. Most of these are minor handicaps, but for the most part these malpositions impose varying degrees of difficulty in management and at times make therapy useless, since they are entirely recalcitrant.

One such problem is the long contact point with approximating roots. These usually occur in anterior teeth because of the nature of the crown and their relation to each other. The long contact point alone is not an insurmountable problem because correction is often possible by prosthetic remedies if other means are ineffective. Food impaction into the contact area and injury to the interdental tissue can be controlled and eliminated. The really difficult aspect of the problem is that these long contact areas sometimes involve roots so closely approximating through much of their length as to preclude any appreciable amount of bone between them. In a previous portion of this chapter a general principle was stated that the closer together the roots, the higher the interproximal tissue. In light of this principle, consider the anatomic features of such an area as was just described. The approximating roots promote a long, narrow papilla, but the long contact of the crowns provides practically no embrasure.

This inconsistency results first in a mushrooming of both labial and lingual peaks, each hyperemic and flaccid, strangulated by the absence of embrasure space. Soon the col area degenerates further, and a crater remains. The gingival contour is absent in the interproximal area, and the papillary level of the gingiva is the same as that of the marginal gingiva at either side of the area under discussion. In the usual progress of events the crater becomes exacerbated and begins to break down.

On the surface this would appear to be the usual crater referred to earlier in the chapter. The uninitiated therapist would fail to recognize the peculiar character of the lesion and would perhaps attempt gingivoplasty to correct the deformity. In this direction lies disaster because these craters do not heal in the normal manner. The result of surgical interference is an enlarged crater with more prodigious food entrapment and more serious exacerbations. Repeated dressings are to no avail. The large, cyanotic, open-mouthed, funnel-shaped crater with the sharply delimited marginal hyperemia is the usual result of surgical interference.

Since the roots approximate so closely for most of their length, there is no need for going apically with surgical methods to find interproximal bone. The truth of the matter is that there is no solution as yet for this problem unless the interproximal area can be widened either by planing the root surfaces of the teeth or by orthodontics. Otherwise the prognosis for one of the teeth is very grave, and if measures are delayed for too long a time, both approximating teeth will most probably be lost.

Some work has been attempted with the placement of a circular wire loop such as orthodontists use in effecting separation. This loop is placed close to the gingiva surrounding the contact area and activated by twisting, thus opening up a space between the crowns. Then a rubber dam elastic is placed around both crowns close to the incisal edge. This is done to attempt bodily movement of the roots by wedging the edges of the crowns, using the wire loop at the cervical contact as a fulcrum. In some instances the procedure meets with success. In other instances excessive scaling (tooth tissue removal) of the proximal surfaces is needed to open up the embrasure space somewhat. This may aid in the correction of the problem.

In such a problem great caution is the rule, with only the most conservative measures in order. These teeth are never to be retained in a restorative treatment plan involving them. It is good judgment to sacrifice one of them, even if bone loss may not be advanced at the time of examination.

OVERLAPPING TEETH

On the surface overlapping teeth would appear to be the same problem as closely approximating adjacent roots with long contact areas. A major problem is plaque control. The overlapped tooth surface is hard to cleanse by toothbrushing. A special effort must be made by the patient to keep areas free of plaque.

There are several important differences between overlapping teeth and those with long proximal contact areas. In the first place the roots are not adjacent with little bone separating them, but are generally divergent. They may be close together at the cervical regions but not so close apically. This is an important factor in therapy. In the second place the faulty contact relationship is correctable either through individual tooth movement or through prosthetic reconstruction.

There is one other point of difference that bears discussion. It has been mentioned earlier that the size and shape of the interproximal tissue depend on the relationship of the roots to each other. In closely approximating roots the interproximal tissue has a tendency to assume a long, narrow form because of lack of embrasure space. The overlapped teeth, on the other hand, frequently have an extremely short, blunt, saddle-type interproximal tissue because the roots are usually some distance apart at the crest of the bone, although they may be fairly close together at the gingival margin. This arrangement frequently provides good embrasure space if the point of contact is not too close to the crestal bone. For this reason it is not unusual to find these areas being maintained in health if the contact is not too inefficient. However, in many instances one tooth serves as a chute for the impact of food against the gingival margin of the other; here a destructive lesion occurs. Also cleansability is markedly hampered.

There are, however, two other contingencies that may arise and cause some breakdown. The first is a poor contact relation that allows the interdental tissue to be traumatized and invaded, and the second is the same situation previously discussed on a constricted embrasure and a deformed topography of the interdental tissue.

The first problem can be solved by standard therapy for the gingival lesion and correction of the contact relationship through minor tooth movement if space permits or through reshaping and securing a proper contact relationship by prosthetic reconstruction; it can also be solved by locking the two crowns together with a solder joint. When overlapping incisors are present and one tooth serves as a chute for food impaction, the remedy lies in the reshaping of the adjacent teeth so that food is deflected in a physiologic manner.

The second contingency requires some evaluation. If there is no embrasure space, we do not face the discouraging situation that we met in the case of the closely approximating roots. The reason that the overlap presents opportunities for management is that the more apical the area, the more divergent the roots. The remedy therefore almost suggests itself. In these areas that break down, the recontouring of the cervical complex of tissues somewhat apically will carry the entire margin to a zone where the roots are wider apart and where adequate embrasure space can be created. This is the key to the solution.

It is perfectly true that sacrifice of marginal tissue is involved, but this is usually in trifling amounts, and the stakes are high. To equivocate on the sacrifice of little tissue to gain the retention of the tooth in health is another example of false conservatism. The dentist must consider the possibility of the patient's cleansing the area of plaque by toothbrushing. The area must be capable of being reached by the bristles to effect plaque removal.

Certain precautions should be observed in operating on such an area. The gingivectomy and gingivoplasty involved are routine enough. Frequently, however, some osteoplastic reshaping is required. The tendency is to remove enough crestal bone either with chisels and files or with a rotary instrument to the desired height and to forget that as we move the crestal margin of the bone apically the process gets thicker. In other words, there is a tendency to create a thick ledge in the interproximal area. This merely substitutes one lesion for another. Care must be taken in these cases to thin carefully all crestal areas in the bone and to hollow out the interradicular areas so that the resultant interproximal tissue is well formed.

It should be remembered also that the more apical the marginal complex is carried, the more blunt the resultant interdental tissue and the less room is needed for it in the embrasure. Therefore too great a change is rarely necessary.

Frequently the two problems appear together; that is, there is the poor contact relationship and a constricted embrasure pattern. In that event both remedial procedures can be carried out together. The periodontist must know that problems in management rarely appear alone, and he must be alert to the opportunity to use several techniques in concert to carry out therapy properly. The more resourceful the operator, the better able he will be to seize therapeutic opportunities to solve his problems.

THERAPY FOR PERIODONTALLY INVOLVED TOOTH IN MALALIGNMENT

Therapy for the periodontally involved tooth in malalignment has two possible variants. The tooth in question may be in either linguoversion or buccoversion. The deformity incident to the malposition will vary, depending on the position. A common situation is the buccoversion of the maxillary second molar; in this instance the contact area of the teeth is not a protective one, and crater formation is commonly found.

TOOTH IN LINGUOVERSION

Although in health the lingually placed tooth may not be involved gingivally, once disease is present this area is far more affected than other areas because of the local environment. In these cases the buccogingival margin is usually thickened and fibrotic. There are cases in which constant irritation of the marginal gingiva will cause edema and cyanosis to be the principal marginal feature. Conservative measures will cause the

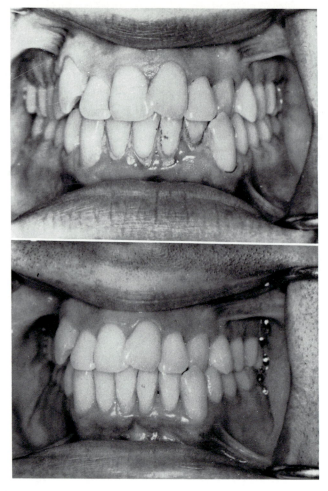

Fig. 28-4. Before and after management of a retruded mandibular lateral incisor with a thickened labial gingiva. Note contour of tissue postoperatively.

edema and cyanosis to be resolved, and, as is usual in long-standing cases, a thickened fibrotic margin will be the result as a later stage of treatment (Fig. 28-4).

To achieve cleansability, soft tissue contouring by gingivoplasty of the thickened margin may be utilized. However, there is frequently a need for marginal osteoplasty, that is, thinning the marginal bone on the buccal and interproximal surfaces of the tooth. The reason for this is that the lingual malposition of the single tooth usually leaves a buccal ledge of thick bone. This is true because the alveolar process maintains a consistent contour that is continuous from the adjacent teeth (both buccal to the tooth in question). This continuity creates the marginal bony ledge that, along with the overlying gingiva, must be thinned marginally. This is performed via a flap procedure.

Not to be overlooked is the reshaping of the crowns of the teeth involved to negate the action of food impaction by means of a chute against the gingiva in chewing. It is this action that usually sets up the chronic irritaiton. Correction usually involves reshaping the buccal contour on proximal surfaces of adjacent teeth to flare out the narrow chutelike contour. The converse of the lingually placed tooth is the one malposed buccally. This usually results in the single prominent tooth with an extensive recession.

In all these malalignments of teeth, deviation from the norm must be minimized in the gingiva and bone, but the crowns of the teeth themselves are just as important. By judicious reshaping much of the malalignment can be minimized, and the bulging contours of the crown in the area of malposition can be reduced; for example, suppose an upper second premolar is malposed palatally; after other procedures are completed, the buccal contour of the first molar and the first premolar are shaved as much as is practicable; then the palatal surface of the second premolar is similarly reduced within limits possible. This is done so that there is a more consistent and physiologic occlusal alignment as well as achievement of cleansability.

TOOTH IN BUCCOVERSION OR LABIOVERSION

The single tooth in buccoversion or labioversion usually shows considerable buccal or labial recession. The reasons for this sudden precipitous gingival recession are twofold: (1) the root of the tooth has no buccal plate of its alveolar process and (2) the root of such a tooth is subject to more than its normal share of abrasion due to the passage of food over it. Even the toothbrush, no matter how careful its application, is bound to come into contact with such a prominence more than with adjacent teeth. The usual result of such stresses, generally physiologic in normally aligned teeth, is enough to send the gingival margin migrating apically. When no buccal plate is present over the buccal surface of the root, the apical migration of the gingival margin is just that much more rapid.

The remedy for this condition is twofold: (1) The gingival marginal level is made more consistent by gingivectomy and, if necessary, by osteoplasty with that of the adjoining teeth. Making the gingival margin consistent does not mean making it exactly like that of its neighbors. It merely means that the degree of difference will be as slight as possible so that cleansing measures can be more effective. (2) The tooth is recontoured so that the food during mastication is deflected by the tooth surface onto the attached gingiva, bypassing the gingival margin over the exposed buccal surface. This entails alteration of the buccal contour so that it does not present a long sloping face but is, on the contrary, interrupted with a short bevel near the occlusal table; this bevel narrows the occlusal table at the same time.

Similar situations exist in many anterior segments in which there has been crowding and overlapping of the teeth and also in deep overbite cases in which traumatization of marginal gingiva by food impaction occurs, with the incisal edges of the teeth of the opposing jaw acting as the plunger mechanism. Exactly the same principles apply here as applied in the malposed premolars. Through gingivectomy and marginal osteoplasty the gingival line should be recontoured, and the level of the margin should be made consistent with that adjacent to the area under scrutiny.

In the case of the deep overbite the usual reaction to the constant traumatizing effect of food impaction is a thick, heavy marginal fibrosis or a severe marginal inflammation. Such a gingiva is easily repositioned somewhat apically so that it is not in the direct path of the incisal edges of the teeth of the oposing jaw. Palatal gingivae of the upper anterior teeth and labial gingivae of the lower anterior teeth are sometimes found so affected.

Particular care must be taken with oral hygiene techniques. All our toothbrushing measures in their standard application are most effective when the gingival margin is level and consistent. Just as soon as there is a sudden departure from that level, the margin will be either traumatized or skipped entirely, depending on the position of the tooth in the arch. It is for this reason that these special cases need individual attention in their care. This usually involves brushing the aberrant tooth individually in a special excursion and not as a unit in a segment.

The repositioning of teeth to correct these local environmental factors is a more permanent method of therapy. This is described in Chapter 21.

GINGIVAL DEFORMITIES
GINGIVAL CLEFT

The gingival cleft is a phenomenon usually found in the anterior segments. Clinically it appears as a vertical split in the gingiva, ending marginally. If the irregular cleft is probed, it can be seen to be intimately associated with pocket formation. If the method in which gingival clefts form is taken into account, the remedy almost suggests itself. The gingival cleft is merely the progression of the periodontal pocket on the labial surface of a tooth over which there is an extremely thin or no labial plate of bone (Fig. 28-5). Incident to pocket formation the very thin labial plate is completely eroded through its entire thickness. This is followed by a splitting of the gingiva overlaying it because of a coalescing of proliferating epithelium. The correction of the cleft is largely dependent on its width and length. If the cleft is quite small and the adjacent periodontal tissues are gingivally affected only, then either (1) curettage followed by gingivoplasty or (2) gingivectomy can be performed to eliminate the cleft. The resultant gingival topography should conform to the adjacent areas; this makes the gingival margins consistent throughout the segment. One word of caution might be useful. In these gingival clefts it is wise to stretch the lips to determine whether there is an abnormal frenum attachment associated with the pocket. This too may require correction that if

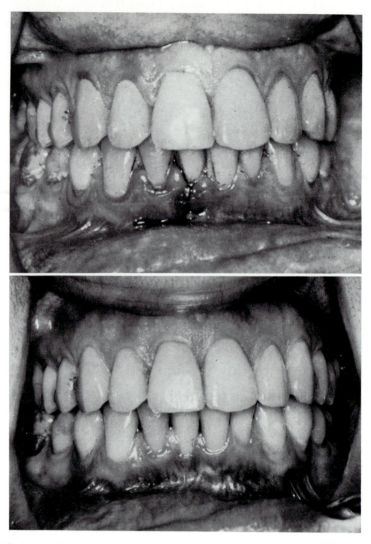

Fig. 28-5. Before and after therapy of a deep gingival cleft extending to mucobuccal fold. Operative procedure consisted of preoperative scaling and mucogingival surgery.

not done will cause a recurrence of the pocket. The method of caring for an aberrant frenum will be discussed later in this chapter. The important aspect to remember is that one is dealing with a pocket or its deformity, and therefore standard therapy for pocket elimination is the method of choice. However, should the cleft be quite deep and wide, then the procedure of choice for correction is the pedicle periosteal graft (see Chapter 26). Dependent on circumstances, the free mucosal graft may be utilized to secure an adequate buffer of "hard" gingival tissue to stop the progression of the pocket-cleft formation. The therapist in this instance must make sure that the best gingival topography is attained under the circumstances.

GINGIVAL CRATER

The gingival crater deformity is a fairly common one in chronic cases of necrotizing ulcerative gingivitis. It consists of an inversion of the interdental col so that there is a funnel-shaped interproximal architecture. Indeed, there are cases in which the peaks are even enlarged. In these cases there seems to be a labial and lingual curtain of gingiva with no interdental connection between the two.

In any case it can be readily seen that these mutilations constitute a serious problem. The actual survival of the natural dentition depends on a solution. The solution is of course gingivectomy and, if necessary, osteoplasty. The important thing to recognize in these cases is that in the true crater the base becomes the coronal tip of a new interdental topography. This of course entails the creation of some gingival recession adjacent to the interproximal area under consideration. The aesthetic results are usually quite good, and the gingival recession created by the gingivectomy is masked by illusion. Observation seems to suggest that the newly created papilla begins to enlarge and push coronally under function, drawing with it the marginal gingiva. Even a single millimeter of coronal proliferation has a profound effect upon the aesthetics of the case.

In performing gingivectomy the operator might do well in these cases to exaggerate somewhat the interdental hollowing out of the labial gingiva to exaggerate the root eminences between them. This makes for aesthetically pleasing contours as well as a functioning interdental area.

The gingivae occasionally break down interproximally even after gingivectomy, when the contact relationship of the adjoining teeth is open or poor. It is felt that the newly created interdental tissue is still to fragile and immature immediately after the removal of the dressing to withstand the traumatizing effect of food impaction. Considerable success in these cases has been attained by creating an immediate contact. A temporary method is an interproximal lacing of wire, which provides enough of a barrier to prevent the direct thrust of food upon the papilla. Hygiene, however, must be more meticulous than ever in these cases.

FLAT PALATE

A local environmental problem influencing therapy is the flat palate interference when pocket depth reaches that proportion where excision of the gingival tissue results in a V-like or wide trough defect. Thus a pocket on the palatal aspect of the maxillary posterior teeth may be complicated by the anatomic topography of the palate. An approach that has been successful in many instances is the flap with an internal bevel. The initial incision is made parallel to the sulcular area down to the alveolar crest region, and the tissue is removed. Vertical relaxing incisions are usually necessary. The flap is then thinned and repositioned against the alveolar margin. The main problem is replacing the flap in the correct position. Of extreme importance is the method of suturing the flap tautly against the bone. The flap must be held securely (Fig. 28-6).

The same problem is also encountered in the anterior portion of the palate. At times this area takes on a flattened appearance, and when there

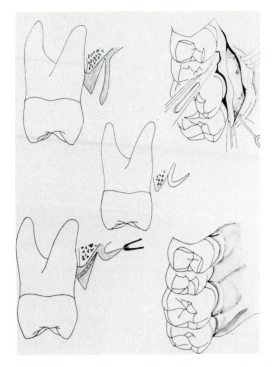

Fig. 28-6. Management of a deep pocket on palatal surface of a maxillary second molar in an instance where a flat palate is present. A partial-thickness split flap is raised and inner portion is removed, thus thinning gingival tissue. This allows for closer adaptation of gingiva to tooth. In this way pocket elimination is accomplished.

are pockets on the palatal aspect of the teeth, routine gingivectomy is difficult or impossible. Here again the internal bevel flap is a useful procedure.

TOOTH STANDING ALONE IN A SADDLE AREA

The single tooth, usually a molar, standing with no adjoining tooth and requiring surgical intervention, poses a problem in dressing the surgical wound. Since the surgical cement used is not adhesive and depends on being locked interproximally, it can be seen that when there is no interproximal lock and the strength of the dressing itself is extremely poor as a cement, the problem of retention is a real one.

This is a very easy problem to solve, however. Bar has developed a technique in which a copper band is fitted to the tooth and then one end of the band is cut in ribbon fashion. The strips are then bent over, resembling an umbrella. Thus a cradle retaining device is produced. The band is placed in position on the tooth, and the occlusion is tested. The pack is put around the tooth, covering the operative site, and is thus held by the umbrella of the band.

Another method to retain a pack is a stent made of quick-setting acrylic. Various designs are possible. The therapist must make sure that excessive pressure does not result on the tissue by the stent.

The key to periodontal surgery is frequently the ability to secure the dressing. The acrylic stent is one effective method of attaining our objective; tinfoil is another.

PERIODONTAL ABSCESS

The periodontal abscess is an acute exacerbation of a periodontal pocket. The usual concept of the periodontal pocket is that of a chronic low-grade inflammatory process, and this is of course the common picture. However, when the mouth of the pocket becomes partially or completely occluded with debris, or when drainage from the wound surface is blocked, a perfect situation for an acute periodontal abscess occurs.

Clinically such an abscess usually gives rise to swelling in the area, extreme tenderness of the tooth to even trifling percussion, sudden loosening of the tooth in the alveolus, and extrusion. There may be some temperature rise. In an acute situation of this kind the patient usually seeks treatment on an emergency basis.

Certain types of periodontal pockets are prone to abscess formation. It can be readily seen that deep infrabony pockets with a narrow aperture marginally can be easily occluded partially or completely. Teeth with bifurcation or trifurcation involvement are also common offenders in this direction (Fig. 28-7).

The tissue reaction to these mechanical blocks is interesting. In contradistinction to other periodontal pockets that are characterized by chronic inflammatory elements, the pocket complicated by abscess formation exhibits all the signs of acute inflammation. This fact brings in its train some unusual phenomena. In the standard periodontal pocket the rate of bone resorption is slow and insidious, whereas in the periodontal abscess the rate of destruction is rapid and fulminating. At times discernible bone loss can be observed roentgenographically in a single day. The response to therapy is just as dramatic when successful.

Treatment of the periodontal abscess falls into two general phases. The first is concerned with reduction of the acute signs that constitute the emergency, and the second consists of standard therapy for the elimination of the pocket. Both aspects have special problems.

The first task confronting the operator is the establishment of drainage for the entrapped purulent exudate and the concomitant relief of pain and extrusion of the tooth. Wherever possible, this is best done through the lumen of the pocket. Since the blocking of this opening is the initiating cause of the periodontal abscess, it can be seen readily that finding this aperture may often be difficult. Curets are usually much too large to search out this point, and so the periodontal probe is usually the instrument of choice. This is moved circumferentially in the pocket with a gentle probing pressure, seeking the opening. It is well to attempt several angles of entry when the slightest dip in the attachment level is encountered. Any small-headed instrument, for example, a file, may be used to enter the pocket. The file does very nicely in slipping through the still constricted marginal opening, and some débridement and evacuation may begin. After several passages of the instrument, enlarging the pocket orifice, the purulent exudate should be freely flowing, and some of the tension of the area can be relieved. At this point a small curet can be easily inserted, and definitive, careful curettage can be instituted (Fig. 28-8).

It must be remembered that the tissues with which we are dealing are excruciatingly painful and great care must be taken, especially at the beginning, to minimize tissue displacement as much as possible. Some pain is unavoidable, and this cannot be eliminated by local anesthesia, since injection into the area is not desirable. However, some palliation of the pain may be achieved by local application of ethyl chloride if available or by premedication with one of the more effective sedatives and analgesics.

Frequently teeth so involved are extruded and mobile and are painful when percussed. Adjustment of the occlusal relationship on the basis of the individual tooth is necessary. In grinding, bracing the tooth by finger support minimizes the pain caused by the vibration of the stone.

On occasion a situation will be enountered in which the swelling from the abscess is removed some distance from the opening of the pocket. Spiral pockets and pockets of bizarre configuration are not at all unusual around teeth involved with periodontal abscess formation. In fact, the very tortuousness of the neck of the pocket often predisposes it to obstruction and abscess formation. Such a pocket will be extremely difficult to explore and open through its orifice at the gingival margin. It is for this reason that the acute phase of

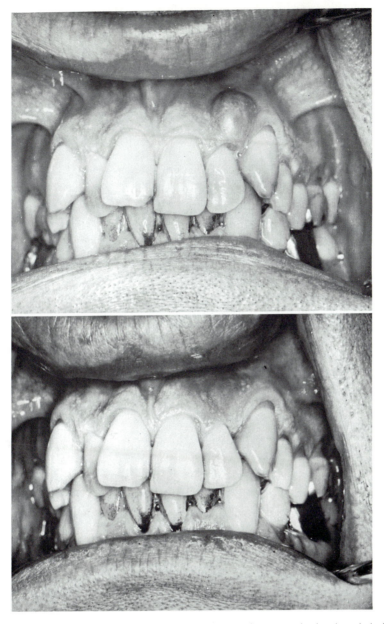

Fig. 28-7. Management of acute periodontal abscess. Area was incised and drained. In lower photograph, note results 1 week after operation.

the periodontal abscess is often managed in a different fashion.

The alternate method of evacuating the purulent exudate is by the standard technique in abscess formation: direct incision and drainage. This method has several advantages that may apply in the given case. If the abscess is pointing and ripe for entry, a generous incision, beginning with a stab of a sharp-pointed scalpel, effects a very quick evacuation of the contents of the abscess. Judicious curettage through the incision of the under-lying tissues may at times be effective if the destruction of the labial plate exposes the root and the fundus of the abscess. This procedure is known as the buttonhole approach. Caution must be used in attempting it, since unless the actual abscess cavity is open and accessible to the curet, one may be poorly advised to curet healthy tissues indiscriminately under these circumstances.

During the emergency or initial phase of periodontal abscess therapy it is entirely rational to administer antibiotic therapy. The only precaution

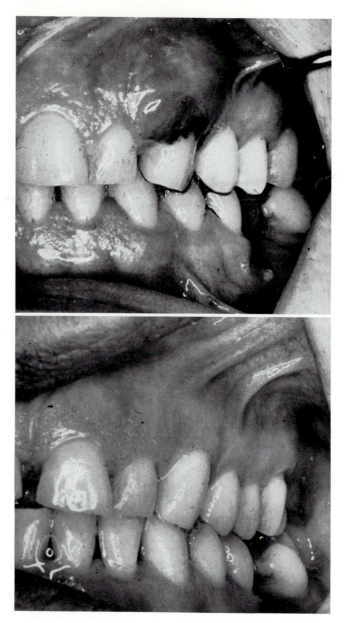

Fig. 28-8. Management of acute periodontal abscess around cuspid. Patient was diabetic. Note postoperative results. Abscess was opened for drainage.

necessary is to adhere to sound principles of administration on dosage and standard methods.

The results of the incision and drainage are very quickly realized. The pain and extrusion are soon relieved, and the abscess becomes quiescent. Similar results are obtained with entry through the mouth of the pocket when feasible.

When the acute phase has subsided and the patient is once again comfortable, the initial phase of treatment has been completed. Unfortunately, too often the absence of signs and the dramatic results of emergency treatment lull the operator into a false sense of security. There still remains, however, the treatment of the underlying cause. Unless this phase of therapy is performed, the abscess will be reexacerbated, and the very rapid bone loss will continue unabated.

The treatment of the periodontal pocket may properly be called the definitive phase of therapy. Here again some evaluation is in order to place the problem in proper perspective. Ordinarily, periodontal pockets exhibit all of the aspects of chronic inflammation, and, on the whole, the process of resorption is a slow one. Pockets involved with a periodontal abscess, on the contrary, show an acute inflammatory response, and bone loss is much more rapid. As is usually the case, the more acute the exacerbation, the more rapid will be the response. Pockets involved in abscess formation are no exception to this general rule. Not only does the acute phase yield dramatically but even the second phase of pocket therapy also is more rewarding than usual.

One type of pocket is somewhat more prone to periodontal abscess formation, and that is the infrabony pocket. Not only are those pockets infrabony in character, but they also often assume rather bizarre forms. The spiral pocket, the flask-shaped pocket, and even long narrow pockets with two terminal processes have been recorded. It can be surmised that these are lesions that because of their form frequently are exacerbated into becoming acute periodontal abscesses.

These pockets have normally a good prognosis for reattachment attempts, especially those completely encompassed by bone. However, the rate of success is distinctly higher in these pockets after they have been involved in abscess formation than in those that have never been so involved. This statement is based on clinical observation and is not the result of controlled experiment, so it is subject to some question. Nevertheless, it has been the clinical experience of a large number of therapists and thus cannot be waved aside as a mere subjective opinion of a single observer. Prichard has recorded a number of these cases in the sequence of their appearance over many months and has reported a large number of successes.

These observations give rise to a number of conjectures. First, it is possible that the acute process, which subsequent drainage, evacuates the contents of the pocket more completely than would be possible in the usual curettage procedure. There is of course the possibility that the acute periodontal abscess has somewhat altered the metabolism of the region, permitting a more favorable response to therapy than would otherwise be the case. Possibly this is due to the introduction of the cellular elements of acute inflammation. Second, the acute inflammatory process causes such a rapid rate of bone loss that the denuded root surface is not exposed to the destructive tendency of the exudate. Also the acute process destroys the transseptal collagen fibers that run between tooth and bone in the infrabony pocket, thus evacuating the tissue in the area. Thus the chances for repair are greater.

In any event the procedure for treating these lesions is fairly well standardized into a two-phase procedure. The second phase consists of the accepted therapy for pocket elimination, depending on the nature of the lesion with which we are dealing. The flap method provides the best access for root and soft tissue curettage in tortuous pockets. This is exactly like any other pocket that requires the open approach for therapy.

Lest it be surmised that all periodontal abscesses can be resolved successfully, it might be well to mention that abscess formation is frequently the terminal exacerbation of a tooth hoeplessly involved with an intractable trifurcation involvement or a similar situation. Many of these teeth are inevitably lost, but it must be kept in mind that the hoeplessness of the situation is not due to the periodontal abscess per se.

ACUTE MARGINAL PERIODONTITIS

Acute marginal periodontitis is not commonly encountered. Recognition and prompt and thorough therapy are of utmost importance, however, if the teeth in the involved area are to be salvaged. Clinically it is a sharply localized, acute inflammatory process, involving the interproximal and marginal areas of two or more adjacent teeth. Acute pain with slight purulent exudate from edematous, inflamed gingiva marks the appearance of this syndrome. There are usually more evidences of a general systemic reaction than the appearance of the local findings would indicate. A general malaise with slight temperature rise is not uncommon. In the later stages crestal sequestra of various dimensions are formed, depending on the severity of the case. The gingiva of the involved area is intensely painful to probing.

Acute marginal periodontitis may be easily differentiated from necrotizing ulcerative gingivitis by the absence of necrotic ulcers and by the presence of exudate. It is felt that the syndrome is an acute localized osteitis of a not too well-established etiology.

Thereapy is more or less symptomatic. The acute phase is reduced by the use of adequate dosage of antibiotics and warm irrigation. After the reduction of the acute stage the area is debrided of sequestra with an open flap approach with the patient under block anesthesia or general anesthesia. The debriding procedures are best carried out during a second course of antibiotic administration as a prophylactic measure. Recovery is uneventful, with some edema and pain to be expected. Often bone regeneration is amazing.

With prompt and thorough therapy bone loss is minimized, and healing is quite good. There are, however, always recalcitrant or difficult cases in which the amount of bone loss is considerable.

ACUTE PERICORONITIS

Acute pericoronal infections are common around teeth that are incompletely erupted or that because of their location in the arch cannot be completely freed of enveloping gingiva up to or even over the occlusal surface. Lower third molars and often second molars are commonly found partially covered by flaps of gingival tissue. That is not to imply that other teeth are immune, but the most common finding of acute pericoronitis involves the lower third molar.

In acute exacerbation the flap of gingiva is violently inflamed and edematous. Often it is associated with a necrotizing ulcerative gingivitis. Trismus is a common finding, making access difficult. Neglected cases have been known to result in a peritonsillar abscess with possible serious consequences. Fatality as a result of such a pericoronal infection with such a course has been seen.

Treatment of the acute phase is much the same as that of any other similar infection. *Proper antibiotic administration with lavage with warm water is effective.* In some acute attacks the patient may experience such a severe degree of trismus and external swelling that the introduction of appropriate intraoral treatment has to be suspended temporarily. When the external swelling subsides in response to antibiotic therapy and there is less interference with mouth opening, it then becomes possible to institute the full regimen of relevant local measures. The occluding tooth on the opposing jaw must be checked to see whether it impinges on the flap. It must be ground if it does. Besides the use of lavage by the therapist in cleansing out the area under the flap the use of methylene blue (2%) is of benefit. The solution is picked up with cotton pliers, and the drug is diffused under the flap into the wound site. A variety of other drugs can be used. A bulb syringe of a fine gauge is extremely useful as a nontraumatizing debriding technique when used frequently by the patient at home. He should be instructed in the method of inserting the tip of the syringe under the flap to reach the involved area most effectively.

When the acute phase has subsided and the area is perfectly comfortable, a decision must be made regarding disposition of the tooth. Resection of the offending flap covering the crown, especially the mandibular second molar, is the best course to follow if the crown of the tooth

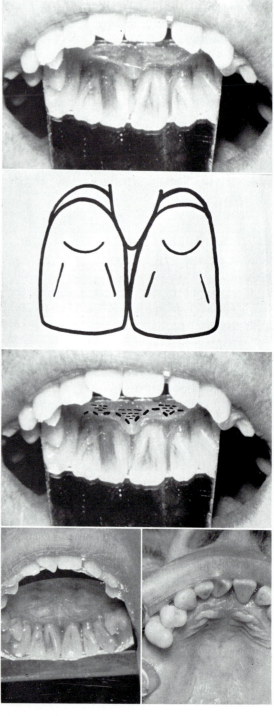

Fig. 28-9. Management of pockets extending below papilla palatina. Note resultant gingival form in bottom photographs.

can be well freed from the new margin of the gingiva. In lower third molars the tooth is so far distal in the arch that frequently the third molar invades the ramus of the mandible partially so that the soft tissue covering it encroaches on the occlusal surface of the tooth. There is no room distal to the tooth to free it properly. In other words, there should be the possibility of a short saddle area distal to the crown of the molar before success can be expected. If this is not the case, such a tooth should be extracted because it will be reexacerbated in the future and is functionally useless in any event.

If the operator wishes, he may observe the area for a period of time to see whether it breaks down again. In this way some compromise may be arrived at. However, repeated exacerbations should be solved by extraction.

PALATINE PAPILLA AND RUGAE

The palatine papilla fills the interdental embrasure of the two upper central incisors from the palatine aspect. Occasionally this area becomes extremely tender from invasion either by food debris and retention or by direct trauma from the lower incisors in a deep overbite. Very frequently it is in the line of routine surgical correction of the upper anterior segment (Fig. 28-9) (see Chapter 25).

This area is usually no problem, but careless overextensive resection will on occasion encounter some difficulty so that minor precautions should be taken into account. In contouring the palatine papilla either because of a deep pocket in the area or because of proliferation of the papilla due to trauma, the therapist should be careful to preserve the general form of the papilla in surgery. In other words, it is not advisable to resect this area with a blunt horizontal incision but rather to shape the incision so that the midline will form a small tip or papilla. The reason for this is that there is cartilage in this area, and invasion of the deepest portion of the area would expose it in the surgical wound.

As in all other surgical situations, the usual standards of correct form should be set so that knifelike margins are created and the line of incision blends with the surrounding palatine anatomy. Since the tissue here is sometimes thick, this is a reconstructive problem. Rotary abrasives have been found to be particularly effective here.

In many instances palatine rugae interfere with the initial beveling incision in the gingivectomy procedure. Care should be exercised that a gentle slope is created. This may mean that the nearby rugae will have to be contoured to blend in with the topography set up for the gingival tissue. Here again, sharp cutting or rotary abrasive stones are useful.

Part II
MANAGEMENT OF FURCA INVOLVEMENT OF MOLAR TEETH

For many years the accepted method of treating osseous defects located in interradicular areas was to expose the furcation via surgical procedures so that patients could cleanse the area and maintain a healthy attachment apparatus. This limited the number of teeth that could be treated because of the restricting anatomic requirements for successful therapy. If teeth had widely divergent, long roots and a favorable relationship to the mucogingival complex of tissues, the osseous defect in the interradicular area could be eliminated by ostectomy-osteoplasty procedures, and the tooth maintained. There are many problems inherent in this philosophy of furcation treatment, and a compromise in treatment goals frequently had to be accepted. The majority of teeth requiring treatment for lesions in interradicular areas do not possess the necessary anatomy required in the tooth structure, contiguous bone, and mucogingival tissues for treatment by ostectomy-osteoplasty procedures.

If the bone loss in the interradicular area is extensive, the amount of bone and attachment apparatus that must be sacrificed to attain physiologic contours in the bone and overlying soft tissues is excessive and weakens the support of the affected tooth and adjacent teeth.

Plaque and calculus accumulate on the interradicular surfaces of teeth that have been treated for furcation defects by exposing the area through osseous resection techniques. This area poses a considerable challenge to even the most dedicated patients to maintain the interradicular tooth surfaces free of bacterial plaque. The irritants from the plaque cause the gingival tissues to proliferate and obliterate the access to the furcation area created by the surgical procedure. The inflamed, hyperplastic tissue prevents cleansing of the interradicular area, and the disease process becomes progressively worse.

A second and allied problem is the initiation of root caries on the root surfaces adjacent to the interradicular area. The carious lesions are hard to detect and, practically speaking, impossible to restore. It is the experience of many clinicians that molars so treated are retained for an average period of about 5 years, after which they must be extracted because of advanced periodontal destruction, excessive mobility, or pulpitis resulting from a carious exposure.

The current trend in therapy is to eliminate the osseous defect in the interradicular area by (1) new attachment procedures, (2) root amputation, hemisection procedures, or trisectioning, and (3) root division procedures. If teeth with furcation lesions are to be utilized as abutment teeth in fixed prosthetic appliances, it is advisable that the tooth and associated osseous defect receive definitive treatment (Nyman and Lindhe, 1976 a and b).

PROGNOSIS

The prognosis for teeth that have sustained bone loss and loss of attachment apparatus in the interradicular area depends on a number of factors:

1. Extent of tissue destruction in three dimensions in the interradicular area
2. Morphology of the interradicular surface, and the number of roots involved
3. The length, shape, and divergence of the roots, furcal ridges, and grooves (Fig. 26-30)
4. Relationship of the adjacent osseous tissues and mucogingival complex of tissues
5. Access for surgical correction
6. Access for oral hygiene procedures
7. Possibility for gaining a new attachment
8. Possibility for elimination by odontoplasty, osteoplasty, and ostectomy
9. Vitality of the tooth
10. Extent of coronal and root caries
11. Possibility of root amputation or hemisection
12. Strategic importance of the tooth
13. Cost factor for endodontic and restorative procedures

In maxillary molars the anatomy of three roots must be considered. Usually a pathway exists between the two buccal roots, extending toward either the mesial or the distal aspect of the palatal root. Any topographic variation may exist—the two buccal roots may be involved or the mesial or distal surface of the palatal root may extend toward or fuse with the two buccal roots. Another type of involvement may exist only on the proximal aspect of the tooth, extending to the opposite side. This is commonly seen in the maxillary first premolar area. As a rule the prognosis for maxillary

first premolar teeth with osseous defects in the interradicular area is poor.

MANAGEMENT OF FURCA INVOLVEMENT OF MAXILLARY MOLARS: COMBINED ENDODONTIC-PERIODONTIC TREATMENT

Furca involvement of the maxillary molars may be classified as incipient, cul-de-sac, or complete (through-and-through) involvement. Combined endodontic-periodontic therapy offers a solution. This is an excellent procedure for use when destruction of the supporting structures is limited to a single root, with the remaining portion of the tooth in relatively sound periodontal health. Removal of one buccal root, or even the two buccal roots and in some instances the palatal root, may be performed. Much of course depends upon the condition of the interradicular bone (Fig. 28-10).

Also it must be emphasized that these problems can be complicated, because a bone deformity may result if no planning is made for osseous therapy. Treatment may consist of reshaping of the tooth and also of the alveolar crest; such a

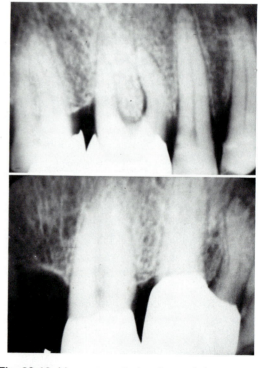

Fig. 28-10. Management of molar teeth by contouring of osseous tissue and adaptation of flap tautly against teeth. Full veneer crowns were subsequently made. These radiographs were taken 19 years apart. Patient was able to cope with furca openings by meticulous oral hygiene.

procedure results in an acceptable topography without much bone loss. However, in instances where an osseous defect is present, the defect becomes larger once the root is removed. The therapist must take into consideration the possibility of reconstructive repair. Bone or periosteum may be utilized (Fig. 28-11).

MANAGEMENT OF MAXILLARY MOLARS WITH CLOSE APPROXIMATION OF BUCCAL ROOTS

Very often the distobuccal root of the maxillary first molar lies close to the mesiobuccal root of the second molar. Tissue loss is often exaggerated in this area because of the small dimensions of the interdental septum. In many instances the proximal entrance to the furca may be opened by loss of bone. Removal of one of the buccal roots after endodontic therapy of the tooth offers a solution, since the interdental septum is widened by this procedure. The interdental tissue can be contoured to a desired topography. Should a defect be left after the removal of the root, the therapist must take into consideration bone healing and the resultant topography (Fig. 28-12).

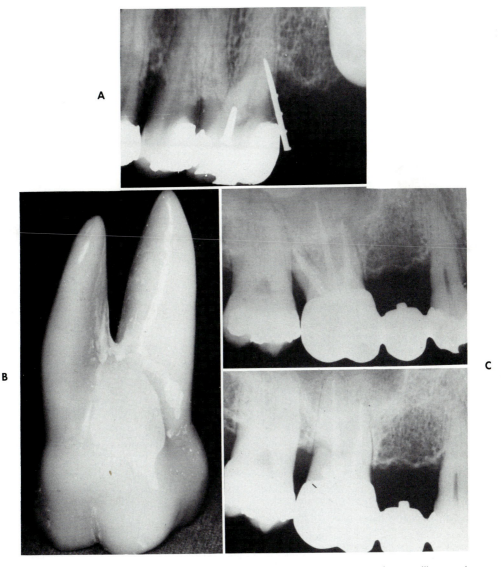

Fig. 28-11. A, Radiograph of silver points extending into furca area of a maxillary molar tooth. Distal furca is associated with an osseous defect on distal aspect of tooth. It is important to ascertain in examination extent and boundaries of lesion. **B,** Model illustrating removal of buccal root and how surface is contoured. **C,** Before and after radiographs showing removal of distal buccal root. Note cortical layer of bone interproximally after healing.

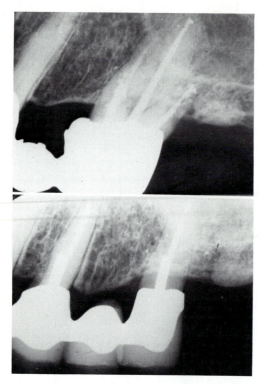

Fig. 28-12. Before and after radiographs in a case showing removal of two buccal roots of a maxillary molar, leaving palatal root to serve as an abutment for a fixed partial prostheses. (Operator must make sure that there is sufficient bone on buccal aspect of palatal root; therefore it is imperative that examination be thorough to ascertain bone loss present.) After radiograph was taken 6 years postoperatively.

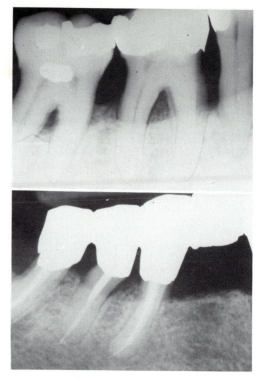

Fig. 28-13. Before and after radiographs of management of furca of first and second mandibular molar teeth. First molar was hemisected, and both roots were retained. Mesial root of second molar was retained, and distal root was removed. Note interproximal septal width postoperatively.

MANAGEMENT OF FURCA INVOLVEMENT OF MANDIBULAR MOLARS

Extensive involvement of the interradicular area of mandibular molars requires careful consideration in treatment planning. Surgical exposure and maintenance of an open furca should be limited to those patients capable of carrying out an adequate cleansing of the area. Patient motivation and cooperation are necessary to prevent caries in the furca from occurring as well as further destruction of the periodontal tissues. The roots cannot be close together since there will be insufficient access for cleansing; also there should be an adequate zone of attached gingiva to allow the toothbrush and other cleansing instruments to be used (Fig. 28-13).

Hemisection—splitting of the tooth into two parts—allows for molars to be treated as premolars. The roots must be moved apart to allow for sufficient interdental space. This is accomplished by a simple orthodontic appliance of which several designs are possible. In many instances one root is removed, leaving the other in place. The remaining root must be stable with a good clinical crown–clinical root ratio. If both roots remain, when the roots are moved apart the crestal area may be lower than either the mesial or distal crest. A flap procedure is generally utilized with either reconstructive, reparative techniques or with osteoectomy-osteoplasty should an insignificant amount of bone need to be removed (Fig. 28-14).

Mandibular molars with interradicular osseous defects often have a more favorable prognosis than maxillary molars because of the positioning of the two roots versus three roots. Mandibular first molars usually have a more favorable prognosis than second molars. The roots of mandibular second molars are not as divergent as first molars, and

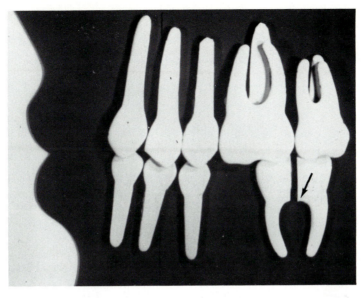

Fig. 28-14. One major problem in hemisection of mandibular molar, after endodontics, is that usually mesial and distal bone crests of tooth may be occlusally placed in relation to interradicular crest. Once roots are separated and move apart orthodontically, therapist must take into account osseous topography of area. It is important that osseous structure be level mesially, interradicularly (new septum), and distally. Vital area is interradicular bony crestal relationship to mesial and distal aspects *(arrow)*. This illustration depicts use of either one or two roots of a lower molar to serve as an abutment for a fixed partial prosthesis. A major factor in therapy that one must consider in addition to the above is position of oblique ridge of mandible. Oftentimes it rides extremely high; as a result a shallow vestibule is formed. In such an instance there may be an insufficient zone of attached gingiva; therefore therapy must include management of a variety of problems.

the furcation is usually located at a more apical position on the root in relationship to the crown of the tooth than on adjacent first molar teeth.

THERAPY

Management of osseous defects located in interradicular areas includes the following therapy:

1. Ostectomy-osteoplasty procedures for elimination of shallow osseous defects located in the buccal and lingual interradicular areas of mandibular molars and the interradicular areas of maxillary molars
2. Odontoplasty procedures for recontouring the tooth in conjunction with ostectomy-osteoplasty procedures to increase access for thorough cleansing
3. Lateral sliding mucoperiosteal flaps for new attachment procedures in cul-de-sac–type osseous defects in the interradicular area of maxillary and mandibular molars
4. Osseous tissue autografts for new attachment in cul-de-sac–type osseous defects in the interradicular area of maxillary and mandibular molars

5. Endodontic hemisection of mandibular molars, separation of roots, or removal of one root
6. Endodontic procedures and removal of buccal or palatal roots to eliminate interradicular osseous defects in maxillary molars
7. Maintenance by repeated scaling and curettage

Management of shallow osseous defects. If pocket depth is minimal and a wide band of attached gingiva exists, the pocket in the interradicular area may be eliminated by recontouring the gingival tissues and the tooth, which makes up one of the walls of the pocket. Gingivectomy-gingivoplasty procedures are used to contour the gingiva, and osteoplasty-odontoplasty procedures are used to recontour the osseous margin and furcation area of the tooth. Rotary diamond stones are used to cut the bony margin through the overlying soft tissue or through a short vertical incision made over the interradicular area. The same diamond stone is used to recontour the tooth surface. The amount of tooth substance that may be removed by odontoplasty to produce smooth contours in the

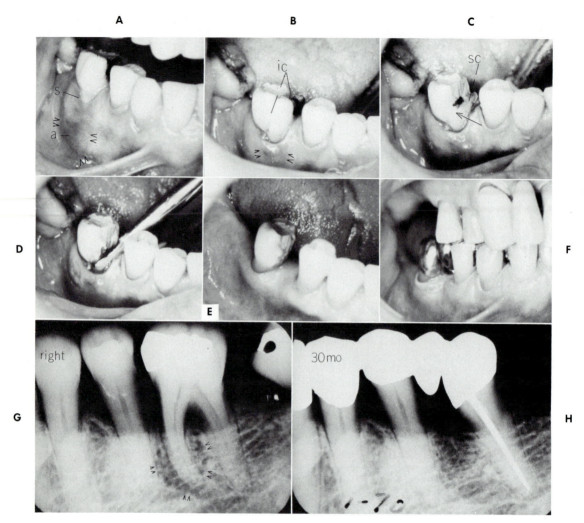

Fig. 28-15. A, Interradicular osseous defect and acute abscess, *a,* with suppuration, *s,* surrounding mesial root of first molar *(arrows).* Third molar hopelessly involved and indicated for extraction. Distal root of first molar desired for use as an abutment. **B,** After root canal therapy on distal root, initial cut, *ic,* has been made to hemisect tooth. **C,** Secondary cut, *sc,* made to obtain vision and room for instrumentation. Care must be taken not to overcut distal root portion that is to be crowned. **D,** Sectioning completed. Mesial root "floated out" in suppuration. Area curetted. **E,** Three months after hemisection. Occlusion closely checked on distal portion of tooth. **F,** Restoration completed. **G,** Pretreatment roentgenogram; note interradicular bone loss and area of abscess *(arrows).* **H,** Thirty months after treatment. (Endodontics by Dr. E. Kozel and prosthesis by Lt Col L. Lewis, U.S. Army Dental Corps.)

furcation area is limited. The age of the patient and presence of existing cervical sensitivity must be critically evaluated. Although root sensitivity may be less severe in older individuals, the acute and persisting cervical sensitivity that is produced by the odontoplasty procedure may prove to be a greater problem than the original shallow osseous defect that existed in the interradicular area.

If the volume of the interradicular osseous defect (depth, width, height) exceeds the amount of gingival tissue that can be removed by gingivectomy, an internally beveled flap must be created for access to the defect and apical positioning of the gingiva at the termination of the procedure. Ostectomy and osteoplasty procedures are utilized to contour the bone and eliminate the osseous defect in the interradicular area. Adjacent soft tissue anatomy and the relationship of the base of the defect in the interradicular area to adjacent bony landmarks such as the external oblique ridge govern the extent to which the defect can be eliminated by osseous resection and mucogingival surgical techniques.

The infrabony pocket on the mesial of the maxil-

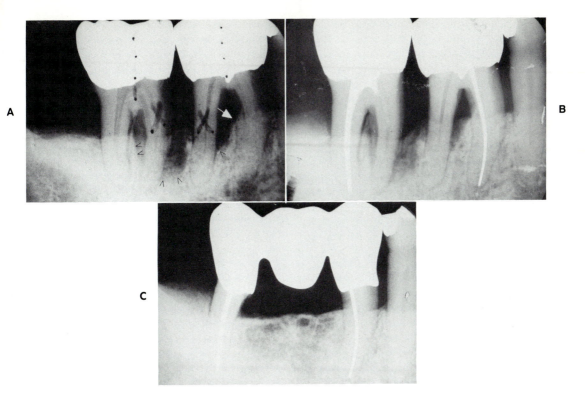

Fig. 28-16. A, Deep interradicular osseous defects *(arrows),* 65-year-old man. Root and bone morphology favorable for hemisection procedure. Distal root of first molar and mesial root of second molar to be extracted to eliminate osseous defects and save roots for abutments in periodontal prosthesis. **B,** Endodontics completed. **C,** Thirty-six months after treatment. (Endodontics by Dr. E. Kozel and prosthesis by Dr. P. Crowe, U.S. Army Dental Corps.)

lary second molar in Fig. 27-7, *KK* to *VV*, is a good example of the limitations of osseous resective surgery to completely eliminate the osseous defect that remains at the mesial entrance to the trifurcation of the molar. If further bone were removed it would unnecessarily deprive the distobuccal and palatal roots of needed bone, while further reducing the bone on the distal of the first molar. The osseous defect penetrated deeply into the mesial furcation, and in order to make the base of the defect the tip of the new osseous crest, too much bone would have to be sacrificed. The tooth was removed from its socket in Fig. 27-7, *QQ,* to show the full extent of the defect. By resecting the mesial buccal root and markedly enlarging the interdental area, a gradual slope could be produced in the osseous topography from the distal of the first molar to the mesial of the altered second molar (Fig. 27-7, *OO* to *TT*). Healing of the extraction socket and natural remodeling of the osseous crest may suffice to produce the desired osseous and soft tissue contours. If not, a second-stage flap procedure after complete healing of the socket area may be required to further contour the embrasure between the molars (Fig. 27-7, *UU* and *VV*).

New attachment procedures. New attachment procedures may be utilized to eliminate the interradicular osseous defect if the topography of the defect is favorable. If the osseous defect does not communicate with another tooth surface and forms a cul-de-sac, an osseous tissue autograft may be utilized to eliminate the interradicular osseous defect. These defects resemble a three-wall osseous defect, but the roots of the tooth comprise the greater proportion of the calcified tissues surrounding the defect. The avascular root surfaces limit the healing potential in this type of a defect if the flap-curettage method of new attachment procedure is utilized to gain a new attachment. Osseous tissue autografts offer a greater potential for gaining a new attachment in cul-de-sac–type defects.

Through-and-through defects. Despite the advances made in surgical therapy, the through-and-through type of interradicular osseous defect remains a challenging problem in therapeutic management. One of the fundamental goals of therapy is to create contours in the tissues that permit oral hygiene procedures to be accomplished effectively and simply. The unfavorable contours in bifurcation and trifurcation areas hinder the accomplishment of this basic objective. Patients eventually become lax in their use of pipe cleaners, interradicular brushes, three-ply yarn, or water irrigating devices, and plaque accumulation increases in the interradicular area. Root decay and exacerbation of acute periodontal disease are the usual sequelae of teeth treated by exposing the area for maintenance by hygiene procedures. Many clinicians have documented evidence that teeth can be treated in this manner and maintained for decades, but it appears that the average life span of teeth so treated approximates 5 years or less.

New attachment procedures employing osseous tissue autografts of oral bone have not proved satisfactory for treatment of through-and-through interradicular osseous defects. Schallhorn (1967), Schallhorn et al. (1970), and Schallhorn and Hiatt (1972) have demonstrated the most favorable results in grafting class III furcations by using frozen autogenous hip marrow. Autogenous bone from oral sites has not usually worked as well as frozen hip marrow. The reasons for this are not clear. It may well be that calculus deposits or plaque were not completely removed from the tooth surface in the interradicular area or granulomatous tissue remained in the depths of the osseous defect. Mechanical access for adequate instrumentation of the interradicular area is severely limited in most instances (Fig. 28-14), and it is difficult to seal off

the site of the implant with the flaps at the termination of the procedure. Greater success has been attained by sectioning the teeth, which permits a radical change to be made in the anatomy of the interradicular area (Fig. 28-15).

Hemisection and root amputation procedures. Interradicular osseous defects that communicate from one tooth surface to another may be treated by the following methods:

1. Hemisectioning of mandibular molars to create two ''premolars'' or extraction of the most involved root and creation·of the single ''premolar'' out of the remaining root
2. Amputation of the mesial, distal, or palatal roots of maxillary molars—any combination of the three roots may be retained, and a trifucation may be turned into a bifurcation or a single palatal, distal, or mesial buccal rooted tooth
3. Amputation of the buccal or palatal root of maxillary first premolars

Endodontic therapy is accomplished prior to surgical therapy to ensure that it is possible to completely instrument the root canals in the portions of the tooth to be retained. Although vital root amputation and hemisections have been successfully accomplished when it was discovered during periodontal surgery that the pocket and osseous defect could not be eliminated by any other method, one runs the risk of later failure because of an inability to successfully complete the endodontic portion of the treatment procedure.

Restorative procedures are usually necessary to restore and splint the coronal portions of the remaining root or roots to neighboring teeth in the dental arch. Care must be exercised not to overcut the portion of the tooth that is to be retained when the teeth are sectioned. Overcutting of the crown and root greatly complicates the restorative phase of treatment for the involved tooth (Figs. 28-15, *D,* and 28-16).

MANAGEMENT OF PALATAL AREA

Friedman's early description of palatal flap management and the palatal approach to osseous surgery designed by Ochsenbein and Bohannan offers a sound rationale for elimination of the osseous interproximal defects as well as conservation of the buccoradicular bone.

The partial-thickness palatal flap offered by Corn is a further modification of the soft tissue management of this area, based on the same rationale (Figs. 28-18 and 28-19). This approach, although managed from the palate, has as its primary concern the conservation of the alveolar pro-

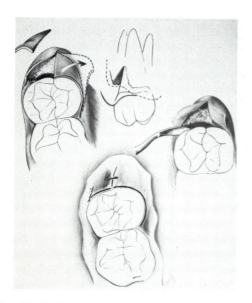

Fig. 28-17. Wedge procedure for maxillary tuberosity. In this instance a two-wall osseous defect is present, extending from buccal to palatal aspect of tooth. There is no furca entrance. After contouring bone as much as possible, with limitations of topography, flaps are collapsed as closely to bone as possible.

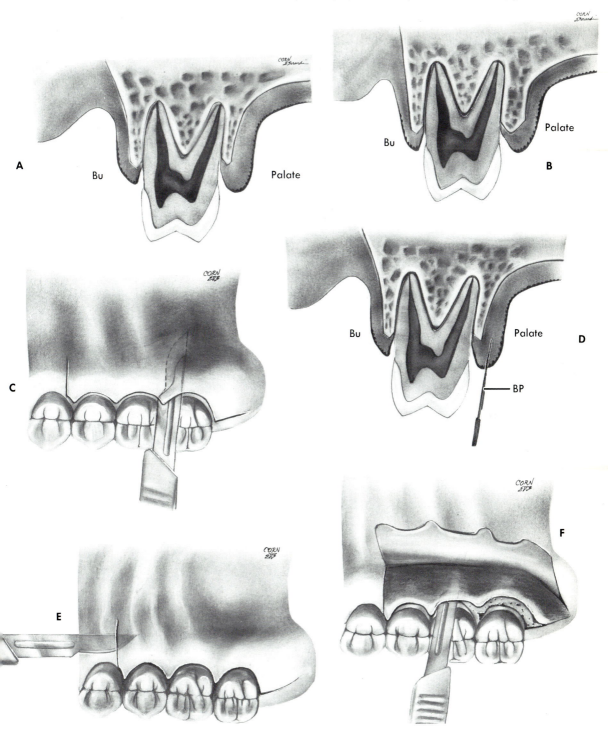

Fig. 28-18. Palatal flap surgery. **A** and **B,** Thickness of palatal tissue may be due to thick soft tissue and thin alveolar process, or vice versa. *Bu,* Buccal aspect. **C** and **D,** If tuberosity needs surgical correction, procedures are combined and first palatal incision is initiated along palatal aspect of tuberosity as a partial-thickness dissection (see Fig. 28-22). Bard-Parker handle, *BP,* with a no. 15 blade enters tissue approximately 1.5 mm. Dissection is repeated using same tissue entry. It becomes an undermining incision to create a thin primary flap. Blade *should not* dissect deeply as shown in interrupted outline of blade, **C. E,** A convenient way to finalize thin primary flap is to make a vertical incision along distopalatal line angle of most anterior tooth in surgical area. To maintain easy visibility, dissection is in an apicocoronal direction. Tissue forceps or a periosteal elevator create slight marginal tension to facilitate dissection.

Continued.

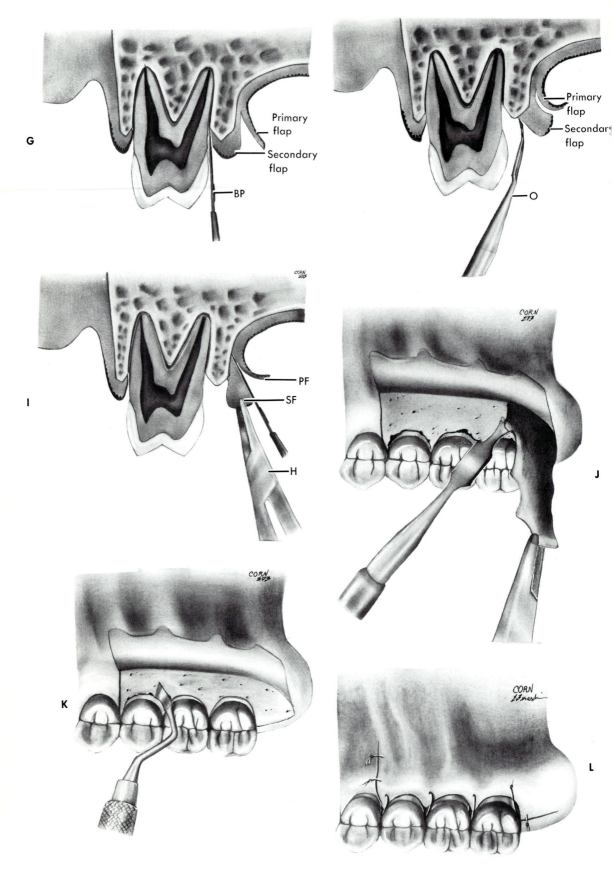

Fig. 28-18, cont'd. For legend see opposite page.

cess on the buccal aspect of the teeth. Experience has shown that many complications arise with the apical placement of the buccoradicular alveolar process.

Key decisions must be made as to the extent of apical contouring of the radicular bone in an effort to eliminate conceptually interproximal craters and yet not expose the furca:

1. The palatal tissues must be raised in order to gain a relationship of the palatal bone with the buccal bone.
2. The interproximal defects must be explored.
3. The anatomy of the distobuccal root of the first molar and its proximity to the mesiobuccal root of the second molar must be ascertained.
4. The extent to which radicular bone can be removed and yet not involve the furca must be determined.

The furca is generally around 4 mm apical to the cervical line on the first molar and 5 or 6 mm from the cementoenamel junction on the second molar. Therefore more radicular bone can be removed on the second molar than on the first molar to correct an interproximal defect without involving the furca unnecessarily.

The roentgenogram is a guide to the distal curvature flare of the distobuccal root of the first molar toward the mesiobuccal root of the second molar. As the osseous defects extend apically, these two root surfaces approximate each other more closely and create technical difficulties in establishing a physiologic gingival and osseous environment.

The depth of the craters must be measured interproximally. Judgment must be used in combining all of this information. It is best to avoid the level to which the furca would be approached; bone should be removed only to this height. The balance of the defect is ramped on the palatal aspect. This, of course, is correlated with the curvature of the distobuccal root of the first molar and communication with the distal furcation. This is most carefully examined by using a no. 17 explorer.

The use of a palatal flap has offered access to osseous defects not formerly visualized. One common osseous problem is that of a high incidence of large exostoses present on the palatal alveolar process, extending from the mesial aspect of the maxillary first molar distally to the terminus of the tuberosity (Fig. 28-20) (Corn, 1968; Larato, 1972; Nery et al., 1977). This finding correlates with the reported comments that palatal gingivectomies in the molar area frequently heal more slowly than they do in other areas. In all probability the reason for this is that the palatal osseous tissue is exposed with the resection of the palatal tissue. This coincides with the frequent observation of palatal exostoses. If deep pockets exist in the molar areas requiring osseous correction or if one can anticipate the exposure of the palatal bone, a palatal flap should be utilized.

The advantages of the palatal flap modification include the following:

1. Greater ease of performance
2. Better control of flap thickness
3. More precise control of the final gingival margins covering the alveolar crest
4. Smoother blending with the management of the tuberosity

As one moves anteriorly from the premolars forward in the palatal area (provided that infrabony pockets are not present), the use of resection techniques is advisable, since the osseous morphology seems to mimic the conceptual osseous form.

The palatal flap is not a mucogingival flap but a gingival flap (masticatory mucosa). Because we are involved with the submucosal structures of the palata, the glandular and fatty tissues, and the loose alveolar connective tissue, the scope of mucogingival surgery will encompass this type of procedure.

In designing palatal flaps one must salvage as much of the gingiva as practical. With a primary incision into the lamina propria of the gingiva and

Fig. 28-18, cont'd. F to I, Following elevation of primary flap, scalpel is directed to bony crest in tuberosity area and marginal bone at base of pocket to free attachment of secondary flap from tooth. Ochsenbein chisel no. 2 is convenient to elevate secondary flap, *SF.* Tissue can be held with a hemostat, *H,* to facilitate its dissection and removal. By directing scalpel away from palatal aspect toward alveolar process, branches of greater palatine artery can be avoided. Thin primary flap, *PF,* is not traumatized. *O,* Ochsenbein chisel. **J** and **K,** Any residual attachment to tooth or palatal exostosis can be released by Ochsenbein chisel. Marginal osseous correction is finalized with a Rhodes chisel (Hartzell no. 36/37). **L,** Flap is held with a tissue forcep (Hu-Friedy no. 34) and contoured so that gingiva covers alveolar crest between 1 and 2 mm. Continuous suturing is used to adapt graft to hard tissues. Interrupted sutures are used as shown.

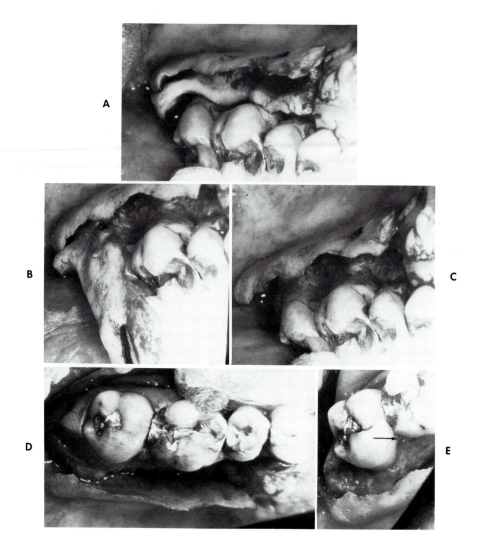

Fig. 28-19. Combined procedures of palatal flap and management of tuberosity. **A,** Primary and secondary incisions, originating at falloff of tuberosity, enable demonstration of primary (outer) partial-thickness flap and secondary (inner) mucoperiosteal flap. Note vertical incisions at terminus of tuberosity and distal aspect of first premolar. If vertical incision was to terminate at mesial line angle of second premolar, access to interproximal crestal bone between premolars would be limited and blending of interproximal correction with palatal radicular bone of first premolar would result in a denudation. **B,** Thin primary flap remains. Secondary mucoperiosteal flap, as held by mosquito hemostat, is being removed. Extension of dissection of secondary flap includes mucoperiosteal tissue of tuberosity. **C,** Complete removal of secondary flap, leaving interproximal and marginal pocket tissue as well as crestal tissue at tuberosity. **D,** Crestal pocket tissue on distal aspect of second molar. Partial-thickness internal beveled incision on buccal aspect originates at falloff of tuberosity, proceeds along buccal incline of tuberosity, and connects with internal beveled incision on buccal aspect. Note common finding of an exostosis on palatal alveolar process opposite second molar (mirror view). **E,** Soft tissue has been removed, and a wide osseous defect is visualized on distal aspect of second molar. Note osseous crater between molars *(arrow)* (mirror view).

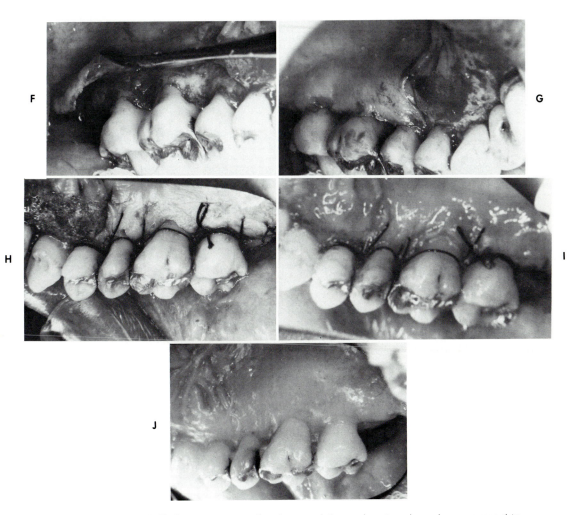

Fig. 28-19, cont'd. F, Osseous correction is complete, and craters have been ramped to palate. **G,** Anterior palatal gingivectomy blends with palatal flap, which is excessive in length. **H,** Palatal marginal tissue is scalloped and sutured over the crest by continuous sutures. Note complete closure of tuberosity area (mirror view). **I,** Palatal healing in 10 days. Note accurate control of scalloped flap. Note also that healing is advanced for this period of time. Were there no control of flap, proliferative granulation tissue would be seen beyond margin of the flap (mirror view). **J,** Six months' healing on palate, with blending of interproximal tissue toward palate as well as response in tuberosity area (mirror view).

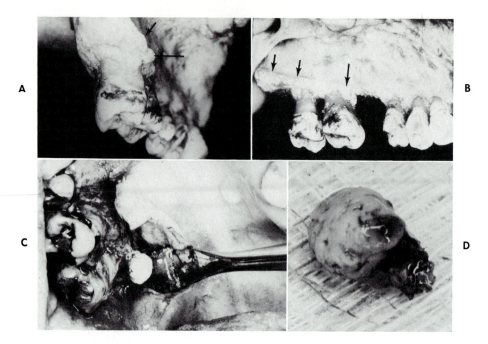

Fig. 28-20. A, Buccolingual view of tuberosity. Note exostosis on palatal alveolar process. This is common with use of flap procedures. **B,** Exostosis extends from terminus of tuberosity to mesial aspect of maxillary first molar. **C,** Another form of exostosis is this pedunculated form. **D,** A rongeur has removed this exostosis.

superficial layers of the submucosa, the primary flap is a partial-thickness flap. The tissue remaining against the tooth and laveolar process contains the pocket. This tissue (the secondary flap), including the periosteum, is elevated after a marginal incision and is subsequently discarded. In reality, it is a submucous resection including the periosteum. Removal of the secondary flap permits access to the underlying osseous tissue, while retention of the primary flap permits the closure of the operative field, utilizing a thin retained flap (Fig. 28-21).

The flaps are positioned to cover the crest or to remain 1 or 2 mm coronal to it and are sutured by continuous suturing (3-0 or 4-0 black silk suture). The dressing is applied and changed at 10-day intervals as in other flap procedures. Postoperative instructions include the use of an ice pack. Analgesics are prescribed for pain.

One can anticipate rapid healing and an uneventful postoperative course following this modification as outlined. The facility with which this approach can be blended with the management of the tuberosity defects (Corn, 1968) (Figs. 28-22 and 28-23) offers a reliable, predictable, and thoroughly planned solution to a most common clinical situation.

Fig. 28-24 illustrates the palatal flap design in detail, combining the blending of the tuberosity correction.

Fig. 28-25 demonstrates the access gained to a distal furcation involvement as well as the use of a partial-thickness apical positioned flap on the buccal surface to avoid destruction of the long connective tissue attachment on the first premolar. A fenestration on the mesiobuccal root of the first molar is avoided. The obvious advantage of the access to the palatal osseous defect is shown.

MANAGEMENT OF MAXILLARY TUBEROSITY

The responsibility of the therapist is to treat all the surfaces of the gingival attachment to the tooth. A difficult and frequently compromised area is the distal aspect of the terminal maxillary second or third molar (Fig. 28-17 and Fig. 28-22).

In the past the use of the resection technique was often disappointing because frequently pocket depth was not eliminated because of anatomic limitations realized only after the use of a complete visualization approach, as in the flap techniques.

Goldman's suggestion for treatment of pockets extending into the tuberosity was to make a horizontal incision at the distal end of the tuberosity and to resect all the tissue to the base of the pocket.

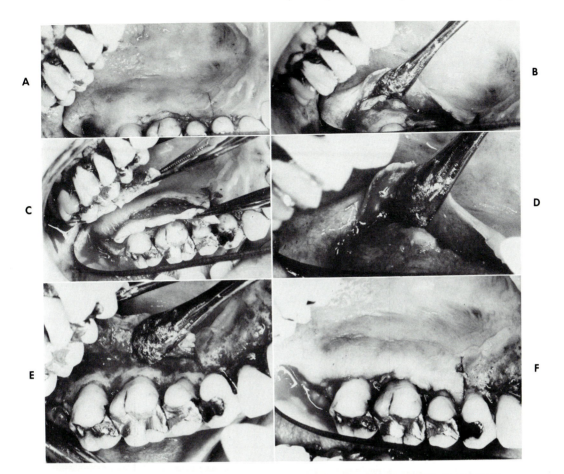

Fig. 28-21. Combined procedures to eliminate a large palatal exostosis. **A,** In palatal view a fine incision initiates at falloff of tuberosity and extends as a partial-thickness gingival flap along palatal aspect of tuberosity and cervical area of second premolar and molars. Anterior terminus of operative site is completed by a vertical incision along distal line angle of first premolar. It is essential to include entire gingival papilla within the primary flap so that access can be gained to entire crestal embrasure between premolars. **B,** Elevation of thin primary flap and exposure of large palatal exostosis. **C,** Hemostat aids removal of secondary flap, including palatal pocket walls. Excision extends to include palatal aspect of tuberosity. **D,** Complete exposure of exososis can be seen. **E,** Completion of osseous correction is viewed. **F,** Palatal flap is too long and must be scalloped to configuration of alveolar margin.

Continued.

This was indicated when no osseous lesion was present. However, often different types of infrabony pockets and furcation involvements on the distal aspect of the terminal tooth are found. Should a resection be done and an osseous defect be found, the defect will remain uncovered. Under these circumstances a flap procedure should be performed.

Certain anatomic limitations are peculiar to the tuberosity area. Roentgenograms may evidence communication between an impacted third molar and the distal pocket of the second molar. Removal of the third molar aids in the pathogenesis of a pocket in this area (Fig. 28-19). Even with a congenitally missing third molar the gingival morphology is one of bulbous, fibrotic tissue which is 3 or 4 mm coronal to the cementoenamel junction. The development of a pocket in this area becomes significantly heightened, with food retention and food impaction. Add a shallow palatal vault, a high mucogingival junction on the buccal aspect, a close proximity of the tuberosity to the terminus, and the climate is set for resection failure. Unrecognized palatal exostoses and an enlarged maxillary process in the tuberosity area further impede pocket elimination by the gingivectomy technique (Figs. 28-20 to 28-22).

All these anatomic limitations have been over-

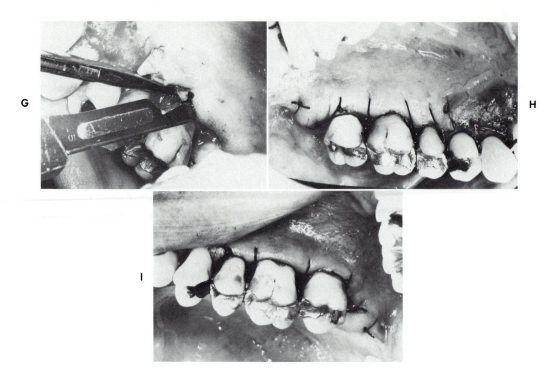

Fig. 28-21, cont'd. G, Using a mosquito hemostat as a guide, radicular alveolar crest is determined and gingival flap is held 1 mm from osseous tissue and no. 15 Bard-Parker blade excises excess tissue to tip of hemostat. **H,** Tissue involving premolar, second premolar, and molars is adapted to roots of teeth by means of continuous suturing. Because tuberosity profile was apical to alveolar outline, a vertical incision on distal of second molar was made in tuberosity area buccally and lingually so that close adaptation of gingival flap could be carried out by interrupted sutures. This closely adapts tissue to tuberosity. Anterior area was treated by a resection technique. **I,** Buccal full-thickness mucogingival flap is adapted by continuous sutures, and this view shows complete closure of tuberosity area along with buccal vertical incision, allowing mucogingival tuberosity flap to be closely adapted to alveolar ridge.

come by the tuberosity flap approach. Oral surgery texts have described the tuberosity flaps for the submucous resection of soft tissue overgrowth in preparation for dentures. An increase in intermaxillary space is required to allow for the maxillary and mandibular denture material in this area. Corn suggests the periodontal adaptation of this approach in the use of partial-thickness flaps that are integrated with the apically positioned flap approach on the buccal and palatal flap design.

The objectives of the tuberosity flap procedure are as follows:

1. To retain and preserve mature masticatory mucosa
2. To gain access to the underlying osseous defects as well as exostoses that interfere with the integrity of the periodontium
3. To protect the osseous defect that is being treated by new attachment procedures, autogenous bone implants, osseous surgery, or a combination of these

4. To eliminate all pockets by coaptation of the thin partial-thickness flaps
5. To facilitate rapid healing
6. To minimize pain

A comprehensive understanding of incisional design will allow a uniform blending of these procedures, permitting adequate access for each discrete area involved. One must realize that the use of the internal beveled incision is essential to the development of the thin partial-thickness flap.

There are two components to the tuberosity flap preparation. The buccal portion is a mucogingival flap, and the palatal portion is a gingival and masticatory mucosal flap. The tuberosity flap approach is usually combined with quadrant surgery and blended so that there is a precise continuity of the internal beveled incisions. The technical aspects of this procedure are illustrated in Figs. 28-22 and 28-23.

The buccal incision is initiated at the terminus of the tuberosity. A partial-thickness dissection

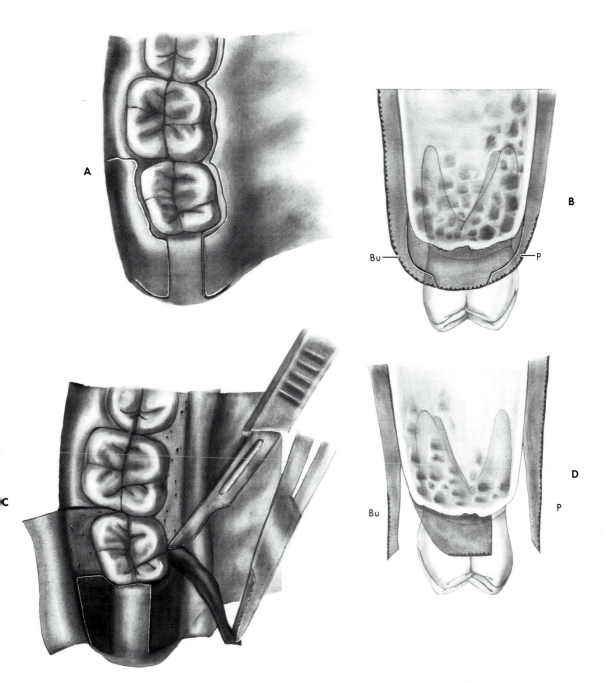

Fig. 28-22. Management of tuberosity. **A,** Incisional outline for surgical entry of tuberosity area. Buccal and palatal incisions initiate from terminus of tuberosity and extend forward. Palatal incision includes surgical field of palatal flap approach. Vertical incisions extend from distobuccal line angle of first molar (includes entire papilla) and terminus of tuberosity on buccal and palatal aspects. Tuberosity is relatively flat and does not have a fall-off to hamular notch. Distance between incisions in tuberosity is dependent upon thickness of soft tissue and bulk reduction of osseous form required. **B,** After initial incision to reduce thickness of tuberosity flaps, incisions continue as "undermining" incisions to outer edge of bony crest of tuberosity. *Bu,* Buccal aspect; *P,* palatal aspect. **C,** A full-thickness flap is raised on buccal surface. Dissection continues as a partial-thickness flap on palate. Removal of secondary flap of palate is continued anteroposteriorly. **D,** An incision along epithelial margin of tuberosity to bone facilitates removal of secondary flap. Full-thickness portion of flap is shown on buccal surface.

Continued.

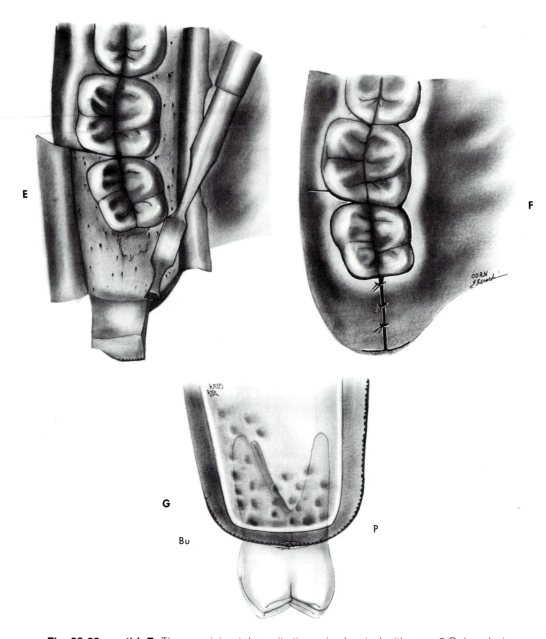

Fig. 28-22, cont'd. E, The remaining tuberosity tissue is elevated with a no. 2 Ochsenbein chisel, held with a hemostat, and excised. Osseous corrections are made. **F** and **G,** Complete closure of tuberosity area using interrupted sutures or continuous locked sutures. Thinness of flaps helps to avoid pocket recurrence. Any excess tissue should be removed so that coaptation can be completed without soft tissue overlap or space between tissue margins.

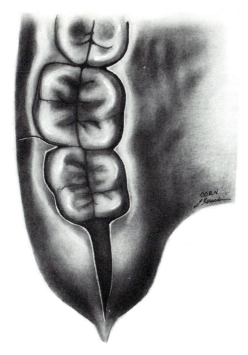

Fig. 28-23. If there is a falloff to tuberosity, distal vertical incisions are not necessary.

along the buccal incline of the tuberosity, extending to the distal aspect of the terminal tooth, prepares a thin buccal flap. The Bard-Parker no. 15 blade extends into the lamina propria of the gingiva and the submucosa of the alveolar mucosa. A vertical incision buccopalatally at the terminus of the tuberosity provides mobility to the flaps. A similar incision extends along the palatal incline of the tuberosity to the terminal tooth. It continues along the palatal gingiva of the molar teeth, blending into the palatal flap. The resection of the secondary underlying mucoperiosteal flap provides the flexibility needed for the palatal portion of the flap. With the elevation of these two flaps a fibrotic mass of gingiva, including the soft tissue pocket wall, remains on the tuberosity crest (Figs. 28-18, *I;* 28-19, *C;* 28-22, *D* and *E*).

The entire block of tissue, extending from the terminal vertical incision to the distal surface of the last tooth, is resected at the crest of the alveolar process. The removal of this tissue is achieved with the use of either a spear-shaped knife or the Ochsenbein chisel (Star Dental Manufacturing Co., Philadelphia). Subsequent to the osseous corrections the thin buccal and palatal flaps adapt to the newly established osseous form of the tuberosity and can be tightly sutured at the middle of the alveolar ridge. Vertical incisions at the distal line angles of the terminal teeth ensure complete closure of the tuberosity flaps

(Fig. 28-25, *I* and *P*). The mobility of the mucosal base of the buccal flap permits accurate approximation of the two flaps. Unless the resistant palatal portion is undermined correctly, adaptation to the alveolar ridge is incomplete. This surgical plan for the management of the tuberosity can be employed even under the most limited access situation. A smooth saddlelike gingival surface is formed on the distal surface of the terminal tooth.

Robinson (1966) has developed the distal wedge procedure to treat a similar clinical problem. However, the removal of a wedge may leave a troughlike soft tissue form prone to breakdown and to retaining debris. Braden (1969) and Tibbetts and Ochsenbein (1976) also have described procedures for tuberosity management.

The design and blending of the tuberosity flaps with adjacent plastic surgery procedures are seen in Figs. 28-24 and 28-25.

Pocket elimination should include the therapy of large edentulous ridge areas in preparation for restorative dentistry. Fig. 28-26 includes this principle combined with the removal of a retained deciduous root during palatal flap surgery.

A modification of the edentulous area pedicle graft preparation in the tuberosity area salvages the entire edentulous ridge of soft tissue (Corn, 1968; Tibbetts and Ochsenbein, 1976). The purpose of this surgical design is to retain a thin flap in this area to protect an autogenous bone implant on the distal of the terminal molar or avoid an oral antral communication when osseous defects are in close proximity to the maxillary sinus (Fig. 28-27).

MANAGEMENT OF RETROMOLAR AREA

In the past the area that is distal to the terminal mandibular second or third molar has been considered impractical, too painful, or anatomically unrealistic for complete pocket elimination. Heroic attempts at pocket elimination have included denudation procedures, with protracted healing periods.

Factors that preclude success with the resection technique include the following:

1. The retromolar tissue itself is usually bulbous. It can be composed of dense enlarged gingiva or pendulous alveolar mucosa with a minimal collar of gingiva.
2. The pocket depths are exaggerated and extend beyond the level of the gingiva.
3. The close proximity of the ascending ramus to the terminal tooth limits surgical access

Text continued on p. 1046.

Fig. 28-24. For legend see opposite page.

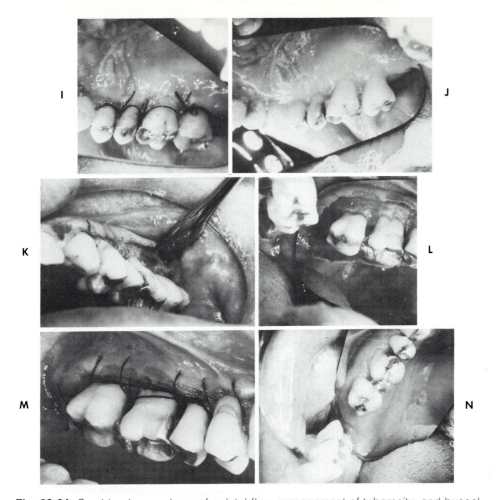

Fig. 28-24. Combined procedures of palatal flap, management of tuberosity, and buccal apically positioned flap. **A,** Primary and secondary incisions, originating at falloff of tuberosity, enable demonstration of primary (outer) partial-thickness flap and secondary (inner) mucoperiosteal flap. Note vertical incisions at the terminus of the tuberosity and the distal aspect of first premolar. If vertical incision was to terminate at mesial line angle of second premolar, access to interproximal crestal bone between premolars would be limited and blending of interproximal correction with palatal radicular bone of first premolar would result in a denudation. **B,** Thin primary flap remains. Secondary mucoperiosteal flap, as held by mosquito hemostat, is being removed. Extension of dissection of secondary flap includes mucoperiosteal tissue of tuberosity. **C,** Complete removal of secondary flap, leaving interproximal and marginal pocket tissue as well as crestal tissue at tuberosity. **D,** Crestal pocket tissue on distal aspect of second molar. Partial-thickness internal beveled incision on buccal aspect originates at falloff of tuberosity, proceeds along buccal incline of tuberosity, and connects with internal beveled incision on buccal aspect. Note common finding of an exostosis on palatal alveolar process opposite second molar (mirrow view). **E,** Soft tissue has been removed, and a wide osseous defect is visualized on distal aspect of second molar. Note osseous crater between molars (arrow) (mirror view). **F,** Osseous correction is complete, and craters have been ramped to palate. **G,** Anterior palatal gingivectomy blends with palatal flap, which is excessive in length. **H,** Palatal marginal tissue is scalloped and sutured over the crest by continuous sutures. Note complete closure of tuberosity area (mirror view). **I,** Palatal healing in 10 days. Note accurate control of scalloped flap. Note also that healing is advanced for this period of time. Were there no control of flap, proliferative granulation tissue would be seen beyond margin of the flap (mirror view). **J,** Six months' healing on palate, with blending of interproximal tissue toward palate as well as response in tuberosity area (mirror view). **K,** Thick buccal bone after elevation of full-thickness flap. **L,** Buccal osseous correction. Note elimination of tuberosity defect, ramping of interproximal craters to palate, and interproximal and interradicular osseous morphology. An important preparation of soft tissue form is level radicular osseous margins at furca (mirrow view). **M,** Buccal flap is positioned over crest and sutured. Continuity of area is blended with tuberosity. **N,** Six-month postoperative view, buccal aspect. Note gingival form achieved in molar area and contours of tuberosity (mirror view).

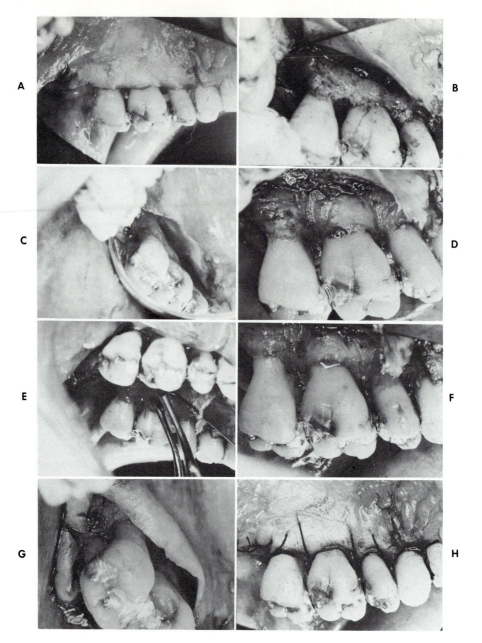

Fig. 28-25. Blending of several plastic surgery procedures—palatal flap, management of tuberosity, and partial-thickness apically positioned flap. **A,** Path of initial incision of primary gingival flap, originating at falloff of tuberosity along palatal incline of crest of tuberosity and marginal gingiva (palatal mirror view). A maximum of gingiva is retained. Vertical incisions on distal aspect of first premolar and at terminus of tuberosity permit access to underlying osseous defects. **B,** Secondary underlying flap has been removed, exposing osseous craters between molars and premolars and distal furcation involvement of second molar. **C,** Distal furcation involvement of second molar. Note delicate nature of primary gingival flap. **D,** Craters have been ramped to the palate. Note reverse osseous architecture. **E,** A Hu-Friedy no. 8 spoon curet corrects osseous irregularities. **F,** Completion of osseous surgery. Note osseous configuration and ramping on palate. Note also early furcation involvement of mesial furca of second molar. **G,** Correction of distal furcation involvement of second molar. Note planning and coordination of thin buccal flap and its vertical incision on distobuccal line angle of second molar in preparation for coaptation with a palatal flap for closure of tuberosity area. **H,** After scalloping of palatal margin primary gingival flap is sutured tightly at crest. Note palatal vertical incision at distopalatal line angle of second molar to allow complete closure of tuberosity area.

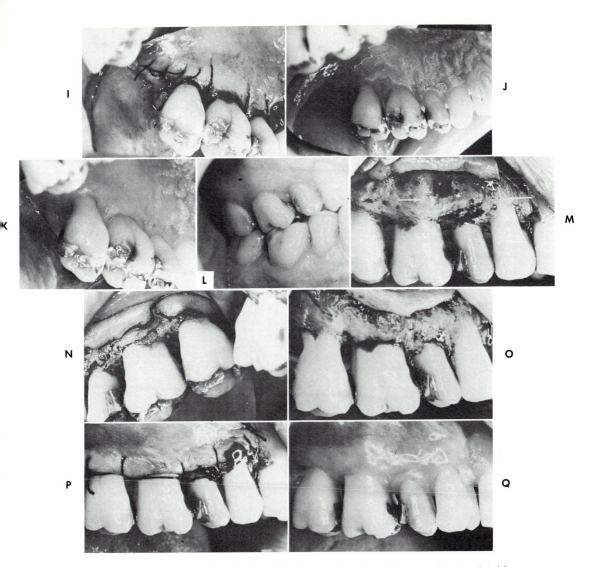

Fig. 28-25, cont'd. I, Coaptation of tuberosity tissues. Note how tissues relate to distal furcation of second molar. Palatal gingival flap is sutured to mucogingival flap on buccal aspect to close completely tuberosity saddle area. Vertical incisions at distobuccal and distopalatal line of second molar permit this complete soft tissue closure. **J,** Palatal healing and level of tuberosity tissue. Note ramp of soft tissue to palate. **K,** Gingival form in distal furca area. Pockets have been eliminated. **L,** Preoperative view. Maxillary right posterior quadrant. Note prominence of mesiobuccal root of first molar and first premolar as well as effect of frenum pull. **M,** Partial-thickness mucogingival flap on buccal aspect avoids destroying connective tissue attachment to teeth, particularly mesiobuccal root of first molar and first premolar. These areas show a high incidence of fenestrations and dehiscences. Note connective tissue covering fenestration on mesiobuccal root of first molar and dehiscence on first premolar *(arrows).* **N,** Osseous craters between premolars and molars (mirrow view). **O,** Connective tissue attachment on first premolar has not been disturbed. Radicular bone was exposed only where osseous corrections were necessary on first and second molars. Note that connective tissue remains attached apical to 1 mm or so of marginal bone on mesiobuccal root of first molar that required therapeutic correction. Alveolar margin of second molar is blended apically toward distal aspect and is kept level with cervical line in furca area. **P,** Suturing of partial-thickness apically positioned flap over crest on buccal aspect of molars. Note suturing of vertical incision at distal aspect of lateral incisor and adaptation of tissue in tuberosity. One millimeter or more of connective tissue is exposed on first and second premolars (mirror view). **Q,** Three months' healing on buccal aspect. Note increase in dimension of gingiva in premolar area. Contour of tissue blends smoothly into tuberosity area (mirror view).

4. The external oblique ridge may be level with the osseous margin of the terminal tooth, or it may be coronal to the osseous margin, creating a trough on the distobuccal aspect of the last molar.

5. The heavy ledge of lingual bone has a variety of osseous molar defects.

The use of partial-thickness mucogingival flaps in the retromolar area (Fig. 28-28) offers versatility of access to and protection of osseous therapy; reduction of tissue thickness permits accurate coaptation of flaps, thus eliminating pockets; and primary retention healing minimizes patient discomfort.

Corn (1968) suggests a procedure so that the design of the incisions for the partial-thickness flaps beyond the terminal molar compensates for the anatomic limitation of the area. Here again, treatment of this area is blended with quadrant surgery. The original internal beveled incision begins at the buccal incline of the crest of the retromolar ridge. The incision extends forward and around the distal surface of the terminal tooth into the sulcular area on the buccal surface. Similarly an internal beveled incision is planned to originate on the lingual incline of the crest of the retromolar ridge. This incision extends forward and around the lingual surface of the last molar (Fig. 28-28, A).

These incisions on the distal retromolar areas are partial-thickness dissections that leave the greater bulk of fibrous tissue remaining attached to the alveolar crest and the tooth. (Fig. 28-28, C). As these incisions are extended forward, they can continue as partial-thickness dissections (as might be found on the buccal surface) or as a full-thickness flap (as found on the lingual surface). The full-thickness flap is achieved by changing the path of the scalpel from within the soft tissue to direct contact with the bone so that a mucoperiosteal flap can be raised.

The forward course of the incision on the lingual or buccal surface is dependent on the amount of gingiva present. If there is minimal gingiva present, as is frequently observed on the buccal surface of the second or third molar, sulcular curettage and a sulcular incision, with a scalloped design, can salvage all of the gingiva for apical positioning. If, however, an abundance of gingiva is available on the lingual surface, the course of

Text continued on p. 1052.

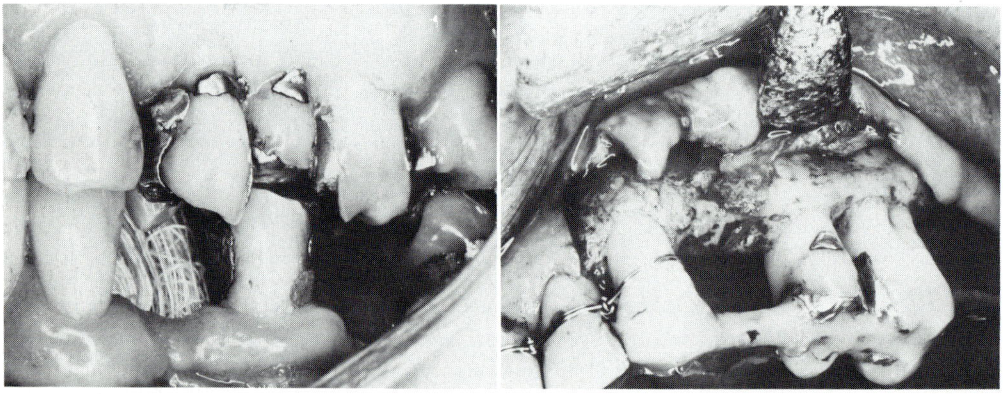

Fig. 28-26. Combined surgical procedures managing retained palatal deciduous roots and correcting a large edentulous tuberosity area. **A,** Buccal pretreatment view. **B,** Partial-thickness and full-thickness mucoperiosteal flap reveals osseous profile. Partial-thickness mucogingival flaps in edentulous and tuberosity areas have been carried out, and large block of dense fibrous tissues dissected from alveolar crest has been removed. **C,** Secondary flap has been removed on palate, and with reflection of primary flap that is preserved a retained deciduous root is exposed *(arrow).* Correction of osseous contour has been completed prior to removal of deciduous root. **D,** Another view of corrected osseous form. Mesial furcation of molar cannot be probed. Deciduous root has been removed. **E,** Osseous correction has been completed on buccal. **F** to **H,** Complete closure of surgical site with mucogingival flaps closely adapted to alveolar crests and tuberosity area. Flap margins are between 1 and 2 mm coronal to alveolar crest on roots of teeth. Note continuous locked suture. **I** to **K,** Two-year restorative view of buccal, palatal, and tuberosity areas. (In conjunction with Dr. Manuel H. Marks, Levittown, Pa.; restorative dentistry procedure by Dr. Herman Press, Fairless Hills, Pa.)

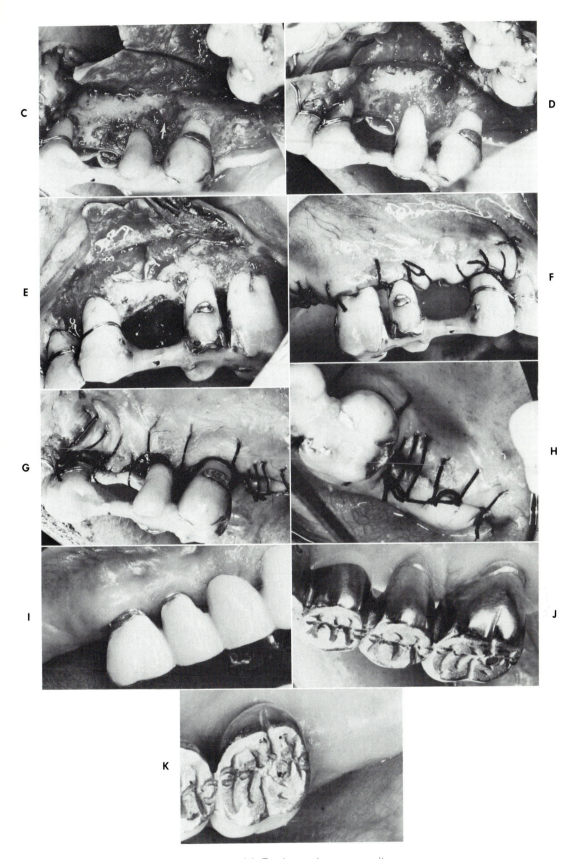

Fig. 28-26, cont'd. For legend see opposite page.

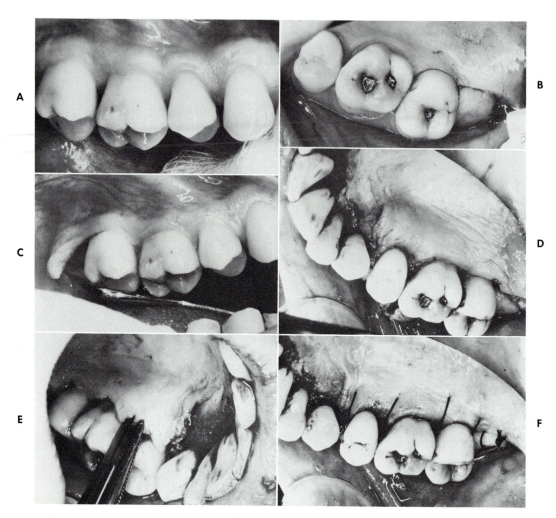

Fig. 28-27. Modification of tuberosity approach combined with quadrant surgery. This modification is utilized to protect autogenous bone implants on distal aspect of second molar and when maxillary sinus is in close proximity to alveolar crest. **A,** Pretreatment view. **B,** Partial-thickness incision is made posteroanteriorly to palatal line angle on distal of second molar, preserving entire tuberosity tissue as one flap. Vertical incision at distal terminus of operative site facilitates elevation of flap. **C,** Entire tuberosity tissue is reflected toward buccal aspect. **D,** Completion of surgical procedure. Autogenous bone implant has been inserted, and entire tuberosity flap protects implant. Primary gingival flap of palate extending to distal line angle of canine must be contoured. Flap is too long; it must be scalloped to cover alveolar crest. **E,** Gingival margin for each tooth must be managed separately. A mosquito hemostat is used to feel alveolar crest and is moved 1 mm coronally from crest and gingival flap, then is held serving as a guideline for no. 15 Bard-Parker blade to remove excess gingival tissue. Blade creates a scalloped gingival margin as seen on first and second molars. Excision extends to tip of mosquito hemostat. **F,** Closure of palatal flap by continuous sutures is seen as well as closure of tuberosity by means of interrupted sutures. Anterior area was treated by resection technique.

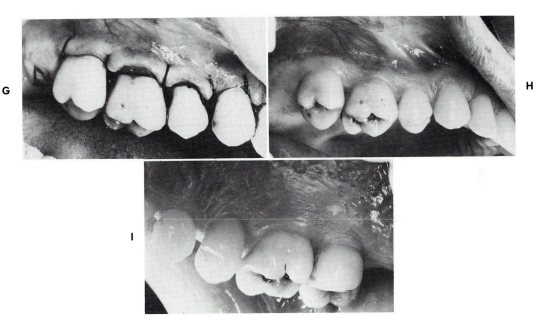

Fig. 28-27, cont'd. G, Scalloped buccal mucogingival flap is coapted by continuous suturing technique. Closed tuberosity area can be viewed. **H** and **I,** Two-year postoperative healed result. All pockets have been eliminated.

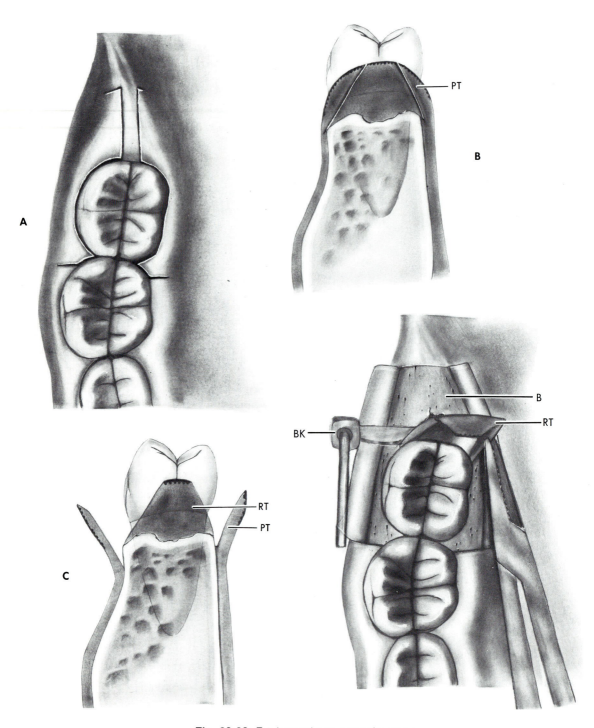

Fig. 28-28. For legend see opposite page.

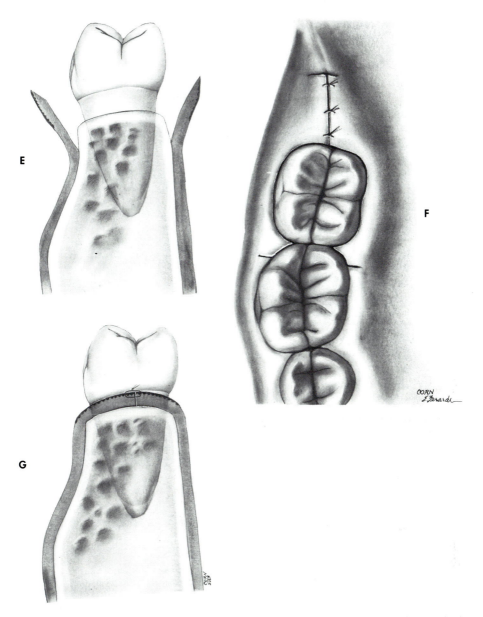

Fig. 28-28. Management of retromolar pad area. **A** and **B,** Incisional outline for surgical entry of retromolar area. Angle of incision (accomplished with Blake handle [ash] and no. 15 blade) creates a partial-thickness, *PT,* flap. Distolingual vertical incision does not extend beyond mucogingival junction. **C,** Elevation of partial-thickness flaps that become full-thickness flaps where dissection meets bone. Entire connective tissue mass of retromolar tissue, *RT,* can be removed to expose osseous defect. Extension of distal vertical incision on buccal surface aids in access for buccal osteoplasty. Note full-thickness flaps on buccal and lingual of second molar. **D** and **E,** Removal of retromolar tissue, *RT,* using Blake knife, *BK.* All is accessible for osseous correction. Hemostat may be needed to remove tissue. *B,* Buccal aspect. **F** and **G,** Tissue closure following surgery with interrupted sutures. Interrupted sutures are needed between first and second molars.

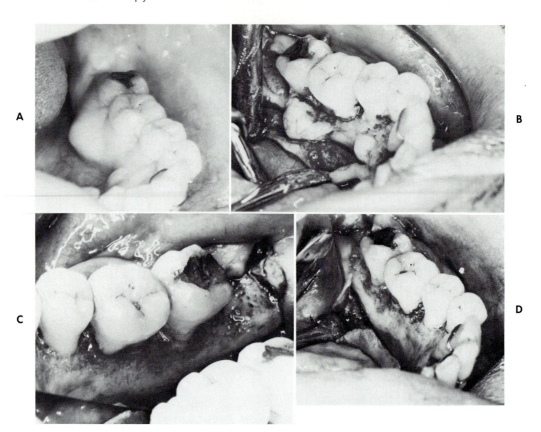

Fig. 28-29. Management of pocket elimination in retromolar pad area combined with full-thickness apically positioned flaps on lingual aspect for correction of lingual tori. **A,** Pretreatment view. Bulge of lingual tissue is related to thickened underlying osseous tissue. **B,** Full-thickness flap is raised, exposing a heavy lingual ledge of bone and mandibular tori that interfere with correction of interproximal and lingual craters. A buccal flap has been raised. Osseous defects involving retromolar can be seen from lingual view. **C,** Thin buccal and lingual flaps are initiated as a component of retromolar flaps about 10 mm distal to second molar. Portion of flaps involving retromolar area is partial thickness in design, leaving greater bulk of fibrous tissue remaining attached to alveolar crest and tooth. Original internal beveled incisions begin at buccal and lingual inclines of retromolar crest. Incisions extend forward and around distal surface of terminal tooth. In this case continuity of incisions is maintained by extending blade of scalpel to contact osseous tissue, which permits elevation of full-thickness flaps on buccal and lingual aspects. Space in retromolar area indicates where block of retromolar tissue was removed. Elimination of osseous defects is carried out in following manner: (1) no. 8 carbide bur grooves large bony mass as suggested by Ochsenbein; (2) Chandler no. 1 chisel can remove sectioned cortical bone, eliminating bulk of overgrowth; and (3) final contouring is accomplished with a Fox F3 diamond stone; this blends retromolar area with lingual osseous reshaping. **D,** Anteroposterior view of corrected osseous form.

the incision retains 3 or 4 mm of this gingiva for apical positioning, covering the crest of the bone or remaining 1 mm coronal to it (Fig. 28-29).

Ideally the length of the incision within the retromolar area should be at least 5 mm or more. However, several factors limit the extent of the original incision on the distal surface of the second molar. They are tooth position, degree to which the mouth can open, proximity of the ascending ramus, height of the external oblique ridge, and the amount of soft tissue recession and osseous defects on the lingual surface. Recently Tibbetts and Ochsenbein (1976) discussed the rationale of lingual osseous surgery.

At the point of the original incision on the distal aspect of the retromolar area a vertical incision is made through the tissue to the bone. The vertical incision extends along the crestal incline buccally

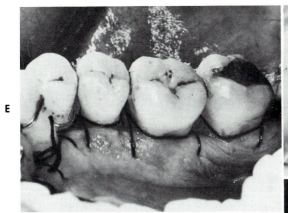

E

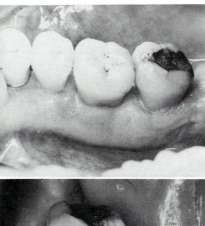

F

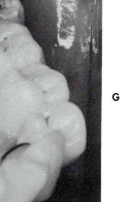

G

Fig. 28-29, cont'd. E, Note vertical incision on distal aspect of retromolar area. Because third molar is missing, vertical incision is made about 10 mm beyond second molar, enabling a gradual flow of tissues in this area. Continuous suturing positions retained gingiva of lingual flap over crest of bone. Closure of thin partial-thickness mucogingival flaps in retromolar area is by individual surgical knots, which permit close adaptation to bone. **F,** One-year postsurgical appearance of lingual tissue and elimination of pockets in retromolar area. **G,** Gingival profile in 1 year is maintained similar to alveolar contour corrected by osseous surgery.

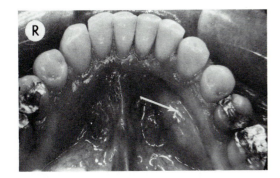

Fig. 28-30. Mandibular torus should be removed only if it interferes with pocket elimination. Similar tori existed on right and left sides on lingual aspect. Right torus, *R,* required correction as part of periodontal therapy, while left torus remained untouched, since pocket elimination did not involve this overgrowth of bone *(arrow)* (mirror view).

and lingually so that the flaps can be easily raised, avoiding laceration of the tissue. The vertical incision on the lingual aspect *must not* penetrate beyond the gingiva; otherwise there is danger of involvement of lingual vessels. The raised flaps provide access for the total excision down to the bone of the trapezoidal pad of tissue, which remains on the retromolar ridge. A spear-shaped knife or Ochsenbein chisel is used. Thus there are partial-thickness flaps on the buccal and lingual surfaces of the retromolar pad and full-thickness flaps on the buccal and lingual surfaces of the molars, both of which expose the bone that must be therapeutically managed (Figs. 28-29 and 28-30).

By coaptation of the thin buccal and lingual flaps and with removal of the fibrous tissue in the retromolar area, the height of the retromolar pad can be lowered several millimeters. Having flaps available for coaptation, treated osseous defects can be protected conveniently (Fig. 28-31). Suturing is achieved by both individual surgical knots on

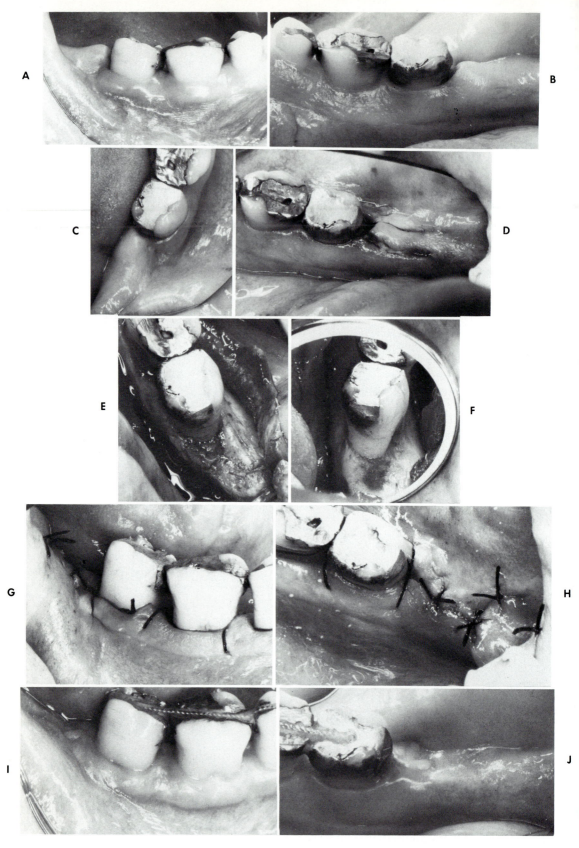

Fig. 28-31. Retromolar area surgery. Preoperative buccal, **A,** lingual, **B,** and occlusal, **C,** views. All show need for correction. **D,** Partial-thickness mucogingival flap incisions. Distance between buccal and lingual incisions is determined by thickness of tissue and bulk reduction of osseous defects required. **E,** Exposure of retromolar osseous defect. **F,** Following osteoplasty. **G** and **H,** Interrupted sutures in retromolar area. **J,** 18-month healing response.

the distal saddle area and continuous suturing on the buccal and lingual flaps. Occasionally, redundant tissue remaining beyond the retromolar incisions requires reduction. This area is treated as a submucous resection and blended with the level of the retromolar tissue anteriorly located.

All the cases described within this section have been those in which adequate gingiva has been preserved, allowing for the correction of underlying osseous defects, the elimination of pockets, and the reestablishment of an intact functional gingival unit.

GENERAL CONSIDERATIONS

In all these difficult areas problems in therapy are met by a variety of solutions. For the most part standard methods serve, although on occasion special techniques have been devised to meet the situation. Of greatest importance are not the techniques themselves but the recognition of the problems. When this is done, the way is open to find a method to accomplish the desired end. This is the meaning of rational therapy. The consideration of the area in which the problem exists and of the demands made upon that area in function, together with an intimate knowledge of the nature and composition of the tissues to be dealt with, is the cornerstone of resourceful therapy. It has been the aim in this chapter to discuss the reasoning behind each decision more fully than the decision itself. In this direction lies the solution to problems not discussed or not yet attempted.

REFERENCES

Amen, C.: Hemisection and root amputation, Periodontics **4**:197, 1966.

Amsterdam, M., and Rossman, S.: Technique of hemisection of mutirooted teeth, Alpha Omegan **54**:4, 1960.

Bar, U.: Personal communication.

Beube, F. E.: Interdental tissue resection; an experimental study of a surgical technique which aids in repair of the periodontal tissues to their original contour and function, Am. J. Orthod. **33**:497, 1947.

Braden, B. E.: Deep distal pockets adjacent to terminal teeth, Dent. Clin. North Am. **13**:161, 1969.

Bradin, M.: Precautions and hazards in periodontal surgery, J. Periodontol. **33**:154, 1962.

Corn, H.: Mucogingival surgery and associated problems. In Goldman, H. M., and Cohen, D. W., editors: Periodontal therapy, ed. 4, St. Louis, 1968, The C. V. Mosby Co.

Corn, H.: Edentulous area pedicle grafts in mucogingival surgery, Periodontics **2**:229, 1964.

Friedman, N.: Mucogingival surgery; the apically repositioned flap, J. Periodontol. **33**:328, 1962.

Goldman, H. M.: Therapy of the incipient bifurcation involvement, Oral Surg. **29**:112, 1958.

Gottsegen, R.: Frenum position and vestibule depth in relation to gingival health, Oral Surg. **7**:1069, 1954.

Haskell, E. W., and Stanley, H. P.: Vital root resection on a maxillary first molar, Oral Surg. **33**:92, 1972.

Larato, D. C.: Palatal exostosis of the posterior maxillary alveolar process, J. Periodontol. **43**:486, 1972.

Nery, E. B., Corn, H., and Eisenstein, I. L.: Palatal exostosis in the molar region, J. Periodontol. **48**:663, 1977.

Ochsenbein, C.: The double-flap approach to mucogingival surgery, Periodontics **1**:17, 1963.

Ochsenbein, C., and Bohannan, H. M.: The palatal approach to osseous surgery. II. Clinical application, J. Periodontol. **35**:54, 1964.

Ochsenbein, C., and Bohannan, H. M.: The palatal approach to osseous surgery. I. Rationale, J. Periodontol. **34**:60, 1963.

Pfeifer, J. S.: The growth of gingival tissue over denuded bone, J. Periodontol. **34**:10, 1963.

Prichard, J. F.: Various techniques in periodontal case management, J. Mich. Dent. Assoc. **40**:179, 1958.

Prichard, J. F.: Management of the periodontal abscess, Oral Surg. **6**:474, 1953.

Robinson, R. E.: The distal wedge operation, Periodontics **4**:256, 1966.

Sibley, L., and Prichard, J.: Etiologic factors contributing to bony deformities in the mandibular cuspid-lateral incisor area, J. Periodontol. **34**:101, 1963.

Simon, H. S., Glick, D. H., and Frank, A. L.: The relationship of endodontic-periodontic lesions, J. Periodontol. **43**:202, 1972.

Sorrin, S.: A method of treating the parodontal abscess, N.Y. J. Dent. **13**:387, 1943.

Staffileno, H., Jr.: Palatal flap surgery: mucosal flap (split thickness) and its advantages over the mucoperiosteal flap, J. Periodontol. **40**:547, 1969.

Sternlicht, H.: A new approach to the management of multirooted teeth with advanced periodontal disease, J. Periodontol. **34**:151, 1963.

Tibbetts, L. S., Ochsenbein, C., and Loughlin, D. M.: Rationale for the lingual approach in mandibular osseous surgery, Dent. Clin. North Am. **20**(1):61-78, 1975.

Tibbetts, L. S., and Ochsenbein, C.: Management of problems in the posterior maxilla. In Clark, J. W. editor: Clinical Dentistry, vol. 3, New York, 1976, Harper & Row, Publishers.

Yeretsky, W.: Acute fulminating suppurative periodontitis, J. Periodontol. **23**:52, 1952.

29 Gingivoplasty

The interdependence of gingival form and periodontal health has been widely accepted. As in all other biologic areas, form may be expressed as a range rather than as a fixed point. In such a physiologic range, contour, sluiceways, and festoons do not conform to a single monolithic configuration, but rather they fall into general patterns.

Nowhere is the regard for topography expressed more clearly than in the objectives of therapy. Aside from débridement, all our therapeutic efforts are directed in part to the correction of aberrant form. In fact, the sequelae of periodontal disease are described in terms of deviation from normal form.

Methods were required to deal with these deviations from normal form both in the gingiva and in the underlying bone. Gingivoplasty was introduced to facilitate dealing with abnormal form in gingiva and was essentially a surgical procedure designed to reshape the gingiva without necessarily reducing sulcular depth after curettage. Its principles were soon included in gingivectomy, and both approaches were blended into one more often than not. It soon also became obvious that gingival form was intimately related to the bone housing of the tooth and that it was necessary to reshape the outer portions of the alveolar process to secure the thin margin and spillways for protection of the gingiva. Thus osteoplasty as a technical procedure in therapy came into being. Gingival form that allows for cleansibility must be a prime goal of therapy. Thick, irregular gingival margins are obstacles in cleansing of the cervical margins of the teeth. The therapist cannot expect individuals with such gingival topography to be able to cleanse their teeth properly.

Thus in addition to other major requirements the aims of periodontal therapy should be to achieve physiologic gingival form. *The operative procedure to achieve this, should adequate gingival form not result after definitive periodontal therapy, may be termed ''gingivoplasty'' —an operative technique to contour the gingiva.*

Festooning of the gingiva to obtain interdental grooves is an important feature in reestablishing gingival physiology. These grooves are in the attached gingiva and are depressions over the indentations of the alveolar process between the root eminences of the teeth. It is necessary to blend the form of the interdental papillae onto the interdental grooves so that the resultant shallow depressions act as spillways for food.

Thus gingivoplasty as a periodontal technique consists of the shaping of gingival tissue as a plastic procedure and may be performed with a blade scalpel or electrosurgical scalpel. Diamond rotary abrasive stones and nippers are also utilized as an adjunct to the scalpel or the sole instruments for the execution of this procedure.

INDICATIONS

After periodontal therapy there are many instances in which tissue topography is so altered from the acceptable ''norm'' that it becomes advisable to change the gingival architecture. These instances may be encountered when (1) thickened gingival margins are present, (2) there are varying levels of the gingival margins in adjacent areas, (3) minor reverse gingival architecture is present, and (4) after the healing of a necrotizing ulcerative gingivitis (NUG) that still has clinical evidence of minor gingival alterations. Thus the consideration of gingival architecture after all procedures, for example, subgingival curettage, gingivectomy, flap procedures, and grafts, must be entertained, and correction by gingivoplasty must be performed if necessary. Such an instance may be cited when after curettage and despite an apparent gingival healing with a shallow sulcus a resultant improper contour with thickened interproximal papillae has resulted. Another example is the result of a deviation in gingival topography after a flap procedure. Here again, contouring of the gingival tissue is the advisable procedure to follow.

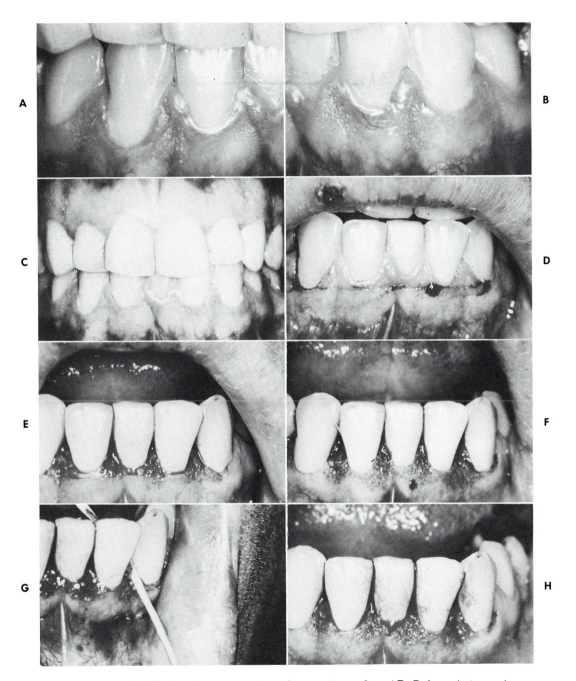

Fig. 29-1. A to **F,** Gingivoplasty procedure after curettage. **A** and **B,** Before photographs. **C,** Curettage was performed, and results can be seen. Gingivoplasty procedure consisted of beveled cut at base of interdental papillae. Interproximal cut was then made toward center of tooth, creating an interdental pyramid. With nippers, tissue was contoured. **F,** Results. In this series design of gingivoplasty was to conform tissue topographically; it did not concern itself with pocket elimination. **G** to **J,** Continuation of **A** to **F.** To eliminate any tissue tabs, twisted dental floss was utilized. Note that in **G** a small section of tissue is being engaged and removed. Once contouring of tissue has been accomplished, it is covered with a periodontal pack and allowed to heal.

Continued.

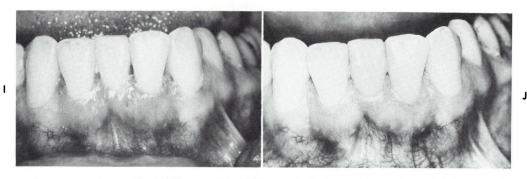

Fig. 29-1, cont'd. I, Healing in 1 week. **J,** Healing in 3 months. Note how keratinization of gingival tissue has taken place.

No form of periodontal therapy will create lasting physiologic contours in the presence of detrimental environmental changes that cause periodontal breakdown as a result of the collection of plaque in uncleansible areas. Thickened margins preclude easy access for cleansing by oral hygiene techniques.

The most common indication for gingivoplasty is the need for correction of the grossly thickened gingival margin. It should be stated at the outset that when any deformity is mentioned it connotes that *preliminary scaling followed by definitive therapy* has been performed. This means that edema and frank clinical inflammation have been resolved and therefore no longer play an active part in the deformity. It also means that any thickening and enlargement or other gross distortion from normal form is due for the most part to collagenous deposition, which is nature's attempt at healing. This is particularly common in long-term chronic irritants. These facts have important clinical implications (Fig. 29-1). (1) The density and toughness of the tissue make it more easily carved and contoured with some preoperative preparation. (2) Any surgical correction is likely to be permanent, since the tissue is a comparatively stable complex and is not so variable as inflamed edematous gingiva, provided that the local environment is favorable.

TECHNIQUE

After the operative field has been prepared for gingivoplasty, the operation may proceed immediately. Using the Goldman-Fox no. 7 scalpel or any similar instrument, the operator carves the marginal and attached gingiva with a long, sloping bevel and contours it to the desired form. In reality he slices the tissue. Some reduction of the gingival mass in the attached gingiva between the root

eminences is occasionally possible. The marginal tissue, however, must always be knifelike, and special attention must be paid to the interproximal papilla. Not only must it be shaped to the desired form, but it should also if at all possible be carved to a concave form from the labial aspect. The cut is made in the center of the col area. This excises most of the peak. In the posterior regions the cut is usually flatter because of the broader buccolingual interdental area.

As much as possible of the procedures mentioned is done by incision, since that is the quickest, least traumatic method of reducing tissue. Added rigidity in the gingival mass stands the operator in good stead at this point as well as in later stages. Rigid tissue can be incised and split so much more easily than can movable gingiva.

When the tissue has been contoured as much as practicable with scalpels of various shapes and sizes, it may be further contoured and shaped by the use of nippers or by rotary abrasives. Another modality is the use of the short-wave electronic scalpel.

NIPPERS

Nippers have become an important part of the armamentarium. These are small rongeurs capable of excising small sections of gingiva and bone as well, if it is necessary. They are small enough to insert interdentally to shape the papilla. With the advent of nippers, contouring of tissue has not only been facilitated but also is less time consuming. They can be manipulated so that the interproximal area is easily reached, and at the same time the spillway is carved and the tissue is left smooth. One distinct advantage is that a large section of tissue can be contoured with but a few nips. A disadvantage is the difficulty in their manipulation on the lingual surfaces.

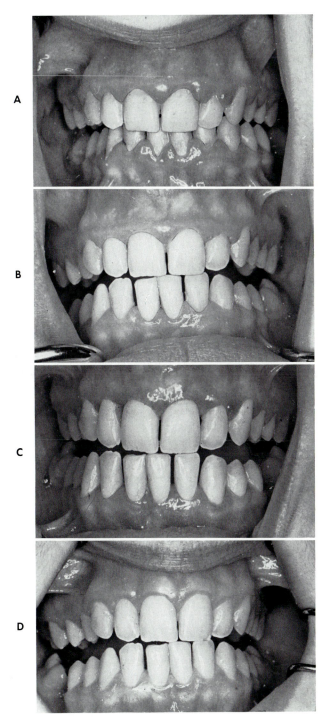

Fig. 29-2. Step-by-step procedure in a case in which gingivoplasty was utilized to achieve gingival architectural form. **A** and **B,** Results of scaling and curettage. **C,** Postoperative views 2 weeks later. **D,** Six months later. Rotary abrasive method was used to perform gingivoplasty.

SCRAPING

Using a scalpel as a hoe and passing the instrument lightly but firmly over a firm, tough tissue surface will result in a shaving of that surface. Because the blade, which should be large enough to ensure against gouging small serrations, will ride partially on the labial surfaces of the teeth, the contour created will have a tendency to conform to the general dental alignment and arrangement, with large undulant curves and a textured surface. Very gratifying results are attainable by this method. It is of course equally useful in the posterior areas both buccally and lingually. The palatal tissue yields to its recontouring when too great a mass of tissue is not involved. Since it is a shaving technique it should be reserved for small alterations. It serves excellently in finishing a gingivoplasty that was performed by incision.

ROTARY ABRASIVES

The use of rotary abrasives consists essentially of abrading tissue until it has assumed the desired form. It is not indigenous to dentistry. Dermatologists use sandpaper either manually operated or spun by motor, wire wheels, and other abrasive techniques with outstanding success in the plastic correction of heavy scarring in old cases of acne. Strangely enough, gingivoplasty is also used most often to correct scarring (or heavy deposition of collagen) elicited by a longstanding low-grade infection and inflammation (Fig. 29-2).

The rules governing the application of the rotary abrasive to soft tissue are exactly those that apply to hard tissue. A stream of water on the instrument expedites the procedure immeasurably just as it does on bone, enamel, or dentin. Accelerated speed ensures a smooth, rapid operation while the stream of water provides temperature control and prevents clogging of the instrument.

The texture of the abrasive instrument, be it the diamond stone or the sandpaper point, should be somewhat coarser than the grit used on enamel. The therapist should keep in mind that the soft tissue must be engaged by the grit to be reduced. This brings up the point of the preparation of the soft tissue for this procedure. Naturally the closer the resemblance between soft and hard

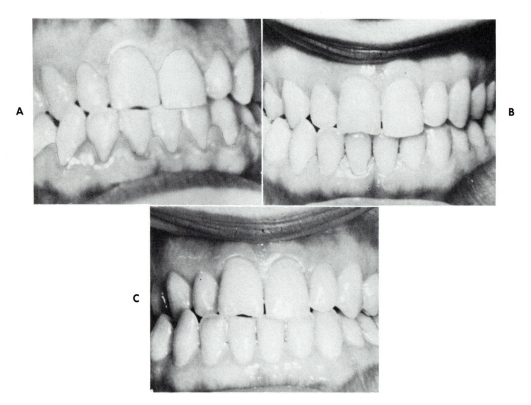

Fig. 29-3. Gingivoplasty may be utilized after gingivectomy. **A,** Preoperative findings. **B,** Changes that have occurred after gingivectomy. In evaluation of typography of lower gingiva it was noted there was thickening in lower areas. Gingivoplasty was performed; note architectural pattern postoperatively in **C.**

tissue, the closer their behavior will resemble each other in management by similar agencies. It is in this sort of situation that the injection assumes some importance. The combining of anesthesia and tissue preparation merits some attention, in the rotary method particularly. Although it is highly useful in gingivoplasty by incision, it appears to be even more so with abrasives (Fig. 29-3).

The actual abrasive points found useful are shown in Fig. 29-4. It will be noted that the grit of these points is somewhat coarser than usual; this is an important consideration. In using them we want cutting with a minimum of heat and burnishing. So far as shape is concerned, the reader may prefer others. Throughout this work the technique is the important factor and certainly not the instrument. Proper understanding of the technique enables us to operate in an extremely wide range of instrument choice.

The application of the abrasive point to the tissue is with a light intermittent pressure under water. Constant appraisal is made of the form and nature of the cut so that overcontouring is avoided.

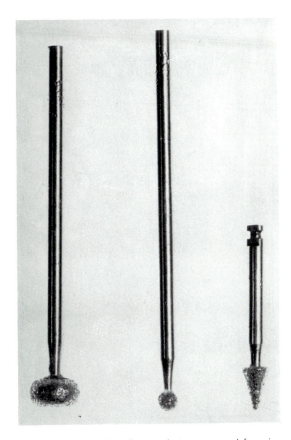

Fig. 29-4. Abrasive diamond stones used for gingivoplasty and osteoplasty.

Hollowing out the tissues between the root eminences is particularly satisfactory with this method because, should the mucosal sheath be pierced and the actual alveolar process be exposed to the stone, no difference in technique is necessary, nor is any change in instrument required. This presents us with as close an approximation of a universal instrument as can be imagined. In addition it is an instrument with which every dentist is most familiar from other aspects of practice.

Heavy and thickened gingival margins are easily contoured and thinned with a diamond stone in the handpiece by the same method of application. This is true of heavy squared ledges of palatal mucosa as well. Frequently in the performance of gingivectomy it will be found impossible to apply the scalpel in such a manner as to achieve a long, sloping bevel so necessary to the good architectural postoperative result. In those cases a bevel may be procured by either nippers or the scraping method, using the sharp blade of the scalpel as a hoe, or by a diamond stone. The stone is particularly successful in this indication. A rather large, rapidly acting stone is the instrument of choice. Needless to say, the same rules apply here as elsewhere in tissue preparation and management (Fig. 29-5).

The important thing to remember is that these techniques are either primary or adjunctive, and the operator must always be careful to avoid thinking of any of these methods in a vacuum. They are all ideally used in combination with the other methods presented. For the most part, nippers or the smaller diamond points will be used to finish what the scalpel cannot do as a cutting instrument. However, the abrasive diamond stone used either as a finsihing tool or as a primary modality is employed for the same reason: achievement of physiologic form.

It may be found that immediately after the use of a rotary abrasive the resultant soft tissue shows minute shreads of incompletely removed tissue. These are quite simply removed by applying the aspirator tip to them from a distance of 1 or 2 cm, which makes them stand up at right angles to the tissue. In such a position they are easily trimmed with fine surgical shears. When this has been done, the operative field is ready for the dressing.

The dressing is applied with a technique similar to that described for gingivectomy. Often when the gingivoplasty has produced a comparatively slight alteration in mass so that the interproximal tissue has been merely thinned, it will be found

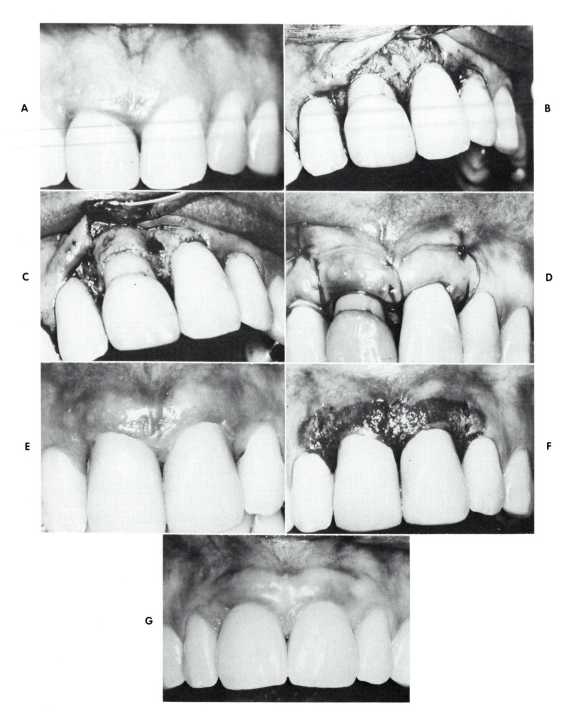

Fig. 29-5. Gingivoplasty after flap operation. **A,** Preoperative condition. Note that right central incisor has a jacket crown and that gingival margin is apically positioned in relation to left incisor tooth. **B,** Flap raised. Bone was contoured and leveled to correspond to left central incisor, **C. D,** Flap has been sutured back into position. **E,** Healing occurred but contour was not acceptable. Gingivoplasty was performed. Note thin margin and anatomic contour developed, **F. G,** Condition 2 years postoperatively. Note that gingivae of two maxillary central incisors coincide.

that the cement must be applied *over* this area, not *through* it, so that a firm lock for the dressing is not present. This occurs most frequently when only the labial area or only the lingual area is reshaped. Despite the seemingly precarious perch enjoyed by the dressing on the tissues, it seems to do quite well and is usually retained for the 4 to 7 days required for initial healing.

In all these surgical procedures we cover and protect the operative field until the area has been epithelized. The rate of healing shows a wide range of variation, with much depending on the nature and extent of the surgical interference as well as the inherent quality of the tissue operated upon.

Some indications for the rotary abrasive are the following:

1. Lingual or palatal areas inaccessible to incision or scraping
2. Tough fibrotic tissue that does not yield to scraping
3. Definitive carving between root eminences — difficult with scraping and impossible with incision except in the crudest outline
4. Contouring of thickened marginal gingiva into the dimple of a bifurcation where quarters are confined — requirements for a nonelectronic method because of proximity to bone or to a metallic restoration

ELECTROSURGICAL SCALPEL

In discussing techniques for the electronic knife one must keep in mind that here is an instrument that can affect tissues with or without the knowledge or desires of the operator. Therein lies its greatest weakness. The skillful operator will soon learn the limitations and possibilities of his instrument and will use it with a maximum of efficiency and a minimum of undesirable side effects.

With this technique certain methods of application are important. It is vital that the weakest effective cutting current be used. The reasons for this are obvious. The heavier the current, the greater will be the side effects. Therefore some trial is necessary on each machine before it can be used routinely. It also must be kept in mind that on the depression of the foot pedal, activating the current, a surge of power into the electrode is experienced that is nearly *double* that of the ordinary continuous flow. For this reason the electrode should be kept away from contact with the tissues when the foot pedal is just depressed. And, too, even with a minimal cutting current,

lengthy static application of the electrode to a given area will result in deep penetration of the current. Therefore it is important that smooth, continuous movement of the electrode be maintained on the tissues. Since it is electric current and not actual pressure by the electrode that does the cutting, one can see that the most efficacious way of using the electrode is to handle it as if painting with a fine brush.

The consequence of an application that is too lengthy or of a penetration of current that is too deep is a slow shower of bone sequestra. The electrode must never be allowed to come into contact with bone or even come near bone for any but the most fleeting motions. Constant penetrating probing is a prime necessity for establishing the thickness of the mucosa. It will be found that even with all of the usual precautions an occasional small sequestrum may be noticed.

Bone is not our only concern in the use of the electronic scalpel. Care must be taken in touching metallic fillings with the electrode because any electrical conductor in contact with the electrode becomes itself an electrode. Therefore inlays or foil fillings or amalgam restorations may cause the death of the pulp if the electrode is used indiscriminately in their presence. In fact, even a mouth mirror is avoided, and a wooden tongue blade is used for retraction because of this property.

The greatest advantage of the electrosurgery electrode is its ability to incise or shave minute masses of gingival tissue. In addition, since no force is required to do the cutting, it can be used in restricted and inaccessible areas where the steel scalpel would be immobilized and useless. For this reason it functions ideally in the carving and reshaping of fibrotic tissue, especially if the gross reshaping is done by steel scalpel so that the electrode is functioning for the minimum time.

Using the anterior gingiva as a sample area upon which to operate, we will assume that the tissues have been reshaped to a limited degree with standard steel scalpels. At this point a small round loop electrode is inserted into the cutting handle, and the minimum cutting current is activated, with the electrode held clear of tissue. With the current already flowing the electrode is used in a delicate, deliberately moving, but never quite still, manner that resembles fine painting strokes. The thickened gingiva is thinned appropriately, the thickened mucosa between root eminences is thinned, and the lingual or palatal fibrosis is reduced to conform to our concept of physiologic form. The interproximal tissue is properly contoured. The loop electrode is then changed to a needle electrode, and the interproximal tabs and inaccessible shreds of tissue are removed. The area then is generally debrided of scorched tissue remnants with scraping scalpel or curet and is dressed with a periodontal pack.

The odor of burned tissue is sometimes offensive to the patient, but deodorizing chemicals are available to make these odors inoffensive. The dressing is allowed to remain a week, and the area is inspected. On occasion it will be found to be sufficient. However, if the operative field is still not epithelized, another dressing should be applied until inspection of the field proves further dressing unnecessary.

Healing after the use of the electronic scalpel may be slower than after the use of any other method mentioned. The postoperative dressing usually is not required after 2 weeks or so, depending on the degree of epithelization of the incised tissues.

REFERENCES

Carranza, F. A.: Cuándo y por qué sacrificar hueso en el tratamiento de la paradentosis, Odontol. Rev. (Malmo) **30:**646, 1942.

Carranza, F. A., and Carranza, F. A., Jr.: The management of the alveolar bone in the treatment of the periodontal pocket, J. Periodontol. **27:**29, 1956.

Fox, L.: Rotating abrasives in the management of periodontal soft and hard tissues, Oral Surg. **8:**1134, 1955.

Friedman, N.: Periodontal osseous surgery; osteoplasty, osteoectomy, J. Periodontol. **26:**257, 1955.

Friedman, N., and Levine, H. L.: Mucogingival surgery, Dent. Clin. North Am., p. 63, Mar. 1964.

Friedman, N., and Levine, H. L.: Mucogingival surgery, current status, J. Periodontol. **35:**5, 1964.

Goldman, H. M.: The development of physiologic gingival contours by gingivoplasty, Oral Surg. **3:**879, 1950.

Lobene, R., and Glickman, I.: The response of alveolar bone to grinding with diamond stones, J. Periodontol. **34:**105, 1963.

Matherson, D.: An evaluation of periodontal osseous surgery, master's thesis, University of Rochester, N.Y. 1963.

Ochsenbein, C.: Rationale for periodontal osseous surgery, Dent. Clin. North Am., p. 27, Mar. 1960.

Ochsenbein, C.: Osseous resection in periodontal surgery, J. Periodontol. **29:**15, 1958.

Ochsenbein, C., and Bohannan, H. M.: The palatal approach to osseous surgery. I. Rationale, J. Periodontol. **34:**60, 1963; II. Clinical application, J. Periodontol. **35:**54, 1964.

Ogus, W. I.: Electrosurgery in dentistry, Dent. Dig. **48:**411, 1942.

Ogus, W. I.: Electrosurgery, Am. J. Orthod. **27:**93, 1941.

Orban, B.: Clinical and histological study of the surface characteristics of the gingiva, Oral Surg. **1:**827, 1948.

Pfeifer, J. S.: The growth of gingival tissue over denuded bone, J. Periodontol. **34:**10, 1963.

Pollock, S.: Gingivoplasty technique using rotary diamond stones at ultra speed, Dent. Clin. North Am., p. 99, Mar. 1964.

Prichard, J.: Gingivoplasty, gingivectomy, and osseous surgery, J. Periodontol. **32:**275, 1961.

Robinson, R. E., and John, R.: A simplified method for ramping interproximal bone in conjunction with a gingivoplasty, Periodontics **1:**215, 1963.

Schluger, S.: Surgical techniques in pocket elimination, Tex. Dent. J. **70:**246, 1952.

Schluger, S.: Osseous resection—a basic principle in periodontal surgery, Oral Surg. **2:**316, 1949.

Sibley, L., and Prichard, J.: Etiologic factors contributing to bony deformities in the mandibular cuspid-lateral incisor area, J. Periodontol. **34:**101, 1963.

Wilderman, M. N., Wentz, F. M., and Orban, B.: Histogenesis of repair after mucogingival surgery, J. Periodontol. **31:**283, 1960.

Zander, H., and Matherson, D.: The effect of osseous surgery on interdental tissue morphology in monkeys, Abstract no. 58, I.A.D.R. Program and abstract of papers, 1963.

30 Occlusal adjustment

Selective grinding of the natural dentition may be defined as a method of correcting the function, aesthetics, or destructive effects of an injurious occlusal arrangement by means of reshaping the teeth.

Occlusal adjustment is utilized as a modality in periodontal therapeutics. However, the therapist must realize that the grinding of the teeth to achieve a functional relationship is combined with other modalities such as temporary splinting, tooth movement, and permanent stabilization.

IMPORTANCE OF STABILITY OF TEETH DERIVED FROM GINGIVAL FIBER APPARATUS

Stability of the teeth is derived from two systems: the gingival fiber apparatus and the attachment apparatus (cementum, periodontal ligament, and alveolar and supporting bone). The dentist must recognize that mobility may come about from loss of gingival fibers due to gingival disease and a functional state too great for the supporting tissue to withstand. Therein lies a problem in diagnosis, since the dentist must be capable of establishing causation of mobility. Thus it is important that gingival disease be overcome before assaying mobility. Teeth frequently become much firmer after scaling in initial preparation and certainly become firmer after definitive treatment, even though the functional state of the teeth has not changed.

It is therefore most important that occlusal adjustment be performed once healing of the marginal gingival and periodontal disease is attained. Certainly there are many instances where the clinical crown is so much greater than the clinical root that the functional aspect is important regardless.

The dentist must be cognizant that changes in function affect the supporting structure of the teeth. The changes take place in the periodontal ligament, the alveolar bone (lamina dura), and the supporting bone. As indicated in Chapter 9, the tissue changes in hypofunction are a thinning of the periodontal ligament space with loss of principal fibers, some thinning of the alveolar bone, and loss of supporting bone. However, because of the narrow width of the periodontal ligament space the tooth is not mobile, especially if the gingival fiber apparatus is intact. On the other hand, the changes in hyperfunction are located in the same tissues, but are opposite in reaction, namely, a wider periodontal ligament, more principal fibers, and more bone trabeculae in the supporting bone area. Since the periodontal ligament area is wider, there is usually some mobility; therein lies a dilemma for the dentist since he as a rule associates mobility with occlusal trauma.

The differentials in diagnosis are the essential features. Hyperfunction shows a thicker lamina dura in the radiograph and a more solid-appearing supporting bone. In occlusal trauma the lamina dura is broken and thinned in localized areas and there is evidence of rear resorption in the radiograph. In occlusal trauma the functional range is such that the periodontal tissues are damaged (see Chapter 9).

Mobility of teeth may arise as a result of excessive loss of crestal bone. In these instances the clinical crown becomes greater than the clinical root. This has been termed ''secondary occlusal trauma.'' In these instances occlusal adjustment will make little improvement; splinting may be necessary even if the marginal structures become intact.

If mobility, however, is the result of the tissue changes occurring in the attachment apparatus, then occlusal adjustment is of value to change the functional aspects.

• • •

It is necessary to review those diseases of the masticatory system that can definitely be attributed to occlusal disorders before a discussion of the indications and rationale of occlusal adjustment procedures can be presented.

DISEASES OF MASTICATORY SYSTEM DEFINITELY ATTRIBUTABLE TO OCCLUSAL ABNORMALITIES

The masticatory system can be defined as a functional unit composed of diverse anatomic structures whose combined activity results in performing those functions normally ascribed to the oral cavity. The masticatory system includes the dentition, the periodontium, the tongue, lip, and cheek system, the salivary system, the neuromuscular system, the osseous structures, the temporomandibular joint, and the musculature necessary to move the mandible and stabilize the cranium. For purposes of a clinically oriented discussion of dental occlusion the masticatory system can be divided into three subdivisions:

1. *Periodontium.* The periodontium is composed of the attachment apparatus and gingival units.
2. *Teeth.* The teeth are composed of both calcified and soft tissues (pulp).
3. *Temporomandibular joint and associated structures.* The temporomandibular joint and associated structures include the muscles of mastication and head posture and the investing structures of the joint proper.

Disorders that are definitely caused by faulty dental occlusion are best described by reviewing the relation of the three clinical divisions of the masticatory system to occlusal activity.

Occlusal activity and periodontium
ATTACHMENT APPARATUS

The attachment apparatus is the tissue group whose apparent primary function is to sustain the root of the tooth against forceful displacement. Hypofunction is commonly encountered; the tissue changes comprise thinning of the periodontal ligament width with a diminished number of fibers extending from tooth to bone and loss of trabeculae in the supporting bone. Hyperfunction, seen in some instances, is characterized by a thickened periodontal ligament with an increased number of principal fibers, a thicker alveolar plate, and more

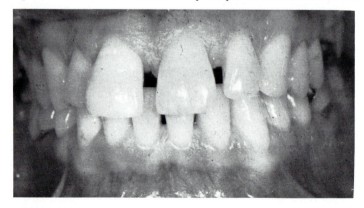

Fig. 30-1. Spreading of anterior teeth caused by posterior bite collapse after posterior tooth loss. This type of anterior tooth migration is a symptom of posterior occlusal disorder.

condensed supporting bone. Abnormal forces that exceed the physiologic tissue limits may result in the change known as occlusal traumatism. The lesion of occlusal traumatism may be defined as a destructive, dystrophic response of the attachment apparatus to adverse occlusal load. Symptoms and changes associated with the lesion of primary occlusal traumatism have been discussed his-

tologically, clinically, and roentgenographically in previous chapters but will be reviewed now.

Histologic changes include thrombosis of the vessels, ischemia of the periodontal ligament, hyalinization of the principal fibers, necrosis of the periodontal ligament, absorption of the alveolar bone, absorption of the root of the tooth, and cemental tears.

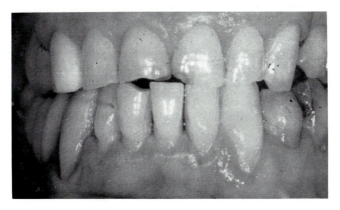

Fig. 30-2. Foreign object-to-tooth parafunction. Irregular wear of anterior teeth is due to upholsterer's tacks that were held in mouth.

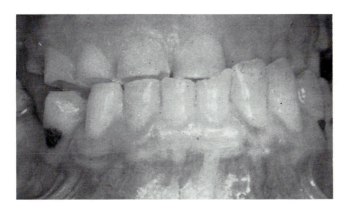

Fig. 30-3. Tooth-to-tooth parafunction. Severe pernicious retrograde wear is due to a grinding habit.

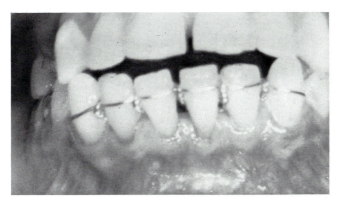

Fig. 30-4. Oral musculature-to-tooth parafunction. Anterior open bite is caused by a retained infantile swallow.

Clinical signs include increased mobility of the tooth, tenderness of the tooth, migration of the tooth (Fig. 30-1), and incomplete or complete fracture of the crown or root.

Roentgenographic signs include thickening of the periodontal ligament space, loss of definition of the periodontal ligament space, loss of continuity of the osseous tissue wall lining the alveolus (so-called lamina dura), root resorption, and osseous resorption.

Primary occlusal traumatism. The term "primary occlusal traumatism" is generally reserved for the condition wherein the lesion of occlusal traumatism is due to forces that are greater than those experienced in normal function.

Fig. 30-5. Testing tooth relationships.

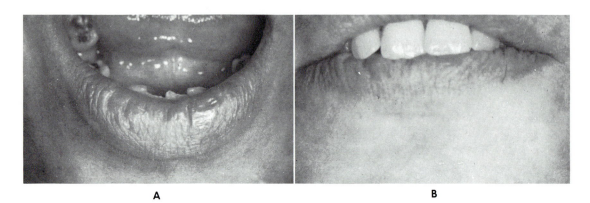

A   B

Fig. 30-6. Oral musculature-to-tooth parafunction. **A,** Indentations in lower lip. **B,** Lip biting habit.

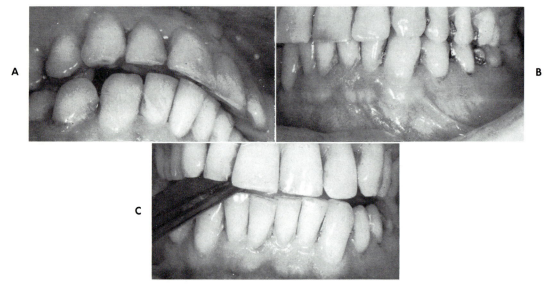

A   B

C

Fig. 30-7. Foreign object-to-tooth habit. **A,** Large overjet of canines, with wear of incisal edges. **B,** Slight overjet of opposite side of mouth. **C,** Pipestem fits overjet area exactly.

Origin of forces in primary occlusal traumatism: parafunction. Functions of the masticatory system that normally may require tooth contact or occlusal pressure are the acts of mastication, deglutition, and speech. It is the consensus of opinion that occlusal loading in the mastication of food is not the cause (except under very un-

usual conditions) of primary occlusal traumatism in the dentition that has a fairly intact periodontium.

Belief for this has been based on the fact that masticatory activity is intermittent and sufficient time for repairs is present to overcome any destruction that might occur during this function. Tooth

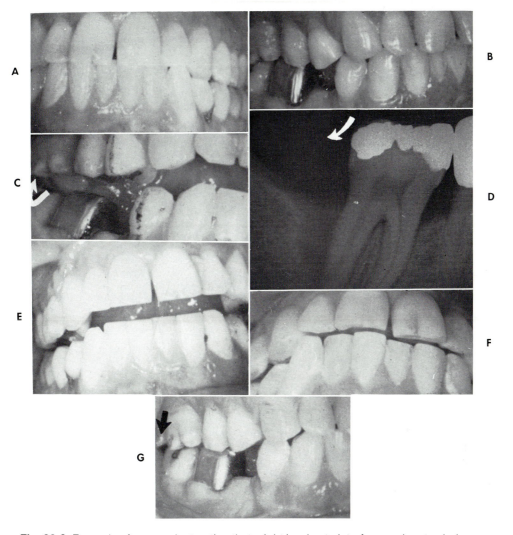

Fig. 30-8. Example of severe destruction that might be due to interference in retruded contacting position. **A,** Intercuspal position. Note spreading of anterior teeth, a symptom of posterior occlusal disorder. **B,** Intercuspal position, right side. **C,** Retruded contacting position, right side. Note contact of distal marginal ridge of lower second molar with extruded upper third molar *(arrow)*. **D,** Roentgenogram of lower second molar, showing tremendous distal bone loss. Note direction of tooth movement *(arrow)* that was most probably responsible for osseous change. Only time that lower second molar could be moved in the direction shown is during contact in the intercuspal position. **E,** Retruded contacting position, showing a negative free-way space. It is quite possible that this interference could have obliterated free-way space. **F,** Anterior tooth arrangement after occlusal adjustment by selective grinding, showing alleviation of pressure on upper incisors. **G,** After correction of occlusion. Extruded molar *(arrow)* has been corrected. (Courtesy Morton Amsterdam, Philadelphia.)

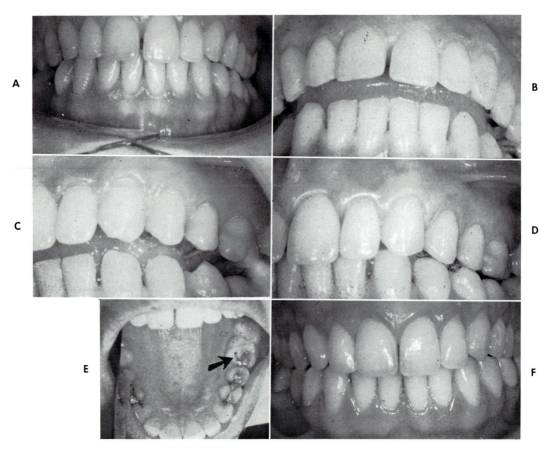

Fig. 30-9. Example of early posterior bite collapse. **A,** Spreading of anterior teeth due to increased distance between retruded contacting and intercuspal positions caused by early posterior tooth loss. **B,** Intercuspal position, showing secondary tongue thrust necessary to seal space between upper anterior teeth. This was responsible for spreading of lower incisors. **C,** Retruded contacting position, left side. **D,** Intercuspal position, left side. **E,** Mirror view, showing location of first interference of extruded molar *(arrow)*. **F,** Postocclusal adjustment by selective grinding and restoration by mandibular fixed bridges. Note reduction in anterior tooth spacing created by making intercuspal and retruded contacting positions the same by adjustment. *No tooth movement procedures were performed.* (Courtesy Morton Amsterdam, Philadelphia.)

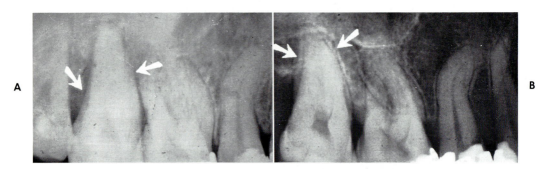

Fig. 30-10. Healing of primary occlusal traumatism after occlusal adjustment. **A,** Preoperative roentgenogram. Note thickening of periodontal ligament space *(arrows)*. **B,** Seven years after selective grinding procedures were performed. Note thinner more distinct periodontal ligament space *(arrows)*.

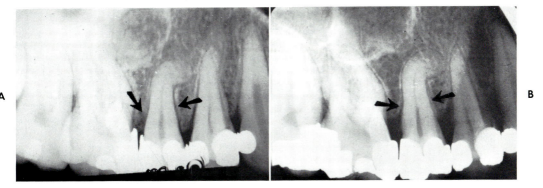

Fig. 30-11. Healing of primary occlusal traumatism after occlusal adjustment. **A,** Preoperative roentgenogram. Note thickening of periodontal ligament space *(arrows).* **B,** Seven years after selective grinding procedures were performed. Note thinner, more distinct periodontal ligament space *(arrows).*

OCCLUSAL TRAUMATISM

	PRIMARY	SECONDARY
1. Etiologic forces	Forces greater than normal	Normal forces
2. Condition of periodontium	Usual periodontium	Far less than usual periodontium
3. Healing	Potential for reversibility	No potential for reversibility Treatment is splinting

Fig. 30-12. Comparison between primary and secondary occlusal traumatism.

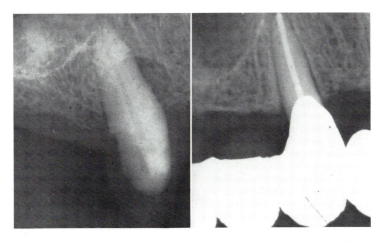

Fig. 30-13. Secondary occlusal traumatism, with severe intraosseous defect. Treatment required fixation (splinting of tooth) on a permanent basis after free osseous tissue autograft was used in infrabony defect. (Courtesy D. Walter Cohen, Philadelphia.)

contact rarely if ever occurs during mastication of foods. As Anderson, Manly, and Yurkstas each have brought out, there is strong evidence to suggest that the occlusal loading in mastication is far less than the individual's maximum biting force. The term "parafunction" is used to describe activities of the masticatory system that are outside the range of normal function, that is, the so-called occlusal neuroses and habits. Parafunctional states are believed to be initiating causes of primary occlusal traumatism because of the duration and severity with which the loads are applied. Parafunctional activity can be classified most simply in terms of the object responsible for transmitting the destructive force to the tooth.

A classification of tooth parafunction (Figs. 30-2 to 30-7) reads as follows:

I. Tooth-to-tooth habits
   A. Clenching
   B. Grinding
   C. Doodling
II. Oral musculature tooth habits
   A. Lip biting
   B. Cheek biting
   C. Abnormal tongue behavior
      1. Retained infantile swallowing
      2. Adult tongue thrusting
         a. Anterior tongue thrust
         b. Anterior tongue thrust secondary to acquired tooth spacing
         c. Lateral tongue pressure
III. Foreign object-to-tooth habits
   A. Smoking habits
   B. Finger-mouth habits
   C. Occupational habits
   D. Other habits

Tooth-to-tooth parafunctional states are perhaps the most widespread of destructive habits. Control of the habit is often difficult and requires removal of tooth interference as a secondary cause.

Nonmasticatory or empty mouth swallowing occurs throughout the day to void the mouth of saliva. The frequency of nonmasticatory swallowing appears to be directly related to the rate of saliva flow. Because empty mouth swallowing can occur quite frequently and in most cases requires tooth contact, tooth interference during nonmasticatory swallowing may also be responsible for initiating the changes of primary occlusal traumatism (Fig. 30-8).

Healing of primary occlusal traumatism after treatment. The histologic, clinical, and roentgenographic changes of the lesion of primary occlusal traumatism have the potential for reversibility if the irritant can be controlled. *Signs of healing after occlusal adjustments for primary occlusal traumatism are as follows:*

   I. Clinical changes
      A. Decrease in tooth mobility
      B. Maintenance of the migrated tooth in the corrected position (Fig. 30-9)
      C. Disappearance of pain or tenderness
   II. Roentgenographic changes, a reconstruction of what appears to be normal healthy attachment apparatus architecture on the roentgenogram
      A. Periodontal ligament space becoming thin
      B. Periodontal ligament space becoming distinct
      C. Alveolar periphery (so-called lamina dura) becoming distinct and intact (Figs. 30-10 and 30-11)

Secondary occlusal traumatism. It is important that clinical distinction between primary and secondary occlusal traumatism be understood, and it is important to note some of the salient features. Secondary occlusal traumatism may be defined as a condition of occlusal traumatism, secondary to previous periodontal disease both inflammatory and dystrophic, resulting in severe bone loss and reversal of the crown-to-root ratio. Teeth affected with secondary occlusal traumatism are so mobile that continued injury can occur in normal forces of mastication, deglutition, and pressures of the lip, cheek, and tongue.

In most cases of secondary occlusal traumatism, control of the clinical symptoms requires fixed stabilization (splinting) procedures of a permanent nature (Figs. 30-12 and 30-13).

GINGIVAL UNIT

Although occlusal forces directed on a tooth do not cause gingival change, occlusal activity will certainly have a definite effect on gingival health because of the direction of force given to foods during mastication. When there is unilateral mastication, marginal gingivitis with edema, bleeding, and increased plaque deposition due to lack of function is generally observed on the unused side (Fig. 30-14, *A* and *B*). Food impaction and food retention are related to occlusal activity. Tooth impingements (Fig. 30-14, *C* to *E*) on the maxillary and mandibular gingiva in deep overbite cases, resulting in pathologic changes in the tissues, are examples of gingival changes related to occlusal activity.

Although occlusal trauma has no direct influence on the gingiva, the reverse is true. The gingiva contributes to the stability of the teeth. Should there be a gingival inflammation present, then that stability provided by the fiber apparatus of the gingiva is lost. Thus mobility from attach-

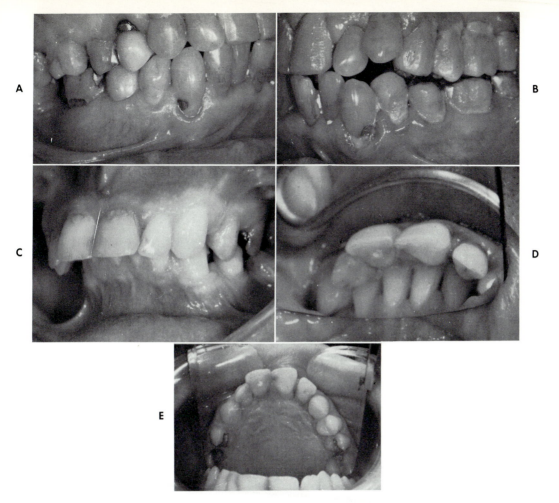

Fig. 30-14. Comparison of used and unused sides of mouth in mastication in a patient who does not brush his teeth. **A,** Used side. Note reduced plaque and absence of gingival caries and gingival disease. **B,** Unused side. Note accumulation of materia alba and severe gingival inflammation. **C** to **E,** Gingival destruction due to occlusal activity. Note extruded incisors, causing severe palatal destruction because of direct soft tissue impingement.

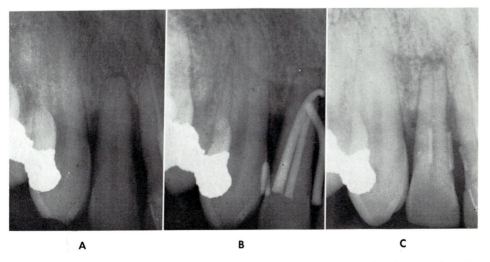

Fig. 30-15. Infrabony pocket associated with periodontitis and occlusal traumatism. **A,** Preoperative roentgenogram. **B,** Same teeth with gutta-percha points in place. **C,** Three months after operation with gutta-percha points in place. Treatment consisted of selective grinding for isolated tooth and curettage procedure.

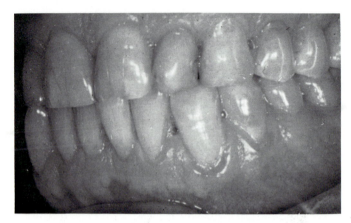

Fig. 30-16. Normal, physiologic, and ideal occlusion, age 66 years. This is an ideal arrangement of teeth for age 66. Masticatory system is free of disease. Note moderate cuspal and interproximal attrition in harmony with age of patient.

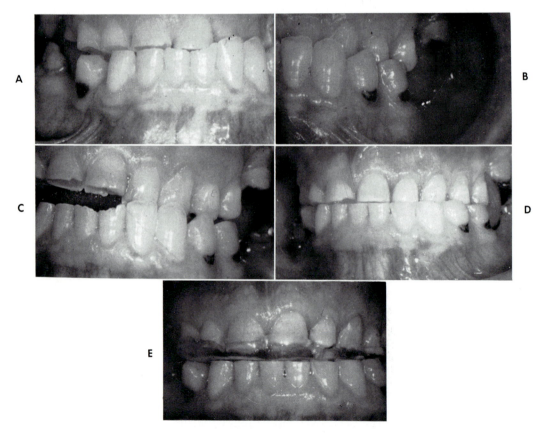

Fig. 30-17. Cusp-to-plane grinding. **A** and **B,** Preoperative intercuspal position. **C,** Retruded contacting position. **D,** Correction of occlusion, grinding to a harmonious plane. **E,** Bite guard in place.

ment apparatus change can be augmented from loss of fiber apparatus of the gingiva as a result of inflammation (Fig. 30-15).

Occlusal activity and teeth: calcified tissues

Symptoms of abnormal occlusal activity found in the calcified hard tissues of teeth are in the form of retrograde pernicious wear caused by parafunctional tooth-to-tooth behavior. Extreme occlusal attrition is generally difficult to control and may take place in the absence of advanced periodontal disease. A distinction should be made between advanced wear caused by tooth-to-tooth contact and wear caused by an interspersed abrasive medium such as coarse foods (found especially in some parts of the world), chewing tobacco, and foreign objects. Although occlusal and interproximal attrition of teeth may be considered a physiologic necessity to maintain arch continuity, wear of teeth should be in harmony with the age of the individual (Fig. 30-16).

Retrograde pernicious wear that can definitely be attributed to occlusal activity of the teeth must be considered a disease of the masticatory system that requires early treatment. Therapy may often be rendered by the removal of occlusal interferences and the fabrication of a bite guard (Fig. 30-17).

Occlusal activity and temporomandibular joint with its associated structures

Myofascial pain dysfunction syndrome, characterized by severe craniofacial pain radiating to the neck and shoulder, limited movement of the mandible, inability to perform various masticatory functions, crepitus, and subluxation, is generally multifactorial in its etiology. The common causative ingredients generally found in varying proportions are occlusal interference, emotional anxiety, heavy parafunctional activity, and muscular spasm (Fig. 30-18).

It is interesting to note that the following types of occlusal interferences appear with great frequency in myofascial pain dysfunction syndrome:

1. Nonworking interference that prevents contact on the working side (Fig. 30-19)
2. Posterior protrusive interference that prevents incisive contact of the anterior teeth
3. Intercuspal interferences that are unilateral and prevent full intercuspal contact for the opposite side of the mouth

Treatment must be directed toward overcoming each of the etiologic agents and will generally require occlusal adjustment, aspirin or muscular relaxant physical therapy and drugs, tranquilizers, and occlusal retainers. It is further emphasized that presence of the above occlusal contacts are not themselves to be considered disease entities.

INDICATION FOR OCCLUSAL ADJUSTMENT
NORMAL VERSUS PHYSIOLOGIC OCCLUSION

The term "normal occlusion" has been defined by Strang as follows:

. . . that structural composite consisting fundamentally of the teeth and jaws and characterized by a normal relationship of the so-called occlusal incline planes of teeth that are individually and collectively located in architectural harmony with their basal bones and with cranial anatomy, exhibit correct proximal contacting and axial positioning and have associated with them a normal growth, development, location, and correlation of all environmental tissues and parts. [Strang, 1938]

In reality a normal occlusion is an ideal occlusion and is the hypothetical arrangement of teeth believed to be most correct for humans. This preconceived dental ideal does not represent a norm in a statistical sense. There is little evidence

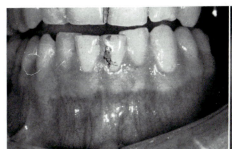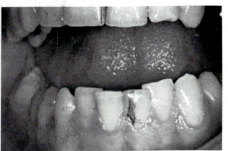

Fig. 30-18. Myofascial pain dysfunction syndrome. **A,** Slight opening. **B,** Maximum opening showing deviation of mandible to left.

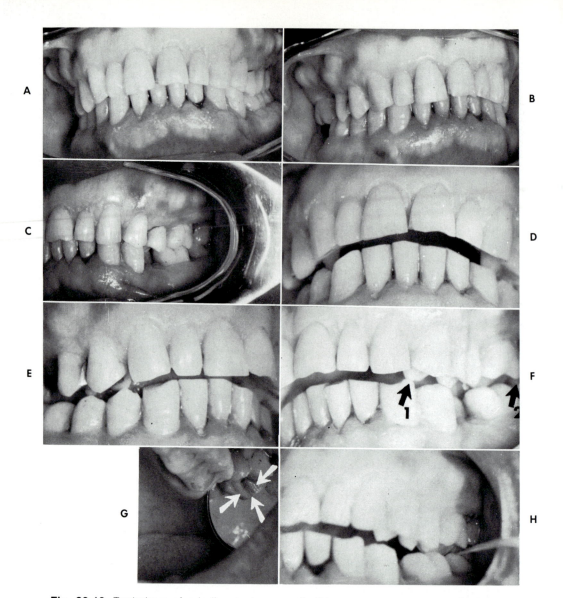

Fig. 30-19. Technique of grinding to improve (in this case a severe nonworking interference) other mechanical problems while establishing landmark correction in stage one of a cusp-to-landmark correction. **A** to **C,** Intercuspal position, preoperative views. **D,** Retruded contacting position, anterior view. **E,** Retruded contacting position, right side. Note total lack of occlusal contact. **F,** Retruded contacting position, left side. Note that initial interference is in lower canine, *1,* and that next interfering contact is in second molar area, *2.* This means that if care is exerted in grinding procedure the very same inclinded planes that interfere in nonworking contacts (Fig. 30-9) can be selectively ground while landmark relations are corrected. **G,** Typical direction and marking of a nonworking interference *(arrows).* **H,** Locating second molar nonworking interference, using dental floss to encircle discrepancy. **I** to **Q,** Postocclusal adjustment. **I,** Intercuspal position is in harmony with retruded contacting position. **J,** Protrusive glide, showing anterior teeth in group function necessary for this case. **K,** Right side, corrected intercuspal position, with correct landmark arrangement of teeth. **L,** Right side, lateral working glide, with buccal cusp contact. **M,** Left side, corrected intercuspal position with correct landmark arrangement of teeth. **N,** Left side, lateral working glide with buccal cusp contact. **O,** Left side, lateral glide. Nonworking side was free of contact. Nonworking interference was corrected during landmark correction of retruded contacting position. **P,** Markings of left upper second molar, showing supporting contact in absence of nonworking contact. **Q,** Markings of left lower second molar, showing supporting contact in absence of nonworking contact. **R,** Preoperative roentgenogram of lower second molar that was in constant pain. Note periapical thickening. There was complete remission of pain after occlusal adjustment. **S,** Postoperative roentgenogram showing periapical improvement in same tooth.

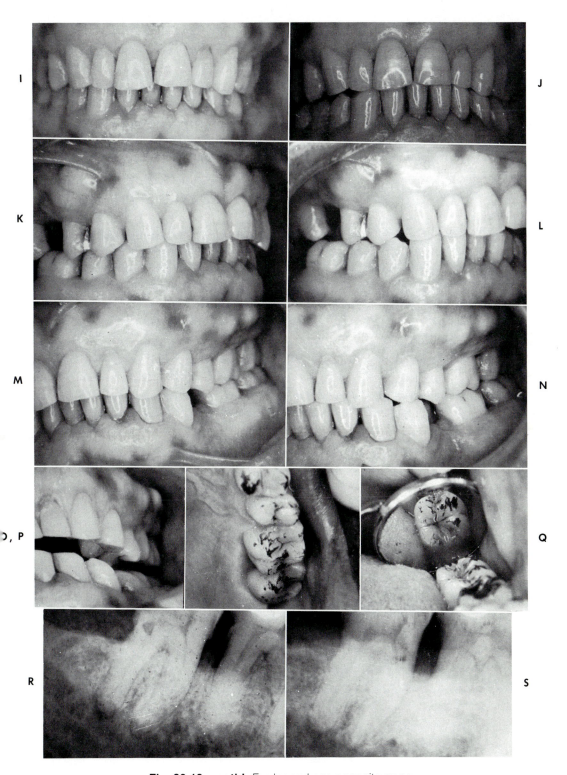

Fig. 30-19, cont'd. For legend see opposite page.

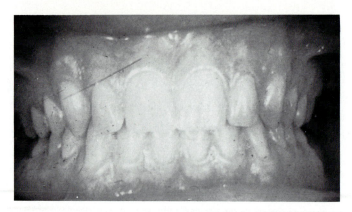

Fig. 30-20. Normal occlusion, age 18 years. This conforms to hypothetical ideal. (Courtesy D. Walter Cohen, Philadelphia.)

to tell us of the precise and exact manner in which teeth should be aligned in *Homo sapiens*. If a normal occlusion (Fig. 30-20) were used as a yardstick to determine the need for treatment in the adult, at least 90% of the general population would require occlusal correction.

PHYSIOLOGIC OCCLUSION

Physiologic occlusion refers to the dentition in the adult that has demonstrated its ability to survive despite its deviation from a preconceived hypothetical ideal of normal (Figs. 30-16 and 30-21 to 30-23). This is the masticatory system that is symptom free. There is no evidence of occlusal traumatism, retrograde wear, pulpal disturbance, or temporomandibular joint pain dysfunction syndrome. This is the dentition that chews comfortably and adequately, with an acceptable cosmetic arrangement, and requires no therapeutic change for the existing occlusal arrangement. The physiologic occlusion is a dentition, therefore, that seems to be in harmonious function with its environment.

The ability to determine clinically the presence of a physiologic occlusion is necessary in occlusal adjustment to isolate those individuals who should not receive therapeutic changes in their occlusal arrangement despite the mechanical deviation from a preconceived norm.

PATHOLOGIC OCCLUSION

Pathologic occlusion is the masticatory system that presents evidence of disease that can definitely be attributed to hyperocclusal activity. These symptoms can occur at any one or more subdivisions of the masticatory system. In order for the dentition to qualify as a pathologic occlusion one must be able definitely to ascertain the pres-

ence of a cause-and-effect relation between symptoms and occlusal activity; for example, the presence of mobility, a common symptom of occlusal traumatism, does not necessarily imply that occlusal interference is the responsible agent. Mobility can also be produced by a periodontitis or certain physiologic alterations such as pregnancy. To render a positive indictment of the occlusal discrepancy (a necessary prerequisite to occlusal correction) one must be able definitely to visualize a link between the location of the tooth interference and the mobile tooth.

The concept of prophylactic occlusal adjustment of the adult dentition is based on very little rational biologic evidence. If dentistry were called upon to adjust every occlusion that did not conform to a preconceived hypothetical dental arrangement, it would be obliged to rearrange the occlusion of the overwhelming majority of adults seen in general practice. From a practical point of view this is absolutely impossible. Furthermore, one aspect of disease with respect to occlusal change is the resistance of the host. Since this facet of periodontal pathology is one that is little understood, it becomes rather difficult to predict the initiation of disease, at least with respect to occlusal interference.

The risks of occlusal adjustment in the symptom-free adult mouth are many, but the most important is *induced dental awareness*. Induced dental awareness, or the so-called positive occlusal sense, is a high state of occlusal anxiety triggered by disturbing the existing occlusion and thereby altering the patient's accustomed reflex functions to functions of higher cortical awareness. From a psychologic point of view it may represent a great threat to a patient in terms of loss of self. The risk of inducing dental awareness rests on the therapist

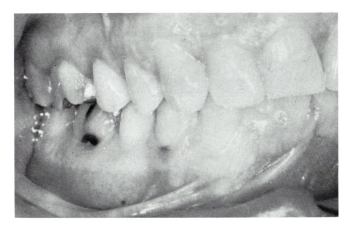

Fig. 30-21. Physiologic occlusion, age 50 years. Note that anterior overbite exceeds ideal. Despite this, dentition has survived.

A 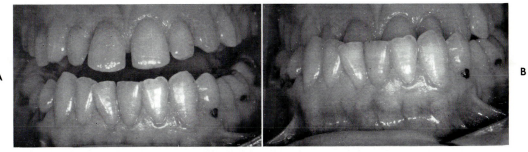 B

Fig. 30-22. Physiologic occlusion, age 45 years. **A,** Open position. **B,** Closed position, showing skeletal class III occlusion. Despite severe deviation from a class I arrangement this masticatory system is free of disease.

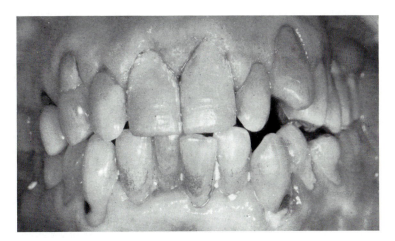

Fig. 30-23. Physiologic occlusion, age 85 years. Although there is gingivitis due to poor oral hygiene, there is no evidence of disease caused by occlusion. This mouth has given overwhelming evidence of survival despite its enormous deviation from a normal occlusion.

and deserves special attention because symptom release is therapeutically very difficult to obtain.

Interfering with the physiologic occlusion that might be individually normal for a given patient may also upset a delicate state of occlusal homeostasis that exists for the individual.

Since at this time there is division of opinion regarding the question of the exact arrangement of teeth in the ideal state, any correction of a healthy mouth is somewhat presumptuous in terms of the objectives of therapy.

A pathologic occlusion is a dentition that requires treatment. A pathologic occlusion is diagnosed only after a careful survey of the symptoms and an accurate analysis of the dynamic aspects of occlusal function and activity have been obtained.

RATIONALE OF UTILIZING A GIVEN JAW POSITION AS A THERAPEUTIC REFERENCE POINT

When the occlusion is therapeutically altered, there is an important responsibility placed on the clinician. The newly created intercuspal position must be physiologically acceptable and reliably reproducible, and it must not create an induced dental awareness.

All physiologic movements of the mandible have a definite distal closing component toward a posterior intercuspal position. The act of incision is accomplished by the mandible's closing into the food in either a protrusive or lateral protrusive position and then moving toward the intercuspal position. In masticatory cycles the mandible also moves distally toward the intercuspal position after opening and closing on the bolus of food in a lateral position. The act of masticatory and nonmasticatory deglutition requires that the mandible be braced against the maxilla in a posterior position so that the hyoid bone can be elevated while the base of the tongue is positioned posteriorly.

The terminal hinge pathway of closure is a relatively reliable, reproducible movement formed by the points of the most posterior mandibular position in each level of vertical opening. Patients can be trained to move the mandible in a terminal hinge arc as a reference pathway, and unlike any other jaw closure the terminal hinge arc does not vary with body posture (Figs. 30-24 and 30-25).

It is recognized that a posterior jaw position is necessary for the establishment of a corrected intercuspal position. Is it then possible to use the terminal hinge arc of closure as a reference position for the establishment of a therapeutically

created intercuspal position? Can the resultant occlusion be physiologically acceptable? The terminal hinge arc stands alone in its reliability as a reproducible reference area. It is our opinion that the intercuspal position can be created on the terminal hinge reference arc and be physiologically acceptable with the absence of induced dental awareness, providing that three important conditions for mandibular climate are mechanically fulfilled: (1) the occlusal vertical dimension must be acceptable; (2) the intercuspal position must be in harmony with the retruded contacting position in a stabilized manner; and (3) there must be total mandibular freedom from restraint.

Acceptable occlusal vertical dimension. That the occlusal vertical dimension must be acceptable implies that an adequate free-way space must be present in the mouth. Interocclusal clearance is necessary for the muscles of mastication to perform their functional activities. The so-called physiologic rest position of the mandible is in reality the postural position of the mandible. This is the position of mandibular tonus when the individual is either standing or seated erect. The postural position of the mandible varies with changes in body posture and will also vary with particular states of muscular contraction relative to fatigue and anxiety.

Although no fixed dimension can be given as an average free-way space, the therapist cannot arbitrarily alter this dimension. Any change in either increasing or decreasing free-way space must be approached experimentally for a trial period of time.

Harmony of therapeutically created intercuspal position and retruded contact position. In order for the intercuspal position to provide proper support to the occlusal vertical dimension in the therapeutically altered occlusion, there must be bilateral, simultaneous contacts of the posterior teeth. The nature of the tooth contacts must be of a stable form.

Mandibular freedom from restraint. That there must be mandibular freedom from restraint implies that the mandible must move in either a cyclic or a gliding manner to and from the therapeutically created intercuspal position without restraint. For this to happen, *no* cusp, inclined plane, or tooth must act as an impediment or locking device against the mandibular movement. Although the mandible may appear to have total freedom in its movement, it must not do so at the expense of a tooth or group of teeth being displaced out of their alignment in the arch. During

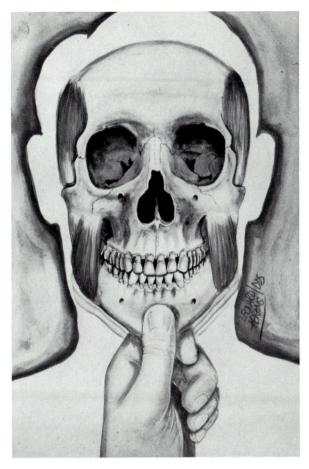

Fig. 30-24. Diagrammatic representation of location of reproducible retruded path of mandibular closure (terminal hinge). When patient is trained in this movement there should be bilateral symmetric muscular activity. (Courtesy Morton Amsterdam, Philadelphia.)

glide movements there must be little or *no fremitus* of the maxillary teeth.

OBJECTIVES OF OCCLUSAL ADJUSTMENT

The occlusal adjustment must achieve the following objectives:

1. Promote healing of the attachment apparatus
2. Promote gingival health through changes of impingement against gingiva by tooth
3. Create occlusal support for jaw positions that will be compatible with requirements of the temporomandibular joint and associated structures
4. Control tooth-to-tooth parafunction
5. Satisfy functional and aesthetic requirements of the patient
6. Maintain or create a negative occlusal sense

In promoting healing of the attachment apparatus in primary occlusal traumatism the occlusal adjustment must do the following:

1. Reduce tooth interference in basic jaw positions and distribute the load over an acceptable number of teeth
2. Direct occlusal forces axially where they will be best withstood
3. Attempt to position teeth over their alveolar housing
4. Establish correct buccolingual dimension to the occlusal table and thereby contain forces within the alveolar housing
5. Reduce grasping contacts of the teeth

In promoting gingival health the occlusal adjustment must accomplish the following:

1. Restore lost function to unused portions of the dental arch
2. Create contours of teeth that will reduce plaque deposit in the gingival sulcus
3. Correct food impaction
4. Provide for maintenance of interproximal stabilization of the teeth through proper embrasure form

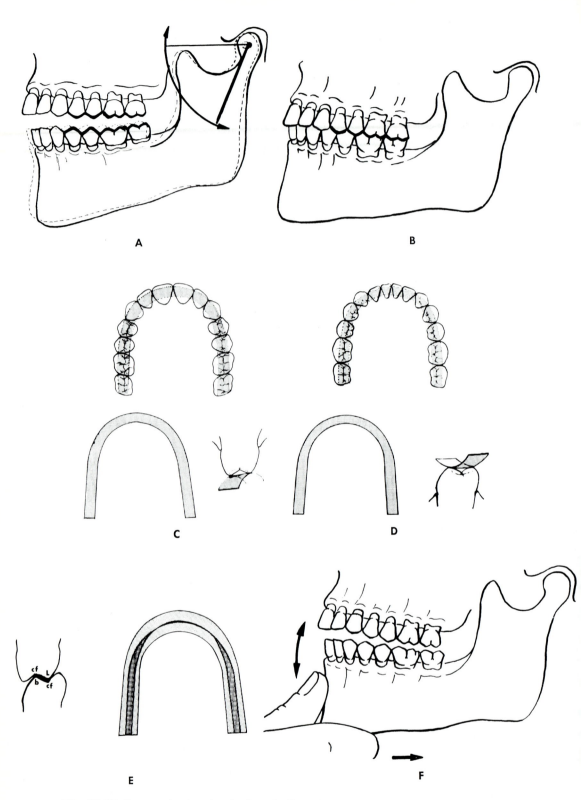

Fig. 30-25. Cusp-to-landmark grinding. **A,** Retruded path of closure (dark outlined mandible). Dotted line represents postural position. **B,** Mandible in intercuspal position. **C,** Imaginary bite block created by upper occlusal table. **D,** Imaginary bite block created by lower occlusal table. **E,** Teeth in the intercuspal position, with occlusal landmarks in correct position. *b,* Bucco-occlusal line of lower posterior tooth; *cf,* central fossa line; *L,* linguo-occlusal line of upper posterior tooth. Overlap of bite blocks shows shaded area of supportive contact. **F,** Mandible closed *(vertical arrow)* in retruded path *(horizontal arrow).*

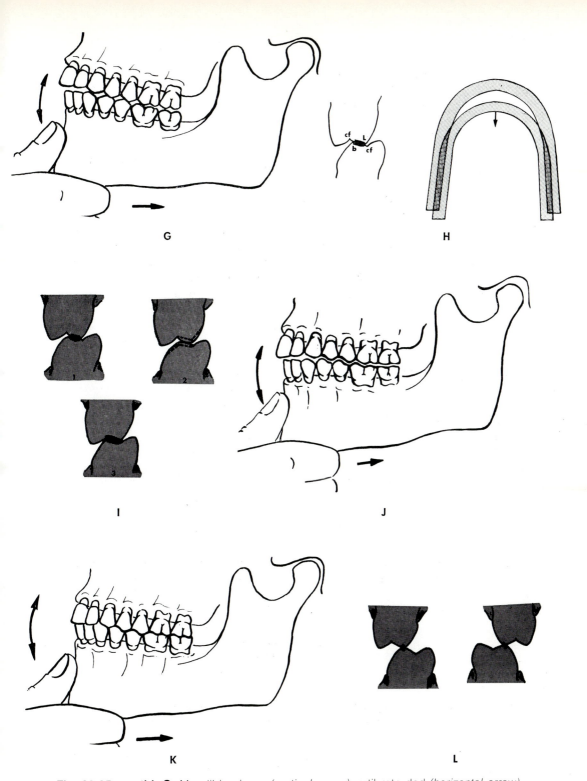

Fig. 30-25, cont'd. G, Mandible closes *(vertical arrow)* until retruded *(horizontal arrow)* contacting position is reached. **H,** Change in landmarks when mandible is moved from retruded contacting to intercuspal position. Note that bucco-occlusal line of lower posterior tooth, *b,* is now lingual to upper central fossa line, *cf.* Upper linguo-occlusal line, *L,* is buccal to lower central fossa line, *cf.* Note also that overlap of bite blocks is diminished so that area of occlusal support is greatly diminished. **I,** *1,* initial interference with landmarks not on target; *2,* initial grinding to widen teeth to achieve correct landmark positioning. This will be followed by a compensatory narrowing only after correct landmark relations are ensured, as seen in *3.* **J,** Correction of mesiodistal landmarks. Note concave inclined planes—distal lower and mesial upper—in order to give proper support to occlusion. **K,** Final landmark correction. Thus one is ready to proceed to stage two of adjustment. **L,** If in retruded contacting position this is relation of landmarks, obviously no correction by grinding is possible. (Courtesy Morton Amsterdam, Philadelphia.)

In creating occlusal support for jaw positions compatible with the 'requirements of the temporomandibular joint the following conditions must be met:

1. The occlusion must be at an acceptable occlusal vertical dimension, with adequate free-way space.
2. The intercuspal position must be in harmony with the retruded contacting position, with stabilized occlusal support.
3. There must be total mandibular freedom from restraint so that (a) the mandible may close in cyclic or glide movement to and from the intercuspal position with mechanical ease; (b) posterior protrusive and nonworking occlusal contact may be eliminated; and (c) the anterior teeth may be prevented from parting in protrusive and lateral glide movement.

In controlling tooth-to-tooth parafunction the adjustment will eliminate occlusal interference in the form of locking or deflective contacts. Restraining contact has been considered by Fox, Ramfjord, and Posselt as a secondary and sometimes a primary cause of tooth-to-tooth parafunctional activity. It is believed that patients under these conditions are attempting to grind out the occlusal and incisal prominences. The removal of tooth interference is important in controlling clenching, grinding, and doodling habits.

In satisfying functional and aesthetic requirements of the patient, especially when there is a deepened vertical overlap of anterior teeth, some aesthetic benefit can be given by reshaping and shortening the incisors and canines. If the cementoenamel junction is exposed, the tooth can be reshaped to give the illusion of a slightly longer anatomic crown. Care must be taken not to destroy the incisive guide function of the anterior teeth.

In maintaining or creating a negative occlusal sense during the adjustment the following will be necessary:

1. Occlusal adjustment will be performed only where indicated.
2. Bite plane appliances will be used frequently if the patient seems overly aware of the adjustment procedures.
3. The occlusal arrangement will never be drastically altered too suddenly.
4. Careful discussion of the occlusal adjustment procedure with the patient will take place prior to treatment.

METHODS OF OCCLUSAL ADJUSTMENT

The pathologic occlusion is treated by methods of occlusal adjustment that can be likened unto forms of "clinical arithmetic." Occlusal adjustment may take place as a "subtraction" procedure, which is selective grinding or the extraction of an extruded tooth; it may take place as an "addition" procedure, which is restorative dentistry; or it may take place as a "multiplication or division" procedure, which would be orthodontics or minor tooth movement. The selection of the definite kind of arithmetic necessary for a given situation is based on a twofold analysis: (1) the needs of the dentition with respect to the nature of the symptom complex must be determined and (2) the mechanical arrangement of the teeth must be dynamically examined. When selective grinding is to be employed as the occlusal adjustment method of choice, it requires the ability to predict a reasonable mechanical result by this approach. An analysis and understanding of the landmarks of teeth give us a definite clue as to the kind of occlusal adjustment procedure that is to be performed.

DENTAL ARTICULATION AND LANDMARKS OF TEETH

Before any discussion of occlusal analysis can take place, a brief review of the possibilities of tooth contact, the incline plane arrangements of teeth, and their relation to the spatial aspects of jaw kinematics is necessary.

Groups of teeth

Two groups of teeth, the posterior and the anterior teeth, are the focus of the ensuing discussion (Figs. 30-26 and 30-27).

The posterior teeth should be responsible for sustaining the forces necessary to support the occlusal vertical dimension. These groups of teeth, composed of premolars and molars, have occlusal surfaces that appear to be well designed to sustain occlusal load in an apical direction (assuming that tooth alignment is in harmony with basal bone).

The anterior teeth have the capacity to separate the posterior teeth during mandibular glide movements. This group is composed of canines and incisors and provides the so-called incisal guidance. They are ideally suited for this role by virtue of their anterior position in the arch and the design of their biting surfaces.

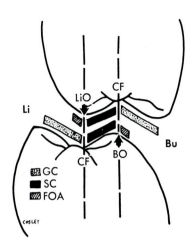

Fig. 30-26. Buccolingual landmark relations. *Li,* Lingual; *Bu,* buccal. Note the following: *BO,* bucco-occlusal line angle of lower posterior tooth; *CF,* central fossa line of upper posterior tooth and lower posterior tooth; *LiO,* linguo-occlusal line of upper tooth; *GC,* guiding incline of upper posterior tooth and lower posterior tooth; *SC,* supporting cusp of upper tooth and lower tooth; *FOA,* functional outer aspect of upper or lower teeth. (Courtesy Morton Amsterdam, Philadelphia.)

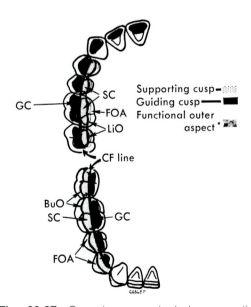

Fig. 30-27. Cuspal groups include supporting cusps, guiding inclines (note that this includes lingual surface of upper anterior teeth), and *FOA* (note that this includes incisal edges of lower anterior teeth). Landmarks of teeth include bucco-occlusal line, central fossa line, and linguo-occlusal line. (Courtesy Morton Amsterdam, Philadelphia.)

CUSPAL GROUPINGS OF POSTERIOR TEETH

The posterior occlusal surfaces are divided into two classes of cusps: (1) supporting and (2) guiding. Supporting cusps perform the supportive role of posterior teeth with respect to the occlusal vertical dimension. They are the buccal cusps of the mandibular teeth and the lingual cusps of the maxillary teeth. The supporting cusps function in their capacity by contacting the opposing occlusal surfaces. Guiding cusps have the potential for occlusal contact only when the mandible moves out of the intercuspal position in glide movements. The guiding cusps are composed of the buccal cusps of the maxillary teeth and the lingual cusps of the mandibular teeth. They differ from the supporting cusps in that they do not oppose the central portions of the opposite occlusal tables.

RULES FOR LANDMARK RELATIONS OF POSTERIOR TEETH

The rules for landmark relations of the posterior teeth are as follows:

1. *Buccolingual landmarks* (Fig. 30-26). (a) The bucco-occlusal line angle of the mandibular posterior teeth is related to the central fossa line of the maxillary posterior teeth, and (b) the linguo-occlusal line angle of the maxillary posterior teeth is related to the central fossa line of the mandibular posterior teeth.

2. *Mesiodistal landmark.* In a quadrant all supporting cusps, except two, are cradled on interproximal marginal ridge areas. The exceptions are the mesiolingual cusps of the maxillary molars and the distobuccal cusps of the mandibular molars. These cusps are cradled by opposing central fossa areas (Fig. 30-28).

Functional outer aspect (FOA) areas of supporting cusps

For the supporting cusps to be properly cradled by the opposing occlusal table a portion of the outer aspects must be included in its supporting contacting role. This is 1 mm of the outer aspect and is referred to as the functional outer aspect of the supporting cusps. Although depicted diagrammatically as a separately inclined plane situation, it is in reality a roundness of cuspal form that is present without distinct boundaries and that ensures the total cradling of a cusp by its opposing occlusal relief. The functional outer aspect area has a second role that is quite important, for this is the area on the outer aspect of the supporting cusp that has the potential for contact with the opposing

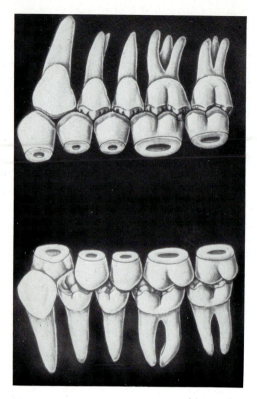

Fig. 30-28. Mesiodistal landmarks of teeth in inter-cuspal position. All supporting cusps fit between opposing teeth except mesiolingual cusps of upper molars and distobuccal cusps of lower molars. (Courtesy Morton Amsterdam, Philadelphia.)

guiding inclines during mandibular glide. In the adjusted occlusion, contact of the mandibular FOA with the maxillary guiding inclines may be required.

Since the mandibular anterior teeth have potential for contact with the lingual surfaces of the maxillary anterior teeth, there is a conceptual continuation of the functional outer aspect area of the lower posterior teeth along the incisal edges of the mandibular anterior teeth. The FOA area can be considered as an area that runs from the second molar on one side of the mandibular arch around and across the incisal edges of the mandibular canines and incisors to the second molar on the opposite side. The FOA ribbon is an area of approximately 1 mm in width. The outer aspects of the guiding cusps fall outside the occlusal table and as such do not have functional areas.

The lingual surfaces of the maxillary canine and incisors are mechanically similar to the guiding inclines of the guiding cusps and are part of the guiding incline group. It is interesting to note that the anterior teeth retain certain features present

in the posterior teeth. The mandibular anterior teeth have functional outer aspect areas found in supporting cusps. The maxillary anterior teeth have guiding inclined areas found on guiding cusps.

Landmark relations in adjusted occlusion

Landmark relations in the adjusted occlusion are as follows:
1. The buccolingual occlusal landmarks must be coordinated in the corrected intercuspal position (Fig. 30-25, *I*).
2. The mesiodistal landmarks must be modified so that a marginal ridgelike concavity can be created on the cuspal incline to allow proper platform stability to the supportive cusp in the corrected intercuspal position (Fig. 30-25, *J* and *K*).
3. In glide movements the anterior teeth will be called upon to separate the posterior teeth. This will be accomplished by the following:
   a. The lower incisor, canine, and first premolar FOA will contact the upper incisor and canine guiding inclines.
   b. In lateral glide only the FOA of the mandibular supporting cusps of the working side will be permitted to contact the guiding inclines of the upper guiding cusps.
   c. Every effort is made to avoid or eliminate nonworking or posterior protrusive contacts (Figs. 30-29 and 30-30).
   d. The final design of the corrected occlusion will be dependent on the mechanical arrangement of the teeth, the relative health of the periodontium of the various teeth present, and the number and distribution of teeth.

EXAMINATION OF OCCLUSION

Examination of the occlusion is preceded by a thorough periodontal charting of mobility, pocket formation, and roentgenographic findings. The actual examination of the occlusion is divided into three phases:
1. Occlusal history
2. Examination of the study casts in both guided and unguided function
3. Direct examination of the dynamic aspects of the mouth in both guided (passive) and unguided (active) function

A specific chart has been designed for use in recording the occlusal findings and is currently in

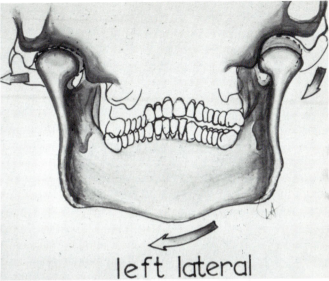

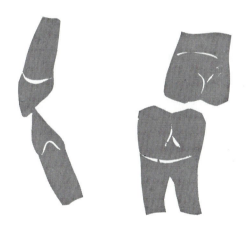

Fig. 30-29. In adjusted occlusion there might be contact of buccal cusps on working side only. Note that *there is no* cross tooth and cross arch balancing contact. (Courtesy Morton Amsterdam, Philadelphia.)

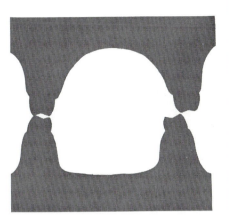

Fig. 30-30. In adjusted occlusion anterior teeth separate posterior teeth in protrusive mandibular glide. (Courtesy Morton Amsterdam, Philadelphia.)

use at the School of Dental Medicine, University of Pennsylvania. The purpose of any chart is that of a mnemonic device to train the practitioner to follow a thorough and orderly course in detailing specific findings to aid in the diagnosis and treatment. The chart to be described is redundant by intent so that certain aspects of occlusal function will be emphasized.

Occlusal history

Patient evaluation of aesthetics, function, and comfort. The patient evaluation portion of the occlusal history chart is concerned with whether there is adequate function in the present dental arrangement and attempts to evaluate the feelings of the patient with respect to subjective symptoms of the masticatory system in terms of the patient's ability to function comfortably.

Aesthetics may be extremely important to the patient and will be significant to the therapist only if the patient is not happy with the way his teeth look. Many patients will develop parafunctional oral musculature activities to hide missing teeth in the anterior portion of the mouth. These lip and cheek habits could be significant etiologic factors of occlusal disease. Patients will tend to become overly aware of their teeth if there is an aesthetic problem. Anterior tooth spacing must be differentiated between eruptive and secondary as relates to posterior bite collapse.

During the occlusal examination the patient is asked, "What do you think about how your teeth look?" It is important to remember that although the dentition may not satisfy the examiner's eye for aesthetics, the patient may be unaware of a cosmetic liability, in which case it would be poor clinical judgment to alter the anterior arrangement without prior discussion (Fig. 30-32).

If there are a sufficient number of teeth absent, phonetics may be impaired. This occurs primarily with anterior tooth loss. To check the possibility of a phonetic problem, the operator asks the patient whether there are difficulties in pronouncing any words. Here again the value judgment is in the hands of the patient, not the operator.

The ability to chew certain types of foods is primarily important to the patient. Subjective complaint of an inability to chew properly may be the first sign of occlusal disorders that do not allow the teeth to function properly. Many times these discrepancies can be easily corrected, resulting in a return of masticatory function. In the presence of missing teeth it is important to ask the patient about his feelings with respect to masticatory

---

I. *Occlusal history*

A. Patient evaluation of aesthetics, function, and comfort

	Yes	No
1. Aesthetics		
2. Phonetics		
3. Mastication		
List foods difficult to chew		
4. Tooth sensitivity		
Location		
5. Food impaction		
Location		
6. Missing teeth		
Location		
Duration		
7. Spacing of teeth		
Location		
Duration		

B. Habit history

	First visit	Second visit
1. Tooth-to-tooth contact		
Clenching		
Grinding		
Doodling		
2. Oral musculature– to–tooth contact		
Adult tongue thrust		
Infantile tongue thrust		
Lip biting		
Cheek biting		
3. Foreign object–to– tooth contact		
Notes		

II. *Examination of study casts*

A. Examination of each arch

	Continuity; rhythmicity	Contact areas	Marginal ridges	Malposed teeth	Food impaction	Wear patterns	Plane of occlusion; curve of Spee
1. Maxilla							
2. Mandible							

B. Examination of study casts in the intercuspal position

1. Angle classification _____

2. Overbite _____ mm

3. Overjet _____ mm

4. Landmark relations: mesiodistal _____ buccolingual _____

5. Severe deformities: postbite collapse _____

   Migration of anterior teeth _____ Open bite _____

C. Examination of study casts in the retruded contacting position

1. Location of initial interferences _____

2. Mandibular deflection: direction _____ distance _____

3. Landmark relations: mesiodistal _____ buccolingual _____

Chart 30-1. Occlusal history and examination. (Courtesy Department of Periodontics, School of Dental Medicine, University of Pennsylvania.)

ability to determine the need for replacement services.

The patient is asked if he is aware of any teeth being sensitive to hot or cold or to touch. A sensitive tooth may be directly under trauma from the occlusion, or it may be sensitive due to a pulpitis of another etiologic cause. The patient may avoid this tooth, resulting in an abnormal mandibular movement that will place other teeth under severe occlusal stress.

Subjective awareness of the location of a food impaction may also result in abnormal mandibular movements during the masticatory cycle. This is primarily due to a plunger cusp on improper embrasure form.

Missing teeth and spacing of teeth can best be recorded from examination of models; however, the duration of loss and the spacing of teeth can be significant. A tooth that does not have an antagonist will have the tendency to erupt continuously, while teeth proximal to an extraction site will tend to drift. Subtle changes in tooth position resulting from the loss of one tooth can adversely affect the entire dentition. For this reason early or immediate replacement of missing teeth is highly recommended, especially in the young adult. However, often an elderly patient will present himself with a missing tooth that has been absent for 10 or more years, yet the proximal teeth and the antagonist will not have drifted or supererupted. Obviously this patient has been able to resist the adverse effects that usually occur when a missing tooth is not immediately replaced. In this case no restorative service is indicated.

Habit history (Figs. 30-2 to 30-7). The examiner at this point should have a good evaluation of the patient's opinion of the dentition and relative state of occusal awareness. Most individuals are

---

III. *Examination of dynamic aspects of the mouth in both unguided and guided functions*

  A. Unguided (active) function

    1. Postural position: free-way space _____ mm

    2. Swallowing, normal _____ Adult tongue thrust _____

       Infantile tongue thrust _____ Tooth displacement _____

    3. Maximum opening _____ mm: deviation _____ direction _____

    4. Fremitus in habitual closure: location _____ magnitude _____

    5. Horizontal mandibular glide: fremitus _____

Interference	Right	Left
Working		
Balancing		
Protrusive		

  B. Guided (passive) function

    1. Initial interference at retruded contacting position

      Location _____

      Buccolingual landmark relations _____

      Mesiodistal landmark relations _____

      True free-way space _____ mm

    2. Mandibular movement from retruded contacting to intercuspal position

      a. Distance of mandibular deflection _____ mm

      b. Direction of mandibular deflection _____

IV. *Diagnosis*

V. *Treatment plan*

Chart 30-1, cont'd. Occlusal history and examination.

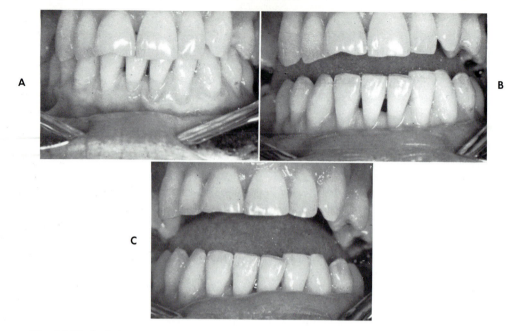

Fig. 30-31. A, Chipped anterior tooth in full occlusion. **B,** Mouth in open position, showing severity of overbite that will tolerate aesthetic shortening. **C,** After aesthetic shortening of anterior teeth. Note that prominence of cementoenamel junction of upper right central and lateral incisors (exposed by gingival surgery) is reduced by so-called odontoplasty.

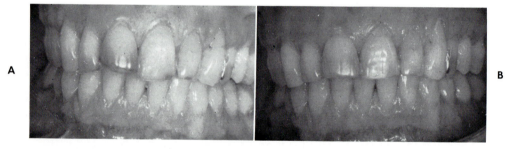

Fig. 30-32. A, Prior to aesthetic correction of anterior teeth. **B,** After correction. Note that amount of overbite permits such a correction.

unaware of parafunctional habits, since they are initiated at the unconscious level.

During the occlusal examination the patient may appear to be extremely apprehensive. He may unconsciously perform an oral habit in the examiner's presence that he will deny when specifically asked about it. The chart is therefore arranged so that the questions are asked at the first and second visits.

Parafunctions associated with tooth-to-tooth contact, for example, clenching, doodling, and bruxing, are important potential etiologic factors of occlusal traumatism. Although the patient may not be aware of any such habit, the examiner may suspect abnormal occlusal activities by the pa-

tient's emotional state or by the presence of wear facets on the study casts.

The patient is requested to report any habits of which he may become aware between the first and second visit. The examiner must be extremely careful, however, not to make the patient overly aware of the occlusion, especially if he senses that the patient is under emotional stress or anxiety.

Recording of an oral musculature–to–tooth contact habit must be done during direct examination of the patient. The patient is asked to swallow as he normally would, and the examiner observes the activity of the oral musculature. In normal swallowing there should not be any tongue thrust. In the infantile tongue thrust there is great activity or contraction of the orbicularis oris and facial muscles during the swallowing tongue thrust. In the adult tongue thrust this muscle activity is absent, yet the tongue is thrust between the anterior teeth. In the occusal examination we are recording only the presence or absence of a tongue thrust, not its etiology. In many patients with advanced periodontal disease in which fanning of the anterior teeth is associated with loss of the posterior support and a decrease in the vertical dimension, tongue thrusting may be secondarily present to seal the spaces between teeth during the swallowing act. If the teeth are in secondary occlusal traumatism, this tongue thrust becomes an important etiologic factor that must be considered and treated during therapy.

Recording habits of lip biting and cheek biting can be done by examining the mucosa of the lip and cheeks for hyperkeratinized areas at the level of the occlusal plane. If such areas are present the patient should be asked to demonstrate the habit to verify the etiology of the hyperkeratinized areas.

Foreign object–to–tooth contact, for example, biting pencils, pens, the ends of eyeglass frames, fingernails, and pipestems, may be elicited. Occupational habits such as holding nails between the teeth in the case of carpenters and upholsterers may account for traumatism of the teeth.

The presence of chipped or bizarre wear of the incisal edges of teeth generally implies foreign object biting.

Examination of study casts

Examination of each dental arch. Intra-arch form and alignment provide important information and may strongly foreshadow occlusal functional disturbances. This portion of the chart is arranged primarily to aid the examiner in thinking in terms of a comparison between the patient's dentition and an image of harmonious tooth alignment. Although deviations from a preconceived image do not automatically infer disease, the examiner is better able to analyze the functional dynamics of the dentition when he can recognize these differences, that is, improper continuity of tooth alignment, contact areas, marginal ridges, and so on.

Examination of study casts in intercuspal position. The angle classification is indicated on the chart, the overbite is measured, and the overjet is evaluated. Our concept of overjet is slightly different from the definition usually found in various texts. Overjet is the distance from the in-

cisal edge of the mandibular incisors to the palatal surface of the maxillary incisors. Using this description of overjet, one finds that it is possible to have a 0.0 mm overjet in the natural dentition even though the maxillary incisors are properly aligned and present a normal overbite relation. Recording the overjet in this manner is only a tool in understanding the potential of occlusal traumatism in the anterior segments of the mouth.

Examination of study casts in retruded contacting position. To observe the behavior of the interarch tooth relations in the retruded contacting position one must properly mount the study casts on a semi- or fully adjustable articulator. This requires a facebow orientation of the upper cast and a positional record of the lower cast on the retruded path. So that errors can be avoided, the cast mountings must be authenticated by comparison with the intraoral situation with respect to the accurate duplication of both the intercuspal and retruded contacting positions.

The following observations must be made:
1. Buccolingual landmark relations in the retruded contacting position
2. Mesiodistal landmark relations in the retruded contacting position
3. Spatial relations in the mouth in terms of the teeth free of contact in the retruded contacting position
4. Anterior tooth relations (incisal guidance) in the retruded contacting position
5. Location of the initial interference and the amount and direction of deflection of the mandible to full closure

Examination of dynamic aspects of occlusion in both guided and unguided function

The free-way space is recorded in millimeters (Fig. 30-33). Although it may seem adequate in the convenience position, there may be impingements on the free-way space when the mandible is placed in the retruded position. It is possible to have a normal free-way space of 3 mm in the incisor area from the convenience position; yet when the mandible is retruded and there is a posterior interference in the retruded path of closure, the amount of separation between the teeth in the incisor region may be 4 or 5 mm. In this case there is truly a negative free-way space of 1 or 2 mm, which occurs at the point where the mandible makes initial contact in hinge closure. The negative free-way space is potentially a very serious source of trauma.

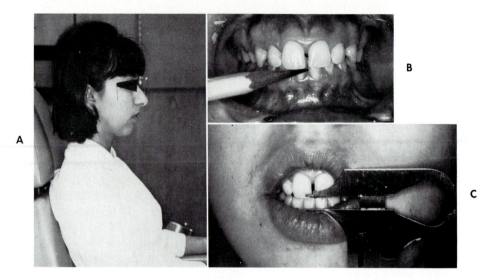

Fig. 30-33. Examination of postural position. **A,** Patient seated erect, head unsupported. **B,** Marking vertical overlaps of incisors. **C,** Measuring free-way space, using incisal overlap line when mandible is in postural position.

The landmark relations mesiodistally are examined at this time in both the intercuspal and retruded contacting positions. If the teeth are properly aligned in the intercuspal position, the landmark relations previously described in the chapter should apply. Any deviation from these landmark relations either mesiodistally or buccolingually should be noted (Fig. 30-34).

The presence of severe deformities such as posterior bite collapse and migration of the anterior teeth is noted.

Review of the swallowing pattern is an integral part of normal function evaluation. Tooth displacement during swallowing indicates that oral musculature to tooth contact is producing a damaging effect upon the supporting structures of the teeth. At this point in the examination there should be little concern as to whether the damage to the periodontium is the result of a primary effect of the tongue or of another source which has weakened the support of the teeth to the extent that the tongue is secondarily causing a pathologic condition.

Determination of maximum opening gives a rough idea of the state of health of the muscles of mastication. The maximum mandibular opening range is 35 to 50 mm. If the opening is small in a patient who otherwise seems normally developed, there may be muscle spasm present that inhibits normal mandibular opening. Deviation of the direction of the mandibular opening path is also indicative of muscular spasm. Unilateral muscle dysfunction may produce an S-shaped opening. This could also be caused by posterior crossbite interferences in closure.

Fremitus (Fig. 30-34, *C* and *D*) as it applies to dentistry is the vibrating patterns of teeth. The maxillary teeth are examined for fremitus by placement of the examiner's index finger (which is moistened with the patient's saliva) on the maxillary teeth. The patient is instructed to tap in habitual closure. The index finger of the examiner is slowly moved over the maxillary teeth until all the teeth have been tested. A record is made of any tooth that is felt to move during habitual closure. The magnitude of fremitus is subjective, but a guide that the examiner can use is as follows:

1. One-degree fremitus is recorded when only slight movement can be felt in the involved tooth.
2. Two-degree fremitus is recorded when the tooth is clearly palpable but movement is barely visible.
3. Three-degree fremitus is recorded when visual movement is clearly observed.

Fremitus is also checked in horizontal mandibular glides. This is extremely important since doodling, working, and nonworking interferences can be observed in many cases to produce displacement of the maxillary posterior teeth. Displacement of the maxillary incisors during protrusive and lateral protrusive movements must also be recorded. The fremitus record is important also because it is used as a guide for the amount of correction that is necessary.

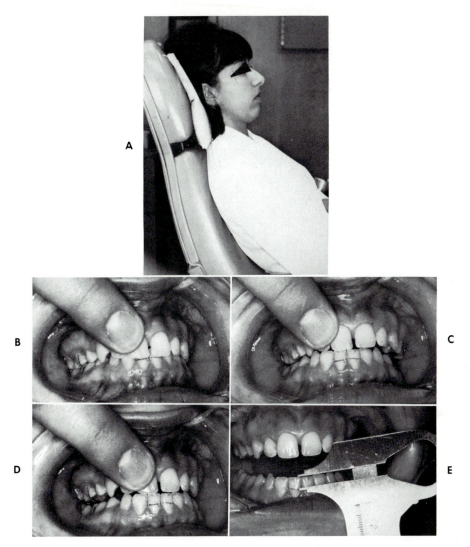

Fig. 30-34. Examination of intercuspal position and active unguided function. **A,** Patient is seated upright, and head is supported. **B,** Testing for fremitus in closure to intercuspal position. **C,** Testing for fremitus in lateral mandibular glide. **D,** Testing for fremitus in protrusive mandibular glide. **E,** Measuring vertical overlap of maxillary incisors over mandibular.

As stated earlier in the chapter, the mandible must have freedom from restraint. It is extremely important to record any interference that restrains the mandibular glides. An interference in the glide to the working position may frequently occur during posterior tooth crossbite relations. The interference usually is a result of a cross tooth contact on the inner incline of the lingual cusp of the mandibular tooth in crossbite with the inner incline of the buccal cusp of the maxillary tooth in crossbite. The mandible must open to clear the interference in order to complete the working glide.

The interference on the nonworking (balancing) side is checked by use of the dental floss encircling method (see discussion on Occlusal Indicators, Marking Devices, and Diagnostic Aids).

The most common area of contact in the nonworking interference is the inner incline of the mesiolingual cusp of the maxillary molar with the inner aspect of the distobuccal cusp of the mandibular molar. When this contact is made, there is a palatal thrust placed upon the maxillary tooth and a buccal thrust placed upon the mandibular tooth. Nonworking interferences have a great potential for producing pathologic changes in the periodontium of the involved teeth.

When the patient moves into the protrusive po-

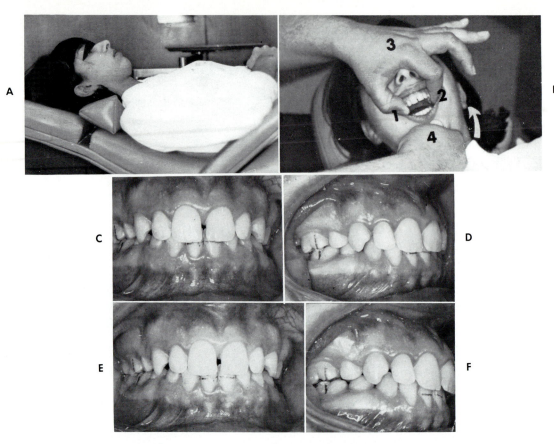

Fig. 30-35. Examination of retruded contacting position. **A,** Patient placed horizontally to facilitate posterior mandibular closure. **B,** Retruding mandible by so-called jiggling method. Note that thumb, *1,* and index finger, *2,* separate occlusal surfaces of posterior teeth while heel of hand, *3,* stabilizes forehead. Other hand, *4,* holds chin and begins opening and closing movements. **C** and **E,** Teeth in intercuspal position. **D** and **F,** Teeth in retruded contacting position.

sition, there should be incisive function in the absence of contact in the posterior teeth. If contacts in the posterior teeth are present during the protrusive glide, the clashing and bumping of the posterior teeth, until incisal contact is made, can be destructive to the periodontium as well as to the temporomandibular joint.

Arch relations in the retruded occlusal contacting position are recorded (Fig. 30-35). The mandible is retruded, using the technique described elsewhere in the chapter. When the first tooth contact is sensed by the patient, the closing movement is stopped, and the location of the contact is made. Most often the contact will be in the premolar area unilaterally or bilaterally. The patient is then instructed to squeeze tight, and in the majority of cases an anterior slip will be observed as the mandible slides from the retruded contacting position to the slightly anterior intercuspal position. The direction and distance of the deflection are

recorded. The significance of the anterior displacement is that the patient has an interference in the retruded path of closure (usually on one or two teeth) that is reflexly avoided, allowing the patient to close directly into the intercuspal position.

In the examination of the intercuspal position a patient may have had a 0.0 mm overjet (contacts between anterior incisors present), while in the retruded contacting position the overjet may be 1 or 2 mm. Closure of this case in the intercuspal position results in the maxillary and mandibular incisors' taking the full force of mandibular closure. If fremitus is recorded in these teeth during habitual closure and if there is other clinical evidence of occlusal traumatism present, the occlusion can be indicated as the cause of the symptoms.

The mesiodistal and buccolingual landmark relations in the retruded contacting position are compared with those recorded in the intercuspal position. If there is only a slight deviation of the ideal landmark relations in the retruded contacting position, occlusal adjustment by selective grinding can be performed. If, however, there is a great discrepancy in and landmark relations in the retruded contacting position, selective grinding may not be feasible as a method of adjusting the occlusion. Orthodontic treatment, utilizing either minor or major tooth movement techniques, is indicated before this dentition can be finally adjusted by the selective grinding technique.

It is only after a detailed occlusal examination that the practitioner can arrive at a specific diagnosis and treatment plan. Not only does the teaching occlusal examination chart indicate when an occlusal adjustment, utilizing selective grinding techniques, can be done; it also indicates when such a technique cannot possibly fill the requisites for returning a pathologic occlusion to health and function. Perhaps this is one of the most important benefits to be derived from a complete examination of the occlusion.

TECHNIQUES OF SELECTIVE GRINDING
Cusp-to-landmark grinding

The cusp-to-landmark form of occlusal adjustment is the most desirable, for it allows the therapist to obtain proper landmark relations of teeth in harmony with jaw position and movement. When the landmark areas of teeth are properly related, there is the best possibility for occlusal stability and freedom. This type of grinding is performed in three stages (Figs. 30-9, 30-19, 30-25, and 30-36).

STAGE ONE: CORRECTING LANDMARK RELATIONS OF TEETH IN RETRUDED CONTACTING POSITION

The first stage of the cusp-to-landmark grinding procedure is to remove the discrepancies in the retruded path of closure (Fig. 30-25, *1*). The objective in this phase is properly to relate the landmark relations of teeth. The decision as to what marking to grind on an interfering tooth is based on the disparity between opposing landmark areas. As a practicality most grinding procedures will be performed to alter the positions of the supporting occlusal line angles. Occasionally the central fossa line will require repositioning either buccally or lingually in a malposed tooth, but this is usually difficult to do.

In the description of selective grinding procedures that usually appears in most texts the first

stages are outlined as follows: (1) round off all wear facets, (2) level marginal ridges, and (3) narrow buccolingual diameters. From a mechanical point of view this could lead to gross errors. If the wear facets are reduced first, it is possible to destroy a portion of the tooth that might be necessary for the establishment of a supportive landmark. When the mandible is moved to the retruded contacting position, the wear facets may no longer be operational in terms of grasping contacts.

The fallacy of first leveling marginal ridges is that at this point in the procedure it is not known whether the depressed or elevated marginal ridge will be needed as a supporting area. Proper correction may require restoration of the depressed marginal ridge. It is possible that the elevated marginal ridge might prove interfering in the retruded path, and it should therefore be reshaped. In grinding for landmark stability the operator must make the decision where to grind and must take into consideration the leveling of marginal ridges wherever possible without compromising occlusal function.

It has long been recognized that narrow buccolingual dimensions of the occlusal tables tend to center the forces in the root support of the tooth. One philosophy of adjustment holds that most teeth have widened buccolingual diameters because of the so-called disproportional wear of teeth and that since these areas are potential interferences and will require correction anyway, teeth should be narrowed to their correct buccolingual dimension as a means of expediting the adjustment. This type of grinding is extremely presumptuous because it may result in eliminating areas that are very necessary for landmark coordination.

Buccolingual occlusal widths should be made narrow wherever possible but *not at the expense of a stabilized and free occlusion*. The decision of where to grind, therefore, will be related to the ability to keep teeth narrow and at the same time to permit reasonable landmark coordination.

The objectives of stage one—correction of landmarks in the retruded path of closure—are as follows:

1. To create a stable intercuspal position in harmony with the retruded path of the mandible. In so doing the operator will properly coordinate the landmarks and thereby allow the FOA areas of the supporting cusps to be cradled by the opposing teeth. The FOA must be in a place of readiness to make immediate contact with guiding

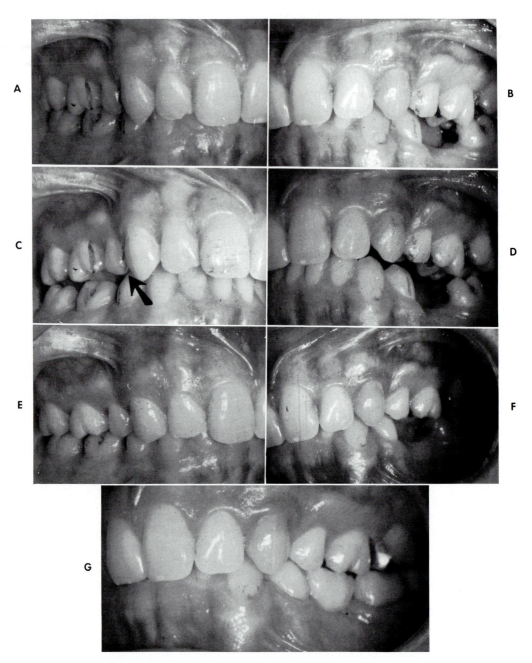

Fig. 30-36. Selective grinding preparatory to fixed bridge prosthesis. **A** and **B,** Right and left side in intercuspal position. **C** and **D,** Retruded contacting position. Arrow shows initial interference. **E** and **F,** Results of selective grinding. Note that left side extruded molar has been leveled into plane and that proper landmarks have been carved on occlusal surface to facilitate fixed bridge construction. Note also prominent canines that should not be reduced. Prominent canines will be only teeth in contact during lateral mandibular glide. **G,** Fixed bridge 3 years after operation. Note that a mesio-occlusal onlay restoration was necessary to help create a symmetric plane of occlusion.

inclines for future freedom in glide movements.

2. To establish as narrow buccolingual dimensions to the occlusal tables as possible without compromising landmark relations.

3. To correct the form and function of teeth relative to food impaction and retention (leveling marginal ridges, removing plunger cusps, and improving on crown contour) without compromising landmark relations.

4. To grind to improve other mechanical problems (Fig. 30-19). When, for example, severe nonworking interference portions of the inner aspect of the supporting cusps are at fault, occasionally the very same nonworking interfering cusps become the second, third, or fourth line interferences during correction in retruded closure. If, when these very same cusps do appear as interferences, the grinding is concentrated on the cusp

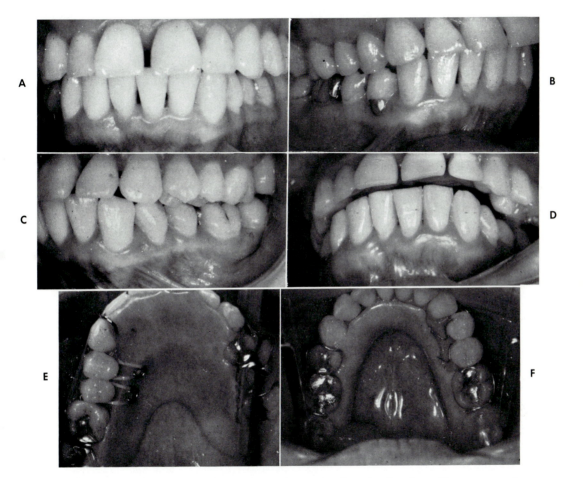

Fig. 30-37. Problem of occlusal adjustment in mouth where landmark positions are poorly related. **A,** Spreading of anterior teeth, age 26 years. Anterior view of intercuspal position. **B,** Left side, intercuspal position. Note that bucco-occlusal line of lower is buccal to central fossa line of upper. **C,** Left side, intercuspal position. Note premolar buccal crossbite with the lower bucco-occlusal line lingual to upper occlusal table. Note also tight contact between lower and upper incisors. **D,** Retruded contacting position, showing unilateral contact on right side and relation of lower premolars completely lingual to upper premolars. As mandible moved laterally to contact left side in intercuspal position, jaw also moved anteriorly. As outer aspects of premolars became worn, mandible required greater anterior displacement to intercuspal position and caused lower incisors to help displace upper incisors because of increased pressure. So that occlusion can be treated, landmarks of opposing teeth must be properly correlated, which requires upper left premolars to be positioned palatally and lower left premolars buccally. **E,** Mirror view of a maxillary bite plane with palatal cleats used as anchorage to move left upper premolars palatally. **F,** Mirror view of a lower lingual appliance with finger springs exerting pressure on premolars for buccal displacement.

Continued.

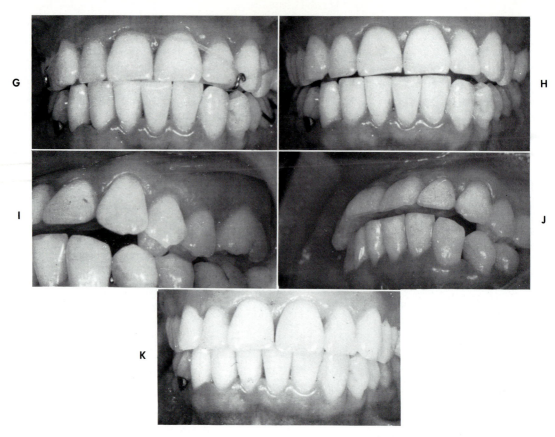

Fig. 30-37, cont'd. G, Anterior view of a bite plane in mouth after 3 months. **H,** After bite plane is removed, newly positioned premolars are only teeth in contact in retruded contacting position. This will require that selective grinding procedure be started on these teeth. **I,** Retruded contacting position. Note that bucco-occlusal line of lower is still *not* in correct relation with respect to upper central fossa line. Grinding procedure will not suffice to give proper stability, and as a result this patient will require indefinite retention in form of bimaxillary night guards. **J,** Intercuspal position in harmony with retruded contacting position after adjustment. Note that lower incisors are no longer traumatizing upper incisors. Note also that landmark relations of left side are still adequate. **K,** Anterior view after adjustment, with anterior teeth together.

heights, the ability of the retruded contacting interfering cusps to act as interferences on the nonworking side will be eliminated. The same principle for any severe glide discrepancy involving a supporting cusp applies.

When correcting in stage one, the operator should bear in mind that the buccolingual landmark relations must be correct. If occlusal stability is to be achieved, the bucco-occlusal line angle of the mandibular arch must be related and positively cradled by the central fossa line of the maxillary arch. This, of course, holds true for the maxillary linguo-occlusal line and its relation to the mandibular central fossa line. The mesiodistal landmarks, on the other hand, may never be reestablished for most corrections. Once the mandible has been moved from the intercuspal position to the retruded contacting position, and the distance exceeds 2 mm, the cusps can no longer be corrected to fit between one another. It is important, therefore, that a platform be created on the supportive cuspal incline to simulate the effect of the marginal ridge area so that the opposing supportive cusps can be properly held. In order that this may be accomplished, the involved cuspal inclines in many instances must be carved somewhat concave. If it is discovered in the intercuspal position that the difference between the landmark positions is very great, it may not be possible to treat adequately the occlusion by means of selective grinding procedures. Selective grinding procedures require the ability to predict proper and stable landmark positioning (Fig. 30-37).

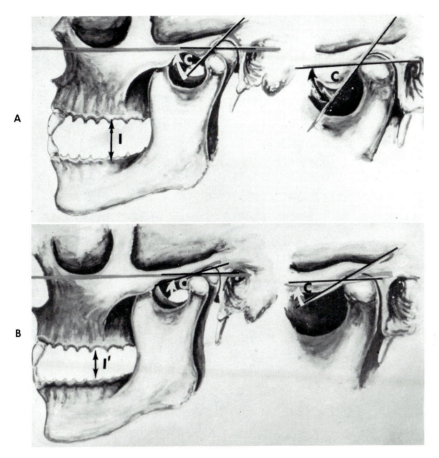

Fig. 30-38. Relation between condylar guidance and molar clearance. For a given incisal guidance amount of interocclusal clearance in molar area is a product of anterior condylar guidance. With a steep anterior condylar guidance, *c,* interocclusal clearance, *1,* in **A** is greater than interocclusal clearance, *1',* in **B,** which has a reduced condylar guidance. (Courtesy Morton Amsterdam, Philadelphia.)

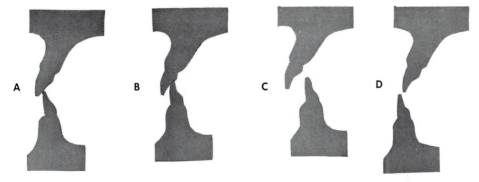

Fig. 30-39. Incisal guidance. **A,** Moderate incisal guidance. **B,** Steep incisal guidance. This will allow for a steeper posterior cuspal form. **C,** Ineffective incisal guidance. This will require a very shallow posterior cuspal form. **D,** Edge-to-edge 0-degree incisal guidance. This requires a nearly flat posterior cuspation. (Courtesy Morton Amsterdam, Philadelphia.)

STAGE TWO: DEFINING FOA AREAS

When the landmarks of teeth have been correctly related in the retruded contacting position, the operator must stop and proceed toward defining the portion of the outer aspect of the supporting cusps that will function as the FOA. One need not wait until all the interferences in the retruded path of closure have been eliminated. All that is required is that the landmarks be correlated with a minimum of mandibular displacement. To define the FOA area the operator places an occlusal marking device of his own choosing in the patient's mouth, and the patient is allowed to slide into various horizontal mandibular glide movements. These movements will produce markings on the outer aspects of the supportive cusps and on the mandibular incisal edge. At this point a determination is made of the amount of area that is to function as the FOA. All other outer tooth surfaces containing markings are reduced until the marked area resembles a 1 mm ribbon running from second molar to second molar across the central incisors. The FOA area, once created, is never adjusted again.

The guiding inclines are adjusted at this point, using the FOA areas as a carving device.

STAGE THREE: GRINDING GUIDING INCLINES

In protrusive glide (Figs. 30-30 and 30-38 to 30-40). The lower incisor and canine FOA areas will be responsible for marking the guiding incline of the upper incisors and canines. Removal of tooth structure here is performed only on the guiding inclines of the upper anterior teeth. Occasionally it will be necessary to modify the FOA of an extruded or lingually positioned incisal edge during the protrusive and lateral glides.

Care must be taken to avoid posterior tooth contact in the protrusive mandibular glide. It is important that an anlaysis be made of the amount of interocclusal space that is present between the premolars and molars during protrusive glide prior to any grinding procedure. The amount of grinding that can be performed in the anterior region will be directly related to the amount of posterior interocclusal space that is present during protrusive glide. Correction of protrusive glide must take into consideration the patient's cosmetic needs—the so-called lip line aesthetics—and his phonetic pattern. It is important to consult with the patient if a drastic alteration of the anterior tooth length is to be performed. It is also wise to instruct the patient that some speech adjustment with sibilant sounds may be necessary after the grinding has been performed.

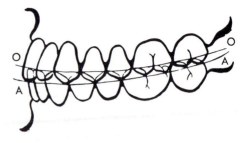

Fig. 30-40. Relation between anterior incisal guidance and posterior cuspation must be harmonious so that there is a gradual diminution in overbite (vertical overlap of teeth), cusp height, and cusp width from anterior to posterior portion of mouth. (Courtesy Morton Amsterdam, Philadelphia.)

In lateral mandibular glide (Fig. 30-29). In lateral horizontal mandibular glide the FOA areas of the lower anterior and posterior teeth will mark the guiding incline of the upper buccal cusps and the upper anterior teeth. Care is taken to reduce the interfering areas to allow for a smooth, unimpeded glide. The FOA areas of the upper lingual cusps will mark the guiding inclines of the lower lingual cusps. Every effort will be made to reduce tooth contact of the lower lingual cusps to avoid cross tooth balance. A strong limiting factor to lateral horizontal glide correction will be the possibility of creating nonworking interferences on the opposite side of the mouth (Fig. 30-41). The same type of relation exists between the working and nonworking sides of the mouth as exists between the anterior and posterior portions of the mouth in the protrusive glide. The examiner must be especially careful to note the amount of interocclusal clearance that is present on the nonworking side. The amount of lateral correction will vary for each patient. The guide to the amount of grinding will be the fremitus patterns of the maxillary teeth. Once the state has been reached whereby the mandible can move from the corrected retruded contacting position into a lateral glide and return with a minimum of fremitus and with a smooth even glide, grinding can be stopped. If in one case we have contacting teeth only in the incisors and canines, but the above conditions are fulfilled, then this would be correct for that patient. On the other hand, if fremitus were present in the incisors and canines, then continued grinding would be necessary to reduce the steepness of the guiding incline so as to direct forces more apically and perhaps to bring more teeth in contact on the working side. It is important again to reemphasize that the amount of grinding that is to be done for a given mouth is dependent on

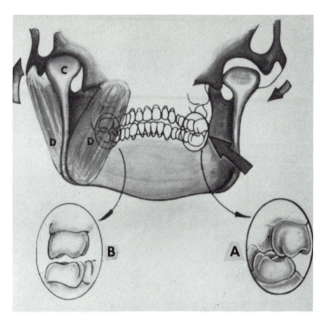

Fig. 30-41. Hypothetical relation between interference on nonworking side and muscular spasm and pain on working side. Nonworking interference, *A (large diagonal arrow),* prevents teeth from contacting on functional working side, *B.* As patient attempts to bring working teeth into occlusion, there is a tendency for working condyle, *C,* to be displaced superiorly *(vertical arrow).* So-called splinting reflex tends to limit condylar displacement, with possible joint and ligament injury by means of spasm in working-side musculature, *D.* (Courtesy Morton Amsterdam, Philadelphia.)

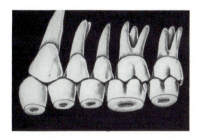

Fig. 30-42. Buccal cusps on working side in lateral mandibular glide have capacity to slide through one another. Amount of group function needed will be related to amount of periodontal destruction. (Courtesy Morton Amsterdam, Philadelphia.)

a total knowledge of the mechanical and functional factors that are present (Fig. 30-42).

All patients cannot be stamped into a single occlusal pattern. The idea of the so-called canine protected occlusion or, on the other hand, the group function protected occlusion to be applied to all patients is physiologically incorrect. If the canine tooth is quite prominent, is in position to receive the horizontal glide load, and is in periodontal condition to sustain the load, then it would be incorrect drastically to reduce a prominent canine just to conform the occlusion to a group function concept. On the other hand, if such a

prominent canine were mobile and unable to sustain the load, then it would be equally incorrect to force the occlusal pressures on such a tooth. In the latter case continued grinding of the canine would be necessary to bring more teeth into play and to reduce the steepness of the incline plane relations of the teeth. Because of the very limited nature of selective grinding our objectives must be obtainable under the circumstances that exist.

FINALIZING ADJUSTMENT

Since teeth tend to shift when their occlusal contact has been altered, it is important to allow for shifting in the selective grinding procedure. It is strongly recommended that selective grinding procedures be performed in short visits at intervals of 1 week to 10 days between visits. In our experience most selective grinding procedures are performed in three to five visits. At the completion of selective grinding techniques the teeth must be carefully polished. For polishing, ultraspeed alpine stones and slow-speed rubber abrasive wheels are used with a copious flow of water. It is possible to perform the selective grinding procedure in the absence of water with ultraspeed and airspray so long as the operator does not penetrate the dentoenamel junction. However, the stones must be passed rapidly across the teeth. In most adults this type of grinding can be done without any discomfort to the patient. One advantage of the technique is that there is no loss of visibility on the part of the operator.

Cusp-to-plane grinding

Cusp-to-plane grinding (Fig. 30-17) is necessary to overcome situations of severe bilateral crossbite, cusp tip–to–cusp tip relations, unilateral crossbite, or anterior crossbite. In this type of grinding the operator attempts to acquire as many supportive contacts as possible along an imaginary plane that intersects the junction of the two opposing arches. In order to grind to this hypothetical plane he must proceed slightly differently from the way he did in the previous category. Grinding here is accomplished by placing the mandible in the retruded contacting position and allowing the patient to engage in mandibular glides both in protrusive and lateral movements. The teeth are first ground to conform to these glide movements. The decision to grind in this instance is based on interference with this continuous, harmonious plane that intersects the arches. The technique for this type of grinding follows.

Technique
1. Horizontal mandibular glide grinding—in both protrusive and lateral glides
2. Grinding in the retruded contacting position, obtaining supportive contacts where they can be found (There must be a resultant harmony between the intercuspal and retruded contacting positions.)
3. Polishing the teeth

Objective. The objective here is to allow for a harmonious mandibular glide in all directions that is free of nonworking contact and molar protrusive contact. Each glide, right to left, must be directed so that there is no vertical opening or parting of the anterior teeth during the total length of the glide. The protrusive glide is handled by attempting to place contact as close as possible to the front of the mouth, preferably in the canine or first premolar areas. The arrangement of these contacts must occur on the working side in such a manner that the glide movement is free and easy. Caution must be taken in crossbite situations because the lower buccal and upper lingual cusps are potential nonworking interferences. This type of grinding is similar to the kind that is performed in correcting the occlusion of a night guard.

Grinding from intercuspal position

In those clinical situations where the discrepancy between the intercuspal and the retruded contacting positions is so great that it is impossible for a correction to be performed by selective grinding, a clinical compromise is necessary. If in the opinion of the operator the basic cause of occlusal disease is due to mandibular glide contact, it is possible in this type of mouth to correct the lateral and protrusive glides starting only from the intercuspal position. *Every attempt is made not to interfere with the intercuspal position.* This is a case where there might be a severe nonworking interference or a severe working or protrusive interference. In any event, this type of grinding can represent an intelligent compromise with the usual grinding techniques.

Grinding isolated tooth or group of teeth

In a mouth that has an intact dentition with symptoms of occlusal traumatism that appear to be isolated in one or two teeth, sometimes it is advantageous only to correct the contacting areas on the affected teeth. This is a technique that is frequently employed, particularly in those cases where an acute periodontal abscess has formed.

Grinding procedures necessary in preparation for various restorative approaches

Full denture. When a single intact arch opposes an edentulous ridge, it is important that the operator attempt to position and accentuate the occlusal landmark so as to facilitate the placement of denture teeth. This means that the bucco-occlusal line angle will be aligned in a continuous fashion and the central fossa line will be cleanly defined and leveled in a harmonious fashion. The bucco-lingual dimension of the posterior teeth will be compatible with the alveolar root support. All this serves to facilitate and simplify denture construction. The result will be a denture that functions harmoniously against the natural dentition and minimizes the amount of destruction to the natural teeth.

Removable partial denture. In grinding preparatory to a removable partial denture it is important that the natural teeth opposing the partial edentulous ridges simulate the case of the full denture; for example, if the occlusal table of the partial denture is to reside over the crest of the ridge, it is important that the opposing central fossa line be directed over this area. It is also essential in preparation for a removable partial prosthesis to establish as many natural tooth contacts as possible.

Preparation for fixed partial prostheses (Fig. 30-36). In preparation for fixed partial prosthesis the grinding that is done preparatory to the fixed bridge is performed to rectify the discrepancies in the retruded contacting position and to create a harmonious opposing platform by reshaping extruded and malposed teeth. However, this type of selective grinding cannot be sufficiently amplified because of limited space. The therapist should be aware of this problem and consult other texts on this subject.

METHODS OF LOCATING VARIOUS JAW POSITIONS AND MOVEMENT

Intercuspal position (Fig. 30-34). The intercuspal position is the usual position of maximal occlusal contact, generally referred to as centric occlusion or the position of convenience, and is the most closed occlusal contacting position. The intercuspal position can be located for most patients by placing the *study casts* into the tightest contacting arrangement. Those individuals with open bite or prognathic situations may present occlusal arrangements that do not allow for intercuspal examination by hand held study casts. However, these patients are in the minority.

Of great interest is the fact brought out by Brenman that habitual closure into intercuspal position varies with change in body posture. For this reason it is essential that when the intercuspal position is evaluated in the mouth the patient be seated upright in the dental chair. Further, the operator's hands must touch the teeth or chin very slightly, if at all, so as not to influence or deflect closure. When testing fremitus in maximum closure, the examiner places a moistened fingertip over the facial surfaces of the maxillary teeth, and the patient is instructed to tap his teeth together quite hard.

Postural position (Fig. 30-33). The postural position, sometimes referred to as the physiologic rest position of the mandible, is a position of mandibular tonus—the position of mandibular posture when the individual is either standing or seated erect. The postural position for the patient is located, with the patient seated in an erect position and the head unsupported. An effort is made to get the patient to relax his jaw by having his moisten his lips and swallow a few times and engage in some phonetic activity such as humming or repeating various syllables like m-l-m and Mississippi. A line is scribed on the lower incisors at the level of the upper anterior overbite so that it is visible to the eye. When the examiner is confident that the patient is in postural position with the lips parted, the measurement is taken between the incisal edge of the upper anterior teeth and the line that has been scored on the mandibular incisors. This measurement is referred to as the *apparent* free-way space. When the mandible is placed in the retruded contacting position, another measurement can be taken between these same measuring points. The difference between the two measurements is sometimes referred to as the *true* free-way space.

Retruded contacting position (Fig. 30-35). The retruded contacting position is determined by first locating the terminal hinge of the retruded path of closure for the mandible. To facilitate this determination the patient's chair is placed almost at a horizontal position. This tends to encourage closure of the mandible in the posterior area. The technique requires directed opening and closing movements. The fingers are placed between the teeth, preventing them from contacting—the thumb on one side and the index finger on the other. The mandible is elevated and depressed in a rhythmic manner in what is sometimes referred to as a jiggling movement. The mandible is directed in this open and closed manner with no distal thrust. The amount of opening is 2.5 cm or less. When the examiner has ascertained that the mandible is opening and closing in a free and easy manner, a slight posterior thrust is placed on the mandible. It is easy to determine that the mandible is opening in this hingelike rhythmic manner. The mandible is allowed to close in this posterior path until pressure of the mandible against the inserted fingers is encountered. The mandible is slowly allowed to close, with the fingers supporting the mandibular position, until initial tooth contact is made. If, during the procedure, resistance is encountered from the musculature in the form of either deviation or protrusion, or stiffness or tightness, some technique will probably have to be employed to free the musculature. The most frequently employed technique is the use of a Hawley bite plane appliance to reduce the afferent impulses of tooth contact and to allow the muscles to come to some state of rest. On rare occasions various muscular relaxants or sedatives may be employed to facilitate this determination. The location of the retruded contacting position and the retruded path of closure is actually performed by training the patient to close in this manner. The patient is trained by digital manipulation. On many occasions the patient can be aided in this closing movement by being told to place the tip of the tongue on the roof of the mouth as far posteriorly as possible. Once the patient has been trained in this closure, there is generally no problem encountered in reproducing the movement. One merely holds the mandible and asks the patient to close easily.

Glide movements from intercuspal position (Fig. 30-34). Glide movements from the intercuspal position should be observed in the absence of any digital manipulation on the part of the operator. If the patient is unable to make a given glide movement, it must be concluded that this is due to locking of the occlusion. On occasion a lateral glide movement or a protruded glide movement

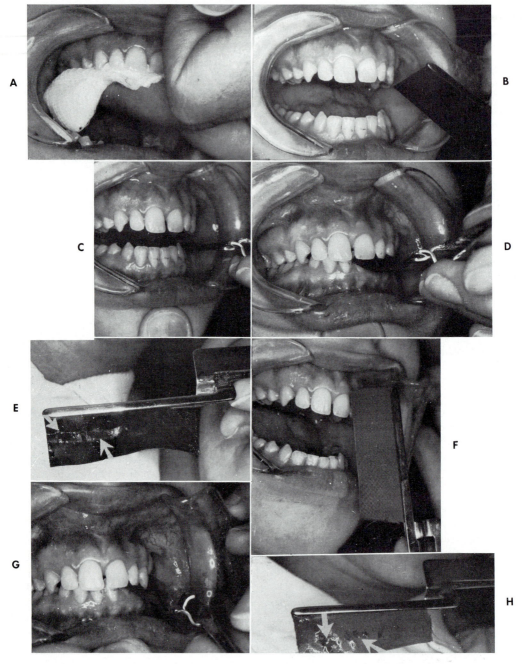

Fig. 30-43. Marking teeth in retruded contacting position. **A,** Drying teeth with a gauze sponge. **B,** Warmed, thick articulating paper about to be placed in mouth. **C,** Placing articulating paper in mouth, with chin held in retruded position. **D,** Closing rhythmically into retruded contacting position upon paper. **E,** Indentations *(arrows)* can be observed in thick articulating paper, showing interfering contact. **F,** Red typewriter ribbon. **G,** Closing into retruded contacting position on red typewriter ribbon. **H,** Blue markings can be observed on red typewriter ribbon at points of interfering contact *(arrows).*

can be facilitated if the patient will start with either the incisor tip–to–tip arrangement or lateral cusp tip–to–tip arrangement and slide back to the intercuspal position.

Glide movements from retruded contacting position. Glide movements from the retruded contacting position are of little diagnostic value, but they are of great benefit in reinforcing the occlusal marking made for the retruded contacting posi-

tion. In doing so the examiner directs the patient to close lightly in the retruded contacting position and, with the patient's teeth together and with guided support to the mandible, asks the patient to make a slight lateral glide to the right and to the left. This not only serves to reinforce the marking in the retruded contacting position but also helps to give a good approximation of the direction of the mandibular glide from this position.

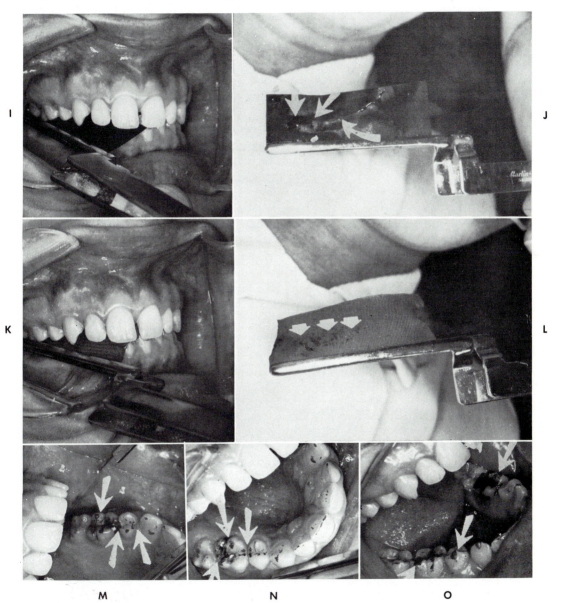

Fig. 30-43, cont'd. I, Thick articulating paper on right side in retruded contacting position. **J,** Indentations *(arrows)* in thick articulating paper at points of interference. **K,** Articulating paper on right side in retruded contacting position. **L,** Blue markings *(arrows)* on red articulating paper. **M,** Mirror view of left side, showing occlusal markings *(arrows).* **N,** Mirror view of right side, showing occlusal markings *(arrows).* **O,** Direct view of lower arch, showing markings *(arrows).* Note that in all cases markings coincide with indentations on thick marking paper and blue markings on typewriter ribbon.

OCCLUSAL INDICATORS, MARKING DEVICES, AND DIAGNOSTIC AIDS

Marking paper
Typewriter ribbon
Dental floss
Wax recording
Sound
Direct inspection of teeth
Finger pressure upon teeth
Dental articulator and face bow

Marking paper (Fig. 30-43, A to E). The dental supply market is flooded with a variety of marking papers of varying thicknesses and degrees of markability. We will discuss only those papers that are commonly used, and their teaching situations.

The preferred paper is one that is thick and rather smudgy, gives a definitive sound when teeth strike it, and allows for comparative imprints in the paper itself that can be read as a wax bite. It is desirable that this paper be able to locate not only the initial interference but the second and third as well.

The paper should be warmed slightly either over a flame or in some cases over the dental unit light. The amount of warming depends on the severity of biting pressure of a given individual. The teeth to be marked are dried, and the paper is introduced. It is helpful in recording glide movements not only to obtain a reading of the marking of the glide contacts but also to reemphasize the marking by taking the paper out of the mouth and having the individual move into lateral glides so that the scraping teeth create white streaks within the smudgy areas.

Typewriter ribbon (Fig. 30-43, F to H). The typewriter ribbon that is used is a finite marker that will locate only the first interference in the retruded contacting position. Because of the ribbon's slight faint mark the marking is difficult to locate by it-self and therefore is used immediately on top of the previous blue paper marking. The typewriter ribbon serves to amplify the blue marking so that the red center is present in a blue field. It is further useful in that one is able to read the location of interferences in the form of blue marks on the red ribbon.

Dental floss (Fig. 30-44). Dental floss can be used to encircle a variety of interferences. It is placed around a given mandibular quadrant, and the mandible is placed in the jaw position or movement to be examined. At the desired point both ends of the floss are brought forward until the interference is encircled. This technique is especially useful in locating the nonworking interferences.

Wax recording. The use of wax is an important adjunct to the study of occlusal contacts. The wax (S. S. White no. 7) is slightly warmed and placed and molded over the maxillary teeth. The mandible occludes against the maxilla, causing an imprint in the wax. In this way the exact contact of the teeth can be determined. A premature contact will cause complete displacement of the wax, whereas teeth that do not occlude have a thickness of wax denoting that they are not in contact.

Sound. The sound of a properly adjusted occlusion is distinct, crisp, and clear and is caused by all teeth striking simultaneously in the correct retruded contacting position. When interference is present in closure, the sound is somewhat mushy and prolonged. The ear of the therapist can be trained to hear this sound of residual interference in retruded contacting adjustments. The differences in the sound of teeth unilaterally contacting thick marking paper can be an aid in locating the side of the mouth wherein the initial interference resides. When the initial interference is present on one side, a crisp clean (although faint) sound of tooth contact will be heard as an overtone to the sound of tooth striking paper on the opposite side.

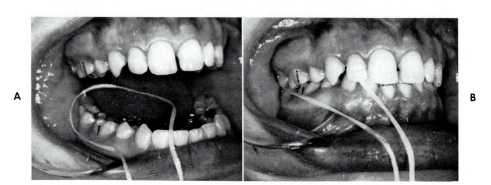

Fig. 30-44. Use of dental floss to encircle interference. **A,** Placing floss around quadrant. **B,** Two ends of floss are pulled tight after teeth are closed.

When only the sound of tooth striking paper is heard, then the interference is on the same side. This is a technique that can be mastered easily and can be of great help.

Direct inspection of teeth. During the final stages of retruded contacting adjustment there are minute discrepancies that cause the mandible to slip an extremely small amount. If one concentrates his vision in the second premolar area, directing his line of view from below the occlusal level, the amount of displacement can be seen. If the interference is located on one side of the mouth, the amount of displacement on that side will be less than on the opposite side. Therefore the side that seems to have the greatest amount of displacement is the side free of initial interference.

Digital pressure (Fig. 30-34, *B* to *D*). A moistened fingertip placed over the labial surfaces of the teeth becomes an indispensable tool in adjusting the occlusion. The determination of fremitus is not only important from a diagnostic point of view but is also the most desirable means of determining an end point to the occlusal adjustment procedure. The techniques of grinding in the glide movements are employed to reduce fremitus.

Dental articulator. The dental articulator, which has always been an important tool to prosthodontists, can be of great help to the periodontist as well. If casts are properly mounted and oriented to the terminal hinge pathway of closure, great benefits in determining the mechanical possibilities of a grinding procedure can be obtained. The novice is strongly urged to mount the study casts and set the semiadjustable articulator for a practice grinding session before any occlusal adjustment is attempted. Although the dental articulator can be extremely accurate for purposes of restorative dentistry, it has certain important, distinct limitations with respect to the selective grinding procedure. It is extremely important that these differences be emphasized. Fremitus, which is an essential diagnostic guide for the need of adjustment and a key determining factor for the completion of adjustment, cannot be observed on casts mounted on the dental articulator. The end point of grinding on the dental articulator will always take on the shape of a prosthetic type of occlusion because of the degree of friction that is present between the models and the fact that there is no fremitus to guide the operator. Further it is possible to overgrind the occlusion of the study casts and obtain a result not possible in the mouth. If one is careful to recognize the limitations of the use of an ar-

ticulator, he will definitely find it to be of great benefit in planning the adjustment.

SPECIAL PROBLEMS

Treatment of induced dental awareness. The condition of dental awareness is accompanied by a high state of emotional anxiety and distress. The technique for handling this clinical situation follows.

1. *Reassurance.* The patient must be reassured that the condition he has is real and can be controlled. Furthermore the patient should be told that he is not alone in this respect and that other patients have had similar conditions and have been helped.

2. *Use of an interocclusal clearing appliance.* An interocclusal clearing appliance that will keep the teeth apart and reduce afferent proprioceptive stimuli is to be fabricated and inserted in the patient's mouth. The design of the appliance is based entirely upon the mechanical arrangement of the teeth present. It is important that this appliance have the following properties: (a) It must be very stable and not be displaced during occlusal contact. (b) It must fit securely. (c) It must offer minimal interference in the free-way space. (d) It must be of the simplest mechanical design to allow for stable contact in the retruded path and for freedom of movement. The patient is told that this is a "forgetting appliance" and that it will help him forget that he has teeth. The appliance is worn continuously for 4 to 6 weeks except during meals. When the patient has become comfortable and has lost the awareness and anxiety, the next phase of treatment begins.

3. *Occlusal adjustment phase.* Before the occlusal clearing appliance can be withdrawn from the patient the occlusion must be completely adjusted. The adjustment is performed over a prolonged period, approximately 3 to 5 weeks, with short weekly visits. At the close of each adjustment period the teeth must be meticulously polished. The patient is told to continue to wear this appliance until the therapist believes that the occlusion has been adjusted to its ultimate corrected state.

For some patients a period of withdrawal is necessary because the patient becomes extremely dependent on the appliance. In these cases the appliance is taken out of the mouth experimentally at first during the day. After this has been successful, it is then removed during the night as well. Before the patients are dismissed they are told that this condition might occur at any time in the future with dental procedures and that, if it should re-

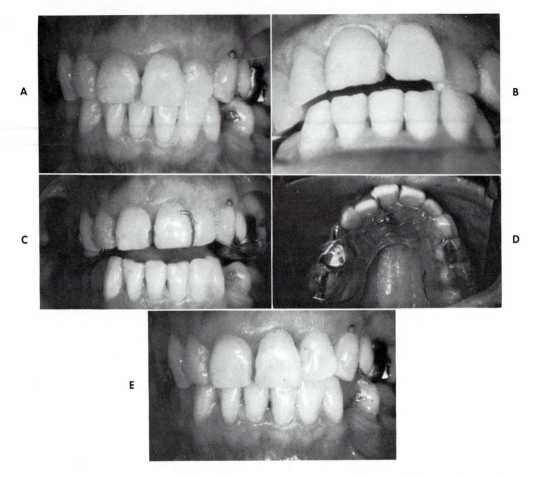

Fig. 30-45. Correction of anterior tooth of initial interference with retruded contacting position. **A,** Intercuspal position. **B,** Retruded contacting position, with initial interference in left lateral incisor. **C** and **D,** Tooth movement appliance. **E,** Final correction.

cur, not to become alarmed because the appliance will be kept in readiness for them.

Interference in retruded path located in anterior tooth (Fig. 30-45). When a crossbite anterior tooth interferes with the retruded closure, tooth movement procedures must be performed prior to selective grinding.

In the anterior crossbite the degree of postoperative retention is directly related to the vertical overlap of the malposed tooth. The tooth movement may require contraction of the lower anterior segment, expansion of the upper anterior segment, or both. Sufficient interocclusal clearance must be created with some type of appliance.

Once the anterior tooth preventing posterior tooth contact in the retruded path has been repositioned, grinding procedures can be performed.

Nonworking interference. The nonworking interference deserves special attention because the cusps that interfere on the nonworking side are the same cusps that are responsible for supporting the occlusal vertical dimension. It one were arbitrarily to remove nonworking interferences without regard to support of the occlusion, it would be possible to eliminate the supportive capacity of a number of teeth. The nonworking interference has been recognized as perhaps the most destructive of all grasping interferences in periodontics.

In correcting the nonworking interference the operator makes every effort not to eliminate the supportive capacity of the supporting cusps. The methods of eliminating a nonworking interference are as follows:

1. *Correction of part of the grinding for landmark relations in the retruded path.* Here the nonworking interfering cusps are reduced as part of stage one in cusp-to-landmark correction (Fig. 30-19). This is the most ideal method for obtaining such a correction.

2. *Establishing a groove for the movement paths of the opposing supporting cusps.* Recordings of the nonworking movement paths of the supporting

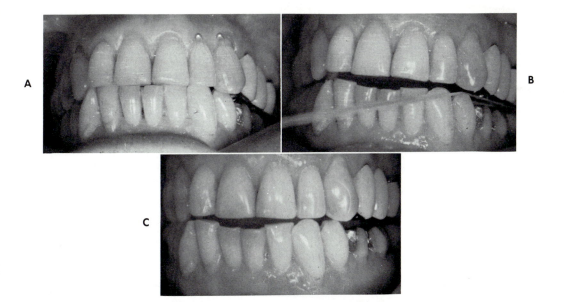

Fig. 30-46. Extruded lower third molar, preventing anterior incisive function with temporo-mandibular joint pain. **A,** Intercuspal position. **B,** Protrusive glide. Note lack of anterior contact. Note also dental floss locking on extruded third molar. **C,** Anterior incisive contact possible after third molar extraction.

cusps and of their opposing occlusal tables are made. The correction takes place by carving a groove to coincide with the movement path of the supporting cusps. Every care is taken so as not to reduce the supporting capacity of the cusp tips.

3. *Restoration.* The restoration to eliminate the nonworking interference may be on the working side so as to increase the function of the working cusp by restoring the guiding incline or the lower FOA; or the restoration may be in the central fossa area to take up the slack in the reduction of a prominent supporting tip. In either case this can be a successful means of adjustment.

4. *Reduction of the noncontacting cusp.* When only one supporting cusp is actually functioning in support, the cusp that is out of contact is further reduced to eliminate its nonworking potentials.

The nonworking interference requires constant surveillance because one of the more frequent causes of the nonworking interference is overzealous grinding on the working side. The operator must be ever mindful of the dangers of inducing nonworking interferences.

Extruded molar that prevents incisive function. Occasionally an extruded mandibular third molar may prevent the anterior teeth from coming together in incisive function. When this occurs, the only effective treatment of choice is removal of the third molar. Unfortunately and in many instances this type of problem goes unnoticed. When incisive function is prevented from occurring, the pos-

sibility of temporomandibular joint problems is quite great (Fig. 30-46). In this case we see that the incisive function is restored by extracting the third molar.

Use of Hawley appliance to induce posterior eruption and to gain mechanical advantage. If in the course of the grinding technique anterior teeth are caused to strike quite heavily, the grinding procedure must stop, for this indicates that a closure in the occlusal vertical dimension past the original opening has taken place. At this point it is suggested that a Hawley bite plane appliance be introduced to induce posterior tooth eruption. Although the induced posterior eruption will not be of a permanent nature, it will allow further selective grinding of the posterior teeth without reducing the occlusal vertical dimension. This allows for better mechanical advantage in carrying out a more complete and thorough adjustment of the occlusion. Unfortunately the nature of this text does not permit elaboration of the technique in great detail at this time. The reader is referred to Chapter 21 for further amplification.

SUMMARY

The limitations of occlusal adjustment must be thoroughly understood if the reshaping procedures are to offer their maximum therapeutic effect. Thorough examination of the symptoms present, together with a complete and meticulous evaluation of the dynamic mechanical and physiologic aspects of the occlusion, are mandatory to determine whether an occlusal adjustment is necessary and whether selective grinding will be able to obtain a desired result. It is our strong belief that selective grinding procedures should never be employed prophylactically in the adult. The differences between the physiologic and pathologic occlusion must be thoroughly understood.

GLOSSARY
Jaw position

apparent free-way space Amount of space between teeth in postural position; this distance may not be the true free-way space.

cyclic movements of mandible Masticatory cycles that are tear drop chewing strokes made by mandible during mastication.

free-way space Space between teeth when mandible is in postural position.

glide movement of mandible Horizontal mandibular movement with teeth in contact.

intercuspal position Habitual end contact of teeth that gives maximum support to lower teeth; it may or may not be in harmony with terminal hinge area; it is the most closed occlusal contacting position.

lateral mandibular glide Glide movement of mandible moving laterally with teeth in contact to the right or left.

nonworking side Side of mandible opposite direction to which mandible has been moved in lateral glide movement.

occlusal vertical dimension Vertical dimension of face when teeth are in intercuspal position.

postural position of mandible Position of mandible when individual is erect, in which the only work being done by muscles of mastication is to support weight of mandible; these muscles maintain tonus in this position and are not truly at rest; this is position of mandibular tonus also referred to as physiologic resting position of mandible.

postural vertical dimension Vertical dimension of face when jaw is in postural position; postural vertical dimension is dimension that is not fixed for each individual and may be anywhere from 1 to 11 mm.

protrusive mandibular glide Glide movement of mandible whereby mandible moves forward and incisors are brought together edge to edge.

retruded contact position Most superior position along retruded path of closure; initial contact of teeth during terminal hinge arc of closure.

retruded path of mandible Terminal hinge arc of mandibular closure.

true free-way space Difference between vertical dimension recorded in retruded contact position and vertical dimension recorded in postural position.

working side Side to which mandible has been moved in lateral glide movement.

Landmarks of teeth

buccolingual landmarks Bucco-occlusal line angle of mandible will be related to central fossa line of maxillary teeth; linguo-occlusal line of maxilla will be related to central fossa line of mandibular teeth.

bucco-occlusal line Imaginary line that is formed by junction of occlusal surface with outer aspect of buccal cusps of lower posterior teeth; in treatment this landmark must be related to central fossa line of opposing arch.

central fossa line Imaginary line (continuous with all posterior teeth in well-aligned dentition) that runs through center of teeth; it is not necessarily straight line.

continuity of the arch Appearance of posterior teeth, demonstrating that bucco-occlusal line and linguo-occlusal line angles are continuous and connecting; central fossa line should be uninterrupted; proper continuity of arch requires marginal ridges to be at same level and positioned in relation to supporting cusp tips; axial positioning of teeth should enhance this aspect; continuity of arch must be evaluated as part of examination of study casts.

guiding cusps Have potential for contact when mandible moves in glide movement; guiding cusps are inner aspects of mandibular lingual cusps and inner aspects of maxillary buccal cusps; lingual inclines of incisors and canines in maxillary arch must also be considered gliding inclines because they function together with guiding cusps.

linguo-occlusal line In upper arch is equivalent to lower bucco-occlusal line angle; it is formed by junction of occlusal surfaces and outer surfaces of upper supporting cusps.

mesiodistal landmark relations All supporting cusp tips articulate with interproximal marginal ridge areas except two—mesiolingual cusps of maxillary molars and distobuccal cusps of mandibular molars; these fall in central fossa areas.

normal width to the occlusal table Rarely if ever exceeds 55% of the overall tooth width; thus, under normal circumstances, natural tooth is quite narrow; when teeth are narrowed in therapy, they are narrowed to reestablish this relation.

occlusal table Width of occlusal surface of tooth; it is formed by inner aspects of cusps.

overbite Vertical overlap of teeth; distance from incisal edge of maxillary incisors to incisal edge of mandibular incisors when teeth are in intercuspal position.

overjet Horizontal overlap of teeth; when measured in incisor region, it is distance from incisal edge of mandibular incisors to lingual surface of maxillary incisors, when teeth are in intercuspal position.

rhythmicity of the arch Appearance of posterior cuspation; when cusps are aligned with rhythmic pattern, there is diminution in cusp height from anterior to posterior part of mouth, with gradual decrease in cusp width.

supporting cusps Portions of teeth that are responsible for support of force of occlusion; supporting cusps are comprised of lower buccal cusps and upper lingual cusps; they are distinctive in that they articulate with central fossa line areas of opposing teeth; supporting cusps are able to perform their function because of cradling action of opposing areas.

Tooth interference

fremitus Vibratory patterns of teeth; it is examined by placing index finger over maxillary teeth and feeling degree of vibration present during various jaw and glide movements; classified as class I, II, or III.

grasping contact Type of tooth interference whereby there is wide facetlike wear, with great friction between opposing parts; it is perhaps most destructive, since it offers greatest amount of friction between contacting surfaces.

Diagnosis

induced dental awareness Situation whereby positive occlusal sense has been caused by dental manipulation.

negative occlusal sense Lack of dental awareness; in healthy masticatory system the property of physiologic occlusion.

pathologic occlusion Refers to dentition that shows evidence of disease definitely attributable to occlusal abnormality; it can also refer to dentition in which there is inadequate function or cosmetic satisfaction; refers to mouth that requires treatment.

physiologic occlusion Refers to masticatory system that is free of disease attributed to occlusal abnormality; refers to mouth that can function comfortably and chew adequately, with no interference in either cosmetic or phonetic patterns; physiologic occlusion is one that has demonstrated ability to survive despite deviation from preconceived ideal.

positive occlusal sense Pathologic condition whereby patient is completely aware of arrangement of teeth and the way in which teeth strike; it usually carries with it a great deal of emotional anxiety.

REFERENCES

Amsterdam, M., and Abrams, L.: Periodontal prosthesis. In Goldman, H. M., Schluger, S., Fox, L., and Cohen, D. W.: Periodontal therapy, ed. 3, St. Louis, 1964, The C. V. Mosby Co.

Anderson, D. J.: A method of recording masticatory loads, J. Dent. Res. **32:**785, 1953.

Brenman, H., and Millsap, J.: A "sound" approach to occlusion, Bull. Phila. Cty. Dent. Soc. **24:**1, 1959.

Cohen, D. W.: Changes in the attachment apparatus in occlusal trauma, Alpha Omegan **45:**117, 1951.

Fox, L.: The occlusal factor in periodontal disease, Alpha Omegan **43:**124, 1949.

Manly, R. S.: Factors affecting masticatory performance and efficiency among young adults, J. Dent. Res. **30:**874, 1951.

Manly, R. S., and Braley, L. C.: Masticatory performance and efficiency, J. Dent. Res. **29:**448, 1950.

Manly, R. S., and Vinton, P.: The prosthodontist's problem patients, N.Y. Dent. J. **18:**113, 1952.

Manly, R. S., Yurkstas, A., and Reswick, J. B.: An instrument for measuring tooth mobility, J. Periodontol. **22:**148, 1951.

Posselt, U.: Recent trends in the concept of occlusal relationship, Int. Dent. J. **11:**331, 1961.

Posselt, U.: Range of movement of the mandible, J. Am. Dent. Assoc. **56:**10, 1958.

Posselt, U.: Studies in the mobility of the human mandible, Acta Odontol. Scand. **10**(supp. 10):19, 1952.

Strang, R. H. W.: Discussion of paper by Hemley, Am. J. Orthod. **24:**721, 1938.

31 Periodontal considerations in restorative dentistry

The problem
Priority
Realignment of teeth
Recontouring of ridges
Readjustment of occlusion
Restoration of teeth

The problem

Dental disease, neglect, and ill-conceived intervention often adversely affect the contour, alignment, and occlusion of the teeth and in the end seriously impair the health and integrity of the supporting tissues. This is strikingly exemplified by the changes that follow the premature removal of a tooth. In this situation the teeth that oppose the edentulous area extrude, and their alveolar housing and supporting tissues extrude with them. The interproximal contacts shift their position. Teeth adjacent to the edentulous area tip into the space (Fig. 31-1).

As a result there is a loss of protective coronal contour, of proper occlusal relationship, and of appropriate mutual support and alignment. Loose contacts and improper papilla and embrasure form then allow food impaction and retention that frequently predispose to the formation of osseous defects (Fig. 31-2). Poorly designed fixed restorations not only impose further stress on abutment teeth, but may also seriously injure the mucosa and bone of the intervening ridge (Fig. 31-3).

Priority

Under problem conditions, normal form, alignment, and occlusion of the teeth must be restored to ensure recovery and continued function of the supporting tissues. Tooth position, alignment, and contact should be adjusted first. When necessary, edentulous ridges should be recontoured. Soft tissue lesions must be removed, and the integrity of the gingival unit regained. Occlusal disharmony must be corrected to better distribute occlusal forces and to eliminate occlusal prematurities. Finally, the surfaces of those teeth destroyed because of disease processes or excessive wear should be restored and missing teeth replaced.

Realignment of teeth

The teeth should be so positioned that they have maximum resistance to the axial forces of occlusion. Such forces are best received when the teeth have proper interarch and intra-arch alignment and contact, when the buccolingual width of the food table is within the alveolar housing, and when the teeth are correctly positioned over basal bone.

Teeth that have become malaligned after premature tooth loss can ordinarily be uprighted or repositioned by minor tooth movement. Such procedures utilize tipping or tilting actions and involve uprighting or regrouping of anterior teeth. Moving teeth bodily may also be necessary. Such major orthodontic correction becomes essential when cusp tips occlude with each other in the terminal position or when the lower teeth fall entirely within the upper arch (Fig. 31-4).

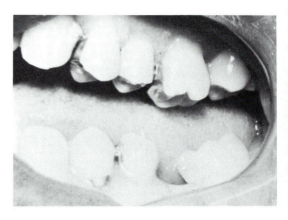

Fig. 31-1. Typical case of posterior bite collapse. Note extruded upper molar, drifting of teeth adjacent to edentulous space, uneven marginal ridges, poor contacts, and lingual position of lower second molar.

1112

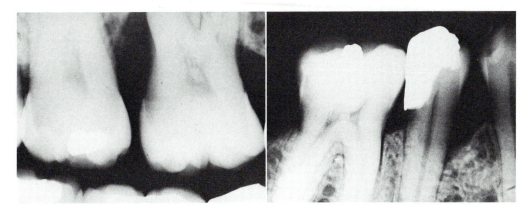

Fig. 31-2. Open contacts and associated osseous lesions.

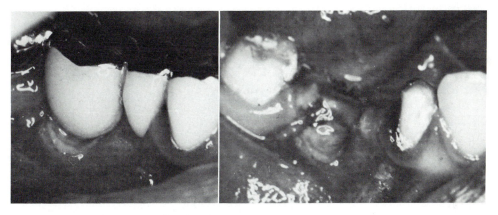

Fig. 31-3. Overextended pontic impinging on mucosal tissue. Note ulceration and osseous exposure when bridge is removed.

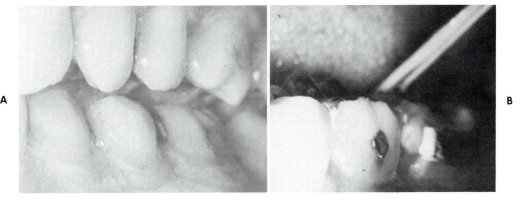

Fig. 31-4. A, Tips of lower buccal cusps with mandible positioned to coincide with terminal axis. **B,** Cross arch elastic bands utilized to upright teeth.

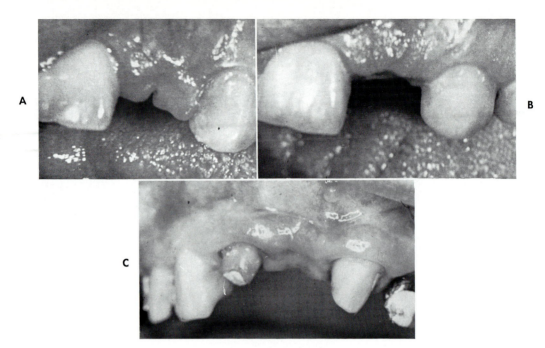

Fig. 31-5. A, Ridge immediately after poorly designed and unglazed porcelain trupontic was removed. **B,** Ridge 2 weeks later. **C,** Improper ridge form. It would be difficult to adapt a pontic to this ridge and maintain it in health.

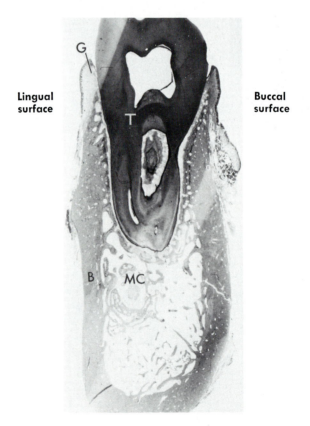

Fig. 31-6. Buccolingual section of mandibular first molar, showing thinner buccal plate in marginal area. *T,* Tooth; *B,* bone; *G,* gingiva; *MC,* mandibular canal.

Recontouring of ridges

Edentulous areas often need surgical intervention to ensure firm attachment of soft tissues to the bone. Often it is necessary to increase the zone of keratinized attached gingiva over the buccal aspect of the edentulous ridge. Surgical recontouring of osseous tissues may also be required to establish compatible ridge form in these same areas. Such recontouring should provide normal papillary form between the abutment and pontic in fixed restorations (Fig. 31-5).

Readjustment of occlusion

Occlusal discrepancies can frequently be corrected by selective grinding. Occlusal adjustment should precede the restorative phase. Such procedures accomplished prior to tooth preparation not only aid in estimating an adequate thickness of restorative material, but also allow for better final anatomic relationships between teeth. Reshaping the teeth that oppose a restoration will also permit better occlusal dimension and contour in the restored area.

The amount of grinding is related specifically to the interarch and intra-arch tooth position in centric occlusal relation. Selective grinding is contraindicated when relocation of the mandible to the terminal position relates the posterior teeth more than half a tooth distally. In these instances other procedures are indicated.

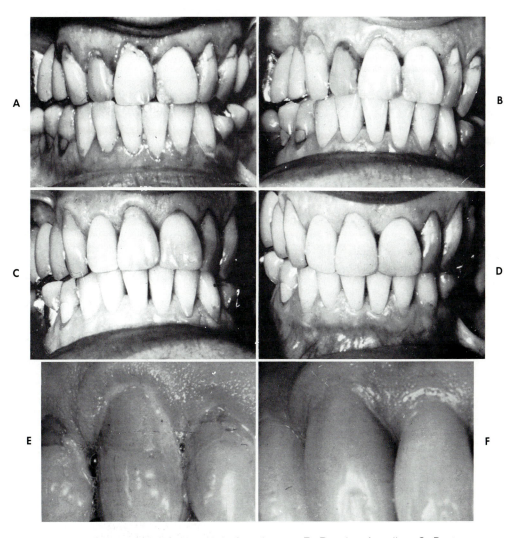

Fig. 31-7. A, Status of gingival health before therapy. **B,** Results of scaling. **C,** Postoperative results of periodontal therapy. Note poorly contoured silicate filling on labial surface of maxillary right central incisor. **D,** Change in gingival tissue after correction of this restoration. **E,** Inflammation around teeth because of insufficient subgingival contour. **F,** Healthy gingival tissue after restoration of proper subgingival form.

Restoration of teeth

Health of investing tissues is predicated upon a normal occlusal load and may necessitate restorative intervention. Sound intervention of course must guard the supporting tissues during the preparation and fabrication of the restoration. Favorable tissue response depends on the delicacy and respect with which the tissues are handled in each procedure.

During the preparation of a crown, for example, the supragingival area must be adequately prepared to allow subgingival preparation without mutilation of the keratinized epithelial cuff. Again, when drugs are carried subgingivally to retract the gin-

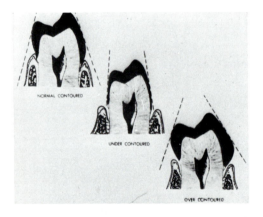

Fig. 31-8. Desired or normal crown contour, undercontour, and overcontour. With undercontoured crown, food in mastication is impacted into gingival sulcus. With an overcontoured crown, there is a marked tendency for plaque accumulation.

gival unit, they must be thoroughly controlled so that ischemia and gingival sloughing do not result.

All restorative procedures conducted on buccal and labial surfaces must be managed with the utmost care for the gingivae because of the delicate morphologic structure of the supporting tissues in these areas (Fig. 31-6). Where indicated, partial coverage restorations are used to avoid these facial gingival tissues.

Many times, however, because of inadequate contour the buccal or labial subgingival tissues need additional support to hold the gingival cuff securely to the subjacent tooth. When adequate subgingival tissue is not present, the gingival unit collapses and assumes the appearance of a worn-out elastic band. Subsequent proper subgingival contour can restore this tissue to health (Fig. 31-7).

The importance of buccal and labial supragingival contour cannot be overemphasized. These surfaces must be contoured sufficiently to prevent food impaction in the gingival sulcus and at the same time allow physiologic stimulation of the gingival unit (Fig. 31-8).

With the widespread use of porcelain and plastic veneer crowns at present, the problem is generally one of overcontour. From a mechanical and aesthetic standpoint, it is difficult not to exceed desired crown contour, so it is essential to make adequate tooth preparation.

The intimate relationship of interproximal tissues, tooth contact, and embrasure form is important to gingival health. Restorative dentists have therefore labored to restore proper interproximal

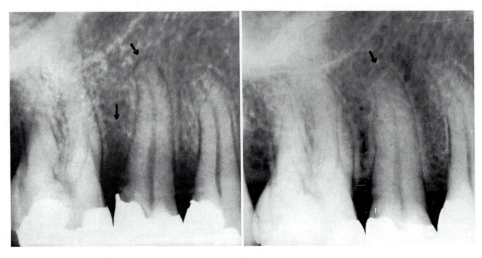

Fig. 31-9. Before and after healing of crestal area between second premolar and first molar. New restorations established proper marginal ridges and contacts. Occlusal adjustment was performed. Note changes in attachment apparatus *(arrows)* and also healing of lamina dura.

form to maintain healthy gingival tissue (Fig. 31-9).

Tooth contacts are definitely positioned both in the buccolingual and the occlusogingival directions. Thus occlusogingival contact occurs about the junction of the occlusal and middle third of the tooth. Except for the upper molars, buccolingual contact occurs approximately at the junction of the buccal and middle thirds of the teeth. Func-

tionally such an arrangement provides room for the gingival papilla and for the escape of food during mastication from the occlusal surface out the lingual spillway. The lingual tissue is much broader and appears more capable of resisting the passage of food (Fig. 31-10).

Finally, attention must be paid not only to tooth preparation and to the contour and contacts of the restoration but also to margins. Margins of resto-

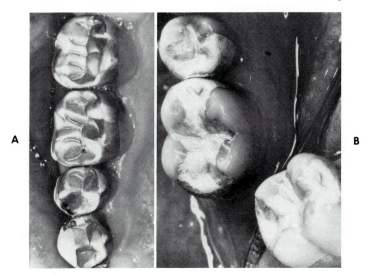

Fig. 31-10. A, Gold inlay restorations for posterior quadrant in position and being checked for occlusal relationships prior to cementation. Note markings on buccodistal marginal ridge of first premolar, tip of mesiobuccal incline of second premolar, and distolingual cusp of second molar. Proximal contacts as well as cervical margins are tested. Proximal contour of restorations should be checked. **B,** Amalgam restorations in position and being checked for proximal contact. Note that proximal marginal ridge of premolar has a crease in it that should be considered as a fault. Food impaction is possible under these circumstances.

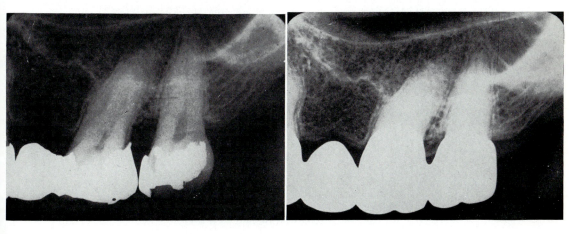

Fig. 31-11. Correction of faulty contact and overhanging restoration between two molars. New bridge was inserted, and two molars were splinted to be utilized as abutments. Note regeneration of interdental crest.

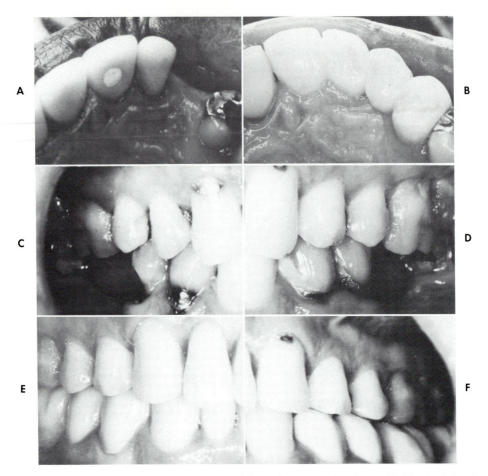

Fig. 31-12. A, Gingival inflammation around lingual aspect of incisors. **B,** Tissue 1 week after provisional restoration was placed. Note absence of inflammation around provisional as compared to unrestored central and lateral teeth. **C** to **F,** Manner in which occlusion has been corrected with provisional restoration. Note correction of extruded upper molars and reestablished occlusal plane.

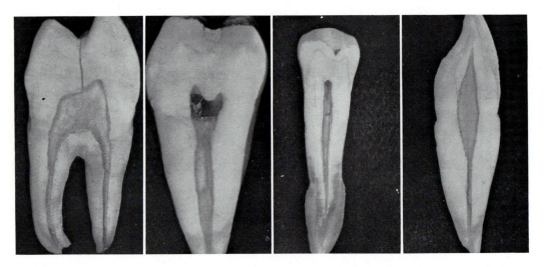

Fig. 31-13. Variation in size and shape of roots of teeth. Length of root is important, but total surface area of root housed by a healthy attachment apparatus is key to selection of abutment teeth.

rations should be placed below the gingival crest to prevent sensitivity and recurrent decay and to provide subgingival support for the gingival unit. The effect of overhanging margins and unpolished surfaces has been obvious to the astute clinician for years. A restoration that thus encroaches on the space occupied by healthy supporting structures must eventually end in failure (Fig. 31-11).

Provisional restorations. Temporary or provisional restorations not only serve to protect prepared teeth during the fabrication of the finished restoration, but they should also maintain occlusal forces, restore buccal, lingual, and interproximal

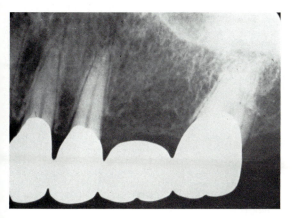

Fig. 31-14. Proper form of crowns and embrasure spaces in a fixed prosthesis.

contours, provide a finite gingival margin and adequate subgingival contour, be smooth and polished to allow keratinization of the gingival sulcus, and replace the missing teeth. This will begin conditioning the periodontal ligament to the increased load. To meet these demands a restoration must be quickly and precisely fashioned.

The gold band acrylic provisional restoration best meets this need in fixed prosthesis. The shell can be fabricated from an impression of a model after occlusion has been altered to meet the functional demands. Utilization of the gold band acrylic technique, in contrast to the alginate impression technique, permits better control of the heat during chemical polymerization of the acrylic and avoids undue tissue damage.

The use of these provisional restorations permits the occlusion to be established on abutment teeth with resilient plastic. Thus an atrophic periodontal ligament can begin to repair, and a normal periodontal ligament can be conditioned to withstand the additional load. The gingival tissues should remain in health. But when the gingival tissues are not healthy because of improper subgingival crown contour, the provisional restoration provides this contour, and the tissues can be returned to health. Furthermore, the entire restoration can be set up and the finished result visualized (Fig. 31-12). Evaluation of the completed pro-

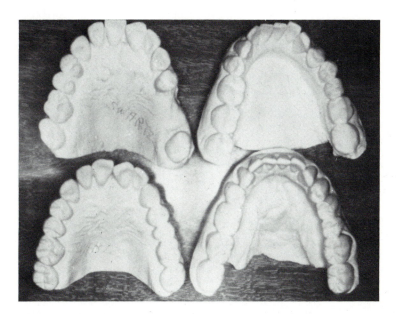

Fig. 31-15. Properly designed restorations and fixed partial prosthesis for maxillary left posterior segment can be seen in lower casts. Upper casts reveal uneven marginal ridges, insecure proximal contacts (for example, maxillary left first and second premolars and maxillary right first and second molars) and a reverse occlusal plane. Note corrections as seen in lower casts.

visional restoration should facilitate a more accurate prognosis of the finished restoration.

Finished restorations. Whenever a choice exists, missing teeth should be permanently replaced with fixed restorations so that the forces transmitted to the abutment teeth might be more adequately controlled. These restorations must be designed, of course, so that the investing tissues can sustain the forces placed upon them by occlusion. Careful assessment must therefore be made of the potential ability of any tooth to support the load of additional tooth replacement. Abutment teeth should either be vital or have successfully received endodontic treatment. They must possess sufficient supragingival tooth structure for retention of the retainer. They must be firmly supported by alveolar bone and periodontal liga-ments in healthy condition. And, finally, the total surface area of healthy attachment apparatus, estimated from the amount of bone and the size and shape of the roots, must be clinically judged sufficient to sustain the occlusal load over the length of the span (Fig. 31-13).

Adequate abutments with pontics properly designed for anatomic form and contour in the critical interproximal areas (Fig. 31-14), for occlusal table, and for joint strength will ensure successful tooth replacement. Such fixed restorations will reestablish arch integrity, correct occlusal disharmonies, and protect the investing tissues (Fig. 31-15). Dental intervention then becomes a therapeutic service restoring tooth form and function and creating a more physiologic periodontium and total oral environment.

32 Periodontal prosthesis

DEFINITION AND CLINICAL GUIDELINES

Periodontal prosthesis may be defined as those restorative and prosthetic endeavors that are indicated and essential in the total treatment of advanced periodontal disease. Whereas specifically it refers to the treatment of the dentition mutilated by the ravages of periodontal disease, in general its concepts, principles, and techniques may be employed in any restorative or tooth replacement service involving the natural dentition.

Restorative dentistry and prosthetic dentistry are primarily concerned with the maintenance of dental health and function. Disease processes that may disturb this status could affect any part of the masticatory organ. These parts are the teeth, their supporting structures (hard and soft), and the temporomandibular articulation and its associated musculature. Although periodontal prosthesis is primarily concerned with the teeth and their supporting structures, at no time should treatment conflict with the function of the temporomandibular joint and its associated musculature. Conversely, any treatment of dysfunction of the temporomandibular joint and associated musculature may not be performed in violation of the health and function of the teeth and their supporting structures.

The two most common diseases that threaten the natural dentition are dental caries and periodontal disease. Although separate and distinct disease entities, they have certain traits in common in that they are both responsible for loss of teeth. Dental caries is primarily a disease of the child and the young adult and is responsible for most teeth that are lost in the first three decades of life. Periodontal disease, although present in the child and young adult, increases in rate and incidence almost proportional to the age of the patient and is responsible for the loss of most teeth after the first three decades of life. In our society the life span of human beings has been increased markedly; it therefore becomes the responsibility of the dental profession to see that the life span of the natural dentition is increased proportionally.

Research endeavors have revealed that periodontal disease is due to microbial masses (plaque) on the teeth. In advanced cases of the results of periodontal disease, not only is it important that the disease process be overcome, but in many instances a periodontal prosthesis may be necessary to control the hypermobility of the teeth that may exist postoperatively. It should be stressed that a carefully designed plaque control program must be followed by the patient. With these therapeutic measures it has been demonstrated that periodontal health can be maintained.

In addition dental caries and periodontal disease are important contributing factors in etiology, one to the other. Dental caries is one of the most important etiologic factors in periodontal disease for the following reasons:

1. Loss of proximal contact, with resultant food impaction and retention
2. Loss of smooth surface area, with food retention and loss of protective tooth contour
3. Accelerated drift of teeth and bite collapse due to loss of proximal contact and occlusal surface area
4. Disturbance of function and alteration in chewing habits and home care complications
5. Introduction of operative dental procedures or iatrogenic factors
6. Premature loss of teeth, with gross alteration in their form and function resulting from loss of interarch and intra-arch integrity

Periodontal disease contributes as a causative factor to dental caries in the following ways:

1. Increase of bacterial plaque formation due to food impaction and retention

2. Alteration in form and function, that is, embrasures and crown-tissue relations

3. Areas of tooth structure exposed that are more susceptible to dental caries than is enamel

4. Alteration in function and home care resulting from root sensitization

In periodontal disease, as in dental caries, we find that the mutilations of the disease become permanent and are frequently more complicating in therapy than the active disease process itself. In fact, the scars of the disease may become propagating etiologic factors. *Periodontal prosthesis concerns itself with the correction of the mutilating factors of dental disease by attempting to restore alterations in form, particularly as it relates to function* (Fig. 32-1).

One important aspect of reconstruction of the dentition afflicted by periodontal disease and caries to such a degree that healing of the periodontium alone is not sufficient for maintenance of health is the stabilization and replacement of missing teeth.

The therapist must have an understanding of periodontics as well as the knowledge and capability to perform fixed and removable partial prosthetics. He must be capable of performing occlusal adjustment via prosthetic means. Amsterdam reported on 25 years of periodontal prosthesis in retrospect as follows:

In our profession we have very few facts, and therefore much of what we do clinically is conceptual. A valid clinical concept must have at least, a firm foundation in basic science. In addition, what plagues us as clinicians is that we are always treating a statistically insignificant number—one—that particular patient, and we know not where that patient may fall in any statistical study.

With these factors in mind we must observe the following guidelines in practice that are true in any field.

1. The first key to success is the ability to establish a correct diagnosis. *There may be different ways of treating a disease, but there can be but one correct diagnosis.*

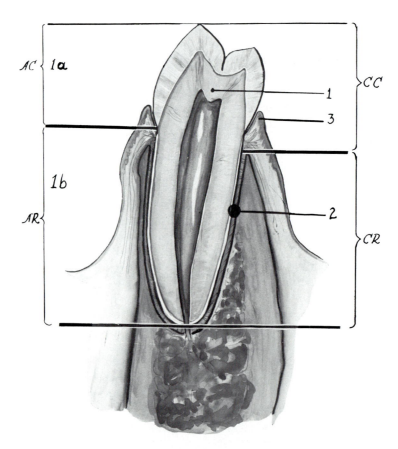

Fig. 32-1. Basic dental unit is composed of the following: *1,* tooth; *2,* attachment apparatus; *3,* gingival unit. Tooth may be further divided into anatomic crown, *1a,* and anatomic root, *1b. AC,* Anatomic crown; *CC,* clinical crown; *AR,* anatomic root; *CR,* clinical root.

2. The basis of all therapy is the identification, elimination, or control of all known etiologic factors.
3. The prognosis will be dependent on the following:
   a. the ability to determine a correct diagnosis
   b. the ability of the therapist to eliminate, control, or modify influential aspects of the contributing etiologic factors
   c. the ability of the patient to understand and cooperate in this endeavor.
4. The more known and recognizable etiologic factors ascertained, the more predictable the prognosis.
5. Most of the known and discernible factors are local.
6. When present and determinable, the significance of systemic factors may be the key to a successful prognosis.
7. More frequently than not, systemic factors are not definable either because of inadequate knowledge or of inadequate available diagnostic tests. One must realize, because of the infrequency of positive systemic findings, that it is easy to overlook or ignore situations where, if proper evaluative methods were used, findings might be positive.
8. The host resistance factor or immunologic factors are the areas most fruitful and logical for basic research, for herein lie most of the critical answers to the problem—"What makes one patient more susceptible to the disease than another?"
9. The patient with a multitude of recognizable causative factors even though in a more advanced state of disease presents a better prognosis than a patient less involved, but with no determined cause.
10. Because of the progressive nature of the disease process, the age of the patient is a peculiarly significant factor in prognosis. Despite possible increased length of healing time, all other factors being equal, *the older the patient the better the prognosis.*

All of these factors must be constantly borne in mind from the inception of treatment and every effort made to keep the scope of therapy within the confines of that which is optimal for that patient.

What may be good treatment for one patient may be poor treatment for another.[Amsterdam, 1974]

COLLECTIVE PROTECTIVE ACTION OF TEETH

In normal function the teeth serve to protect the two basic areas of the periodontium: the gingival tissues and the attachment apparatus.

EFFECTS OF FACIAL AND LINGUAL CONTOURS OF TEETH

The facial and lingual surfaces of the crowns (Fig. 32-2) exhibit convex contours on their gingival third of approximately 0.5 mm (mandibular molars may be as great as 1 mm on the lingual surface).

The convexity is precisely related to the position of the gingival sulcus and directs the passage of food away from the sulcus and onto the attached gingiva. The sulcus therefore is prevented by the coronal convexity from becoming a depository for debris and microbial plaque (Fig. 32-3).

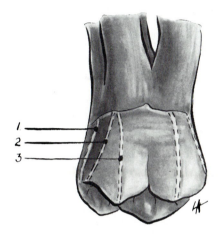

Fig. 32-2. Normal coronal contours of tooth can be divided into three areas: *1,* proximal surface—flat and in some instances concave; *2,* transitional line angle—also very flat; *3,* buccal surface—convex with height of convexity in gingival third of crown.

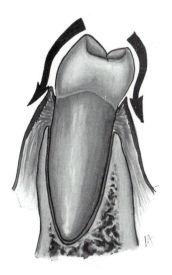

Fig. 32-3. Normal dental unit. Arrows indicate passage of food that is deflected away from sulcus onto attached gingiva.

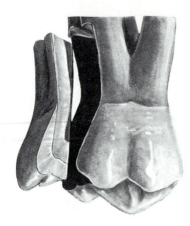

Fig. 32-4. Proximal section of tooth from transitional line angle to transitional line angle has been removed to emphasize flattened design of this area.

EFFECTS OF PROXIMAL CONTOURS OF TEETH

The proximal surfaces of the crowns create the interproximal embrasures that form the canopy that houses the interdental papilla. These surfaces are flattened and in some instances concave (Fig. 32-4).

Under normal circumstances the interdental papilla will completely fill the interproximal embrasure. The flattened proximal contours will permit sufficient room for the interdental papilla to reside in health and at the same time to protect this area from the adversities of food and debris retention.

The interproximal embrasure space created by the correct adjacent contacts of teeth should possess the following properties:

1. Contact areas of the teeth are located in the occlusal fourth and slightly closer to the buccal surface in posterior teeth.
2. Proximal surfaces of adjacent teeth tend to be minor images of each other so that a symmetric canopy is created.
3. Adjacent marginal ridges are of the same height.
4. Contact is sufficiently tight to prevent any food impaction or retention. (It should be noted that the contact surface area widens with age as a result of proximal wear.)

Correct interproximal embrasures result in correct arch alignment that possesses a definite continuity of tooth forms. This continuity is expressed as a gradual change from anterior to posterior teeth and demonstrates a continuous alignment of occlusal tables, central fossae, and cusp tips.

Since the interdental embrasure is a primary site of dental disease, both gingival and carious, it bears close surveillance. As was stated earlier, this area may be considered a canopy that houses the interdental papilla. The roof is created by the very tight positioning of the contact areas of the teeth. The walls are formed by the proximal surfaces of the adjacent teeth. The base is formed by the proximal surfaces of the adjacent teeth. The base is formed by the cementoenamel junctions of the proximal surfaces.

Symmetry to this area is created by the approximating surfaces of the teeth, which will be mirror counterparts of each other. The cementoenamel junctions will be at the same level. It should be noted that crestal bone height parallels the relative heights of the proximal cementoenamel junctions. The distance between the base of the contact areas and the cementoenamel junction will be the same in adjacent teeth. Sufficient room will be created by these symmetric walls to allow for the establishment of an adequate interdental gingival papilla with a minimum of col formation.

The end result of embrasure form therefore will be the establishment of a series of contours that will either prevent debris retention or allow the normal processes of detergent mastication and lip, cheek, and tongue action to render the area clean.

This fine harmony of tooth form and resultant soft tissue protection is predicated not only upon the correct crown contour alignment but also upon the correct architecture and positioning of the gingival tissues.

Even though the dental arch may possess a desirable continuity of tooth forms, all this may be negated by any changes in gingival positioning in either a coronal or a gingival direction.

In summation, therefore, one can say that the teeth protect the gingiva by the correct relations of crown contour, arch continuity, gingival architecture, and gingival position.

ATTACHMENT APPARATUS

The importance of direction in a given occlusal load and its tolerance by the attachment apparatus (Fig. 32-5) has been well established. Forces transmitted in an axial direction are best withstood.

The location and design of the occlusal table of the posterior tooth tend to accomplish this end by the following three means:

1. The buccolingual width of the occlusal table is no more than 60% of the overall buccolingual width of the tooth (Figs. 32-20 and 32-21).
2. The occlusal table is located over the axial center of the root.

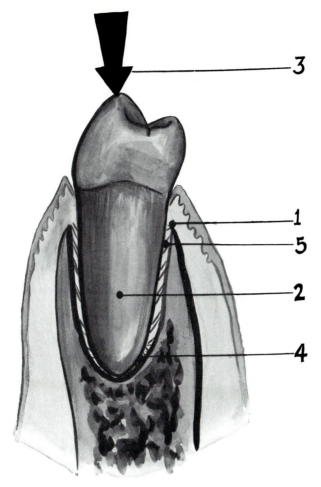

Fig. 32-5. Physiologic occlusal force upon a normal dental unit. *1,* Height of alveolar bone; *2,* fulcrum point; *3,* axially applied force; *4,* area of pressure; *5,* area of tension.

3. The occlusal table is perpendicular to the axial inclination of the tooth.

All this tends to place the force recipient area of the posterior tooth directly over the central axis of the root, which in turn serves to direct the occlusal load vertically within the alveolar housing.

The occlusal tables of posterior teeth perform their protective function during maximum jaw closure in the bracing position. It is at this time that the greatest occlusal load is applied.

Due to the absence of occlusal tables in the maxillary anterior teeth, centric occlusal forces here are not transmitted axially. The maxillary incisors and canines therefore require protection from the possibilities of horizontally directed forces during maximum occlusion. This necessary protection is provided by the posterior teeth, which create the proper stability and support to the mandible during bracing.

The anterior teeth appear to be designed as guideposts to the functional movements of the jaw.

It is suspected that in this role they play a sensory function as well. This affords a reciprocal protective action to the posterior teeth by causing them to be disarticulated when the mandible moves out of the maximum occlusal position.

In summation, we can say that when the mandible is in the bracing position of maximum occlusion only posterior teeth are designed to sustain this load. This in turn protects the anterior teeth from horizontal overloading. When the mandible moves to and from maximum occlusion, the anterior teeth, with their guidances, both mechanical and sensory, reciprocate by disarticulating the posterior teeth and thus prevent their horizontal overloading and excessive wear.

ALTERED FUNCTION OF DISEASED DENTAL UNIT

As stated previously, periodontal disease most frequently results in tissue loss that for the most part cannot be recovered. Only in the instance of

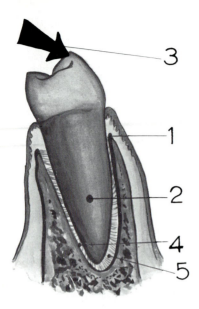

Fig. 32-6. Primary occlusal traumatism. *1,* Height of alveolar bone (normal); *2,* fulcrum point; *3,* horizontally applied pathologic force; *4,* area of pressure; *5,* area of tension.

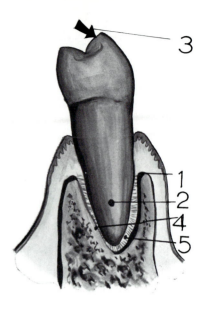

Fig. 32-7. Secondary occlusal traumatism. *1,* Height of alveolar bone (lost due to previous disease); *2,* fulcrum point; *3,* horizontally applied force during normal function; *4,* area of pressure; *5,* area of tension.

gingivitis (Fig. 32-8) and primary occlusal traumatism (Fig. 32-6) is it possible to resolve the lesions without permanent tissue deformity. However, once there is true periodontitis, the resultant apical migration of the epithelial attachment creates exposure of anatomic root surface. The changes that result in a difference between the anatomic crown and the clinical crown and a difference between the anatomic root and the clinical root are most damaging (Fig. 32-9).

As long as the anatomic crown and root and clinical crown and root are identical, the problems in therapy are relatively simple. In this instance dentistry may offer the simplest and most economic treatment with a most favorable prognosis. Conversely, the greater the deviation between the anatomic and clinical counterparts, the less dentistry can offer in prognosis and the more dentistry demands in effort and cost. Unfortunately this is the situation that exists in most cases truly requiring periodontal prosthesis.

However, the important contribution of periodontal prosthesis from a public health standpoint is what has been learned from it. Certainly if its principles, concepts, and techniques can create favorable results in treating the advanced cases, the effects are most beneficial when applied to the incipient or less advanced clinical condition, and the health service is far greater.

An understanding of the known etiologic se-

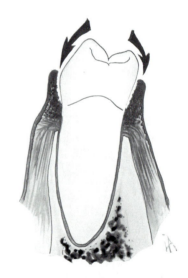

Fig. 32-8. Gingival edema with pseudopocket formation causes a change in position of gingival margin that will negate protective contours of tooth, causing gingival sulcus to become a depository for food debris and plaque.

quence of events in the history of a mouth with advanced periodontal disease makes the importance of early and proper therapeutic intervention quite clear. In the absence of marginal inflammatory disease of the attachment apparatus, as was stated earlier, a dentition may be completely healed without tissue loss after rational therapy. Such is the

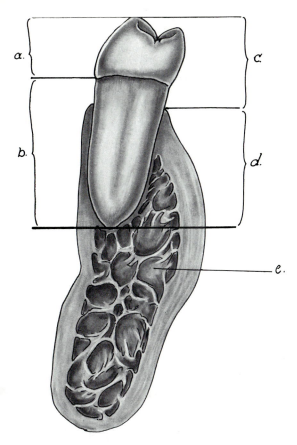

Fig. 32-9. Clinical crown-root ratio. *a,* Anatomic crown; *b,* anatomic root; *c,* clinical crown; *d,* clinical root; *e,* alveolar process. Anatomic crown of tooth is that part covered by enamel. Clinical crown of tooth is that part coronal to epithelial attachment. Anatomic root is that part of tooth covered by cementum or originally covered by cementum. Clinical root is that part of tooth apical to epithelial attachment. Determination and evaluation of crown-to-root ratio are made by roentgenographic interpretation done in conjunction with clinical periodontal probing.

case of primary occlusal traumatism (Fig. 32-5). Here, as a result of excessive force in the presence of a normal amount of supporting tissue, changes in the attachment apparatus are observable as the classic signs and symptoms of the lesion of occlusal traumatism.

In this instance, particularly if arch integrity and interarch relations are correct, occlusal therapy may resolve the problem, and healing will ensue. Occlusal adjustment by selective grinding is most efficient under these circumstances.

When untreated, gingival inflammation, even in the absence of an occlusal irritant, penetrates deeper into the periodontal structures, and the resulting apical migration of the epithelial attach-

ment causes exposure of tooth structure ill designed for the oral environment (Figs. 32-10 and 32-11). The exposed cementum in many instances is soon lost, and dentin is then uncovered. Both dentin and cementum, as discussed earlier, are softer, more conducive to plaque formation, and less resistant to abrasion, erosion, and caries than is enamel. Further, these areas of exposed anatomic root may become hypersensitive and thus alter masticatory and home care habits. This alteration in form and function results in an interruption of the self-protective capacity of the dental unit by creating a disparity of embrasure forms, crown-tissue relations, and marginal gingiva. Root caries present one of the most vexing and insoluble problems to the dentist attempting to use routine restorative procedures.

If allowed to continue, the resultant loss of supporting structure may become so extensive that secondary occlusal traumatism will result. When this phenomenon occurs in the presence of an intact dentition, it is challenging enough; however, if arch integrity is lost and posterior bite collapse is superimposed upon the condition, the results may well be clinically disastrous.

Posterior bite collapse occurs most frequently because of the accelerated mesiodistal drift of teeth, and it results in loss of the stabilizing support of the posterior teeth. This in turn causes the extension of excessive load to the anterior teeth and negates the natural protection that the posterior teeth normally afford. In addition tilting of the posterior teeth prevents optimal transmission of axial forces.

Posterior bite collapse may occur as a result of the following:

1. Premature loss of a posterior tooth or teeth without proper replacement
2. Orthodontic deformity and arch crowding
3. Loss of proximal contact at an excessive rate either through caries or iatrogenic causes
4. Abnormal wear of teeth
5. Reduction of occlusal surface contact areas due to either caries or inadequate operative dentistry

It has been our experience that 95% of all patients requiring periodontal prosthesis have as a common denominator posterior bite collapse. The overwhelming majority of these dental casualties are the result of premature loss of posterior teeth, and the 6-year molar is the usual victim.

Here the result is mesial drift of the distal molars, distal drift of the premolars, and extrusion of the opposing teeth. This gives rise to the de-

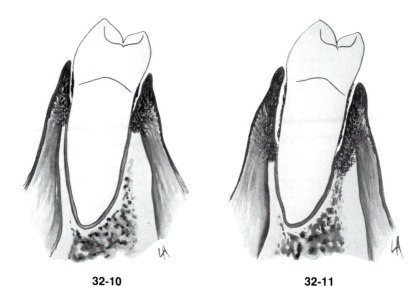

32-10   **32-11**

Fig. 32-10. Periodontitis with true pocket formation, causing a disparity between anatomic crown and root and clinical crown and root.

Fig. 32-11. Further progression of marginal disease, causing further loss of supporting tissue, resulting in secondary occlusal traumatism.

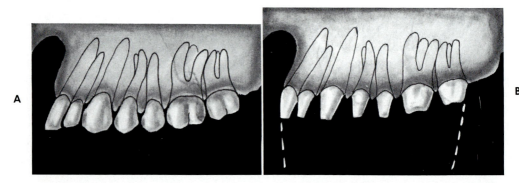

Fig. 32-12. Clinical crown and root and anatomic crown and root are identical. **A,** Prior to tooth preparation. **B,** After tooth preparation, showing relative simplicity of restorative design.

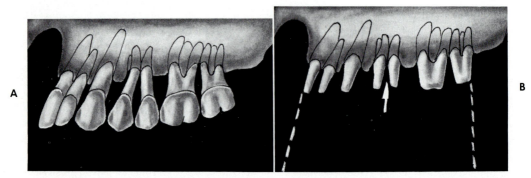

Fig. 32-13. Clinical crown and root are not identical to anatomic crown and root, as in severe periodontal disease. **A,** After periodontal therapy. **B,** Problems in tooth preparation magnified because of increased length of roots, uncovering of flared roots, and convergent roots *(arrow).* Note that parallelism is impossible.

velopment of unlevel marginal ridges and marginal gingiva and altered embrasure forms. For every unlevel marginal ridge there is an unlevel cementoenamel junction. The unlevel cementoenamel junction gives rise to angular crestal formation, which in turn may be responsible for alveolar osseous defects, and thus infrabony pockets may be a common sequela in the presence of gingival inflammation. The mandible usually is displaced anteriorly as a result of interfering occlusal contacts, with an excessive load being placed on the anterior teeth, which ultimately may fan and become mobile. Control of the clinical condition at this point obviously requires the most heroic of dental efforts.

In summation, therefore, it must be reemphasized that the only effective treatment for advanced periodontal disease is prevention or early treatment. This requires a complete and thorough understanding of the self-protective mechanism of the individual dental unit and its application to the collective mutual protective action of the dentition, which after all is the sum total of the individual dental units. It would seem therefore that the key to prevention of irreversible ravages of dental disease is the maintenance of the integrity of this system on an individual and collective basis.

In the case of dental caries, if the invasion of decay is through enamel and dentin, not only must the active disease process be removed, but form must also be replaced to restore function and to protect against further progression of the disease. Admittedly there is little problem in removing the active disease process; the difficulty lies in doing it in such a way that functional form can be restored. Such is also the case in the treatment of periodontal disease. Removal of the diseased gingival attachment is not difficult, but to do so and to restore proper form and function may be quite complicated and often impossible without the aid of restorative dentistry.

BASIC RESTORATIVE PRINCIPLES OF OCCLUSION
Physiologic versus pathologic occlusion

Angle has defined normal occlusion as the structural composite of teeth and jaws arranged in a harmonious relationship of the occlusal inclined planes of the teeth individually and collectively located in architectural harmony with their basal bones and with cranial anatomy. The teeth should exhibit correct proximal contacting and axial positioning and should be associated with a normal growth and developmental pattern in correlation with their environmental tissues.

This is the picture of a set of conditions that is rarely seen in clinical practice. When the dentist is confronted with deviations from this pattern, he must evaluate the conditions carefully and must determine whether a pathologic occlusion is present. It is imperative that the dentist recognize the basic fact that even though occlusal relations do not conform to a preconceived standard, the patient may still present a physiologic occlusion, an occlusion that is *individually normal for him*. A "physiologic occlusion" may be defined as one in which the system of forces acting on the teeth during occlusion is in a state of equilibrium and will not change the healthy relation existing between the teeth and their supporting structures.

In evaluating the occlusion of a patient the dentist must use the criteria of health, function aesthetics, and comfort, which follow:

1. Can the patient chew adequately?
2. Is he aesthetically satisfied?
3. Does he have a good phonetic pattern?
4. Is he in good periodontal health?
5. Is he free from subjective and objective temporomandibular joint symptoms?
6. Is there an absence of retrograde wear patterns of the teeth?
7. Is there a negative occlusal sense present?

If the patient affirmatively meets these criteria, the clinician must use good judgment lest he interfere with a state of conditions to which the patient has comfortably and adequately become adapted. A "pathologic occlusion" is one that does not meet these requirements. It should be kept in mind, however, that functional, aesthetic, and phonetic standards will vary with each patient and must be handled accordingly.

Objectives of occlusal intervention

The treatment of the pathologic occlusion and the control of its associated symptom complex demand utmost attention to the therapeutic principles involved. The corrected occlusion, particularly in those cases requiring periodontal prosthesis, must fulfill the following six objectives that are conducive but not necessarily prerequisite to health:

1. The teeth should be in maximum occlusion when the jaws are in centric relation at an acceptable vertical dimension, allowing for an adequate interocclusal distance.
2. The mandible should have freedom to move to and from centric relation without restraint.
3. The crown-to-root ratio must be at the opti-

mal level permissible under the existing clinical conditions.

4. The teeth should be so positioned and axially inclined that their roots are located within the confines of their periodontal structures.

5. The coronal forms and the proximal contacting relationships of the teeth should be such as to provide maximum protection to the investing structures.

6. The aesthetic pattern should satisfy the needs of the patient.

OPTIMAL OCCLUSION IN CENTRIC RELATION

Centric relation* is that maxillomandibular relationship in which all the muscles and their ligaments on each side of the temporomandibular articulation are in a state of balance when the condyles are rested terminally and in which position the maximum interocclusal relation of the teeth is achieved.

Centric relation would not exist or certainly could not be recognized in the absence of teeth or their counterpart. It is therefore a three-dimensional phenomenon, having a mediolateral, an anteroposterior, and a vertical dimension.

The genesis of centric relation is associated with the eruption of teeth and the establishment of facial height. The anteroinferior limit to centric relation is the mandibular postural position (physiologic rest position). The posterosuperior limit is the terminal hinge position. It has been well established that the occlusal vertical dimension must be created at a facial height that will allow for sufficient interocclusal clearance (interocclusal distance).

The only known functions that may occur in centric relation are a phase of the swallowing reflex and, infrequently, the fleeting termination of the masticatory cycle. All functional masticatory and deglutitory movements of the mandible are distal and retrusive in direction. The most posterior mandibular position is located on the terminal hinge arc of closure. This is a reproducible posterior border movement and as such is determined by the action of the temporomandibular and capsular ligaments. In functional movements the proprioceptive action of muscle spindles and Golgi tendon organs of the associated musculature probably function to limit distal superior condylar movements before tension on the ligaments becomes extreme. Therefore, conceptually, centric

relation must be slightly anterior to the extreme condylar position as ultimately determined by the distensibility of ligaments. *The distance between the extreme, strained terminal condylar position and the one in which the musculature and the ligaments are in a state of balance is usually not clinically measurable.* The conceptual difference between the strained and the unstrained position must be kept in mind when one is attempting to locate the ideal harmonious relation between the temporomandibular articulation and the maximum intercuspation of the teeth.

Although the terminal hinge position may be employed as a guide in attempting to locate and transfer centric relation to an articulator, the final adjustment and acceptance of centric relation must be made in the mouth. Usually this is accomplished by a series of remount procedures that bring the registration closer and closer to the desired position. Correct centric relation must demonstrate a simultaneous articulation of all the individual centric holding surfaces of the posterior teeth in total harmony with bilateral symmetric neuromuscular activity in the absence of any proprioceptive action of the ligaments.

In the therapy of a pathologic occlusion it is important that a positive centric relation be established for the following reasons:

1. Centric relation is the only position that is both reliably reproducible and physiologically acceptable.

2. Centric relation is the only functional bilateral tooth contacting position of the mandible. This position allows for maximum bracing of the mandible by the teeth during the initiation and termination of the swallowing reflex. This reflex is initiated in the most posterior mandibular position and always terminates in the maximum intercuspal position.

3. Correct centric relation is essential in the control of parafunctional mandibular movements (bruxing and grinding habit patterns). Parafunctional tooth contacts are believed to be the initial insult in the origination of the lesion of primary occlusal traumatism. Although this action is complex, being of both local and emotional origin, the consensus of clinical investigators is that local tooth interferences play an important role in the initiation of these destructive habits.

The most important occlusal discrepancies are those that interfere with the reflex jaw closure in both conscious and preconscious swallowing. These tooth interferences are observable when centric occlusion is incorrect and mandibular displace-

---

*We have taken the liberty of making the terms "centric occlusal relation" and "centric relation" synonymous.

ment is present. Therefore occlusal adjustment for the purpose of establishing a correct and positive centric relation will tend to eliminate or minimize the triggering action of occlusal interference. This is indispensable to the clinical control of the destructive effects of parafunction.

4. Correct centric relation is particularly necessary if the patient clenches in this position. To overcome the effects of the isometric contraction of the muscles of mastication, there must be an optimum distribution of this maximum force in a direction that is most favorable to the supporting structures.

FREEDOM OF MANDIBULAR MOVEMENT

The cuspal relations of the teeth in both an anterior and a posterior direction should allow the mandible to move to and from centric relation without restraint. There should be a coordinated anterior and posterior overbite. The Bennett movement should be a noninterfering factor.

It is especially important that mandibular freedom be created during glide movements in the complete absence of a so-called bilaterally balanced occlusion. Contacts of the teeth on the nonworking or balancing side can be extremely detrimental, have little or no application in the treatment of the natural dentition, and should be avoided.

Inclined plane control of mandibular excursive movements should be supplied by the anterior teeth (especially the canines) and the buccal cusps unilaterally on the working side. No posterior tooth contact is required or desired during protrusive movements.

The temporomandibular joint serves as a limiting factor in the final occlusal design and does not function as the prime dictating agent in the articulation of the cusps.

The recording of the anterior condylar guidance is important only insofar as it relays to the clinician the degree of flatness of the condylar paths. This information is helpful in keeping the nonworking and posterior segments free of contact during lateral and protrusive mandibular glide movements. A recording of the direction of the Bennett component of lateral jaw movement is essential in permitting the buccal cusp tips on the working side to slide through one another without impeding or restraining jaw movements. Occlusal discrepancies that do not serve as an impediment to mandibular freedom but that cause rocking of the teeth or of the fixed or removable restorations must of course be eliminated.

OPTIMAL CROWN-TO-ROOT RATIO: MODIFICATION IN CASES REQUIRING PERIODONTAL PROSTHESIS

The relation of the clinical crowns to the clinical roots of the teeth is probably one of the most important considerations in diagnosis and treatment planning. It has great bearing on the establishment of a prognosis for both individual teeth as well as the total mouth.

Actually the most serious consequence of periodontitis is the loss of supporting tissues, resulting in an adverse leverage factor on the remaining alveolar housing of the teeth. Here the deformity of the disease process results in the phenomenon of secondary occlusal traumatism. In this condition even forces normally well tolerated, for example, those generated during mastication, may become excessively destructive due to the inadequate mechanical resistance of the attachment apparatus. If this should occur in the presence of parafunctional traumatic influences such as clenching and grinding, the problem becomes quite difficult.

In considering the crown-to-root ratio one must evaluate not only the vertical aspect but also the following factors:

1. Size, shape, and form of the crown as it relates to the size, shape, form, number, and position of roots
2. Axial inclination of the tooth as it relates to its housing
3. Number and distribution of the remaining teeth
4. Quality as well as quantity of the remaining bone and attachment

Teeth with large bulbous crowns and short tapering roots seem to be predestined to periodontal disease, particularly occlusal traumatism.

Whereas the total area of attachment is an important consideration, of greater importance is its architectural form. A short broad root is less supporting than a long narrow root, total surface area being equal.

The unfavorable factors of crown-to-root ratio that exist in most cases requiring periodontal prosthesis are important influences on the development of an occlusion modified to satisfy the mechanical requirements of the case (Figs. 32-14 to 32-16).

Reducing the vertical aspects of the crown-to-root ratio is a limited procedure, particularly in the *posterior teeth*. Exceptions to this are extruded teeth and raised cusps on tilted teeth. Any gain in leverage here is usually offset by the fact that the length of the lowered cusps of the tilted

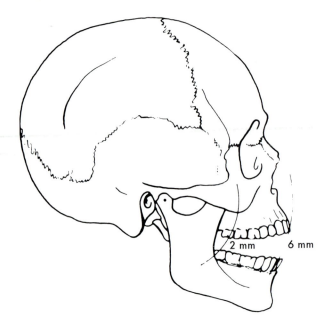

Fig. 32-14. Reduction in clinical crown length. Note relative difference between opening in interior part of mouth and that in posterior area. Ratio is approximately 3:1. (From Bohannan, H., and Abrams, L.: J. Prosthet. Dent. **11:**781, 1961.)

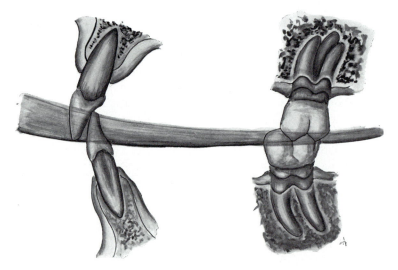

Fig. 32-15. Reduction in clinical crown length. Difference between amount of overbite in anterior and posterior areas of mouth is shown as a shaded band. Any decrease in clinical crown length of posterior teeth will have a threefold effect upon anterior teeth.

teeth must be raised as the occlusal form is developed.

In fact in most instances, as we correct centric occlusion, the mandible moves downward and backward so that the occlusal vertical dimension is usually increased. In the corrected jaw position, teeth that formerly were interposed in the acquired occlusion are now directly apposed, and space for rebuilding the occlusion becomes limited. It must be remembered that a 1 mm reduction in posterior

height results in a 3 mm increase in anterior overbite. Reducing the posterior crown height would therefore aggravate this problem as well as cause a further deepening of the anterior overbite. The resultant excessive interocclusal distance may also create functional problems.

There are certain instances in which it is not only possible but desirable to effect marked reduction in posterior crown height. Such an instance would be in cases of anterior open bite.

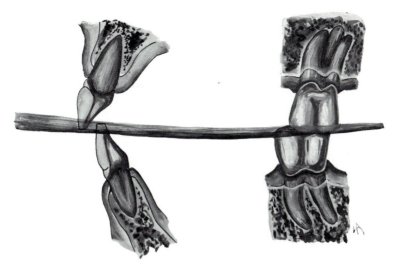

Fig. 32-16. Clinical crown length in final restoration. Anterior teeth have been shortened considerably, with a resultant improvement in crown-to-root ratio and a decrease in incisal guidance. Note that posterior crown length has not been shortened and that any attempt to decrease this crown length would result in a drastic decrease in occlusal vertical dimension.

It is often quite possible as well as desirable to reduce the height of the *anterior teeth*. In fact most cases of posterior bite collapse result in a deepening of the overbite and a fanning of the anterior teeth. The reduction in length of the clinical crown is quite effective in reducing the overbite. Fanned incisors become longer relative to the occlusal plane and therefore usually must be shortened as they are repositioned lingually.

Another result of the scarring of periodontal disease is the creation of an aesthetic deformity in the form of exceptionally long anterior teeth. Shortening these teeth usually results in a restoration of a more functional and aesthetic pattern.

The limitations to the extent of anterior crown height reduction are lip line aesthetics, phonetics, pulpal proximity, and the need for a definite anterior incisal guidance.

As one can see from this discussion, reduction of clinical crown length is frequently limited, inadequate, or impossible as a therapeutic means of overcoming the adverse leverage factors of poor crown-to-root ratio. Mechanical modification of the total occlusal restorative design is mandatory in the execution of periodontal prosthesis. These modifications have as a basic intent the reduction and control of occlusal leverage and the axial radicular transmission of occlusal load.

The mechanical modifications of occlusal design are therapeutic splinting of teeth, alteration in incisal guidance and reduction of anterior crown length, reduction of cusp height, and maintenance of proper buccolingual diameters of occlusal tables.

Therapeutic splinting of teeth (Figs. 32-17 to 32-19). Teeth are normally stabilized in a mesiodistal direction by the proximal contact of the teeth within the arch when proper tooth alignment and arch form are present. Buccolingual stabilization is possible only when the opposing teeth occlude in a correct fashion. However, in cases of secondary occlusal traumatism much of the damage occurs when the teeth are not in full occlusion. Further, rare is the instance in which periodontal prosthesis is required in the presence of a fully intact dentition. This necessitates additional stabilization procedures.

Teeth may demonstrate mobility in one or more of several directions: mesiodistally, buccolingually, circumferentially, and axially. The prognosis of a tooth will be proportionate to the ability of the treatment to minimize or negate movement in all these directions. It has been said that so-called physiologic movement of teeth is requisite to the health of the supporting tissues. However, although admittedly our ability to determine the extent of mobility accurately is limited, it should be stated emphatically that any movement perceptible to the eye is pathologic. A possible exception to this statement is the lower anterior teeth.

It may be emphasized again that only axial resultant forces transmitted to the periodontium pro-

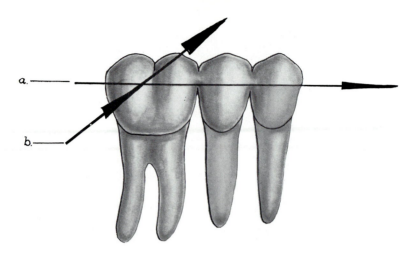

Fig. 32-17. Therapeutic splinting of teeth, showing a unilateral splint that has excellent resistance to mesiodistal displacement but less resistance to buccolingual movement. *a,* Forces applied mesiodistally; *b,* forces applied buccolingually.

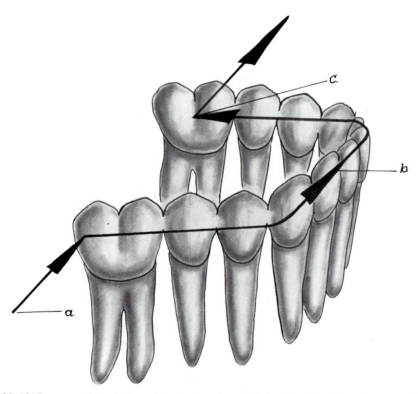

Fig. 32-18. Therapeutic splinting of teeth, showing a bilateral splint with resistance to force in all directions. *a,* Forces applied buccolingually; *b,* transmission of forces around anterior segment of arch; *c,* point of resistance to forces applied to opposite side of arch.

duce true physiologic stimulation of the fiber apparatus.

Splinting action is the joining of two or more teeth to increase resistance to applied force by a stabilization effect and a reorientation of force and stress.

Stabilization is an increase in patterns of resis-

tance to mesiodistal, buccolingual, and apical force vectors by increasing the root area of resistance and by providing reciprocal antagonisms to force patterns. In pure stabilization procedures the force may remain the same, but the resistance to force is increased.

The reorientation of force and stress on the teeth

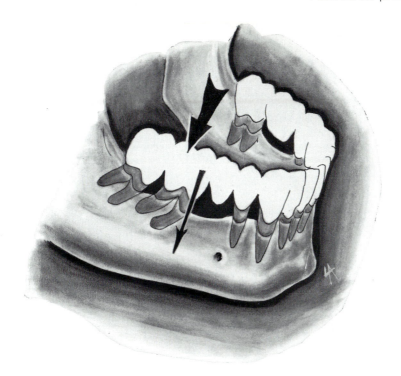

Fig. 32-19. Therapeutic splinting of teeth, showing use of splint to offset occlusal load placed on tilted molars. Here large occlusal force *(large arrow)* is converted to a much lessened stress *(small arrow)* in attachment apparatus.

is possible through splinting action because of the following:

1. The unit area of resistance to force and stress is increased.
2. The direction of force is altered.
3. The total force may remain the same, but the areas of application may be altered.

Splinting has an effect similar to increasing the number of roots per tooth, thus changing the fulcrum point so that forces are more favorably received and dissipated.

Unilateral splinting is the joining of two or more teeth on one plane of an arch segment. In this type of splint the resistance is primarily against mesiodistal force action. The only buccolingual resistance is that afforded a weakened abutment by its firm neighbors.

Bilateral splinting, or cross arch splinting, involves the inclusion of teeth on two or more segments of an arch up to and including the entire arch. In this type of splint action the resistance to force is in all directions, and weakened or mobile teeth can actually give support to other mobile abutments.

The concept of splinting is a very important adjunct in therapy. *However, its advantages should not be abused, nor should its presence be substituted for proper occlusal relations.*

Alteration in incisal guidance and reduction of anterior crown length. The anterior overbite relation must conform to the patient's aesthetic and phonetic needs. As stated earlier, the shortening of anterior teeth serves to reduce crown-to-root ratio and overcome cosmetic deformities associated with the treated periodontal lesion. Generally the result will be to shallow the overbite present. This reduction in incisal guidance may also be accomplished by changes in the occlusal vertical dimension. In many instances, when the occlusion has been established in centric relation, there is an increase in the anterior overjet so that the same tooth length is responsible for creating a decreased incisal guide angle. Reduction of the incisal guide angle will tend to decrease the horizontal overloading of the anterior teeth.

Care must be taken to prevent undue shallowing of the overbite that will cause the anterior teeth to be parted during mandibular glide movements. This creates the undesirable situation of posterior tooth contacts during lateral and protrusive jaw movements.

The incisal guidance probably affords the greatest influence upon the form that the final occlusion will assume. Consequently, reductions of the anterior overbite must precede any attempts to shallow posterior cusp height.

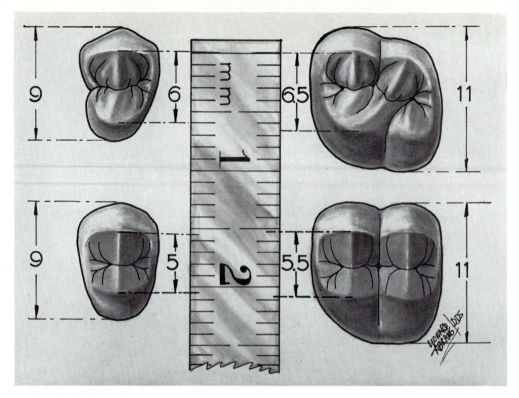

Fig. 32-20. Figs. 32-20 to 32-24 show mechanical modifications in occlusal form utilized as a modified cusp in periodontal prosthesis. Note comparison between buccolingual width of occlusal table of unworn tooth and that of restored tooth. Ideally restored occlusal table should not exceed this width.

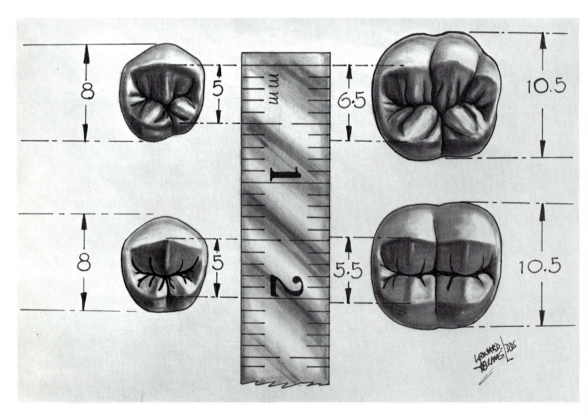

Fig. 32-21. Comparison in a lower posterior tooth between unworn natural tooth and restored tooth with therapeutic cuspal modifications.

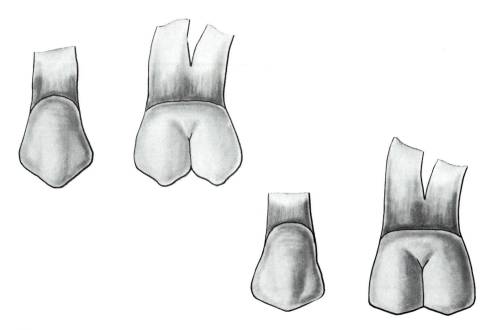

Fig. 32-22. Comparison of cusp height of natural unworn tooth and that of restored dentition. Note that in most instances it is necessary to decrease posterior cusp height to accommodate decrease in incisal guidance.

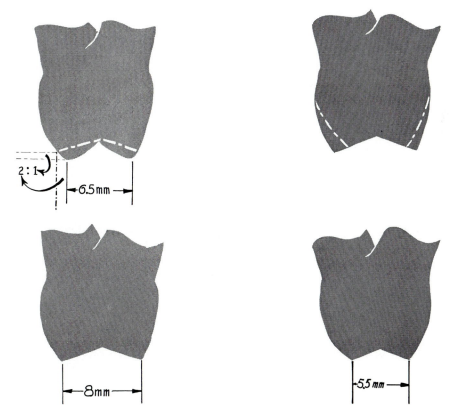

Fig. 32-23. Any attempt to decrease posterior cusp height causes occlusal table to be widened.

Fig. 32-24. After cuspal height reduction a compensatory narrowing of occlusal table is necessary.

Reduction of cusp height (Figs. 32-22 to 32-24). Reduction of horizontal overloading of the posterior teeth may be greatly enhanced by shortening cusp height. This modification must conform to the limitations imposed by the incisal guidance, curve of Spee, and condylar factors. The centric occlusion must be supported by natural posterior teeth. This point cannot be overemphasized. Although a splint can greatly contribute to the stability of the remaining teeth, it must be stressed that the teeth themselves, however aided, ultimately support the occlusion just as any foundation supports the structure. The occlusal design should provide a decrease in the height of buccolingual cuspal angulations and at the same time present the proper form necessary to do the following:

1. Permit the posterior teeth to stabilize the mandible in centric relation
2. Permit the occlusal load to be transmitted axially
3. Permit mandibular freedom of movement to and from centric relation
4. Prevent nonfunctional or balancing occlusal contact in lateral jaw movement
5. Prevent posterior occlusal contact in protrusive jaw movement
6. Prevent parting of the anterior teeth during all mandibular glide patterns

The modified cuspal form is an indispensable part of the mechanical design of the restoration. Cuspal occlusal arrangements are a therapeutic convenience that permits the fabrication of a stable occlusion with a minimum increase in the occlusal vertical dimension and at the same time allows for the control of posterior aesthetic patterns. However, the most important factor is that correct cuspal inclinations form the tool with which the clinician directs mandibular freedom in the absence of undesirable posterior tooth contacts.

Maintenance of proper buccolingual diameters of occlusal tables (Figs. 32-20 to 32-24). Accurate control of the width and position of the occlusal tables (the force recipient areas of the teeth) will increase the ability of the teeth to transmit occlusal forces axially within their alveolar housing. The buccolingual diameters of the occlusal tables, as was stated earlier, should not exceed 60% of the overall buccolingual width of the normal posterior tooth.

In those frequently encountered situations of bulbous and extremely large crowns it is obvious that the 60% formula would result in an occlusal form that would still be too wide. If at all possible the molar occlusal table width should fall within the 6 to 6.5 mm range. This poses a special problem in maxillary molars because of the extreme flair of the palatal roof.

At no time should excessive narrowing of the occlusal tables pose a threat to the ability of these teeth to stabilize centric relation or to prevent balancing contact.

Tooth preparation must allow for the final crown width. This can be accomplished best by preshaping the tooth prior to final tooth preparation.

The occlusal table must be positioned over the kernel of the root and may require the utilization of tooth movement procedures. However, there are those instances in which orthodontics is not feasible, and it may be necessary to widen an occlusal table to create occlusal contacts. If at all possible this unfavorable compromise should be avoided.

LOCATION OF ROOTS WITHIN PERIODONTAL STRUCTURES

For optimal distribution of force and stress to the remaining root support, teeth should be positioned centrally within their alveolar housing. Those teeth that have migrated or tilted to unfavorable positions should be realigned so that it is possible by occlusal design to direct forces in a favorable direction.

When gross distortions of occlusal tables are utilized to compensate for severe orthodontic deformities and poor arch-to-arch relations, the force recipient areas of the restored teeth are located poorly with respect to their root support. This generally results in an increase in horizontal overloading of the abutment teeth, which can be remedied only by a change in tooth position. Tooth preparation is a poor substitute for correct tooth position.

Minor tooth movement procedures to position teeth properly with respect to their support are the rule rather than the exception in the execution of the periodontal prosthetic treatment plan. In many instances major orthodontic intervention is required to remedy the more severe malocclusions. With rare exceptions, age is no contraindication to advanced full mouth–banded orthodontic therapy.

Of great importance is the effect of severely tilted and malposed teeth on gingival architecture and embrasure form. Proper tooth position is therefore essential for the establishment of physiologic tooth form and embrasure patterns as well as for the more obvious reasons of force control and aesthetics.

MAXIMUM PROTECTION TO INVESTING STRUCTURES

The gingival third of the restored tooth regardless of whether it covers exposed root surfaces must be contoured to imitate true anatomic crown form if it is to be compatible with the gingiva. The facial and lingual surfaces in this area should be slightly convex to prevent food retention. When determining the degree of convexity necessary for a given restoration, the clinician should consider that the faciolingual diameter of the widest portion of the crown is only 1 to 1.5 mm. greater than the faciolingual diameter of the cervical line.

The proximal surfaces, on the other hand, should be flat and somewhat concave. This permits adjacent teeth to form adequate embrasure spaces to house the interdental papilla properly.

The clinician should further protect the gingival margin by not permitting any portion of the fixed or removable restoration to rest, regardless of how lightly, on this area. This prohibition also applies to mechanical devices such as solder joints, pontic areas, retainers, connectors, and denture bases.

Subgingival restorative margins must not impinge on the epithelial attachment. Any prosthesis that is constructed must minimize or eliminate areas that will tend to lodge residual food debris. Furthermore the design of the restoration should permit ready access to the patient for simplified oral hygiene techniques. One must be ever mindful that the basis of any periodontal maintenance program is a thorough and effective oral physiotherapeutic regimen.

To create the required restorative atmosphere for gingival health the telescope crown principle in many instances becomes a necessary part of the final treatment plan. This innovation of an older idea enables the clinician to restore proper form to the individual dental units being treated and at the same time to fulfill the aesthetic, functional, and occlusal requirements of the total prosthesis.

SATISFACTORY AESTHETIC PATTERNS

The final restoration must fulfill the patient's aesthetic needs. These requirements vary among different individuals and will influence ultimate case design a great deal. Again, emphasis must be placed on the importance of correct tooth position and axial inclination in gaining control of aesthetic patterns.

Strategic also is the avoidance of anterior teeth in the restorative plan if they are aesthetically satisfactory. In many instances mandibular incisors may be maintained unrestored in the presence of moderate mobility if the following clinical conditions are met:

1. The lower incisors must be correctly positioned and axially inclined over their root attachments.
2. The mandibular anterior teeth must be shortened to the fullest extent possible to reduce the clinical crown-to-root ratio.
3. The incisors must exhibit proper tight proximal alignment.
4. Complete stability and support to the maximum occlusal portion must be maintained by the posterior teeth and canines.

These considerations generally limit the amount and direction of occlusal load to which the lower incisors will be subjected.

In those situations in which the periodontal disease has extensively involved the posterior teeth, bilateral splinting is indicated; the clinician is justified in his reluctance to implicate the anterior teeth if they are relatively free of caries and bone loss. In selected cases it may be possible to achieve bilateral splint action by means of a removable palatal strap instead of the customary anterior fixed splint. This permits bilateral stabilization of the posterior occlusal segments in the absence of anterior tooth restoration.

The final prosthesis must take into consideration the most intelligent compromise of the case versus the aesthetic desires of both the patient and the dentist. A leading pitfall for many practitioners is encountered in the attempt to minimize the display of metal in the fabrication of extensive fixed restorations. Very often this necessitates the injudicious use of either porcelain or acrylic, which may result in the creation of additional problems such as extreme wear, fracture of materials, inadequate interproximal embrasures, and faulty margins.

Special consideration of distal extension problem

In those instances in which all the teeth of one or more posterior sections of the mouth are missing, the anterior teeth are called on to support the forces of centric occlusion. As stated previously, the maxillary anterior teeth are ill designed for this purpose.

The resultant effect is increased trauma and possibly accelerated fanning of the maxillary anterior teeth, particularly in the presence of periodontal disease.

This situation requires the following special considerations in planning the restorative treatment:

1. Teeth should be realigned so as to be positioned over basal bone.
2. The form of the canine or canines, if the situation is bilateral, should be modified on the lingual cingulum to enable the forces to be directed axially.
3. If the canine is missing, the lateral incisor should be modified in the same fashion. When this is necessary, the lateral incisor should be splinted bilaterally. Where the lateral incisor is the terminal abutment, it is often judicious to extirpate the pulp intentionally and to place the attachment directly over the root. Thus if the lateral incisor, a poor abutment risk, is ever lost, a split lingual cantilever attachment is still present.
4. The palatal tissues surrounding the canine receive this modification in coronal form quite well. The tissues around the incisors are not so receptive, however, and should not be so treated unless absolutely necessary.
5. Certain patients should be handled with a fixed cantilever attachment provided that the following conditions are met:
   a. Functional and aesthetic needs must be fulfilled.
   b. Bilateral splinting must be used to support the cantilever.
   c. Adequate support must surround the abutment teeth.
6. Where a fixed removable prosthesis is indicated in a situation that is to be both tooth and tissue borne, the following are recommended:
   a. The forces of occlusion must be carried by the natural abutment teeth.
   b. Centric occlusal forces on anterior teeth must be directed axially (modified canine hold).
   c. Tissue-borne cases must ultimately settle until support is again on natural abutment teeth.
   d. A double impression technique must be utilized in relating the denture base to the abutment teeth. This entails a casting made from an impression of the tissues of edentulous areas at rest. The casting is then related to the abutments under compression.
   e. The split lingual attachment should be used as a retaining device, provided that the abutments are bilaterally splinted, which accomplishes the following:

(1) Additional area of fixed support in centric occlusion
(2) Longer precision attachment utilized without disturbing embrasure form
(3) Male attachments less subject to wear
(4) Female attachments less likely to spread and hence more durable
   f. The telescopic removable attachment may also be utilized as a retaining device.
   g. When sufficient length of terminal abutments will permit, a conventionally distally placed precision attachment may be used.
   h. Properly designed clasps may also be utilized if necessary. In this instance the rest should be designed to form the modified centric holding surface.

TREATMENT PLANNING AND SEQUENCE OF THERAPY

It should now be quite apparent that the various phases of clinical dentistry are intimately related to their ultimate objective, the preservation and maintenance of the natural dentition in health. Endodontics, periodontics, orthodontics, and prosthodontics by themselves may be nonentities —it is only how they alone or in combination fulfill the ultimate objective that is significant.

The actual life or vitality of a mature tooth is not dependent on the vitality of the pulp but on the health and integrity of the attachment apparatus. An attachment apparatus that supports a root without a crown is meaningless. A tooth by itself is nothing unless it is related to the entire dentition and its associated structures, providing a system capable of adequate function.

This realization necessitates the establishment of a treatment plan based on an orderly sequence of therapy that will remove all known etiologic factors, restore proper form and function, and establish the conditions necessary to create and maintain a healthy masticatory organ.

Periodontal prosthesis cannot be considered a sure cure and should not be contemplated until the alternative measures have been explored so that every reasonable attempt has been made to avoid it. However, once committed, the clinician must be prepared to follow the restoration through to its ultimate completion with painstaking attention to detail. There are no effective halfway measures.

In most instances the need for extensive restorative dentistry should be evident during the diagnostic and treatment planning procedures. When periodontal prosthesis is indicated, it should appear as an integral phase of the total periodontal treatment plan. The extent and sequence of periodontal therapy for the same patient will differ, depending on whether the restorative need is to be fulfilled. Unfortunately there are those situations in which the patient has been informed for the first time, following the completion of periodontal surgery, that reconstruction or splinting is indicated. Unless a rare contingency arises during periodontal therapy, the need for restorative dentistry should have been apparent to the clinician and explained to the patient prior to the onset of treatment.

Many clinical situations demand that pocket elimination be modified, curtailed, or delayed until such time as the patient is either emotionally, physically, or financially able to make the necessary restorative commitment. This is especially applicable to those cases in which the exposure of root surface created by the correction of periodontal deformities causes a much greater problem than the disease that has been treated.

The total treatment plan can be divided into three phases: the preparatory phase, the restorative phase, and the maintenance phase. The preparatory phase consists of all of the diversified procedures necessary to prepare the mouth for restorative dentistry.

The following is a brief outline of the usual order of therapy:

I. Preparatory phase
  A. Initial stage
    1. Emergency care for acute complaints
    2. Reduction of gingival inflammation and bleeding by the following:
      a. Scaling and limited curettage
      b. Home care instruction
      c. Removal of irritating portions of restorations (fixed and removable)
    3. Caries removal and temporary restoration
    4. Predictable endodontic therapy for the following:
      a. Known carious exposures
      b. Pulpal disease
      c. Pulpless teeth
      d. Periapical involvement
      e. Teeth to be treated by hemisection
    5. Occlusal adjustment
      a. Bite plate therapy (modified Hawley type) —appliances used for many different purposes, which they can fulfill singly or at the same time, but mainly to:
        (1) Free the posterior occlusion and prevent further trauma by locking type occlusal interferences
        (2) Allow for eruption of depressed premolars and molars

        (3) Serve as an important diagnostic and therapeutic aid in the treatment of temporomandibular joint pain dysfunction syndrome (as such, used in the first step to relieve acute pain)
        (4) Disarticulate the teeth to facilitate minor tooth movement procedures or to supply anchorage for the orthodontic force
      b. Removal of gross occlusal interferences
      c. Minor tooth movement—realignment of individual teeth by means of tipping actions
    6. Temporary stabilization of mobile segments of teeth

In many instances it may be necessary to ligate severely mobile teeth prior to scaling and certainly prior to surgical procedures. The design of the temporary splint must be such that it supplies rigid fixation of mobile teeth and at the same time does not interfere with gingival healing and oral hygiene. The provisional restoration should not be used at this time to supply the needed temporary fixation unless necessary, for it may have to be remade after periodontal surgery. Generally this complicates therapy and may be responsible for problems during healing. The recommended splinting techniques are the following:

      a. Wire and plastic ligation—when ligation used preparatory to restorative dentistry; procedure facilitated by cutting horizontal grooves in the teeth to correspond to positions of wire placement
      b. Embedded twisted wire-and-acrylic splint—an excellent means of splinting posterior teeth because the resulting rigidity is created without interfering with the embrasure space, an added advantage here in that this may be used to establish additional anchorage for minor tooth movement procedures
      c. Orthodontic band splint—of limited usefulness in the absence of minor tooth movement techniques
    7. Strategic extraction and hemisection

In an intact segment of the dentition this includes the removal of teeth or roots (hemisection of multirooted teeth) that have severe infrabony pockets that threaten the bony support of adjacent roots either by extension or by the therapeutic ostectomy pocket elimination procedure. The teeth that should be included in this category are those that pose a severe problem in overcrowding or, because of the severity of their periodontal involvement, are responsible for the gingival zone of an entire quadrant to be placed much farther beyond the mucogingival junction. This should be performed early enough in treatment to allow for complete osseous healing of the extraction site prior to mucogingival and osseous surgery.

8. Major orthodontics or continuation of minor tooth movement

When extensive tooth movement is to precede osseous and mucogingival surgery, time must be permitted to elapse after final orthodontic stabilization so that complete organization and calcification of the newly positioned root attachments can take place.

B. Final stage
1. Reevaluation

The response of the patient to removal of local environmental factors is observed, and the final periodontal surgical procedures are designed.

2. Periodontal surgery

The procedure must be specifically designed to prepare the dentition for extensive restoration. Whenever possible it is advisable to wait until final healing has occurred at the sites of previous strategic extractions and hemisection. Surgical preparation for restorative procedures must include the following:
   a. Correct osseous contouring—osseous compromise to conserve root support to be avoided
   b. Pocket elimination to be complete with the preservation or creation of an adequate zone of attached gingiva that exhibits correct architectural form
   c. In cases of subgingival caries or previous restorations osseous tissue to be removed to provide sufficient sound tooth structure for tooth preparation
   d. Pontic areas to be prepared properly by the adequate reduction of hard and soft saddle tissue so that the replacement tooth can be compatible aesthetically and functionally with the restored tooth—dangerous situation created by insufficient saddle reduction in that there is inadequate room for a strong solder joint and proper embrasure form

3. Observation of healing

Sufficient time must elapse after periodontal surgery before the final restorative phase can commence. This waiting period, which lasts 2 to 3 months, is essential for complete healing and maturation of the newly constituted tissues formed at the surgical site. Since healing time varies considerably among different individuals, care must be taken to avoid hasty restorative intervention that will jeopardize the periodontal result and lead to recurrence of pocket depth and chronically inflamed gingival tissues. The zero gingival sulcus will remain for a longer time after mucogingival and osseous surgery. It is advisable, therefore, to wait for the return of a normal sulcular depth.

II. Restorative phase
A. Provisional restoration
1. Fabrication

The provisional restoration must be executed with sufficient care so that it approximates as much as possible the environment to be established by the final restoration. The provisional restoration of choice is the metal band acrylic restoration that has been described in the literature. A new improvement, however, is the introduction of the gold band as a substitute for the copper band. The gold bands have been prepared by the manufacturers for this purpose and have the advantage of greater marginal stability and better adaptation and resistance to oxidation.

2. Final tooth positioning

This is accomplished by using the provisional restoration to restore lost occlusal vertical dimension and as anchorage for rubber dam elastics.

3. Intentional vital extirpation

During construction of the provisional restoration the teeth are evaluated as to their needs for intentional extirpation. This is not haphazard operative pulpal exposure but is a very definitive procedure necessary to the successful execution of treatment. The indications are the following:
   a. Extruded teeth
   b. Very poor crown-to-root ratio of anterior teeth
   c. Severely malposed teeth not amenable to tooth movement
   d. Hemisection of involved root or roots of multirooted teeth

B. Evaluative period—establishment of the final prognosis
1. Periodontal response to the provisional restoration

Frequently it is difficult to establish a prognosis for certain teeth until they have been treated and until sufficient time has elapsed so that the response to therapy can be evaluated properly. The acrylic and gold band splint is so designed that it can be utilized for a sufficient period of time to allow for tissue response in teeth or tissues presenting this problem. This use of the splint is of particular importance when a key abutment tooth is involved because very often the entire treatment plan may be changed, pending the response to treatment of a key tooth.

The following results in response to therapy must be achieved during the provisional splinting stage before the clinician can proceed to completion of the case:
   a. Mobile teeth to become more stable
   b. Soft tissues to present a normal physiologic state, particularly as it affects the character of healthy attached gingiva
   c. Periodontal ligament, where thickened, now to approach a more proportional state and a well-defined lamina dura to be evident roentgenographically

d. Periapical areas of rarefaction that have received endodontic therapy to exhibit signs of healing
e. Patient to be free of any subjective symptoms
2. Extraction of all teeth that have not responded to therapy
3. Final determination of acceptability of the occlusal vertical dimension established by the provisional restoration
4. Temporomandibular joint symptoms at this time to be under control—certainly no new complaints to appear during the provisional restorations
5. Evaluation of function
   a. Aesthetics—provisional restoration offered as acceptable solution to patient's aesthetic problems
   b. Phonetics—no alteration of or impediment to patient's speech
   c. Chewing ability—decision to utilize either a fixed cantilever or a distal extension removable tooth replacement made at this time and a provisional restoration

provided for the patient as a means of acceptable masticatory performance
C. Finished restoration
   After prognosis has been established, the design of the finished restoration is finalized, and the necessary mechanical steps in the form of impressions, registrations, and remount procedures follow. Strict attention to minutiae is absolutely mandatory.
III. Maintenance phase
A. Oral health
   Upon satisfactory completion of the periodontal prosthesis the patient should be placed upon a normal periodontal recall maintenance program. At these visits scaling-curettage procedures are performed, and patient home care is evaluated and revised. Care must be taken not to injure the junctions of the veneering material and the fine metal restorative margins during this procedure. The use of ultrasonic scaling devices is contraindicated in the presence of restorative dentistry. The occlusion and integrity of the cement seal of the restorations must also be evaluated carefully at this time. If necessary, the restoration may require recementation during the recall visit.
B. Mechanical maintenance
   The final restorations must be designed to permit ready repair or alteration in the event of any future mechanical contingency. Temporary cementation and telescope crowns play an indispensable role toward this end.
   After 5 to 10 years the veneer may need reprocessing. This is usually not a difficult step if the final restoration has been designed to allow for its future maintenance.

CHOICE OF ABUTMENT RESTORATION
CLINICAL CROWN AND ANATOMIC CROWN THE SAME

All or most teeth present; mobility not significant (Fig. 32-12). When the clinical crown and the anatomic crown are the same, general dentistry is most efficient, and periodontal therapy is quite simple. The choice of restoration is varied as all requisites of cavity preparation, according to Black, may be accomplished. The use of inlays, overlays, amalgams, and so on and porcelain jacket crowns with full shoulder preparation is ideal. Fixed bridge prosthesis and even splinting, if indicated (this is rare), present no particular problem. Coronal contours are guided, embrasure forms are preestablished, and adequate amounts of attached gingiva and adequate vestibular depth should be present.

This is an ideal set of circumstances and the situation in which dental therapy can accomplish the most when properly executed, particularly when the concept of the individual dental unit and arch integrity is maintained.

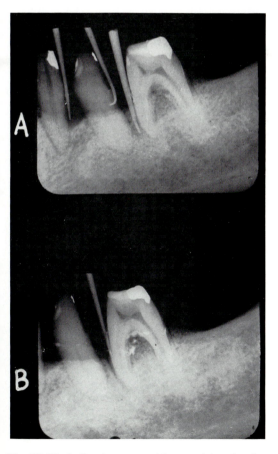

Fig. 32-25. A, Teeth prepared for provisional splinting, 1952. Points in place, showing infrabony pocket depth, class II mobility. **B,** Eight years later, 1960, prosthesis was removed for recementation. Note healing, with no mobility present.

Periodontal therapy needs consist usually of scaling and curettage, home care program, and possibly gingivoplasty. Occlusal adjustment by selective grinding, unless orthodontics is indicated, offers its greatest potential as a therapeutic entity.

Unfortunately, and this is the great tragedy of dentistry, either through neglect or through inadequate dental diagnosis, improper treatment planning, and improper therapy, too many individuals are allowed to progress beyond this state.

CLINICAL CROWN AND ANATOMIC CROWN DISSIMILAR

More advanced cases; missing teeth; mobility of teeth a significant factor (Fig. 32-13). When the clinical crown and the anatomic crown are not the same, which incidentally is the category into which most cases requiring periodontal prosthesis must be placed, there is not a great latitude in the choice of restoration.

Full coverage is the usual basic unit of restoration for the following reasons:

1. It provides the best mechanical retention for splinting.
2. It provides the best mechanical retention for abutment teeth to be used as retainers for both fixed and removable prosthesis.
3. It offers the best means of reshaping coronal form to satisfy occlusal needs.
4. It affords the best opportunity to restore the relation of the clinical crown to the surrounding tissues.
5. It provides maximum protection of the exposed root structure to recurrent caries.

6. In cases in which root caries or erosion are present, it is the only well-conceived means of treatment.
7. Properly used, it offers the maximum in aesthetics under all these circumstances.
8. It allows for a nonpermanent cementation procedure so that extensive restorations may be removed later, if necessary, for purposes of case alteration and maintenance.

The full-coverage restoration, however, is not without its disadvantages, and the operator should be well aware of these. They are as follows:

1. Operative trauma to pulp
2. Reaction of tissues to marginal contours and fit
3. Washout of cement medium whether temporary or permanent
4. Inability to test for vitality of pulp

The greatest disadvantage to the use of full coverage restoration and of splinting has been their abuse. For some unknown reason and particularly with the advent of high-speed instrumentation it has been treated as an easy or simple operative technique. Nothing could be further from the truth.

Full coverage and splinting of teeth are two of the most difficult procedures to perform well. Both require the utmost in precision from diagnosis and treatment planning to sequence of therapy and mechanical execution.

Whereas it is difficult to speak of precision under these circumstances, everything must be done to minimize error. Unfortunately both full coverage and splinting have been utilized to cover a multitude of sins.

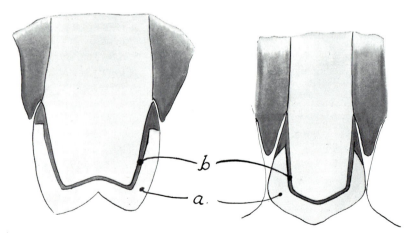

Fig. 32-26. Figs. 32-26 to 32-32 show design of telescopic crown used in fixed restoration. Note contours of telescopic coping shoulder related to gingival sulcus (buccal and proximal). *a,* Overcasting or superstructure; *b,* undercasting or telescopic coping. (Courtesy Morris Feder, Philadelphia.)

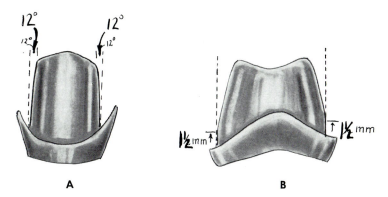

Fig. 32-27. Mechanical form of telescopic coping. **A,** Proximal walls have a 12-degree taper. **B,** Buccal and lingual walls are parallel in gingiva 1.5 mm (Courtesy Morris Feder, Philadelphia.)

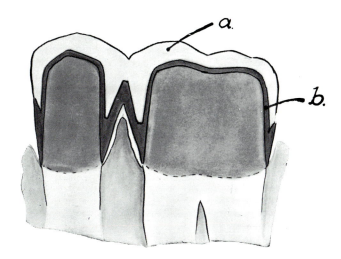

Fig. 32-28. Design of interproximal embrasure, with adjacent telescopic coping. Note that proximal shoulders are contacting and that they design embrasure form, providing needed protection for underlying papilla. Overcasting should not exceed normal coronal contours and width. *a,* Overcasting (telescopic); *b,* coping. (Courtesy Morris Feder, Philadelphia.)

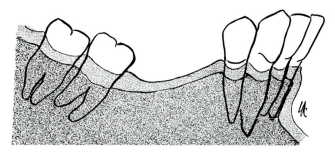

Fig. 32-29. Figs. 32-29 to 32-32 show use of telescopic crown to restore severely tilted posterior abutments. Note extensive edentulous area, with remaining posterior teeth severely tipped mesially.

Many of the problems seen in the past few years relating to the maintenance and survival of extensive restorations have led to a condemnation of the procedures employed. In most instances this reaction has been based upon incorrect conclusions and evaluation of the circumstances.

Careful assessment on the part of interested and able investigators has resulted in the following evaluation as to the causes of failure:

1. Improper case selection relative to patient type, that is, emotional stability, intellectual approach to problem, and ability to appreciate responsibilities of home care

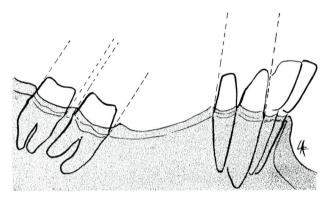

Fig. 32-30. Tooth preparation of abutment teeth. Note that molars have been repaired as true standing teeth, with due regard for conservation of tooth structure but not for parallelism.

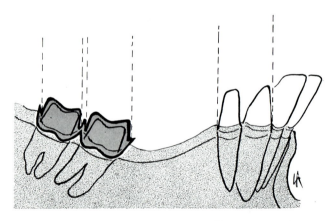

Fig. 32-31. Telescope coping restoration of molars. These restorations are permanently cemented in place and create necessary gingival and subgingival contours. Cemented telescopes allow for a path of insertion of final appliance.

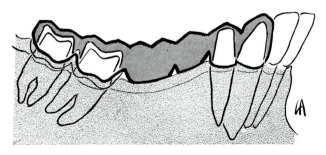

Fig. 32-32. Final appliance cemented with a nonpermanent cement. Overcasting forms a continuous correct contour with cemented undercasting.

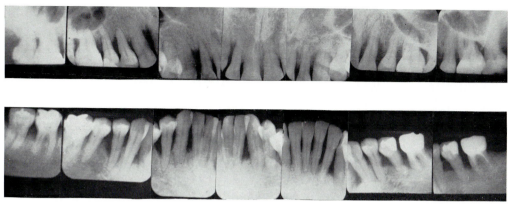

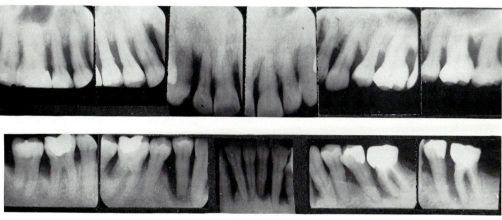

A (1948)

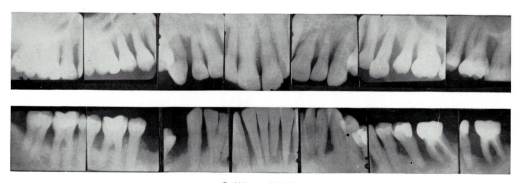

B (1951)

C (Mar. 1952)

Fig. 32-33. A, Roentgenograms taken in 1948, 4 years preoperatively, showing extent of periodontal disease in a 48-year-old white woman. **B,** 1951, 1 year before operation. Note rate of progress of disease. **C,** March 1952, immediately before operation. Note the following: loss of mandibular left premolar; hopeless involvement of mandibular right molars and incisors; prevalence of infrabony pockets. Patient was accepted for treatment on the basis of number and distribution of remaining teeth and type of osseous lesions believed to be three wall in nature and suitable for a new attachment procedure and diagnosis of periodontitis and secondary occlusal traumatism.

Continued.

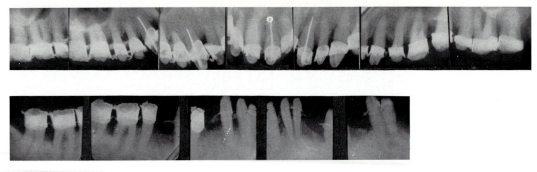

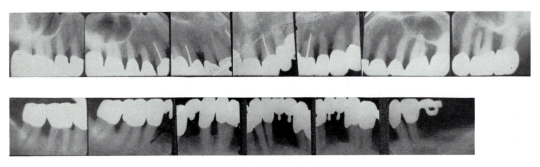

D (Nov. 1952)

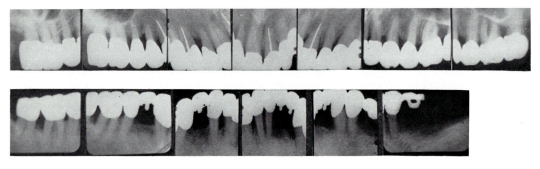

E (Mar. 1953)

F (1960)

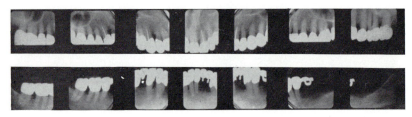

G (1962)

Fig. 32-33, cont'd. D, Nov. 1952. Note response to periodontal therapy and provisional restoration. Periodontal therapy was performed in conjunction with provisional splinting. It consisted of an open flap approach and curettage for infrabony pocket therapy. Note also healing of infrabony lesion. **E,** March 1953, immediately after insertion of finished restoration, which consisted of the following: bilateral splinting using full-coverage restoration of abutment teeth; fulfillment of therapeutic occlusal objectives; cantilever used to replace lower right second premolar. Opposing teeth are prevented from erupting because of splint action. Patient's requirements for masticatory performance were met. **F,** 1960, showing the 8-year follow-up and continued healing. **G,** 1962, 10 years after operation. Note maintenance of case and continued thinning of periodontal ligament space. Re-formation of lamina dura shows principal fibers receiving functional stimulation.

2. Improper case selection as to prognosis potential
3. Poor treatment planning
   a. Inadequate periodontal therapy
   b. Orthodontic needs
4. Inadequate mechanical execution
   a. Poor tooth preparation
   b. Inadequate impression techniques, resulting in marginal failures of teeth and tissues
   c. Improper composite fit of splinted restoration, resulting in washout of cement medium regardless of type
   d. Lack of proper occlusal form and relations

Time does not permit a full discussion of tooth preparation and impression techniques or of the means of handling the technical aspects in the establishment of a functional occlusion. However, one major advancement that must be mentioned is the use of the telescope crown, for it has greatly enhanced the ability to overcome many of the problems confronted despite the attention paid to the details discussed.

TELESCOPE CROWN

Even after the maximum has been gained in tooth movement and preparation procedures, it is still impossible to achieve an individual and composite fit to the restoration due to the flaring of roots and so on. This may result in springing of the appliance, wedging of the teeth, opening of the margins, and rocking fit of the restoration. Properly designed undercastings reshape the anatomic

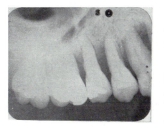 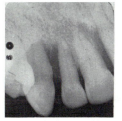 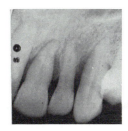 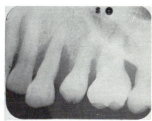

H (Mar. 1952)

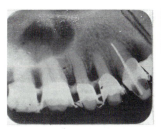 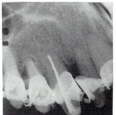 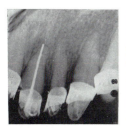 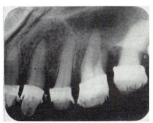

I (Nov. 1952)

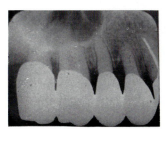 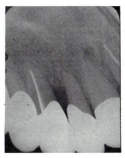 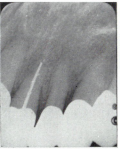 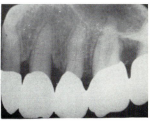

J (1960)

Fig. 32-33, cont'd. H, Close-up of roentgenograms taken in March 1952. **I,** Nov. 1952. **J,** 1960.

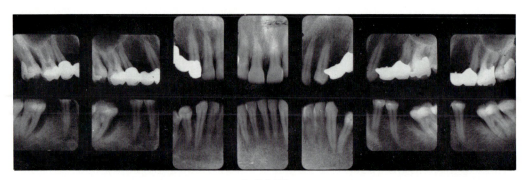

A (1952)

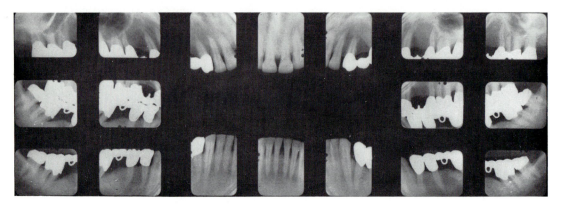

B (1954)

C (1952)

D (1952)

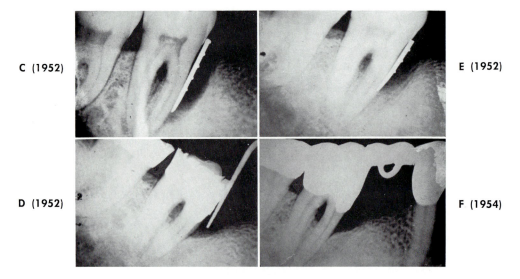

E (1952)

F (1954)

Fig. 32-34. A, Typical pattern of posterior bite collapse. Note mesial drifting of distal molars, distal drifting of premolars, extrusion of opposing molars, deepening of overbite, and fanning of anterior teeth. Note also pattern of bone loss on distal surface of maxillary molars and on mesial surface of mandibular molars. **B,** Ten years later, after treatment. **C,** Close-up view of lower left molar area. A Hirschfeld point in place indicates depth of infrabony pocket. **D,** Postinfrabony pocket therapy. Note that healing has occurred before splinting. Therapy performed by D. Walter Cohen. **E,** Provisional restoration in place. **F,** Ten years after operation. Note maintenance of healed situation.

roots so that the superstructure represents a restoration of the anatomic crowns (Figs. 32-26 to 32-36).

Each undercasting is seated and cemented individually so that the superstructure is placed in position without restriction or torque and does not interfere with individual and composite fit. Further, it is thus possible to contour and finish the margins better, to establish embrasure forms, and to maintain them.

It might also be stated that when necessary, the superstructure can be removed with relative ease. Washout as a result of improper composite fit is

not a usual problem, and when it does occur the tooth is still protected by the undercasting.

Properly handled and with proper respect paid to detail, splinting, with the full cast crown as the abutment retainer, provides the most excellent and proper means of treating the complexity of problems faced in periodontal prosthesis.

SUMMARY

The purpose of this chapter has been to define the philosophy, concepts, and principles of periodontal prosthesis. It was our intent to introduce this phase of clinical dentistry into the scheme of

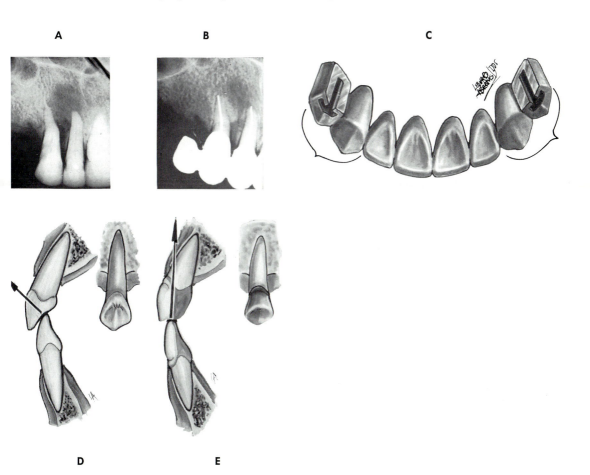

Fig. 32-35. A, Preoperative roentgenogram of maxillary left canine key terminal abutment tooth for a distal extension restoration. Note the following: marked mobility (class III); mesial infrabony pocket; both lateral incisor and canine are nonvital, with area of rarefaction at apex. **B,** Eight years after operation. Note the following: healing of periapical area after endodontic therapy; healing of infrabony pocket; teeth now firm; canine forms modified so that functional cingulum enables centric forces to be directed axially; split lingual attachments used as retainer for cast gold base of partial denture fabricated by double impression technique. **C,** Split lingual precision attachment built into cantilevered first premolars. **D,** Occlusal relations of unrestored canine. Note direction of transmission of occlusal load, which in this case is predominantly horizontal *(arrow)*. **E,** Centric hold created in restored canine permits occlusal load *(arrow)* to be transmitted axially. Note that exaggerated cingulum does not interfere with normal gingival coronal contour.

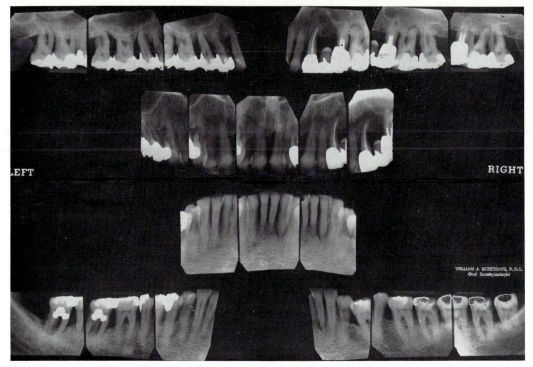

A (1959)

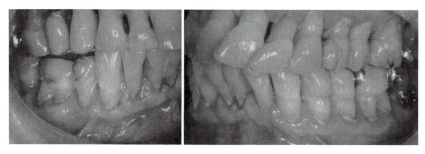

B (1959)

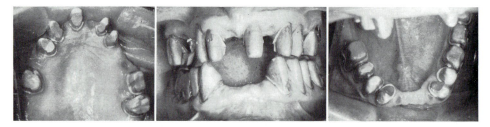

C (1959)

Fig. 32-36. A, Complete roentgenographic survey taken in 1959 after many years of inadequate dental treatment. Severity of bone loss, with no apparent potential for new attachment, in addition to extent of pocket depth on clinical probing made prognosis negative. **B,** Clinical photographs taken at same time as roentgenograms. Note marked discrepancy between anatomic and clinical crown, alteration in embrasure form and bifurcation and trifurcation involvements, accelerated mesial drift resulting in fanning and crowding of anterior teeth, and also marginal areas with multitudinous debris and plaque formation. This occurred despite tremendous effort in home care and frequent scaling and curettage. Clinical probing demonstrated pockets extending within 1 to 2 mm of apex on buccal and labial aspects.

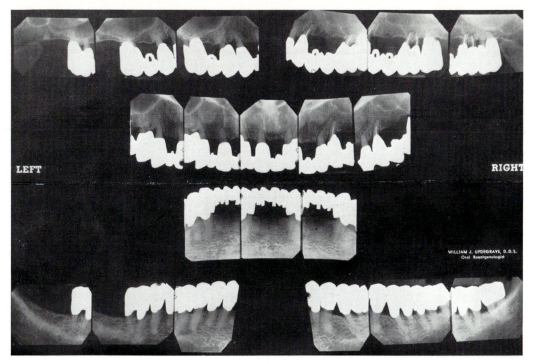

D (1963)

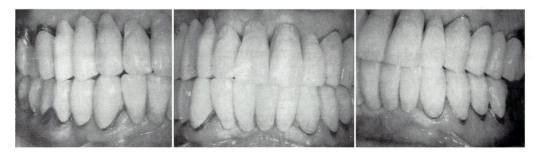

E (1963)

Fig. 32-36, cont'd. Despite negative prognosis, this case was treated on a provisional basis because of patient's insistence. Periodontal surgery was contraindicated, since all incisions would have been in alveolar mucosa, and osseous exposure, resulting in any resorption, would have been disastrous. Diamond stone curettage was done at time of tooth preparation, and provisional gold band–and–acrylic splint was fabricated. Response to this therapy in first area was so dramatic that entire case was treated. The following teeth were extracted:

$$
\begin{array}{c|c}
\text{R} & \text{L} \\
5\ 1 & 2\ 5\ 7 \\
\hline
2\ 1 & 1\ 2\quad 7
\end{array}
$$

Palatal root of 6 | was removed. **C,** Telescopic restorations cemented in position. Note the following: conversion of clinical root to simulate anatomic root with exception of anterior teeth, which were compromised for aesthetic reasons; even and parallel path of insertion; finished embrasure forms and marginal areas; superstructure then to simulate anatomic crowns and when in place to provide bilateral splint action. **D,** Four years later, 1963. Note maintenance of bone height and improvement in quality of attachment. **E,** Four years after operation. Superstructure is in position, demonstrating response of tissue to therapy. Note the following: tissue tone and form; amount of attached gingiva; embrasure form; coronal contours (double deflecting contours) used because of coronal length—done for the purpose of better aesthetics as well as to minimize protective contours (there is too great a tendency to overcontour restorations in this critical area); and ease of home care with excellent results—patient now able to take care of her mouth.

the text on periodontics, but to have attempted this would have made it necessary to review certain basic fundamentals that have been described in detail elsewhere in the text. It was felt that not to review these fundamentals would have prevented the development of the entire concept that gives the biomechanical basis for diagnosis and treatment.

REFERENCES

Abrams, L., and Feder, M.: Periodontal considerations of removable prosthesis, Alpha Omegan **55:**123, 1962.

Amsterdam, M.: Periodontal prosthesis: twenty-five years in retrospect, Alpha Omegan, December, 1974.

Amsterdam, M.: The distal extension problem. Presented to to the Northeastern Society of Periodontology, New York, 1961.

Amsterdam, M.: Periodontal considerations in the selection and treatment of abutment teeth. Presented to the Centennial Meeting of the A. D. A., New York, 1959.

Amsterdam, M.: Postgraduate and graduate notes, University of Pennsylvania, School of Dental Medicine, 1957.

Amsterdam, M., and Fox, L.: Provisional splinting—principles and technics, Dent. Clin. North Am., p. 73, Mar. 1959.

Amsterdam, M., and Grossman, L.: Handbook of dental practice, ed. 3, Philadelphia, 1958, J. B. Lippincott Co.

Amsterdam, M., and Rossman, S. R.: Technique of hemisection of multirooted teeth, Alpha Omegan **53:**4, 1960.

Angle, E. H.: Malocclusion of the teeth, ed. 7, Philadelphia, 1907, S. S. White Dental Mfg. Co.

Atwood, D. A.: A cephalometric study of the clinical rest position of the mandible, J. Prosthet. Dent. **6:**504, 1956.

Bennett, N. G.: A contribution to the study of the movements of the mandible, Proc. R. Soc. Med. **1:**79, 1908.

Bohannan, H., and Abrams, L.: Intentional vital pulp extirpation in periodontal prosthesis, J. Prosthet. Dent. **11:**781, 1961.

Cohn, L. A.: Occluso-rehabilitation and the periodontal problem. In Glickman, I., editor: Clinical periodontology, ed. 2, Philadelphia, 1958, W. B. Saunders Co.

Cohn, L. A.: Integrating treatment procedures in occluso-rehabilitation, J. Prosthet. Dent. **7:**511, 1957.

Cohn, L. A.: The physiological basis for tooth fixation in precision attached partial dentures, J. Prosthet. Dent. **6:**220, 1956.

Geiger, A., Hirschfeld, L.: Minor tooth movement in general practice, ed. 3, St. Louis, 1974, The C. V. Mosby Co.

Goldman, H. M., and Cohen, D. W., editors: Periodontal therapy, ed. 5, St. Louis, 1973, The C. V. Mosby Co.

Hindels, G. W.: Load distribution in extension saddle partial dentures, J. Prosthet. Dent. **2:**92, 1952.

Hirschfeld, I.: Food impaction, J. Am. Dent. Assoc. **17:**1504, 1930.

Jankelson, B.: Physiology of human dental occlusion, J. Am. Dent. Assoc. **50:**664, 1955.

Jankelson, B.: Physiology of stomatognathic system, J. Am. Dent. Assoc. **46:**375, 1953.

Lindhe, J., and Nyman, S.: The role of occlusion in periodontal disease and the biological rationale for splinting in treatment of periodontitis, Oral Sci. Rev. **10:**11, 1977.

Maynard, J. G., and Wilson, R. D. R.: Physiologic dimension of the periodontium significant to the restorative dentist, J. Periodontal. **50:**170, 1979.

McCollum, B. B., and Stuart, C. E.: A research report, South Pasadena, Calif., 1955.

Peeso, F.: Crown and bridge work for student and practitioners, ed. 2, Philadelphia, 1924, Lea & Febiger.

Posselt, U.: Physiology of occlusion and rehabilitation, Philadelphia, 1962, F. A. Davis Co.

Ramfjord, S.: Bruxism, a clinical and electromyographic study, J. Am. Dent. Assoc. **62:**21, 1961.

Schweitzer, J. M.: Oral rehabilitation, St. Louis, 1951, The C. V. Mosby Co.

Sicher, H.: The biologic significance of hinge axis determination, J. Prosthet. Dent. **6:**616, 1956.

Thompson, J. R.: Concepts regarding function of the stomatognathic system, J. Am. Dent. Assoc. **48:**626, 1954.

Valderhaug, J., and Berkeland, J. M.: Periodontal conditions in patients 5 years following insertion of fixed prostheses, J. Oral Rehab. **3:**237, 1976.

Valderhaug, J., and Helpe, L. A.: Oral hygiene in a group of supervised patients with fixed prostheses, J. Periodontol. **48:**221, 1977.

Wheeler, R.: Textbook of dental anatomy and physiology, Philadelphia, 1958, W. B. Saunders Co.

33 Maintenance of the periodontally treated patient

Examination
Ascertaining quality of patient's PPC
Scaling and root planing
Adjunctive procedures
Reinforcement of patient's PPC efforts
Continued motivation during maintenance phase

Once the periodontal patient has been treated, his need for continued periodontal therapy will exist as long as his dentition remains with him. The successful initial periodontal treatment can and often does yield remarkable results, but the problem lies in maintaining these results. The maintenance phase of treatment follows the definitive therapy and will continue through the life of the patient. The prevention of a remission, or the development of new disease, is primarily the responsibility of the patient, but the practitioner has an obligation to help the patient in this responsibility.

Unfortunately the guiding role assumed by the practitioner is not always adequate to maintain the results of treatment. Too often the therapist fails to impress upon the patient the need for continued vigilance. Furthermore, the practitioner is often hindered by the inertia or that innate lack of motivation possessed by the average patient. The problem of achieving productive motivation appears to be more readily surmountable during the initial therapy, but becomes increasingly more difficult as time passes, comfort ensues, and absence from the therapist's office dims the memory of the patient. Part of the problem is a residual from the past, when our profession failed to place adequate emphasis on the patient's therapeutic duties. The profession compounded its error and complicated his duties with terminology. The most common expression used to describe the activities to be accomplished by the patient in his home has been "home care." Two other phrases, "oral physiotherapy" and "oral hygiene" are used, but do not enjoy a widespread acceptance. The term "home care" is so inexact that it allows an interpretation relating it to the care of the home and not to the care of the mouth.

It should simplify the patient's recognition of his therapeutic responsibility by replacing our ambiguous phrases with the self-explanatory term "plaque control." It is accepted that plaque is a major causative agent in the etiology of periodontal disease. Patients must be educated to the realization that plaque is their problem and that plaque control constitutes a lifetime assignment.

Part of the problem of both the initial and the continued motivation of the periodontal patient can be solved by the use of semantically correct terminology to describe his personal therapeutic endeavors. Rather than home care, oral physiotherapy, or oral hygiene, the therapist should substitute the terms "plaque control" and "periodontal care."

Plaque control consists of procedures done by the patient and the therapist to control the population of microorganisms around the teeth. To the patient this means a daily habit pattern whereby he can mechanically remove plaque utilizing the various oral hygiene instruments. To the therapist this means allocating adequate instructional periods so that each patient understands the significance of plaque and the rationale for its reduction or elimination.

The term "plaque control" is synonymous with periodontal care. However, the benefits of plaque control extend to the management of dental caries as well as periodontal disease. Plaque accumulation contributes to the decay of teeth as well as initiating periodontal inflammation. The periodontal care program designed with a primary objective of plaque elimination will concomitantly benefit the dental caries problem.

Hence the terms "plaque control" and "periodontal care" can be used interchangeably. If we place the word patient or personal in front of plaque control or periodontal care, we generate the phrases "personal plaque control," "patient plaque control," "personal periodontal care," or "patient's periodontal care." An abbreviation of all these phrases would be PPC (Robinson; Robinson et al.). The term "preventive plaque control" can be utilized for instructing the nonperiodontal and treated periodontal patients.

PPC would then aptly define those measures employed by the patient on a daily basis to reduce or eliminate the accumulation of plaque. The term "oral physiotherapy" could be used during active treatment by those individuals who feel that massage of the gingivae is desirable. "Oral hygiene" could be used as a term to include the cleansing of

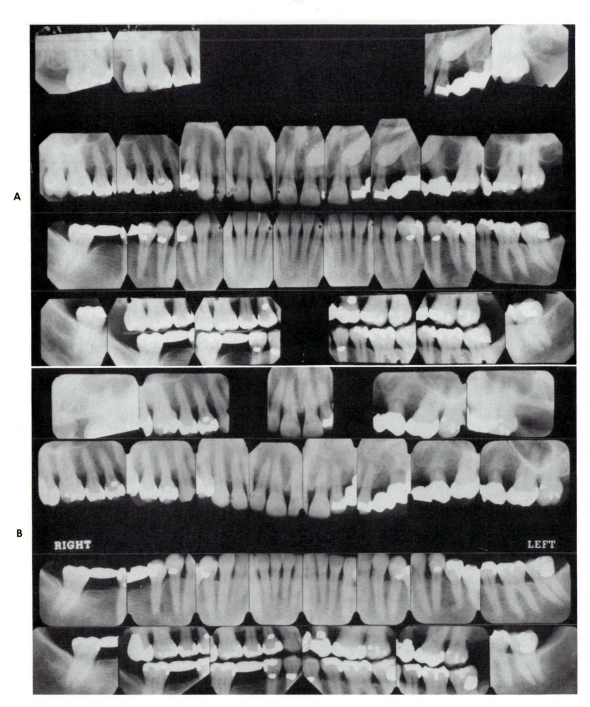

Fig. 33-1. A, Pretreatment roentgenograms. **B,** Posttreatment roentgenograms 17 years later. Bone level held and in some areas improved.

the tongue and the use of mouthwashes to improve the odor of the breath.

But the specific effort to reduce plaque accumulation around the teeth designed to prevent periodontal disease and dental caries, reduce or reverse inflammation, and maintain the established equilibrium after treatment should be called "plaque control."

The effect of this change in terminology would serve as a constant reminder to the patient that plaque is his problem. This change also aids in correlating therapy to disease, disease to prevention, and prevention to maintenance.

It is often difficult initially to motivate some patients to establish a good plaque control program,

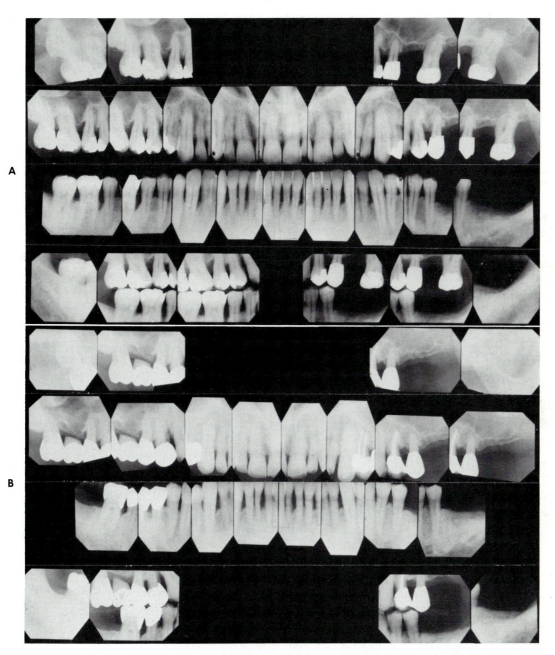

Fig. 33-2. A, Pretreatment roentgenograms, 1955. Severe mobility in lower central incisors and maxillary left second bicuspid. **B,** Sixteen years later, 1971. No mobility present. Note mandibular right central incisor root defect from use of toothpicks. Maxillary left bicuspids were splinted. Lower anterior wire splint was discarded 6 months after therapy. Several periodontal pockets were maintained on recall visits.

Continued.

and even more difficult to sustain this motivation over a lifetime. Nevertheless, *it is the continual reinforcement of this motivation that is the single most important criterion in maintaining the periodontally treated patient.* A good plaque control program will include the initial instruction of the patient and those periodic check-ups utilized by the therapist to remove calculus, reinforce the patient's motivation, and identify for the patient those areas of incomplete plaque removal. After a patient has been treated for periodontal disease, the follow-up, or maintenance, phase has been called the recall system.

The periodontal recall should be part of the plaque control program in the treated case. Even though the result of initial therapy might be judged successful, changes in a patient's local or systemic balance may occur along with decreased personal periodontal care. Therefore to minimize remissions and to prevent new disease entities, supervision of the patient on a periodic basis is essential. This supervision at recall affords the therapist the opportunity to reinforce the patient's PPC, judge the results of treatment on a continuing basis, intervene when new disease processes develop, and aid in a team effort approach to maintain the patient's functional dentition throughout life.

Such an approach is valuable in terms of the disease prevention for the patient with a healthy mouth, but it is mandatory for the patient who has periodontal disease. This maintenance approach serves to preserve teeth where the prognosis had been regarded as hopeless. Examples of this spectrum of therapy can be seen in Figs. 33-1 to 33-12.

The recall system consists of appointing the patient to a periodic visit at the dental office. The time interval between appointments can range from 1 to 12 months, but it is most often 2 to 4 months. In the past the profession and the public came to believe the optimum recall interval to be 6 months, based on the advertising of toothpaste companies who advocated the concept and introduced the phrase, ''Brush twice a day and see your dentist twice a year.''

Based on recent studies the optimum recall interval is much more frequent and is dependent on each patient's periodontal disease and caries problem, personal plaque control, and immunologic response to plaque by-products. The decision as to the proper interval rests with the therapist. After the first year of recall appointments the therapist should know the approximate needs of the patient for remotivation and reinforcement of his plaque control program. The time required for each appointment can also be determined after 1 to 4 re-

C

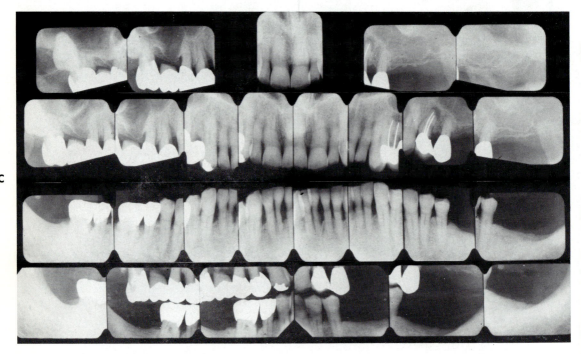

Fig. 33-2, cont'd. C, Twenty-two years after operation. Patient is being maintained on 3-month recall schedule. Periapical involvement on maxillary first bicuspid is asymptomatic and is being watched by an endodontist. Patient refused partial dentures.

call sessions. The therapist can then ascertain the need for calculus removal, polishing, occlusal adjustment, an inspection of night guards, retainers, splints or prosthetic appliances, a caries check-up, and a plaque control review. The patient should develop an appreciation for the recall appointment and, with instruction, understand the facts of plaque and periodontal disease. The patient should visually, and with the aid of his tactile sense, recognize and feel plaque and calculus

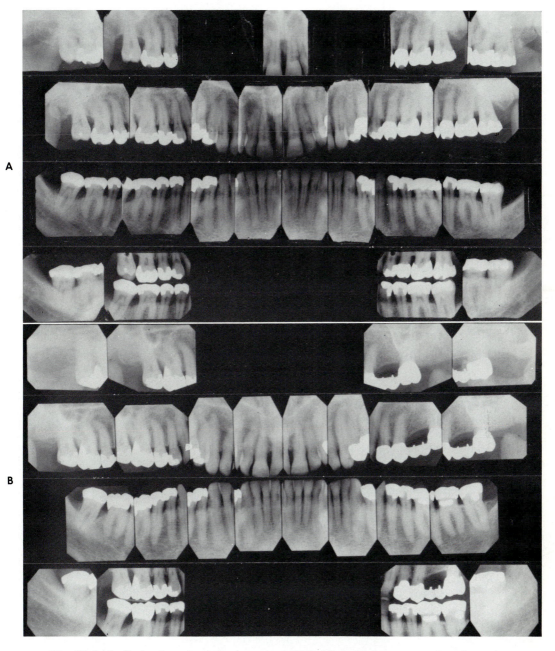

Fig. 33-3. A, Pretreatment roentgenograms, 1953. Minor tooth movement performed on maxillary centrals. Left maxillary first molar lost because of subsequent endodontic problems. Initial treatment was followed by routine recall visits for 10 years. Recurrence of periodontal pockets on distal aspect of maxillary second molars required surgical intervention. Original therapy consisted of gingivectomies and occlusal adjustment; 10 years later, distal wedge procedures and osseous recontouring were accomplished. Patient continued recall visits for another 13 years; pockets remained present but stable on right second molars. Total treatment period was 23 years. **B,** Eighteen years after initial treatment.

Continued.

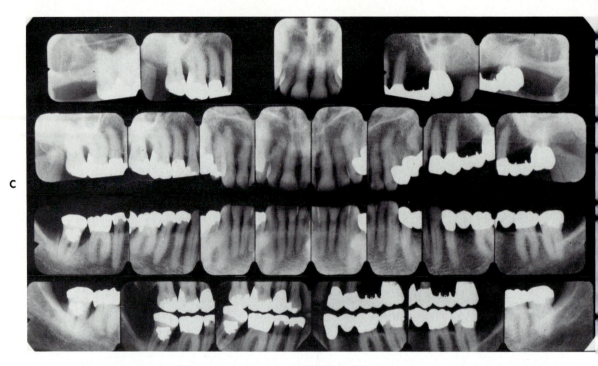

Fig. 33-3, cont'd. C, Twenty-three years after initial treatment periodontal pockets still present on right second molars, but pocket depth remained unchanged. Success of treatment and longevity of teeth due to consistent recall program. (Restorative work by Dr. Raleigh Davies.)

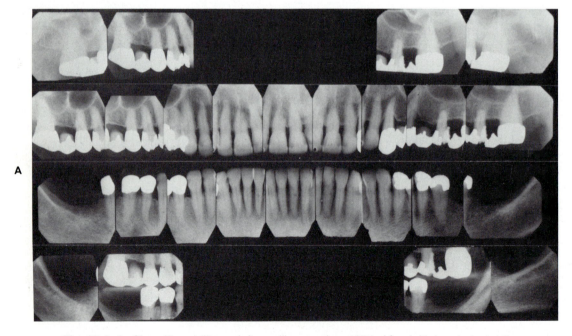

Fig. 33-4. A, Class III mobility on left maxillary canine, 1954. After initial periodontal therapy, including extraction of left maxillary bicuspid, a removable prosthetic appliance was constructed with a rest on canine.

accumulation and even be able to notice any changes in the color or texture of the gingival tissue. A well-trained patient can help the therapist decide to accelerate the recall period or to extend it.

The findings of Lovdal et al., Theilade et al., Socransky, Suomi et al., and Lindhe and Nyman add to the considerable evidence that bacterial plaque is the primary agent in the initiation of periodontal disease and show it to be the primary

Text continued on p. 1166.

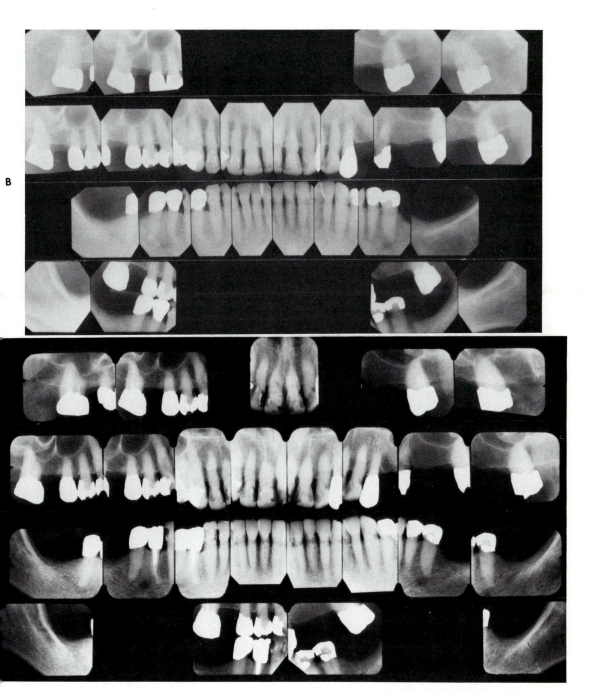

Fig. 33-4, cont'd. B, Seventeen years later, 1971. Maxillary left canine still presents an unfavorable crown-root ratio, but no mobility or pockets are present. **C,** Twenty-three years later. Periodontal disease under good control, but note patient's caries problem, resulting in multiple reconstructive restorations.

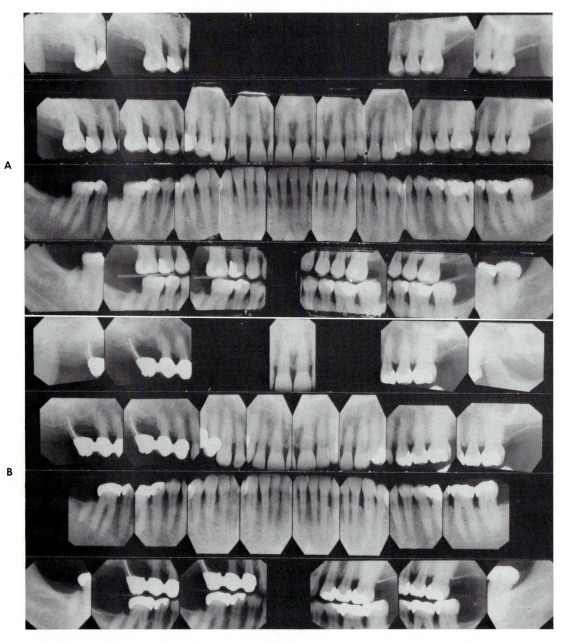

Fig. 33-5. A, After initial therapy, 1954. Four-year postoperative roentgenograms show failure of initial therapy on maxillary right posterior segment. Note trifurcation involvement accentuated on maxillary right first molar, dental caries present on mesial aspect of maxillary left first molar, calculus present on mesial aspect of left mandibular canine, and poor overall plaque control. Patient refused extraction, but accepted root amputation and fixed prosthesis. **B,** Plaque control improved, 1966. Recall visits were more consistent, but patient developed periapical problems on right maxillary bicuspids. Splinting of mandibular left molars was accomplished to prevent extrusion.

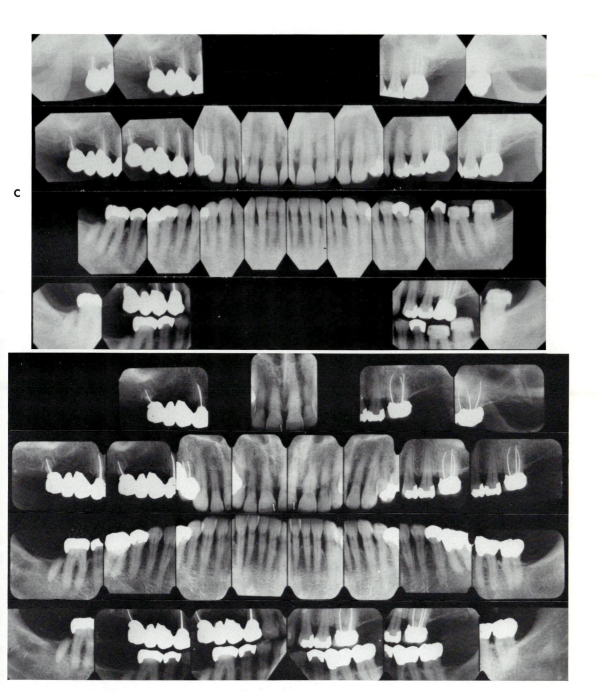

Fig. 33-5, cont'd. C, Seventeen years after initial therapy, 1971. Endodontics required on right maxillary bicuspids and left maxillary first molar. New fixed prosthesis was constructed on maxillary right posterior segment, and at time of periodontal recall a new splint was in progress for mandibular left molars. This patient was maintained on recall and aptly demonstrates need for vigilance. Case points out that combined therapy (periodontics, endodontics, and restorative dentistry) is oftentimes necessary in overall patient management. It shows too that a root tip may be beneficial to an adjacent tooth. **D,** Twenty-three years later. A continuing periapical problem resulted in root amputation of maxillary right second bicuspid. Bridge was preserved and is entirely functional. (Endodontic therapy by Dr. John Greco; restorative dentistry by Dr. Raleigh Davies.)

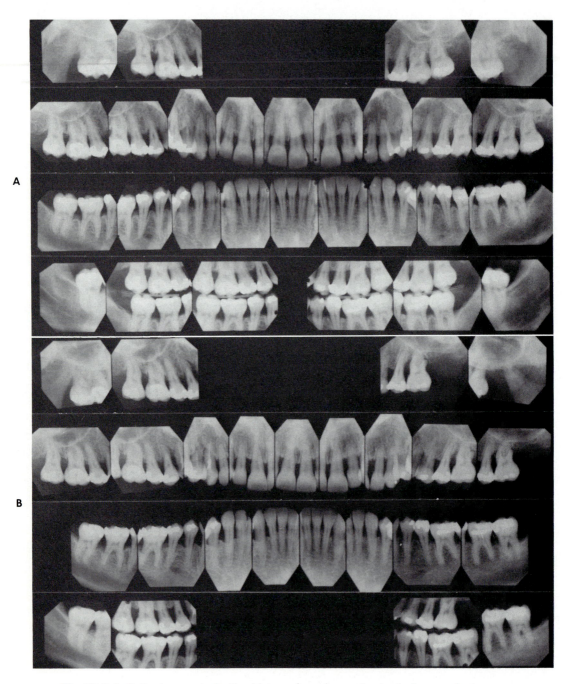

Fig. 33-6. A, Patient presented with a history of previous orthodontic therapy, large crowns, poor root structure, and a generalized periodontitis with multiple furcation involvements, 1956. **B,** After 6 years of initial periodontal therapy and recall visits, 1962. Roentgenograms show progression of disease. Severe mobility continued because of poor overall crown-root ratio. Left maxillary second molar was lost, and left maxillary first molar and right first bicuspid were beyond repair. At this time fixed periodontal prosthesis was prescribed.

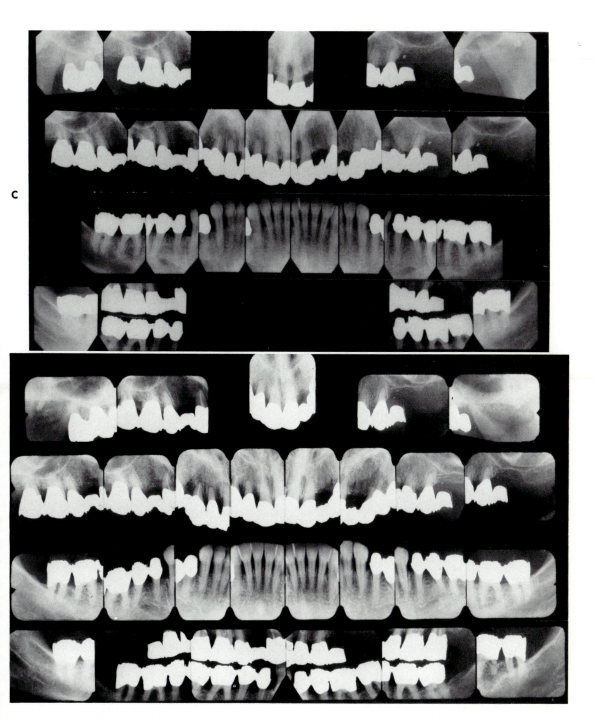

Fig. 33-6, cont'd. C, Posttreatment roentgenograms 15 years after initial periodontal therapy and 9 years after periodontal prosthesis, 1971. Patient was maintained on a 4-month periodontal recall schedule for 19 years and then lost motivation. After an absence of 2 years she returned with several pocket areas out of control. **D,** Twenty-two years after initial therapy. Note increased severity around maxillary right first and second molars. Root amputation is now indicated. This case demonstrates value of periodontal recall schedule. An absence from maintenance program ensures further progression of disease and possibly more complicated treatment procedures. (Prosthesis by Dr. Dan Feder, Beverly Hills, Calif.)

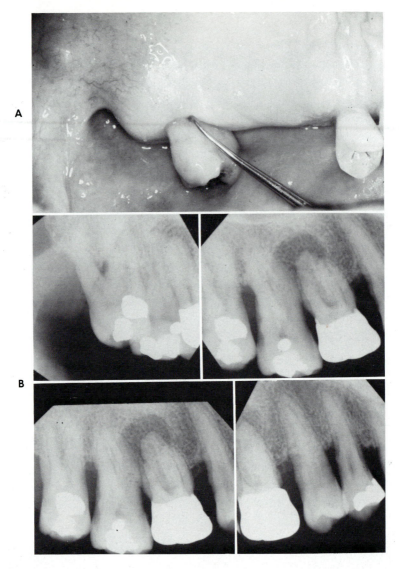

Fig. 33-7. A, Trifurcation involvement on recall visit. Patient is maintained with root curettage and plaque control. Curved explorer can be seen entering furcation. Eleven years after initial therapy. Note stain before prophylaxis. **B,** Roentgenogram of **A** trifurcation, 1960. First and second molars extracted because of severe involvement.

agent in the continuation and progression of the disease throughout life as well. Even though host response to injury has a significant role in disease, the actual continued mechanical removal of plaque on a daily basis is mandatory in the maintenance of a treated case. The challenge of the maintenance program is in the constant and forceful reminder to the patient of the role that plaque plays and of the need for him to control plaque at home. Plaque removal on the part of the patient, however, is not always successful; therefore the periodontal recall system may be the most important part of therapy for some patients.

It has been felt in the past by many clinicians

that frequent recall visits in the first year after therapy were most important, because any failures that might occur would occur in this period. It might be possible to overlook a bruxing habit or periodontal traumatism resultant from an occlusal discrepancy, but most probably any failure would be the failure of the patient to accept and to perform plaque breakup and removal procedures taught during the active phase of treatment.

Discovery of this failure and reinstruction of plaque-removal methods as well as reinforcement of motivation can take place during the frequent recall visits in the first year. Some therapists place such a value on this approach that they include

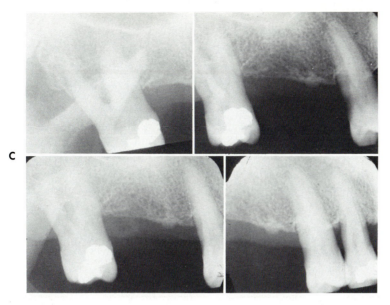

Fig. 33-7, cont'd. C, Roentgeongram of **A** trifurcation 19 years later, 1979. Very little change can be noted. Tooth supports removable prosthesis.

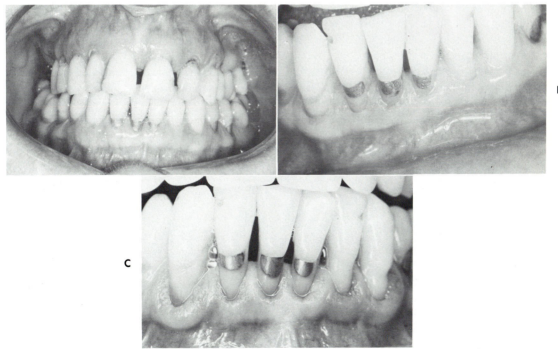

Fig. 33-8. A, Incisors quite mobile prior to gingivoplasty. **B,** Postgingivoplasty before prophylaxis; mobility still present, **C,** Ten-year postsurgical therapy. Patient on a consistent recall schedule and a compulsive personal plaque control program. Patient rejected splinting and overcompensates in plaque control measures. Teeth extremely mobile, and yet no pockets. Note recession and fibrotic appearance of gingiva probably due to excessive PPC.

these first-year visits in their original fee. Certainly the other advantages of frequent recall appointments in the first year are (1) to help the doctor determine future recall needs and (2) to help educate the patient about a recall appointment pattern. It is during this time that therapist and patient can come to an understanding of actual recall needs.

However, at the initial consultation, before active therapy takes place, the therapist should state that upon completion of the initial phase, there will be a recall visit once every 2 or 3 months for the first year. It should be explained that some patients will need this schedule throughout life; others will need to return every 4 months, every 6 months, or every 12 months after the first year. If the schedule is established at the initial visit, it is easier to create an understanding of the recall need and to foster loyalty to the program. Such is often not the case, and misunderstanding can ensue, resulting in a lapse of recall visits and a potential recurrence of the patient's problem. If the recall aspect of treatment is understood from the beginning of therapy and reinforced at the end of therapy, then continuation of the established or the revised recall program will become an accepted fact. Reduction of the frequency of recall visits is dependent upon the individual's severity of disease and his daily personal plaque control measures.

Economics often influence dental treatment, and unfortunately this includes the periodontal recall. With the advent of the third party in the delivery of dental care (insurance companies), it has been very difficult to have preventive plaque control instruction included in dental benefits. Similarly, the insurance industry has followed the statement, "Brush twice a day, and see your dentist twice a year." Most insurance companies will not cover more than 2 recall visits a year. They have not accepted the fact that some patients in a preventive program might need 4 or 6 periodontal recall visits a year. However, such frequent recall appointments would save the insurance companies enormous sums of money over the years.

Patients with advanced periodontal disease, multiple furcation involvements, and extensive reconstruction and even those patients who are unable or unwilling to develop a good home program of plaque control should be placed on a 1- or 2-month recall schedule. Where plaque control on the part of the patient fails, the therapist must remove the plaque and any deposits for the patient. Rosling et al. have suggested that with the use of 2-week coronal scalings and interproximal taping, regardless of the type of surgical therapy employed, periodontal disease can be cured and further progression of periodontitis stopped. It should be noted that in the Rosling et al. study chlorhexidine digluconate rinses were used for 2 weeks following surgical therapy. The significance of this study seems to be that even though plaque control was taught and encouraged, superior oral hygiene was actually ensured by the dental hygienist once every 2 weeks. It is this plaque control that stops the progression of periodontal disease. However, a 2-week recall visit to the dental hygienist is not feasible at this point in routine practice. Economics, lack of patient interest, failure of patient motivation, space, personnel, and

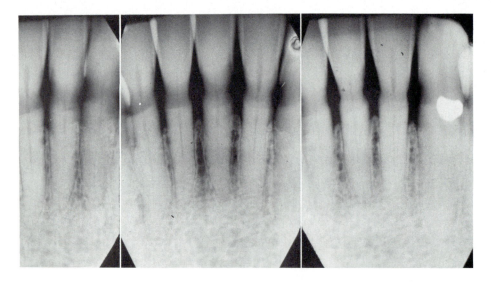

Fig. 33-9. Many years of root curettage have caused an hourglass appearance of these teeth.

other factors preclude this kind of approach in the present dental care delivery system. However, in certain selected cases, it is possible to recall a patient once a month or once every 2 months in the average practice.

Ramfjord has also maintained that regardless of the kind of initial therapy that has been employed, with or without the surgical elimination of pockets, the 2-month recall schedule substantially retards the destruction of the periodontium from periodon-

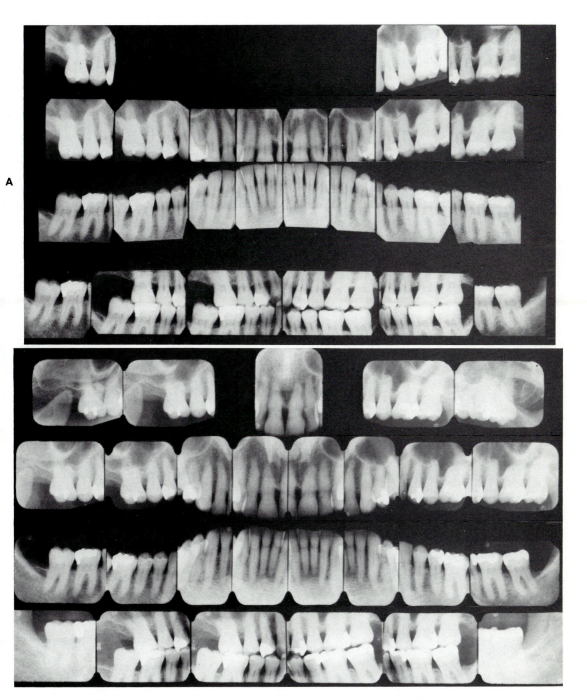

Fig. 33-10. A, Long-term cases of periodontal maintenance. Initial therapy was subgingival curettage. Patients were recalled once every 2 or 3 months for 25 years. **B,** Twenty-five years after initial therapy. Note closure of diastema between maxillary central incisors. Very little extrusion took place on lower right second molar. Patient had good plaque control and never missed a recall appointment.

tal disease. If recalls were based on an average of once every 2 months following initial therapy, an additional incentive might develop on the part of the patient if it became known that the better his PPC, the longer his recall interval. The prospect of increasing the recall interval from 2 to 3 months, from 3 to 4 months, or even from 4 to 6 months would afford the patient a participatory goal.

The method of recalling the patient is up to the individual practitioner. Three approaches are most generally in use today: (1) the utilization of a card

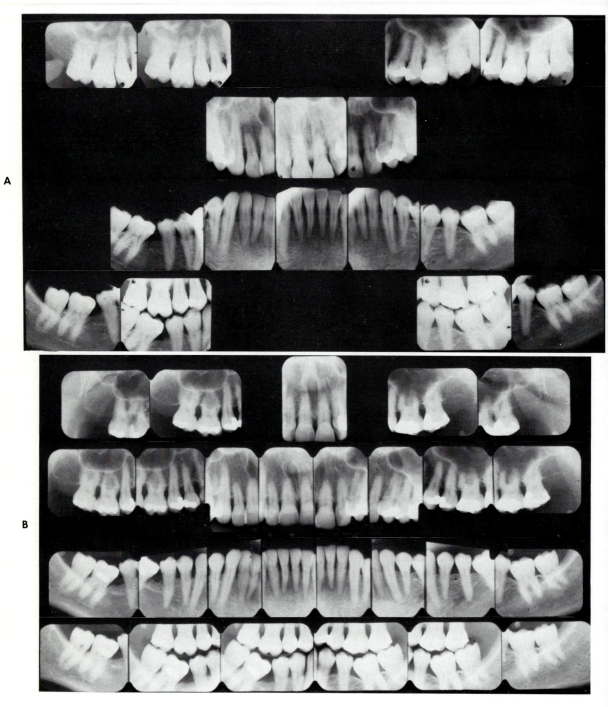

Fig. 33-11. A, Twenty-five year periodontal case treated by gingivectomies on maxillary posteriors and curettage on remainder of teeth. Patient taught plaque control and maintained on a 4-month consistent recall program. **B,** Twenty-five years later.

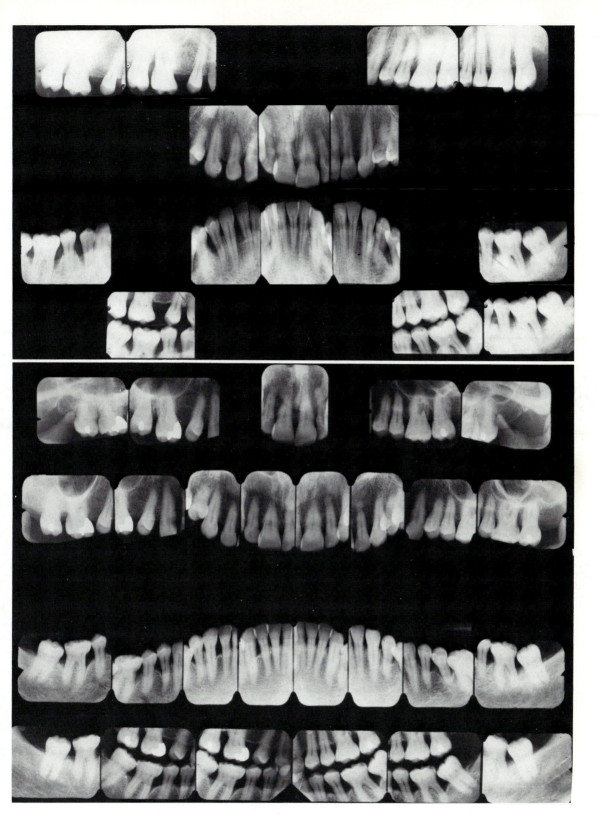

Fig. 33-12. A, Twenty-five year periodontal case treated by multiple flap surgeries for new attachment. **B,** After initial therapy, 25 years later. Patient had a severe malocclusion that did not lend itself to adjustment or correction. Initial new attachment flap surgery, training in flossing and brushing, and consistent 3-month recall visits were sole therapy over 25 years. Note that some intrabony defects present but improved, some pockets are still present but greatly reduced, and patient has maintained mouth as is for all these years.

that states that the recall period is up and suggests that the patient call the office for an appointment; (2) a telephone call to the patient at the end of the recall period at which time the appointment is made; and (3) appointing the patient in advance for the next recall session; 1 week before the appointment either a reminder card is mailed, or the patient is telephoned as a direct reminder. The last approach seems to be the most effective because it establishes a continuity in therapy and imparts to the patient the knowledge and security of continued maintenance.

A recall card suggesting the patient call the office is the least effective method and the easiest to ignore. Advance appointments and a telephone reminder of the date and the time of the visit seem to be the protocol most appreciated by the patient and the most efficient method of follow-up of treated patients.

The recall appointment consists of the following procedures: (1) examination, (2) ascertaining the quality of the patient's PPC, (3) scaling, root planing, and polishing, (4) adjunctive procedures, (5) reinforcement of the patient's PPC efforts, (6) continued motivation, and (7) advance appointment.

Examination

The first consideration in a recall appointment is the same as in an initial examination of a patient. The entire oral cavity will receive a most careful scrutiny, and this will include the lips, the buccal mucosa, the palatal mucosa, the vestibular trough, the tongue, the soft palate, and the throat. Any soft tissue changes noted should be recorded and, if significant, managed. The patient should be asked if there has been any change in his medical history since the last recall visit, and if so it should be recorded.

Examination of the gingiva follows, and the dentist meticulously observes the color and texture of the tissues—always looking for signs of inflammation, bleeding, exudate, and enlargements. With a periodontal probe or explorer all gingival crevices should be checked, and if pockets are present, they should be checked against previous markings and significant changes recorded. Examination of all bifurcation and trifurcation entrances is important, and if furcation involvement is present, the current status should be checked against previous charting. Mobility of teeth must be tested and compared to previous values.

In a long-standing periodontal practice there will be individual periodontal pockets present that are

accepted as relatively stable or quiescent, bifurcation or trifurcation involvements (Fig. 33-7) that are maintained, and occasionally loose teeth that have stabilized with continued mobility but are maintained without splinting (Fig. 33-8). Fortunately, these are the exceptions rather than the rule and are only possible if the patient has an exceptional personal plaque control program and is faithful to the periodontal recall system.

All too often when concentrating on tissue texture, color, and architecture, periodontal pockets, and tooth mobility, the therapist may overlook dental caries. Specifically, any sign of root caries should be detected and recorded, and interproximal areas thoroughly checked. When the periodontal recall is handled by a specialist, dental caries must be prominently noted on the outgoing recall report.

Roentgenograms should be taken every 2 or 3 years for most periodontal patients. Bite-wing films every 6 months are helpful, particularly with patients who are prone to dental caries. An occasional single film may be desired to check an infrabony defect that has had new attachment therapy or an osseous graft. Kodachromes can be taken at various intervals as an optional procedure, dependent upon the persuasion of the operator and the individual case. If the patient is a tongue thruster and exhibits signs of incipient diastemata, serial Kodachromes can afford the operator a record of the most subtle change. In addition, Kodachromes can be a learning device for the therapist as well as a teaching aid to the patient. Utilization of Kodachromes and plaque-staining techniques can be a valuable aid in the patient's plaque control program, since the photographic slides can readily show the improvement or failure of his plaque removal technique.

Ascertaining quality of patient's PPC

The ability of the patient to properly perform plaque control procedures away from the dental office is the most important single aspect in the maintenance of the periodontally treated case. A detailed description of the methods of personal periodontal care and personal plaque control will be found in Chapter 18.

The recall appointment is the time to observe the end result of the training period in personal plaque control that the patient received during initial treatment. Utilization of a dye to stain plaque is an effective way to show the patient deficiencies in plaque removal techniques. A high percentage of pocket formation and bone loss occurs interproximally, and yet the dental profession continues to overemphasize the use of the toothbrush. The toothbrush used in the best possible fashion will not clean the interprosimal areas of the teeth. A simple experiment will verify this statement. Have the patient brush and subsequently use a stain to reveal plaque. In most cases the disclosing stain will allow visualization of the intact interproximal plaque.

The patient who only brushes his teeth is unable to attain the desired end result—good personal plaque control. The additional use of interproximal cleaners such as dental floss, the Perio-Aid, the Plaque Pik, the D-Plak-R, Stim-U-Dents, the rubber tip, the interproximal brush, or just plain yarn must be stressed by the therapist until such time as a patient understands that their incorporation into the PPC program is mandatory. Several plaque-staining techniques are available. Numerous companies produce chewable tablets and small bottles of liquid dye that stain plaque readily. Another technique is the use of a fluorescent dye (Brillant), which requires a special lamp that effectively discloses plaque. Most of the dyes stain plaque red. The two-tone dye stains new plaque red and older plaque blue. This is now produced by several companies. All methods are excellent adjuncts to plaque control training.

Block and Derdivanis did an 18-day study on a patient who was instructed not to perform plaque control procedures on the lower anterior teeth. The patient was also instructed not to use the anterior teeth for incisal mastication. After initial scaling and polishing, the two-tone dye was used at various intervals to record photographically the areas of thin or early plaque and the subsequent development of areas of thick or older plaque. The thin plaque stains red and the thick plaque stains blue. Samples of red and blue plaque were taken at intervals and examined by phase-contrast microscopy. Plate 2 shows the 1- to 18-day test. The changes in the hue and intensity of the color of the stain over a period of time suggests that this technique may demonstrate the aging of the plaque and the development of plaque architecture.

Red plaque revealed the following information:
1. Extreme thinness
2. No evidence of orderly architecture
3. Filaments, spirochetes, and vibrios not present
4. Motility not noted

Blue plaque revealed the following:
1. A considerably greater thickness
2. A well-organized architecture

3. Great numbers of filaments
4. Motility often present
5. Spiral organisms and vibrios present
6. Increased cocci and rods

It was found that zones of light blue to purple appeared between the red and blue. The investigators found this light blue-to-purple zone to look microscopically more like blue plaque than red and that this intermediate color represented a transition from red to blue plaque.

After the detection of plaque and the determination of the effectiveness of the patient's personal plaque removal efforts, consideration of the formation of calcareous deposits must be made. Although periodontal disease can exist without calculus, the importance of calculus as a factor in periodontal disease must not be minimized. Calculus forms subsequent to plaque accumulation and provides a favorable environment for further plaque formation. Its removal is necessary in the maintenance of the periodontally treated patient. Unfortunately, patients cannot remove calculus as they can remove plaque; hence, the technique of calculus removal lies in the hands of the therapist.

The rate of calculus formation varies from patient to patient, and even though numerous articles on calculus can be found in the literature, not too much is known about this phenomenon. It is known, however, that the better the plaque control, the more effective the inhibition of calculus formation. And the better the personal plaque control and inhibition of calculus formation, the better the periodontal health status of the patient. Scaling and prophylaxis at recall appointments is not as effective a preventive measure as is the daily regimen of personal periodontal care that removes plaque and inhibits the early formation of calculus. The exception to this last statement might be coronal polishing and interproximal taping once every 2 weeks (Rosling et al.).

Not only are there variations in the rate of calculus deposition, but there are individual differences in the inflammatory response to the presence of plaque and calculus. This varied response is undoubtedly partially due to a resistance factor on the part of the patient, but the pathogenicity of the microorganisms may also be an operative factor. Plaque is discussed in detail in Chapter 3.

An interesting experiment was performed by one of the editors of this text. Eight individuals with healthy mouths and twelve individuals with periodontal disease were selected and assigned to participate in a toothbrush study. Each patient was instructed to brush one side of his mouth once daily and the alternate side three times daily. At the conclusion of the study there was no observed variation in the amount of accretions on any of the teeth in the control group, that is, those with a "normal" dentition. In the periodontally involved group, however, there was a markedly greater accumulation of accretions on those teeth that were brushed only once a day. The periodontal patient must be impressed with the critical necessity for individualized periodontal care, since the dental health conditions he presents may be at least partially dependent on his rate of calculus deposition and his salivary chemistry.

It is believed by some periodontists that the physical quality of the diet is an important factor in the inhibition of plaque and calculus formation. Many therapists believe that during the active treatment phase the patient should be placed on a low-carbohydrate, high-protein diet with the abundant incorporation of detergent foods such as raw vegetables and raw fruit. Although there is little doubt that a detergent diet reduces the accumulation of food debris in the mouth, it is a difficult aspect to control. After the active treatment has been completed and the patient is no longer under the close supervision of the therapist, he has a tendency to revert to previously established dietary habits. If that diet has been of a consistency and quality that favors food retention and the accumulation of materia alba, very possibly plaque and calculus will occur much more rapidly. Plaque buildup occurs much more rapidly in patients who have a high sugar intake. It is very disconcerting to the therapist to find root caries at recall appointments. In such cases the patient often has a candy habit, which he is not likely to admit. Certain patients suck hard candies, which bathes the dentition continually with sucrose throughout the day. This can have a disastrous effect on the teeth in spite of plaque control measures. Part of the recall responsibility of the therapist should be to encourage the patient to maintain a high-protein, high-detergent diet free of refined sugars.

In such cases where the patient's diet is one prescribed by a physician for a gastroenterologic disease, the patient's plaque control program must be accelerated. A soft nondetergent ulcer-type diet requires more frequent plaque removal activity. The same would apply to those patients who for various reasons have a low-protein, low-detergent diet.

Scaling and root planing

One would hope that after periodontal therapy and with an adequate personal plaque control pro-gram, the accumulation of calcareous deposits would be kept to a minimum. Nonetheless, calculus does form, and as mentioned above the rate varies from patient to patient. The rate of deposition is governed by the plaque control program, salivary chemistry, and diet and is influenced by the frequency of recall appointments. The periodontal patient who misses several recall appointments will oftentimes eventually return to the periodontal office with what the therapist classifies as remarkable amounts of calculus. Poor plaque control by the patient, along with a failure to appear for recall appointments, invariably leads to further periodontal breakdown.

During the examination of the recall patient, the periodontal health status is reviewed and any pocket formation is noted. Therapy for these areas is made on the basis of elimination or control. Therefore treatment can range from curettage to complicated surgical procedures. At recall visits the process of cleansing the root surfaces must be fastidious and handled with an expertise based on clinical judgment. It must be kept in mind that the root surfaces are much softer than the enamel portion of the tooth. Sometimes, because of prior therapy, the cementum has been removed and dentin is exposed. In any case both the cementum and dentin are readily subject to nicking and grooving in scaling. In theory, nicked or grooved cemental and dentinal surfaces would expedite the accumulation of plaque. Nicks and grooves can be detected by the development of a good sense of touch, and the judicious use of the curet will prevent overscaling and grooving. Overscaling can cause needless cervical hypersensitivity, and many years of overscaling will cause an hourglass design of the tooth (Fig. 33-9).

Eminent clinicians of the past, such as Dixon Bell of San Francisco and Isadore Hirschfeld of New York, looked upon the recall curettage as both an art and a science. Their ability to curet a root surface without overscaling, nicking, and grooving, along with patient cooperation, permitted the long-term maintenance of periodontally treated cases for periods extending to 40 and 50 years. To their students and the profession these men left a legacy of documented proof that patients with periodontal disease, once treated, could be maintained successfully for many decades. This was possible because these therapists were able to secure patient cooperation, which included good personal periodontal care and faithfulness to the periodontal recall. There is also evidence that once a patient with periodontal disease is treated, and regardless of the type of treatment, a success-

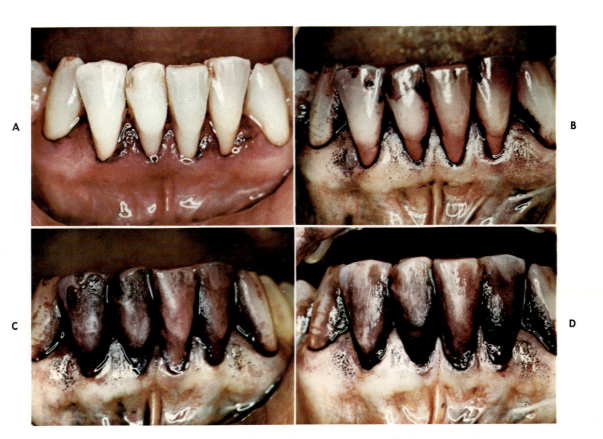

Plate 2. Use of two-tone dye (Dis-Plaque) disclosing solution. Oral hygiene methods were not used by this patient. **A,** Immediately after prophylaxis. **B,** Two days after prophylaxis. **C,** Nine days after prophylaxis. **D,** Eighteen days after prophylaxis. (Courtesy P. Block and J. Derdivanis and Dis-Plaque Co.)

ful maintenance program can result with good PPC and consistent recalls (Oliver).

Three maintenance cases, each of 25-years' duration, are presented. The patient in Fig. 33-10 was treated by initial therapy that consisted of sub-gingival curettage, plaque control, and occlusal adjustment. The patient in Fig. 33-11 was treated by initial therapy that consisted of gingivectomy-gingivoplasty on the maxillary posterior sextants and plaque control. The patient in Fig. 33-12 was treated by flap surgery with bone regeneration and new attachment attempts as well as with plaque control. All three cases were maintained satisfactorily over the 25-year span with 3- and 4-month consistent recall visits.

The time factor in a periodontal recall is a vexing one. The average periodontal recall, including examination, inspection of the patient's personal plaque control, and root curettage, demands not less than a 30-minute appointment. If one adds reinforcement of the plaque control program and polishing, an additional 30 minutes may be required. Patients who smoke or drink coffee and tea often have a severe stain problem and should expect their periodontal recall appointment to take longer than the usual 30 to 60 minutes. The therapist should not be penalized for working with individuals who volunteer to subject their teeth to these staining habits, and the patient should be aware that such habits require the extra service and time of the dentist. Variation in time taken to perform the periodontal recall is often dependent on the patient's personal plaque control program, frequency of recall visits, dietary habits, and habits conducive to staining such as smoking and the use of coffee or tea.

Adjunctive procedures

It is important to understand that the periodontal recall is not just scaling and polishing teeth. The patient's role in plaque control has been mentioned, and the need to reinforce it on recall will follow. But in addition the recall must encompass observation and detection of dental caries. It has been previously specified that roentgenograms should be taken every 2 or 3 years, and bite-wing films every 6 months. Bite-wing examinations aid in the detection of interproximal caries as well as showing the level of crestal bone. They will also show the periodontal space at the crestal margin of the bone and the contact relationship of adjacent teeth. Bite-wing roentgenograms will oftentimes show the crestal margin bone more accurately than do regular periapical films. The horizontal angle at which the bite-wing roentgenogram is

taken will sometimes reveal much that the standard method conceals. With the advent of the single film full-mouth survey (Fig. 33-13, *A*), it should be pointed out that for periodontal purposes these are not as desirable as a complete roentgenographic survey (Fig. 33-13, *B*). In addition complete periapical x-ray surveys better aid in the supervision of operative and restorative procedures done subsequent to the periodontal therapy. Where periodontal prosthesis has been accomplished, careful observation and scrutiny is mandatory in proper maintenance. Roentgenographic changes of any kind must be noted, recorded, and acted upon. The periapical region must be checked carefully to detect any developing endodontic problems.

General observation of the periodontal prosthesis must include a careful inspection of the tissues. The most excellent restorations may on occasion cause a marginal gingival problem, and the therapist should be prepared to make note of this and institute corrective procedures. If the therapist accomplished both the periodontics and the periodontal prosthesis, he has a very real responsibility toward the patient to maintain the prosthetic appliance in proper function. If a periodontist did the periodontics, he too must accept some of the responsibility of this prosthetic maintenance. Most often in such cases the periodontist has worked with the referring dentist in the planning and design of the periodontal prosthesis, and it is at this time that a thorough understanding of a shared responsibility should be assumed. An alternate recall between the two therapists is probably the best approach. However, the periodontist must be allowed to increase the frequency of recall if the case requires additional activity or services such as the reinforcement of personal plaque control or root curettage.

An alternating recall form for the periodontal specialist is on p. 1177. Three copies should be made; one is retained, one is sent to the referring dentist, and the third is given to the patient. In this way a fairly good communication system is begun. In many treated cases the best maintenance approach is a shared recall system between the periodontal office and the dental office.

When temporary or provisional splints are used in therapy, the patient should be seen every 2 or 3 months. At this time the temporarily cemented appliances should be tapped off, the tissues carefully inspected, and the crown preparations checked for dental caries. Active therapy may be reinstituted to care for any return of periodontal disease. This is one of the advantages of provisional splinting. Some therapists employ a temporary cement for permanent restorations in order that they may tap them off with relative ease for examination and inspection at the recall appointment; there are both advantages and hazards inherent in this modus operandi.

Routine operative dentistry must be clinically checked in the maintenance phase. This type of treatment is necessary on a continuing basis in many patients, and as a consequence must not be overlooked in the periodontal recall. New inlays or crowns are checked for occlusal anatomy and marginal ridge form, and contact points should be tested with dental floss. Vigilance is necessary to prevent interproximal food impaction, food wedging in contact points, or poor food flow patterns resulting from faulty anatomic design. In amalgams, inlays, and crowns both the unintentional overhang and inadequate margins will function as plaque traps. Other plaque traps will occur with washed-out synthetics or plastic restorations. Removable prosthetic appliances often attract plaque, and patients should be instructed in an appropriate cleaning method for these appliances.

Any change in the crown-root ratio should be

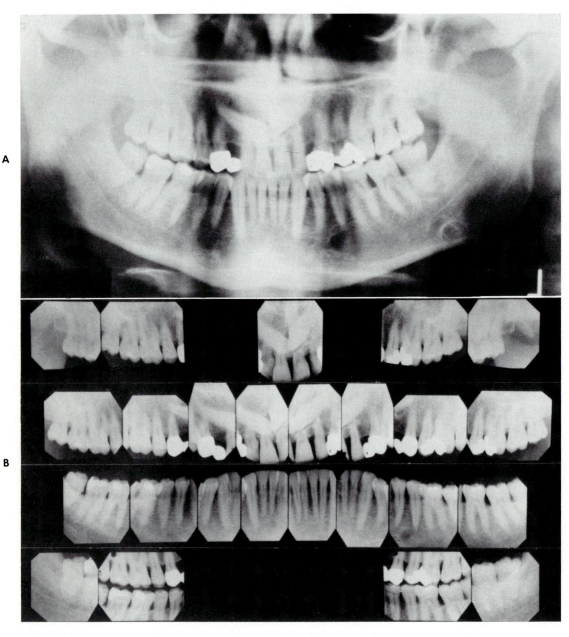

Fig. 33-13. A, Single film full-mouth roentgenogram. Note lack of detail. **B,** Same case showing improved detail.

PERIODONTAL ALTERNATING RECALL PROGRAM

Patient _____

Date of completion of initial periodontal therapy _____

Optimum recall period _____

Date of first recall at periodontal office _____

Estimated date of first recall at dental office _____

cc: _____
      (referring dentist)

cc: _____
      (patient)

---

noted. As an example, a new crown on a tooth with a poorly formed root could cause periodontal trauma and, in effect, actually shorten the life span of that tooth.

Patients with a history of tongue thrusting or bruxism often have appliances constructed to control these habits during active therapy. Minor tooth movement is often done in periodontal therapy, and retainers are constructed to maintain this tooth repositioning. Sometimes these retainers are temporary and utilized only before permanent splinting or permanent retention is instituted. On occasion the patients will wear a removable retainer for a long time, either because of economics or by personal preference. They may prefer to wear their retainer at night, rather than having fixed permanent splinting. These retainers need to be checked periodically for wear and possible traumatic effects on either the teeth or soft tissues. Night guards for bruxism often wear rapidly on the occlusal surface because of the habit patterns of the patient and will require resurfacing or replacement. Likewise, night guards can create trauma to the teeth, which can produce undesirable orthodontic forces.

In some instances cast chrome splints, wire-and-acrylic splints, intercoronal splints, and orthodontic bands are constructed or fabricated to help stabilize mobile teeth. These too must be checked on a periodic basis, and the dentist should ascertain such factors as the patient's utilization of the appliance, the continued necessity of using the appliance, physical damage to the appliance itself, wear of the teeth, or the deterioration of their supporting structures. Irreversible damage to the teeth and the periodontium can occur without proper supervision.

Occlusal adjustment is often done as part of the active phase of treatment. Ideally one would hope that a harmonious relationship will be achieved and self-maintained. Such is not always the case, and vigilance at recall is necessary to observe and correct all significant occlusal changes that may be detrimental to the periodontal health of the patient. Attrition of teeth, shifting of the teeth from occlusal and proximal wear, and parafunctional habits may all have an effect on the occlusal status.

Reinforcement of patient's PPC efforts

It has been said that plaque is our plague (Cohen). The control of plaque by the periodontally treated patient is probably the most important variable in the maintenance of the treatment result. For those patients who do not have periodontal disease, the control of plaque is a truly preventive measure. Patients who have had periodontal disease represent a population group whose vulnerability to further periodontal breakdown is more than that of the average individual. Whatever the reason, those people who succumb to the pathogenicity of the organisms in the microbiota by developing marginal gingivitis or periodontitis appear to remain more susceptible to periodontal disease even after "successful" treatment. The rate of the inflammatory response may in some way be regulated by the individual's resistance factor. We see this clinically from patient to patient. The individual's response to plaque varies from individual to individual, just as the rate of calculus deposition varies from individual to individual. In addition, changes in the resistance factors may occur from time to time in a patient's life span. There is no guarantee that periodontal disease will not recur in the susceptible patient, and the susceptible patient is that one with a history of periodontal disease.

The only positive thought that can sustain the motivation and morale of a periodontally treated patient is that with good PPC the inflammatory response to the microcosm can be kept to a minimum.

Ogilvie has stated that the periodontal patient can be likened to the treated diabetic or tubercular patient who must guard his health and give it continued regard if he is to survive. In the same sense the treated periodontal patient must maintain a good PPC program if he wants his teeth to survive. The periodontal recall then must be a period in which the patient's efforts at plaque control be recognized, encouraged, and fortified. The educational efforts in establishing a personal periodontal care or PPC program that were undertaken during the initial or active therapy must be continued throughout the maintenance phase. Patients forget details readily, and they also forget terminology and techniques. One of the values of a consistent recall program after therapy is the reinforcement of the knowledge imparted about plaque and the techniques to be used in its visualization and removal.

Continued motivation during maintenance phase

Motivation is discussed in detail in Chapter 19. It should be recognized that motivation attempts undertaken by the therapist during initial therapy should be continued during the maintenance phase. Because every patient is different, the key to an individual's motivation factor must be searched out before it can be utilized. The motivation must be directed toward two goals: (1) to establish and maintain personal plaque control and (2) to establish the desire to participate in a continued supervisory program (the periodontal recall). Not all patients can be motivated, nor do all patients maintain a consistent motivation over a long period of time. But those who do represent that group of patients whose therapy can be termed a success.

REFERENCES

Arnim, S. S.: Prevention of dental disease, Pediatr. Clin. North Am. **10**:275, 1963.

Arnim, S. S.: The use of disclosing agents for measuring tooth cleanliness, J. Periodontol. **34**:227, 1963.

Bass, C. C.: An effective method of personal oral hygiene, J. La. Med. Soc. **106**:100, 1954.

Block, P., and Derdivanis, J.: The two-tone dye. Presented at the Western Society of Periodontology, San Diego, May, 1971.

Block, P., Lobene, R., and Derdivanis, J.: A two-tone dye test for dental plaque, J. Periodontal. **43**:423, 1972.

Brillant, H.: In Goldman, H. M., and Cohen, D. W., editors: Periodontal therapy, ed. 4, St. Louis, 1968, The C. V. Mosby Co.

Chace, R.: The maintenance phase of periodontal therapy, J. Periodontol. **22**:234, 1951.

Cohen, D. W.: Periodontics: reflections and projections, Alpha Omegan **2**:173, 1969.

Glickman, I.: Preventive periodontics. In Bernier, J. L., and Muhler, J. C., editors: Improving dental practice through preventive measures, ed. 2, St. Louis, 1970, The C. V. Mosby Co.

Goldman, H. M., and Cohen, D. W., editors: Periodontal therapy, ed. 5, St. Louis, 1973, The C. V. Mosby Co.

Grant, D. A., Stern, I. B., and Everett, F. G.: Orban's periodontics, ed. 4, St. Louis, 1972, The C. V. Mosby Co.

Lindhe, J., and Nyman, S.: The effect of plaque control and surgical pocket elimination on the establishment and maintenance of periodontal health. A longitudinal study of periodontol therapy in cases of advanced disease. J. Clin. Periodontol. **2**:67-79, 1975.

Lovdal, A., Arno, A., Schei, O., and Waerbaug, J.: Combined effect of subgingival scaling and controlled oral hygiene on the incidence of gingivitis, Acta Odontol. Scand. **19**:537-55; 1961.

Nyman, S., Rosling, B., and Lindhe, J.: Effect of professional tooth cleaning on healing after periodontal surgery, J. Clin. Periodontol. **2**:80-86, 1975.

Ogilvie, A. L.: Recall and maintenance of the periodontal patient, Periodontics **3**:198, 1967.

Oliver, R.: Tooth loss with and without periodontal therapy, Periodont. Abstr. **17**:8, 1969.

Pritchard, J. F.: Advanced periodontal disease, Philadelphia, 1965, W. B. Saunders Co.

Ramfjord, S. P., Knowles, J. W., Nissle, R. R., Shick, R. A., and Burgett, F. S.: Longitudinal study of periodontal therapy, J. Periodontol. **44**:66-77, 1973.

Robinson, R. E.: How patients are motivated and taught to practice effective oral hygiene, Periodont. Abstr. **16**:100, 1968.

Robinson, R. E.: Practice management problems with the referred patient, Periodont. Abstr. **8**:1, 8-9, 1960.

Robinson, R. E., Derdivanis, J., and Block, P.: P.P.C. and the third party world. Presented to the American Academy of Periodontology, Montreal, September, 1970.

Rosling, B., Nyman, S., Lindhe, J., and Jesn, B.: The healing potential of the periodontal tissues following different techniques of periodontal surgery in plaque free dentition, J. Clin. Periodontol. **3**:233-250, 1976.

Socransky, S. S.: Relationship of bacteria to the etiology of periodontal disease, J. Dent. Res. **49**:203, 1970.

Suomi, J. D., Green, J. C., Vermillien, J. R., Doyle, J., Chang, J. J., and Heatherwood, E. C.: The effect of controlled oral hygiene procedures on the progression of periodontal disease in adults: results after third and final year. J. Periodontol. **42**:152-160, 1971.

Theilade, E., Wright, W. H., Borglum-Jensen, S. and Low, H.: Experimental gingivitis in man. II. A longitudinal clinical and bacteriological investigation: Journal Periodont. Res. **1**:1-13, 1966.

Thomas, B. O. A.: What is periodontal maintenance care and whose responsibility is it? J. West. Soc. Periodont. **11**:8, 1963.

Index